Mosby's

HANDBOOK OF HERBS AND SUPPLEMENTS AND THEIR THERAPEUTIC USES

WITHDRAWN

Mosby's

HANDBOOK OF HERBS

AND SUPPLEMENTS AND THEIR

THERAPEUTIC USES

Steven Bratman, MD
Consulting Editor to Complementary and Alternative
Medicine for HealthGate Data Corp
Fort Collins, Colorado

Andrea M. Girman, MD, MPH
Fellow, Integrative Medicine
Continuum Center for Health and Healing
Beth Isreal Medical Center
New York, New York

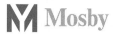 Mosby

An Affiliate of Elsevier Science
St. Louis   London   Philadelphia   Sydney   Toronto

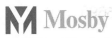

An Affiliate of Elsevier Science

11830 Westline Industrial Drive
St. Louis, Missouri 63146

MOSBY'S HANDBOOK OF HERBS AND SUPPLEMENTS AND
THEIR THERAPEUTIC USES   ISBN 0-323-02015-1
Copyright © 2003, Mosby, Inc. All rights reserved.

NOTICE

Knowledge regarding the proper use of herbs and supplements is ever
changing. Standard safety precautions must be followed, but as new research and clinical experience broaden our understanding, changes in
use may become necessary or appropriate. Readers are advised to check
the most current product information provided by the manufacturer of
each product to be administered to verify the recommended dose, the
method and duration of administration, and contraindications. It is the
responsibility of the treating licensed practitioner, relying on experience and knowledge of the patient, to determine dosages and the best
treatment for each individual patient.

This publication is not intended as a substitute for medical therapy nor
as a manual for self-treatment. Readers should seek professional advice
for any specific medical problems.

Neither the Publisher nor the author assumes any liability for any injury
and/or damage to persons or property arising from this publication.

International Standard Book Number 0-323-02015-1

Publishing Director: Linda L. Duncan
Acquisitions Editor: Kellie F. White
Associate Developmental Editor: Jennifer L. Watrous
Publishing Services Manager: Linda McKinley
Project Manager: Rich Barber
Designer: Julia Dummitt
Cover Art: Sheilah Barrett

TG/QWF

Printed in the United States

9 8 7 6 5 4 3 2 1

CONTENTS

INTRODUCTION

Alternative medicine has captured the public's interest to such an extent that, regardless of its fundamental merits, no healthcare provider can safely ignore it. Perhaps the most significant issue is that the overwhelming majority of individuals who use alternative therapies such as herbs do not report it to their healthcare professionals.[1] This creates a real risk of drug-herb or drug-nutrient interactions, as well as interference with procedures such as surgery. Second, many individuals who desire information about using natural products do not expect a conventional healthcare provider—whether physician, nurse, physician's assistant, or pharmacist—to possess adequate education in the field. Thus they conduct their own research—often from questionable sources—or seek out alternative care practitioners whose medical education may be insufficiently comprehensive to ensure patient safety.

Mosby's Handbook of Herbs & Supplements and Their Therapeutic Uses is designed to help the healthcare provider address these problems. The handbook has two sections, the first covering 76 common medical conditions and the second covering 163 popular herbs and supplements. Each section has a particular role to play in patient care.

The condition articles address the first problem noted above: patients failing to inform healthcare providers regarding their use of alternative therapies. Using this book, the practitioner can look up a patient's medical condition and immediately discover which specific herbs and supplements that individual might be using. The practitioner can properly assess the scientific evidence (if any) of the use of a particular treatment and, based on the patient's answers to detailed and specific questions, can then provide expert advice regarding potential drug interactions and other safety issues.

This handbook also helps solve the second problem. If a patient inquires about natural remedies for a given medical condition or wishes to know more about a specific herb or supplement, both the condition and herb/supplement articles will supply detailed and scientifically credible information. This allows the conventional healthcare practitioner to be once again the primary and most reliable source of medical advice.

The Clinical Evidence Ratings Scale

To enable the healthcare provider to rapidly assess the strength of the evidence for alternative therapies and thereby make rational treatment recommendations, this handbook provides a rating scale for each treatment.

The research record on alternative therapies is uneven. Some therapies have relatively strong scientific support, others have little, and a few have been proven ineffective. The following scale is designed to rate the current knowledge of therapeutic efficacy.

[+4]	Multiple double-blind trials of satisfactory design and size, leading to mainstream medical acceptance of the evidence as meaningful
[+3]	Moderate-sized, positive, double-blind, placebo-controlled trials (at least one with n > 100) or double-blind, comparative studies when comparator drug is well-established
[+2]	Small, positive, double-blind, placebo-controlled trials (n < 100)
[+1]	Animal data, epidemiologic studies, uncontrolled clinical trials, in vitro studies, or indirect evidence
[0]	No evidence
[−1]	Small, negative, double-blind, trials (n < 100) or other forms of negative evidence
[−2]	Moderate to large, negative, double-blind trials (at least one with n > 100)
X modifier	Conclusions challenged in a study of similar design and size

(For easy, quick reference, this information can also be found on the inside front cover.)

In general, a +4 and in some cases a +3 rating indicate a level of evidence similar to that of a pharmaceutical before U.S. Food and Drug Administration (FDA) approval. A +2 ranking suggests preliminary evidence only. A +1 rating has little predictive value; research is best considered to fall in the category of basic science.

A rating of 0 indicates no evidence one way or the other, the state of affairs for many alternative treatments. Below this lies −1, indicating preliminary evidence that a treatment is not effective. Finally, a rating of −2 reports meaningful evidence that a treatment does not work.

The X rating can modify both positive and negative ratings. For example, a +3X rating indicates that the evidence is generally positive and includes at least one moderate-sized, double-blind trial, but another study of comparable size returned negative results. A −2X rating would also indicate mixed results but with a preponderance of negative outcomes.

Keep in mind that the ratings used here are not formal, rigid analyses of the literature. Rather, they are intended primarily as a guide to the clinician, and as such we have felt free to alter a strict use of the definitions above to consider potential mitigating factors, such as differences in dosage or trial length, study power, use of secondary outcome measures, and study quality.

Drug Interactions

Drug interactions probably represent the greatest safety risk with the use of herbs and supplements. This book addresses this problem in several ways.

Each herb and supplement article discusses relevant interactions between the subject of the article and drugs used to treat the condition under discussion. Similarly, each condition article also discusses drug-herb and drug-nutrient interactions, using two distinct tables.

The first table summarizes known drug interactions with each principal natural treatment described in the article. (For example, if the condition in question is Hypertension, the article includes a brief summary of drug interactions with such putative antihypertensives as garlic and CoQ_{10}) More detailed information regarding a potentially important interaction may be found in the full article on that herb or supplement.

The second table takes a different perspective. It is organized by drug and drug class commonly used for the condition under discussion, listing potential interactions with *any* herb and supplement. Using the Hypertension example again, suppose a hypertensive patient takes calcium channel blockers. This second table suggests herbs and supplements that might present risk of interaction with that drug category, whether or not those therapies are proposed as treatments for hypertension itself.

Positive Interactions

The term "drug interaction" ordinarily implies harmful interactions. However, there are numerous known or hypothesized positive interactions between drugs and herbs or supplements. These too are introduced in this handbook.

The most important type of positive interaction involves relative or absolute depletion of a nutrient by drug therapy. Patients using a drug that causes such depletion might benefit from general supplementation with that nutrient. Individuals interested in alternative medical treatment will likely appreciate receiving such suggestions when warranted. Again, the condition article offers a summary of the positive interaction, whereas the herb or supplement article in question provides more information.

Important Information on Herbs and Supplements

Herbs and supplements present some issues that differ from those of over-the-counter and prescription drugs. We briefly summarize them here.

Legally, herbs and supplements fall under the general category of "dietary supplements." This vague term includes vitamins, minerals, amino acids and food extracts, herbs, and other plant-derived substances. The metabolites, constituents, and extracts of these substances can be classed as dietary supplements as well.

With a few exceptions (e.g., folate for the prevention of neural tube defect) a product sold as a dietary supplement cannot be labeled in such a way to indicate it as a treatment for any medical condition. Instead, vague "structure-function" claims must be used. Examples listed by the FDA as permitted include the following: "calcium builds strong bones," "antioxidants maintain cell integrity," and "fiber maintains bowel regularity." In contrast, a phrase such as "treats depression" or "cures arthritis" is a disease claim and is forbidden.

Manufacturers of dietary supplements do not need FDA approval to use such structure-function claims. However, labels using such structure-function claims must include the disclaimer "This statement has not been evaluated by the Food and Drug Administration. This product is not intended to diagnose, treat, cure, or prevent any disease." Because the precise distinction between a permitted structure-function claim and a forbidden disease claim is not always clear, much litigation is expected.

Another consequence of this peculiar legal standing is that there is little to no governmental supervision of herb or supplement quality. Content labeling may be inaccurate or misleading; in addition, products of undetermined safety may be legally marketed until danger is shown.

Although they fall under the same legal definition, crude or near-crude medicinal herbs present significantly different issues from other dietary supplements. For this reason, they will be discussed separately under the somewhat artificial headings of "Herbs" and "Food Supplements."

Herbs

There are two major problems specific to herbs: reproducibility and adulteration. In addition, herb-drug interactions can be expected, and an increasing number have been reported.

Reproducibility Herbs contain innumerable natural constituents that can be present in unpredictable quantities. The nature of the soil, the extent of exposure to the sun, the season's weather—all these factors can markedly influence the constituents of a batch of herb.

This problem of reproducibility was the original motivation for finding the active principles of herbs, such as foxglove, and purifying them into single-chemical drugs (e.g., digoxin). However, most of the common herbs that possess an identifiable active ingredient have long since been transformed into pharmaceuticals; for example, vincristine from periwinkle and scopolamine and atropine from belladonna. In most of the remaining therapeutic herbs, no single active ingredient has been identified to account for the observed effects. Most likely, two or more ingredients are involved, exponentially magnifying the difficulties presented to the analytic chemist who wants to isolate the bioactive constituents. Unfortunately, asserting sample interchangeability is difficult without such identification. Two batches of the identical herb might possess radically different pharmaceutical potency.

Both the efficacy and safety of herbal products are complicated by this issue of multiple varying ingredients. In Europe, manufacturers attempt to partially circumvent the problem by creating herbal extracts standardized to a fixed percentage of one ingredient or class of ingredients. For example, *Ginkgo biloba* extract is typically standardized to contain 24% ginkgo-flavone glycosides. It is not that the glycosides are proven to be the active components in ginkgo; rather, they are used as a standardization handle to bring along numerous other constituents in relatively fixed proportions.

However, many problems exist with this method. One of the most important difficulties is that two different extraction methods (e.g., alcohol and water vs. acetone and water) can be adjusted to yield identical levels of inactive marker chemicals while causing differing levels of other, more important, but unidentified constituents. A related problem is that once a substance is chosen as a marker, manufacturers begin to tune their efforts to producing maximal levels of that ingredient, again possibly at the expense of unidentified but potentially more bioactive ingredients.

For all these reasons, it simply is not possible at the present time to assert bioequivalence between two batches of herbs. For this reason, double-blind evidence for an herb's effectiveness applies only to the particular form of herb used in the study. For example, nearly all the meaningful studies of St. John's wort for depression used a particular methanol and water extract known as LI 160. The manufacturing process for this product specifies total darkness and temperatures that are raised only briefly to 60 to 80 degrees Celsius. If another manufacturer sells a St. John's wort formulation that has been produced according to different specifications, there is no guarantee that it will be equally effective as LI 160. After all, the active ingredients are unknown, and small differences in extractive processes can radically alter the proportions of these numerous ingredients. Unfortunately, this second manufacturer might still cite the results of studies of LI 160 as evidence for the effectiveness of its own product. In the natural products industry, this practice is called "borrowing science," and it is widely criticized yet widely practiced.

Adulteration   Herbs are harvested, not manufactured. This, along with weak governmental oversight, creates a significant potential for adulteration. For example, samples of the herb plantain were found to contain cardiac glycosides.[2] Because these substances do not exist in plantain, an investigation ensued, ultimately demonstrating inadvertent adulteration with a similar-appearing foxglove species. A related problem has been associated with herbs manufactured in China: potential contamination with pesticides and heavy metals.

Potential adulteration has another consequence besides potential toxicity: it can also lead to an incorrect assignment of cause in case reports. Thus one report of coma purportedly induced by kava turned out to involve a toxic product containing no kava at all.

At present, there is no absolute safeguard available against adulteration. However, using products manufactured by reputable companies, especially those whose products have undergone double-blind testing, should tend to decrease the risk.

Herb-Drug Interactions   Herbs and drugs must necessarily impact overlapping physiologic systems, whether it is the target organ or liver cytochromes. The herb St. John's wort is the most extensively investigated for drug interactions, but there is little doubt that numerous herb-drug interactions exist.

The FDA has now begun to encourage practitioners to report herbal adverse drug reactions (ADRs) to their MEDWATCH drug surveillance program (tel: 800-332-1088). Conversely, clinicians should be encouraged to report clinical data on the absence of potential herb-drug interactions as data become available from practice.

Food Supplements

The term "food supplements" is usually taken to apply to vitamins, minerals, amino acids, or other substances found in plant or animal products commonly consumed as a food. Unlike herbal products, most food supplements contain one or at most a few related compounds, essentially eliminating the problems of standardization and batch-to-batch variability.

It is a matter of considerable historical irony that vitamins and food supplements have come to be considered staples of alternative medicine. Until the early 1950s, vitamins and other food supplements were more the province of conventional than alternative practitioners. Early naturopathic writers derided vitamins as a futile attempt by scientists to outdo nature, condemning vitamins as synthetic and unnatural. Adelle Davis and, later, Linus Pauling changed these attitudes, and soon the alternative camp embraced food supplements as the mainstay of treatment. Excesses of this enthusiasm led to a counterreaction in conventional medicine.

The use of food supplements is commonly called "nutritional therapy." However, this term is only a fair description when using vitamins and minerals at levels approximating recommended daily intake. Oral supplementation with calcium and vitamin D to help prevent osteoporosis falls in this category. The use of supplements at supranutritional doses is properly regarded as pharmacologic treatment. Vitamin E at 400 IU daily, commonly (and probably inappropriately) recommended for heart disease prevention, is a good example of pharmacologic treatment. The use of supplements can be described as quasinutritional when they are taken to correct local tissue deficiencies caused by disease or drug treatment. The supplement CoQ_{10} illustrates such use; numerous drug classes as well as congestive heart failure itself may lead to an absolute or relative depletion of CoQ_{10} levels, making oral supplementation a potentially valuable repletion therapy.

Making Rational Recommendations

A rapid perusal of this text will show that numerous herbs and supplements have significant scientific evidence behind them, but many more do not.

Recommending a trial of an evidence-based herb or supplement treatment to a patient may be appropriate for conditions that do not require definitive and immediate care. However, the healthcare provider will also be faced with situations in which a patient wishes to try an unproven treatment.

If the treatment is thought to be safe, physician support for a patient wishing to try an unproven approach may be acceptable, but it does veer from the current standard of evidence-based medicine. This presents an ethical issue that each provider will have to evaluate.

One analogy to consider when facing this ethical issue is off-label use of FDA-approved medications. In some cases, such uses are based on anecdote rather than double-blind trials. Use of unproven herbs and supplements presents a similar situation. However, if carried too far, the philosophy "it couldn't hurt, so why not try it" could lead to a premodern form of medicine in which entirely unproven therapies proliferate.

Therefore a balanced and prudent attitude is recommended when considering treatment with herbs or supplements. This handbook will provide the raw information necessary to tread this fine line.

CONDITIONS

ACNE

Principal Proposed
Natural Therapies

Zinc [+2X]

Niacinamide gel [+2]

Tea tree oil *(Melaleuca alternifolia)* [+1]

(Higher numbers indicate stronger evidence; X modifier indicates contradictory results. See page xviii of the Introduction for details of the rating scale.)

Approach to the Patient

Some evidence suggests that oral zinc may be modestly helpful for acne. One study suggests that niacinamide gel may be effective, and indirect evidence supports the use of topical tea tree oil.

Other natural treatments your patients may be using include burdock, chromium, red clover, selenium, and vitamin E. For potential safety risks with the more common of these substances, see the full herb/supplement articles.

In addition, many patients interested in alternative medicine believe that accumulated toxins are the cause of acne and that this can be corrected through "detoxification." The latter may involve dietary changes, "colon cleansing," and supplementation with specific herbs and supplements. Malnutrition can occur in the more extreme forms of this approach.

Caution: The recommended dosages of zinc for acne are high enough to present risk of toxicity from copper depletion as well as, perhaps, direct effects.

Zinc   +2X

Evidence of low serum zinc in individuals with acne[1-3] led to therapeutic trials of zinc supplementation. Several small double-blind studies involving a total of more than 300 individuals have returned somewhat conflicting results, but on balance the evidence suggests modest benefit.

In one of these trials, 54 individuals with acne were given either placebo or 135 mg daily of zinc as zinc sulfate for a period of 6 weeks. Zinc produced slight but measurable benefits.[4] Similar results have been seen in most but not all studies using 90 to 135 mg of zinc daily.[5-10] Zinc in the form of gluconate has been found effective at the lower (and safer) dose of 30 mg daily.[11]

Two small double–blind trials compared zinc with tetracycline. One 12-week trial found that zinc (45 mg three times daily) was as effective as tetracycline (250 mg three times daily, then twice daily, then once daily),[12] but another trial found the antibiotic significantly more effective when taken at 500 mg daily.[13]

A 3-month, dose-determination trial found no benefit in the use of a loading dose of zinc as opposed to continuous treatment with 30 mg daily.[14]

Note: Zinc can be toxic at high dosages, primarily by causing copper deficiency. Concurrent administration of copper at a dose of 1 to 3 mg daily can counteract this effect.

For more information, including dosage and safety issues, see the **Zinc** article.

Niacinamide Gel   +2

In a double-blind trial, 76 individuals with moderate inflammatory acne were treated with either 4% niacinamide gel or 1% clindamycin gel.[15] Both treatments produced statistically similar improvements in acne symptoms over the 8-week trial period.

Tea Tree Oil   + 1

A single-blind, randomized, comparative trial of 124 patients with mild to moderate acne evaluated the efficacy and skin tolerance of 5% tea tree oil gel compared with 5% benzoyl peroxide lotion.[16] This study found that benzoyl peroxide was more effective than tea tree oil. Significant improvements from baseline were seen in the tea tree oil group as well, but the lack of a placebo group makes these apparent benefits difficult to interpret.

For more information, including dosage and safety issues, see the **Tea Tree Oil** article.

Other Proposed Natural Therapies

A preliminary controlled trial suggests that oral **gugulipid** (50 mg of guggulsterones twice daily) might be helpful for acne.[17]

Other commonly mentioned natural treatments for acne include burdock, chromium, red clover, selenium, and vitamin E. However, there is no clinical evidence for any of these treatments at this time.

Drug Interactions

See the article on each individual supplement for a full description of the interactions summarized here.

Principal Natural Therapies for Acne: Interactions with Pharmaceuticals		
Natural Therapy	**Pharmaceutical**	**Interaction**
Zinc	Amiloride	Possible elevated serum zinc
	Fluoroquinolones, pencillamine, tetracyclines	Mutual absorption interference

Pharmaceuticals Used for Acne: Possible Harmful Interactions with Natural Therapies

Pharmaceutical	Natural Therapy	Interaction
Isotretinoin	Vitamin A	Potentiation of drug toxicity
Sulfonamides	PABA	Reduced drug effectiveness
	Potassium	Possible hyperkalemia
	Dong quai, St. John's wort	Possible increased risk of photosensitivity
Tetracyclines	Mineral supplements	Mutual absorption interference
	Potassium citrate	Decreased serum tetracycline levels
	Dong quai, St. John's wort	Possible increased risk of photosensitivity

Pharmaceuticals Used for Acne: Natural Therapies with Potential Supportive Interactions

Pharmaceutical	Natural Therapy	Interaction
Sulfonamides	Folate	Correction of possible drug-induced deficiency

ALLERGIC RHINITIS

Principal Proposed
Natural Therapies

Butterbur [+2]

Freeze-dried nettle leaf [+2]

(Higher numbers indicate stronger evidence; X modifier indicates contradictory results. See page xviii of the Introduction for details of the rating scale.)

Approach to the Patient

There are not many options for allergy relief with dietary supplements, but two have some supporting evidence.

One double-blind, comparative study suggests that the herb butterbur (*Petasites* spp.) may have antiallergy effects that are equivalent to those of cetirizine. In addition, freeze-dried nettle leaf *(Urtica dioica)* has been widely promoted as a treatment for allergic rhinitis based on one poorly reported study.

The bioflavonoid quercetin has been marketed as an allergy treatment on even less evidence: primarily in vitro findings of basophil and mast cell stabilization.

Other natural treatments your patient may be using for allergies include bee pollen, betaine hydrochloride, cat's claw, *Coleus forskohlii,* fish oil, GLA (gamma-linolenic acid), MSM (methyl sulfonyl methane), oligomeric proanthocyanidins (OPCs; grape seed or Pycnogenol), spirulina, and vitamins B_6, B_{12}, or C.

Some patients interested in alternative medicine may believe that allergies are caused by "adrenal exhaustion." Treatments for this purported condition include various herbs and supplements, among them ginseng and B vitamins; most are, at least, relatively benign.

Butterbur   + 2

The herb butterbur (*Petasites* spp.) is best known as a migraine prophylaxis. However, it has also been proposed as a treatment for allergies and asthma.

A 2-week, double-blind study of 125 individuals with seasonal allergic rhinitis compared a standardized butterbur extract against cetrizine (10 mg daily).[16] Treatment effectiveness according to the primary outcome measure, Medical Outcome Health Survey Questionnaire (SF-36), indicated that both treatments were equally effective. Equivalent effectiveness was also seen on the Physician's Clinical Global Impression score.

For more information, including dosage and safety issues, see the **Butterbur** article.

Freeze-Dried Nettle Leaf   + 2

A double-blind, placebo-controlled trial enrolled 98 individuals with allergic rhinitis.[1] Each participant received gelatin capsules containing either 300 mg of freeze-dried stinging nettle leaf or placebo and was instructed to take two capsules at the onset of symptoms. Assessment was based on diary notes 1 hour after taking the capsules, as well as on a global assessment questionnaire. A total of 69 individuals completed the study. Global assessments showed clear benefit; symptom diaries showed a marginal difference. However, analysis of statistical significance was not reported.

For more information, including dosage and safety issues, see the **Nettle** article.

Other Proposed Natural Therapies

In vitro studies suggest that flavonoids such as **quercetin** may reduce histamine release from mast cells and basophils.[2-10] Similar effects may be seen with **spirulina**.[11,12] However, clinical trials have not been performed.

Preliminary evidence suggests that **vitamin C** might reduce nasal and pulmonary responses to histamine provocation.[13,14] Vitamin B_6, vitamin B_{12}, cat's claw, *Coleus forskohlii*, GLA, fish oil, MSM, and betaine hydrochloride are sometimes recommended, but there is as yet no significant evidence that they are effective for allergic rhinitis.

Although bee pollen is sometimes suggested for treating allergic rhinitis on the theory it might help the body build up resistance to local pollens, there is no evidence that it works, and in some cases severe allergic reactions to the bee pollen itself might occur.

An 8-week, double-blind trial of 49 individuals found no benefit with **grapeseed extract**, a source of **OPCs** (dose not stated).[15]

Drug Interactions

See the article on each individual supplement for a full description of the interactions summarized here.

Principal Natural Therapies for Allergic Rhinitis: Interactions with Pharmaceuticals
None known.

Pharmaceutical Used for Allergic Rhinitis: Possible Harmful Interactions with Natural Therapy		
Pharmaceutical	Natural Therapy	Interaction
Pseudoephedrine	Ephedra (ma huang)	Potentiation of effects and side effects

ALTITUDE SICKNESS

Principal Proposed
Natural Therapy

Ginkgo biloba [+2]

(Higher numbers indicate stronger evidence; X modifier indicates contradictory results. See page xviii of the Introduction for details of the rating scale.)

Approach to the Patient

A preliminary study suggests that the herb *Ginkgo biloba* might be helpful for preventing altitude sickness. Other natural treatments your patient may be trying for altitude sickness include antioxidants, magnesium, glutamine, and silymarin (a constituent of the herb milk thistle). For potential safety risks with the more common of these substances, see the full herb/supplement articles.

Ginkgo biloba +2

A placebo-controlled study (practitioner blinding not stated) of 44 mountaineers on a Himalayan expedition found that 80 mg twice daily of standardized ginkgo extract significantly reduced the incidence of mountain sickness.[1] Symptoms related to cold extremities were also reduced.

The presumed mechanism of action of ginkgo is increased cerebral and peripheral oxygen flow.

For more information, including dosage and safety issues, see the **Ginkgo** article.

Other Proposed
Natural Therapies

A double-blind trial of 18 mountaineers climbing to the Mt. Everest base camp found that use of antioxidant vitamin supplements (100 mg vitamin C, 400 IU vitamin E, and 600 mg of lipoic acid daily) significantly improved symptoms of altitude sickness as compared with placebo.[2] Treatment was begun 3 weeks before ascent and continued during the 10 days of climbing.

Magnesium, glutamine, and silymarin, alone or in combination, have also been suggested for preventing altitude sickness. However, there is no real evidence as yet that any of these treatments are effective for this purpose.

Drug Interactions

See the article on each individual supplement for a full description of the interactions summarized here.

Principal Natural Therapy for Altitude Sickness: Interaction with Pharmaceuticals		
Natural Therapy	Pharmaceutical	Interaction
Ginkgo	Anticoagulant and antiplatelet agents	Possible increased risk of bleeding complications

Pharmaceuticals Used for Altitude Sickness: Interactions with Natural Therapies
None known.

ALZHEIMER'S DISEASE, NON-ALZHEIMER'S DEMENTIA, ORDINARY AGE-RELATED MEMORY LOSS

Principal Proposed Natural Therapies

Ginkgo biloba

Alzheimer's disease or non-Alzheimer's dementia   [+4]

Ordinary age-related memory loss   [+3]

Improving memory and mental function in the young   [+2X]

Phosphatidylserine

Dementia   [+3]

Mild to moderate cognitive impairment   [+3]

Huperzine A   [+3]

Vinpocetine   [+3]

Ginseng   [+3]

Vitamin E   [+2]

Acetyl-L-carnitine   [−2X]

(Higher numbers indicate stronger evidence; X modifier indicates contradictory results. See page xviii of the Introduction for details of the rating scale.)

12

Approach to the Patient

Significant evidence supports the use of ginkgo, phospha-tidylserine, huperzine A, and vinpocetine for treatment of Alzheimer's and non-Alzheimer's dementia. German physicians use ginkgo as frequently as more standard pharmaceutical treatments and consider it equally effective.

Lesser evidence supports using ginkgo and phosphatidylserine for ordinary age-related memory loss, technically known as age-related cognitive decline (ARCD) or age-associated memory impairment (AAMI). Still weaker evidence suggests that ginkgo may improve memory or mental function in the young.

Vitamin E may slow the progression of Alzheimer's disease.

Most of these treatments have potential interactions with anti-coagulant or antiplatelet agents.

Other natural treatments your patient may be using for demen-tia or memory loss include acetyl-L-carnitine; *Bacopa monniera;* bee pollen; dehydroepiandrosterone (DHEA); inositol; magne-sium; nicotinamide adenine dinucleotide (NADH); phos-phatidylcholine; pregnenolone; vitamins B_1, B_{12}, and C; and zinc. For potential safety risks with the more common of these substances, see the full herb/supplement articles.

Caution: A case report suggests that the herb St. John's wort may not be safe for individuals with Alzheimer's disease. Use of St. John's wort was associated with acute delirium with psychotic features in a 76-year-old woman with Alzheimer's disease.[77]

Ginkgo biloba

Ginkgo biloba has been studied in dementia and in age-associated memory impairment. For more information, including dosage and safety issues, see the **Ginkgo** article.

Alzheimer's Disease or Non-Alzheimer's Dementia   +4

A well-regarded, double-blind, placebo-controlled study of *Ginkgo biloba* in dementia (primarily Alzheimer's), involving 309 patients in a 52-week parallel-group multicenter trial, found significant improvement in a performance-based test of memory and language (the cognitive subscale of the Alzheimer's Disease Assessment Scale [ADAS-Cog]) and a caregivers' evaluation (the Geriatric Evaluation by Relative's Rating Instrument [GERRI]).[1]

Other European studies have evaluated the effectiveness of ginkgo in Alzheimer's and non-Alzheimer's dementia and also found benefit.[2,3] In addition, more than 40 other double-blind, controlled trials had evaluated the benefits of ginkgo in "cerebral insufficiency" (dementia) before 1992.[4] Of these, eight were rated of good quality, involving a total of about 1000 patients, and results were positive in all but one of these studies.

However, a 24-week, double-blind, placebo-controlled study of 214 participants found no benefit with ginkgo extract at a dose of 160 or 240 mg daily.[5] This study enrolled both individuals with mild to moderate dementia and those with ordinary age-associated memory loss.

Ordinary Age-Related Memory Loss   +3

The results of six double-blind studies suggest that ginkgo might be useful for age-associated memory impairment (AAMI) and other forms of fairly mild memory loss, although a seventh study found no benefit. In a double-blind, placebo-controlled trial, 241 seniors complaining of mildly impaired memory were given placebo, low-dose ginkgo, or high-dose ginkgo for 24 weeks.[6] The results showed modest improvements in certain types of memory, especially in the low-dose ginkgo group. Benefits were also seen in three other double-blind, placebo-controlled trials of continuous ginkgo use[7-10] and in two double-blind trials that used one-time dosing.[9,11]

However, set against these positive findings is the 24-week study mentioned above, which found no benefit in ordinary age-associated memory loss.[5] The reason for this discrepancy is unclear.

Improving Memory and Mental Function in the Young   +2X

A 30-day, double-blind, placebo-controlled trial that enrolled 61 healthy men and women evaluated the effects of 120 mg of gingko extract daily.[78] The 50 completers ranged in age from 18 to 40 years old (average 30.4 years). The results of the per-protocol evaluation showed significant improvements in some measures of memory function, including digit span backwards and working memory speed; an intention-to-treat (ITT) analysis was not performed.

In addition, in a double-blind, placebo-controlled, crossover trial, 20 individuals aged 19 to 24 years received a one-time dose of either placebo or ginkgo at 120, 240, or 360 mg.[12] The results showed improvement in various measures of mental performance, most dramatically in one that measured ability to rapidly perform attention-related tasks. Mixed results were seen in two smaller double-blind, placebo-controlled, crossover trials.[13,14]

Phosphatidylserine

Phosphatidylserine has been studied in both dementia and mild to moderate cognitive impairment.

For more information, including dosage and safety issues, see the **Phosphatidylserine** article.

Dementia   +3

Nine double-blind studies, enrolling more than 1000 individuals with Alzheimer's and other types of age-related dementia, have found phosphatidylserine beneficial.[15-23] For example, one double-blind, placebo-controlled trial of 494 older subjects found treatment for 6 months with phosphatidylserine, 300 mg/day, improved behavior, mental function, and depression.[15]

Mild to Moderate Cognitive Impairment   +3

Like ginkgo, phosphatidylserine might also be helpful for AAMI. A double-blind, placebo-controlled study enrolling 149 individuals with cognitive impairment memory loss short of dementia found significant benefits with phosphatidylserine treatment.[24]

H u p e r z i n e   A   + 3

Huperzine A is a purified alkaloid derived from a particular type of club moss *(Huperzia serrata)*. A highly specific acetylcholinesterase inhibitor, huperzine is really more a drug than an herb; however, it is sold over-the-counter as a dietary supplement for memory loss and mental impairment, for use in both healthy individuals and those with dementia.

Many research papers report that huperzine A can improve memory skills in older animals as well as in younger animals whose memories have been deliberately impaired.[25-41] All human trials of huperzine were performed in China and reported in Chinese.

A double-blind, placebo-controlled study evaluated 103 individuals with Alzheimer's disease who received either huperzine A or placebo twice daily for 8 weeks.[17] According to the English abstract, about 60% of the treated participants showed improvements in memory, thinking, and behavioral functions compared with 36% of the placebo-treated group, a significant difference.

Benefits were also seen in an earlier double-blind trial using injected huperzine in 160 individuals with dementia or other memory disorders.[42]

However, another double-blind trial of 60 individuals with Alzheimer's disease found no significant difference in symptoms between the group treated with oral huperzine and the placebo group.[43] Huperzine is also reportedly helpful for improving memory in healthy individuals. A double-blind trial of 34 matching pairs of adolescent students reported memory improvements in the treated group.[44] For more information, including dosage and safety issues, see the **Huperzine** article.

Vinpocetine   +3

Vinpocetine is a chemical derived from vincamine, a constituent in the leaves of common periwinkle as well as in the seeds of various African plants. Developed in Hungary more than 20 years ago, vinpocetine is sold in Europe as a drug under the name Cavinton, used for dementia as well as ordinary age-related mental impairment. In the United States, vinpocetine is available as a dietary supplement.

A review of the literature found a total of three meaningful double-blind, placebo-controlled trials of vinpocetine extract for the treatment of dementia, enrolling a total of 327 patients.[45,46,49,79] Benefits were seen in each trial. Other positive studies have been reported as well.[47,48,50,51]

The largest of these, a 16-week, double-blind, placebo-controlled trial of 203 individuals with mild to moderate dementia, found significant benefit in the vinpocetine-treated group as compared with placebo.[45]

For more information, including dosage and safety issues, see the **Vinpocetine** article.

Ginseng   +3

Several studies have found evidence that ginseng can improve mental function, but the effects seen are inconsistent among trials.

In a 22-month, double-blind, placebo-controlled study, 112 healthy, middle-aged adults were given either ginseng or placebo.[52] The results showed that ginseng improved abstract thinking ability. However, there was no significant change in reaction time, memory, concentration, or overall subjective experience between the two groups. In contrast, a double-blind, placebo-controlled study of 120 individuals found that ginseng gradually improved reaction time over a 12-week treatment period among those 40 to 60 years old.[53]

Another double-blind, placebo-controlled trial of 60 elderly individuals found that 50 or 100 days of treatment with *Panax ginseng* produced improvements in numerous measures of mental function, including memory, attention, concentration, and ability to cope.[54] Benefits were still evident at the 50-day follow-up. However, virtually no improvement was seen in the placebo group, a result that is highly unusual and raises doubts about the accuracy of the study. An 8-week, double-blind, placebo-controlled study enrolled 50 men and found that treatment with a ginseng extract improved ability in completion of a detail-oriented editing task.[55] Benefits were also seen in a double-blind trial of 16 healthy males.[56]

For more information, including dosage and safety issues, see the **Ginseng** article. One study evaluated combined treatment with ginseng and ginkgo[57]; see the **Ginkgo** article for more information.

Vitamin E   +2

A 2-year, double-blind, placebo-controlled trial of 341 individuals with Alzheimer's disease found evidence that high-dose vitamin E, 2000 IU (dl-alpha-tocopherol) daily, may slow the progression of the disease.[58] However, because of an accident of randomization, the three groups were not equivalent, and statistical adjustment was required to reach a statistically significant outcome.

Associations have also been found between vitamin E intake and decreased risk of vascular dementia.[59]

For more information, including dosage and safety issues, see the **Vitamin E** article.

Acetyl-L-Carnitine   −2X

Numerous double- or single-blind studies involving a total of more than 1400 patients have evaluated acetyl-L-carnitine in the treatment of Alzheimer's disease and other forms of dementia.[60-70] Although some reported positive results in some measures of mental function, the balance of the evidence is negative. One of the largest double-blind, placebo-controlled studies, observing 431 patients with mild to moderate probable Alzheimer's for 1 year, found no significant improvement with supplemental carnitine.[71] Based on benefits seen in subgroup analysis, the same researcher performed a subsequent study to evaluate whether acetyl-L-carnitine was useful in young-onset Alzheimer's disease.[72] In this 1-year, double-blind, placebo-controlled trial of 229 patients, no benefits were seen. For more information, including dosage and safety issues, see the **Carnitine** article.

Other Proposed Natural Therapies

In a 1-year, double-blind, placebo-controlled trial of 86 healthy elderly individuals, use of a **vitamin and mineral supplement** significantly improved cognitive function.[73]

A 12-week, double-blind, placebo-controlled trial evaluated the possible cognitive benefits of the herb *Bacopa monniera* in 46 healthy adults.[74] *B. monniera* is an herb used widely in Ayurveda, the traditional medicine of India. A total of 16 measures of cognitive function were used. Of these, five showed statistically significant improvement compared with placebo after 12 weeks of treatment with the herb. These included speed of visual processing, learning rate, and memory consolidation. The large number of measurements, however, raises concerns about "data dredging."

Marginal vitamin B_{12} deficiency might cause cognitive impairment.[75]

Bee pollen, DHEA,[76] inositol, magnesium, NADH, phosphatidylcholine, pregnenolone, vitamin B_1, vitamin C, and zinc
are also sometimes recommended for Alzheimer's disease, but
there is no evidence as yet that they are effective for this or related conditions.

Drug Interactions

See the article on each individual supplement for a full description of the interactions summarized here.

Principal Natural Therapies for Alzheimer's Disease, Non-Alzheimer's Dementia, and Ordinary Age-Related Memory Loss: Interactions with Pharmaceuticals		
Natural Therapy	Pharmaceutical	Interaction
Ginkgo, vitamin E	Anticoagulant and antiplatelet agents	Possible increased risk of bleeding complications
Phosphatidylserine	Anticoagulants	Possible increased risk of bleeding complications
Vinpocetine	Anticoagulants	Possible antagonism of drug action

Pharmaceuticals Used for Alzheimer's Disease, Non-Alzheimer's Dementia, and Ordinary Age-Related Memory Loss: Interactions with Natural Therapies		
Pharmaceutical	Natural Therapy	Interaction
Donepezil, tacrine, rivastigmine	Acetyl-L-carnitine, huperzine A	Possible potentiation of side effects because of similar mechanism of action

AMYOTROPHIC LATERAL SCLEROSIS

Principal Proposed Natural Therapies

BCAAs [+2X]	**Creatine** [+1]
L-Threonine [+2X]	**Vitamin E** [−2]

(Higher numbers indicate stronger evidence; X modifier indicates contradictory results. See page xviii of the Introduction for details of the rating scale.)

Approach to the Patient

Because amyotrophic lateral sclerosis (ALS) appears to involve impaired glutamate metabolism, amino acids necessary for glutamate metabolism have been proposed as treatments. However, the results of preliminary studies have been mixed. The sports supplement creatine has also been tried for ALS, with some promising results. However, in order not to raise false hopes, keep in mind that none of these treatments has shown more than marginal benefits.

Other natural treatments your patient may be using for ALS include amino acids, adenosine monophosphate (AMP), antioxidants, coenzyme Q_{10} (CoQ_{10}), genistein, guanidine, multivitamins, octacosanol, and vitamins B_{12} and E. For potential safety risks with the more common of these substances, see the full herb/supplement articles.

Branched-Chain
Amino Acids   +2X

Branched-chain amino acids (BCAAs) are most well-known as
a sports supplement but have also been tried as a treatment for
ALS based on their role in glutamate metabolism. However,
study results have been mixed.[1-6] For example, one very small
double-blind, placebo-controlled study found that individuals
treated with BCAAs for 1 year maintained muscle strength and
the ability to walk longer than those on placebo.[3] However,
other controlled trials found no effect,[1,2] and one actually found
a slight increase in deaths during the study period as compared
with placebo.[5]

For more information, including dosage and safety issues, see
the **Branched-Chain Amino Acids** article.

L-Threonine   +2X

L-Threonine, an essential amino acid that also affects glutamate
metabolism, has been the subject of preliminary investigation.
Open trials and one double-blind study found some short-term
improvement in symptoms, but in other research the results
have not been impressive.[2,7-9] A typical dosage of L-threonine is
1 g taken four times daily.

Although extensive safety studies have not been performed, current data suggest that L-threonine is generally well-tolerated
and causes no more than nonspecific side effects.[2,5,7]

Creatine   +1

Evidence from animal and open human trials suggests that the
sports supplement creatine may improve strength and slow the
progression of the disease.[10-12]

For more information, including dosage and safety issues, see
the **Creatine** article.

Vitamin E   −2

A 1-year, double-blind, placebo-controlled trial of 289 individuals with ALS found that treatment with alpha-tocopherol (500 mg twice daily) combined with rituzole produced no effect on primary outcome measures (change in functional status).[13] In addition, use of vitamin E failed to alter most secondary measures. Vitamin E did appear to increase the time participants remained in the milder state of the disease as measured by the ALS Health State Scale (AHSS), but only when researchers collapsed the two milder AHSS states into state A and the two more severe states into state B.

Other Proposed Natural Therapies

Other nutrients that have been tried for ALS with some promising results include **vitamin B_{12}, CoQ_{10}, genistein,** and **guanidine.**[14-18] Numerous other nutritional supplements have been tried for ALS but appear to be ineffective; these include **multivitamins, AMP,** and **octacosanol.**[19,20]

One very small trial tested a combination pill containing **amino acids, antioxidants,** and **nimodipine,** finding suggestive evidence that it might slow the progression of the disease.[21]

Drug Interactions

See the article on each individual supplement for a full description of the interactions summarized here.

Principal Natural Therapies for Amyotrophic Lateral Sclerosis: Interactions with Pharmaceuticals		
Natural Therapy	**Pharmaceutical**	**Interaction**
BCAAs, threonine	Levodopa	Impaired action of drug-based amino acid/levodopa interaction

ANGINA

Principal Proposed Natural Therapies

N-Acetyl cysteine (NAC)   [+3X]

Hawthorn   [+2]

Carnitine   [+2]

Magnesium   [+2]

(Higher numbers indicate stronger evidence; X modifier indicates contradictory results. See page xviii of the Introduction for details of the rating scale.)

Approach to the Patient

Preliminary evidence suggests that hawthorn, L-carnitine or L-propionyl carnitine, and magnesium may be useful adjuvant therapies in the treatment of angina. *N*-acetyl cysteine (NAC) appears to improve the effectiveness of nitroglycerin but may cause severe headaches.

Other natural treatments your patient may be using for angina include coenzyme Q_{10}, *Coleus forskohlii*, khella, oral magnesium, and vitamin E. Also ask your patient about beta-carotene ingestion, which may actually increase angina symptoms. For a full description of potential safety risks with the more common of these substances, see the full herb/supplement articles.

Chromium and coenzyme Q_{10} may be helpful for individuals taking beta-blockers. Beta-blockers can reduce high-density lipoprotein (HDL) levels as a side effect; chromium supplements may reverse this. Beta-blockers also impair CoQ_{10}-containing enzymes; taking supplemental CoQ_{10} might therefore be a form of repletion therapy (see the full articles on **Chromium** and **Coenzyme Q_{10}** for more information).

Caution: Patients may need to be counseled that angina is too serious a condition for self-treatment.

N-Acetyl Cysteine (NAC)   +3X

A 4-month, double-blind, placebo-controlled study of 200 individuals with unstable angina found that the combination of nitroglycerin and NAC was more effective than either drug alone in preventing death, myocardial infarction (MI), or the need for revascularization.[1] The mechanism of action is not clear. Unfortunately, combined treatment was also associated with a high rate of severe headaches. This side effect has been seen in other studies as well.[2] One small study found that NAC helped prevent nitrate tolerance, although another found no benefit.[3,4]

For more information, including dosage and safety issues, see the **N-Acetyl Cysteine** article.

Hawthorn   +2

One double-blind study of 60 patients with angina found that treatment for 3 weeks with 180 mg/day of hawthorn extract increased exercise tolerance.[5]

For more information, including dosage and safety issues, see the **Hawthorn** article.

Carnitine   +2

A controlled (but not blinded) study enrolled 200 patients with exercise-induced angina.[6] All were maintained on standard therapy, but one half were also given an additional 2000 mg/day of L-carnitine and observed for 6 months. The carnitine-treated group showed significant improvements in various cardiac parameters: the most dramatic was ST-segment depression during maximal effort, which fell from 0.5 mm to 0.15 mm in the treated group but did not change significantly in the untreated group ($P < 0.0001$). There were smaller but statistically significant improvements in exercise tolerance, number of premature ventricular contractions (PVCs), maximum cardiac frequency, double cardiac product, and maximum systolic pressure.

Clinical improvement was also marked in the treated group. At the onset of the study, the percentage of patients rated at New York Heart Association (NYHA) class II failure was about 40%, but by the end of the study only 10% were so rated, the rest having improved to stage I. There were no such changes in the control group (P value not stated). Medication needs also declined significantly in the treated group, as follows: nitroglycerides 60%, other nitro derivatives 40%, nifedipine 33%, diltiazem 47%, beta-blockers 36%, antihypertensives 44%, cardiac glycosides 35%, diuretics 34%, anticoagulants 44%, antiarrhythmics 70%, and hypolipidemics 61%. There were only minor declines in drug use in the control group (P value not stated). The treated group also showed a decrease in plasma cholesterol from 230 to 208 and of triglycerides from 174 to 154. There was no significant change in the control group. HDL cholesterol did not change significantly in either group.

A smaller but double-blind, placebo-controlled trial enrolled 52 individuals with stable angina and also found benefits.[7] Benefits have also been seen in similar-sized or smaller single- and double-blind studies using propionylcarnitine.[8-11] However, in one comparative study, L-propionylcarnitine appeared to be less effective than diltiazem.[10]

For more information, including dosage and safety issues, see the **Carnitine** article.

Magnesium   +2

A double-blind, placebo-controlled trial of 50 individuals with stable coronary artery disease (CAD) found that supplementation with magnesium at 730 mg daily significantly improved exercise tolerance, apparently by improving endothelial function.[12] In addition, the same research group conducted a 3-month, double-blind, placebo-controlled trial of 42 individuals with CAD and found that magnesium supplementation at 800 to

1200 mg daily inhibited platelet-dependent thrombus formation.[13] The effect appeared to be independent of platelet aggregation and activation and was additive with aspirin.

For more information, including dosage and safety issues, see the **Magnesium** article.

Other Proposed Natural Therapies

Coenzyme Q$_{10}$ as well as oral **arginine** may offer some benefits as well.[14,15,18] **Vitamin E** has been found only slightly effective at best, and **beta-carotene** may actually increase angina.[16] Oral **magnesium** has shown some promise.[17]

The herbs khella and *Coleus forskohlii* are also sometimes recommended, but as yet little clinical evidence supports their use in angina.

Drug Interactions

See the article on each individual supplement for a full description of the interactions summarized here.

Principal Natural Therapies for Angina: Interactions with Pharmaceuticals		
Natural Therapy	**Pharmaceutical**	**Interaction**
NAC	Nitrates	Increase of headache side effect

Pharmaceuticals Used for Angina: Possible Harmful Interactions with Natural Therapies		
Pharmaceutical	Natural Therapy	Interaction
Anticoagulant and antiplatelet agents	Garlic, ginkgo, high-dose vitamin E, policosanol, others	Possible increased risk of bleeding complications
Beta-blockers	Calcium	Absorption interference
Calcium channel-blockers	Combined high-dose calcium and vitamin D, grapefruit juice	Possible antagonism of drug action
Nitrates	NAC	Increase of headache side effect

Pharmaceuticals Used for Angina: Natural Therapies with Potential Supportive Interactions		
Pharmaceutical	Natural Therapy	Interaction
Beta-blockers	Coenzyme Q_{10}	Possible correction of drug-induced relative deficiency
	Chromium	Increased HDL levels
Nitrates	Folate, NAC, vitamin C, vitamin E	Possible prevention of nitrate tolerance

ANXIETY AND PANIC ATTACKS

Kava [+3]   **Melatonin** [+2]

5-HTP [+2]   **Valerian** [+2]

Multivitamin/mineral   **Passion flower** [+2]
supplement [+2]

Inositol [+2]

(Higher numbers indicate stronger evidence; X modifier indicates contradictory results. See page xviii of the Introduction for details of the rating scale.)

Approach to the Patient

Preliminary evidence suggests that the herb kava possesses anxiolytic effects of benefit in individuals with anxiety disorders. However, reports of liver failure from use of kava have made this herb substantially less appealing as an option.

Aside from kava, other potential treatment options have relatively minimal supporting evidence. Some research results suggest that the serotonin precursor 5-HTP (5-hydroxytryptophan) and the B vitamin inositol might have some benefit in anxiety disorders as well. Multivitamins plus specific minerals appear to reduce anxiety symptoms in healthy individuals. Melatonin may be helpful in preoperative anxiety, valerian might help in social stress situations, and passion flower may be useful for generalized anxiety disorder.

Other natural treatments your patient may be using include ash-wagandha, chamomile, GABA, gamma-oryzanol, gotu kola, hops, lemon balm, skullcap, and suma. For potential safety risks with the more common of these substances, see the full herb/supplement articles.

Caution: Herbs with anxiolytic properties might potentiate the effects of pharmaceutical anxiolytics and sedatives; this is a poorly studied area with possible risks.

Kava   + 3

Double-blind studies involving a total of about 400 participants suggest that kava is an effective treatment for symptoms of anxiety.

The best study to date is a 6-month, double-blind, placebo-controlled trial of 100 individuals with various forms of anxiety.[1] The results showed significant comparative improvement in Hamilton Anxiety (HAM-A) scale scores after 8 weeks of treatment with kava. Previous placebo-controlled studies (two involving menopausal anxiety) found a more rapid response to kava.[2-4]

A double-blind, placebo-controlled, crossover trial of 40 individuals with various anxiety disorders found that kava facilitated withdrawal from benzodiazepine therapy, reducing withdrawal symptoms and maintaining control of anxiety.[5]

A double-blind comparative study conducted in 1993 observed 174 patients with anxiety symptoms for a period of 6 weeks.[6] Patients received either kava (100 mg/day with 70% kavalactone content), 15 mg/day of oxazepam (a subtherapeutic dose), or 9 mg/day of bromazepam (a full therapeutic dose). Similar improvement in HAM-A scores were seen in all groups, but no intergroup statistical analysis was reported.

For more information, including dosage and safety issues (e.g., reports of fulminant hepatic failure from kava use), see the **Kava** article.

5-HTP   +2

The serotonin precursor 5-HTP is best-known as a proposed treatment for depression. However, an 8-week, double-blind, placebo-controlled study compared 5-HTP and clomipramine in 45 individuals with anxiety disorders.[7] The results showed that clomipramine was more effective than 5-HTP, but 5-HTP was more effective than placebo.

For more information, including dosage and safety issues, see the **5-HTP** article.

Multivitamin/ Mineral Supplement   +2

A double-blind, placebo-controlled trial of 80 healthy male volunteers found that 28 days of treatment with a multivitamin and mineral supplement (containing calcium, magnesium, and zinc) significantly reduced perceived anxiety and stress.[8]

Inositol   +2

A double-blind, placebo-controlled, crossover study of 21 individuals with panic disorder found that those given 12 g of inositol daily had fewer and less severe panic attacks compared with the placebo group.[9]

In addition, a double-blind, crossover study of 20 individuals compared inositol (up to 18 g daily) with fluvoxamine (up to 150 mg daily).[10] The results over 4 weeks of treatment with each agent suggest that inositol was at least as effective as fluvoxamine.

For more information, including dosage and safety issues, see the **Inositol** article.

Melatonin   +2

In a randomized, double-blind, placebo-controlled study, perioperative effects of melatonin compared to midazolam were evaluated in 75 women.[11] Patients who received either midazolam or 5 mg melatonin had a significant decrease in anxiety levels before and after surgery, as compared with placebo. Except for greater preoperative sedation in the midazolam group, the two drugs were equally effective. Similar results were seen in a subsequent double-blind trial conducted by the same researcher with 84 women.[12]

For more information, including dosage and safety issues, see the **Melatonin** article.

Valerian   +2

A double-blind, placebo-controlled crossover study of 48 participants placed under social stress situations evaluated the effects of valerian and propranolol, as well as their combination.[13] Although propranolol reduced both physical and subjective sensations of stress, valerian improved subjective sensations only. No potentiation was seen when the two treatments were combined.

For more information, including dosage and safety issues, see the **Valerian** article.

Passion Flower   +2

The herb passion flower *(Passiflora incarnata)* has a long traditional history of use as a mild sedative.

A double-blind, placebo-controlled trial of 36 individuals compared a passion flower extract (45 drops per day) with oxazepam (30 mg/day) for the treatment of generalized anxiety disorder.[15] Oxazepam showed a more rapid onset of action, but by the end of the 4-week trial, both treatments resulted in statistically equivalent improvements in HAM-A scores. Oxazepam use was associated with more problems relating to job performance.

Other Proposed Natural Therapies

A double-blind, placebo-controlled trial of 40 individuals found that **gotu kola** reduced the startle response to sudden loud noises.[14] The authors interpreted these findings to suggest that gotu kola may have anxiolytic effects.

Ashwagandha, chamomile, GABA, gamma-oryzanol, hops, lemon balm, skullcap, and suma are sometimes recommended, but no clinical evidence supports these treatments for anxiety at this time.

Drug Interactions

See the article on each individual supplement for a full description of the interactions summarized here.

Principal Natural Therapies for Anxiety and Panic Attacks: Interactions with Pharmaceuticals		
Natural Therapy	Pharmaceutical	Interaction
5-HTP	SSRIs, other serotonergic drugs	Possible risk of serotonin syndrome
	Levodopa-carbidopa	Possible increased risk of scleroderma-like syndrome
Kava	Antipsychotics	Increased risk of dystonic reactions
	Benzodiazepines	Possible facilitation of benzodiazepine withdrawal
	Benzodiazepines, other sedatives	Possible potentiation of sedation
	Levodopa	Possible antagonism of drug action
Valerian	Sedatives	Possible potentiation of sedation

Pharmaceuticals Used for Anxiety and Panic Attacks: Possible Harmful Interactions with Natural Therapies		
Pharmaceutical	Natural Therapy	Interaction
Benzodiazepines	Kava, valerian, other sedative herbs	Possible potentiation of sedative effects
SSRIs, tricyclic drugs	5-HTP, SAMe, St. John's wort	Possible risk of serotonin syndrome

Pharmaceuticals Used for Anxiety and Panic Attacks: Natural Therapies with Potential Supportive Interactions		
Pharmaceutical	Natural Therapy	Interaction
Benzodiazepines	Kava	Possible facilitation of drug discontinuation
SSRIs	Ginkgo	Possible reversal of SSRI-induced sexual dysfunction

APHTHOUS ULCERS

Principal Proposed Natural Therapies

Deglycyrrhizinated licorice (DGL)   [+1]

Chamomile   [–2]

(Higher numbers indicate stronger evidence; X modifier indicates contradictory results. See page xviii of the Introduction for details of the rating scale.)

Approach to the Patient

Deglycyrrhizinated licorice (DGL), a form of licorice not likely to cause systemic effects, is widely used for the symptomatic treatment of aphthous ulcers. Although there is little evidence to support this use, there is little harm in trying it either.

Chamomile mouthwash has been tried and found ineffective in treating the aphthous ulcers from 5-FU chemotherapy.

Other natural treatments your patient may be using for mouth sores include *acidophilus, Calendula,* and vitamin B_1. For potential safety risks with the more common of these substances, see the full herb/supplement articles.

Caution: The leaves of the herb feverfew can cause a significant incidence of aphthous ulcers when chewed. Encapsulated feverfew (typically used in the treatment of migraines) does not appear to cause this problem.

Deglycyrrhizinated Licorice (DGL)   +1

An open trial suggests that deglycyrrhizinated licorice (a modified form of licorice without aldosterone-like effects) may help relieve the discomfort of aphthous ulcers.[1]

For more information, including dosage and safety issues, see the **Licorice** article.

Chamomile   −2

A double-blind, placebo-controlled trial of 164 individuals found that chamomile mouthwash was not effective for treating the mouth sores caused by 5-FU.[2]

For more information, including dosage and safety issues, see the **Chamomile** article.

Other Proposed Natural Therapies

Other treatments recommended for aphthous ulcers include *acidophilus*, *Calendula*, and vitamin B_1, but there is no clinical evidence to support these uses.

Drug Interactions

None known.

ASTHMA

Principal Proposed
Natural Therapies

Tylophora [+3X]   **Vitamin B$_6$** [+2X]

Boswellia [+2]   **Fish oil** [−1]

(Higher numbers indicate stronger evidence; X modifier indicates contradictory results. See page xviii of the Introduction for details of the rating scale.)

Approach to the Patient

Although the Indian herb tylophora has shown some promise in treating asthma, the best-designed study found no benefit. No other proposed natural treatments for asthma have any significant documentation.

Patients interested in natural medicine are frequently concerned about taking inhaled corticosteroids, failing to differentiate their side effects from those of oral corticosteroids. This point may be worth addressing at some length.

Other natural treatments your patient may be using for asthma include *Aloe vera*, antioxidants (e.g., vitamin E, vitamin C, beta-carotene, selenium), betaine hydrochloride, chamomile, *Coleus forskohlii*, damiana, elecampane, garlic, grindelia, licorice, lobelia, ma huang (ephedra), magnesium, marshmallow, mullein, onion, quercetin, reishi, vitamin B$_{12}$, and yerba santa.

Some patients interested in alternative medicine may believe that asthma is caused by "adrenal exhaustion." Treatments for this purported condition include various herbs and supplements, including ginseng and B vitamins; most are at least relatively benign.

Tylophora   +3X

In a double-blind, placebo-controlled, crossover study of 195 individuals with asthma, participants showed significant improvement in symptoms when given 40 mg of a tylophora alcohol extract daily for 6 days as compared with placebo.[1] Reportedly, the comparative benefit between tylophora and placebo was even more marked months after use of the herb was stopped. Although it seems difficult to believe that only 6 days of treatment could produce such enduring benefits, similarly long-lasting results were reported in two other double-blind, placebo-controlled studies involving more than 200 individuals with asthma.[2,3]

However, the design of most of these studies was convoluted and the reporting incomplete. A better-reported, double-blind, placebo-controlled study that enrolled 135 individuals and followed a more straightforward design found no benefit of tylophora in asthma.[4]

For more information, including dosage and safety issues, see the **Tylophora** article.

Boswellia   +2

Boswellia is best known as a purported treatment for rheumatoid arthritis. A 6-week, double-blind, placebo-controlled study of 80 individuals with relatively mild asthma found that treatment with boswellia at a dose of 300 mg three times daily reduced the frequency of asthma attacks and improved objective measurements of breathing capacity.[5]

For more information, including dosage and safety issues, see the **Boswellia** article.

Vitamin B$_6$ +2X

Although one double-blind study of high-dose vitamin B$_6$ in 76 asthmatic children found significantly reduced use of bronchodilators and steroids after the second month of therapy,[6] another double-blind study of 31 adults who also used either in-haled or oral steroids failed to find benefit.[7]

For more information, including dosage and safety issues, see the **Vitamin B$_6$** article.

Fish Oil   −1

Because of their antiinflammatory effects in rheumatoid arthri-tis, fish oil supplements have been tried for asthma.[8-15] However, a review of clinical trials found no consistent evidence that fish oil is effective for this purpose.[16] One study found that fish oil can actually worsen aspirin-related asthma.[10]

For more information, including dosage and safety issues, see the **Fish Oil** article.

Other Proposed Natural Therapies

Preliminary evidence suggests that treatment with the AMP-stim-ulating herb *Coleus forskohlii* may improve asthma symptoms.[17-19]

The Chinese herb **ma huang** (ephedra) is definitely effective for mild asthma because it contains ephedrine. However, because of the difficulty of assuring appropriate ephedrine dosing, the possibility of dangerous drug interactions, and the outdated na-ture of ephedrine as an asthma treatment, ma huang cannot be recommended.

In vitro studies suggest that the flavonoid **quercetin** may inhibit the release of pro-inflammatory substances from mast cells; how-ever, no clinical trials of quercetin in asthma have been performed.

Other herbs and supplements sometimes recommended for asthma include aloe, antioxidants (including beta-carotene, sele-nium, and vitamins C and E), betaine, chamomile, damiana, elecampane, garlic, grindelia, hydrochloride, licorice, lobelia, magnesium, marshmallow, mullein, onion, reishi, vitamin B$_{12}$, and yerba santa. However, no real evidence supports these treatments at this time.

Drug Interactions

See the article on each individual supplement for a full description of the interactions summarized here.

Principal Natural Therapies for Asthma: Interactions with Pharmaceuticals		
Natural Therapy	Pharmaceutical	Interaction
Fish oil	Anticoagulant and antiplatelet agents	Possible increased risk of bleeding complications
Vitamin B_6	Levodopa	Reduction of efficacy (N/A if carbidopa taken as well)

Pharmaceuticals Used for Asthma: Possible Harmful Interactions with Natural Therapies		
Pharmaceutical	Natural Therapy	Interaction
Beta$_2$-agonists	Ephedra	Possible increased stimulant side effects
Oral and topical corticosteroids	Licorice	Potentiation of drug action
Theophylline	Black pepper	Increased serum levels of drug
	Ipriflavone, St. John's wort	Decreased serum levels of drug

Pharmaceuticals Used for Asthma: Natural Therapies with Potential Supportive Interactions		
Pharmaceutical	**Natural Therapy**	**Interaction**
Oral and inhaled corticosteroids	Combined high-dose calcium and vitamin D	Counter corticosteroid-induced osteoporosis
	Chromium	Counter corticosteroid-induced diabetes

ATTENTION DEFICIT HYPERACTIVITY DISORDER (ADHD)

Principal Proposed Natural Therapies

DMAE (2-dimethylamin oethanol) [+2]

Essential fatty acids [–1X]

(Higher numbers indicate stronger evidence; X modifier indicates contradictory results. See page xviii of the Introduction for details of the rating scale.)

Approach to the Patient

Many patients have come to believe that numerous alternative treatments for ADHD are highly effective. However, there is little to no scientific support for any of these widely advocated options. Conversely, many believe that methylphenidate (Ritalin) and related drugs are profoundly dangerous; this topic should be approached with delicacy.

Scant preliminary evidence suggests that treatment with DMAE benefits ADHD.

Other natural treatments your patient may be using for ADHD include essential fatty acids; combinations of amino acids (usually GABA, glycine, L-glutamine, L-phenylalanine, L-tyrosine, taurine); blue-green algae; calcium; inositol; iron; magnesium; St. John's wort; combinations of the polysaccharides (fucose, galactose, glucose, mannose, N-acetylneuraminic acid, N-acetylgalactosamine, N-acetylglucosamine, xylose); trace minerals; vitamin B_3 (niacin); vitamin B_6; or zinc.

For potential safety risks with the more common of these substances, see the full herb/supplement articles.

DMAE   +2

A 1974 article reviewed two 10-week, double-blind, placebo-controlled studies enrolling a total of 124 children with ADHD-related diagnoses, and reported that treatment with DMAE (2-dimethylaminoethanol) significantly improved test scores,[1] comparably to methylphenidate (Ritalin) in one of these trials.[1] Positive results were also seen in a small open study.[2]

Manufacturers' recommended dosages and those used in clinical studies vary between 400 mg and 1800 mg daily.

Although most clinical investigations using DMAE report that participants experienced no side effects, enough researchers have found adverse reactions to suggest that some caution is appropriate in using this supplement. Reported adverse effects include increased confusion, drowsiness, and elevated blood pressure,[3] as well as headache and muscle tension.[4] At least one other paper suggests that weight loss and insomnia may accompany use of DMAE.[5] There is also one case report of a woman who developed severe tardive dyskinesia after long-term DMAE use for a hand tremor.[4] In addition, a number of manufacturers warn against the use of DMAE in individuals with a history of seizures.

Maximum safe dosages for young children, pregnant or lactating women, or individuals with severe hepatic or renal disease have not been established.

Essential Fatty Acids   −1X

Omega-3 and omega-6 fatty acids are widely marketed as effective treatments for ADHD. However, the evidence base for this usage is unimpressive at best.

DHA has been tried as adjuvant therapy for ADHD. In a double-blind trial, 63 children with ADHD and stabilized on stimulant therapy were additionally given either DHA (345 mg/day, from an algae source) or placebo for 4 months.[6] The results showed no difference between the groups.

A 12-week, double-blind, placebo-controlled trial of 41 children found weak evidence that a combined fish oil and evening primrose oil might improve ADHD symptoms.[7] However, a high dropout rate and lack of significant differences on many of the scoring systems used mitigate the meaningfulness of the results.

Evening primrose oil failed to show efficacy for attention deficit disorder in a double-blind, placebo-controlled trial.[10] In another small, placebo-controlled, comparative trial, evening primrose oil proved less effective than D-amphetamine.[8]

Other Proposed Natural Therapies

A 1991 review of natural medicine literature found no evidence supporting treatment of ADHD with **vitamin B$_3$ (niacin), vitamin B$_6$,** or **multivitamin** or **mineral supplements.**[9]

Other supplements that are sometimes recommended for ADHD include combinations of amino acids (usually GABA, glycine, L-glutamine, L-phenylalanine, L-tyrosine, taurine); blue-green algae; calcium; inositol; iron; magnesium; St. John's wort; combinations of the polysaccharides (fucose, galactose, glucose, mannose, N-acetylneuraminic acid, N-acetylgalactosamine, N-acetylglucosamine, xylose); trace minerals; and zinc. However, no evidence supports any of these treatments for ADHD at this time.

Drug Interactions

See the article on each individual supplement for a full description of the interactions summarized here.

Pharmaceuticals Used for Attention Deficit Hyperactivity Disorder: Possible Harmful Interaction with Natural Therapy		
Pharmaceutical	Natural Therapy	Interaction
CNS stimulants	Ephedra	Potentiation of action

BENIGN PROSTATIC HYPERPLASIA (BPH)

Principal Proposed Natural Therapies

Saw palmetto [+3]   **Grass pollen** [+3]

Pygeum [+3]   **Nettle root** [+2]

Beta-sitosterol and beta-sitosterolin [+3]

(Higher numbers indicate stronger evidence; X modifier indicates contradictory results. See page xviii of the Introduction for details of the rating scale.)

Approach to the Patient

There is very little doubt at present that the herb saw palmetto is effective for benign prostatic hyperplasia (BPH). It may be equally effective as finasteride in reducing symptoms, although the herb does not shrink the prostate as substantially. One potential advantage over finasteride, however, is that saw palmetto does not alter prostate-specific antigen (PSA) levels. In addition, saw palmetto does not impair sexual function.

Numerous other botanical treatments for BPH have a significant level of evidence behind them as well, such as pygeum, sitosterols, nettle root, and grass pollen. Potentiation of treatment effects through combined therapy has been reported in some preliminary trials.

Except in cases of severe BPH in which urinary retention is a possibility, a trial of one of these options may be reasonable in patients who strongly desire it.

Other natural treatments your patient may be using include flaxseed oil, pumpkin seeds, and zinc. For potential safety risks with the more common of these substances, see the full herb/supplement articles.

Saw Palmetto   +3

At least seven double-blind studies involving a total of more than 475 patients have compared the benefits of saw palmetto with those of placebo over a period of 1 to 3 months.[1-10] In all but one of these studies,[6] the treatment significantly improved urinary flow rate and most other measures of prostate disease.

One 6-month, double-blind study of 1098 men compared finasteride with saw palmetto and found both about equally effective at reducing symptoms.[11] Neither treatment caused significant adverse effects, but one of the reported outcomes suggested that finasteride was more likely to impair sexual function. However, this study has been criticized on the basis that its inclusion criteria and duration precluded maximal efficacy of finasteride.[12,13]

A 48-week, double-blind trial of 543 patients with early BPH compared combined saw palmetto and nettle root with finasteride and found equal benefits.[14] Analysis of a 431-patient subgroup with larger prostate volume (> 40 ml), in which finasteride might be more effective, found similar results.

A 52-week, double-blind study of 811 men compared saw palmetto to the alpha-blocker tamsulosin and found equivalent efficacy in subjective and objective scores of BPH severity.[15] Saw palmetto, however, caused a decrease in prostate volume, whereas tamsulosin caused a small increase. Both treatments were well-tolerated; however, tamsulosin caused a higher incidence of ejaculation dysfunction.

A 6-month, double-blind, placebo-controlled trial of 44 men
given a saw palmetto herbal blend also containing nettle root and
pumpkin seed oil found significant reduction in prostate size.[16]
No significant improvement in symptoms was seen, but the study
size did not have the power to detect any improvement.

For more information, including dosage and safety issues, see
the **Saw Palmetto** article.

Pygeum   +3

More than 10 double-blind, placebo-controlled studies of
pygeum have been published.[17] Duration of these trials ranged
from 6 to 12 weeks using daily doses of pygeum extract from
75 to 200 mg. Quality-of-life and objective measurements (urinary flow rate, residual volume, nocturia) were typically reported to improve by 2 months[17] and remain improved for at
least 1 month after treatment.[18] The best was a double-blind,
placebo-controlled trial of 263 men, which found a reliable, statistically significant improvement in urinary flow rate, voided
volume, residual volume, daytime frequency, and nocturia (no
change in prostate weight was reported in this study).[19]

For more information, including dosage and safety issues, see
the **Pygeum** article.

Beta-Sitosterol and Beta-Sitosterolin   +3

Three out of four randomized double-blind, placebo-controlled
studies enrolling a total of 519 men with benign prostatic hyperplasia found significant benefits with beta-sitosterol.[20-23] The
largest, enrolling 200 men with BPH for a period of 6 months,
showed significant improvements in IPSS (International
Prostate Symptom Score) and modified Boyarsky score in the
treatment group as compared with the placebo group, beginning at 4 weeks.[23] Significant relative improvements were also

seen in peak flow and mean residual urinary volume. Reduction in prostatic volume was not observed. Similar results were seen in a 6-month, double-blind trial of 177 individuals with BPH.[21]

For more information, including dosage and safety issues, see the **Beta-Sitosterol** article.

Grass Pollen   +3

Two double-blind, placebo-controlled studies found that grass pollen extracts can improve symptoms of BPH. The first trial enrolled 103 men with BPH for 12 weeks, and the results showed significant improvements in signs and symptoms.[24] The second observed 57 men for 6 months, with similar outcome; prostate size also decreased significantly.[25]

For more information, including dosage and safety issues, see the **Grass Pollen** article.

Nettle Root   +2

In a 4- to 6-week, double-blind, placebo-controlled study of 72 men, treatment with nettle root produced a 14% improvement in urine flow and a 53% decrease in residual urine, a significant improvement as compared with placebo.[26] Another double-blind study of 40 men found a significant decrease in frequency of urination after 6 months.[27] Finally, a 9-week, double-blind study of 50 men found a significant improvement in urination volume, as well as a decrease in sex hormone–binding globulin (SHBG).[26-28]

At least three double-blind studies of nettle root for BPH, ranging in length from 4 weeks to 6 months, and including a total of about 150 men, have reported significant improvement in various urodynamic parameters and symptoms.[26-28]

For more information, including dosage and safety issues, see the **Nettle** article.

Other Proposed Natural Therapies

Pumpkin seeds, zinc, and flaxseed oil are sometimes recommended for BPH, but there is no evidence supporting these treatments at this time.

Drug Interactions

None known.

BIPOLAR DISORDER

Principal Proposed
Natural Therapy

Fish oil   [+2]

(Higher numbers indicate stronger evidence; X modifier indicates contradictory results. See page xviii of the Introduction for details of the rating scale.)

Approach to the Patient

Highly preliminary evidence suggests that high doses of fish oil might help maintain euthymia in bipolar disease.

Other natural treatments your patient may be using include choline, flaxseed oil, folate, lecithin, and vitamins B_{12} and C, but these have little supporting evidence for use in bipolar disorder. Inositol has been tried as an add-on treatment for the depressive phase of bipolar disorder.[1] For potential safety risks with the more common of these substances, see the full herb/supplement articles.

Caution: Case reports of manic episodes have also been reported with the use of other herbs and supplements thought to possess antidepressant properties, such as inositol,[2] St. John's wort, fish oil, and SAMe. The supplement L-glutamine has also been implicated.[3]

Fish Oil   +2

Preliminary evidence suggests that fish oil, a source of omega-3 fatty acids, may be helpful for bipolar disorder. In a double-blind study, 30 individuals with bipolar disorder were given either placebo or fish oil capsules for 4 months, in addition to their existing treatment.[4] The results showed longer symptom-free periods in the treated group.

This trial employed rather high doses of fish oil: seven capsules twice daily, each capsule containing 680 mg of omega-3 fatty acids (440 mg of EPA, 240 mg of DHA). By comparison, most fish oil capsules contain no more than 300 mg of total omega-3 fatty acids.

For more information, including dosage and safety issues, see the **Fish Oil** article.

Other Proposed Natural Therapies

The same researchers who conducted the fish oil study have also experimented informally with **flaxseed oil** for bipolar disorder.[5] Flaxseed oil contains alpha-linolenic acid (ALA), an omega-3 fatty acid upstream from DHA and EPA.

Weak evidence suggests that **choline** and **lecithin** (a source of phosphatidylcholine) may be helpful for bipolar illness.[6,7]

Two poorly reported and designed double-blind trials found some evidence to suggest that **vitamin C** might be useful for bipolar disorder.[8,9]

A pilot study suggests that **inositol** may be helpful in conjunction with standard treatment for the depressive phase of bipolar disorder, although the use of this supplement has also been associated with the occurrence of manic episodes.[1]

Folate deficiency has been associated with poor response to lithium therapy.[10] However, a 1-year, double-blind trial of 75 individuals taking lithium for a variety of disorders found no difference between those given folate and those given placebo.

Vitamin B_{12} has also been proposed as a treatment, but there is no real evidence to turn to.

Drug Interactions

See the article on each individual supplement for a full description of the interactions summarized here.

Principal Natural Therapy for Bipolar Disorder: Interaction with Pharmaceuticals		
Natural Therapy	**Pharmaceutical**	**Interaction**
Fish oil	Anticoagulant and antiplatelet agents	Possible increased risk of bleeding complications

CERVICAL DYSPLASIA

Principal Proposed Natural Therapies

Folate

Prevention [+1]

Treatment [−2]

Vitamin C, beta-carotene

(treatment) [−2]

(Higher numbers indicate stronger evidence; X modifier indicates contradictory results. See page xviii of the Introduction for details of the rating scale.)

Approach to the Patient

Nutritional deficiencies may be associated with the development of cervical dysplasia, and on this basis prophylactic treatment with a general multivitamin and mineral supplement, especially including folate, may be warranted. However, nutrients have not been found effective for cervical dysplasia once it has occurred. Other natural treatments your patient may be using for prevention or treatment of cervical dysplasia include herbs known as emmenagogues, such as black cohosh, blessed thistle, false unicorn, motherwort, true unicorn, and squaw vine.

Caution: Patients may need to be reminded that follow-up testing is essential; they may believe that these natural treatments will definitely cure cervical dysplasia.

Folate (Prevention) +1, (Treatment) − 2

Folate deficiency may act as a co-carcinogen during the initiation of cervical cancer.[1] However, in a 6-month, double-blind trial of 235 women with existing grade 1 or 2 cervical interepithelial neoplasia, folate supplements did not alter the course of the disease.[1]

For more information, including dosage and safety issues, see the **Folate** article.

Vitamin C, Beta-Carotene (Treatment)   − 2

Studies have found that women with cervical dysplasia are likely to have general nutritional deficiencies, as many as 67% of patients in one survey.[2] Particular vitamin deficiencies commonly associated with cervical dysplasia include beta-carotene, vitamin C, vitamin B_6, selenium, and folate,[3,4] which suggests that multivitamin and mineral supplements may be beneficial. However, a double-blind, placebo-controlled study of 141 women found that neither vitamin C nor beta-carotene supplements reversed cervical dysplasia.[5] In addition, a 9-month, double-blind, placebo-controlled study of 98 women with moderate CIN found no benefit with beta-carotene alone.[7] Lack of benefit with beta-carotene alone was also seen in a 2-year, double-blind, placebo-controlled trial of 103 women with high-grade CIN,[8] and in a 12-month, double-blind, placebo-controlled trial of 117 women with abnormal cervical morphology of various types.[9]

For more information, including dosage and safety issues, see the **Vitamin C** and **Beta-Carotene** articles.

Other Proposed Natural Therapies

Indole-3-carbinol (I3C) is a substance found in the broccoli family of vegetables that has been extensively investigated for possible chemopreventive effects. A double-blind trial of 30 women with biopsy-proven CIN II-III compared placebo with 200 mg/day and 400 mg/day of I3C for a period of 12 weeks.[6] No regressions occurred in the placebo group, but four of eight patients in the 200-mg group and four of nine patients in the 400-mg group did experience complete regression.

Emmenagogic herbs, including squaw vine, motherwort, true unicorn, false unicorn, black cohosh, and blessed thistle, are reputed to be helpful in cervical dysplasia, but no evidence supports these treatments at this time.

Drug Interactions

See the article on each individual supplement for a full description of the interactions summarized here.

Principal Natural Therapy for Cervical Dysplasia: Interaction with Pharmaceuticals		
Natural Therapy	Pharmaceutical	Interaction
Vitamin C	Acetaminophen	Possible increased serum levels of drug

CHOLELITHIASIS

Principal Proposed Natural Therapies

There are no evidence-based herbs or supplements for cholelithiasis.

Approach to the Patient

Although there is no real evidence to support their use, your patients may be using natural therapies such as betaine hydrochloride, fumitory, milk thistle, and peppermint. For potential safety risks with the more common of these substances, see the full herb/supplement articles.

Patients interested in alternative medicine may believe that removing the gallbladder deprives the body of an essential organ and is therefore fundamentally wrong. Because this concept invokes a larger belief system concerning "supporting the body," direct contradiction of the patient's beliefs will likely cause a breakdown of communication. Delicacy is advised.

Caution: Certain herbs might present risk by stimulating gallbladder contraction. These include artichoke leaf, boldo, celandine, and turmeric (or curcumin).

Other Proposed Natural Therapies

Highly preliminary studies suggest that formulas containing **peppermint** and related terpenes may help dissolve gallstones.[1] **Milk thistle,** standardized to silymarin content, has been found to improve the liquidity of bile,[2] although its actual effects on gallstones are unknown.

The herb fumitory is said to relieve spasms of the sphincter of Oddi, although no real evidence supports this belief. Herbs sometimes used to expel gallstones include artichoke leaf, boldo, greater celandine, and turmeric, all thought to increase gallbladder contraction. However, if active in this manner, they could create risk of gallbladder rupture, bile or hepatic duct obstruction, or intestinal obstruction.

A large 10-year observational study found that regular **coffee** drinking can reduce the risk of developing gallstones, at least in men aged 40 to 75 years.[3] Those who drank more coffee had an even greater reduction of risk. Observational evidence also suggests that regular use of **vitamin C** supplements might help prevent gallstones in women.[4]

Drug Interactions

None known.

CHRONIC FATIGUE SYNDROME (CFS)

Principal Proposed
Natural Therapies

**NADH (nicotinamide
adenine dinucleotide) [+2]**

**Essential fatty acids (GLA,
fish oil) [+2X]**

(Higher numbers indicate stronger evidence; X modifier indicates contradictory results. See page xviii of the Introduction for details of the rating scale.)

Approach to Patient

There are no well-documented therapies for CFS, but NADH and essential fatty acids have minimal supporting evidence.

Some patients may believe that their condition is due to yeast overgrowth (the "*Candida* syndrome"), food allergies, intestinal dysbiosis, mercury filling sensitivity, or multiple chemical sensitivities (environmental allergies). Although there is no scientific basis for any of these hypotheses, many patients subscribe to these beliefs with a semireligious fervor; it is essential to approach the subject delicately.

Other natural treatments your patient may be using for chronic fatigue include beta-carotene, carnitine, DHEA, echinacea, ginseng, licorice, or multivitamin/mineral supplements.

NADH +2

More often used by athletes, NADH (nicotinamide adenine dinucleotide) supplements have also been tried for CFS. A double-blind, placebo-controlled, crossover trial that observed 26 individuals with CFS given 10 mg of NADH for a 4-week period found some improvement in symptoms during NADH treatment as compared with the period of placebo treatment (31% vs. 8%).[1]

For more information, including dosage and safety issues, see the **NADH** article.

Essential Fatty Acids (GLA, Fish Oil)   +2X

In a 3-month, double-blind, placebo-controlled study, 63 individuals were given either a combination of essential fatty acids containing evening primrose oil (a source of the omega-6 fatty acid GLA) and fish oil, or liquid paraffin placebo.[2] Significant improvements were seen at 1 and 3 months; in addition, the researchers also found at the beginning of the study that many participants had abnormal essential fatty acid levels and that these improved with treatment.

However, a more precisely structured replication of this study in 1999 found no benefit.[3] In addition, this investigation showed no difference in fatty acid levels between individuals with CFS and individuals without CFS who served as comparison. For more information, including dosage and safety issues, see the articles on **Gamma-Linolenic Acid** and **Fish Oil.**

Other Proposed Natural Therapies

A poorly designed trial found weak evidence that **carnitine** might be helpful for CFS.[4] Both **beta-carotene** and **DHEA** have also been suggested as treatments, but the supporting evidence for their use in CFS is exceedingly preliminary.[5-7]

An in vitro trial of **echinacea** and **ginseng** found that both herbs increased cellular immune function in cells taken from individuals with CFS.[8] However, many herbs and supplements cause measurable changes in immune function, and such observations do not correlate well with clinically significant results.

Based on a theory that CFS might be related to low blood pressure, some herbalists have recommended licorice. The herb has mineralocorticoid effects and raises blood pressure when taken long-term in high doses. However, there is no evidence that it works for CFS, and other treatments to raise blood pressure have proven ineffective for CFS.[9]

Although some alternative practitioners have suggested that CFS might be caused by deficiencies of multiple vitamins and minerals, a double-blind, placebo-controlled study of 42 individuals found no significant improvement in CFS symptoms when a **multivitamin/mineral supplement** was given four times daily after meals for 3 months.[10]

Drug Interactions

See the article on each individual supplement for a full description of the interactions summarized here.

Principal Natural Therapy for Chronic Fatigue Syndrome: Interaction with Pharmaceuticals		
Natural Therapy	**Pharmaceutical**	**Interaction**
Fish oil	Anticoagulant and antiplatelet agents	Possible increased risk of bleeding complications

Pharmaceuticals Used for Chronic Fatigue Syndrome: Possible Harmful Interactions with Natural Therapies		
Pharmaceutical	**Natural Therapy**	**Interaction**
Selective serotonin reuptake inhibitors (SSRIs), tricyclic antidepressants	5-HTP, SAMe, St. John's wort	Possible risk of serotonin syndrome
Tricyclic anti-depressants	Dong quai, St. John's wort	Possible increased risk of photo-sensitivity

Pharmaceuticals Used for Chronic Fatigue Syndrome: Natural Therapies with Potential Supportive Interactions		
Pharmaceutical	**Natural Therapy**	**Interaction**
SSRIs	Ginkgo	Possible reversal of SSRI-induced sexual dysfunction
Tricyclic anti-depressants	Coenzyme Q_{10}	Possible correction of drug-induced relative deficiency

CHRONIC OBSTRUCTIVE PULMONARY DISEASE (COPD)

Principal Proposed Natural Therapies

N-Acetyl cysteine (NAC)   [+3]

Carnitine   [+2]

(Higher numbers indicate stronger evidence; X modifier indicates contradictory results. See page xviii of the Introduction for details of the rating scale.)

Approach to the Patient

Reasonably good evidence suggests that *N*-acetyl cysteine (NAC), a modified form of the dietary amino acid cysteine, may be helpful for chronic bronchitis associated with COPD. The mechanism of action may not involve thinning of secretions. The use of carnitine in COPD is also supported by some evidence.

Other natural treatments your patient may be using for COPD include fish oil, antioxidants (e.g., beta-carotene, vitamins A, C, and E), and coenzyme Q_{10}. For potential safety risks with the more common of these substances, see the full herb/supplement articles.

Caution: Patients may need to be advised that these treatments have been researched as adjunctive therapies rather than as substitutes for conventional care.

N-Acetyl Cysteine (NAC)   +3

A metaanalysis of available research focused on eight reasonably well-designed, double-blind, placebo-controlled trials of NAC for chronic bronchitis, involving a total of about 1400 individuals.[1-9] The results of these studies suggest that a daily dose of NAC at 400 to 1200 mg can reduce the number of acute exacerbations of chronic bronchitis.

For more information, including dosage and safety issues, see the **N-Acetyl Cysteine** article.

Carnitine   +2

Evidence from three double-blind, placebo-controlled studies enrolling a total of 49 individuals suggests that L-carnitine can improve exercise tolerance in COPD, presumably by improving muscular efficiency in the lungs and other muscles.[10-12]

For more information, including dosage and safety issues, see the **Carnitine** article.

Other Proposed Natural Therapies

Based on observational studies,[13-18] **fish oil,** as well as the antioxidant supplements **beta-carotene** and **vitamins A, C,** and **E,** has been recommended for the treatment of COPD. However, there is no direct evidence that they are effective against the condition, and one study found that vitamin E and beta-carotene supplementation had no effect on COPD symptoms.[19]

A small open trial suggests that **coenzyme Q_{10}** might improve pulmonary function in individuals with COPD.[20]

Drug Interactions

See the article on each individual supplement for a full description of the interactions summarized here.

Principal Natural Therapy for Chronic Obstructive Pulmonary Disease: Interaction with Pharmaceuticals		
Natural Therapy	Pharmaceutical	Interaction
NAC	Nitrates	Increase of headache side effect

Pharmaceuticals Used for Chronic Obstructive Pulmonary Disease: Possible Harmful Interactions with Natural Therapies		
Pharmaceutical	Natural Therapy	Interaction
Beta$_2$-agonists	Ephedra	Possible increased stimulant side effects
Oral and topical corticosteroids	Licorice	Potentiation of drug
Theophylline	Black pepper	Increased serum levels of drug
	Cayenne	Increased serum levels of drug
	Ephedra, green tea, guarana	Potentiation of stimulant side effects
	Ipriflavone, St. John's wort	Decreased serum levels of drug

Pharmaceuticals Used for Chronic Obstructive Pulmonary Disease: Natural Therapies with Potential Supportive Interactions		
Pharmaceutical	**Natural Therapy**	**Interaction**
Oral and inhaled corticosteroids	Chromium	Counter corticosteroid-induced diabetes
	Combined high-dose calcium and vitamin D	Counter corticosteroid-induced osteoporosis
Theophylline	Vitamin B_6	May reduce side effects

CIRRHOSIS

Principal Proposed
Natural Therapies

Milk thistle [+3X]

SAMe [+1]

(Higher numbers indicate stronger evidence; X modifier indicates contradictory results. See page xviii of the Introduction for details of the rating scale.)

Approach to the Patient

Mixed evidence suggests that the hepatoprotective herb milk thistle may offer some benefit in cirrhosis. Much weaker evidence suggests that the supplement SAMe (S-adenosylmethionine) might be useful as well.

Other natural treatments your patient may be using include BCAAs (branched-chain amino acids), betaine glucuronate, choline, diethanolamine, inositol, methionine, OPCs (oligomeric proanthocyanidins), phosphatidylcholine, and taurine. For potential safety risks with the more common of these substances, see the full herb/supplement articles.

Caution: Use of arginine might cause hyperkalemia in individuals with advanced hepatic disease.

Milk Thistle   +3X

A large body of evidence suggests that milk thistle possesses hepatoprotective properties. In Europe, it is used to treat poisoning by the deathcap mushroom as well as viral hepatitis, alcoholic fatty liver, alcoholic hepatitis, and drug- or chemical-induced hepatotoxicity.

However, studies of milk thistle for cirrhosis have returned inconsistent results.

A double-blind, placebo-controlled study of 170 individuals with alcoholic or nonalcoholic cirrhosis found that in the group treated with milk thistle, the 4-year survival rate was 58% as compared with only 38% in the placebo group.[1] This difference was statistically significant.

A double-blind, placebo-controlled trial that enrolled 172 individuals with cirrhosis and observed them for 4 years found reductions in mortality that just missed the conventional 0.5% cutoff for statistical significance.[2]

Finally, a 2-year, double-blind, placebo-controlled study of 200 individuals with alcoholic cirrhosis found no reduction in mortality attributable to the use of milk thistle.[3] Other double-blind studies of cirrhotic individuals have found reductions in liver enzymes and serum bilirubin,[14,15] although one did not.[16]

For more information, including dosage and safety issues, see the **Milk Thistle** article.

SAMe   +1

A 2-year, double-blind, placebo-controlled study of 123 individuals with alcoholic cirrhosis found a statistically insignificant trend toward improvement in the verum group as compared to the placebo group; post-hoc analysis found significant differences in the subgroup with less advanced disease.[4] Small trials, some of which were double-blind, found possible value in oral contraceptive hepatotoxicity, intrahepatic cholestasis of pregnancy, and Gilbert's syndrome.[5-9]

For more information, including dosage and safety issues, see the **S-Adenosylmethionine** article.

Other Proposed
Natural Therapies

BCAAs have been tried in hepatic encephalopathy, but there is no real evidence as yet that they produce any benefit.[10]

Preliminary evidence suggests that **OPCs** might improve capillary fragility in cirrhosis.[11]

The amino acid **taurine** might help reduce muscle cramps in individuals with cirrhosis.[12]

Preliminary evidence from animal studies suggests that supplemental **phosphatidylcholine** might help protect against the development of alcoholic cirrhosis.[13] Betaine glucuronate, diethanolamine, choline, methionine, and inositol are also sometimes proposed, but there is no real evidence that they are helpful in cirrhosis.

Drug Interactions

See the article on each individual supplement for a full description of the interactions summarized here.

Principal Natural Therapy for Cirrhosis: Interactions with Pharmaceuticals		
Natural Therapy	**Pharmaceutical**	**Interaction**
SAMe	Levodopa or levodopa-carbidopa	Possible increased "wearing off" effect
	Serotonergic drugs (case report involved tricyclic antidepressant)	Possible risk of serotonin syndrome

Pharmaceuticals Used for Cirrhosis: Possible Harmful Interactions with Natural Therapies

Pharmaceutical	Natural Therapy	Interaction
Potassium-sparing diuretics	Arginine	Possible increased risk of hyperkalemia
	Licorice	Antagonism of drug action
	Magnesium	Risk of hyper-magnesemia
	White willow	Salicylate content might interfere with spironolactone action
	Zinc	Excessive zinc levels with spironolactone

Pharmaceuticals Used for Cirrhosis: Natural Therapy with Potential Supportive Interactions

Pharmaceutical	Natural Therapy	Interaction
Potassium-sparing diuretics	Folate	Correction of possible drug-induced depletion

COLIC

Principal Proposed Natural Therapies

There are no evidence-based herbs or supplements for colic.

Approach to the Patient

Infantile colic is a troublesome problem with an unknown cause, for which treatment is unsatisfactory. Although dimethicone is sometimes recommended for colic, evidence suggests that it does not work.[1]

There are no well-documented alternative therapies for colic. Nevertheless, your patient may be trying such natural treatments as various herbs, "gripe water" (which contains a high level of alcohol), and salt substitutes.

Other Proposed Natural Therapies

One small double-blind, placebo-controlled study found that an herbal tea eliminated colic in 57% of 33 infants in the treatment group, as opposed to only 26% in the placebo group (a significant difference).[2] The tea contained extracts of chamomile, vervain, licorice, fennel, and lemon balm—herbs with an antispasmodic reputation. However, the safety of this herbal combination in infants has not been established.

Other herbs sometimes recommended for colic include angelica, cardamom, peppermint, and yarrow, but no scientific evidence as yet supports their use.

In Britain, a preparation called **"gripe water"** is widely sold for the treatment of colic.[3] Varying formulations exist; however, all include aromatic oils such as dill, spearmint, or caraway, combined with alcohol, sucrose, and sodium bicarbonate. There is no scientific evidence for or against the use of gripe water in colic. It should be noted that at the recommended dosage, the infant would receive the equivalent of five shots of whiskey.

In the past, the use of **salt substitutes** containing potassium has been recommended for infants with colic, but at least one case of clinically dangerous hyperkalemia in an infant has been attributed to this treatment.[4]

Studies evaluating the effects of carrying a colicky child more, or using a **motion-simulation device,** have not found benefit.[5,6]

Drug Interactions

None known.

CONGESTIVE HEART FAILURE (CHF)

Principal Proposed Natural Therapies

Coenzyme Q$_{10}$ [+3]	**Arginine** [+2]
Hawthorn [+3]	**Creatine** [+2]
Carnitine [+2]	**Vitamin B$_1$** [+1]
Taurine [+2]	**Vitamin E** [−1]

(Higher numbers indicate stronger evidence; X modifier indicates contradictory results. See page xviii of the Introduction for details of the rating scale.)

Approach to the Patient

Considerable evidence supports the use of coenzyme Q$_{10}$ as adjuvant treatment for CHF. Hawthorn is used as monotherapy in Germany for mild to moderate CHF; however, in contrast with conventional therapies such as ACE inhibitors, hawthorn has not been evaluated for potential long-term reductions in mortality and morbidity. Other supplements of potential value include arginine, carnitine, creatine, taurine, and vitamin B$_1$.

Other natural treatments your patient may be using include magnesium and Chinese herbal medicine. For potential safety risks with magnesium, see the full **Magnesium** article.

Caution: Patients may need to be advised that, unlike ACE inhibitors, hawthorn has not been shown to reduce mortality and morbidity.

Coenzyme Q$_{10}$ +3

Reasonably good evidence supports the use of CoQ$_{10}$ as adjuvant therapy. It is thought to work by improving the efficiency of cardiac muscle.

A double-blind, multicenter study observed 641 patients with New York Heart Association (NYHA) class III or IV failure for 1 year.[1] Half were given CoQ$_{10}$, 2 mg/kg, orally and the rest placebo. Conventional therapy was continued. In the treated group, there was a progressive and statistically significant reduction, in CHF class over the course of the study. There was also a statistically and clinically significant reduction in incidence of acute pulmonary edema, cardiac asthma, and hospitalizations for worsening heart failure in the treated group. In addition, there was a statistically significant difference in the percentage of patients who required one or more hospitalizations during the trial period, from 40% in the control group to about 20% in the treated group.

Benefits have been seen in other studies as well.[2-4] However, a 6-month, double-blind study of 45 individuals with CHF found no benefit.[5]

For more information, including dosage and safety issues, see the **Coenzyme Q$_{10}$** article.

Hawthorn   +3

Since 1981, at least 14 controlled clinical studies (most of them double-blind) were published on the therapeutic efficacy of hawthorn (WS 1442) in CHF.[6-10] Most of the approximately 800 patients participating in these studies had NYHA class II CHF. Significant improvement was generally (but not uniformly) noted in exercise tolerance, anaerobic threshold, ejection fraction, and subjective complaints. The doses of hawthorn used in these studies ranged from 180 to 900 mg/day taken for a period of 21 to 84 days (most studies lasted 42 or 56 days).

There is no evidence that hawthorn reduces CHF morbidity or mortality.

For more information, including dosage and safety issues, see the **Hawthorn** article.

Carnitine   +2

Like coenzyme Q_{10}, carnitine may have value in the adjuvant treatment of CHF.

A double-blind, placebo-controlled study observed 50 patients with NYHA class II CHF for a period of 6 months.[11] Each received 1.5 g of L-propionylcarnitine or placebo daily. At the end of the trial period, exercise duration increased by 1.4 minutes in treated patients vs. 0.36 minutes in controls. Also, as compared with the placebo group, there was a statistically significant improvement in left ventricular shortening fraction, left ventricular ejection fraction, stroke volume index, systemic vascular resistance, cardiac index, and clinical ratings. Improved heart function has also been seen in other studies.[12-15] In one trial, improvements were maintained for 60 days after treatment with carnitine was stopped.[12]

For more information, including dosage and safety issues, see the **Carnitine** article.

Taurine   +2

Research (primarily by one group) including small double-blind studies, open trials, and animal experiments suggests that taurine may be useful adjuvant therapy in class II, III, and IV CHF.[16-22]

For more information, including dosage and safety issues, see the **Taurine** article.

Arginine   +2

Small double-blind trials indicate that arginine may improve some CHF symptoms.[23-25]

For more information, including dosage and safety issues, see the **Arginine** article.

Creatine   +2

Patients with CHF experience muscle fatigue caused by loss of skeletal muscle mass and strength, altered fiber composition, decreased oxidative capacity, and other abnormalities of muscle metabolism. For this reason, creatine (best known as a sports supplement) has been tried as a treatment for CHF. Small double-blind trials suggest that creatine may improve skeletal muscle exercise tolerance in patients with CHF.[26,27]

For more information, including dosage and safety issues, see the **Creatine** article.

Vitamin B_1 +1

Evidence suggests that individuals with CHF are commonly deficient in vitamin B_1, presumably because of the use of loop diuretics.[28] A small, double-blind study found that intravenous administration of thiamine followed by oral supplementation could improve heart function in individuals with CHF.[29]

For more information, including dosage and safety issues, see the **Vitamin B_1** article.

Vitamin E   −1

A double-blind, placebo-controlled trial of 56 individuals found vitamin E ineffective for the treatment of CHF.[30]

Other Proposed Natural Therapies

Magnesium is often recommended as a treatment for CHF, but there is no real evidence that oral supplementation is helpful.

Traditional Chinese herbal medicine utilizes numerous herbs to treat CHF symptoms, but there has been no significant scientific evaluation of these treatments.

Drug Interactions

See the article on each individual supplement for a full description of the interactions summarized here.

Principal Natural Therapy for Congestive Heart Failure: Interaction with Pharmaceutical		
Natural Therapy	Pharmaceutical	Interaction
Coenzyme Q_{10}	Warfarin	Possible antagonism of drug action

Pharmaceuticals Used for Congestive Heart Failure: Possible Harmful Interactions with Natural Therapies		
Pharmaceutical	Natural Therapy	Interaction
ACE inhibitors	Arginine, potassium	Possible hyperkalemia
	Dong quai, St. John's wort	Possible increased risk of photosensitivity
	Iron	Mutual absorption interference
	Licorice	Antagonism of drug action

Pharmaceuticals Used for Congestive Heart Failure: Possible Harmful Interactions with Natural Therapies—cont'd		
Pharmaceutical	**Natural Therapy**	**Interaction**
Digitoxin, digoxin	*Eleutherococcus* (Siberian ginseng)	Interference with laboratory measurement of digoxin levels
	Horsetail, licorice	Possible hypokalemia leading to increased drug toxicity
	St. John's wort	Decreased serum levels of drug with possible rebound toxicity if herb is stopped
Loop diuretics	Dong quai, St. John's wort	Possible increased risk of photosensitivity
	Licorice	Potentiation of hypokalemic action of drug
Potassium-sparing diuretics	Arginine	Possible increased risk of hyperkalemia
	Licorice	Antagonism of drug action
	Magnesium	Risk of hypermagnesemia
	White willow	Salicylate content might interfere with spironolactone action
	Zinc	Excessive zinc levels with spironolactone
Thiazide diuretics	Calcium	Potential risk of hypercalcemia
	Dong quai, St. John's wort	Possible increased risk of photosensitivity
	Licorice	Potentiation of hypokalemic action of drug

Pharmaceuticals Used for Congestive Heart Failure: Natural Therapies with Potential Supportive Interactions

Pharmaceutical	Natural Therapy	Interaction
ACE inhibitors	Zinc	Correction of possible drug-induced depletion
	Iron	Possible reduction of ACE inhibitor–induced cough
Digitoxin, digoxin	Calcium	Correction of possible drug-induced depletion
	Magnesium	Correction of possible drug-induced depletion; separate dose by 2 hr to avoid absorption interference
	St. John's wort	Reduced serum levels because of P-glycoprotein interactions, with possible rebound toxicity if herb is continued
Hydralazine	Vitamin B_6	Correction of possible drug-induced depletion
Loop diuretics	Magnesium, potassium, vitamin B_1	Correction of possible drug-induced depletion
Potassium-sparing diuretics	Folate	Correction of possible drug-induced depletion
Thiazide diuretics	Magnesium, potassium, zinc	Correction of possible drug-induced depletion

CONJUNCTIVITIS (VIRAL)

Principal Proposed Natural Therapies

There are no evidence-based herbs or supplements for conjunctivitis.

Approach to the Patient

In the traditional treatment of conjunctivitis, herbal teas have been applied to the eyes directly or in compress or poultice form.

Caution: Use of herbal teas as eye wash presents risks of infection and allergic reaction.

Other natural treatments your patient may be using for conjunctivitis include topical use of barberry, calendula, chamomile, eyebright, goldenseal, and Oregon grape, and oral use of andrographis, echinacea, vitamins A and C, and zinc. For potential safety risks with the more common of these substances, see the full herb/supplement articles.

Other Proposed Natural Therapies

As the name suggests, eyebright is a traditional herbal treatment for eye conditions; however, this recommendation was based on the supposed "blood-shot" appearance of its petals rather than any observed medicinal effect.

The herbs barberry, Oregon grape, and goldenseal contain **berberine,** a substance with antimicrobial and antibacterial properties. Purified berberine is used as a pharmaceutical treatment for conjunctivitis in Germany but is not available in the United States. The herb calendula may possess antiinflammatory and antiseptic properties and has been used traditionally as an eye compress, as has chamomile tea.

Herbs and supplements that are generally recommended for respiratory infections, such as andrographis, echinacea, vitamin C, and zinc, might also be tried for conjunctivitis.

Finally, based on the role of vitamin A in vision, vitamin A supplements have been recommended in the lay press as a treatment for conjunctivitis.

Drug Interactions

None known.

CROHN'S DISEASE

Principal Proposed Natural Treatments

General nutritional support   [+4]

Fish oil   [−2X]

(Higher numbers indicate stronger evidence; X modifier indicates contradictory results. See page xviii of the Introduction for details of the rating scale.)

Approach to the Patient

There are no well-documented natural treatments for Crohn's disease, although probiotics have shown some promise. (Probiotics have been more intensively investigated for ulcerative colitis.)

Patients interested in alternative medicine will likely appreciate focused attention on correcting the nutritional deficiencies that are common in this condition.

Other natural treatments your patient may be using include fish oil, glutamine, and boswellia. For potential safety risks with the more common of these substances, see the full herb/supplement articles.

General Nutritional Support   + 4

Deficiencies of numerous nutrients are well-known in individuals with Crohn's disease. Malabsorption, decreased appetite, drug side effects, and increased nutrient loss through the stool may lead to mild or profound deficiencies of protein; vitamins A, B$_{12}$, C, D, E, and K; folate; calcium; copper; magnesium; selenium; and zinc.[1-10] Supplementation to restore normal nutriture is advisable.

For more information, including dosage and safety issues, see the appropriate supplement articles.

Fish Oil   − 2 X

Fish oil has been tried for Crohn's disease but with mixed results. In a 1-year, double-blind, placebo-controlled trial that observed 120 individuals in remission, treatment with fish oil (3.3 g EPA, 1.8 g DHA, non–enteric coated, daily) failed to reduce the relapse rate,[11] and negative results were also seen in a smaller double-blind trial.[12] However, a 1-year, double-blind, placebo-controlled trial involving 78 participants with Crohn's disease in remission who were at high risk for relapse found that enteric-coated fish oil capsules (1.8 g EPA, 0.9 g DHA daily) helped to keep the disease controlled.[13]

For more information, including dosage and safety issues, see the **Fish Oil** article.

Other Proposed Natural Therapies

Glutamine is believed to play a role in intestinal wall integrity and on this basis has been studied as a treatment for Crohn's disease; however, the clinical evidence regarding its effectiveness is still highly preliminary.[14-16]

The **probiotic** yeast *Saccharomyces boulardii* has also been the subject of preliminary investigations[17]; other probiotics have been tested with some success in ulcerative colitis.

Preliminary evidence suggests that the herb **boswellia** *(Boswellia serrata)* may also be helpful for inflammatory bowel disease.[18-20]

Drug Interactions

See the article on each individual supplement for a full description of the interactions summarized here.

Principal Natural Therapy for Crohn's Disease: Interaction with Pharmaceuticals		
Natural Therapy	Pharmaceutical	Interaction
Fish oil	Anticoagulant and antiplatelet agents	Possible increased risk of bleeding complications

Pharmaceuticals Used for Crohn's Disease: Possible Harmful Interactions with Natural Therapies		
Pharmaceutical	Natural Therapy	Interaction
NSAIDs	Dong quai, St. John's wort	Possible increased risk of photosensitivity
	Feverfew	Possible increased risk of gastritis
	Garlic, ginkgo, high-dose vitamin E, policosanol, others	Possible increased risk of bleeding complications
	Potassium citrate	Possible decreased serum levels of salicylates
	White willow	Additional salicylates may increase risk of all side effects
Oral and topical corticosteroids	Licorice	Potentiation of drug action

Pharmaceuticals Used for Crohn's Disease: Natural Therapies with Potential Supportive Interactions		
Pharmaceutical	**Natural Therapy**	**Interaction**
NSAIDs	Cayenne, colostrum, licorice	Possible cytoprotection
	Folate, vitamin C	Correction of possible drug-induced deficiency
Oral and inhaled corticosteroids	Chromium	Counter corticosteroid-induced diabetes
	Combined high-dose calcium and vitamin D, ipriflavone	Counter corticosteroid-induced osteoporosis

CYSTITIS

Principal Proposed Natural Therapies

Cranberry (Prophylaxis of Acute UTI)   [+3], (Chronic Bacteruria/ Pyuria)   [+2X]

Uva Ursi (Treatment) [+1]

(Higher numbers indicate stronger evidence; X modifier indicates contradictory results. See page xviii of the Introduction for details of the rating scale.)

Approach to the Patient

Some evidence supports the use of cranberry juice for preventing urinary tract infections (UTIs). Tablets are more convenient than cranberry juice (which is very bitter). Cranberry juice cocktail contains little cranberry juice.

Caution: The herb uva ursi is believed to have urinary antiseptic properties but may present risk of toxicity if taken long-term.

Other natural treatments your patient may be using include probiotics, buchu, cleavers, dandelion, goldenrod, horsetail, juniper, and parsley. For potential safety risks with the more common of these substances, see the full herb/supplement articles.

Cranberry (Prophylaxis of Acute UTI)   +3, (Chronic Bacteriuria/Pyuria)   +2X

Evidence suggests that cranberry juice interferes with the adherence of bacteria to the epithelial cells of the bladder by acting on bacterial adhesins that attach to oligosaccharide or monosaccharide receptors.[1-6] Such inhibition has been documented in *Escherichia coli*, *Proteus*, *Klebsiella*, *Enterobacter*, and *Pseudomonas*. Because bacteria have been noted to adhere particularly easily to the bladder wall of women who experience recurrent bladder infections,[7] cranberry juice might be an etiologically appropriate treatment for this condition.

An unpublished trial presented at the June 2001 meeting of the American Urological Association provides the only real evidence for the use of cranberry as prophylaxis for acute UTIs. This 1-year, double-blind, placebo-controlled study of 150 sexually active women compared placebo with both cranberry juice and cranberry tablets.[8] Both forms of cranberry significantly reduced the number of episodes of symptomatic UTI; however, cranberry tablets were more cost-effective.[9]

A widely reported year-long open trial of women with recurrent UTIs found that a cranberry-lingonberry combination exerted superior prophylaxis as compared with probiotics or no treatment; but given the reputation of cranberry, the placebo effect and observer bias cannot be excluded.[10]

A double-blind, placebo-controlled study observed 153 women with a mean age of 78.5 years for a period of 6 months.[11] The study was designed to examine the effects of cranberry on bacteriuria/pyuria, whether symptomatic or not. One half of the participants were given a standard commercial cranberry drink and the other half a placebo drink prepared to look and taste the same. Both treatments contained the identical amount of vitamin C to eliminate the possible antibacterial influence of that supplement. Despite the weak preparation of cranberry used, the results showed a 58% decrease in bacteriuria with pyuria compared with the control group. Further, in women who were initially bacteriuric/pyuric, their chance of remaining so was 73% less in the treated than in the control group. However, subsequent responses to this report called it into question on statistical and methodologic grounds.[12,13]

A double-blind, placebo-controlled crossover study of 15 children with neurogenic bladder reported no reduction in bacteriuria attributable to the cranberry concentrate used.[14]

For more information, including dosage and safety issues, see the **Cranberry** article.

Uva Ursi   +1

Uva ursi contains arbutin, a urinary antiseptic once widely used in conventional medicine. Arbutin is thought to work by liberating hydroquinone in the bladder. Because of the toxic risk of hydroquinone, uva ursi and arbutin are generally recommended only for short-term use. However, a 1-year, double-blind, placebo-controlled study of uva ursi (in combination with dandelion leaf) in 57 women showed a lower incidence of bladder infection in the treatment group.[15]

For more information, including dosage and safety issues, see the **Uva Ursi** article.

Other Proposed Natural Therapies

Probiotics are sometimes recommended for the treatment of cystitis, based on their potential for reducing intestinal carriage of pathogenic bacteria. However, a 1-year open trial found no benefit.[10] The supplement methionine may decrease bacterial adherence to the bladder wall.[16]

Herbs with diuretic reputation are also sometimes recommended for urinary infections as adjuvant treatment. These include buchu, cleavers, dandelion, goldenrod, horsetail, juniper, parsley, and many others.

Drug Interactions

See the article on each individual supplement for a full description of the interactions summarized here.

Principal Natural Therapy for Cystitis: Interaction with Pharmaceuticals		
Natural Therapy	Pharmaceutical	Interaction
Cranberry	Antipsychotics, morphine-based analgesics, some antidepressants	Increased urinary excretion because of acidification

Pharmaceuticals Used for Cystitis: Possible Harmful Interaction with Natural Therapies		
Pharmaceutical	Natural Therapy	Interaction
Antibiotics, macrolides, sulfonamides, tetracyclines	Dong quai, St. John's wort	Possible increased risk of photosensitivity

DEPRESSION (MILD TO MODERATE)

Principal Proposed Natural Therapies

St. John's wort [+3X]	**Acetyl-L-carnitine** [+2]
SAMe [+2X]	**Ginkgo** [+2]
Phenylalanine [+2]	**Phosphatidylserine** [+2]
5-HTP [+2]	**Inositol** [+2]

(Higher numbers indicate stronger evidence; X modifier indicates contradictory results. See page xviii of the Introduction for details of the rating scale.)

Approach to the Patient

Strong clinical evidence indicates that St. John's wort is an effective treatment for major depression of mild to moderate severity, comparable to conventional antidepressant drugs, with negligible side effects. (Contrary to widespread incorrect publicity, St. John's wort has been studied almost exclusively in major depression, not in more minor conditions such as dysthymia or generic "depression.") However, St. John's wort has significant interaction with several important drugs and drug categories and presents other potential safety risks. In addition, St. John's wort is not believed to be effective for major depression of high severity. As with all herbs, various products may not be equally effective regardless of label claims; using the actual brands that have been studied in double-blind trials is advisable.

Much weaker evidence supports the use of phenylalanine, 5-HTP, SAMe, acetyl-L-carnitine, ginkgo, phosphatidylserine, and dehydroepiandrosterone (DHEA). In addition, the nutrient folate may augment the antidepressant effects of selective serotonin reuptake inhibitors (SSRIs).

Other natural treatments your patient may be using include beta-carotene, damiana, fish oil, inositol, nicotinamide adenine dinucleotide (NADH), pregnenolone, tyrosine, and vitamins B_6 and B_{12}. For potential safety risks with the more common of these substances, see the full herb/supplement articles.

St. John's Wort   + 3 X

St. John's wort has been extensively evaluated as a treament for major depression of mild to moderate severity, as determined by HAM-D scores and other measures. Numerous double-blind comparative or placebo-controlled trials in this population have been reported, enrolling a total of more than 2000 individuals.[1-10,49-51]

Only two of the placebo-controlled trials failed to find St. John's wort effective.[5,50] It is worth noting that 35% of all double-blind studies comparing pharmaceutical antidepressants with placebo have failed to find the active agent significantly more effective; in the more recent of the two negative trials of St. John's wort, sertraline also failed to demonstrate more effectiveness than placebo on any primary outcome measure. (The presumed causes of this relatively high rate of negative outcomes in studies of drugs known to be effective include the high rate of placebo effective in depression and the relative imprecision of the HAM-D rating scale.)

Comparative trials using appropriate doses of the pharmacologic agent found St. John's wort equally as effective as conventional antidepressants.[5-8,10,52] For example, an 8-week, double-blind trial of 263 individuals compared a St. John's wort product standardized to hyperforin content against placebo and imipramine.[6] Participants were diagnosed with major depression by ICD-10 criteria and had average baseline 17-item HAM-D scores of 22.6, representing a moderate level of disease severity. The results showed St. John's wort more effective at reducing HAM-D scores than placebo and as effective as imipramine, 100 mg/day.

St. John's wort has also been compared with SSRIs. A 6-week, double-blind trial of 240 individuals with mild to moderate depression compared St. John's wort with fluoxetine, 20 mg daily.[8] The results showed that St. John's wort was equally effective on the Hamilton Depression (HAM-D) scale, more effective on the Clinical Global Impressions (CGI) scale, and significantly superior in type and number of adverse events. Another 6-week, double-blind study of 149 seniors with mild to moderate depression (HAM-D average about 19) also found St. John's wort equally effective to 20 mg of fluoxetine.[4,7] A small trial found it equally as effective as sertraline.[5] In addition, St. John's wort has been found equivalent to imipramine for mild to moderate depression[3,6,7,10] but not for severe depression.[53]

For more information, including dosage and safety issues, see the **St. John's Wort** article.

S-Adenosylmethionine (SAMe)   + 2 X

The research record for SAMe in depression is modest, contradictory, and marked by numerous flaws; further, many studies involved IV or IM administration.

Three double-blind, placebo-controlled studies including a total of 135 patients with major, postmenopausal, or postpartum depression found significant improvements in depressive symptoms in those treated with oral SAMe as compared with placebo.[11-13] However, one double-blind, placebo-controlled study of 32 patients found no significant difference between treatment and control groups.[14] These studies were generally marred by poor reporting and unusually wide variation in the placebo group response (0% to 65%).

Further, in a double-blind, placebo-controlled study of 133 depressed patients, the effects of intravenous SAMe, 800 mg/day, failed to achieve significance over placebo, unless subgroup analysis or secondary outcome measures were employed.[15]

Comparative trials of oral SAMe have also been reported. The largest was a 6-week, double-blind trial of 281 individuals that compared oral SAMe (1600 mg/day) with imipramine (150 mg/day).[16] Patients had all received the diagnosis of major depressive episode, with baseline HAM-D (21-item) of greater than 18. Using CGI (final score < 2) and HAM-D score (decrease of 50%) as the efficacy criteria, intention-to-treat analysis showed no differences in outcome. Note that a 21-item HAM-D score of 18 is a very mild level of depression; in the absence of a placebo group, it is impossible to rule out nonspecific effects as the primary source of improvement.

Equivalent benefits were also seen in an otherwise similar trial using IM SAMe (400 mg/day) vs. oral imipramine (150 mg/day) in a double-dummy design.[17]

Other small studies have also compared the benefits of oral or IV SAMe with those of tricyclic antidepressants, finding generally equivalent results, although again poor reporting and study design (e.g., inadequate trial length) mar the meaningfulness of the outcomes.[18-20]

For more information, including dosage and safety issues, see the **S-Adenosylmethionine** article.

Phenylalanine   +2

Small comparative studies suggest that D-phenylalanine[21] or DL-phenylalanine[22,23] may be comparably effective to imipramine, 100 mg, for relief of depression symptoms. No placebo-controlled trials have been reported.

For more information, including dosage and safety issues, see the **Phenylalanine** article.

5-HTP   +2

There have been several preliminary studies of 5-HTP for depression.[24] The best of these was a 6-week comparative study of 63 individuals given either 5-HTP (100 mg three times daily) or fluvoxamine (50 mg three times daily), which found these treatments equally effective.[25]

For more information, including dosage and safety issues, see the **5-HTP** article.

Acetyl-L-Carnitine   +2

A double-blind study of 60 seniors with dysthymia found that treatment with acetyl-L-carnitine, 3 g/day, over a 2-month period significantly improved symptoms as compared with placebo.[26] Improvements in affective symptoms have also been observed in trials of individuals with dementia.[27-29]

For more information, including dosage and safety issues, see the **Carnitine** article.

Ginkgo   +2

As with acetyl-L-carnitine, many studies of ginkgo in dementia have noted improvement in affective symptoms. In addition, two studies have directly evaluated this potential benefit. In an 8-week, double-blind, placebo-controlled trial, 40 depressed patients over the age of 50 years who showed incomplete response to tricyclic or tetracyclic antidepressants were given adjuvant treatment with either placebo or ginkgo extract at 80 mg three times per day.[30] Patients in the treated group demonstrated significantly improved outcomes compared with the placebo group.

In another double-blind, placebo-controlled trial, 60 inpatients with "cerebral insufficiency" (a purported condition involving impaired cerebral blood supply) manifesting primarily as depression were given either placebo or 160 mg of ginkgo extract daily for 6 weeks.[31] The results showed significantly greater improvements in the treated group.

For more information, including dosage and safety issues, see the **Ginkgo** article.

Phosphatidylserine   +2

Phosphatidylserine is another treatment for dementia found incidentally to improve affective symptoms. One small double-blind, crossover study found direct evidence that phosphatidylserine can be useful in geriatric patients with depression.[32]

For more information, including dosage and safety issues, see the **Phosphatidylserine** article.

Inositol   +2

Several small double-blind studies suggest that inositol may be helpful for depression.[18,19,33] For example, in a parallel-group, double-blind, placebo-controlled trial, 28 depressed individuals were given a daily dose of 12 g of inositol for 4 weeks.[19] By the fourth week, the group receiving inositol showed significant improvement compared with the placebo group. The only negative result was a double-blind, placebo-controlled study of 42 patients with severe depression not responding to SSRIs.[34] No improvement was seen when inositol was added.

For more information, including dosage and safety issues, see the **Inositol** article.

Other Proposed Natural Therapies

DHEA is also sometimes proposed for depression, on the basis of one small double-blind study and one observational study.[35,36]

An intriguing body of preliminary evidence suggests that **folate** deficiency may contribute to depression and that folate supplements might produce clinical improvement.[37-44] The best evidence is for using folate to augment SSRI therapy. A 10-week, double-blind, placebo-controlled trial of 127 individuals with severe major depression (average HAM-D score above 26) found that folate supplements at a dose of 500 μg daily significantly improved the effectiveness of fluoxetine in female participants.[45] An intention-to-treat analysis showed a higher rate of responders as well as lower HAM-D scores in those who received fluoxetine plus folate as compared with fluoxetine alone. Improvements in male participants were not statistically significant. However, measurements of serum homocysteine in males showed no change, suggesting that the dose of folate was inadequate.

Highly preliminary evidence suggests that deficiencies in essential fatty acids may increase the risk of depression and that **fish oil** supplements could help prevent depression.[46,54] Although diets low in **vitamin B_6** or **vitamin B_{12}** have been associated with symptoms of depression,[47,48] there is little direct evidence that B_6 or B_{12} supplements can treat depression.

Other natural treatments including beta-carotene, damiana, NADH, pregnenolone, and tyrosine are also recommended for depression, but there is no evidence supporting these treatments.

Drug Interactions

See the article on each individual supplement for a full description of the interactions summarized here.

Principal Natural Therapies for Mild to Moderate Depression: Interactions with Pharmaceuticals		
Natural Therapy	Pharmaceutical	Interaction
5-HTP	SSRIs, other serotonergic drugs	Possible risk of serotonin syndrome
	Levodopa-carbidopa	Possible risk of scleroderma-like syndrome
Ginkgo	Anticoagulant and antiplatelet agents	Possible increased risk of bleeding complications
Phenylalanine	Levodopa	Possible impaired action of drug based on amino acid/levodopa interaction
	Neuroleptics	Possible increased risk of tardive dyskinesia
Phosphatidylserine	Anticoagulants	Possible increased risk of bleeding complications
SAMe	Levodopa or levodopa-carbidopa	Possible increased "wearing off" effect
	Serotonergic drugs (case report involved tricyclic antidepressant)	Possible risk of serotonin syndrome
St. John's wort	Clomipramine, clozapine, cyclosporine, digoxin, imipramine, oral contraceptives, olanzapine, protease inhibitors, theophylline, warfarin, others	Reduced serum levels because of CYP and other interactions, with possible rebound toxicity if herb is discontinued

Principal Natural Therapies for Mild to Moderate Depression: Interactions with Pharmaceuticals—cont'd		
Natural Therapy	**Pharmaceutical**	**Interaction**
St. John's wort—cont'd	Doxorubicin, etoposide, mitoxantrone, teniposide	Possible antagonism of drug action
	SSRIs, other serotonergic agents	Possible risk of serotonin syndrome

Pharmaceuticals Used for Mild to Moderate Depression: Possible Harmful Interactions with Natural Therapies		
Natural Therapy	**Pharmaceutical**	**Interaction**
SSRIs	5-HTP, SAMe, St. John's wort	Possible risk of serotonin syndrome
Tricyclic antidepressants	Dong quai, St. John's wort	Possible increased risk of photosensitivity
	St. John's wort	Decreased serum levels of drug, with possible rebound toxicity if herb is stopped

Pharmaceuticals Used for Mild to Moderate Depression: Natural Therapies with Potential Supportive Interactions		
Pharmaceutical	**Natural Therapy**	**Interaction**
SSRIs	Ginkgo	Possible reversal of SSRI-induced sexual dysfunction
Tricyclic antidepressants	Coenzyme Q_{10}	Possible correction of drug-induced relative deficiency

DIABETES

(Higher numbers indicate stronger evidence; X modifier indicates contradictory results. See page xviii of the Introduction for details of the rating scale.)

Approach to the Patient

The nutrient chromium appears to play a physiologic role in glucose metabolism and, when taken as a supplement, may improve glucose control. Weaker evidence suggests efficacy for ginseng (*Panax* spp.). Numerous other natural agents have weak supporting evidence.

The supplements lipoic acid, evening primrose oil, and vitamin E may be beneficial in diabetic autonomic and peripheral neuropathy. Some evidence suggests that use of niacinamide or vitamin D supplements may reduce risk of childhood-onset diabetes.

Other natural treatments your patient may be using include acetyl-L-carnitine, *Aloe vera*, bilberry leaf, bitter melon, CLA (conjugated linoleic acid), *Coccinia indica*, fenugreek, garlic, glucomannan, gymnema, holy basil, nopal cactus, onion, pterocarpus, salt bush, vanadium, and vitamin C. For potential safety risks with the more common of these substances, see the full herb/supplement articles.

Caution: There is some evidence that the supplement glucosamine, used for osteoarthritis, may increase the risk of diabetic cataracts[1] and possibly worsen glycemic control.[2-6]

One study in postmenopausal women found evidence that melatonin might impair insulin sensitivity and glucose tolerance.[7]

Glycemic Control

Chromium   +3

A 4-month study reported in 1997 observed 180 Chinese men and women with type 2 diabetes, comparing the effects of 1000 μg of chromium daily, 200 μg of chromium, and placebo.[8] HbA1c values improved significantly in the group receiving 1000 μg after 2 months and in both chromium groups after 4 months. Fasting glucose was also lower in the higher-dose chromium group.

Another double-blind trial compared placebo with chromium from Brewer's yeast (23.3 μg chromium daily) and chromium chloride (200 μg chromium daily) in 78 individuals with type 2 diabetes.[9] This rather complex crossover study consisted of four 8-week intervals of treatment in random order. The results in the 67 completers showed that both active treatments significantly improved glycemic control. However, other smaller studies found little to no effect.[10,11]

One placebo-controlled study of 30 women with pregnancy-related diabetes found that supplementation with chromium at a dosage of 4 or 8 μg of chromium picolinate/kg body weight significantly improved blood sugar control.[12] Some evidence suggests that chromium might be helpful for corticosteroid-induced diabetes.[13,14]

Chromium may also be helpful in impaired glucose tolerance short of actual diabetes.[9,15-17]

For more information, including dosage and safety issues, see the **Chromium** article.

Ginseng   +2

A double-blind, placebo-controlled study evaluated the effects of ginseng (Dansk Droge, Copenhagen; 100 or 200 mg daily) on 36 newly diagnosed type 2 diabetes patients over an 8-week period.[18] The results showed reduction in fasting serum glucose and glycosylated hemoglobin.

The effects of American ginseng *(Panax quinquefolius)* have also been evaluated in two double-blind trials. The first, a double-blind, placebo-controlled, crossover study of nine subjects with type 2 diabetes, found that a single ginseng dose of 3 g significantly reduced postprandial glycemia.[19] The other study looked at longer-term control of glycemia.[20] In this 8-week trial, American ginseng decreased fasting plasma glucose 9.4% more than placebo.

Indirect support for ginseng as an antidiabetic agent comes from a double-blind study of 12 healthy individuals.[21] Ginseng at a dose of 1 g to 3 g administered 40 minutes before glucose challenge reduced postprandial glycemia. The effects were time-dependent (administration at 20, 10, or 0 minutes before the challenge failed to produce any effect) but were not dose-dependent.

For more information, including dosage and safety issues, see the **Ginseng** article.

Vanadium   +1

Studies in rats with and without diabetes suggest that vanadium may have an insulin-like effect, reducing blood glucose levels.[22-32] Most studies involve vanadium (IV)—that is, oxidation state IV vanadium—but vanadium (V) has also been found effective in at least one animal trial.[33]

Based on these findings, preliminary studies involving human subjects have been conducted, with mostly positive results.[34-39] However, the doses of vanadium used, 100 to 125 mg/day, may present significant toxic risk. There may be some benefit in use of nutritional doses of vanadium, 10 to 30 μg daily.

For more information, including dosage and safety issues, see the **Vanadium** article.

Diabetic Neuropathy

Lipoic Acid (Intravenous)   +3, (Oral)   −2

Oral lipoic acid may be beneficial for cardiac autonomic neuropathy. The DEKAN (Deutsche Kardiale Autonome Neuropathie) study observed 73 diabetics with symptoms of cardiac autonomic neuropathy for a period of 4 months. Treatment with oral alpha-lipoic acid, 800 mg/day, yielded statistically significant but modest improvement compared with placebo.[40]

There is some evidence that IV lipoic acid can reduce symptoms of diabetic peripheral neuropathy in the short term. However, a large study of oral lipoic acid found it ineffective.[41] The positive evidence for oral lipoic acid is limited to open trials or trials with inadequate sample size.[40,42-45]

For more information, including dosage and safety issues, see the **Lipoic Acid** article.

Evening Primrose Oil   +3

Evening primrose oil, a source of GLA, may be helpful for diabetic peripheral neuropathy. A multicenter, double-blind trial enrolling 111 diabetics found that treatment with evening primrose oil for 1 year improved pain and numbness as well as objective signs of nerve injury.[46] This study is in agreement with an earlier double-blind study.[47]

For more information, including dosage and safety issues, see the **Gamma-Linolenic Acid** article.

Vitamin E   +2

A 4-month, double-blind, placebo-controlled trial found that vitamin E at a dose of 600 mg daily improves the ratio of cardiac sympathetic to parasympathetic tone.[48]

For more information, including dosage and safety issues, see the **Vitamin E** article.

Nutrient Deficiencies

Certain nutrient deficiencies may be associated with diabetes. Supplementation may be warranted on general principles, especially for nutrients (e.g., magnesium, zinc) where marginal nutriture is common in the population at large.

Magnesium deficiency appears to be common in diabetes.[49,50] Supplementation may therefore be indicated. However, magnesium appears to increase absorption of oral hypoglycemics, potentially causing a risk of hypoglycemia.[51,52] Individuals with either type 1 or type 2 diabetes may also be deficient in **zinc**.[53-55] **Vitamin C** levels have been found to be low in many diabetics taking insulin, even though they were consuming seemingly adequate amounts in their diets.[56-58] Some individuals with type 1 diabetes appear to be deficient in **taurine**.[59] **Manganese** deficiency reportedly can also occur.[60] Finally, metformin and phenformin may cause **vitamin B$_{12}$** malabsorption; interestingly, this appears to be correctable through calcium supplementation.[61]

For more information, including dosage and safety issues, see the full articles on each nutrient mentioned above.

Prevention

Niacinamide (Vitamin B$_3$)   [+2X]

Two studies found that niacinamide (vitamin B$_3$) may delay or prevent the onset of type 1 diabetes. In a population-based study of more than 20,000 children, treatment of islet cell antibodies (ICA)-positive children with niacinamide for 7 years reduced the incidence of diabetes.[62] Niacinamide might also prolong the "honeymoon period" in type 1 diabetes.[63] However, the German portion of the ongoing European Nicotinamide Diabetes Intervention Trial has failed to demonstrate prevention of diabetes with regular use of niacinamide.[64]

In addition, a small double-blind, controlled trial evaluated niacinamide plus antioxidant vitamins and minerals given at onset of childhood diabetes.[65] No effects on the course of the disease were seen.

For more information, including dosage and safety issues, see the **Vitamin B₃** article.

Vitamin D   [+1]

A Finnish observational trial of 12,231 children suggests that use of vitamin D supplements reduces risk of type 1 diabetes.[122] Similar results were seen in other observational trials.[123,124]

Other Proposed Natural Therapies

Preliminary studies including controlled trials suggest that the herbs **gymnema,**[66-68] *Aloe vera,*[69-74] and **fenugreek**[75-77] may improve glycemic control. Highly preliminary evidence suggests possible benefit with the herbs **bilberry leaf, bitter melon,** *Coccinia indica,* **garlic, guggul,**[78] **holy basil, maitake, nopal cactus, onion, pterocarpus,** and **salt bush,** and with the supplements **zinc, CLA (conjugated linoleic acid), arginine,** and **glucomannan.**[79-108,125]

Other herbs traditionally used for diabetes include alfalfa, *Anemarrhena asphodeloides,* banana, *Catharanthus roseus,* cucumber, *Cucurbita ficifolia,* cumin, damiana, *Euphorbia prostrata, Guaiacum coulteri, Guazuma ulmifolia, Lepechinia caulescens,* neem, *Psacalium peltatum,* red mangrove, spinach, string bean, and *Tournefortia hirsutissima.*[109-117]

The supplement **acetyl-L-carnitine** has shown some promise for cardiac autonomic neuropathy,[118,119] and high-dose zinc might offer benefits for peripheral neuropathy.[108]

A metaanalysis of published studies suggests that **fish oil** can improve hypertriglyceridemia in diabetics without altering glycemic control.[120] Similarly, even when taken in hypolipidemic doses, niacin does not appear to raise serum glucose in diabetics.[121]

In a double-blind, crossover trial of 30 type 2 diabetics with microalbuminemia or macroalbuminuria, use of vitamin C (1250 mg) and vitamin E (680 IU) over a period of 4 weeks significantly reduced urinary albumin excretion rate.[126]

Drug Interactions

See the article on each individual supplement for a full description of the interactions summarized here.

Principal Natural Therapies for Diabetes: Interactions with Pharmaceuticals		
Natural Therapy	**Pharmaceutical**	**Interaction**
Chromium, ginseng,	Hypoglycemic agents and any other agent noted above that may improve glycemic control	Possible risk of hypoglycemia
Niacinamide	Anticonvulsants	Possible increase in serum levels of drug
Vitamin E	Anticoagulant and antiplatelet agents	Possible increased risk of bleeding complications

Pharmaceuticals Used for Diabetes: Possible Harmful Interactions with Natural Therapies

Pharmaceutical	Natural Therapy	Interaction
Oral hypoglycemics	Chromium, ginseng, other herbs and supplements with putative hypo-glycemic effects	Possible increased risk of hypoglycemia
	Dong quai, St. John's wort	Possible increased risk of photosensitivity
	Ipriflavone, magnesium	Possible increased serum levels of drug
	Potassium citrate	Possible decreased serum levels of drug

Pharmaceuticals Used for Diabetes: Natural Therapy with Potential Supportive Interaction

Pharmaceutical	Natural Therapy	Interaction
Oral hypoglycemics	Coenzyme Q_{10}	Possible correction of drug-induced relative deficiency

DYSMENORRHEA

Principal Proposed
Natural Therapies

Fish oil [+2] **Vitamin E** [+2]

Magnesium [+2]

(Higher numbers indicate stronger evidence; X modifier indicates contradictory results. See page xviii of the Introduction for details of the rating scale.)

Approach to the Patient

Because of its effects on prostaglandin production, fish oil has been tried as a treatment for dysmenorrhea, with some evidence of success. Magnesium and vitamin E may be helpful as well.

Other natural treatments your patient may be using include black cohosh, bromelain, Chinese herbal medicine, *Coleus forskohlii*, cramp bark, dong quai, manganese, turmeric, and white willow. For potential safety risks with the more common of these substances, see the full herb/supplement articles.

Fish Oil +2

A double-blind, crossover trial of 42 adolescents with dysmenorrhea compared fish oil (1080 mg EPA, 720 mg DHA with 1.5 mg vitamin E as stabilizer, daily) for 2 months with 2 months of placebo treatment.[1] A total of 37 participants were included in the final analysis. Evaluation of menstrual symptom scores showed significant improvement after fish oil treatment but not after placebo. No order effect was seen.

Another double-blind study observed 78 young women with dysmenorrhea divided into four groups: fish oil, seal oil, fish oil with vitamin B_{12} (7.5 μg daily), or placebo.[2] Treatment lasted three full menstrual periods. Significant improvements were seen in all treatment groups, but the fish oil plus B_{12} proved most effective, and its benefits endured for the longest time after treatment was stopped (3 months). The researchers offered no explanation why vitamin B_{12} should be helpful for dysmenorrhea.

For more information, including dosage and safety issues, see the **Fish Oil** article.

Magnesium   +2

A 6-month, double-blind, placebo-controlled study of 50 women with menstrual pain found that treatment with magnesium significantly improved symptoms.[3] The researchers reported evidence of reduced levels of prostaglandin F_2-alpha. Similarly positive results with magnesium were seen in a double-blind, placebo-controlled study of 21 women.[4]

For more information, including dosage and safety issues, see the **Magnesium** article.

Vitamin E   +2

In a double-blind, placebo-controlled trial, 100 young women with significant menstrual pain were given either 500 IU vitamin E or placebo for 5 days.[5] Treatment began 2 days before and continued for 3 days after the expected onset of menstruation. Although both groups showed significant improvement in pain over the 2 months of the study, pain reduction was significantly greater in the treatment group as compared with the placebo group.

Other Proposed Natural Therapies

Numerous other herbs and supplements are sometimes suggested for dysmenorrhea, including black cohosh, bromelain, *Coleus forskohlii*, cramp bark, dong quai, manganese, turmeric, and white willow. However, no direct evidence supports these treatments at this time. Chinese herbal medicine has a strong anecdotal reputation for effectiveness in dysmenorrhea, but again, there is no evidence supporting its use.

Drug Interactions

See the article on each individual supplement for a full description of the interactions summarized here.

Principal Natural Therapies for Dysmenorrhea: Interactions with Pharmaceuticals		
Natural Therapy	**Pharmaceutical**	**Interaction**
Fish oil	Anticoagulant and antiplatelet agents	Possible increased risk of bleeding complications
Magnesium	Amiloride	Possible hypermagnesemia
	Digitoxin, digoxin	Absorption interference
	Fluoroquinolones, tetracyclines	Mutual absorption interference
	Oral hypoglycemics	Possible potentiation of drug action leading to risk of hypoglycemia

Pharmaceuticals Used for Dysmenorrhea: Possible Harmful Interactions with Natural Therapies

Pharmaceutical	Natural Therapy	Interaction
NSAIDs	Dong quai, St. John's wort	Possible increased risk of photosensitivity
	Garlic, ginkgo, high-dose vitamin E, policosanol, others	Possible increased risk of bleeding complications
	Feverfew	Possible increased risk of gastritis
	Potassium citrate	Possible decreased serum levels of salicylates
	White willow	Additional salicylates may increase risk of all side effects
Oral contraceptives	Androstenedione	Possible elevation of estrogen levels
	Copper	Possible hypercupremia
	Dong quai, St. John's wort	Possible increased risk of photosensitivity
	Licorice	Possible increased fluid retention and other side effects
	Milk thistle, St. John's wort	Possible reduced effectiveness of drug

Pharmaceuticals Used for Dysmenorrhea: Natural Therapies with Potential Supportive Interactions

Pharmaceutical	Natural Therapy	Interaction
NSAIDs	Cayenne, colostrum, licorice	Possible cytoprotection
	Folate, vitamin C	Correction of possible drug-induced deficiency
Oral contraceptives	Magnesium, vitamin B$_2$, vitamin C, zinc	Correction of possible drug-induced depletion

DYSPEPSIA

Principal Proposed
Natural Therapies

Curcumin [+2]   **Pancreatic enzymes** [−1]

**Combination herbal
treatments** [+2]

*(Higher numbers indicate stronger evidence; X modifier indicates contradic-
tory results. See page xviii of the Introduction for details of the rating scale.)*

Approach to the Patient

In Europe, herbs that stimulate gallbladder contraction are
often used for the treatment of nonulcer dyspepsia; these include artichoke leaf, boldo, celandine, and curcumin (also
known as turmeric). Another family of herbs, carminatives (gas
releasing), is also used for dyspepsia; these include caraway oil
and peppermint.

Keep in mind that the placebo effect is particularly strong in this
condition; one study of 30 individuals with dyspepsia found that
after 8 weeks of treatment with placebo, 80% reported their
symptoms had improved.[1]

Other natural treatments your patient may be using for dyspepsia include angelica root, anise seed, banana powder, bitter
orange peel, blessed thistle, caraway, cardamom, cayenne, centaury, chamomile, chicory, cinnamon, cloves, coriander, dandelion root, devil's claw, dill, fennel, gentian, ginger, horehound,
juniper, lemon balm, milk thistle, parsley seed, radish, rosemary,
sage, St. John's wort, star anise, valerian, wormwood, and
yarrow. For potential safety risks with the more common of
these substances, see the full herb/supplement articles.

Curcumin   +2

Curcumin, a component of the spice turmeric, stimulates contraction of the gallbladder.[2,3] A double-blind, placebo-controlled study including 106 individuals compared the effects of 500 mg curcumin four times daily with placebo (and with a locally popular over-the-counter treatment) on dyspepsia. After 7 days, 87% of the curcumin group experienced full or partial symptom relief as compared with 53% of the placebo group.[4]

For more information, including dosage and safety issues, see the **Curcumin** article.

Combination Herbal Treatments   +2

Combinations of various herbs are frequently used in Germany for the treatment of dyspepsia.

A double-blind trial of 60 individuals given either an artichoke leaf–boldo–celandine combination or placebo found improvements in symptoms of indigestion after 14 days of treatment.[5] Similarly positive effects were seen in a double-blind trial of 76 individuals given a combination treatment containing turmeric and celandine.[6] However, there are several case reports of hepatotoxicity attributed to use of products containing celandine.[7-9]

A double-blind, placebo-controlled study of 39 individuals found that an enteric-coated peppermint–caraway oil combination taken three times daily for 4 weeks significantly reduced dyspepsia pain.[10] In addition, a double-blind, comparative study of 118 individuals found that the combination of peppermint and caraway oil is comparably effective to cisapride.[11] Finally, in a double-blind trial of 60 individuals, a preparation of peppermint, caraway, fennel, and wormwood oils compared favorably with metoclopramide.[12]

For more information, including dosage and safety issues, see the appropriate herb articles.

Pancreatic Enzymes   − 1

Digestive enzymes are often recommended for indigestion; however, one placebo-controlled, crossover study enrolling 37 individuals found no significant difference between the effects of digestive enzymes and placebo on dyspepsia symptoms.[13]

Other Proposed Natural Therapies

In an open trial, **banana powder,** a traditional Indian food, improved dyspepsia symptoms.[14]

Herbs with a reputation for relaxing a nervous stomach, such as chamomile, lemon balm, and valerian, are sometimes recommended for dyspepsia. Numerous other herbs are used for dyspepsia as well, including angelica root, anise seed, bitter orange peel, blessed thistle, cardamom, centaury, chicory, dandelion root, cinnamon, cloves, coriander, devil's claw, dill, gentian, ginger, horehound, juniper, milk thistle, parsley seed, radish, rosemary, sage, St. John's wort, star anise, and yarrow.

Capsaicin, the "hot" constituent of all hot peppers, is sometimes recommended for indigestion; however, in a small placebo-controlled, crossover study of 11 individuals, 5 mg capsaicin taken before a high-fat meal did not improve dyspepsia symptoms.[15]

Drug Interactions

See the article on each individual supplement for a full description of the interactions summarized here.

Pharmaceuticals Used for Dyspepsia: Possible Harmful Interaction with Natural Therapy		
Pharmaceutical	Natural Therapy	Interaction
H_2 blockers, proton pump inhibitors	St. John's wort	Possible increased risk of photosensitivity

Pharmaceuticals Used for Dyspepsia: Natural Therapies with Potential Supportive Interaction		
Pharmaceutical	Natural Therapy	Interaction
H_2 blockers, proton pump inhibitors	Folate, iron, vitamin B_{12}, zinc, other minerals	Correction of possible drug-induced deficiency

EASY BRUISING

Principal Proposed Natural Therapies

Diosmin/hesperidin and other bioflavonoids [+2]   **Vitamin C** [+2]

(Higher numbers indicate stronger evidence; X modifier indicates contradictory results. See page xviii of the Introduction for details of the rating scale.)

Approach to the Patient

In European medicine, a variety of bioflavonoids (and other agents such as anthocyanosides, oligomeric proanthocyanidin complexes [OPCs], oxerutins, and rutin) are thought to decrease capillary permeability and strengthen capillary structure. Although these substances are widely used in the treatment of individuals with an unexplained tendency to bruise, the evidence for their effectiveness is stronger in the treatment of sports injuries, venous insufficiency, varicose veins, and hemorrhoids.

After ruling out identifiable causes of easy bruising, it might be reasonable to suggest a trial of citrus bioflavonoids or related substances.

Other natural treatments your patient may be using for easy bruising include arnica, bilberry fruit, butcher's broom, collinsonia, topical comfrey, grape seed, horse chestnut or its constituent escin, pine bark, Pycnogenol, sweet clover, and vitamin C. For potential safety risks with the more common of these substances, see the full herb/supplement articles.

Other substances are used for the treatment of bruising caused by minor injuries but are probably not appropriate for prevention of bruises in general. (See the article on **Minor Injuries**.)

Diosmin/Hesperidin and Other Bioflavonoids   +2

A double-blind, placebo-controlled trial of 96 individuals with evidence of fragile capillaries found that a combination of the two citrus bioflavonoids diosmin and hesperidin decreased the tendency toward capillary rupture.[1] In addition, two studies from the 1960s suggest benefits with a combination of citrus bioflavonoids taken with vitamin C.[2]

Other bioflavonoids or bioflavonoid-like substances, such as anthocyanosides (from bilberry fruit), OPCs (from pine bark or grape seed, often sold as Pycnogenol), oxerutins, and rutin, also appear to stabilize capillaries and are used for the treatment of venous insufficiency; however, they have not been investigated for the prevention of bruising.

For more information, including dosage and safety issues, see the **Diosmin/Hesperidin** article.

Vitamin C   +2

Vitamin C is essential for healthy collagen; severe vitamin C deficiency is marked by easy bruising, among other symptoms. Although scurvy is extremely rare in Western countries today, marginal vitamin C deficiency is not rare and might lead to increased risk of bruising.

A 2-month, double-blind study of 94 elderly individuals with marginal vitamin C deficiency found that vitamin C supplementation decreased their tendency to bruise.[3]

For more information, including dosage and safety issues, see the **Vitamin C** article.

Other Proposed
Natural Therapies

The herbs arnica, comfrey, and sweet clover are widely used externally on bruises and other minor injuries, but no real scientific evidence supports these traditional treatments.

Other herbs taken internally for varicose veins or hemorrhoids might also be tried for easy bruising. These include butcher's broom, collinsonia, horse chestnut, and sweet clover.

Drug Interactions

See the article on each individual supplement for a full description of the interactions summarized here.

Principal Natural Therapies for Easy Bruising: Interactions with Pharmaceuticals		
Natural Therapy	**Pharmaceutical**	**Interaction**
Diosmin/hesperidin, other bioflavonoids, horse chestnut, bilberry fruit, grape seed, pine bark	Anticoagulant or antiplatelet agents	Possible increased risk of bleeding complications

ECZEMA

Principal Proposed
Natural Therapies

Probiotics [+3]

Chamomile (topical) [+1]

Evening primrose oil [−2X]

(Higher numbers indicate stronger evidence; X modifier indicates contradictory results. See page xviii of the Introduction for details of the rating scale.)

Approach to the Patient

Use of probiotics by mother and newborn may help prevent or treat eczema.

Although early evidence suggested that oral evening primrose oil (EPO), a source of gamma-linolenic acid (GLA), improved symptoms of eczema, more recent studies have found little to no benefit. Chamomile cream has also been studied in controlled trials, but these study reports failed to include statistical analysis of the results.

Other natural treatments your patient may be using include probiotics; the herbs burdock, *Coleus forskohlii*, and red clover; and supplemental chromium, quercetin, vitamin B_6, and zinc. For potential safety risks with the more common of these substances, see the full herb/supplement articles.

In addition, many patients interested in alternative medicine believe that accumulated toxins are the cause of eczema and that this can be corrected through "detoxification." The latter may involve dietary changes, "colon cleansing," and supplementation with specific herbs and supplements. Malnutrition can occur in the more extreme forms of this approach.

Probiotics   +3

Use of probiotics during pregnancy and after childbirth may reduce risk of childhood eczema. In a double-blind, placebo-controlled trial that enrolled 159 women, participants received either placebo or *Lactobacillus GG* capsules beginning 2 to 4 weeks before expected delivery.[1] After delivery, breast-feeding mothers continued to take placebo or the probiotic for 6 months; formula-fed infants were given placebo or probiotic orally for the same period of time. The results showed that use of *Lactobacillus GG* reduced risk of eczema developing in offspring by approximately 50%.

According to two small double-blind, placebo-controlled trials in infants, probiotics (*Bifidobacterium lactis* or *Lactobacillus GG*) may be helpful for reducing existing eczema symptoms as well.[2,3]

Chamomile (Topical)   +1

A partially blinded trial (blindness weakened by difference in color and smell of treatments used) compared chamomile cream with 0.5% hydrocortisone cream and placebo in 69 previously untreated individuals with eczema.[4] The authors reported that after 2 weeks, chamomile was slightly superior to hydrocortisone and marginally superior to placebo (strangely, placebo outperformed hydrocortisone). However, statistical analysis was not given.

A controlled trial (blinding not stated) observed 146 individuals with eczema who had previously been treated with 0.1% difluocortolone valerate.[5] Over a period of 3 to 4 weeks, affected right extremities were treated with one of three maintenance therapies: 0.25% hydrocortisone, 0.75% fluocortin butyl ester, or 5% bufexamac. Left extremities were treated with chamomile cream. The study authors concluded that chamomile cream was as effective as 0.25% hydrocortisone, more effective than 0.75% fluocortin butyl ester, and clearly superior to 5% bufexamac; but again, no statistical analysis of the results was presented.

For more information, including dosage and safety issues, see the **Chamomile** article.

Evening Primrose Oil   − 2 X

A 1989 review by Morse et al. of published and unpublished trials concluded that evening primrose oil frequently reduced the symptoms of eczema after several months of use, with the greatest improvement noticeable in pruritus.[6] However, this review has been sharply criticized for including poorly designed studies and possibly misinterpreting study results.[7]

A more recent 16-week, double-blind, placebo-controlled trial of EPO in 58 children with eczema found no significant differences between the treated and placebo group.[8] Negative results were also seen in a 16-week, double-blind, placebo-controlled study of 102 individuals with eczema.[7] In addition, a 24-week, double-blind study of 160 adults with eczema found no benefit of GLA from borage oil over placebo.[9]

One double-blind, placebo-controlled trial of 51 children did find a therapeutic benefit with EPO; but in contrast to the Morse review, pruritus was not significantly improved.[10]

For more information, including dosage and safety issues, see the **Gamma-Linolenic Acid** article.

Other Proposed Natural Therapies

One uncontrolled study suggests that topical **cayenne** might be helpful for prurigo nodularis.[11]

A mixture of **Chinese herbs** sold as Zemaphyte has been popular in the United Kingdom for the treatment of eczema, but a 20-week, double-blind, placebo-controlled trial of 40 individuals found it ineffective.[12]

A small 30-day, double-blind, placebo-controlled trial failed to find vitamin B_6 (at a dose of 50 mg daily) helpful for eczema.[15] Similarly, an 8-week, double-blind, placebo-controlled trial of zinc at the somewhat high dose of 67 mg daily failed to find any benefit for eczema symptoms.[16] The herbs burdock, red clover, and *Coleus forskohlii*, as well as the supplements chromium and quercetin have also been suggested for eczema, but no evidence supports these treatments at this time.

Breast-feeding or use of purified amino acid infant formula may reduce risk of eczema.[13,14]

Drug Interactions

See the article on each individual supplement for a full description of the interactions summarized here.

Pharmaceutical Used for Eczema: Natural Therapy with Potential Supportive Interaction		
Pharmaceutical	Natural Therapy	Interaction
Corticosteroids (topical creams)	Topical licorice	Possible potentiation of drug action

ERECTILE DYSFUNCTION

Principal Proposed Natural Therapies

L-**Arginine** [+2X]   **DHEA** [+1]

Yohimbe [+2]   **Ginkgo** [+1]

(Higher numbers indicate stronger evidence; X modifier indicates contradictory results. See page xviii of the Introduction for details of the rating scale.)

Approach to the Patient

Preliminary evidence suggests that arginine might have some utility in erectile dysfunction. Yohimbine is known to be marginally effective, although use of yohimbe herb may present safety risks. Weak evidence supports the use of the hormone DHEA. Ginkgo may be useful for selective serotonin reuptake inhibitor (SSRI)–induced impotence, but there have been no blinded studies.

Other natural treatments your patient may be using include abuta, ashwagandha, catuaba bark, chuchuhuasi bark, codonopsis, damiana, *Eurycoma longifolia*, gamma-linolenic acid, ginseng (*Panax* spp.), *Lepidium sativum*, lipoic acid, maca (horny goat weed), *Muira puama*, *Pimpinella pruacen*, pygeum africanus, royal jelly, saw palmetto, schisandra, suma, *Tribulus terrestris*, and zinc. Based on intensive marketing efforts, your patient may have heard that many of these treatments have been proven effective; tactfully explaining the weakness of "test tube" and animal studies as a source of evidence might prove helpful. For potential safety risks with the more common of these substances, see the full herb/supplement article.

Caution: The herb licorice may reduce testosterone levels in men and thus may exacerbate impotence.[1] Chewing tobacco is a little-known source of licorice.

L-Arginine   +2X

One double-blind, placebo-controlled trial of 50 patients with erectile dysfunction found subjective improvement in sexual function after 6 weeks with arginine, 5 g/day, as compared with placebo.[3] Those men who improved initially had low urinary nitrate levels, which doubled by the end of the study.

However, a double-blind, crossover trial of 32 men using a much lower dose of arginine (1.5 mg/day) for 17 days found no effect.[11]

Animal studies lend some support for this use as well.[12]

For more information, including dosage and safety issues, see the **Arginine** article.

Yohimbe   +2

Yohimbe is a source of the drug yohimbine. Several small double-blind, placebo-controlled trials have found evidence that yohimbine is modestly effective in the treatment of erectile dysfunction.[4] However, yohimbine presents significant toxicologic risk; the indeterminate yohimbine content in yohimbe, as well as the possible presence of other constituents, makes use of the herb unsafe. It is not recommended.

For more information, including dosage and safety issues, see the **Yohimbe** article.

DHEA   +1

The hormone DHEA (dehydroepiandrosterone) may be helpful for erectile dysfunction, although the evidence is weak.

A double-blind, placebo-controlled study enrolled 40 men with erectile dysfunction and low DHEA levels and found that DHEA at a dose of 50 mg daily improved sexual performance; however, the authors did not undertake a statitistical analysis of the data.[2]

For more information, including dosage and safety issues, see the **DHEA** article.

Ginkgo   +1

Several reports suggest that ginkgo *(Ginkgo biloba)* may reverse the impotence caused by SSRI drugs.[5-9] An open study of ginkgo in 60 men with vascular erectile dysfunction reported a 50% success rate after 6 months.[10] One open trial found no benefit, but it used a nonstandard form of the herb that does not closely resemble typical ginkgo extract.[13] Double-blind trials have not been reported.

For more information, including dosage and safety issues, see the **Ginkgo** article.

Other Proposed Natural Therapies

A double-blind, placebo-controlled study performed in China reported evidence that *Panax ginseng* can improve symptoms of male sexual dysfunction.[14]

Zinc deficiency is one of the most common mineral deficiencies and is known to exacerbate sexual dysfunction; therefore it is logical to assume that supplementation with zinc may be helpful for some men. However, this treatment has not been studied to date.

Other herbs and supplements reputed to improve sexual function, but which lack any substantiation, include abuta, ashwagandha, catuaba bark, chuchuhuasi bark, codonopsis, damiana, *Eurycoma longifolia*, gamma-linolenic acid, *Lepidium sativum*, lipoic acid, maca (horny goat weed), *Muira puama*, *Pimpinella pruacen*, pygeum africanus, royal jelly, saw palmetto, schisandra, suma, and *Tribulus terrestris*. However, at this time no evidence supports these treatments.

Drug Interactions

See the article on each individual supplement for a full description of the interactions summarized here.

Principal Natural Therapies for Erectile Dysfunction: Interactions with Pharmaceuticals		
Natural Therapy	**Pharmaceutical**	**Interaction**
Arginine	Agents causing gastric irritation	Possible increased risk of gastritis or ulceration
	Potassium-sparing diuretics	Possible increased risk of hyperkalemia
Ginkgo	Anticoagulant and antiplatelet agents	Possible increased risk of bleeding complications

FIBROMYALGIA

Principal Proposed Natural Therapies

SAMe (S-adenosyl-methionine)   [+2]

5-HTP (5-hydroxy-tryptophan)   [+2]

Capsaicin   [+2]

Blue-green algae   [+2]

(Higher numbers indicate stronger evidence; X modifier indicates contradictory results. See page xviii of the Introduction for details of the rating scale.)

Approach to the Patient

Although less popular a self-diagnosis than it was in the 1990s, fibromyalgia continues to be an overused term, particularly among those interested in alternative medicine. Nonetheless, there is clearly a real syndrome of muscle tenderness, pain, and fatigue accompanied by unrestful sleep. Conventional treatment for this syndrome remains unsatisfactory.

Highly preliminary evidence suggests that the supplements SAMe, 5-HTP, capsaicin, and the blue-green algae *Chlorella pyrenoidosa* might be helpful for fibromyalgia. The first two are proposed treatments for depression, and therefore their use in fibromyalgia might be somewhat similar to conventional treatment with antidepressants. The third may act as a topical analgesic; the potential mechanism of action of *Chlorella* is unclear.

Other treatments your patients may be using for fibromyalgia include malic acid (which has been found ineffective in one double-blind trial), magnesium, vitamin B_1, vitamin E, selenium, and spirulina. For potential safety risks with the more common of these substances, see the full herb/supplement articles.

Caution: See Drug Interactions for a summary of the extensive potential interactions among pharmaceutical and natural therapies for fibromyalgia.

SAMe   +2

S-adenosylmethionine (SAMe) is an active methyl donor that has been tried as a treatment for both depression and osteoarthritis. Four double-blind trials have studied the use of SAMe for fibromyalgia.[1-4] Three used injectable SAMe; however, only the trial using oral SAMe found positive results.[3] In this trial, 44 subjects with fibromyalgia were given 800 mg SAMe or placebo daily for 6 weeks. Use of SAMe was associated with improvements in pain, fatigue, and morning stiffness.

For more information, including dosage and safety issues, see the **SAMe** article.

5-HTP   +2

5-Hydroxytryptophan (5-HTP) is a serotonin precursor that has been tried for the treatment of depression as well as migraine headaches and obesity.

A double-blind, placebo-controlled study of 50 subjects with fibromyalgia found evidence of benefit with 300 mg of 5-HTP given for 30 days.[5]

For more information, including dosage and safety issues, see the **5-HTP** article.

Capsaicin   +2

Capsaicin, the "hot" constituent of all hot peppers, is a U.S. Food and Drug Administration (FDA)–approved treatment for postherpetic neuralgia. One supposedly double-blind study of 45 individuals found that capsaicin may be beneficial for fibromyalgia as well.[6] In this study, participants used either capsaicin cream or placebo four times per day for 4 weeks, rubbing it into the tender points on one side of their body. Those who used the real treatment reported less tenderness in their tender points than those using placebo. Interestingly, the points on their untreated sides were also less tender. It must be noted, however, that it is difficult to understand how blinding could have been maintained, considering the burning sensation caused by capsaicin.

For more information, including dosage and safety issues, see the **Cayenne** article.

Blue-Green Algae   +2

A double-blind, placebo-controlled, crossover trial of 37 individuals found evidence that the blue-green algae *Chlorella pyrenoidosa* might reduce symptoms of fibromyalgia.[7]

For more information, including dosage and safety issues, see the **Spirulina** article.

Other Proposed Natural Therapies

Malic acid, a substance in apple juice and other plant foods, has been aggressively marketed as a treatment for fibromyalgia, often in combination with **magnesium.** However, in the only published double-blind trial of this treatment, 1200 mg of malic acid and 300 mg of magnesium taken daily for 4 weeks were no more effective than placebo.[8]

Other proposed natural treatments include selenium, vitamin B_1, and vitamin E, but there is no real evidence as yet that they are effective for fibromyalgia.

Drug Interactions

See the article on each individual supplement for a full description of the interactions summarized here.

Principal Natural Therapies for Fibromyalgia: Interactions with Pharmaceuticals		
Natural Therapy	Pharmaceutical	Interaction
5-HTP	Levodopa-carbidopa	Possible increased risk of scleroderma-like syndrome
	Selective serotonin reuptake inhibitors (SSRIs), other serotonergic drugs	Possible risk of serotonin syndrome
SAMe	Levodopa or levodopa-carbidopa	Possible increased "wearing off" effect
	Serotonergic drugs (case report involved tricyclic antidepressant)	Possible risk of serotonin syndrome

Pharmaceuticals Used for Fibromyalgia: Possible Harmful Interactions with Natural Therapies

Pharmaceutical	Natural Therapy	Interaction
NSAIDs	Dong quai, St. John's wort	Possible increased risk of photosensitivity
	Garlic, ginkgo, high-dose vitamin E, policosanol, others	Possible increased risk of bleeding complications
	Feverfew	Possible increased risk of gastritis
	Potassium citrate	Possible decreased serum levels of salicylates
	White willow	Additional salicylates may increase risk of all side effects
SSRIs, tramadol, tricyclics	5-HTP, SAMe, St. John's wort	Possible risk of serotonin syndrome

Pharmaceuticals Used for Fibromyalgia: Natural Therapies with Potential Supportive Interactions

Pharmaceutical	Natural Therapy	Interaction
NSAIDs	Cayenne, colostrum, licorice	Possible cytoprotection
	Folate, vitamin C	Correction of possible drug-induced deficiency
SSRIs	Ginkgo	Possible reversal of SSRI-induced sexual dysfunction
Tricyclic antidepressants	Coenzyme Q_{10}	Possible correction of drug-induced relative deficiency

GOUT

Principal Proposed Natural Therapies

There are no evidence-based herbs or supplements for gout.

Approach to the Patient

At present, natural therapies have little to add to conventional treatment of gout. However, individuals interested in natural medicine particularly appreciate receiving the standard purine-reducing dietary instructions.

Natural therapies your patients may be using include aspartic acid, bromelain, devil's claw, celery juice, cherries, fish oil, folate, selenium, and vitamins A and E. For potential safety risks with the more common of these substances, see the full herb/supplement articles.

In addition, many patients interested in alternative medicine believe that accumulated toxins are the cause of gout and that this can be corrected through "detoxification." The latter may involve dietary changes, "colon cleansing," and supplementation with specific herbs and supplements. Malnutrition can occur in the more extreme forms of this approach.

Other Proposed Natural Therapies

Although high-dose **folate** has been recommended as a preventive for gout, the scant scientific evidence on this treatment is contradictory, and a contaminant (pterin-6-aldehyde) found in some folate sources may actually be responsible for any therapeutic effects.[1-3]

The herb **devil's claw** *(Harpagophytum procumbens)* is sometimes recommended as an analgesic for gout, based on evidence for its effectiveness in various forms of arthritis.[4]

No evidence at this time supports the effectiveness of aspartic acid, bromelain, fish oil, selenium, vitamin A, or vitamin E for either the prevention or treatment of gout.[5] Traditional remedies for gout include cherries[6] and celery juice; however, studies of these have not been reported to date.

Drug Interactions

See the article on each individual supplement for a full description of the interactions summarized here.

HEMORRHOIDS

Principal Proposed
Natural Therapies

Diosmin/hesperidin [+3]

Oxerutins [+2X]

Mesoglycans [+1]

(Higher numbers indicate stronger evidence; X modifier indicates contradictory results. See page xviii of the Introduction for details of the rating scale.)

Approach to the Patient

A fixed micronized combination of the citrus bioflavonoids diosmin and hesperidin is an accepted European treatment for hemorrhoids. The semisynthetic bioflavonoids known as oxerutins also appear to be safe and effective.

Other natural treatments your patient may be using include mesoglycans (glycosaminoglycans derived, usually, from porcine sources), butcher's broom, topical calendula cream, collinsonia root (or stone root), gotu kola, horse chestnut, oligomeric proanthocyanidins (OPCs), and slippery elm. For potential safety risks with the more common of these substances, see the full herb/supplement articles.

Diosmin/Hesperidin   +3

Meaningful evidence suggests that a micronized combination of the citrus bioflavonoids diosmin (90%) and hesperidin (10%), sold as Daflon, is safe and effective for the treatment of hemorrhoids.

A 2-month, double-blind, placebo-controlled trial of 120 individuals with recurrent hemorrhoid flare-ups found that treatment with combined diosmin and hesperidin significantly reduced the frequency and severity of hemorrhoidal exacerbations.[1] Another double-blind, placebo-controlled trial of 100 individuals found that the same bioflavonoid preparation relieved symptoms once an exacerbation of hemorrhoid pain had begun.[2] Benefits were also seen in a 90-day, double-blind trial of 100 individuals with bleeding hemorrhoids.[3] In another trial, this bioflavonoid combination was found to compare favorably with rubber band ligation.[4] However, in a trial where both treated and placebo groups received soluble fiber, intergroup differences were small.[5]

For more information, including dosage and safety issues, see the **Diosmin/Hesperidin** article.

Oxerutins   + 2 X

A double-blind study enrolling 97 pregnant women found oxerutins significantly more effective than placebo in reducing the pain, bleeding, and inflammation of hemorrhoids.[6] Earlier double-blind trials also found oxerutins effective, although one did not find benefit.[7]

For more information, including dosage and safety issues, see the **Oxerutins** article.

Mesoglycans   + 1

Preliminary evidence suggests that mesoglycans (glycosaminoglycans most commonly extracted from pig intestines) can improve the symptoms of hemorrhoids.[8,9] The usual dosage of mesoglycans is 100 mg daily. Because they are essentially processed porcine intestines, they are probably a safe supplement, even in large quantities. However, concerns have been raised regarding a potential anticoagulant effect; therefore they should be used with caution by individuals taking anticoagulant or antiplatelet medications. In addition, prion infection is at least a theoretic possibility. Maximum safe dosages for young children, pregnant or lactating women, or those with severe hepatic or renal disease have not been determined.

Other Proposed Natural Therapies

Diosmin/hesperidin and oxerutins are also used for the treatment of varicose veins and chronic venous insufficiency. Based on similarities in activity, other natural substances clinically tested for varicose veins and venous insufficiency have been proposed for hemorrhoids: these include butcher's broom, gotu kola, horse chestnut, and OPCs. Collinsonia root, calendula cream, and slippery elm are also sometimes recommended for hemorrhoids; however, there is no supporting evidence for this use.

Drug Interactions

See the article on each individual supplement for a full description of the interactions summarized here.

Principal Natural Therapies for Hemorrhoids: Interactions with Pharmaceuticals		
Natural Therapy	Pharmaceutical	Interaction
Mesoglycans	Anticoagulant or antiplatelet agents	Possible increased risk of bleeding complications

HEPATITIS (VIRAL)

Principal Proposed
Natural Therapies

Milk thistle [+2]

Taurine [+2]

Phyllanthus amarus [−1X]

(Higher numbers indicate stronger evidence; X modifier indicates contradictory results. See page xviii of the Introduction for details of the rating scale.)

Approach to the Patient

Preliminary evidence suggests that the hepatoprotective herb milk thistle may be helpful for chronic and acute hepatitis. The supplement taurine may be useful for acute viral hepatitis. Your patients may wish to use these therapies along with standard treatments; it may be worth explaining that antagonism rather than synergism is possible (although there is no meaningful evidence either way).

Despite one promising study, the herb *Phyllanthus amarus* appears to be ineffective.

Other natural treatments your patient may be using include astragalus, lecithin, liver extracts, reishi, schisandra, thymus extract, and high-dose vitamin C. For potential safety risks with the more common of these substances, see the full herb/supplement article.

Caution: Ask your patient about use of potentially hepatotoxic herbs, including kava, comfrey, chaparral, coltsfoot, and pennyroyal.

Milk Thistle +2

Small double-blind studies of patients with *chronic* viral hepatitis have found significant improvement in symptoms and signs in milk thistle–treated groups.[1-3]

A 21-day, double-blind, placebo-controlled study of 57 patients with *acute* viral hepatitis found significant improvements in the group receiving milk thistle.[4] A 35-day study of 151 patients with acute hepatitis failed to find benefit with milk thistle as compared with no treatment, but this study has been criticized for failing to document that the participants actually had acute viral hepatitis.[5]

For more information, including dosage and safety issues, see the **Milk Thistle** article.

Taurine +2

A double-blind, placebo-controlled study of 63 individuals with *acute* viral hepatitis (type not specified) evaluated the effects of 12 g of taurine daily or placebo.[6] The results showed significant improvements in liver function tests in the treatment group compared with the placebo group. However, a small double-blind, placebo-controlled study found no effect of taurine therapy on liver function tests (LFTs) in individuals with *chronic* hepatitis.[7]

For dosage and safety information, see the **Taurine** article.

Phyllanthus amarus −1X

The herb *Phyllanthus amarus* has been extensively studied as a treatment for chronic hepatitis, but the balance of evidence suggests that it is not effective.[8]

For more information, including dosage and safety issues, see the **Phyllanthus** article.

Other Proposed
Natural Therapies

In Japan, an injectable combination of **licorice** and certain **amino acids** is used for chronic hepatitis, with some success.[9] However, it is not clear that oral licorice is equally effective, and the high dosages used for treatment of chronic hepatitis may cause hypertension.

The **traditional herbal medicines of Japan and China** typically use combinations of herbs. At present, there is no conclusive evidence that any of these combinations are effective for the treatment of hepatitis B.[10] **Thymus extract** has been tried as a treatment for hepatitis B and C. However, the results of small double-blind trials have not been positive.[11-14]

Other treatments sometimes recommended for hepatitis include astragalus, lecithin, liver extracts, reishi, schisandra, taurine, and high-dose vitamin C. However, there is as yet no real clinical evidence that these approaches work.

Drug Interactions

See the article on each individual supplement for a full description of the interactions summarized here.

Principal Natural Therapy for Viral Hepatitis: Interaction with Pharmaceuticals		
Natural Therapy	Pharmaceutical	Interaction
Milk thistle	Oral contraceptives	Theoretic interference with action of drug

HERPES SIMPLEX

Principal Proposed
Natural Therapies

**Topical lemon balm
(treatment)** [+3]

L-Lysine (prevention)
[+2X]

**Topical aloe
(treatment)** [+2]

**Topical zinc/glycine
(treatment)** [+2]

**Eleutherococcus
(prevention)** [+2]

**Echinacea
(prevention)** [−1]

(Higher numbers indicate stronger evidence; X modifier indicates contradictory results. See page xviii of the Introduction for details of the rating scale.)

Approach to the Patient

Preliminary evidence suggests that acute herpes infections may respond to topical treatment with any one of the following: lemon balm cream, *Aloe vera*, and a mixture of topical zinc and glycine. Oral use of the herb eleutherococcus (*Eleutherococcus senticosus*, or Siberian ginseng) has shown some promise for prevention. Lesser evidence suggests that oral L-lysine may also have prophylactic effects when taken in sufficient doses.

Caution: Patients may incorrectly believe that these treatments will prevent transmission of genital herpes.

Other natural treatments your patient may be using include astragalus, bee propolis, cat's claw, elderberry, licorice, tea tree oil, and vitamin C. For potential safety risks with the more common of these substances, see the full herb/supplement articles.

Topical
Lemon Balm (Treatment)   +3

A double-blind trial evaluated 116 patients with genital or oral herpes given either lemon balm cream or placebo for a period of 5 days.[1] The largest intergroup differences were seen at day 2 of treatment, showing statistically significant improvements in favor of the treated group. In addition, the total number of patients who were completely recovered on day 5 was significantly higher in the treated group than in the placebo group. Physician and patient evaluation of the course of the outbreak was also strongly in favor of the treated group.

Another double-blind, placebo-controlled study observed 66 individuals at the onset of oral herpes.[2] Treatment with lemon balm cream again produced significant, benefits on day 2, reducing intensity of discomfort, number of blisters, and size of the lesions. Researchers specifically looked at day 2 because of the previous study's results, as well as their belief that day 2 is the point of maximum symptomatology. Long-term informal follow-up suggested to the researchers that continuous lemon balm application also delayed the next herpes flare-up.

For more information, including dosage and safety issues, see the **Lemon Balm** article.

Topical Aloe (Treatment)   +2

A 2-week, double-blind, placebo-controlled trial enrolled 60 men with active genital herpes (mean 4.1 days after lesion onset).[3] Participants applied aloe cream or placebo cream three times daily for 5 days. Use of aloe cream resulted in a reduced mean time to healing and total number of healed patients.

A previous double-blind, placebo-controlled study by the same author enrolled 120 men with genital herpes and compared aloe cream and aloe gel with placebo.[4] Aloe cream proved most effective.

Eleutherococcus (Prevention)   + 2

A 6-month, double-blind, trial of 93 men and women with recurrent herpes infections found that treatment with oral eleutherococcus (2 g daily) significantly reduced the frequency of flare-ups.[5]

For more information, including dosage and safety issues, see the **Eleutherococcus** article.

L-Lysine (Prevention)   + 2 X

L-Lysine may have a dose-dependent effect on herpes prophylaxis, with benefits seen at 1250 to 3000 mg daily.

A double-blind, placebo-controlled study observed 52 participants with a history of recurrent herpes.[6] While receiving 3 g of L-lysine daily for 6 months, the treatment group experienced an average of 2.4 fewer herpes infections than the placebo group—a significant difference. When infections did occur, those in the lysine group were significantly less severe and healed faster.

A double-blind, placebo-controlled, crossover study (two 6-month treatment periods) of 41 subjects also found improvements in the frequency of infections with 1250 mg of lysine daily but not with 624 mg daily.[7] However, another double-blind, placebo-controlled, crossover study (two 3-month treatment periods) observed 65 patients and found no benefit with 1000 mg of lysine daily.[8] Negative results were also seen using 1200 mg of lysine daily in a small parallel-design trial with 21 subjects.[9]

Lysine has not been found effective for treating acute herpes attacks.[10]

For more information, including dosage and safety issues, see the **Lysine** article.

Topical Zinc/Glycine (Treatment)   + 2

In a double-blind, placebo-controlled trial, 46 individuals with active facial or circumoral herpes lesions were treated with a zinc oxide cream or placebo every 2 hours until cold sores resolved.[11] The results showed a significant reduction in severity and duration of symptoms in the treated group as compared with the placebo group. Some temporary burning and irritation from the zinc treatment were observed.

As with topical zinc treatment of upper respiratory infections (URIs), proper design of the zinc formulation to release zinc ions is believed to be necessary. This trial used a zinc oxide/glycine formulation.

For more information, including dosage and safety issues, see the **Zinc** article.

Echinacea (Prevention)   − 1

In a 1-year, double-blind, placebo-controlled, crossover trial of 50 individuals with frequently recurrent genital herpes, treatment with oral *Echinacea purpurea* extract (Echinaforce, 800 mg twice daily) failed to impact disease recurrence.[12]

For more information, including dosage and safety issues, see the **Echinacea** article.

Other Proposed Natural Therapies

One study suggests that topical treatment with a **vitamin C** solution may speed healing of herpes outbreaks,[13] and another suggests that oral vitamin C may also be useful, especially when combined with **bioflavonoids.**[14]

One preliminary study suggests **bee propolis** may be helpful for treating herpes.[15] A small study using tea tree oil found statistically insignificant trends toward benefit.[16]

Although the herbs astragalus, cat's claw, elderberry, and licorice are sometimes recommended for herpes, currently no clinical evidence supports these treatments.

Drug Interactions

See the article on each individual supplement for a full description of the interactions summarized here.

Principal Natural Therapy for Herpes Simplex: Interaction with Pharmaceuticals		
Natural Therapy	**Pharmaceutical**	**Interaction**
Eleutherococcus	Digitoxin, digoxin	Interference with determination of serum levels of drug

HERPES ZOSTER

Principal Proposed
Natural Therapies

Proteolytic enzymes   [+2]

(Higher numbers indicate stronger evidence; X modifier indicates contradictory results. See page xviii of the Introduction for details of the rating scale.)

Approach to the Patient

Double-blind, comparative trials suggest that oral proteolytic enzymes are equally as effective as acyclovir for the treatment of acute herpes zoster. However, placebo-controlled trials of proteolytic enzymes in herpes zoster are lacking.

Other natural treatments your patient may be using for herpes zoster include adenosine monophosphate (AMP), vitamin B_{12}, and vitamin E. For potential safety risks with the more common of these substances, see the full herb/supplement articles.

Proteolytic Enzymes   +2

Although best known as replacement therapy in pancreatic insufficiency, proteolytic enzymes are also thought to have systemic effects. Treatment with proteolytic enzymes may be as effective as acyclovir for acute herpes zoster, but placebo-controlled trials have not been performed.

A double-blind, trial of 192 individuals with acute herpes zoster compared the effect of a proprietary proteolytic enzyme mixture with acyclovir.[1] Participants were given four capsules five times daily until the disappearance of symptoms (maximum 14 days), and their pain was assessed at intervals. Each enzyme capsule contained 30 mg trypsin, 30 mg chymotrypsin, and 75 mg papain, as well as 30 mg thymus extract (a purported immune stimulant); the acyclovir tablets contained 200 mg of the drug. Statistically equivalent pain relief was documented for both groups, but the acyclovir group had more side effects (primarily mild gastrointestinal disturbance).

Equivalent benefits between drug and supplement were also seen in another double-blind trial.[2] Ninety subjects were given an initial injection of acyclovir or proteolytic enzymes, followed by a 7-day course of oral medication, four tablets five times daily. In this case, each enzyme tablet contained 40 mg trypsin, 40 mg chymotrypsin, and 100 mg papainases.

For more information, including dosage and safety issues, see the **Proteolytic Enzymes** article.

Other Proposed Natural Therapies

Injectable adenosine monophosphate (AMP) has been studied as a possible treatment for acute herpes zoster as well as for preventing postherpetic neuralgia. In a double-blind, placebo-controlled study of 32 individuals with acute herpes zoster, AMP was injected three times per week for 4 weeks.[3] At the end of the treatment period, 88% of the treated individuals were pain-free, as opposed to only 43% in the placebo group; all patients with continuing discomfort were then given AMP, and no recurrence of pain was reported in the 3 to 18 months of follow-up. Oral AMP has not been studied for this condition.

Vitamins E and **B$_{12}$** have also been suggested as possible treatments for postherpetic neuralgia, but the evidence that they work for this condition is extremely weak.[4-6]

Drug Interactions

See the article on each individual supplement for a full description of the interactions summarized here.

Principal Natural Therapy for Herpes Zoster: Interaction with Pharmaceuticals		
Natural Therapy	Pharmaceutical	Interaction
Papain	Anticoagulants	Possible increased risk of bleeding complications

HIV SUPPORT

Principal Proposed Natural Therapies

Boxwood extract [+3]

Carnitine [+1]

(Higher numbers indicate stronger evidence; X modifier indicates contradictory results. See page xviii of the Introduction for details of the rating scale.)

Approach to the Patient

Surveys have shown that individuals with human immunodeficiency virus (HIV) or acquired immunodeficiency syndrome (AIDS) often take natural remedies in addition to multiple medications. Some of these may present significant risks: see especially the discussion of St. John's wort and garlic in Herbs to Avoid, below. Others might offer benefits, although the evidence is not strong. A special extract of the herb boxwood has shown some promise in one study. The supplement carnitine may also be useful as adjunctive therapy. In addition, routine multivitamin/mineral supplementation may be advisable.

Numerous other natural treatments have limited or no evidence behind them. Discussed under several separate headings below, they include aloe; andrographis; astragalus; bacailin; beta-carotene; bitter melon; bovine colostrum; boxwood extract; Chinese herb combinations; cinnamon; coenzyme Q_{10}; curcumin, dehydroepiandrosterone (DHEA); echinacea; elderberry; fish oil; garlic (see Herbs to Avoid); ginseng *(Panax ginseng, P. quinquefolius)*; glutamine; glutathione; glycyrrhizin; iron; lipoate; maitake; medium-chain triglycerides (MCTs); multivitamins; *N*-acetyl cysteine (NAC); niacin; omega-6 fatty acids; propolis; proteolytic enzymes; reishi; schisandra; sele-

nium; spirulina; tea tree oil; trichosanthin (compound Q); vitamins A, B_1, B_2, B_6, B_{12}, C, and E; and whey protein.

Boxwood Extract   +3

Preliminary research suggests that an extract of the leaves and
stems of the boxwood shrub may delay the progression of HIV
disease.[2]

In a double-blind, placebo-controlled study of 145 HIV patients, French researchers studied the effects of two doses of an
extract from evergreen boxwood: 990 mg and 1980 mg per day
for periods ranging from 4 to 64 weeks.[2] At the beginning of the
trial, participants had no symptoms, and none were given HIV
medications throughout the trial. The trial end point was therapeutic failure, defined as the development of AIDS or AIDS-
related complex (ARC) or CD4 counts below 200×10^6 on two
occasions. The results showed significantly fewer therapeutic
failures in the 990-mg group.

No severe side effects were reported in this study, and the individuals taking boxwood had the same overall rate of side effects
as those taking placebo.[2] However, there are some safety concerns with this herb, mostly relating to one of its presumed active ingredients, cycloprotobuxine.[3] High doses of this substance
can cause vomiting, diarrhea, muscular spasms, and paralysis.
Safety of boxwood extract in pregnant or lactating women,
young children, or individuals with hepatic or renal disease has
not been established. In addition, touching fresh boxwood leaves
can occasionally cause skin irritation.[4]

Only a special boxwood extract has been studied as a treatment
for HIV infection, not raw boxwood leaf.

The potential benefits of combination treatment with boxwood
extract and standard HIV therapy have not been systematically
explored.

Carnitine   +1

Preliminary evidence suggests that L-carnitine may diminish the mitochondrial toxicity associated with zidovudine (AZT) and other nucleoside analogs, exert independent positive effects on HIV infection parameters, and complement traditional chemotherapeutic regimens in HIV-infected patients.

AZT therapy causes a mitochondrial myopathy characterized by depletion of mitochondrial deoxyribonucleic acid (DNA) and other destructive changes that has been associated with a reduction of muscle carnitine levels.[5] Based on the observation that L-carnitine plays a major role in long-chain fatty acid transport and facilitates the beta-oxidation of fatty acids, it has been proposed as a treatment for these AZT side effects.[6]

Other preliminary evidence suggests that L-carnitine may also enhance immune function in HIV-infected individuals.[7-9]

For more information, including dosage and safety issues, see the **Carnitine** article.

Other Proposed Natural Therapies

The following inadequately documented treatments are categorized by intended use.

For more information, including dosage and safety issues, see the applicable articles.

Viral Suppression

Numerous natural substances or their constituents have been investigated for possible viral suppression, including aloe, astragalus, bacailin, curcumin, elderberry, licorice, maitake, propolis, reishi, schisandra, and spirulina. However, there is no clinical evidence as yet that they are effective for this purpose.

The herb **St. John's wort** contains hypericin, a substance that has been investigated for possible antiretroviral effects. However, studies have concluded that it is not clinically useful. In addition, St. John's wort seriously impairs the activity of protease inhibitors and might lead to treatment failure (see Herbs to Avoid).

Wasting

Medium-chain triglycerides (MCTs) are more easily absorbed than ordinary fats (long-chain triglycerides) and may help decrease diarrhea and wasting. Two small double-blind trials enrolling a total of about 50 individuals with HIV or AIDS found that MCTs were more easily absorbed by the participants than long-chain triglycerides.[10,11] However, there is no direct evidence as yet that MCTs actually help HIV-positive patients gain weight.

A double-blind, placebo-controlled study of 21 individuals with AIDS-related weight loss found that a combination of **glutamine** and **antioxidants** (vitamins C and E, beta-carotene, selenium, NAC) led to significant weight gain.[12] Another small double-blind trial (n = 68) found that combination treatment with glutamine, **arginine,** and **hydroxymethyl butyrate (HMB)** could increase muscle mass and possibly improve immune status.[13]

Whey protein and **fish oil** are also sometimes tried for weight gain in HIV, but evidence for their effectiveness is minimal at best.[14,15,75]

Immune Function Support

Preliminary human trials of **NAC** for maintaining CD4+ counts in HIV-infected individuals have had mixed results.[16-18] A pilot study suggests that an ingredient of andrographis, andrographolide, might increase CD4+ counts.[19]

Other natural treatments purported to boost immunity in HIV include bitter melon, coenzyme Q_{10}, DHEA, echinacea, ginseng, glycyrrhizin (a component of licorice), lipoate, maitake, omega-6 fatty acids, proteolytic enzymes, and trichosanthin (compound Q). However, there is no real evidence as yet that these treatments actually work for this purpose.

Garlic is sometimes recommended as well; however, for safety reasons, garlic should be avoided in HIV infection (see Herbs to Avoid).

Fish oil is also sometimes recommended for enhancing immunity in HIV infection. However, one 6-month double-blind trial of 64 individuals found that a combination of the omega-3 fatty acids in fish oil plus the amino acid arginine was no more effective than placebo.[20]

Miscellaneous Symptoms of HIV

Bovine colostrum has been suggested for the chronic diarrhea that commonly occurs in HIV and AIDS, but the evidence that it offers benefit remains weak at best.[21-23] **Tea tree oil** and **cinnamon** have been suggested as treatments for oral thrush.[24]

Levels of **dehydroepiandrosterone (DHEA)** appear to decrease in HIV infection, possibly because of malnutrition and/or stress,[25,26] and there is some evidence that decreased serum levels of DHEA correlate with more rapid progression of the disease.[76,77] One small double-blind trial suggests that DHEA (50 mg/day) may improve mood and fatigue scores in individuals with HIV.[78] However, another small trial found inconclusive results.[27]

A standardized mixture of **Chinese herbs** including astragalus, andrographis, and more than 30 others was no more effective than placebo at reducing HIV symptoms in either a pilot study or in a larger double-blind study involving 68 individuals.[28,29]

Side Effects of AZT

Zidovudine (AZT) therapy may deplete body **zinc** stores, an effect that appears to diminish drug effectiveness and impair immune function.[30-32] For this reason, zinc supplementation may be warranted. However, see discussion of zinc below under General Nutritional Support for cautions.

Based on highly preliminary evidence, **vitamin B$_{12}$** has been suggested as a preventive for neutropenia caused by AZT.[33]

Side Effects of TMP-SMX (Trimethoprim-Sulfamethoxazole)

It has been suggested that the supplement **NAC** might help prevent side effects caused by long-term use of TMP-SMX. However, two randomized controlled studies found that NAC did not significantly decrease adverse reactions to TMP-SMX compared with placebo.[34,35]

TMP-SMX may impair **folate** activity to some extent; folate supplements might counteract this effect.[36]

General Nutritional Support

Individuals infected with HIV may be particularly vulnerable to malnutrition because of decreased appetite, poor absorption, or possibly increased requirements for specific nutrients.

Vitamin A/Beta-Carotene

An observational study suggests that **vitamin A** deficiency may be linked to lower CD4+ counts as well as higher death rates among HIV-infected individuals.[37]

A few preliminary studies have raised hopes that **beta-carotene** supplements might increase or preserve immune function or decrease symptoms.[38-41] One small double-blind study involving 21 individuals suggested that taking beta-carotene might raise white blood cell counts in individuals with HIV.[41] However, two subsequent larger, randomized, controlled trials involving a total of 124 individuals found no significant differences between those taking beta-carotene or placebo in CD4+ count or other measures of immune function.[42,43]

Two observational studies lasting 6 to 8 years suggest that higher intakes of vitamin A or beta-carotene may be helpful, but they also found that caution is in order with regard to dosage.[44] This group of researchers generally linked higher intake of vitamin A or beta-carotene to lower risk of AIDS and lower death rates, with an important exception: individuals with the highest intake of either nutrient (more than 11,179 IU per day of beta-carotene, or more than 20,268 IU per day of vitamin A) did worse than those who took somewhat less.

Despite hopes that vitamin A given to pregnant HIV-positive women might decrease the infection rate of their infants, two double-blind studies enrolling a total of more than 1500 HIV-positive mothers found no significant differences between infants of mothers given vitamin A and those given placebo.[45,46]

B Vitamins

An observational study found that HIV-positive men with the highest intakes of **vitamins B_1, B_2, B_6**, and **niacin** had significantly longer survival rates. For example, men who, early in the course of their disease, took supplements of vitamin B_1, B_2, or B_6 at several times higher than the respective recommended daily allowances (RDAs) had lower death rates 8 years later.[47] A similar study found that those taking the most B_1 or niacin had a significantly lower rate of developing AIDS.[44] **Vitamin B_{12}** deficiencies in HIV have been linked to neurologic symptoms, including slower processing of information in studies of cognitive functioning; early research suggests that restoring B_{12} levels to normal may decrease these symptoms.[48,49] Vitamin B_{12} deficiency has also been linked to lower CD4+ counts and more rapid development of AIDS.[50,51]

Vitamins C and E

Massive doses of **vitamin C** have at times been popular among individuals with HIV infection, based on highly preliminary evidence.[52,53]

An observational study linked high doses of vitamin C with slower progression to AIDS.[44] High intake of **vitamin E** was also linked to decreased risk of progression to AIDS in a different observational study.[54] However, a double-blind study of 49 HIV-positive individuals who took combined vitamins C and E or placebo for 3 months did not show any significant effects on viral load or frequency of opportunistic infections.[55]

It has been suggested that vitamin E may enhance the antiviral effects of AZT, but evidence for this is minimal.[56]

Selenium

Selenium is required for a properly functioning immune system.[57,58] Observational studies have linked higher blood levels of selenium with higher CD4+ counts[57] and reduced risk of mortality from HIV disease.[59,60]

However, in a randomized controlled study of 52 individuals with HIV, selenium did not improve clinical conditions or raise CD4+ counts any more than no treatment did.[43] A prospective controlled trial of randomized partial crossover design studied selenium combined with NAC, with mixed results: the combination affected T cell counts in some participants but not others.[17] Selenium has also been proposed as a preventive or treatment for AIDS-related cardiomyopathy, but evidence so far is weak.[61,62] Some evidence does suggest that selenium deficiency may increase vaginal viral shedding in women with HIV-1.[63]

Zinc

Some, but not all, observational studies have found that HIV-positive individuals tend to be deficient in **zinc,** with levels dropping lower in more severe disease.[50,64-68] Higher zinc levels have been linked to better immune function and higher CD4+

cell counts, whereas zinc deficiency has been linked to increased risk of dying from HIV.[50,69] (See also the discussion of zinc and AZT above.)

One preliminary study among individuals taking AZT found that 30 days of zinc supplementation led to decreased rates of opportunistic infection over the following 2 years.[32] However, an observational study linked higher zinc intake to more rapid development of AIDS.[44] In another observational study of HIV-positive individuals, those with higher zinc intake or those taking zinc supplements in any dosage had a greater risk of death within the following 8 years.[47]

Other Nutrients

A study of 71 HIV-positive children noted a high rate of **iron** deficiency.[70] One observational study of 296 men with HIV infection linked high intake of iron to a decreased risk of AIDS 6 years later.[54]

In addition, evidence suggests that individuals with HIV who are low in choline may experience more rapid disease progression.[71]

Multivitamins

Because so many nutrients are affected by HIV infection and treatments, **multivitamin** supplements are a logical choice in HIV support.

Researchers interviewed 296 men with HIV (but not AIDS) about their diets and multivitamin use and then observed their progress for 6 years.[54] Statistical analysis correcting for confounding factors concluded that those participants who took a daily multivitamin had a significantly lower risk of developing AIDS.

Herbs to Avoid

Because of interactions with CYP enzymes, **St. John's wort** markedly reduces serum levels of indinavir and presumably other protease inhibitors.[72] St. John's wort may also interact with nonnucleoside reverse transcriptase inhibitors.[1] Each of these effects could lead to treatment failure as well as the emergence of resistant strains of HIV. In addition, St. John's wort, along with dong quai, might also present increased risk of photosensitivity if combined with zidovudine.

Garlic may also present risks. Two individuals with HIV experienced severe gastrointestinal toxicity from ritonavir after taking garlic supplements.[73] In addition, garlic has been found to reduce plasma concentrations of saquinavir.[74]

Drug Interactions

See the article on each individual supplement for a full description of the interactions summarized here.

Pharmaceuticals Used for HIV: Possible Harmful Interactions with Natural Therapies		
Pharmaceutical	Natural Therapy	Interaction
Azathioprine	Dong quai, St. John's wort	Possible increased risk of photosensitivity
Protease inhibitors	Garlic	Possible increased gastrointestinal distress
	Grapefruit juice	Increased serum levels of drug
	St. John's wort	Reduced serum levels of drug
Sulfonamides	Dong quai, St. John's wort	Possible increased risk of photosensitivity
	Potassium	Possible hyperkalemia

Pharmaceuticals Used for HIV: Natural Therapies with Potential Supportive Interactions		
Pharmaceutical	**Natural Therapy**	**Interaction**
Azathioprine	Carnitine	Possible enhanced action of drug and reduced side effects
Sulfonamides	Folate	Correction of possible drug-induced deficiency
Protease inhibitors and nonnucleoside reverse transcriptase inhibitors	St. John's wort	Reduced serum levels because of CYP and other interactions, with possible rebound toxicity if herb is discontinued

HYPERLIPIDEMIA

Principal Proposed Natural Therapies

Vitamin B₃ (niacin) [+4]	**Garlic** [+3X]
Fiber [+4]	**Artichoke leaf** [+3]
Stanol esters [+3]	**Red yeast rice** [+2]
Soy protein/ isoflavones [+3]	**Guggul** [+2]
Policosanol [+3]	

(Higher numbers indicate stronger evidence; X modifier indicates contradictory results. See page xviii of the Introduction for details of the rating scale.)

Approach to the Patient

Good evidence supports the beneficial effects of niacin, fiber, stanol esters, soy protein, and policosanol in improving lipid profiles. Other treatments with some supporting evidence include artichoke leaf, garlic, red yeast rice (off the market at press time), and guggul. Weaker evidence supports the use of calcium, chromium, curcumin, creatine, fenugreek, flaxseed oil, L-carnitine, lecithin, mesoglycans (glycosaminoglycans extracted from pig intestines), probiotics, and spirulina. Fish oil and pantethine may primarily reduce triglycerides.

Other natural treatments your patient may be using include ashwagandha, bilberry leaf, chondroitin, copper, curcumin (extract of turmeric), gamma-oryzanol, grass pollen, He shou wu, lecithin, and maitake. For potential safety risks with the more common of these substances, see the full herb/supplement articles.

Caution: Combination therapy with garlic and policosanol, intended to magnify hypolipidemic effects, might potentially cause significant impairment of hemostasis.

Vitamin B₃ (Niacin)   +4

Niacin is a well-known treatment for hyperlipidemia. Niacin lowers total and low-density lipoprotein (LDL) cholesterol by 15% to 25%, lowers triglycerides by 2% to 50%, and raises high-density lipoprotein (HDL) by 15% to 25%.[1-5]

For more information, including dosage and safety issues, see the **Vitamin B₃** article.

Fiber   +4

Numerous studies have shown that water-soluble fiber lowers cholesterol.[6]

Stanol Esters   +3

At least 14 double-blind, placebo-controlled studies, ranging in length from 30 days to 12 months and involving a total of about 1000 individuals, have found stanol esters (and related sterols) effective for improving cholesterol levels.[7-20] The combined results suggest that stanols can reduce total and LDL cholesterol by about 10% to 15%. Stanols did not have any significant effect on HDL or triglycerides in most of these studies.[21] When combined with a standard NCEP step-1 diet, use of a spread enhanced with plant sterols improved total cholesterol, LDL cholesterol, HDL cholesterol, and triglycerides as compared with a normal reduced-fat spread.[22]

In one of the best of the double-blind, placebo-controlled studies, 153 individuals with mildly elevated cholesterol were given margarine with or without sitostanol ester (at a dose of 1.8 or 2.6 g of sitostanol per day) for a total of 1 year.[12] The results in the treated group receiving 2.6 g per day showed that total cholesterol was reduced by 10.2% and LDL by 14.1%—

significantly better than the results in the control group. Neither triglyceride nor HDL cholesterol levels were affected.

Two studies found stanols to be safe and effective for lowering cholesterol levels in individuals with type 2 diabetes.[7,23] In one of these studies, pravastatin plus sitostanol was more effective at lowering total cholesterol and LDL levels than the drug treatment alone.[23] Additive benefits were also seen in a study of nondiabetics taking statin drugs who began taking stanols as well.[10]

The suggested dosage of stanol esters varies depending on the product and the quantity of sitostanol ester per serving. Typical dosages of stanols to lower cholesterol range from 3.4 to 5.1 g per day.[10] One manufacturer of a commercially prepared margarine recommends taking 3 teaspoons per day (1.5 g of sitostanol ester per teaspoon). A substantial decrease in total cholesterol may take up to 3 months to become evident.[12]

Stanols are considered safe because they are not absorbed.[10,24] No adverse effects have been reported in any of the studies on lowering cholesterol, with the exception of one that reported mild gastrointestinal complaints in a few preschool children.[25] In addition, no toxic signs were observed in rats given stanol esters for 13 weeks at levels comparable to or exceeding those recommended for lowering cholesterol.[26]

Although concerns have been expressed that stanols might impair absorption of the fat-soluble vitamins A, D, and E, this does not seem to occur at the dosages of stanols required to lower cholesterol.[11] Stanols might, however, interfere with absorption of alpha- and beta-carotene,[8,15] although some studies have found no such effect.[12,13] Until more is learned, it may be reasonable for individuals using stanol products to make sure to consume carotenoid-rich vegetables (yellow/orange and dark green vegetables).[13]

Soy Protein/Isoflavones   +3

In 1995, a review of 38 controlled studies on soy and heart disease concluded that soy is effective at reducing total cholesterol (TC), LDL, and triglycerides,[27] and the U.S. Food and Drug Administration (FDA) approved a "heart-healthy" label for foods containing significant soy protein content.

There is conflicting evidence regarding whether soy isoflavones are the active hypocholesterolemic ingredient in soy protein,[28-30,124] although other studies disagree with this assertion.[31-34,125] Inaccurate label claims for isoflavone content of soy products, as well as differences in the distribution of various isoflavones among products, may account for some of these contradictions.[35]

Although they are similar to soy isoflavones, red clover isoflavones were found ineffective for lowering cholesterol in a 12-week, double-blind study of 66 women.[36]

For more information, including dosage and safety issues, see the **Soy Protein** and **Isoflavones** articles.

Policosanol   +3

Fifteen double-blind, placebo-controlled trials, involving more than 1000 individuals and ranging in length from 6 weeks to 12 months, have found the sugar cane extract policosanol effective for improving total and LDL cholesterol levels, as well as LDL/HDL and TC/HDL ratios.* Effects on HDL cholesterol and triglycerides have been less consistent. All but one of these studies was conducted in Cuba by one research group.

The largest of these trials was a double-blind, placebo-controlled study that enrolled 437 individuals with type 2 hypercholesterolemia.[47] Participants were first placed on a step-1

---

*References 37-42, 44-49, 134, 138, 140.

diet for 5 weeks. Lipid profiles were taken twice within the next 2 weeks and averaged to provide a baseline value. Then, participants received either placebo or policosanol at 5 mg/day for 12 weeks. At that point, the dosage was doubled to 10 mg/day in the treated group, and the study continued for an additional 12 weeks. The results showed significant improvements with both policosanol doses, but greater improvement at the end of the higher-dose period. By the conclusion of the trial, LDL cholesterol in the treated group improved by 25.6%, total cholesterol by 17.4%, HDL cholesterol by 28.4%, and triglycerides by 5.2%. These results were statistically significant from baseline as well as compared with the outcome in the placebo group.

Seven other double-blind trials enrolling a total of about 400 individuals compared policosanol with pravastatin, fluvastatin, simvastatin, and lovastatin and found these agents to be essentially identical in effect on lipid parameters.[50-55,142] One of these trials was reported by a different Cuban research group.[51]

For more information, including dosage and safety issues, see the **Policosanol** article.

Garlic +3X

Despite extensive German literature finding garlic effective for hypercholesterolemia,[56-59] most more recent trials have found no benefit.[60-65] The explanation may lie in garlic's apparently modest effect. A metaanalysis that accepted 13 trials found evidence of cholesterol reduction in the range of 5% compared with placebo.[66] Negative trials lacked study power to identify a benefit this small.

For more information, including dosage and safety issues, see the **Garlic** article.

Artichoke Leaf   +3

In a 6-week, double-blind, placebo-controlled study of 143 individuals with hyperlipidemia, artichoke leaf extract significantly
improved lipid profiles.[67] Total cholesterol fell by 18.5% as
compared with 8.6% in the placebo group; LDL by 23% vs.
6%; and LDL/HDL ratio decreased by 20% vs. 7%.

An earlier double-blind, placebo-controlled study of 44 healthy
individuals failed to find any improvement in cholesterol levels
attributable to artichoke leaf.[68] However, because average baseline cholesterol levels of the study participants were lower than
normal, reduction would not be expected.

For more information, including dosage and safety issues, see
the **Artichoke** article.

Red Yeast Rice   +2

The evidence from preliminary studies suggests that red yeast
rice can reduce levels of total cholesterol, LDL, and triglycerides in subjects with hyperlipidemia. It contains several naturally occurring substances in the statin drug family (including
mevinolin, identical to lovastatin).

A 12-week, double-blind, placebo-controlled trial of 83 subjects
evaluated red yeast rice for hyperlipidemia.[69] At 8 weeks, mean
total cholesterol in the red rice group decreased significantly
compared with placebo (208 mg/dL vs. 254 mg/dL). At 12
weeks, LDL was 135 mg/dL for the treated group vs. 175 for
the placebo group , and triglyceride levels were 124 mg/dL vs.
146 mg/dL. However, no significant differences were noted in
HDL levels from baseline or between groups.

Benefits were also seen in U.S. and Chinese open trials.[70,71]

For more information, including dosage and safety issues, see
the **Red Yeast Rice** article.

Guggul   +2

A double-blind, placebo-controlled study enrolled 61 hyperlipidemic individuals and observed them for 24 weeks.[72] After 24 weeks of treatment, the results showed that the treated group experienced an 11.7% decrease in total cholesterol, a 12.7% decrease in LDL, a 12% decrease in triglycerides, and an 11.1% decrease in the total cholesterol/HDL ratio. These improvements were significantly greater than those seen in the placebo group.

Similar results were seen in a double-blind, placebo-controlled trial of 40 individuals.[73] In a double-blind, comparative trial, equivalent hypolipidemic effects were seen in 228 individuals given either guggul or clofibrate.[74]

For more information, including dosage and safety issues, see the **Guggul** article.

Other Proposed Natural Therapies

Limited and sometimes contradictory evidence supports the use of esterin processed alfalfa,[75] mesoglycans,[76-78] calcium,[79,80] chitosan,* chromium,[91-94] combined chromium and grapeseed,[94] curcumin,[95-98] caigua,[99] *Achillea wilhelmsii*,[100] creatine,[101] flaxseed oil,[102-105] fenugreek,[131-133,135-137] L-carnitine,[106] probiotics,[107-112] spirulina,[113-115] and tocotrienols[116,117] for dyslipidemia. **Fish oil**[105] and **pantethine**[118-121] appear to primarily lower triglycerides. A 24-week, double-blind, placebo-controlled trial found that use of fish oil enhanced the hypotriglyceridemic effects of simvastatin.[122] However, gemfibrozil appears to be more effective than fish oil.[123]

Lecithin is widely recommended for reducing cholesterol. However, this idea appears to rest entirely on studies of unac-

---

*References 13-19, 21, 81-90, 139, 141.

ceptably low quality.[156] The best-designed studies failed to find any evidence of benefit.[43,126-130]

Other treatments sometimes recommended for lowering cholesterol, but with no meaningful supporting evidence, include ashwagandha, bilberry leaf, chondroitin, copper, gamma-oryzanol, grass pollen, He shou wu, and maitake.

Drug Interactions

See the article on each individual supplement for a full description of the interactions summarized here.

Principal Natural Therapies for Hyperlipidemia: Interactions with Pharmaceuticals		
Natural Therapy	Pharmaceutical	Interaction
Garlic	Anticoagulant and antiplatelet agents	Possible increased risk of bleeding complications
Niacin	Statin drugs	Possible risk of liver enzyme elevations and rhabdomyolysis
Red yeast rice	Azole, antifungals, cyclosporine, fibric acid derivatives, erythromycin, high-dose niacin, warfarin	Possible interactions identical to those of statin drugs
Soy	Thyroid hormone	Possible impaired action of drug

Pharmaceuticals Used for Hyperlipidemia: Possible Harmful Interactions with Natural Therapies

Pharmaceutical	Natural Therapy	Interaction
Fibric acid derivatives	Red yeast rice	Possible increased risk of rhabdomyolysis
Niacin	Red yeast rice	Possible increased risk of liver enzyme elevations and rhabdomyolysis
Statins	Chaparral, coltsfoot, other liver-toxic herbs	Possible increased risk of liver inflammation
	High-dose niacin	Possible increased risk of liver enzyme elevations and rhabdomyolysis
	Grapefruit juice	Increased serum levels of drug
	Red yeast rice	Increased drug levels because of statins in supplement
Simvastatin, lovastatin, atorvastatin (but not pravastatin)	St. John's wort	Reduced drug levels

Pharmaceuticals Used for Hyperlipidemia: Natural Therapies with Potential Supportive Interactions

Pharmaceutical	Natural Therapy	Interaction
Bile acid sequestrants	Folate, possibly other nutrients	Correction of possible drug-induced deficiency
Statins	Coenzyme Q_{10}	Possible correction of drug-induced deficiency

HYPERTENSION

Principal Proposed
Natural Therapies

Stevia [+3]

Garlic [+2]

Coenzyme Q₁₀ [+2]

**Minerals:
calcium, magnesium,
potassium** [+2X]

Fish oil [+2X]

Vitamin C [+2X]

(Higher numbers indicate stronger evidence; X modifier indicates contradictory results. See page xviii of the Introduction for details of the rating scale.)

Approach to the Patient

Relatively weak evidence supports the use of a few natural treatments for hypertension. In practice, all are unlikely to prove effective on their own in any but the mildest hypertension. The best evidence is for the herb stevia, followed by garlic and coenzyme Q₁₀. Supplemental magnesium, potassium, and calcium as well as fish oil and vitamin C might offer some antihypertensive benefits, but study results are inconsistent.

Other natural treatments your patient may be using include glucomannan, chitosan, hibiscus tea, kelp, astragalus, *Coleus forskohlii*, hawthorn, maitake, beta-carotene, flaxseed oil, and taurine. For potential safety risks with the more common of these substances, see the full herb/supplement articles.

Keep in mind that patients interested in alternative medicine may be particularly willing to make significant lifestyle changes to correct hypertension.

Stevia   + 3

Best known as an herbal sweetener, the herb stevia may also possess antihypertensive effects. A 1-year, double-blind, placebo-controlled trial evaluated the effects of the constituent stevioside (250 mg three times daily) in 106 hypertensive individuals.[1] The results showed a significant reduction of approximately 10% in systolic and diastolic blood pressure (BP), beginning at 3 months.

Stevia is thought to be safe when used at recommended doses.[2]

Garlic   + 2

At least 12 randomized clinical trials have examined the effects of garlic on blood pressure, but only two involved individuals with hypertension.[3] According to these small double-blind, placebo-controlled trials, garlic may mildly reduce blood pressure, approximately 10 mm Hg systolic and 5 mm Hg diastolic, as compared with placebo.[3,4]

For more information, including dosage and safety issues, see the **Garlic** article.

Coenzyme Q_{10} + 2

An 8-week, double-blind, placebo-controlled study of 59 men with hypertension found that adjunctive treatment with 120 mg of CoQ_{10} daily reduced average blood pressure by about 9% as compared with placebo.[5] Significant improvements in systolic and diastolic blood pressure were also seen in a double-blind, crossover study in which 18 hypertensive patients received CoQ_{10}, 100 mg/day, or placebo for 10 weeks, with a 2-week washout period.[6]

In addition, a 12-week, double-blind, placebo-controlled study of 83 individuals with isolated systolic hypertension found that use of CoQ_{10} at a dose of 60 mg daily reduced systolic blood pressure levels by about 10% as compared with placebo.[43]

One animal study suggests that CoQ_{10} might prolong the hypotensive effects of enalapril and nitrendipine without changing their maximal effect.[7]

For more information, including dosage and safety issues, see the **Coenzyme Q_{10}** article.

Minerals: Calcium, Magnesium, Potassium   +2X

There is some evidence that magnesium or potassium supplements might slightly improve blood pressure control.[8-13] However, two large studies found no benefit with potassium supplementation.[14,15]

Observational studies have found associations between calcium deficiency and hypertension.[16,17] However, one double-blind, placebo-controlled study found supplemental calcium ineffective in treating hypertension.[18]

Keep in mind that the use of thiazide or loop diuretics might decrease magnesium levels (as well as, of course, potassium levels); conversely, thiazide diuretics can increase calcium levels.

For more information, including dosage and safety issues, see the **Calcium** and **Magnesium** articles.

Fish Oil   +2X

Evidence from double-blind trials of fish oil for hypertension is mixed, with only slight benefits seen in those trials that had positive results.[19-24] A 6-week, double-blind, placebo-controlled study of 59 overweight men suggests that it may be the DHA (docosahexaenoic acid) in fish oil rather than the EPA (eicosapentaenoic acid) that has an antihypertensive effect.[25]

For more information, including dosage and safety issues, see the **Fish Oil** article.

Vitamin C   +2X

A 30-day, double-blind study of 39 individuals taking antihypertensives found that treatment with 500 mg of vitamin C daily reduced blood pressure by an additional 10%.[26] Lesser benefits were seen in studies of normotensive or borderline hypertensive individuals.[27,28] Other studies found no benefit.[29,30]

For more information, including dosage and safety issues, see the **Vitamin C** article.

Other Proposed Natural Therapies

Several studies have found that **glucomannan,** a dietary fiber derived from the tubers of *Amorphophallus konjac,* may improve high blood pressure.[31-33] Weak evidence suggests that another source of fiber, **chitosan,** may inhibit the expected rise in blood pressure after a high-salt meal.[34]

Highly preliminary evidence suggests that **hibiscus tea,**[35] **blue-green algae,**[36] and **kelp**[37] may possess antihypertensive effects.

Adequate **vitamin D** intake might help prevent the development of hypertension.[38-42]

The herbs astragalus, *Coleus forskohlii,* hawthorn, and maitake and the supplements beta-carotene, flaxseed oil, and taurine are sometimes recommended for hypertension, but there is no real evidence that they work.

Drug Interactions

See the article on each individual supplement for a full description of the interactions summarized here.

Principal Natural Therapies for Hypertension: Interactions with Pharmaceuticals		
Natural Therapy	**Pharmaceutical**	**Interaction**
Calcium	Fluoroquinolones, tetracyclines	Mutual absorption interference
	Levothyroxine	Possible absorption interference
	Thiazides	Potential risk of hypercalcemia
Coenzyme Q_{10}	Warfarin	Possible antagonism of drug action
Combined high-dose calcium and vitamin D	Calcium channel blockers	Possible antagonism of drug action
Fish oil	Anticoagulant and antiplatelet agents	Possible increased risk of bleeding complications
Garlic	Anticoagulant and antiplatelet agents	Possible increased risk of bleeding complications
Magnesium	Amiloride	Possible hypermagnesemia
	Digitoxin, digoxin	Absorption interference
	Fluoroquinolones, tetracyclines	Mutual absorption interference
	Oral hypoglycemics	Possible potentiation of drug action leading to risk of hypoglycemia
Vitamin C	Acetaminophen	Possible increased serum levels of drug
	Anticoagulants	Possible antagonism of drug action
	Iron supplements	Increased iron absorption

Pharmaceuticals Used for Hypertension: Possible Harmful Interactions with Natural Therapies		
Pharmaceutical	**Natural Therapy**	**Interaction**
ACE inhibitors	Arginine, potassium	Possible hyperkalemia
	Dong quai, St. John's wort	Possible increased risk of photosensitivity
	Iron	Mutual absorption interference
	Licorice	Antagonism of drug action
Beta-blockers	Calcium	Absorption interference
Calcium channel blockers	Combined high-dose calcium and vitamin D, grape-fruit juice	Possible antagonism of drug action
Clonidine	Yohimbe	Antagonism of drug action
Loop diuretics	Dong quai, St. John's wort	Possible increased risk of photosensitivity
	Licorice	Potentiation of hypokalemic action of drug
Potassium-sparing diuretics	Arginine	Possible increased risk of hyperkalemia
	Licorice	Antagonism of drug action
	Magnesium	Risk of hypermagnesemia
	White willow	Salicylate content might interfere with spironolactone action
	Zinc	Excessive zinc levels with spironolactone

Pharmaceuticals Used for Hypertension: Possible Harmful Interactions with Natural Therapies—cont'd		
Pharmaceutical	**Natural Therapy**	**Interaction**
Thiazide diuretics	Calcium	Potential risk of hypercalcemia
	Dong quai, St. John's wort	Possible increased risk of photosensivitiy
	Licorice	Potentiation of hypokalemic action of drug

Pharmaceuticals Used for Hypertension: Natural Therapies with Potential Supportive Interactions		
Pharmaceutical	**Natural Therapy**	**Interaction**
ACE inhibitors	Iron	Possible reduction of ACE inhibitor–induced cough
	Zinc	Correction of possible drug-induced depletion
Beta-blockers	Chromium	Increased HDL levels
Beta-blockers, calcium channel blockers, methyldopa, other antihypertensives: hydralazine	Coenzyme Q_{10}	Possible correction of drug-induced relative deficiency
Loop diuretics	Magnesium, potassium, vitamin B_1	Correction of possible drug-induced depletion
Potassium-sparing diuretics	Folate	Correction of possible drug-induced depletion
Thiazide diuretics	Magnesium, potassium, zinc	Correction of possible drug-induced depletion

INFERTILITY (FEMALE)

Principal Proposed Natural Therapies

There are no evidence-based herbs or supplements for female infertility.

Approach to the Patient

Numerous herbs and supplements have been recommended for female infertility, but none have substantial supporting evidence.

Natural treatments your patient may be using include chasteberry, multivitamins, calcium and vitamin D, ashwagandha, beta-carotene, traditional Chinese medicine, and caffeine avoidance. For potential safety risks with the more common of these substances, see the full herb/supplement articles.

Other Proposed Natural Therapies

Chasteberry has been suggested as a fertility treatment because it is known to inhibit prolactin secretion.[1] A double-blind trial of 96 women with fertility disorders compared chasteberry with placebo for 3 months.[2] Although a trend in favor of the verum group was seen, it did not reach statistical significance.

One open study suggests that supplementation with **multivitamins** may improve female fertility.[3]

Preliminary investigation suggests that **vitamin D** and **calcium** supplements may benefit infertility related to polycystic ovary syndrome.[4]

Although ashwagandha, beta-carotene, and traditional Chinese herbal medicine have been suggested as treatments for female infertility, there is no evidence for these approaches.

Drug Interactions

None known.

INFERTILITY (MALE)

Principal Proposed Natural Therapies

Zinc plus folate [+2]   **DHA** [−1]

Vitamin E [+2]   **Vitamin B$_{12}$** [−2]

**Vitamin E plus
vitamin C** [−1]

(Higher numbers indicate stronger evidence; X modifier indicates contradictory results. See page xviii of the Introduction for details of the rating scale.)

Approach to the Patient

Weak evidence suggests that vitamin E, or combined treatment with zinc and folate, might be helpful in asthenospermia.

Although vitamin B$_{12}$ supplements and DHA are often used as natural therapies for male infertility, current evidence suggests that they are not effective. One study failed to find vitamin E plus vitamin C effective.

Other natural treatments your patient may be using include L-arginine, ashwagandha, beta-carotene, L-carnitine or acetyl-L carnitine, coenzyme Q$_{10}$, PABA, *Panax ginseng*, pygeum, selenium, vitamin C, and zinc. For potential safety risks with the more common of these substances, see the full herb/supplement articles.

Caution: Ask about use of licorice: this herb may reduce testosterone levels[1] and thus may exacerbate infertility.

Zinc Plus Folate   +2

A 26-week, double-blind, placebo-controlled trial compared the effects of treatment with zinc (66 mg of zinc sulfate, supplying 15 mg of zinc), folate (5 mg), or zinc plus folate (in the same amounts) against placebo.[13] A total of 108 fertile men and 103 men with impaired fertility ("subfertile") participated in the study. The results indicated that when combined, the two supplements significantly improved the sperm count and the percentage of healthy sperm in the subfertile men; neither supplement alone produced this effect, and there was little effect of the combined therapy on fertile men.

Vitamin E   +2

A double-blind, placebo-controlled study of 87 men with asthenospermia found that treatment with 100 IU of vitamin E daily for up to 6 months resulted in improved sperm activity.[2]

Vitamin E Plus Vitamin C   −1

A 56-day, double-blind study of 31 infertile men found no benefit with combined vitamin C (1000 mg) and vitamin E (800 mg).[3]

For more information, including dosage and safety issues, see the **Vitamin E** article.

DHA   −1

Docosahexaenoic acid (DHA) has been proposed as a treatment for infertility, but a double-blind trial of 28 men with asthenospermia found no benefit.[4]

For more information, including dosage and safety issues, see the **Fish Oil** article.

Vitamin B$_{12}$ −2

Adequate vitamin B$_{12}$ nutritional levels are necessary for normal sperm count and activity, and mild deficiencies of B$_{12}$ are common in individuals over 60 years.[5-8] However, a double-blind study of 375 oligozoospermic men found that vitamin B$_{12}$ supplements produced no benefits.[9] In a questionable post-hoc analysis, B$_{12}$ appeared to be effective in a subgroup of patients who had the lowest sperm counts and motility.

For more information, including dosage and safety issues, see the **Vitamin B$_{12}$** article.

Other Proposed Natural Therapies

Preliminary studies suggested that **vitamin C** may improve sperm count and function[12]; however, as mentioned above, a double-blind study of combined vitamin C and E found no benefit.[3]

One study using an untreated control found indications that *Panax ginseng* might improve sperm count and motility.[14] Uncontrolled studies suggest that L-carnitine or acetyl-L–carnitine may be helpful for improving sperm function as well.[10,11,15-19]

Many other substances have been suggested as treatments for infertility, including the herbs ashwagandha and pygeum as well as the supplements L-arginine, beta-carotene, coenzyme Q$_{10}$, PABA, and selenium. However, the supportive evidence is negligible, and studies on the last three supplements have shown more negative than positive results.

Licorice may reduce testosterone levels in men[1] and thus may exacerbate infertility. Chewing tobacco is a little-known source of licorice.

Drug Interactions

See the article on each individual supplement for a full description of the interactions summarized here.

Principal Natural Therapies for Male Infertility: Interactions with Pharmaceuticals		
Natural Therapy	Pharmaceutical	Interaction
DHA, vitamin E	Anticoagulant and antiplatelet agents	Possible increased risk of bleeding complications

INJURIES (MINOR)

Principal Proposed
Natural Therapies

Proteolytic enzymes   [+2]

Oligomeric proanthocyanidins (OPCs)   [+2]

Horse chestnut/escin   [+2]

Vitamin C and diosmin/hesperidin   [+2]

(Higher numbers indicate stronger evidence; X modifier indicates contradictory results. See page xviii of the Introduction for details of the rating scale.)

Approach to the Patient

There is some evidence that various proteolytic enzyme combinations can improve recovery from minor injuries—presumably through antiinflammatory and antiedematous effects—and they are used for this purpose in Europe.

Another class of treatments with some apparent effectiveness in minor injury includes bioflavonoids and similar substances, which appear to decrease capillary permeability and to strengthen capillary structure. Best investigated for venous insufficiency, they have also been studied in the treatment of minor injuries.

Proteolytic Enzymes   +2

Besides acting in the digestive tract, proteolytic enzymes are absorbed whole and appear to exert systemic effects. A double-blind, placebo-controlled study of 44 individuals with sports-related ankle injuries found that treatment with a proprietary proteolytic enzyme combination called Wobenzym (containing pancreatin, papain, bromelain, trypsin, and chymotrypsin, as well as lipase, amylase, and rutin) resulted in faster healing and reduced the time away from training by about 50%.[1] Three other small double-blind studies, involving a total of about 80 athletes, found that treatment with various proteolytic enzyme combinations significantly sped healing of bruises and other mild athletic injuries as compared with placebo.[2-4] In addition, a double-blind trial of 100 individuals given a subcutaneous injection of their own blood to simulate bruising found that treatment with a proteolytic enzyme combination significantly speeded hematoma resolution.[5]

A double-blind, placebo-controlled trial involving 71 individuals with finger fractures found that treatment with trypsin-chymotrypsin significantly improved recovery rate.[6]

In a controlled study, 74 boxers with facial and/or upper-body bruises were given bromelain until all signs of bruising had disappeared[7]; another 72 boxers were given placebo. Fifty-eight of the group taking bromelain lost all signs of bruising within 4 days, compared with only 10 of the group taking placebo.

Additional evidence for the effectiveness of proteolytic enzymes in healing injuries comes from studies involving surgery (see the **Surgery Support** article).

For more information, including dosage and safety issues, see the **Proteolytic Enzymes** and **Bromelain** articles.

Oligomeric Proanthocyanidins (OPCs)   +2

Oligomeric proanthocyanidins (OPCs), bioflavonoid-like substances found in grape seed and maritime pine bark, may be helpful for injuries as well.

A 10-day, double-blind, placebo-controlled study enrolling 50 participants found that OPCs improved the rate at which edema disappeared following sports injuries.[8] OPCs have also been found helpful following surgery.

For more information, including dosage and safety issues, see the **OPCs** article.

Horse Chestnut/Escin   +2

Escin is the presumed active ingredient in horse chestnut. A double-blind, placebo-controlled trial of 70 individuals found that topical 2% escin gel reduces bruise tenderness.[9]

For more information, including dosage and safety issues, see the **Horse Chestnut** article.

Vitamin C and Diosmin/Hesperidin   +2

A poorly reported, double-blind trial of 40 college football players suggests that a combination of vitamin C and the citrus bioflavonoids diosmin and hesperidin taken before practice can reduce the severity of athletic injuries.[10]

For more information, including dosage and safety issues, see the **Vitamin C** and **Diosmin/Hesperidin** articles.

Drug Interactions

See the article on each individual supplement for a full description of the interactions summarized here.

Principal Natural Therapies for Minor Injuries: Interactions with Pharmaceuticals		
Natural Therapy	Pharmaceutical	Interaction
Bioflavonoids, bromelain, horse chestnut, OPCs, proteolytic enzymes	Anticoagulant and antiplatelet agents	Possible increased risk of bleeding complications

Pharmaceuticals Used for Minor Injuries: Possible Harmful Interactions with Natural Therapies		
Pharmaceutical	Natural Therapy	Interaction
NSAIDs	Dong quai, St. John's wort	Possible increased risk of photosensitivity
	Garlic, ginkgo, high-dose vitamin E, policosanol, others	Possible increased risk of bleeding complications
	Feverfew	Possible increased risk of gastritis
	White willow	Additional salicylates may increase risk of all side effects
	Potassium citrate	Possible decreased serum levels of salicylates

INSOMNIA

Principal Proposed Natural Therapies

Valerian [+3]

Melatonin [+3X]

(Higher numbers indicate stronger evidence; X modifier indicates contradictory results. See page xviii of the Introduction for details of the rating scale.)

Approach to the Patient

Preliminary evidence suggests that the herb valerian *(Valeriana officinalis)* may be an effective sleep aid, although whether it is best used for ongoing sleep problems or occasional insomnia remains unclear.

Melatonin is best established as a treatment for jet lag but may be useful for other forms of insomnia as well. One potential use of melatonin that may interest your patients involves its possible utility as an aid in falling asleep at a reasonable hour on Sunday night after staying up late the two nights before.

Other natural treatments your patient may be using include ashwagandha, chamomile, He shou wu, hops, 5-hydroxytryptophan, kava, lady's slipper, lemon balm, passion flower, skullcap, and St. John's wort. For potential safety risks with the more common of these substances, see the full herb/supplement articles.

Caution: Some of these treatments may potentiate sedative drugs.

Valerian +3

Although valerian appears to be an effective sleep aid, studies conflict on whether it produces immediate benefits or requires several weeks to act.

In the largest trial of valerian for insomnia, 121 patients with a history of significant insomnia were enrolled in a 28-day, placebo-controlled, double-blind trial.[1] Significant improvements in sleep quality were seen at 28 but not at 14 days. The study authors interpreted the results to indicate that valerian is most appropriately used as a long-term treatment for poor sleep rather than for occasional insomnia. However, other studies found more immediate benefits.[2-6]

A 28-day, double-blind trial of 75 individuals with various forms of insomnia compared valerian (600 mg qhs) with oxazepam (10 mg qhs).[7] The results showed no differences in efficacy.

Valerian–lemon balm and valerian-hops combinations have also been found effective in double-blind trials.[8-10]

For more information, including dosage and safety issues, see the **Valerian** article.

Melatonin +3X

The best evidence for efficacy of melatonin is in the treatment of jet lag. Most, but not all, studies of melatonin treatment for this purpose have returned positive results.

In a double-blind, placebo-controlled randomized trial, 320 volunteers who had flights over six to eight time zones received placebo or melatonin in a 0.5-mg fast-release, 5-mg fast-release, or 2-mg controlled-release formulation, once daily at bedtime for 4 days after the flight.[11] The 5-mg dose improved self-rated sleep quality, shortened sleep latency, and reduced fatigue and daytime sleepiness, all significantly. The fast-release doses appeared to be more effective than the slow-release melatonin formulation.

Similar benefits were seen in most, but not all, other studies of melatonin for jet lag.[12-18,35,36] Melatonin appears to be less effective than zolpidem[18] but may be equally effective as zopiclone.[35]

Melatonin may also be helpful for other forms of insomnia, although the evidence is weak or inconsistent in some cases.

Surprisingly, studies of melatonin for the treatment of insomnia related to shift work have yielded relatively unimpressive results.[30-32,37,38]

Other small trials have examined the effects of melatonin in insomnia in the older population, yielding generally positive results.[37,39-41] However, the results have been inconsistent regarding which part of the sleep cycle benefited from treatment.

There is some evidence that melatonin may be beneficial for children with sleep-onset insomnia.[19,20]

Individuals who frequently stay up late on Friday and Saturday nights may find it difficult to fall asleep at a reasonable hour on Sunday. A small double-blind, placebo-controlled trial found that this delayed sleep pattern caused a phase delay in endogenous melatonin secretion and that use of melatonin 5.5 hours before the desired Sunday bedtime improved sleep latency.[21]

In one double-blind, placebo-controlled trial, 34 individuals who regularly used benzodiazepine hypnotics for sleep found that melatonin at a dose of 2 mg nightly (controlled-release formulation) assisted benzodiazepine discontinuation.[22]

Some individuals find it impossible to fall asleep until early morning, a condition called delayed sleep phase syndrome (DSPS). Melatonin may be beneficial for this syndrome.[23]

Small controlled studies have found good results with 2 to 3 mg of controlled-release melatonin in intensive care unit (ICU) patients[25] and schizophrenic patients with disturbed sleep patterns.[26] Evidence from a small double-blind trial in children suggests that quick-release melatonin helps in falling asleep, and slow-release melatonin aids in staying asleep.[33]

For more information, including dosage and safety issues, see the **Melatonin** article.

Other Proposed Natural Therapies

Kava, primarily used for anxiety, is also sometimes recommended for insomnia. However, there is no direct evidence that it is helpful in insomnia.

Based on analogous use to standard antidepressants, **St. John's wort** is sometimes tried for the treatment of insomnia. A double-blind trial of 12 healthy volunteers found no sleep-promoting benefit, but this says little about its effectiveness in individuals with sleep problems.[34]

Other herbs and supplements sometimes recommended include ashwagandha, chamomile, He shou wu, hops, 5-hydroxytryptophan, lady's slipper, lemon balm, passionflower, and skullcap.

Drug Interactions

See the article on each individual supplement for a full description of the interactions summarized here.

Principal Natural Therapy for Insomnia: Interaction with Pharmaceuticals		
Natural Therapy	Pharmaceutical	Interaction
Kava, valerian	Sedatives	Possible potentiation of sedation

Pharmaceuticals Used for Insomnia: Possible Harmful Interactions with Natural Therapies		
Pharmaceutical	Natural Therapy	Interaction
Benzodiazepines	Kava, valerian, other sedative herbs	Possible potentiation of sedative effects
Pyrazolopyrimidines	5-HTP, SAMe, St. John's wort	Possible increased risk of hallucinations
SSRIs	5-HTP, SAMe, St. John's wort	Possible risk of serotonin syndrome
Tricyclic antidepressants	5-HTP, SAMe, St. John's wort	Possible risk of serotonin syndrome
	Dong quai, St. John's wort	Possible increased risk of photosensitivity

Pharmaceuticals Used for Insomnia: Natural Therapies with Potential Supportive Interactions

Pharmaceutical	Natural Therapy	Interaction
Benzodiazepines	Melatonin	Possible facilitation of drug discontinuation
Tricyclic antidepressants	Coenzyme Q_{10}	Possible correction of drug-induced relative deficiency

INTERMITTENT CLAUDICATION

Principal Proposed Natural Therapies

Ginkgo   [+3]   **Mesoglycans**   [+3]

Inositol   **Policosanol**   [+2]
hexaniacinate   [+3]

L-Carnitine   [+3]

(Higher numbers indicate stronger evidence; X modifier indicates contradictory results. See page xviii of the Introduction for details of the rating scale.)

Approach to the Patient

Preliminary evidence suggests that ginkgo, inositol hexaniacinate, carnitine, mesoglycans, and policosanol may be helpful for intermittent claudication. Note, however, that ginkgo, policosanol, and mesoglycans may increase risk of bleeding complications if combined with anticoagulants or antiplatelet agents.

Other natural treatments your patient may be using include arginine and antioxidants. For potential safety risks with arginine as well as specific antioxidants, see the full herb/supplement articles.

Ginkgo   +3

A 2000 metaanalysis of studies of ginkgo in intermittent claudication evaluated eight double-blind, placebo-controlled trials.[1] In aggregate, the results found a modest but statistically significant improvement in pain-free walking distance.

For example, a 24-week, double-blind, placebo-controlled study that enrolled 111 patients found a significant improvement in pain-free walking distance with ginkgo compared with placebo.[2] Similar improvements were also seen in a double-blind, placebo-controlled trial of 60 individuals who had achieved maximum benefit from physical therapy modalities.[3]

A 24-week, multicenter, double-blind, placebo-controlled, dose-comparison study of 74 individuals with intermittent claudication reported that ginkgo at a dose of 120 mg twice daily was more effective than 60 mg twice daily.[4]

For more information, including dosage and safety issues, see the **Ginkgo** article.

Inositol Hexaniacinate   + 3

Double-blind studies involving a total of about 300 individuals have found that inositol hexaniacinate (a form of niacin) can improve walking distance for individuals with intermittent claudication.[5-8] For example, in a 3-month double-blind trial, 100 individuals with intermittent claudication were given either placebo or 4 g of inositol hexaniacinate daily.[5] Over the study period, the treated participants significantly improved in time and total steps to claudication.

For more information, including dosage and safety issues, see the **Vitamin B₃** article.

L-Carnitine   + 3

A 12-month, double-blind, placebo-controlled trial of 485 patients with intermittent claudication found that propionyl-L-carnitine at a dose of 1 g twice daily produced a significant (44%) improvement in maximal walking distance in those with initial maximal walking distance less than or equal to 250 m; however, no response was seen in those with milder disease.[9] Quality of life improvements were also noted. Benefits were

seen in most but not all other studies using L-carnitine or
L-propionylcarnitine,[10-20] including one that observed 245
individuals.[10]

Carnitine is thought to work in intermittent claudication by improving muscle energy utilization.

For more information, including dosage and safety issues, see
the **Carnitine** article.

Mesoglycans   +3

A 20-week, double-blind, placebo-controlled trial that enrolled
242 individuals evaluated the effects of mesoglycans (glycosaminoglycans extracted from pig intestines that have some
anticoagulant effects) in intermittent claudication.[25] Significantly more participants in the mesoglycan group responded to
treatment (response was defined as a greater than 50% improvement in walking distance) than in the placebo group.

Policosanol   +2

A 2-year, double-blind, placebo-controlled study of 56 individuals found that treatment with policosanol (10 mg twice daily)
improved walking distance by more than 50% at 6 months, and
the benefits increased over the course of the study.[21] Similar results were seen in a 6-month, double-blind, placebo-controlled
study of 62 individuals.[22]

For more information, including dosage and safety issues, see
the **Policosanol** article.

Other Proposed
Natural Therapies

Preliminary evidence suggests that **arginine,** a stimulator of va-
sodilating nitric oxide (NO), may increase walking distance in
intermittent claudication.[23]

A large, double-blind, placebo-controlled, trial found no benefit from **vitamin E** (50 mg daily), **beta-carotene** (20 mg daily), or a combination of the two.[24]

Drug Interactions

See the article on each individual supplement for a full description of the interactions summarized here.

Principal Natural Therapies for Intermittent Claudication: Interactions with Pharmaceuticals		
Natural Therapy	Pharmaceutical	Interaction
Ginkgo, mesoglycans	Anticoagulant and antiplatelet agents	Possible increased risk of bleeding complications

Pharmaceuticals Used for Intermittent Claudication: Interactions with Pharmaceuticals		
Pharmaceutical	Natural Therapy	Interaction
Anticoagulant and antiplatelet agents	Garlic, ginkgo, high-dose vitamin E, mesoglycans, policosanol, many others	Possible increased risk of bleeding complications

INTERSTITIAL CYSTITIS

Principal Proposed Natural Therapy

Arginine [−1]

(Higher numbers indicate stronger evidence; X modifier indicates contradictory results. See page xviii of the Introduction for details of the rating scale.)

Approach to the Patient

Because conventional treatment for interstitial cystitis (IC) is often less than satisfactory, patients may actively research alternative treatments. The amino acid arginine has been widely recommended, but there is as yet no meaningful evidence that it is effective.

Other natural treatments your patient may be using include mesoglycan or other glycosaminoglycan supplements and quercetin.

Arginine   −1

Arginine promotes formation of nitric oxide (NO).[1-3] This is the basis for its use in cardiovascular disease and for investigations of its possible utility in IC.

In a 3-month, double-blind, trial of 53 individuals with IC, 27 were given 1500 mg of arginine daily and 26 were given placebo[4]; 21 completed the arginine arm, and 25 completed the placebo arm of the study. Although consistent trends toward superior symptomatic results were seen in the verum group as compared with the placebo group, intention-to-treat (ITT) analysis showed no statistically significant difference in primary outcome measures. A smaller double-blind trial with 16 participants also failed to find evidence of benefit,[5] and one experimental study found no change in bladder NO.[6]

For more information, including dosage and safety issues, see the **Arginine** article.

Other Proposed Natural Therapies

A small, double-blind, placebo-controlled trial found that a supplement containing **quercetin** reduced symptoms of interstitial cystitis.[7]

Some investigations suggest that the surface layer of the bladder in IC is deficient in **glycosaminoglycans (GAGs).**[8] This might lead to inflammation and also expose proteins that initiate autoimmune reactions. However, there is no direct evidence as yet that supplemental GAGs (e.g., as mesoglycans) are helpful for IC.

Drug Interactions

See the article on each individual supplement for a full description of the interactions summarized here.

Principal Natural Therapy for Interstitial Cystitis: Interactions with Pharmaceuticals		
Natural Therapy	Pharmaceutical	Interaction
Arginine	Agents causing gastric irritation	Possible increased risk of gastritis or ulceration
	Potassium-sparing diuretics	Possible increased risk of hyperkalemia

Pharmaceuticals Used for Interstitial Cystitis: Possible Harmful Interactions with Natural Therapies

Pharmaceutical	Natural Therapy	Interaction
Cetirizine, hydroxyzine	Kava, valerian, other sedative herbs	Possible increased sedation
NSAIDs	Dong quai, St. John's wort	Possible increased risk of photosensitivity
	Feverfew	Possible increased risk of gastritis
	Garlic, ginkgo, high-dose vitamin E, policosanol, others	Possible increased risk of bleeding complications
	Potassium citrate	Possible decreased serum levels of salicylates
	White willow	Additional salicylates may increase risk of all side effects

Pharmaceuticals Used for Interstitial Cystitis: Natural Therapies with Potential Supportive Interactions

Pharmaceutical	Natural Therapy	Interaction
NSAIDs	Cayenne, colostrum, licorice	Possible cytoprotection
	Folate, vitamin C	Correction of possible drug-induced deficiency

IRRITABLE BOWEL SYNDROME (IBS)

Principal Proposed Natural Therapies

Peppermint oil [+3X]   **Flaxseed** [+2]

Probiotics (Lactobacillus acidophilus, L. plantarum) [+2]

(Higher numbers indicate stronger evidence; X modifier indicates contradictory results. See page xviii of the Introduction for details of the rating scale.)

Approach to the Patient

Preliminary evidence suggests that peppermint oil, probiotics, and flaxseed may improve IBS symptoms.

Other natural treatments your patient may be using include *Coleus forskohlii*, glutamine, and slippery elm. For potential safety risks with the more common of these substances, see the full herb/supplement articles.

Peppermint Oil   +3X

Menthol, the presumed primary active ingredient in peppermint oil, possesses antispasmodic properties.[1-4]

Several double-blind studies, involving a total of about 240 individuals with irritable bowel syndrome, found evidence that peppermint provides relief from crampy abdominal pain.[5-7,11] In the largest of these, 110 individuals with IBS were given either enteric-coated peppermint oil (187 mg) or placebo three or four times daily, 15 to 30 minutes before meals, for 4 weeks.[4,11] The results in the 101 individuals who completed the trial showed significant improvements in abdominal pain, distention, stool frequency, borborygmi, and flatulence.

However, smaller double-blind studies involving a total of more than 90 people failed to find significant improvement in symptoms as compared with placebo.[8-10]

A metaanalysis concluded that while clinical trials suggest efficacy, the methodologic quality of those trials was, on average, poor, preventing firm conclusions from being drawn.[16]

For more information, including dosage and safety issues, see the **Peppermint** article.

Probiotics (*acidophilus*, other *Lactobacillus* spp.)   +2

The evidence regarding use of probiotics for irritable bowel syndrome is mixed. In a 4-week, double-blind, placebo-controlled trial of 60 individuals with IBS, treatment with *Lactobacillus plantarum* reduced intestinal gas significantly, and the benefits persisted for 1 year after treatment was stopped.[13] In another 4-week, double-blind trial, 40 individuals with IBS also received either *L. plantarum* or placebo.[17] The results showed improvements in pain as well as in overall symptom score.

A small 6-week trial using *L. acidophilus* also found suggestions of benefit.[14] However, in a double-blind, placebo-controlled, crossover study of 24 individuals with IBS, use of *Lactobacillus GG* failed to produce any significant benefit as compared with placebo.[12]

For more information, including dosage and safety issues, see the **Probiotics** article.

Flaxseed   +2

In a double-blind study, 55 individuals with chronic constipation caused by IBS received either ground flaxseed or psyllium seed daily for 3 months.[15] Those taking flaxseed had significantly fewer problems with constipation, abdominal pain, and bloating than those taking psyllium.

For more information, including dosage and safety issues, see the **Flaxseed** article.

Other Proposed Natural Therapies

Coleus forskohlii, glutamine supplements, and slippery elm are sometimes recommended for IBS, but there is no clinical evidence supporting their use in this condition.

Drug Interactions

See the article on each individual supplement for a full description of the interactions summarized here.

Pharmaceuticals Used for Irritable Bowel Syndrome: Possible Harmful Interactions with Natural Therapies		
Pharmaceutical	**Natural Therapy**	**Interaction**
Anxiolytics and sedatives	Kava, lemon balm, valerian, many others	Possible potentiation
	Grapefruit juice	Possible increased or decreased serum levels of drug

MACULAR DEGENERATION

Zinc and zinc plus antioxidant supplements   [+3X]

Antioxidant supplements alone   [−2X]

(Higher numbers indicate stronger evidence; X modifier indicates contradictory results. See page xviii of the Introduction for details of the rating scale.)

Approach to the Patient

Mixed evidence suggests that high-dose zinc supplementation might be helpful for some forms of age-related macular degeneration (ARMD), especially in combination with antioxidant therapies. However, zinc toxicity (primarily caused by copper depletion) is a concern at the recommended dosage. This can be corrected by use of copper supplements at 1 to 3 mg daily.

Other natural treatments your patient may be using include lutein and other carotenoids.

Caution: Patients may need to be advised not to attempt to self-treat exudative macular degeneration.

Zinc and Zinc Plus Antioxidants   + 3 X

A double-blind, placebo-controlled trial evaluated the effects of antioxidants and zinc on the progression of macular degeneration in 3640 individuals with extensive small drusen, intermediate drusen, large drusen, noncentral geographic atrophy, pigment abnormalities in one or both eyes, or advanced ARMD in one eye.[13] Participants were randomly assigned to receive one of the following: antioxidants (vitamin C 500 mg, vitamin E 400 IU, beta-carotene 15 mg), zinc (80 mg), and copper (2 mg); antioxidants plus zinc; or placebo. (Copper was administered along with zinc to prevent zinc-induced copper deficiency.) The results suggest that zinc alone or antioxidants plus zinc can significantly slow the progression of the disease. A previous double-blind, placebo-controlled study of 151 individuals with ARMD observed for 1 to 2 years found that zinc supplements at a dose of 80 mg elemental zinc daily helped preserve vision.[1] However, a 2-year, double-blind study of 112 individuals given the same dose found no reduction in development of macular degeneration in the second eye among individuals with exudative ARMD in one eye.[2]

Note: At these dosage levels, zinc can be toxic. Concurrent administration of copper is essential. For more information, including dosage and safety issues, see the **Zinc** article.

Antioxidant Supplements Alone   − 2 X

Observational studies have found associations between higher dietary intake of vitamin C, vitamin E, carotenes, and wine (a source of numerous antioxidant flavonoids) and decreased incidence of macular degeneration.[3-7] However, most trials of antioxidant supplements have not been encouraging.

A small, 18-month, double-blind, placebo-controlled study found that a daily supplement containing 750 mg of vitamin C, 200 IU of vitamin E, 50 μg of selenium, and 20,000 IU of beta-carotene (along with other ingredients) stabilized, but did not improve, atrophic macular degeneration.[8] Another small, double-blind trial suggests benefit with the flavonoid-rich herb ginkgo *(Ginkgo biloba)*.[9] However, in the much larger double-blind trial described in the previous section, antioxidants alone were not strongly associated with improvement.[13] For more information, including dosage and safety issues, see the article on each individual supplement.

Other Proposed Natural Therapies

In addition to its antioxidant properties, the carotenoid **lutein** is a macular pigment and may help prevent macular degeneration by screening out damaging wavelengths of light.[10,11]

However, one observational study found little association between macular degeneration and intake of lutein (or zeathanthin).[12]

Drug Interactions

See the article on each individual supplement for a full description of the interactions summarized here.

Principal Natural Therapies for Macular Degeneration: Interactions with Pharmaceuticals		
Natural Therapy	**Pharmaceutical**	**Interaction**
Ginkgo, vitamin E	Anticoagulant and antiplatelet agents	Possible increased risk of bleeding complications
Vitamin C	Acetaminophen	Possible increased serum levels of drug
	Anticoagulants	Possible antagonism of drug action
	Iron supplements	Increased iron absorption
Zinc	Amiloride	Possible elevated serum zinc
	Fluoroquinolones, pencillamine, tetracyclines	Mutual absorption interference

MENOPAUSAL SYNDROME

Principal Proposed Natural Therapies

Isoflavone sources

  Soy [+3X]

  Red clover [−1]

Progesterone cream [+3]

Estriol [+4]

Black cohosh [+2X]

Ginseng [−2]

Vitamin E [−1]

Dong quai [−1]

(Higher numbers indicate stronger evidence; X modifier indicates contradictory results. See page xviii of the Introduction for details of the rating scale.)

Approach to the Patient

This article primarily addresses treatments for menopausal symptoms. See the **Osteoporosis** article for natural treatments relating to this complication of menopause.

Increasing evidence suggests that soy isoflavones may reduce vasomotor symptoms of menopause and possibly improve other symptoms as well. It is generally thought that the isoflavones in soy are responsible for these effects, but study results are inconsistent, and similar isoflavones from red clover have not been found effective.

The weak estrogen estriol, although undoubtedly effective for menopausal symptoms, has been marketed with misleading claims that it offers a better safety profile than other estrogens.

The herb black cohosh is not estrogenic, and only weak evidence suggests it might offer symptomatic benefits.

Ginseng (*Panax* spp.), dong quai, and vitamin E do not appear to be effective for menopausal symptoms.

Other natural treatments your patient may be using include alfalfa, bioflavonoids, chasteberry, essential fatty acids, flaxseed, gamma-oryzanol, licorice, St. John's wort, suma, and vitamin C. For potential safety risks with the more common of these substances, see the full herb/supplement articles.

Isoflavone Sources: Soy +3X, Red Clover −1

According to most but not all studies, soy protein (presumably because of its isoflavone content) can reduce vasomotor and other symptoms of menopause.[1,2,4,5,37]

For example, a 12-week, double-blind, placebo-controlled study of 104 women found that soy protein (60 g daily) provided significant relief from vasomotor symptoms as compared with placebo (milk protein).[1] Similarly, a 12-week study that enrolled 114 women found evidence of benefit for hot flashes and vaginal dryness but not for menopausal symptoms as a whole.[2] Reductions in hot flashes were seen in two 6-week, double-blind trials as well.[3,4]

However, one study did not find benefit. This 24-week, double-blind study of 69 women found no benefit with either isoflavone-rich or isoflavone-poor soy.[5] In another possibly relevant double-blind, placebo-controlled trial, use of soy in 123 breast cancer survivors failed to reduce vasomotor symptoms.[6]

In addition, isoflavones from red clover have not shown benefit in studies on menopausal symptoms. A 28-week, double-blind, placebo-controlled, crossover trial of 51 postmenopausal women found no reduction in hot flashes among those given 40 mg daily of red clover isoflavones,[7] nor were benefits seen in another double-blind, placebo-controlled trial involving 37 women given red clover isoflavones at a dose of either 40 mg or 160 mg daily.[8]

For more information, including dosage and safety issues, see the **Isoflavones** article.

Progesterone Cream   + 3

A 1-year, double-blind trial of 102 women given either progesterone cream (providing 20 mg progesterone daily) or placebo cream, along with calcium and multivitamins, found a significant reduction in vasomotor symptoms in the treated group.[9]

For more information, including dosage and safety issues, see the **Progesterone Cream** article.

Estriol   + 4

Controlled and double-blind trials have found oral or vaginal estriol effective for reducing many menopausal symptoms,[10-18] and estriol may cause less vaginal bleeding than other forms of estrogen.[10,11] However, evidence from controlled studies indicates that oral estriol presents risks comparable to those with other forms of estrogen.[10,19-22]

For more information, including dosage and safety issues, see the **Estriol** article.

Black Cohosh   + 2 X

A 12-week, double-blind, placebo-controlled trial of 80 patients at one gynecologic practice compared the effects of black cohosh, conjugated estrogens (0.625 mg), and placebo over a period of 12 weeks.[23] Black cohosh produced significantly greater improvements than placebo in the Kupperman index, the Hamilton Anxiety scale, and the degree of proliferation of the vaginal epithelium. Estrogen proved equivalent to placebo, a result that is somewhat hard to believe.

Further concerns about the validity of this trial come from growing evidence that black cohosh is not estrogenic and does not affect vaginal epithelium.[24-28] In addition, a 2-month, double-blind trial of 85 breast cancer survivors found that use of black cohosh did not reduce menopausal symptoms.[29]

Several open studies found that when black cohosh was given to women, their menopausal symptoms decreased.[27,30-32] These studies are widely cited in favor of black cohosh as a treatment for menopause; however, considering that hot flashes have been reported to improve by an average of 50% in the placebo arm of numerous placebo-controlled trials,[33] these studies indicate little.

Thus on balance the evidence for black cohosh as a treatment for menopausal symptoms is very weak.

For more information, including dosage and safety issues, see the **Black Cohosh** article.

Ginseng   − 2

Although ginseng is sometimes recommended for menopausal symptoms, a double-blind, placebo-controlled study of 384 postmenopausal women evaluated ginseng at a dose of 200 mg daily for 16 weeks.[34] No intergroup differences in primary end points were observed, and there were no estrogenic effects.

For more information, including dosage and safety issues, see the **Ginseng** article.

Vitamin E   − 1

Although vitamin E is often recommended for menopausal hot flashes, a 9-week, double-blind, placebo-controlled trial of 104 women with hot flashes associated with breast cancer treatment found marginal benefits at best.[35]

For more information, including dosage and safety issues, see the **Vitamin E** article.

Dong Quai   −1

A 12-week study compared the effects of dong quai to placebo in 71 postmenopausal women.[36] The results showed no statistically significant differences between groups in endometrial thickness, vaginal maturation index, number of vasomotor flushes, or the Kupperman index.

For more information, including dosage and safety issues, see the **Dong Quai** article.

Other Proposed Natural Therapies

Other natural treatments considered for menopause symptoms—because of phytoestrogen content or for other reasons—include alfalfa, bioflavonoids, chasteberry, essential fatty acids, flaxseed, gamma-oryzanol, licorice, St. John's wort, suma, and vitamin C. However, as yet no substantive clinical evidence supports these treatments.

Drug Interactions

See the article on each individual supplement for a full description of the interactions summarized here.

Principal Natural Therapies for Menopausal Syndrome: Interactions with Pharmaceuticals		
Natural Therapy	**Pharmaceutical**	**Interaction**
Soy products	Thyroid hormone	Impaired action/absorption
Panax ginseng	Monoamine oxidase inhibitor (MAOI)	Multiple symptoms (possibly because of ginseng contamination with caffeine)
	Hypoglycemic agents	Possible hypoglycemia
	Warfarin	Possible interference with action
Vitamin E	Antiplatelet and anticoagulant agents	Possible increased risk of bleeding complications
Dong quai	Photosensitizing agents	Possible increased photosensitization
	Anticoagulants and antiplatelet agents	Possible increased risk of bleeding complications
Ipriflavone	Cytochrome P-450–metabolized drugs: theophylline, caffeine, theobromine, phenytoin, sodium warfarin, tolbutamide, phenacetin, nifedipine	Increased drug metabolism
Ipriflavone	Estrogens	Possible increased uterotropic effects

Pharmaceutical Used for Menopausal Syndrome: Possible Harmful Interaction with Natural Therapies		
Pharmaceutical	Natural Therapy	Interaction
Estrogen	Androstenedione, boron, grapefruit juice	Possible increase of estrogen

Pharmaceuticals Used for Menopausal Syndrome: Natural Therapies with Potential Supportive Interactions		
Pharmaceutical	Natural Therapy	Interaction
Estrogen	Calcium, vitamin D	Enhanced bone-sparing effect
Estrogen	Magnesium	Possible correction of drug-induced nutrient deficiency

MIGRAINE HEADACHES

Principal Proposed Natural Therapies

Feverfew [+2X]

Butterbur [+2]

5-Hydroxytryp-tophan [+2X]

Magnesium [+2X]

Vitamin B$_2$ (riboflavin) [+2]

Fish oil [−2]

(Higher numbers indicate stronger evidence; X modifier indicates contradictory results. See page xviii of the Introduction for details of the rating scale.)

Approach to the Patient

Preliminary evidence suggests that feverfew leaf, butterbur, 5-hydroxytryptophan, magnesium, and vitamin B$_2$ may help prevent migraine headaches. Fish oil appears to be ineffective, according to the largest and most recent trial.

Your patients may not realize that no herbs or supplements have been evaluated for the treatment of acute migraines.

Other natural treatments your patient may be using include calcium, chromium, folate, ginger, and vitamin C. For potential safety risks with the more common of these substances, see the full herb/supplement article.

Feverfew   +2X

Three small, double-blind studies using whole feverfew leaf for migraine prophylaxis returned positive results[1-3]; a trial using an alcohol extract of feverfew found no benefit,[4] and a study using a CO_2 extract found benefits only in a predefined subgroup with more severe symptoms.[21]

The first trial used feverfew leaf from British sources with a parthenolide content of 0.66%.[1] In this 8-month crossover study of 59 patients, treatment with 82 mg feverfew daily was associated with a 24% reduction in the number of migraines, a significant decrease in nausea and vomiting during attacks, and a trend toward reduced severity of headache pain.

In the second study, all 57 migraine patients were initially treated with 50 mg twice daily of an Israeli whole feverfew leaf containing 0.2% parthenolide for 2 months, followed by a 2-month, double-blind, crossover trial.[2] The results showed significant improvement in intensity of headache pain, nausea, vomiting, and photophobia and light sensitivity. Unfortunately, the study did not report whether there was an effect on migraine frequency.

Benefits were also seen in a poorly designed, double-blind, placebo-controlled trial of 17 individuals.[3]

In contrast to these positive results, a randomized, double-blind, placebo-controlled trial of 50 individuals given an alcohol extract of feverfew standardized to its parthenolide content found no benefit.[4] This negative outcome, in conjunction with the positive results of the low-parthenolide study mentioned above, suggests that the identification of parthenolide as the active principle was premature.

In addition, an unpublished, double-blind, placebo-controlled study of 147 individuals found equivocal evidence for a proprietary CO_2 feverfew extract called Mig-99.[5] The primary outcome measure was reduction of migraine incidence during the final 4-week period of the 12-week treatment phase as compared with migraine incidence during a 4-week baseline interval. Three doses of feverfew extract were compared with placebo. No statistically significant differences were seen in the feverfew group as a whole as compared with placebo. However, in a predefined subgroup of 47 individuals with four or more migraines at baseline, the two higher doses of feverfew significantly reduced the number of migraine attacks.

For more information, including dosage and safety issues, see the **Feverfew** article.

Butterbur   + 2

A double-blind, placebo-controlled study involving 60 men and women with a history of at least three migraines per month evaluated the effectiveness of butterbur as a migraine prophylactic.[6] After a 4-week washout period, participants were given either 50 mg of butterbur extract or placebo twice daily for 3 months. The results were positive: both the number of migraine attacks and the total number of days of migraine pain were significantly reduced in the treatment group as compared with the placebo group. Three out of four individuals taking butterbur reported improvement, as compared with only one out of four in the placebo group. No significant side effects were noted.

For more information, including dosage and safety issues, see the **Butterbur** article.

5-Hydroxytryptophan   + 2X

5-HTP may be effective for migraine prophylaxis if taken in sufficient doses. In a 6-month trial that evaluated 85 individuals, prophylactic 5-HTP (600 mg/day) proved equally effective to methysergide in reducing the intensity and duration of migraine attacks.[7] Equal benefits were also seen in a double-blind trial of 66 individuals comparing 5-HTP (400 mg/day) to pizotifen.[8]

However, in a double-blind trial that enrolled 39 individuals, 5-HTP (up to 300 mg/day) was less effective than propranolol.[9] In addition, a double-blind, placebo-controlled, crossover trial in 27 children with migraines failed to demonstrate any benefit.[10]

Other studies that are sometimes quoted as evidence that 5-HTP is effective for migraines actually enrolled adults or children with many different types of headaches, including migraines.[11-13]

For more information, including dosage and safety issues, see the **5-Hydroxytryptophan** article.

Magnesium   +2X

Three small double-blind trials found magnesium effective for prevention of migraines,[14-16] including a 12-week study of 81 individuals with recurrent migraines that found a 41.6% decrease in migraine frequency in the treated group.[14] Another trial failed to demonstrate benefit, but it used unusually strict criteria for evaluating results.[17]

For more information, including dosage and safety issues, see the **Magnesium** article.

Vitamin B$_2$ (Riboflavin)   +2

A 3-month, double-blind, placebo-controlled study of 55 patients with migraines found that vitamin B$_2$, 400 mg/day, significantly reduced the frequency and duration of migraine attacks.[18]

For more information, including dosage and safety issues, see the **Vitamin B$_2$** article.

Fish Oil   −2

A 16-week, double-blind, placebo-controlled study of 167 individuals with recurrent migraine headaches found that fish oil did not significantly reduce headache frequency or severity.[22] These results failed to confirm previous, much smaller trials that did find benefit.[19,20]

Other Proposed Natural Therapies

Although they are sometimes recommended, no evidence supports the use of calcium, chromium, folate, ginger, or vitamin C for migraines.

Drug Interactions

See the article on each individual supplement for a full description of the interactions summarized here.

Principal Natural Therapies for Migraine Headaches: Interactions with Pharmaceuticals		
Natural Therapy	**Pharmaceutical**	**Interaction**
5-HTP	Selective serotonin reuptake inhibitors (SSRIs), other serotonergic drugs	Possible risk of serotonin syndrome
	Levodopa-carbidopa	Possible increased risk of scleroderma-like syndrome
Feverfew	Anticoagulant and antiplatelet agents	Possible increased risk of bleeding complications
	Nonsteroidal anti-inflammatory drugs (NSAIDs)	Possible increased risk of gastrointestinal side effects
Magnesium	Amiloride	Possible hypermagnesemia
	Digitoxin, digoxin	Absorption interference
	Fluoroquinolones, tetracyclines	Mutual absorption interference
	Oral hypoglycemics	Possible potentiation of drug action leading to risk of hypoglycemia

Pharmaceuticals Used for Migraine Headaches: Possible Harmful Interactions with Natural Therapies

Pharmaceutical	Natural Therapy	Interaction
Beta-blockers	Calcium	Absorption interference
Serotonergic agents, sumatriptan and related triptans, SSRI antidepressants, tramadol, tricyclic antidepressants	5-HTP, SAMe, St. John's wort	Possible risk of serotonin syndrome
Tricyclic anti-depressants	Dong quai, St. John's wort	Possible increased risk of photosensitivity

Pharmaceuticals Used for Migraine Headaches: Natural Therapies with Potential Supportive Interactions

Pharmaceutical	Natural Therapy	Interaction
Beta-blockers	Chromium	Increased HDL levels
	Coenzyme Q_{10}	Possible correction of drug-induced relative deficiency
Tricyclic anti-depressants	Coenzyme Q_{10}	Possible correction of drug-induced relative deficiency

MULTIPLE SCLEROSIS (MS)

Principal Proposed Natural Therapies

Manipulation of dietary fatty acids [+3X]

Threonine [+2]

(Higher numbers indicate stronger evidence; X modifier indicates contradictory results. See page xviii of the Introduction for details of the rating scale.)

Approach to the Patient

Although there are no well-documented natural treatments for multiple sclerosis (MS), some evidence supports the use of dietary fat modifications for improving the overall course of the illness and the use of threonine for spasticity.

Other natural treatments your patient may be using include adenosine monophosphate (AMP); bee venom; biotin; calcium; evening primrose oil; fish oil; ginkgo; glycine; magnesium; phenylalanine; proteolytic enzymes; selenium; and vitamins B_1, B_6, B_{12}, C, D, and E. For potential safety risks with the more common of these substances, see the full herb/supplement articles.

Caution: For theoretic reasons, herbs that might activate components of the immune system should probably be avoided in MS. These include echinacea, *Panax ginseng*, and andrographis.

Manipulation
of Dietary Fatty Acids   + 3 X

The Swank diet of physician R.L. Swank is a popular diet for MS in which unsaturated fats replace most saturated fat. However, the only evidence supporting its use is a case series in which Swank reported that those adhering most closely to the diet for 20 to 34 years developed significantly less disability than those who consumed more saturated fat.[1,2]

Supplementation with essential fatty acids has also been tried. The best evidence is for the omega-6 fatty acid linoleic acid, found abundantly in sunflower oil. Of three double-blind trials with olive oil placebo,[3-5] two studies observing a total of about 190 individuals for 2 years found that linoleic acid reduced the duration and severity of MS exacerbations[3,4]; however, the frequency of exacerbation and overall level of disability were not significantly affected. The third study, with 76 participants, found no benefits.[5] Another researcher suggests that these studies were too short; it may take longer than 2 years for linoleic acid to exert its effects on myelin.[6] In addition, olive oil may not be a neutral treatment, since it also contains important fatty acids.

In the three double-blind studies described above, participants received 17 to 20 g of linoleic acid per day, the equivalent of 1 ounce of sunflower seed oil. As a nutrient found in food, linoleic acid is considered to be safe. However, maximum safe dosages for young children, pregnant or lactating women, or individuals with severe hepatic or renal disease have not been determined.

Other fatty acids have also been investigated, including fish oil and gamma-linolenic acid (GLA).[7-11]

However, in a 2-year double-blind study of fish oil for MS with 292 participants, there were no significant differences between the fish oil and olive oil groups.[11]

For more information, including dosage and safety issues, see the **Gamma-Linolenic Acid** and **Fish Oil** articles.

Threonine   +2

Two small double-blind, placebo-controlled studies found a modest but statistically significant improvement in muscle spasticity among individuals given the amino acid threonine.[12,13] In one, an 8-week study of 21 individuals with MS, the improvement was so slight it was detectable by researchers but not by participants.[13] In the other, a 2-week crossover trial of 33 individuals, researchers and a few of the treated participants noted improvement, with some individuals reporting fewer spasms and milder pain.[12] The doses used in these trials were 6 and 7.5 g daily. No significant side effects were noted in either study.

Other Proposed Natural Therapies

Because of some similarities between MS symptoms and symptoms of **vitamin B_{12}** deficiency, B_{12} supplementation has been tried. However, a double-blind trial with 50 individuals found that high doses of injected hydroxocobalamin did not affect the course of disease.[14]

MS is most common in areas with less sunshine, except when residents eat a great deal of fish that is rich in **vitamin D.**[15-18] This has led to a theory that vitamin D might confer some protection against MS, but there is no direct evidence as yet to support this theory.

Phenylalanine combined with transcutaneous nerve stimulation (TENS) has been tried as a treatment for pain and spasticity, with some apparent success.[19]

Other treatments sometimes suggested for MS, with little to no evidence, include AMP, bee venom, biotin, glycine, proteolytic enzymes, selenium, vitamin B_1, vitamin C, and vitamin E. One double-blind trial found that ginkgolide B, a constituent of **ginkgo,** was ineffective in treating MS attacks.[20]

Drug Interactions

See the article on each individual supplement for a full description of the interactions summarized here.

Principal Natural Therapy for Multiple Sclerosis: Interaction with Pharmaceutical		
Pharmaceutical	Natural Therapy	Interaction
Threonine	Levodopa or levodopa-carbidopa	Possible impaired action of drug based on amino acid/ levodopa interaction

NAUSEA

Principal Proposed
Natural Therapies

Vitamin B$_6$ (pregnancy)   [+3]

Ginger (various)   [+3X]

(Higher numbers indicate stronger evidence; X modifier indicates contradictory results. See page xviii of the Introduction for details of the rating scale.)

Approach to the Patient

A large double-blind trial found vitamin B$_6$ effective for the nausea (but not vomiting) of pregnancy. Ginger has shown promise for various types of nausea.

Other natural treatments your patient may be using include chamomile, lemon balm, licorice, and valerian. For potential safety risks with the more common of these substances, see the full herb/supplement articles.

Vitamin B$_6$ (Pregnancy)   +3

In a double-blind trial, 342 pregnant women were given placebo or 30 mg of vitamin B$_6$ daily.[1] Subjects then graded their symptoms by noting the severity of their nausea and recording the number of vomiting episodes. The women in the B$_6$ group experienced significantly less nausea than those in the placebo group. However, vomiting episodes were not significantly reduced.

For more information, including dosage and safety issues, see the **Vitamin B$_6$** article.

Ginger (Various)   + 3 X

Several double-blind, comparative trials observing a total of more than 1500 individuals have found ginger equally effective for motion sickness as standard agents, including cinnarizine, cinnarizine with domperidone, cyclizine, dimenhydrinate with caffeine, meclizine with caffeine, and scopolamine.[2-6] However, three small trials using strong nausea stimuli found no benefit.[7-9]

Evidence regarding postsurgical nausea is also mixed. A double-blind British study of 60 patients compared the effects of 1 g of ginger, placebo, and metoclopramide in the treatment of nausea following gynecologic surgery.[10] The results showed that both treatments produced a similar and statistically significant benefit compared with placebo. Comparable results were seen in a nearly identical study of 120 women.[11] However, ginger produced no benefit in two other studies of similar design and size.[12,13]

A double-blind, placebo-controlled trial of 70 pregnant women evaluated the effectiveness of ginger for morning sickness.[14] Particpants received either placebo or 250 mg of freshly prepared powdered ginger three times daily for a period of 4 days. The results indicated that ginger significantly reduced nausea and number of vomiting episodes.

Benefits were also seen in a double-blind, crossover trial of 27 women.[15]

For more information, including dosage and safety issues, see the **Ginger** article.

Other Proposed Natural Therapies

Various herbs and supplements have an antinausea reputation, including chamomile, lemon balm, licorice, valerian, and vitamins C and K, but there is no real evidence that they are effective.

Drug Interactions

See the article on each individual supplement for a full description of the interactions summarized here.

Principal Natural Therapies for Nausea: Interactions with Pharmaceuticals		
Natural Therapy	Pharmaceutical	Interaction
Ginger	Anticoagulant and antiplatelet agents	Possible increased risk of bleeding complications
Vitamin B_6	Levodopa	Reduction of efficacy; N/A if carbidopa taken as well
Vitamin K	Warfarin-related	Antagonism of drug's anticoagulant action

Pharmaceuticals Used for Nausea: Possible Harmful Interactions with Natural Therapies		
Pharmaceutical	Natural Therapy	Interaction
Phenothiazines	Dong quai, St. John's wort	Possible increased risk of photosensitivity
	Kava	Possible potentiation of sedative effects; also possible increased risk of dystonic reactions
	Phenylalanine	Possible increased risk of tardive dyskinesia
	Yohimbe	Increased risk of yohimbe toxicity
Sedative antihistamines	Sedative herbs such as kava and valerian	Increased sedation

Pharmaceuticals Used for Nausea: Natural Therapies with Potential Supportive Interactions		
Pharmaceutical	**Natural Therapy**	**Interaction**
Phenothiazines	Coenzyme Q_{10}	Correction of drug-induced relative deficiency
	Ginkgo	Possible reduction of sexual dysfunction side effects
	Milk thistle	Possible hepatoprotection
	Vitamin E	Possible reduced risk of tardive dyskinesia

OSTEOARTHRITIS

Principal Proposed
Natural Therapies

Glucosamine [+3X]

Chondroitin sulfate [+3]

S-adenosylmethionine
(SAMe) [+3]

Avocado/soybean
unsaponifiables [+3]

Proteolytic enzymes [+2]

Niacinamide [+2]

White willow [+2]

Dietary factors [+1]

Vitamin E [−1]

(Higher numbers indicate stronger evidence; X modifier indicates contradictory results. See page xviii of the Introduction for details of the rating scale.)

Approach to the Patient

Glucosamine and chondroitin are relatively well-documented treatments for osteoarthritis that offer two potential advantages over conventional treatments: superior side effects profiles and possible disease-modifying activity. Substantial evidence also supports the use of avocado/soybean unsaponifiables and SAMe (S-adenosylmethionine). Weaker evidence supports the use of proteolytic enzymes, niacinamide, and white willow.

Some evidence indicates that vitamin E may be ineffective for the treatment of osteoarthritis.

Other natural treatments your patient may be using include *Alpinia galanga*; beta-carotene; boron; boswellia; bromelain; cartilage; cat's claw; chamomile; copper; dandelion; devil's claw; feverfew; ginger; green-lipped mussel; molybdenum; MSM (methyl sulfonyl methane); D-phenylalanine; selenium; turmeric; vitamins B_1, B_6, B_{12}, C, and E; yucca; and zinc. For potential safety risks with the more common of these substances, see the full herb/supplement articles.

Glucosamine   +3X

A double-blind study compared the effectiveness of glucosamine sulfate and placebo in 252 patients with radiologic stage I to III osteoarthritis of the knee.[3] The participants were treated three times daily with oral glucosamine sulfate, 500 mg, or placebo. At the end of the 4-week study period, ratings on Lequesne's index (a measure of osteoarthritic severity) significantly improved in the treated group as compared with placebo. Smaller double-blind studies performed in the early 1980s reported similar results.[4-6]

However, a 2-month, double-blind, placebo-controlled trial of 98 individuals with osteoarthritis of the knee found no benefit, possibly because the participants had fairly advanced arthritis.[7] A double-blind, placebo-controlled trial of glucosamine chloride also produced negative results.[8]

Comparison trials have also been reported. One double-blind study observed 200 subjects with osteoarthritis of the knee, one half of whom received ibuprofen, 1200 mg/day, and the other one half glucosamine sulfate.[9] Although ibuprofen produced faster results, both groups experienced comparable relief at the end of 4 weeks. In addition, although 35% of the ibuprofen-treated group complained of side effects, only 6% of the glucosamine group did so. Essentially equivalent results were seen in a similar 4-week double-blind trial of 178 patients with knee osteoarthritis.[10] A 3-month, double-blind trial of 45 individuals with temporomandibular joint osteroarthritis found that glucosamine was at least as effective as ibuprofen (400 mg three times daily).[11]

One double-blind, placebo-controlled study of 212 participants over 3 years found radiologic evidence of reduced cartilage loss in the treated group, suggesting that glucosamine is a disease-modifying drug in osteoarthritis.[12]

For more information, including dosage and safety issues, see the **Glucosamine** article.

Chondroitin Sulfate   +3

Double-blind placebo-controlled studies, following a total of several hundred OA patients for a duration of 3 months to 1 year, found significant improvement in subjective pain and variables related to locomotion within 3 to 6 months.[13-17] However, one trial failed to find statistically significant benefits.[18]

A double-blind comparative study of 146 individuals evaluated the effects of chondroitin versus diclofenac sodium.[19] The results suggested that chondroitin acted less rapidly, but its effects continued for at least 3 months after cessation of treatment.

Three double-blind placebo-controlled studies of a total of about 250 patients with OA found radiologic evidence that suggests chondroitin may slow disease progression.[15,17,20] One animal study evaluating the effects of oral and injected chondroitin found significantly more healthy cartilage remaining in the damaged joint of those treated than untreated.[21] Giving chondroitin orally was as effective as giving it by injection.

For more information, including dosage and safety issues, see the **Chondroitin Sulfate** article.

S-Adenosylmethionine (SAMe)   +3

A 4-week, double-blind Italian study involving 732 patients at 33 centers treated OA patients with 1200 mg/day of SAMe (oral dose), 750 mg/day of naproxen, or placebo.[22] The results showed similar benefits in the SAMe and naproxen groups.

A small double-blind study compared 1200 mg/day of oral SAMe with full doses of piroxicam (20 mg), and found similar efficacy.[23]

In other double-blind studies, oral SAMe has also shown equivalent benefits to indomethacin (150 mg/day), ibuprofen (400 mg twice daily, again a low dose), and naproxen (initially 250 mg 3 times daily, then twice daily, a low dose).[24-26]

For more information, including dosage and safety issues, see the **S-Adenosylmethionine** article.

Avocado/Soybean Unsaponifiables +3

Extracts of avocado and soybean oil called avocado/soybean unsaponifiables (ASU) have been investigated as a treatment for osteoarthritis in several double-blind placebo-controlled trials enrolling a total of almost 600 individuals.[35-37]

For example, in a 3-month, double-blind trial, 260 individuals with arthritis of the knee were given either placebo or ASU at 300 or 600 mg daily.[35] The results indicate that use of ASU at either dose significantly improved Lequesne's index scores and reduced the use of NSAIDs and analgesics.

It has been suggested that ASU may also have a disease modifying effect. However, a 6-month, double-blind study of 163 individuals that evaluated ASU to determine whether they limit progression of joint space loss failed to find statistically significant evidence of benefit, except in a post-hoc subgroup with more severe narrowing.[38]

Protelytic Enzymes +2

Proteolytic enzyme combinations may be helpful for osteoarthritis.[39] A 28-day, double-blind trial of 80 individuals with osteoarthritis of the knee compared Wobenzym (7 tablets QID) with diclofenac (50 mg bid) in a double-dummy design.[40] The results showed equivalent improvement in symptoms between the two groups.

Two double-blind trials presented in abstract form evaluated proteolytic enzymes (2 tabs tid, each containing 90 mg bromelain, 48 mg trypsin, and 100 mg of the flavonoid rutoside) in, respectively, 73 individuals with knee arthritis and 40 individuals with shoulder arthritis.[41] Again, benefits were seen with use of proteolytic enzymes.

For more information, including dosage and safety issues, see the **Proteolytic Enzymes** article.

Niacinamide   +2

In a double-blind study, 72 individuals with OA were given either 3000 mg daily of niacinamide (in five equal doses) or placebo for 12 weeks.[27] The treated participants experienced a 29% reduction in symptoms, compared to a 10% increase in symptoms in the placebo group.

For more information, including dosage and safety issues, see the **Vitamin B$_3$** article.

White Willow   +2

The herb white willow contains the substance salicin, a salicylic acid prodrug. A double-blind, placebo-controlled trial of 78 individuals with osteoarthritis of the knee or hip found that white willow at a dose providing 240 mg of salicin daily significantly improved pain levels.[28]

For more information, including dosage and safety issues, see the **White Willow** article.

Dietary Factors   +1

Observational studies suggest that a diet high in foods containing vitamin C, vitamin E, and beta-carotene can slow the progression of OA by as much as 70%.[29]

Vitamin E [−1]

A 6-month, double-blind trial of 77 individuals with osteo-arthritis found no benefit with vitamin E at dose of 500 IU daily compared with placebo.[43]

Other Proposed Natural Therapies

A double-blind trial (published as a doctoral dissertation) of 50 individuals with various types of arthritis found that 10-day treatment with **devil's claw** provided significant pain relief.[30]

Adjunctive use of supplemental **vitamins B_1, B_6, and B_{12}** may enhance NSAID effectiveness.[31]

Animal studies suggests that **green-lipped mussel** may help alleviate OA symptoms.[32-34]

A 6-week, double-blind, placebo-controlled trial evaluated a mixture of ginger and the Asian spice galanga *(Alpinia galanga)* in knee arthritis.[1] (This study was widely misreported as a trial of ginger alone.) A total of 247 individuals were included in the intention-to-treat (ITT) analysis, which found statistically significant evidence of efficacy in the primary outcome measure (pain on standing).

Another trial that did evaluate ginger alone failed to find evidence of benefit except through post hoc exploratory statistical analysis.[2]

Other herbs and supplements sometimes recommended for OA include beta-carotene, boron, boswellia, bromelain, cartilage, cat's claw, chamomile, copper, dandelion, feverfew, MSM, molybdenum, D-phenylalanine, selenium, turmeric, vitamins C and E, yucca, and zinc. However, there is little real evidence supporting these treatments at this time.

Drug Interactions

See the article on each individual supplement for a full description of the interactions summarized here.

Principal Natural Therapies for Osteoarthritis: Interactions with Pharmaceuticals		
Natural Therapy	Pharmaceutical	Interaction
Niacinamide	Anticonvulsants	Possible increase in serum levels of drug
SAMe	Levodopa or levodopa-carbidopa	Possible increased "wearing off" effect
	Serotonergic drugs (case report involved tricyclic anti-depressant)	Possible risk of serotonin syndrome
White willow	Alcohol, anticoagulants, antiplatelet agents, aspirin, methotrexate, metoclopramide, NSAIDs, phenytoin, probenecid, potassium-sparing diuretics, sulfonamides, valproate	Interactions potentially identical to those with aspirin

Pharmaceuticals Used for Osteoarthritis: Possible Harmful Interactions with Natural Therapies

Pharmaceutical	Natural Therapy	Interaction
NSAIDs	Dong quai, St. John's wort	Possible increased risk of photosensitivity
	Feverfew	Possible increased risk of gastritis
	Garlic, ginkgo, high-dose vitamin E, policosanol, others	Possible increased risk of bleeding complications
	Potassium citrate	Possible decreased serum levels of salicylates
	White willow	Additional salicylates may increase risk of all side effects

Pharmaceuticals Used for Osteoarthritis: Natural Therapies with Potential Supportive Interactions

Pharmaceutical	Natural Therapy	Interaction
NSAIDs	Cayenne, colostrum, licorice	Possible cytoprotection
	Folate, vitamin C	Correction of possible drug-induced deficiency
	Vitamins B_1, B_6, and B_{12}	Possible potentiation of drug

OSTEOPOROSIS

Principal Proposed
Natural Therapies

**Calcium and
vitamin D** [+4]

Ipriflavone [+3X]

**Dehydroepiandro-
sterone (DHEA)** [+2]

Isoflavone sources [+2X]

Vitamin K [+1]

Progesterone [−2]

(Higher numbers indicate stronger evidence; X modifier indicates contradictory results. See page xviii of the Introduction for details of the rating scale.)

Approach to the Patient

Calcium supplements slow the progression of various forms of osteoporosis; a combination of calcium and vitamin D appears to be still more effective. Individuals using other antiosteoporotic treatments, such as estrogen-replacement therapy (ERT) and bisphosphonates such as Fosamax, can benefit from such supplementation; indeed, Fosamax has not been shown effective *except* in individuals taking calcium. (However, calcium supplements must not be taken in close proximity to Fosamax.)

Evidence from numerous double-blind studies suggests that ipriflavone may slow disease progression or reverse osteoporosis to some extent; however, there are significant safety concerns with this treatment.

Growing evidence suggests that the hormone dehydroepiandrosterone (DHEA), soy isoflavones, and vitamin K may also be helpful for preventing or treating osteoporosis.

Your patient may have been swayed by proponents of estriol (a weak estrogen) as a "safe" alternative therapy for treating menopausal syndrome and preventing osteoporosis, claiming that it presents a lower cancer risk than stronger estrogens. However, although estriol is probably effective for osteoporosis,[1-6] it appears most likely that it presents the same uterine and breast cancer risk as other forms of estrogen when taken in doses high enough to produce clinical effects.[7-11] See the **Estriol** article for more information.

Similarly, so-called "natural" progesterone has been strongly advocated as a virtual magic cure for osteoporosis. However, these claims, which spawned numerous books, are not justified. See the **Progesterone Cream** article for more details.

Other natural treatments your patient may be using include black tea, boron, copper, folate, horsetail, magnesium, manganese, pregnenolone, strontium, vanadium, and vitamin B_{12}. For potential safety risks with the more common of these substances, see the full herb/supplement articles.

Calcium and Vitamin D   +4

Numerous well-designed studies indicate that calcium supplementation can help prevent and slow nonvertebral bone loss in postmenopausal women.[12-14] Vitamin D in conjunction with calcium supplements may produce better results, slowing both vertebral and nonvertebral bone loss and perhaps reversing the disease to some extent.[15] (Vitamin D deficiency appears to be common among individuals with osteoporosis.[16]) However, calcium and vitamin D use must be continued since improvements in bone rapidly disappear once the supplements are stopped.[17]

This combination may also protect against corticosteroid-induced bone loss.[18-20] Although ERT is more effective than calcium alone, taking calcium in conjunction with estrogen may offer additional benefits.[21] Calcium supplements also appear to build calcium reserves in children and adolescent girls,[22,23] although regular exercise may be more important.[24]

Use of calcium may be enhanced by other nutrients. One study found that calcium citrate malate is more effective in individuals who have a relatively high intake of protein.[72] Adding various trace minerals (15 mg zinc, 2.5 mg copper, 5 mg manganese) along with calcium and vitamin D may also improve the outcome.[25,26] Similarly, essential fatty acid supplementation may enhance the effectiveness of calcium among those who are deficient, but perhaps only among those who are deficient in essential fatty acids.[27-29]

For more information, including dosage and safety issues, see the **Calcium** and **Vitamin D** articles.

Ipriflavone   +3X

Ipriflavone is a semisynthetic isoflavone closely related to soy isoflavones that appears to prevent osteoclastic resorption. Although it is derived from phytoestrogenic compounds, ipriflavone is not a phytoestrogen and its effects appear to be limited to bone. (However, evidence suggests that ipriflavone can reduce lymphocyte count. See the **Ipriflavone** article for details.)

In most of the double-blind, placebo-controlled studies of ipriflavone, involving a total of more than 1700 enrolled subjects, results demonstrated either a significant bone-sparing effect or improvement in bone mineral density measured at the radius, whole body, or vertebrae.[30-41] These studies ranged in length from 6 months to 2 years and involved postmenopausal women (naturally, surgically, or gonadotropin-releasing hormone [Gn-RH]–induced) and women with senile osteoporosis. In those studies that found improvement of bone mineral density in the ipriflavone groups, increases ranged from 0.7% to 7.1% over the course of the study. By comparison, placebo groups had losses as high as 5.0%.

One 2-year, multicenter, double-blind study evaluated ipriflavone's benefit in a group of 453 postmenopausal women (aged 50 to 65 years) with vertebral or radial mineral density 1 standard deviation (SD) below age-matched controls.[35] They received 200 mg ipriflavone three times daily plus 1 g supplemental calcium, or placebo plus calcium. Bone mass was maintained in the ipriflavone group, but the control group exhibited a significant loss in bone density. After 2 years, the results (calculated as a bone-sparing effect) were +1.6% at the lumbar spine (P <0.05) and +3.5% at the radius (P <0.05) compared with placebo.[35]

Evidence also suggests that ipriflavone can reduce the number of bone fractures. A 2-year, multicenter, randomized, double-blind study involving 100 women over 65 years of age found that patients treated with ipriflavone had a significant reduction in new fractures (along with an increase in bone mineral density).[37] A smaller study found a 50% reduction in the rate of new vertebral fractures in the first year of ipriflavone treatment.[38]

However, the most recent double-blind, placebo-controlled study of ipriflavone for osteoporosis found no benefits.[40] In this 3-year trial, 474 postmenopausal women took 500 mg calcium plus either 600 mg ipriflavone or placebo daily. No intergroup differences were seen in spine, hip, or forearm density. The explanation for these negative results may lie in the calcium dosage used: virtually all other studies of ipriflavone used 1 g calcium daily.

Ipriflavone may also protect bone in hyperparathyroidism, during corticosteroid treatment, and in women who are taking leuprolide (Lupron) or corticosteroids.[34,42,43]

There is some evidence that combining ipriflavone with estrogen may improve antiosteoporosis benefits.[44,45] However, it is not currently known whether such combinations increase or decrease the other benefits and/or adverse effects of ERT.

For more information, including dosage and safety issues, see the **Ipriflavone** article.

Dehydroepiandrosterone (DHEA)   +2

Subgroup analysis of a double-blind, placebo-controlled trial with 280 men and women (aged 60 to 79 years) found an improvement in bone turnover in women over 70 years taking 50 mg of DHEA daily for 1 year.[46] However, neither men nor younger women responded to the treatment.

Additional evidence that DHEA might provide a therapeutic benefit in osteoporosis comes from previous smaller clinical trials as well as observational studies.[47,48]

For more information, including dosage and safety issues, see the **Dehydroepiandrosterone** article.

Isoflavone Sources   +2X

In one study evaluating the benefits of isoflavones in osteoporosis, 66 postmenopausal women took either placebo (soy protein with isoflavones removed) or soy protein containing 56 or 90 mg of soy isoflavones daily for 6 months.[49] The high-dose isoflavone group showed significant gains in spinal bone density. There was little change in the placebo or low-dose isoflavone groups. Benefits were also seen in a 24-week, double-blind trial with 69 postmenopausal women.[50]

Similar effects have been seen in animal studies.[51-56] However, several animal studies and one human trial failed to find benefit.[57-59]

Unlike estrogen, which inhibits bone resorption, the soy isoflavone genistein may enhance new bone formation.[52]

For more information, including dosage and safety issues, see the **Isoflavones** article.

Vitamin K   +1

Vitamin K plays a known biochemical role in the formation of new bone. A report from the Nurses' Health Study with 12,700 participants found that higher dietary intake of vitamin K is associated with a significantly reduced risk of hip fracture in women not taking estrogen.[60] There is also evidence from other observational studies that higher vitamin K intake is associated with a reduced incidence of hip fractures.[61]

For more information, including dosage and safety issues, see the **Vitamin K** article.

Progesterone   −2

In vitro studies and other preliminary evidence first suggested that progesterone or progestins stimulate osteoblast activity.[62,63] Subsequently, the results of a series of case histories from one physician's practice were popularized as evidence that progesterone cream can slow or even reverse osteoporosis.[64-66]

However, a 1-year, double-blind trial of 102 women given either progesterone cream (providing 20 mg progesterone daily) or placebo cream, along with calcium and multivitamins, found no evidence of any improvements in bone density attributable to progesterone.[67] Further, in a large 3-year, double-blind trial, combination treatment with estrogen and oral progesterone was no more effective for osteoporosis than estrogen alone.[68]

For more information, including dosage and safety issues, see the **Progesterone Cream** article.

Other Proposed Natural Therapies

On the basis of weak and contradictory evidence,[69,70] the mineral **boron** has become a popular alternative medicine treatment for osteoporosis. However, there are some concerns that boron may raise endogenous estrogen levels, especially in women receiving ERT[69,71] and therefore might present an increased risk of cancer.

A wide variety of other food supplements has also been suggested for the prevention or reversal of osteoporosis, including black tea, copper, folate, horsetail, magnesium, manganese, pregnenolone, strontium, vanadium, and vitamin B_{12}. However, there is as yet little direct evidence that these approaches really work.

Drug Interactions

See the article on each individual supplement for a full description of the interactions summarized here.

Principal Natural Therapies for Osteoporosis: Interactions with Pharmaceuticals		
Natural Therapy	**Pharmaceutical**	**Interaction**
Combined high-dose calcium and vitamin D	Calcium channel blockers	Possible antagonism of drug action
	Flouroquinolones, tetracyclines	Mutual absorption interference
Calcium (especially with vitamin D)	Thiazides	Potential risk of hypercalcemia
Ipriflavone	Cytochrome P-450–metabolized drugs: caffeine nifedipine, phenacetin, phenytoin, S-warfarin, theobromine, theophylline, tolbutamide	Increased drug metabolism
	Immunosuppressants	Possible potentiation of action
	Estrogens	Possible increased uterotropic effects

Pharmaceuticals Used for Osteoporosis: Possible Harmful Interactions with Natural Therapies		
Pharmaceutical	**Natural Therapy**	**Interaction**
Androstenedione, boron, grapefruit juice	Estrogens	Possible increased serum levels of drug
Ipriflavone		Possible increased uterotropic effects

Pharmaceuticals Used for Osteoporosis: Natural Therapies With Potential Supportive Interactions		
Pharmaceutical	**Natural Therapy**	**Interaction**
Combined high-dose calcium and vitamin D	Estrogens	Potentiation of bone-sparing effects
Ipriflavone		Possible increased bone-sparing action
Magnesium		Possible correction of drug-induced depletion

OTITIS MEDIA

Principal Proposed Natural Therapies

Xylitol   [+3]

Probiotic nasal spray   [+3]

Breast-feeding   [+2]

Herbal ear drops (pain reduction)   [+2]

(Higher numbers indicate stronger evidence; X modifier indicates contradictory results. See page xviii of the Introduction for details of the rating scale.)

Approach to the Patient

Routine antibiotic treatment of acute otitis media (AOM) has come under increasing criticism in the lay press, and there is some scientific justification for these concerns.

Evidence suggests that without treatment, most middle ear infections resolve on their own, and antibiotic treatment only slightly improves rate of recovery.[1] Modest benefits with antibiotic treatment were also seen in a more recent trial of 315 children.[2] In addition, early antibiotic treatment has not been found effective in preventing complications such as serous otitis[3] or pneumococcal meningitis[4] or in significantly speeding recovery of hearing.[5] Finally, children with recurrent ear infections do not appear to benefit from prophylactic antibiotic treatment.[6] The benefits of tympanostomy, too, have been questioned.[3,6,7]

However, despite widespread claims by antibiotic opponents that your patients may have heard, early antibiotic treatment does not appear to cause an increased rate of ear infection recurrence.[3]

Patients interested in alternative medicine may accept a compromise solution: watchful waiting with close physician supervision before instituting antibiotic therapy. Use of anesthetic ear drops can alleviate pain during the acute phase of OM; there is some evidence that a traditional herbal ear drop combination may also help.

The natural sugar xylitol, taken in gum, lozenge, or syrup form, may have prophylactic effects against otitis media, as may probiotic nasal spray and breast-feeding.

Other natural treatments your patient may be using include andrographis, arginine, echinacea, ginseng (*Panax* spp.), thymus extract, vitamin C, and zinc. For potential safety risks with the more common of these substances, see the full herb/supplement articles.

Xylitol   +3

A natural sugar found in plums, strawberries, and raspberries, xylitol is used as a sweetener in some "sugarless" gums and candies. Xylitol inhibits the growth and attachment of *Streptococcus pneumoniae* and perhaps the attachment of *Haemophilus influenzae* as well.[8,9] Based on this in vitro evidence, xylitol has been tried as a preventive treatment for AOM, with promising results.

A 3-month, double-blind, placebo-controlled trial of 857 children investigated the prophylactic effects of xylitol taken daily as chewing gum, syrup, or lozenges.[8] Regular use of the gum reduced the risk of developing AOM by 40%. Xylitol syrup was effective to a lesser extent, but the lozenges failed to reduce risk, possibly because of lack of compliance. Similarly positive results were seen in a 2-month, double-blind study by the same researchers, evaluating about 300 children.[10]

In these studies, children given xylitol-sweetened gum received 8.4 g of xylitol daily. Those who took syrup received 10 g daily.

For more information, including dosage and safety issues, see the **Xylitol** article.

Probiotic Nasal Spray   +3

A double-blind, placebo-controlled study of 108 children (mean age 23 months) prone to recurrent otitis media examined the effects of recolonization with probiotic strains of alpha hemolytic streptococci *(S. mitis, S. oralis, S. sanguis)*.[14] These strains were cultured from healthy children and selected for their ability to inhibit *S. pneumoniae, H. influenzae, M. catarrhalis,* and *S. pyogenes.*

Participants received a 10-day course of antibiotic treatment and were then randomized to receive either active or placebo solution for 10 days. Sixty days later, another 10-day course was given. The results showed significantly decreased incidence of otitis media recurrence in the treatment group as compared with the placebo group over the 3-month study period, but the rate of treatment failure was nonetheless high (58%).

However, a smaller double-blind trial found no benefit.[15]

Breast-feeding   +2

Numerous observational studies tracking ear infection frequency in large groups of infants found that those infants exclusively breast-fed had significantly fewer middle ear infections than those fed formula.[11-13]

Herbal Ear Drops
(Pain Reduction)   +2

A randomized, controlled trial of about 100 children and young adults with eardrum pain caused by OM compared the effectiveness of an herbal preparation containing mullein, garlic, St. John's wort, and calendula against an ametocaine and phenazone combination.[16] The results indicated that the two treatments were equally effective.

Other Proposed
Natural Therapies

Herbs and supplements used for colds and flus, including andrographis, arginine, echinacea, ginseng, thymus extract, vitamin C, and zinc, are frequently recommended for AOM as well in the lay press; however, there is no evidence as yet that they are effective for AOM.

Drug Interactions

See the article on each individual supplement for a full description of the interactions summarized here.

Pharmaceuticals Used for Otitis Media: Natural Therapies with Potential Supportive Interactions		
Pharmaceutical	Natural Therapy	Interaction
Amoxicillin, tetracycline	Bromelain	Possible increased absorption of drug
Antibiotics	Probiotics (especially *Saccharomyces*)	May reduce risk of antibiotic-related diarrhea

PARKINSON'S DISEASE

Principal Proposed Natural Therapies

CDP-choline [+2]

SAMe (Parkinson's depression) [+2]

(Higher numbers indicate stronger evidence; X modifier indicates contradictory results. See page xviii of the Introduction for details of the rating scale.)

Approach to the Patient

Although CDP-choline might offer some benefit in Parkinson's disease, the supplement (used as a drug in some countries) is not widely available. SAMe (S-adenosylmethionine) might be helpful for depression in Parkinson's, but there are concerns that long-term SAMe could counter the effects of L-dopa.

Other natural treatments your patient may be using include coenzyme Q_{10}; glutathione; 5-HTP (5-hydroxytryptophan); L-methionine; *N*-acetyl cysteine; NADH (nicotinamide adenine dinucleotide); octacosanol; D-phenylalanine; phosphatidylserine; and vitamins B_6, C, and E. For potential safety risks with the more common of these substances, see the full herb/supplement articles.

Keep in mind that amino acid supplements such as phenylalanine and methionine might act like proteins and impair the action of L-dopa. There are numerous other potential drug interactions with Parkinson's medications as well (see Drug Interactions).

Caution: Individuals with Parkinson's disease sometimes take kava in the belief that it relaxes muscles. However, case reports suggest that kava may have antidopaminergic effects and should therefore be avoided.[1]

CDP-Choline   + 2

Short for cytidinediphosphocholine, CDP-choline (also called citicholine) is an intermediary in the biosynthesis of the phospholipid phosphatidylcholine. Evidence suggests that exogenous CDP-choline may enhance the effects of L-dopa and reduce some symptoms of Parkinson's disease.

In a 4-week, single-blind study of 74 individuals with Parkinson's disease, participants received either their usual daily dose of L-dopa or one half their usual dose, and all participants received 400 mg of oral CDP-choline three times daily.[2] Both groups scored equally well on standardized tests of Parkinson's severity. Other single- and double-blind studies found that intravenous or intramuscular injections of CDP-choline either reduced symptoms or allowed decreased doses of L-dopa without loss of drug effectiveness.[3-6]

In general, CDP-choline appears to be safe.[4] The study of oral CDP-choline for Parkinson's disease reported only occasional mild nonspecific side effects, such as nausea, dizziness, and fatigue.[2] In a 60-day study of 2817 seniors given oral CDP-choline for problems other than Parkinson's disease, side effects were mild and reported in only about 5% of participants[7]; however, the CDP-choline dose in this study was 550 to 650 mg per day, about one half the dose used for Parkinson's disease.

The safety of CDP-choline in pregnant or lactating women, young children, or individuals with severe hepatic or renal disease has not been established.

SAMe
(Parkinson's Depression)   +2

L-Dopa depletes brain levels of SAMe.[8,9] Because exogenous SAMe appears to have antidepressant effects,[10] it has been hypothesized that Parkinson's depression is related to this depletion.

In a double-blind, placebo-controlled trial with 21 individuals taking L-dopa for Parkinson's disease, participants received either placebo or a combination of oral and injected SAMe for 30 days and were then crossed over.[11] The results showed improvements in symptoms of depression without loss of L-dopa efficacy.

However, there are concerns regarding long-term use of SAMe supplements. SAMe participates in metabolic deactivation of L-dopa.[8] It is therefore possible that long-term use of SAMe could lead to decreased effectiveness of L-dopa. SAMe also might interact with selegiline (see Drug Interactions).

For more information, including dosage and safety issues, see the **S-Adenosylmethionine** article.

Other Proposed
Natural Therapies

The serotonin precursor **5-HTP,** another supplement with possible antidepressant effects, has also been tried for Parkinson's depression. However, the evidence that it works is extremely preliminary.[12] In addition, the combination of 5-HTP and carbidopa may lead to a scleroderma-like syndrome.[13-15]

Phosphatidylserine is an important cell membrane phospholipid. Most commonly used as a treatment for Alzheimer's and multiinfarct dementia, it has also been tried for Parkinson's depression, with preliminary indications of success.[16]

Based on the free radical theory of Parkinson's disease, **vitamin E** has been tried for slowing the progression of Parkinson's disease. However, results of large intervention trials have not been encouraging.[17-19]

Vitamin C has been tried as a treatment for L-dopa's "on-off effects" in a small single-blind study,[20] but the benefits were so minimal that the researchers did not feel justified in recommending it.

Other natural treatments sometimes recommended for Parkinson's disease, with minimal or conflicting evidence, include NADH,[21-23] glutathione,[24] octacosanol,[25] and the amino acids D-phenylalanine[26] and L-methionine.[27,28] Caution is advised with the latter two, since they might also interfere with the effectiveness of L-dopa.[25,29]

Treatments sometimes mentioned for Parkinson's, but essentially lacking any scientific data, include N-acetyl cysteine, beta-carotene, coenzyme Q_{10}, the hormone pregnenolone, and vitamin B_6.

Drug Interactions

See the article on each individual supplement for a full description of the interactions summarized here.

Principal Natural Therapies for Parkinson's Disease: Interactions with Pharmaceuticals		
Natural Therapy	Pharmaceutical	Interaction
5-HTP	Levodopa-carbidopa	Possible increased risk of scleroderma-like syndrome
	SSRIs, other serotonergic drugs	Possible risk of serotonin syndrome
SAMe	Levodopa or levodopa-carbidopa	Possible increased "wearing off" effect
	Serotonergic drugs (case report involved tricyclic antidepressant)	Possible risk of serotonin syndrome

Pharmaceuticals Used for Parkinson's Disease: Possible Harmful Interactions with Natural Therapies		
Pharmaceutical	**Natural Therapy**	**Interaction**
Levodopa-carbidopa	5-HTP	Possible increased risk of scleroderma-like syndrome
Levodopa or levodopa-carbidopa	Branched-chain amino acids (BCAAs) methionine, phenylalanine, threonine, other amino acids	Possible impaired action of drug based on amino acid/levodopa interaction
	Iron	Absorption interference
	Octacosanol/policosanol	Possible potentiation of dyskinesia side effect
	SAMe	Possible increased "wearing off" effects
	Vitamin B_6	Impairs effectiveness of levodopa taken alone but does not interact with levodopa/carbidopa combination
Prolactin inhibitors, bromocriptine, pergolide	Bugleweed, chasteberry	Possible potentiation of drug action
Selegiline	5-HTP, SAMe, St. John's wort	Possible risk of serotonin syndrome
	Ephedra, green tea, guarana	Monoamine oxidase inhibitor (MAOI) interaction

PEPTIC ULCER DISEASE

Principal Proposed Natural Therapies

Licorice, deglycyr-rhizinated (DGL) [+1]

Probiotics (adjunctive therapy) [+1]

(Higher numbers indicate stronger evidence; X modifier indicates contradictory results. See page xviii of the Introduction for details of the rating scale.)

Approach to the Patient

Preliminary controlled trials weakly suggest that the licorice derivative DGL may have some utility in ulcer treatment. (DGL is much safer than whole licorice.)

Various probiotics may be useful as adjuncts to triple drug therapy for *Helicobacter pylori*.

Other natural treatments your patient may be using include betaine hydrochloride, bioflavonoids, bovine colostrum, cat's claw, cayenne, garlic, glutamine, marshmallow, MSM (methyl sulfonyl methane), reishi, selenium, suma, turmeric, vitamins A and C, and zinc. For potential safety risks with the more common of these substances, see the full herb/supplement article.

Licorice, Deglycyrrhizinated (DGL)   +1

DGL is a specially processed form of licorice that does not produce pseudohyperaldosteronemia (see Licorice article for more information).

A 12-week, controlled trial (blinding not stated) using endoscopic evaluation compared antacids, cimetidine (220 mg three times daily and 400 mg qhs), geranylferensylacetate (5 mg three times daily), and Caved-S in 874 individuals with duodenal ulcers.[1] No significant differences in outcome were observed. However, considering that Caved-S contains antacids, this study might not actually provide evidence that DGL alone is effective.

In a single-blind trial, 82 individuals with endoscopically healed gastric ulcer were treated for 2 years with cimetidine (400 mg qhs) or DGL. The results showed an equivalent rate of recurrence in the two groups.[2] Again, the effectiveness of DGL alone cannot be determined from this study.

There is no evidence that licorice or DGL eradicates *Helicobacter pylori*. Preliminary evidence suggests that DGL might protect the gastric lining from nonsteroidal antiinflammatory drug (NSAID)–induced gastritis.[3]

For more information, including dosage and safety issues, see the **Licorice** article.

Probiotics
(Adjunctive Therapy)   +1

Probiotics have been found to exert an inhibitory action on *Helicobacter pylori*.[18-22]

Although this action does not appear to be strong enough to eradicate *Helicobacter*, evidence suggests that *Lactobacilli* may be a useful adjunct to standard antibiotic therapy, improving eradication rate and reducing side effects.[4,7,18,23-26]

Unfortunately, the reported studies suggesting benefit were not double-blind.

Other Proposed Natural Therapies

Preliminary studies suggest that various **bioflavonoids** can inhibit the growth of *Helicobacter pylori*.[5] Some evidence suggests that garlic might also act against *H. pylori* when used as a single agent as well as provide synergistic effects when combined with antibiotic therapy.[6] In addition, according to an open controlled trial, *Lactobacillus GG* might help reduce symptoms during triple antibiotic therapy for *H. pylori*.[7]

Some evidence suggests that **cayenne** and **bovine colostrum** can protect the gastric lining against NSAID-induced damage.[8-12]

Contrary to some reports, the herb **turmeric** does not appear to be effective for treating ulcers,[13,14] and it might increase the risk of developing ulcers if taken at excessive doses.[15]

Neither **garlic, fish oil,** nor **cayenne** appears to be helpful against *Helicobacter pylori*.[16,17,27]

Although betaine hydrochloride, cat's claw, glutamine, marshmallow, MSM, reishi, selenium, suma, vitamins A and C, and zinc have also been suggested as aids to ulcer healing, there is no scientific evidence that they are effective.

Drug Interactions

See the article on each individual supplement for a full description of the interactions summarized here.

Pharmaceuticals Used for Peptic Ulcer Disease: Possible Harmful Interactions with Natural Therapies		
Pharmaceutical	Natural Therapy	Interaction
Aluminum antacids	Calcium citrate	May increase aluminum absorption
Proton pump inhibitors, H_2 blockers	St. John's wort	Possible increased risk of photosensitivity

Pharmaceuticals Used for Peptic Ulcer Disease: Natural Therapies with Potential Supportive Interactions		
Pharmaceutical	Natural Therapy	Interaction
H_2 blockers, proton pump inhibitors	Folate, iron, vitamin B_{12}, zinc, other minerals	Correction of possible drug-induced deficiency

PHOTOSENSITIVITY

Principal Proposed Natural Therapies

Beta-carotene [+2X]

Other antioxidants [+2X]

(Higher numbers indicate stronger evidence; X modifier indicates contradictory results. See page xviii of the Introduction for details of the rating scale.)

Approach to the Patient

Based on the theory that free radicals play a role in photosensitivity, a number of antioxidants have been tried, but with contradictory results at best.

Although there are no well-documented natural treatments for *treating* photosensitivity, a number of common herbs and plant products might *increase* the risk. These include oral St. John's wort and dong quai most prominently, as well as topical contact with numerous herbs and essential oils, such as carrot, celery, dill, fennel, fig, lime, parsley, and parsnip, as well as arnica, artichoke, chrysanthemum, dandelion, endive, lettuce, marigold, and sunflower.[1]

Other natural treatments your patient may be using include vitamins B_6, C, and E; epigallocatechin-3-gallate (EGCG from green tea); adenosine monophosphate (AMP); and nicotinamide. For potential safety risks with the more common of these substances, see the full herb/supplement articles.

Beta-Carotene   +2X

Beta-carotene, alone or in combination with other carotenes, might be helpful for polymorphous light eruptions (PLEs) and other forms of photosensitivity, but the evidence is contradictory. Also, high-dose beta-carotene gives a deep yellow color to the skin, which makes it difficult to conduct a long-term, truly double-blind trial.

A 10-week, placebo-controlled study of 50 individuals with PLE found evidence of benefit with beta-carotene plus the carotene canthaxanthin.[2] However, in two other placebo-controlled trials of beta-carotene alone, slight benefits were seen in one study and no significant benefits at all in the other.[3] These trials lasted 12 and 15 weeks, respectively, and the numbers of participants were not reported.

Many uncontrolled studies suggest that beta-carotene extends the time that individuals with erythropoietic protoporphyria (EPP) can safely spend in the sun,[4-6] but a 4-month, placebo-controlled, crossover study of 14 individuals found no effect.[7] In the research on beta-carotene for EPP, adult doses used were 100 to 200 mg per day; in the study with the most positive result, canthaxanthin was given simultaneously at 100 mg per day.[2]

Several studies have found beta-carotene to be helpful in preventing ordinary sunburn,[8-11] but, again, other studies have found no benefit.[12,13]

A few case reports suggest beta-carotene may be helpful in porphyria cutanea tarda (PCT).[6]

For more information, including dosage and safety issues, see the **Beta-Carotene** article.

Other Antioxidants   +2X

Animal studies suggest that topical vitamin C and vitamin E, alone or together, as well as EGCG (from green tea) may help protect against ultraviolet light.[14-19] In addition, two placebo-controlled human studies found that a combination of oral vitamin C and E modestly reduced UV-induced erythema.[20,21] However, placebo-controlled studies of oral vitamin C or E taken alone have found no benefit.[21,22]

Other Proposed Natural Therapies

Vitamin C and **vitamin B$_6$** have been suggested as treatment for EPP, **AMP** has been suggested for PCT,[23-25] and **nicotinamide** has been suggested for PLE. However, there is no real evidence that these approaches are effective. Topically applied extracts of **green tea** might also be helpful.[18,19,26]

Drug Interactions

See the article on each individual supplement for a full description of the interactions summarized here.

Principal Natural Therapies for Photosensitivity: Interactions with Pharmaceuticals		
Natural Therapy	Pharmaceutical	Interaction
Vitamin C	Acetaminophen	Possible increased serum levels of drug
	Anticoagulants	Possible antagonism of drug action
	Iron supplements	Increased iron absorption
	Warfarin-related	Possible antagonism anticoagulants of drug action
Vitamin E	Anticoagulant and antiplatelet agents	Possible increased risk of bleeding complications

PREGNANCY SUPPORT

Principal Proposed
Natural Therapies

Nausea and vomiting

Vitamin B$_6$ [+3]

Varicose veins/venous insufficiency

Oxerutins   [+2]

Hemorrhoids

Oxerutins   [+2X]

Pregnancy-induced hypertension (PIH) and preeclampsia

Calcium   [+3X]

Vitamins C and E   [+3]

Leg cramps

Magnesium   [+2]

Calcium   [−1]

Gingivitis

Topical folate   [+2]

Gestational diabetes

Chromium   [+2]

Preterm birth (prevention)

No rated therapies

Labor and delivery

Raspberry leaf   [+3]

Herbs and supplements to avoid in pregnancy and lactation

See the discussion at the end of the article.

(Higher numbers indicate stronger evidence; X modifier indicates contradictory results. See page xviii of the Introduction for details of the rating scale.)

Approach to the Patient

Although no herbs or supplements (other than vitamins and minerals taken at nutritional doses) have been proven safe in pregnancy, a number are in wide use and may offer some benefits. The best evidence is for vitamin B_6 in treating the nausea and vomiting of pregnancy.

Correcting iron-deficiency anemia in pregnancy is clearly advisable, but research suggests that excess iron may cause an increase in complications of pregnancy and should be avoided.[1-3]

Caution: Numerous herbs may be dangerous in pregnancy. See Herbs and Supplements to Avoid in Pregnancy and Lactation below.

Nausea and Vomiting

Vitamin B_6 +3

A double-blind study of 342 women found that compared with placebo, 30 mg of vitamin B_6 daily led to a significant reduction in nausea, although vomiting episodes were not significantly reduced.[4]

For more information, including dosage and safety issues, see the **Vitamin B_6** article.

Other Proposed Natural Therapies

A double-blind, placebo-controlled trial of 70 pregnant women evaluated the effectiveness of **ginger** for morning sickness.[5] Participants received either placebo or 250 mg of freshly prepared powdered ginger three times daily for a period of 4 days. The results indicated that ginger significantly reduced nausea and number of vomiting episodes. Benefits were also seen in a double-blind, crossover trial of 27 women.[6]

Treatments with minimal to no evidence include a combination of vitamin K (at the enormous dose of 5 mg daily), vitamin C (25 mg),[7] and the herb red raspberry.[8]

Varicose Veins/Venous Insufficiency

Oxerutins   +2

Only one double-blind trial has been performed on pregnant women with varicose veins; this study found oxerutins to be more effective than placebo among 69 women.[9] However, numerous studies have found oxerutins effective for venous insufficiency in nonpregnant individuals.

For more information, including dosage and safety issues, see the **Oxerutins** article.

Other Proposed Natural Therapies

Horse chestnut is a well-established treatment for venous insufficiency, and one small trial found it safe in pregnant women.[10]

Some evidence supports the use of **gotu kola** for venous insufficiency, and it too has been studied in pregnant women.[11]

Hemorrhoids

Oxerutins   +2X

A double-blind study enrolling 97 pregnant women found oxerutins (1000 mg daily) significantly better than placebo at reducing the pain, bleeding, and inflammation of hemorrhoids.[12] Benefits were seen in earlier double-blind trials as well, although one did not find benefit.[13]

For more information, including dosage and safety issues, see the **Oxerutins** article.

Other Proposed Natural Therapies

Meaningful evidence suggests that a micronized combination of the citrus bioflavonoids **diosmin** (90%) and **hesperidin** (10%) is safe and effective for the treatment of hemorrhoids in general. In addition, one trial suggests that the combination is safe to use in pregnancy.[14]

Pregnancy-Induced Hypertension and Preeclampsia

Calcium   +3X

A metaanalysis of 10 studies involving more than 6000 women found evidence that calcium may have a role in preventing pregnancy-induced hypertension and preeclampsia, particularly in women at high risk for hypertension and/or those with low calcium intake.[15,16] However, the largest study in the metaanalysis found no benefits. In this double-blind trial, researchers gave either 2 g of calcium or placebo daily to 4589 women from weeks 13 to 21 of their pregnancy onward. In the end, researchers found no significant decreases in rates of hypertension or preeclampsia, not even among women with the lowest dietary calcium intake.[16]

For more information, including dosage and safety issues, see the **Calcium** article.

Vitamins C and E   +3

A promising preliminary double-blind study of 283 women found that a combination of vitamins C and E might help prevent preeclampsia in women at high risk for the disorder.[17] Subjects took either placebo or a combination of 1000 mg vitamin C and 400 IU vitamin E daily throughout the second half of their pregnancies. Those who were subsequently determined by Doppler ultrasonography to be at low risk before 24 weeks were withdrawn. Only 8% of the treated women developed preeclampsia compared with 17% of those taking placebo, a significant difference.

An earlier double-blind study (n = 56) found that a combination of vitamin C, vitamin E, and allopurinol was no more effective than placebo.[18] However, this trial studied women who were already severely preeclamptic.

For more information, including dosage and safety issues, see the **Vitamin C** and **Vitamin E** articles.

Other Proposed Natural Therapies

Other possible prophylactic treatments for PIH or preeclampsia, with weak or contradictory evidence, include zinc,[19-21] folate,[22] and fish oil.[23-26] Two double-blind trials, one of 400 pregnant women and the other of 568, found magnesium supplements ineffective.[27,28]

Studies of natural treatments for established PIH or preeclampsia have not yielded impressive results. In one double-blind trial of established PIH (n = 58), intravenous and oral magnesium decreased blood pressure compared with placebo, but not enough to reduce the need for antihypertensives.[29] In other double-blind studies, neither evening primrose oil nor calcium supplements were more effective than placebo in treating established preeclampsia among 47 and 75 women, respectively.[30,31]

Leg Cramps

Magnesium   +2

A double-blind study of 73 pregnant women with leg cramps found that oral magnesium was significantly more effective than placebo.[32]

For more information, including dosage and safety issues, see the **Magnesium** article.

Calcium   −1

A double-blind study of 60 pregnant women with leg cramps (using vitamin C as a somewhat questionable placebo control) found no benefits with calcium.[33]

For more information, including dosage and safety issues, see the **Calcium** article.

Other Proposed Natural Therapies

A combination of vitamins B_1 and B_6 has been suggested for leg cramps of pregnancy, but the evidence that it works is minimal.[34]

For more information, including dosage and safety issues, see the **Vitamin B_1** and **Vitamin B_6** articles.

Gingivitis

Topical Folate   +2

Two small double-blind studies suggest that folate mouthwash may help gingivitis in pregnancy.[35,36]

For more information, including dosage and safety issues, see the **Folate** article.

Gestational Diabetes

Chromium   +2

One placebo-controlled study (blinding not stated) of 30 pregnant women suggests that chromium may be useful for gestational diabetes.[37]

For more information, including dosage and safety issues, see the **Chromium** article.

Other Proposed Natural Therapies

Minimal evidence supports the use of **vitamin B_6** for gestational diabetes.[38]

Preterm Birth (Prevention)

Despite numerous studies, there is no definitive evidence that fish oil, calcium, zinc, magnesium, or iron can help prevent premature birth, and folate has been found to be ineffective for this purpose.[19,26-28,39-48]

Labor and Delivery

Raspberry Leaf   +3

Red raspberry is a widely used herb said to make labor "easier." A double-blind, placebo-controlled trial evaluated this traditional treatment in 192 low-risk pregnant women.[49] Treatment (placebo or 2.4 g of raspberry leaf daily) began at the thirty-second week of gestation and was continued until the commencement of labor. No statistically significant differences were seen in length of first-, second-, or third-stage labor; need for augmentation; use of anesthesia; or complications of delivery. The use of raspberry was not associated with any significant adverse effects as compared with placebo.

Herbs and Supplements to Avoid in Pregnancy and Lactation

No herb has been established as safe in pregnancy.

Although it is often recommended to initiate labor, blue cohosh is a toxic herb and should not be used. Case reports have linked maternal use of blue cohosh to neonatal heart failure, hypoxia, seizures, and acute tubular necrosis.[50,51]

Other herbs that should be regarded with particular caution include chasteberry, feverfew, flaxseed, juniper, licorice, nettle, pennyroyal, red clover, shepherd's purse, and yarrow, along with many others.[52,53] The anticoagulant or antiplatelet effects of garlic, ginger, ginkgo, and high-dose vitamin E have also raised concerns. Vitamin A has been implicated in birth defects.

This list is by no means comprehensive.

Drug Interactions

See the article on each individual supplement for a full description of the interactions summarized here.

Principal Natural Therapies for Pregnancy Support: Interactions with Pharmaceuticals		
Natural Therapy	**Pharmaceutical**	**Interaction**
Calcium	Beta-blockers	Absorption interference
	Calcium channel blockers	Possible antagonism of drug action
	Fluoroquinolones, tetracyclines	Mutual absorption interference
	Thiazides	Potential risk of hypercalcemia
	Thyroid hormone	Absorption interference
Chromium	Hypoglycemic agents	Possible potentiation of drug, increasing risk of hypoglycemia
Magnesium	Fluoroquinolones, tetracyclines	Mutual absorption interference
	Oral hypoglycemics	Possible potentiation of drug action leading to risk of hypoglycemia
	Potassium-sparing diuretics, amiloride	Risk of hypermagnesemia
Vitamin B_6	Levodopa	Reduction of efficacy (N/A if carbidopa taken as well)

Continued

Principal Natural Therapies for Pregnancy Support: Interactions with Pharmaceuticals—cont'd		
Natural Therapy	Pharmaceutical	Interaction
Vitamin C	Acetaminophen	Possible increased serum levels of drug
	Anticoagulants	Possible antagonism of drug action
	Nonsteroidal anti-inflammatory drugs (NSAIDs)	Correction of possible drug-induced depletion
	Warfarin-related anticoagulants	Possible antagonism of drug action
Vitamin E	Anticoagulant and antiplatelet agents	Possible increased risk of bleeding complications
	Phenothiazines	Possible reduced risk of tardive dyskinesia

PREMENSTRUAL SYNDROME (PMS)

Principal Proposed Natural Therapies

Calcium [+3]

Chasteberry [+3]

Ginkgo [+3]

Magnesium [+2]

Multivitamin/mineral supplements [+2]

Evening primrose oil (cyclic mastalgia) [+2]

Vitamin B$_6$ [−1X]

(Higher numbers indicate stronger evidence; X modifier indicates contradictory results. See page xviii of the Introduction for details of the rating scale.)

Approach to the Patient

A large trial suggests that calcium supplements may alleviate all the major symptoms of PMS to some extent. Other treatments with significant supporting evidence for PMS symptoms include chasteberry (which has even stronger evidence as a treatment for cyclic mastalgia), ginkgo, magnesium, and multivitamin/mineral supplements. Evening primrose oil appears to be effective for cyclic mastalgia.

Vitamin B$_6$ alone has not been found effective; however, combined treatment with magnesium may lead to synergistic effects.

Other natural treatments your patient may be using include "natural" progesterone cream, red clover isoflavones, St. John's wort, and vitamin E. For potential safety risks with the more common of these substances, see the full herb/supplement articles.

Calcium   + 3

In a double-blind, placebo-controlled study of 497 women, 1200 mg daily of calcium (as calcium carbonate) reduced PMS symptoms over a period of three menstrual cycles.[1] These symptoms included mood swings, headaches, food cravings, and bloating. These results corroborate those of earlier, smaller studies.[2,3]

For more information, including dosage and safety issues, see the **Calcium** article.

Chasteberry   + 3

A double-blind, placebo-controlled study of 178 women found that treatment with chasteberry over three menstrual cycles significantly reduced PMS symptoms.[4] The dose used was one tablet three times daily of the chasteberry dry extract ZE 440. Women in the treatment group experienced significant improvements in symptoms, including irritability, depression, headache, and breast tenderness.

In addition, several double-blind trials have found chasteberry effective for the PMS-related condition cyclic mastalgia.[5-7] For example, a double-blind trial enrolled 160 women with cyclic mastodynia and compared the effects of chasteberry (Mastodynon), a progestin (lynestrenol), or placebo.[6] After four menstrual cycles, the results indicated that both chasteberry and progestin were superior to placebo.

For more information, including dosage and safety issues, see the **Chasteberry** article.

Ginkgo   + 3

One double-blind, placebo-controlled study evaluated the effect of *Ginkgo biloba* extract (80 mg twice daily) on fluid retention and other PMS symptoms over two menstrual cycles.[8] The study evaluated 143 women, 18 to 45 years of age, and observed them for two menstrual cycles. All women admitted to the study had experienced PMS-related congestive symptoms for at least three consecutive cycles. During the study, each woman received either 80 mg ginkgo extract twice daily or a placebo on day 16 of the first cycle. Treatment was continued until the fifth day of the next cycle and resumed again on day 16 of that cycle. Participants could double the dose if they felt they were experiencing inadequate relief. The results showed significant improvement in breast tenderness as well as emotional symptoms.

For more information, including dosage and safety issues, see the **Ginkgo** article.

Magnesium   +2

A double-blind, placebo-controlled study of 32 women found that magnesium (360 mg daily) taken from day 15 of the menstrual cycle to the onset of menstrual flow could significantly improve premenstrual mood changes.[9]

A 2-month, double-blind study of 38 women found that regular use of magnesium could reduce symptoms of PMS-related fluid retention.[10] The results showed no effect after one cycle, but by the end of two cycles, magnesium significantly improved weight gain, swelling of extremities, breast tenderness, and abdominal bloating. Another small double-blind study (20 participants) found that magnesium improved premenstrual symptoms and menstrual migraines.[11]

For more information, including dosage and safety issues, see the **Magnesium** article.

Multivitamin/ Mineral Supplements   +2

Small, double-blind trials have evaluated the effectiveness of a multivitamin/mineral supplement and found some evidence of benefit.[12-14] For example, a randomized, double-blind study evaluated 44 women assigned to receive a placebo or 6 or 12 tablets of the multivitamin/mineral for three menstrual cycles.[14]

The supplement produced significant improvements in PMS symptoms at both dose levels.

The combination of vitamin B_6 and magnesium might offer synergistic benefits for PMS.[15] In a double-blind, crossover trial, 44 women were given the following treatments daily for one menstrual cycle each, in random order: 200 mg magnesium, 50 mg B_6, combined magnesium and B_6, and placebo. The results showed little benefit with any treatment as compared with placebo except in one respect: combined treatment with magnesium and B_6 reduced anxiety-related symptoms.

Evening Primrose Oil (Cyclic Mastalgia)   + 2

Fatty acid metabolism is thought to be disturbed in women with cyclic mastalgia.[16] Evening primrose oil (EPO), a source of GLA (gamma-linolenic acid), may help restore normal levels of fatty acids. However, efficacy has been reported only for mastalgia and then only when significant cysts or fibroadenomas are not present.

In a randomized, double-blind, placebo-controlled, crossover study, 73 patients with cyclic or noncyclic mastalgia (with or without palpable nodularity) experienced significantly less discomfort during the 3-month treatment period with 3 g/day of EPO.[17] However, according to a 1-year, double-blind study of 200 women with cysts large enough to be aspirated, EPO was not more effective than placebo.[18,19] Lack of benefit was also seen in a small, placebo-controlled, 6-month study of 23 women with fibroadenomas.[20]

Although several small studies suggest that EPO is helpful in reducing general PMS symptoms, all suffer from serious flaws.[21]

For more information, including dosage and safety issues, see the **Gamma-Linolenic Acid** article.

Vitamin B$_6$ −1X

A dozen or so other double-blind studies have investigated the effectiveness of vitamin B$_6$ for PMS, but none were well-designed, and overall the evidence for any benefit is weak at best.[22,23] Although it is commonly stated by B$_6$ proponents that the negative results in some of these studies were due to insufficient B$_6$ dosage, in reality there was no clear link between dosage and effectiveness.

A properly designed, double-blind trial of 120 women compared three pharmaceuticals (fluoxetine, 10 mg/day; alprazolam, 0.75 mg/day; and propanolol, 20 mg/day [40 mg/day during the menstrual period]) with vitamin B$_6$ (pyridoxine, 300 mg/day) and placebo.[24] All participants received 3 months of treatment and 3 months of placebo. The best results were seen with fluoxetine; pyridoxine proved no more effective than placebo.

As noted previously, weak evidence suggests that the combination of magnesium and B$_6$ might offer some benefit in PMS.[15]

For more information, including dosage and safety issues, see the **Vitamin B$_6$** article.

Other Proposed Natural Therapies

A small (n = 18) and poorly reported, double-blind, placebo-controlled trial found weak evidence that red clover isoflavones might reduce symptoms of cyclic mastalgia.[25]

Progesterone cream, St. John's wort, vitamin E, and many other herbs and supplements are also commonly recommended for PMS, but there is no evidence that they are effective.

Drug Interactions

See the article on each individual supplement for a full description of the interactions summarized here.

Principal Natural Therapies for Premenstrual Syndrome: Interactions with Pharmaceuticals		
Natural Therapy	**Pharmaceutical**	**Interaction**
Combined high-dose calcium and vitamin D	Calcium channel blockers	Possible antagonism of drug action
	Flouroquinolones, tetracyclines	Mutual absorption interference
	Thiazides	Possible risk of hypercalcemia
Chasteberry	Prolactin inhibitors	Possible potentiation of drug action
Ginkgo	Anticoagulant and antiplatelet agents	Possible increased risk of bleeding complications
Magnesium	Amiloride	Possible hypermagnesemia
	Digitoxin, digoxin	Absorption interference
	Fluoroquinolones, tetracyclines	Mutual absorption interference
	Oral hypoglycemics	Possible potentiation of drug action leading to risk of hypoglycemia

Pharmaceuticals Used for Premenstrual Syndrome: Possible Harmful Interactions with Natural Therapies		
Pharmaceutical	**Natural Therapy**	**Interaction**
Benzodiazepines	Kava, valerian, other sedative herbs	Possible potentiation of sedative effects
Oral contraceptives	Androstenedione	Possible elevation of estrogen levels
	Copper	Possible hypercupremia
	Dong quai, St. John's wort	Possible increased risk of photosensitivity
	Licorice	Possible increased fluid retention and other side effects
	Milk thistle, St. John's wort	Possible reduced effectiveness of drug
Potassium-sparing diuretics	Arginine	Possible increased risk of hyperkalemia
	Licorice	Antagonism of drug action
	Magnesium	Risk of hypermagnesemia
	White willow	Salicylate content might interfere with spironolactone action
	Zinc	Excessive zinc levels with spironolactone
Selective serotonin reuptake inhibitors (SSRIs)	5-HTP, S-adeno-sylmethionine (SAMe), St. John's wort	Possible risk of serotonin syndrome
Thiazide diuretics	Calcium	Potential risk of hypercalcemia
	Dong quai, St. John's wort	Possible increased risk of photosensivitiy
	Licorice	Potentiation of hypo-kalemic action of drug

Pharmaceuticals Used for Premenstrual Syndrome: Natural Therapies with Potential Supportive Interactions		
Pharmaceutical	**Natural Therapy**	**Interaction**
Oral contraceptives	Magnesium, vitamin B_3, vitamin C, zinc	Correction of possible drug-induced depletion
Potassium-sparing diuretics	Folate	Correction of possible drug-induced depletion
SSRIs	Ginkgo	Possible reversal of SSRI-induced sexual dysfunction
Thiazide diuretics	Magnesium, potassium, zinc	Correction of possible drug-induced depletion

PSORIASIS

Principal Proposed
Natural Therapies

Topical *Aloe vera*   [+2]   **Fish oil**   [−2X]

Oregon grape   [+2]

(Higher numbers indicate stronger evidence; X modifier indicates contradictory results. See page xviii of the Introduction for details of the rating scale.)

Approach to the Patient

Preliminary double-blind trials suggest that topical aloe as well as topical Oregon grape may be helpful for psoriasis. However, fish oil does not appear to be effective.

Other natural treatments your patient may be using include shark cartilage; beta-carotene; burdock; chromium; *Coleus forskohlii;* fumaric acid; goldenseal; topical licorice cream; milk thistle; red clover; selenium; taurine; vitamins A, D, and E; and zinc. For potential safety risks with the more common of these substances, see the full herb/supplement articles.

In addition, many patients interested in alternative medicine believe that accumulated toxins are the cause of psoriasis and that this can be corrected through "detoxification." The latter may involve dietary changes, "colon cleansing," and specific herbs and supplements. Malnutrition can occur in the more extreme forms of this approach.

Topical *Aloe Vera*   +2

A double-blind study enrolled 60 individuals with mild to moderate symptoms of psoriasis.[1] Participants were treated with either topical aloe extract (0.5%) or placebo cream, applied three times daily for 4 weeks. Aloe treatment produced significantly better results than placebo. However, the study report lacked many essential details.

For more information, including dosage and safety issues, see the **Aloe** article.

Oregon Grape   + 2

In a double-blind, placebo-controlled, half-side trial of 82 individuals with psoriasis, participants used placebo ointment on one side and Oregon grape on the other.[2] Benefits of Oregon grape were seen in patient, but not physician, assessments. The treatment salve was darker in color than the placebo ointment, possibly breaking the blind.

Another trial (blinding not stated) found evidence that dithranol is more effective than Oregon grape.[3]

For more information, including dosage and safety issues, see the **Oregon Grape** article.

Fish Oil   − 2 X

A 4-month, double-blind, placebo-controlled study followed 145 individuals with moderate to severe psoriasis and found no benefit with oral fish oil treatment.[4]

An 8-week, double-blind, placebo-controlled study followed 28 individuals with chronic psoriasis and found modest improvement in the fish oil group in itching, redness, and scaling, but not in the size of the psoriasis patches.[5]

For more information, including dosage and safety issues, see the **Fish Oil** article.

Other Proposed Natural Therapies

Minimal preliminary evidence suggests that **shark cartilage** might be helpful for psoriasis.[6]

Although beta-carotene; burdock; chromium; *Coleus forskohlii;* fumaric acid; goldenseal; topical licorice cream; milk thistle; red clover; selenium; taurine; vitamins A, D, and E; and zinc are also mentioned as possible treatments for psoriasis, there is no real evidence supporting these treatments at this time.

Drug Interactions

See the article on each individual supplement for a full description of the interactions summarized here.

Principal Natural Therapies for Psoriasis: Interactions with Pharmaceuticals		
Natural Therapy	Pharmaceutical	Interaction
Fish oil	Anticoagulant and antiplatelet agents	Possible increased risk of bleeding complications

Pharmaceuticals Used for Psoriasis: Possible Harmful Interactions with Natural Therapies		
Pharmaceutical	Natural Therapy	Interaction
Methotrexate	Dong quai, St. John's wort	Possible increased risk of photosensitivity
	Potassium citrate	Possible decreased serum levels of drug
	White willow	Possible increased risk of methotrexate toxicity

Pharmaceuticals Used for Psoriasis: Natural Therapies with Potential Supportive Interactions		
Pharmaceutical	**Natural Therapy**	**Interaction**
Methotrexate	Folate	Side effect reduction due to correction of drug-induced relative depletion of nutrient

RAYNAUD'S PHENOMENON

Principal Proposed Natural Therapies

Essential fatty acids [+2]

Inositol hexaniacinate (vitamin B₃) [+2]

(Higher numbers indicate stronger evidence; X modifier indicates contradictory results. See page xviii of the Introduction for details of the rating scale.)

Approach to the Patient

Essential fatty acids, as well as inositol hexaniacinate, have shown some promise in the treatment of Raynaud's phenomenon, but the evidence remains highly preliminary.

Other treatments that patients may be using include ginkgo and vitamin E. For potential safety risks with these treatments, see the full herb/supplement articles.

Essential Fatty Acids   +2

In small double-blind trials, high doses of fish oil (12 g daily) have been found to reduce the severity of Raynaud's phenomenon reactions.[1,2] A small double-blind trial suggests that GLA (gamma-linolenic acid) may have an effect as well.[3]

For more information, including dosage and safety issues, see the **Fish Oil** and **Gamma-Linolenic Acid** articles.

Inositol Hexaniacinate (Vitamin B$_3$)   +2

A double-blind study of 23 patients suggests that inositol hexa-nicotinate (Hexopal, 4 g/day) may be helpful for Raynaud's phenomenon.[4] Patients in the treatment group felt subjectively better and had shorter and fewer attacks of vasospasm during the trial period compared to placebo.

For more information, including dosage and safety issues, see the **Vitamin B$_3$** article.

Other Proposed Natural Therapies

Although no direct evidence shows that **ginkgo** is helpful for Raynaud's phenomenon, it has been found to increase circulation in the fingertips[5] and reduce vascular changes during mountain climbing.[6] This suggests possible utility in Raynaud's as well.

Vitamin E is also sometimes recommended for Raynaud's phenomenon, but there is no evidence that it is effective.

Drug Interactions

See the article on each individual supplement for a full description of the interactions summarized here.

Principal Natural Therapy for Raynaud's Phenomenon: Interactions with Pharmaceuticals		
Natural Therapy	Pharmaceutical	Interaction
Fish oil	Anticoagulant and antiplatelet agents	Possible increased risk of bleeding complications

RESPIRATORY INFECTIONS (MINOR)

Principal Proposed Natural Therapies

Echinacea
(Treatment)   [+3]

Topical zinc
(Treatment)   [+3X]

Vitamin C
(Treatment)   [+3]

Andrographis (Prevention
and Treatment)   [+3]

Garlic (Prevention)   [+3]

Probiotics (Prevention)
[+3]

Ginseng (Prevention)
[+3]

(Higher numbers indicate stronger evidence; X modifier indicates contradictory results. See page xviii of the Introduction for details of the rating scale.)

Approach to the Patient

There are a number of natural supplements for the treatment or prevention of minor respiratory infections that have at least some meaningful supporting evidence.

Reasonably good evidence suggests that echinacea (especially the above-ground portion of *Echinacea purpurea*) can reduce the severity and duration of minor respiratory infections when taken at the onset of symptoms. However, contrary to popular belief, the herb appears to be ineffective for prophylaxis.

A well-designed study found that zinc nasal spray can dramatically reduce the duration of upper respiratory functions; previous studies found less dramatic but still meaningful benefit with zinc lozenges. Regular or acute use of vitamin C also appears to reduce cold severity and duration, but not incidence of colds (with the notable exception of postendurance exercise infection).

Lesser evidence supports both symptomatic and prophylactic usage of the herb andrographis, and prophylactic use of ginseng and garlic. Milk enriched with probiotic bacteria has also been found to provide some protection for children enrolled in daycare.

Other natural treatments a patient may be using include arginine, ashwagandha, astragalus, elderberry, ginger, glutamine, kelp, kudzu, maitake, marshmallow, mullein, multivitamin or multimineral supplements, osha, peppermint, reishi, selenium, suma, thymus extract, vitamin E, and yarrow. For potential safety risks with the more common of these substances, see the full herb/supplement articles.

Caution: High-risk patients may need to be advised not to rely on any natural treatment as a substitute for influenza vaccine.

Echinacea (Treatment)   +3

Numerous double-blind, placebo-controlled trials have found that acute use of echinacea can reduce the severity and duration of minor respiratory infections. However, echinacea has not been found effective for prophylaxis. The best evidence is in regard to use of the above-ground portions of *E. purpurea*, although other preparations and species have also been used.

In a double-blind trial, 246 individuals with recent onset of a respiratory infection were given either placebo or one of three *E. purpurea* preparations: two concentrations of a 95%-herb (leaves, stems, and flowers) and 5%-root combination, and one made only from the roots of the plant.[2] The results showed significant benefit in the two above-ground preparations, but not with the root-only formula.

In a double-blind, placebo-controlled study of 120 patients with acute respiratory infections, use of EchinaGuard (juice extracted from the above-ground parts of *E. purpurea* harvested during the flowering stage, also known as Echinacin and EC3IJ0) resulted in a statistically significant decrease in progression to a "real cold" in the treated group compared to the placebo group, as well as symptomatic benefit in individuals that did develop colds.[6] This included both reduced time to improvement and reduced total duration of cold. Benefits were seen with the same product in a double-blind placebo-controlled trial of 80 individuals.[7]

Another double-blind, placebo-controlled study using *E. pallida* root followed 160 adults with recent-onset URIs.[4] The results showed that treatment significantly reduced the length of illness from presumed bacterial and viral infections compared to placebo.

In a double-blind, placebo-controlled trial of 95 subjects with a new onset respiratory infection, a beverage tea containing above-ground portions of *E. purpurea* and *E. angustifolia* as well as an extract of *E. purpurea* root also has been found effective at reducing duration and severity of infection.[5]

Numerous earlier studies also found benefit, but many used a mixed formulation called Resistan that included other herbs as well as homeopathic preparations.[8]

However, studies of echinacea species for infection prophylaxis have generally failed to find statistically significant benefits.[9-13]

For more information, including dosage and safety issues, see the **Echinacea** article.

Topical Zinc (Treatment)   +3X

Zn^{2+} ions appear to inhibit rhinovirus activity by binding to viral surfaces.[14] Topical zinc acetate and gluconate release Zn^{2+} and have been found effective in the majority of studies; other chemical forms of zinc may be ineffective because of their physical chemistry properties.[15,16] The most recent trials used zinc nasal spray; previous trials used oral lozenges.

In a double-blind, placebo-controlled trial, 213 individuals with recent-onset upper respiratory infections received one inhalation of zinc gluconate or placebo nasal spray per nostril every four hours while awake.[14] The average duration of illness in treated participants was 2.3 days, compared to 9 days in the placebo group. This represents about a 75% reduction in the duration of symptoms. Another double-blind trial found no benefit; however, it used zinc sulfate (a zinc salt that has not been well evaluated) and the dose was 50 times lower.[17]

Less dramatic but still significant reduction in duration or severity of symptoms has been found in most but not all studies of zinc acetate or zinc gluconate lozenges.[15,16,18-20] Other zinc salts appear to be ineffective; in addition, flavoring agents such as citric acid and tartaric acid may impair ion availability and effectiveness.[15,16] Sorbitol, sucrose, dextrose, and mannitol appear to be acceptable, but information on the effect of glycine as a flavoring agent is equivocal.

For more information, including dosage and safety issues, see the **Zinc** article.

Vitamin C (Treatment)   +3

Numerous controlled trials of varying quality, involving a total of several thousand individuals, have found that vitamin C supplements taken at a dose of 1000 mg daily or more can very modestly reduce the duration and severity of cold symptoms.[21-23]

In most of these trials, participants received vitamin C supplements on a daily basis throughout a prolonged study period. A more recent study evaluated the effects of vitamin C use at the onset of infection and found no benefit.[1] This double-blind trial of 400 individuals with new-onset cold symptoms compared the effects of vitamin C at the following daily dosages: 0.03 g daily (placebo), 1 g, 3 g, or 3 g with bioflavanoids. Participants were instructed to take the medication at the onset of cold symptoms and for the following 2 days. The results showed no difference in the duration or severity of cold symptoms between the groups.

In general, regular use of vitamin C does not appear to offer any significant prophylactic benefit against respiratory infections.[24] However, double-blind studies involving a total of more than 200 individuals suggest that vitamin C supplements may reduce the incidence of respiratory infections following acute but not chronic endurance exercise.[25,26] In addition, vitamin C supplementation might also reduce cold incidence in individuals who are ascorbate deficient.[24]

For more information, including dosage and safety issues, see the **Vitamin C** article.

Andrographis (Prevention and Treatment)   +3

The herb andrographis may offer both symptomatic and prophylactic effects in minor respiratory infections.

Three double-blind, placebo-controlled studies enrolling a total of about 250 participants found that andrographis significantly reduces the duration and severity of cold symptoms.[27-29]

In one of these trials, 158 adults with colds received either 1200 mg daily of an andrographis extract (standardized to contain 5% andrographolide) or placebo for 4 days.[27] By day 2 of treatment, and even more by day 4, individuals given andrographis extract experienced significant improvements in symptoms compared to participants in the placebo group. The greatest response was seen in earache, sleeplessness, nasal drainage, and sore throat, but other cold symptoms improved as well.

Similar effects were seen in two double-blind, placebo-controlled studies of an herbal combination treatment containing andrographis and eleutherococcus, enrolling a total of more than 200 individuals.[30]

In a double-blind comparative study, 6 g—but not 3 g—of andrographis proved equally effective to acetaminophen in controlling cold symptoms.[31]

Finally, a 3-month, double-blind, placebo-controlled study of 107 participants found that prophylactic treatment with andrographis at the low dose of 200 mg/day significantly reduced the risk of infection.[32]

For more information, including dosage and safety issues, see the **Andrographis** article.

Garlic (Prevention)   + 3

The herb garlic has a long history of traditional use for treating or preventing colds. The first scientific evidence to support this use appeared in 2001.[3] In this 12-week, double-blind, placebo-controlled trial, 146 individuals received either placebo or a garlic extract between November and February.

Participants receiving garlic were almost two thirds less likely to develop a URI than those who received placebo. Furthermore, participants who did develop a URI recovered about 1 day faster in the garlic group compared to the placebo group.

For more information, including dosage and safety issues, see the **Garlic** article.

Probiotics (Prevention)   + 3

A double-blind, placebo-controlled trial of 571 Finnish children in daycare found that use of milk enhanced with *Lactobacillus GG* modestly but signficantly reduced the rate and severity of minor respiratory infections.[33] Other studies have found evidence that probiotics exert an immunomodulatory effect.[34,35]

Ginseng (Prevention)   + 3

A 12-week, double-blind, placebo-controlled study of 227 individuals evaluated the potential prophylactic and immunization-augmenting effects of *Panax ginseng*.[36] Four weeks into the study, all participants received influenza vaccine. The results showed a statistically significant decline in the frequency of minor respiratory infections (both colds and flus) from weeks 4 to 12 in the treated group compared to the placebo group (15 versus 42 cases). In addition, antibody titers rose to an average of 272 units in the treated group versus only 171 in the placebo group. Natural killer cell activity was twice as high in the ginseng group as in the placebo group.

For more information, including dosage and safety issues, see the **Ginseng** article.

Other Proposed Natural Therapies

There is some evidence that **vitamin E** may improve cellular immunity in the elderly, but whether this translates into an effect on colds has not been determined.[37] Preliminary clinical trials support the use of the herb **elderberry** for reducing the length and severity of flu symptoms[38]; the supplements **arginine** and **thymus extract** for cold prophylaxis[39,40]; and the supplement **glutamine** for preventing post-exercise infections.[41,42]

Use of multivitamin or multimineral supplements or supplements containing zinc and selenium alone may also help prevent infections in elderly individuals.[43-46]

Multivitamin/mineral supplements have also been tried as adjunct therapy to enhance the often inadequate response of elderly individuals to influenza vaccination. Some evidence suggests that combined multivitamin/mineral supplements before vaccination may increase rate of seroconversion and elevate antibody titres.[44,47] However, in one trial, a multivitamin tablet without minerals actually decreased participants' responses to the vaccine.[48]

Various herbs are said to work like ginseng and enhance immunity over the long term, including ashwagandha, astragalus, garlic, maitake, reishi, and suma. However, there is as yet no good evidence that they really work.

Other herbs, including ginger, kudzu, osha, and yarrow, are said to help avert colds when taken at the first sign of infection; but again, there is no scientific evidence that they are effective. Herbs sometimes recommended to reduce cold symptoms include marshmallow, mullein, and peppermint.

Drug Interactions

See the article on each individual supplement for a full description of the interactions summarized here.

Principal Natural Therapies for Minor Respiratory Infections: Interactions with Pharmaceuticals

Natural Therapy	Pharmaceutical	Interaction
Echinacea	Immune suppressants	Theoretical antagonism of drug action
Panax ginseng	Hypoglycemic agents	Possible hypoglycemia
	MAOIs	Tyramine-like syndrome (but might be due to ginseng contamination with caffeine)
	Warfarin	Possible antagonism of drug action
Vitamin C	Acetaminophen	Possible increased serum levels of drug
	Anticoagulants	Possible antagonism of drug action
	Iron supplements	Increased iron absorption
	Warfarin-related anticoagulants	Possible antagonism of drug action
Zinc	Amiloride	Possible elevated serum zinc
	Fluoroquinolones, penicillamine, tetracyclines	Mutual absorption interference

Pharmaceutical Used for Minor Respiratory Infections: Possible Harmful Interactions with Natural Therapies

Pharmaceutical	Natural Therapy	Interaction
Pseudoephedrine	Ephedra (ma huang)	Potentiation of effects and side effects

RESTLESS LEGS SYNDROME

Principal Proposed Natural Therapies

Iron [−1]

(Higher numbers indicate stronger evidence; X modifier indicates contradictory results. See page xviii of the Introduction for details of the rating scale.)

Approach to the Patient

Highly preliminary evidence suggests that symptoms of restless legs syndrome (RLS) may be relieved by supplementation with iron.

Other treatments a patient may be using include folate, magnesium, and vitamins B_6, C, and E. For potential safety risks with the more common of these substances, see the full herb/supplement articles.

Iron −1

A number of studies have linked RLS to low iron stores.[1] In one analysis of the medical records of 27 individuals with RLS, those with the most severe symptoms had lower-than-average levels of serum ferritin.[2] In a case-control study, RLS was again associated with reduced serum ferritin, and iron supplementation appeared to improve symptoms.[3]

However, a double-blind study of 28 individuals with RLS found iron ineffective for individuals with normal iron stores.[4]

For more information, including dosage and safety issues, see the **Iron** article.

Other Proposed Natural Therapies

Based on numerous case reports and one open trial, high-dose **folate** (5 to 30 mg daily) is sometimes recommended for RLS. Folate may be of particular benefit to pregnant women with RLS who are folate deficient.[1]

Preliminary evidence suggests that supplemental **magnesium** might be helpful for RLS, even when magnesium levels are normal.[5,6]

Vitamin E has also been tried for RLS at a dose of 400 to 800 IU daily.[7] Other anecdotal reports suggest that **vitamin C** and **vitamin B$_6$** may be useful.[1,8]

Drug Interactions

See the article on each individual supplement for a full description of the interactions summarized here.

Principal Natural Therapy for Restless Legs Syndrome: Interactions with Pharmaceuticals		
Natural Therapy	Pharmaceutical	Interaction
Iron	ACE inhibitors, levodopa or levodopa-carbidopa, methyldopa, penicillamine, tetracyclines, quinolones, thyroid hormone	Absorption interference

Pharmaceuticals Used for Restless Legs Syndrome: Possible Harmful Interactions with Natural Therapies		
Pharmaceutical	**Natural Therapy**	**Interaction**
Levodopa-carbidopa	5-HTP	Possible increased risk of scleroderma-like syndrome
Levodopa or levodopa-carbidopa	Iron	Absorption interference
	Kava	Possible antagonism of drug action
	Vitamin B_6	Impairs effectiveness of levodopa taken alone, but does not interact with levodopa/carbidopa combination

RHEUMATOID ARTHRITIS

Principal Proposed Natural Therapies

Fish oil [+3]

Gamma-linolenic acid (GLA) [+2]

Devil's claw [+2]

Boswellia [+2X]

Selenium [−1X]

(Higher numbers indicate stronger evidence; X modifier indicates contradictory results. See page xviii of the Introduction for details of the rating scale.)

Approach to the Patient

Although no natural treatment for rheumatoid arthritis (RA) has been found to have disease-modifying effects, evidence suggests that omega-3 fatty acids from fish oil supplements can produce modest symptomatic improvements. Omega-6 fatty acids may be helpful as well. Weaker evidence supports the use of the herbs devil's claw and boswellia. Low selenium status may be a risk factor for RA, but selenium supplements have not been shown effective.

Other natural treatments your patient may be using include curcumin (or turmeric), gamma-linolenic acid (GLA), MSM (methyl sulfonyl methane), *Tripterygium wilfordii*, vitamin E, yucca, and zinc. Numerous other treatments are sometimes recommended as well, including beta-carotene, betaine hydrochloride, boron, burdock, cat's claw, cayenne, chamomile, Chinese herbal combinations, copper, feverfew, folate, ginger, L-histidine, horsetail, magnesium, manganese, molybdenum, pantothenic acid, D-phenylalanine, pregnenolone, proteolytic enzymes, sea cucumber, vitamin C, and white willow. For potential safety risks with the more common of these substances, see the full herb/supplement articles.

Caution: Note that herbs with immune stimulant properties might be contraindicated in RA. This category includes andrographis, echinacea, *Eleutherococcus*, and *Panax ginseng*.

Fish Oil   +3

Thirteen double-blind, placebo-controlled studies involving a total of more than 500 individuals found that the omega-3 fatty acids in fish oil can reduce the symptoms of rheumatoid arthritis.[1,2] However, unlike DMARDs (disease-modifying antirheumatic drugs), fish oil is not thought to slow disease progression.

For more information, including dosage and safety issues, see the **Fish Oil** article.

Gamma-Linolenic Acid (GLA)   +2

GLA, an omega-6 fatty acid found in evening primrose, borage, and currant oils, may be a useful adjunct therapy for RA.

In a double-blind study of 56 patients with RA, 16 of 21 patients treated with GLA for 1 year significantly improved compared to those in the placebo group.[3] This study used very high doses of purified GLA (2.8 g/day, equivalent to about 30 g of EPO daily). Benefits also were seen in other small trials.[4-8]

Devil's Claw   +2

A 2-month, double-blind, placebo-controlled study of devil's claw followed 89 individuals with various rheumatoid disorders and found a significant decrease in joint pain intensity and an improvement in mobility.[9] Another double-blind study of devil's claw in 50 individuals with various types of arthritis showed that 10-day treatment provided significant pain relief.[9]

For more information, including dosage and safety issues, see the **Devil's Claw** article.

Boswellia   + 2 X

According to a review of unpublished studies, preliminary double-blind trials have found boswellia effective in relieving the symptoms of rheumatoid arthritis.[10] However, the information given in this review was insufficient to evaluate the quality of the primary research.

A double-blind placebo-controlled study that enrolled 78 patients found no benefit of boswellia treatment.[11] However, about one half of the patients dropped out, which diminishes the significance of the results.

Other preliminary research has suggested that boswellia may protect cartilage from damage.[12]

For more information, including dosage and safety issues, see the **Boswellia** article.

Selenium   − 1 X

Lower-than-average selenium levels have been found in individuals with rheumatoid arthritis,[13,14] and low selenium status appears to be a risk factor for RH factor–negative RA.[15] However, no improvement was seen in a double-blind study in which 40 patients with severe RA were given placebo or 256 μg of selenium in enriched yeast for 6 months.[13,14] Another double-blind study followed 55 individuals for 90 days and again found no significant improvements attributable to selenium.[29] Similarly negative results were seen in two other small trials.[30,31] Some benefit was seen in a very small double-blind study of mild RA.[16]

For more information, including dosage and safety issues, see the **Selenium** article.

Other Proposed
Natural Therapies

Zinc has yielded mixed results in preliminary trials.[17-19]

Vitamin E might reduce pain in RA, although it does not appear to alter the inflammatory process.[20] In addition, adequate vitamin E intake in general may reduce the risk of developing RA.[15] Preliminary evidence suggests that adjuvant treatment with vitamin E alone or with other antioxidants might improve the results of standard therapy.[21]

Preliminary double-blind trials provide some evidence for benefit with *T. wilfordii*[22] and the herb **yucca.**[23]

Very weak evidence suggests that the supplement **MSM** might be helpful.[24]

A small, double-blind, crossover trial of patients with RA found greater benefits with phenylbutazone than **curcumin.**[25]

Preliminary evidence suggests that a mixture of **poplar, ash,** and **goldenrod** might be helpful for rheumatoid arthritis and related conditions.[26] A 16-week, double-blind, placebo-controlled trial of 182 individuals with active RA evaluated a combination herbal treatment containing **ashwagandha, boswellia, ginger,** and **turmeric,** and found that the herbal treatment was no more effective than placebo in nearly all measurements of disease severity.[27]

Although oral **collagen** has been recommended for the treatment of RA, a small, double-blind, placebo-controlled trial found it ineffective.[28]

The following treatments are also sometimes recommended for RA, but there is as yet little scientific evidence to support them: beta-carotene, betaine hydrochloride, boron, burdock, cat's claw, cayenne, chamomile, Chinese herbal combinations, copper, feverfew, folate, ginger, L-histidine, horsetail, magnesium, manganese, molybdenum, pantothenic acid, D-phenylalanine, pregnenolone, proteolytic enzymes, sea cucumber, vitamin C, and white willow.

Drug Interactions

See the article on each individual supplement for a full description of the interactions summarized here.

Principal Natural Therapies for Rheumatoid Arthritis: Interactions with Pharmaceuticals		
Natural Therapy	Pharmaceutical	Interaction
Fish oil	Anticoagulants	Possible increased risk of bleeding complications
Devil's claw	Anticoagulant or antiplatelet agents	Possible increased risk of bleeding complications

Pharmaceuticals Used for Rheumatoid Arthritis: Possible Harmful Interactions with Natural Therapies		
Pharmaceutical	Natural Therapy	Interaction
Corticosteroids	Licorice	Increased potentiation of action
Methotrexate	Dong quai, St. John's wort	Possible increased risk of photosensitivity
	Potassium citrate	Possible decreased serum levels of drug
	White willow	Possible increased risk of methotrexate toxicity
NSAIDs	Dong quai, St. John's wort	Possible increased risk of photosensitivity

Continued

Pharmaceuticals Used for Rheumatoid Arthritis: Possible Harmful Interactions with Natural Therapies—cont'd

Pharmaceutical	Natural Therapy	Interaction
NSAIDs—cont'd	Feverfew	Possible increased risk of gastritis
	Garlic, ginkgo, high-dose vitamin E, policosanol, others	Possible increased risk of bleeding complications
	White willow	Additional salicylates may increase risk of all side effects
	Potassium citrate	Possible decreased serum levels of salicylates
Penicillamine	Iron, magnesium	Mutual absorption interference

Pharmaceuticals Used for Rheumatoid Arthritis: Natural Therapies with Potential Supportive Interactions

Pharmaceutical	Natural Therapy	Interaction
Corticosteroids	Chromium	Counter corticosteroid-induced diabetes
Methotrexate	Folate	Side-effect reduction due to correction of drug-induced relative depletion of nutrient
NSAIDs	Cayenne, colostrum, licorice	Possible cytoprotection
	Folate, vitamin C	Correction of possible drug-induced deficiency
Penicillamine	Vitamin B_6	Possible correction of drug-induced deficiency

SEXUAL DYSFUNCTION IN WOMEN

Principal Proposed Natural Therapies

Dehydroepiandrosterone (DHEA) **[+2X]**

Ginkgo [+1]

Combination therapies [+2]

(Higher numbers indicate stronger evidence; X modifier indicates contradictory results. See page xviii of the Introduction for details of the rating scale.)

Approach to the Patient

Although there are no well-established treatments for sexual dysfunction in women, there is some evidence that DHEA (dehydroepiandrosterone) may be helpful for the condition in women over 70, as well as in women with adrenal failure.

One promising double-blind trial suggests benefit with a combination therapy containing arginine. There is also some evidence that a combination of yohimbine (a constituent of the herb yohimbe) and arginine might be helpful; however, batches of yohimbe may not be well standardized to yohimbine content and could provide dangerous levels of the drug.

Ginkgo biloba may be helpful for sexual dysfunction induced by SSRIs, but there have not been any blinded trials to evaluate this potential use.

Your patient may have encountered numerous other products on the marketplace, each of which misleadingly claims to have meaningful supporting evidence as treatment for sexual dysfunction. It may be worth explaining that in vitro studies (best described to patients as "test tube studies"), as well as preliminary animal trials, mean little.

DHEA   +2X

A 12-month, double-blind, placebo-controlled trial evaluated the effects of DHEA (50 mg daily) in 280 individuals between the ages of 60 and 79.[1] The results showed that women over 70 years old experienced an improvement in libido and sexual satisfaction. Other participants did not experience benefit. Effects were not seen until the sixth month, which may explain why other trials that only lasted 3 months did not find any effect of DHEA.[2,3]

One 4-month, double-blind, placebo-controlled study of 24 women with adrenal failure found that 50 mg per day of DHEA (along with standard replacement therapy for adrenal failure) improved libido and sexual satisfaction.[4]

In addition, two small, double-blind, placebo-controlled studies tested whether a one-time dose of DHEA at 300 mg could increase sexual arousability in pre- or postmenopausal women, respectively.[11,12] The results again indicate that DHEA is effective for older women but not for younger women.

For more information, including dosage and safety issues, see the **Dehydroepiandrosterone** article.

Combination Therapies   +2

A double-blind, placebo-controlled trial of 77 women (age 22 to 71 years) complaining of low libido tested a combination therapy (ArginMax) containing **L-arginine, ginseng, ginkgo, damiana, multivitamins,** and **minerals.**[9] The results over 4 weeks showed statistically significant improvements in numerous sexual rating scores in the verum as opposed to the placebo group, including improved sexual desire and frequency of intercourse.

A small double-blind study of **yohimbine combined with arginine** found an increase in measured physical arousal among 23 women with female sexual arousal disorder.[10] However, the women themselves did not report any noticeable effects. Only the combination of yohimbine and arginine produced results; neither substance was effective when taken on its own.

Ginkgo   +1

Numerous case reports and open trials suggest that *Gingko biloba* may be an effective treatment for antidepressant-induced sexual dysfunction in women (as well as in men).[5-8] One open trial failed to find benefit, but it used a nonstandard form of the herb that does not closely resemble typical ginkgo extract products.[13] However, in the absence of double-blind trials, it is quite possible that the reported benefits are due to the placebo and related effects.

For more information, including dosage and safety issues, see the **Ginkgo** article.

Other Proposed Natural Therapies

Other herbs and supplements reputed to be helpful for female sexual dysfunction and commonly used in products marketed for this purpose include abuta, ashwagandha, catuaba bark, chuchuhuasi bark, codonopsis, damiana, *Eurycoma longifolia*, gamma-linolenic acid, *Lepidium sativum*, lipoic acid, maca (horny goat weed), *Muira puama*, *Pimpinella pruacen*, royal jelly, saw palmetto, schisandra, suma, and *Tribulus terrestris*.

Drug Interactions

See the article on each individual supplement for a full description of the interactions summarized here.

Principal Natural Therapy for Sexual Dysfunction in Women: Interactions with Pharmaceuticals		
Natural Therapy	Pharmaceutical	Interaction
Ginkgo	Anticoagulant and antiplatelet agents	Possible increased risk of bleeding complications

SUNBURN

Principal Proposed
Natural Therapies

Vitamins E and C   [+2]   **Beta-carotene**   [+2X]

Green tea/EGCG   [+2]

(Higher numbers indicate stronger evidence; X modifier indicates contradictory results. See page xviii of the Introduction for details of the rating scale.)

Approach to the Patient

Because free radicals play a role in sunburn, various oral and topical antioxidants have been tried as preventives; however, the results have not been impressive. Patients can be advised that antioxidants are no substitute for sunblock.

Although topical aloe is popular as a treatment for acute sunburn, there is no evidence that it is effective. Other natural treatments the patient may be using include jojoba and poplar bud.

Vitamins E and C   +2

In several animal studies, topical vitamins E and C reduced ultraviolet damage.[1-4] According to one of these, topical vitamin E was most effective against UVB and topical vitamin C was most active against UVA; combined, the two vitamins offered enhanced effects and also potentiated the effects of sunscreen.[4] In another study, vitamin E produced significant benefits even when applied to mouse skin 8 hours after UV exposure.[2]

Evidence from preliminary double-blind trials suggests that oral use of combined vitamin C (2 to 3 g daily) and E (1 to 2 g daily) may be beneficial as well, perhaps offering benefits equivalent to a sun protection factor of 2.[5,6] However, oral vitamin E or C alone appears ineffective.[6,7]

A small double-blind, placebo-controlled trial suggests that a face cream containing vitamin C improves the appearance of sun-damaged skin.[8]

For more information, including dosage and safety issues, see the **Vitamin E** and **Vitamin C** articles.

Green Tea/EGCG   +2

Epigallocatechin gallate (EGCG), found in green tea, has antioxidant effects. According to several studies, mice given oral or topical green tea were protected against skin inflammation and carcinogenesis caused by exposure to UVB.[9,10] In one controlled human study (blinding and number of participants not stated), topical EGCG (3 mg per square inch) decreased skin inflammation following UVB radiation exposure.[10]

For more information, including dosage and safety issues, see the **Green Tea** article.

Beta-Carotene   +2X

Results with beta-carotene have been mixed. In a double-blind trial, 20 young women were given 30 mg daily of beta-carotene or placebo for 10 weeks before a 13-day stretch of controlled sun exposure at a sea-level vacation spot.[11] Those who had taken the beta-carotene before and during the sun exposure experienced less skin redness than those taking placebo, even when both groups used sunscreen.

Another 10-week study found that high doses of beta-carotene produced only very minor (though statistically significant) protection against sunburn among 30 men exposed to natural sunshine compared to placebo.[12] The study authors didn't feel this small improvement was enough to warrant using beta-carotene to prevent sunburn.

However, in a double-blind trial of 16 older women, beta-carotene taken for 23 days didn't provide any more protection than placebo against simulated sun exposure.[13]

For more information, including dosage and safety issues, see the **Beta-Carotene** article.

Other Proposed Natural Therapies

Despite its popularity, **aloe** does not appear to be helpful for treating sunburn.[14]

Topical jojoba and poplar bud are also sometimes recommended for soothing sunburn pain and itch.

Drug Interactions

See the article on each individual supplement for a full description of the interactions summarized here.

Principal Natural Therapies for Sunburn: Interactions with Pharmaceuticals		
Natural Therapy	Pharmaceutical	Interaction
Green tea	Warfarin	Antagonism of drug action due to vitamin K content
Vitamin C	Acetaminophen	Possible increased serum levels of drug
	Anticoagulants	Possible antagonism of drug action
	Iron supplements	Increased iron absorption
	Warfarin-related anticoagulants	Possible antagonism of drug action
Vitamin E	Anticoagulant and antiplatelet agents	Possible increased risk of bleeding complications

SURGERY SUPPORT

Edema, Lymphedema, Hematoma

Proteolytic enzymes   [+3X]

Oxerutins and other bioflavonoids   [+2]

OPCs   [+2]

Nausea

Ginger   [+3X]

Perioperative Anxiety

Melatonin   [+2]

(Higher numbers indicate stronger evidence; X modifier indicates contradictory results. See page xviii of the Introduction for details of the rating scale.)

Approach to Patient

A number of relatively well-documented natural treatments might be useful for surgery patients.

Proteolytic enzymes (such as bromelain) may help for controlling postoperative inflammation, pain, bruising, and edema. Oxerutins and the citrus bioflavonoid combination diosmin/hesperidin may be helpful for chronic lymphedema as well as for ordinary postoperative edema. Ginger has also been investigated for reducing postoperative nausea, but the most recent trials have found no benefit.

Melatonin has shown promise for reducing perioperative anxiety.

Other natural treatments the patient may be using include bee propolis and horse chestnut.

Caution: Ask the patient about use of herbs and supplements that may possess anticoagulant or antiplatelet effects (see Herbs and Supplements to Avoid). These might increase perioperative bleeding.

Contrary to popular belief, topically applied aloe vera might impair wound healing.[1] See the **Injuries (Minor)** article for other natural treatments a patient might be considering.

Edema, Lymphedema, Hematoma

Proteolytic Enzymes   +3X

Although generally thought of as digestive aids, various proteolytic enzymes are absorbed systemically and may help reduce pain, inflammation, edema, and bruising after surgery.

A double-blind, placebo-controlled study evaluated 160 women postepisiotomy.[2] Participants given 40 mg of bromelain four times daily for 3 days, beginning 4 hours after delivery, showed statistically and clinically significant decreases in edema, inflammation, and pain. However, a similar double-blind study of 158 women failed to find significant benefit.[3]

Another double-blind study used the proteolytic enzyme combination Chymoral in 204 episiotomy patients and found benefit.[4]

Chymoral was also found effective for reducing inflammation in a double-blind, placebo-controlled trial involving 102 surgical removals of impacted wisdom teeth[5] and in a double-blind, placebo-controlled trial of 86 individuals undergoing podiatric surgery.[32] Bromelain showed efficacy at reducing bruising in a controlled study of 53 individuals undergoing nasal surgery.[6] Also, in a double-blind, controlled trial, 95 patients undergoing treatment for cataracts were given 40 mg of bromelain or placebo (along with other treatments) four times daily for 2 days prior to surgery and 5 days postoperatively.[7] The results showed reduced pain and inflammation in the treated group compared to the placebo group.

Benefits were also seen with bromelain in a small double-blind, placebo-controlled, crossover study of individuals undergoing dental surgery.[8] However, no significant benefits were seen in a double-blind, placebo-controlled trial of 154 individuals undergoing plastic surgery of the face.[9]

A proprietary enzyme mixture called Wobenzym (containing pancreatin, papain, bromelain, trypsin, and chymotrypsin, as well as lipase, amylase, and rutin) has also been studied. In a double-blind, placebo-controlled trial involving 80 individuals, treatment with Wobenzym after knee surgery significantly improved the rate of recovery as measured by mobility and swelling.[10] Another double-blind, placebo-controlled trial evaluated the effects of the same enzyme combination in 80 oral surgery patients and also found benefits.[11]

For more information, including dosage and safety issues, see the **Bromelain** and **Proteolytic Enzymes** articles.

Oxerutins and Other Bioflavonoids +2

Natural and synthetic bioflavonoids have been widely used in Europe since the mid-1960s as capillary stabilizers. They have been best investigated as treatments for chronic venous insufficiency but have also been studied for their utility for sports injuries, other minor injuries, hemorrhoids, and surgical support.

Three double-blind, placebo-controlled studies enrolling a total of more than 100 individuals examined the effectiveness of oxerutins in lymphedema following breast cancer surgery.[12-14] In one of these, a 6-month trial, oxerutins proved significantly more effective than placebo in reducing swelling, aiding comfort and mobility, and improving other measures of lymphedema.[14] Two smaller studies also found oxerutins to be more effective than placebo,[12,13] but the researchers were not sure that the improvement was clinically meaningful. In contrast, others who have investigated oxerutins for lymphedema say that this treatment "convert[s] a slowly worsening condition into a slowly improving one."[15]

The citrus bioflavonoid combination diosmin/hesperidin has also been tried in lymphedema, but the results have been less promising.[16]

In addition, oxerutins have been investigated for ordinary post-operative edema. In a double-blind trial with 40 individuals given either oxerutins or placebo for 5 days following minor surgery or other minor injuries, the results showed significant reductions in edema and discomfort.[17]

For more information, including dosage and safety issues, see the **Oxerutins** and **Diosmin/Hesperidin** articles.

OPCs   +2

Oligomeric proanthocyanidin complexes (OPCs) may be helpful for recovery from surgery as well. Like bioflavonoids, OPCs are thought to work by reducing capillary leakage.

A double-blind, placebo-controlled trial involving 63 women found that 600 mg of OPCs daily for 6 months reduced post-mastectomy lymphedema.[19] Additionally, in a double-blind, placebo-controlled study of 32 individuals who were followed for 10 days after cosmetic facial surgery, swelling disappeared more rapidly in the treated group.[19]

For more information, including dosage and safety issues, see the **OPCs** article.

Nausea

Ginger   +3X

Studies evaluating ginger as a treatment for postoperative nausea have returned conflicting results, with the more recent trials failing to find benefit.

A double-blind British study compared the effects of ginger, placebo, and the drug metoclopramide (Reglan) in the treatment of nausea following gynecological surgery.[21] The results in 60 women showed that both treatments produced similar benefits compared to placebo.

A similar British study followed 120 gynecological surgery patients.[21] Whereas nausea and vomiting developed in 41% of participants given placebo, these symptoms developed in only 21% of those treated with ginger and 27% of those treated with metoclopramide.

However, one double-blind study of 108 women and another of 120 women undergoing similar surgery found no benefit of ginger over placebo.[22,23] The explanation for these contradictory results is not known but may be due to different sources of ginger.

For more information, including dosage and safety issues, see the **Ginger** article.

Perioperative Anxiety

Melatonin   +2

In a randomized, double-blind, placebo-controlled study of perioperative effects of premedication in 75 women, patients who received either 15 mg of midazolam or 5 mg of melatonin had a significant decrease in anxiety levels before and after surgery compared to placebo.[24] Except for greater preoperative sedation in the midazolam group, the two treatments were equally effective.

Similar results were seen in a subsequent double-blind trial observing 84 women conducted by the same researcher.[25]

For more information, including dosage and safety issues, see the **Melatonin** article.

Other Proposed
Natural Therapies

Numerous studies have evaluated the relative benefits of various enteral formulation for improving surgical outcomes in high-risk patients. These are beyond the scope of this text. However, an oral supplement containing **arginine, fish oil,** and **yeast RNA** has also been tried for this purpose. In a double-blind, placebo-controlled study, 50 high-risk individuals scheduled to receive coronary artery bypass surgery were given either a placebo liquid nutrient supplement or one enriched with arginine, fish oil, and yeast RNA.[26] Supplementation began 5 to 10 days before surgery and was continued subsequently. The results showed improved measures of immune function in the treated group compared to the placebo group, as well as reduced rate of postoperative infection, improved central and peripheral circulation, and better preservation of renal function.

A highly preliminary placebo-controlled study found that a mouthwash containing the honeybee product **propolis** significantly shortened healing time following oral surgery.[27]

Like OPCs, extracts of **horse chestnut** are sometimes recommended to help reduce swelling after sprains, other athletic injuries, and surgery, based on the known effects of horse chestnut on blood vessels. There is some evidence that these extracts may be effective.[28]

Herbs and Supplements to Avoid

Garlic possesses significant anticoagulant effects, and case reports suggest that it can increase bleeding during or after surgery.[29-31] Because of inadequate data on active ingredients and their half-lives, it is probably reasonably advisable to recommend that patients avoid garlic supplementation for a week prior to surgery and that they not take garlic supplements until the risk of bleeding is past.

In one case report, use of saw palmetto was associated with significantly increased bleeding time and intraoperative hemorrage.[33] PT and PTT were unchanged.

Many other herbs and supplements might increase risk of bleeding, including most prominently ginkgo, policosanol, white willow, and high-dose vitamin E, but also potentially chamomile, devil's claw, fish oil, mesoglycans, papaya, red clover, and reishi, to name only a few. Interestingly, many of the treatments described above for reducing complications of surgery may also possess mild anticoagulant effects.

Drug Interactions

See the article on each individual supplement for a full description of the interactions summarized here.

Principal Natural Therapies for Surgery Support: Interactions with Pharmaceuticals		
Natural Therapy	Pharmaceutical	Interaction
Bioflavonoids, bromelain, ginger	Anticoagulant and antiplatelet agents	Possible increased risk of bleeding complications

Pharmaceuticals Used for Surgery Support: Possible Harmful Interactions with Natural Therapies		
Pharmaceutical	**Natural Therapy**	**Interaction**
Anesthetics and induction agents	Many herbs	Undefined potential interactions

SYSTEMIC LUPUS ERYTHEMATOSUS

Principal Proposed Natural Therapies

DHEA [+3]

Flaxseed (lupus nephritis) [+1]

Fish oil

  overall symptoms [+1]

  lupus nephritis [−1]

Alfalfa (contraindicated)

(Higher numbers indicate stronger evidence; X modifier indicates contradictory results. See page xviii of the Introduction for details of the rating scale.)

Approach to the Patient

Increasingly strong evidence suggests that the hormone dehydroepiandrosterone (DHEA), when used as a part of a comprehensive, physician-directed treatment approach, may be of significant therapeutic utility in systemic lupus erythematosus (SLE). Essential fatty acids, such as those in flaxseed or fish oil, also might offer some benefits.

Other natural treatments a patient may be using include beta-carotene, magnesium, pantothenic acid, selenium, and vitamins B_3, B_{12}, and E. For potential safety risks with the more common of these substances, see the full herb/supplement articles.

Caution: Herbs with putative immunomodulatory effects may be contraindicated in autoimmune diseases. This category includes most prominently andrographis, echinacea, eleutherococcus, and *Panax ginseng*.

DHEA   +3

DHEA appears to improve lupus symptoms and may allow a reduction in corticosteroid dosage.

A 12-month, double-blind, placebo-controlled trial of 381 women with mild or moderate lupus evaluated the effects of DHEA at a dose of 200 mg daily.[1] Although many participants in both groups improved, DHEA was more effective than placebo in overall assessments of disease activity. Similarly positive results were seen in earlier small studies.[2,3]

For more information, including dosage and safety issues, see the **DHEA** article.

Flaxseed (Lupus Nephritis)   +1

Flaxseed, a source of lignans and alpha-linolenic acid, may antagonize the activity of platelet-activating factor (PAF). Because PAF is thought to play a role in lupus nephritis, flaxseed has been investigated for the treatment or prevention of this condition, with some promising results in preliminary animal trials.[4,5]

For more information, including dosage and safety issues, see the **Flaxseed** article.

Fish Oil: Overall Symptoms   +1, Lupus Nephritis   −1

Fish oil does not appear to be helpful for lupus nephritis.[6,7] However, based on its benefits in rheumatoid arthritis, fish oil has been tried for the treatment of overall SLE symptoms, with some success in a very small double-blind trial.[8]

For more information, including dosage and safety issues, see the **Fish Oil** article.

Other Proposed Natural Therapies

Other natural treatments sometimes recommended for SLE include beta-carotene, magnesium, pantothenic acid, selenium, and vitamins B_3, B_{12}, and E. However, there is no real supporting evidence for any of these approaches.

Alfalfa: Contraindicated

The herb alfalfa contains a substance called L-canavanine, which can worsen SLE or bring it out of remission.[9,10]

Drug Interactions

See the article on each individual supplement for a full description of the interactions summarized here.

Principal Natural Therapies for Systemic Lupus Erythematosus: Interactions with Pharmaceuticals		
Natural Therapy	Pharmaceutical	Interaction
Fish oil	Anticoagulant and antiplatelet agents	Possible increased risk of bleeding complications

Pharmaceuticals Used for Systemic Lupus Erythematosus: Possible Harmful Interactions with Natural Therapies		
Pharmaceutical	**Natural Therapy**	**Interaction**
Corticosteroids	Licorice	Increased potentiation of action
Methotrexate	Dong quai, St. John's wort	Possible increased risk of photosensitivity
	Potassium citrate	Possible decreased serum levels of drug
	White willow	Possible increased risk of methotrexate toxicity

Pharmaceuticals Used for Systemic Lupus Erythematosus: Natural Therapies with Potential Supportive Interactions		
Pharmaceutical	**Natural Therapy**	**Interaction**
Corticosteroids	Combined high-dose calcium and vitamin D, ipriflavone	Counter corticosteroid-induced osteoporosis
	Chromium	Counter corticosteroid-induced diabetes
Methotrexate	Folate	Side-effect reduction due to correction of drug-induced relative depletion of nutrient

TARDIVE DYSKINESIA

Principal Proposed Natural Therapies

Vitamin E [−2X]

Choline and related substances [−2X]

(Higher numbers indicate stronger evidence; X modifier indicates contradictory results. See page xviii of the Introduction for details of the rating scale.)

Approach to the Patient

Based on a free radical hypothesis of tardive dyskinesia (TD), vitamin E has been evaluated for both prevention and treatment of the disease with mixed results; the largest and best designed study found no benefit. However, vitamin E might be effective in a subgroup of TD patients.

Supplements thought to increase acetylcholine/dopamine ratios have not proved effective in TD treatment.

Other natural treatments the patient may be using include BCAAs (branched-chain amino acids), essential fatty acids, manganese, melatonin, niacin, and vitamins B_6 and C. For potential safety risks with the more common of these substances, see the full herb/supplement articles.

Caution: Evidence suggests that the amino acid phenylalanine might increase the risk of developing TD or increase the severity of symptoms in existing TD.[1-3]

Vitamin E   − 2 X

A double-blind, placebo-controlled trial of 107 individuals with TD evaluated the effectiveness of 1600 IU of vitamin E given for at least 1 year and found no benefit.[4] However, previous smaller trials in aggregate found evidence that vitamin E might be helpful in individuals with mild or shorter-term TD.[5]

For more information, including dosage and safety issues, see the **Vitamin E** article.

Choline and Related Substances   − 2 X

According to one theory, TD symptoms may be caused by an imbalance between dopamine and acetylcholine. The nutrient choline and several related substances—lecithin, CDP-choline, and DMAE (2-dimethylaminoethanol, also called deanol)—have been suggested as possible treatments in the belief that they might raise acetylcholine levels.

However, the results of small double-blind trials of lecithin and choline are conflicting at best,[6-10] and CDP-choline failed to prove effective in one small trial.[11] The evidence for DMAE is predominantly negative: of 12 double-blind studies reviewed, only one found DMAE to be significantly effective compared to placebo.[12]

Other Proposed Natural Therapies

A 6-week, double-blind, placebo-controlled study of 22 individuals with schizophrenia and TD found that **melatonin** at a dose of 10 mg/day significantly improved TD symptoms.[24]

Highly preliminary evidence suggests that **BCAAs** might decrease TD symptoms.[13] Other proposed treatments include **niacin**,[14] **manganese**,[14] **vitamin B$_6$**,[15-18] and **essential fatty acids**,[19-21] but so far the evidence for their effectiveness is very weak. Two double-blind trials of **GLA** (as evening primrose oil) found that it was not significantly more effective than placebo at reducing TD.[22]

It is sometimes stated that high doses of various **vitamins** can prevent TD, but this belief is based only on an informal and uncontrolled case series.[23] **Melatonin** at 2 mg/day was found ineffective for TD in a small 4-week, double-blind trial.[24]

Drug Interactions

See the article on each individual supplement for a full description of the interactions summarized here.

Principal Natural Therapy for Tardive Dyskinesia: Interactions with Pharmaceuticals		
Natural Therapy	Pharmaceutical	Interaction
Vitamin E	Anticoagulant and antiplatelet agents	Possible increased risk of bleeding complications

Pharmaceuticals Used for Tardive Dyskinesia: Possible Harmful Interactions with Natural Therapies		
Pharmaceutical	**Natural Therapy**	**Interaction**
Levodopa or levodopa-carbidopa	BCAAs, methionine, phenylalanine, threonine, other amino acids	Possible impaired action of drug based on amino acid/ levodopa interaction
	Iron	Absorption interference
	Kava	Possible antagonism of drug action
	Octacosanol/ policosanol	Possible potentiation of dyskinesia side effect
	SAMe	Possible increase of "wearing off" effect
	Vitamin B_6	Impairs effectiveness of levodopa taken alone but does not interact with levodopa-carbidopa combination

TINEA PEDIS

Principal Proposed
Natural Therapies

Tea Tree Oil [+2]

(Higher numbers indicate stronger evidence; X modifier indicates contradictory results. See page xviii of the Introduction for details of the rating scale.)

Approach to the Patient

Tea tree oil has well-established antifungal properties. One double-blind trial suggests topical usage may be effective for tinea pedis, although to a lesser degree than tolnaftate.

Other natural treatments the patient may be using include raw garlic, oil of bitter orange, and other essential oils such as peppermint and eucalyptus.

Tea Tree Oil   +2

Tea tree oil has a long traditional use in Australia for the treatment of skin infections and other infections. This use is supported by evidence that tea tree oil is an effective antiseptic, active against many bacteria and fungi.[1,2]

A 4-week, double-blind, placebo-controlled trial of 104 individuals with tinea pedis compared twice-daily applications of a 10% tea tree oil cream, tolnaftate, and placebo.[3] The results indicate that tea tree oil is more effective than placebo, but less effective than tolnaftate.

Another double-blind study followed 112 individuals with onychomycosis, comparing 100% tea tree oil to clotrimazole, and found equivalent effects.[4] However, because clotrimazole is not particularly effective for onychomycosis, these results mean little.

For more information, including dosage and safety issues, see the **Tea Tree Oil** article.

Other Proposed Natural Therapies

Ajoene is one of the active sulfur compounds in garlic. A 1-week double-blind comparative study of 70 Venezualan soldeirs found that therapy with topical 1% ajoene was equally effective as terbinafine.[5] Ajoene appears to inhibit phosphatidylcholine synthesis in fungi. However, topical garlic has not been tested. Keep in mind that topical garlic can burn the skin.

Preliminary evidence suggests that **oil of bitter orange** (derived from dried bitter orange peel) might have some effectiveness against tinea pedis when applied topically.[6]

More than 120 other plants or plant products (such as essential oils of peppermint and eucalyptus) traditionally used to treat skin diseases have demonstrated antifungal properties in vitro but have yet to be tested clinically.[7-14]

Drug Interactions

None known.

TINNITUS

Principal Proposed
Natural Therapies

Ginkgo   [−2]

(Higher numbers indicate stronger evidence; X modifier indicates contradictory results. See page xviii of the Introduction for details of the rating scale.)

Approach to the Patient

Although *Ginkgo biloba* is widely used, current evidence suggests that the herb is not helpful for tinnitus.

Other natural treatments the patient may be using include glutamic acid, ipriflavone, melatonin, oxerutins, periwinkle *(Vinca major, V. minor)*, vitamin A combined with vitamin E, vitamin B_{12}, and zinc. For potential safety risks with the more common of these substances, see the full herb/supplement articles.

Ginkgo   −2

A 1999 review article found three double-blind, placebo-controlled trials enrolling a total of about 220 individuals that evaluated oral *Ginkgo biloba* extract as a treatment for tinnitus.[1-4]

Although the results were generally positive in these trials, a more recent and much larger study found no benefit. In this double-blind, placebo-controlled trial, 1121 individuals with tinnitus were given 12 weeks of treatment with standardized ginkgo at a dose of 50 mg three times daily.[5] The results showed no difference between the treated and the placebo groups.

Other Proposed
Natural Therapies

Glutamic acid, ipriflavone, oxerutins, periwinkle, vitamins A and E in combination, vitamin B_{12}, and zinc have also been suggested for the treatment of tinnitus.[6-12] However, there is no real evidence for their effectiveness.

Melatonin may improve sleep in individuals with tinnitus but doesn't appear to have any effect on tinnitus itself.[13,14]

Drug Interactions

See the article on each individual supplement for a full description of the interactions summarized here.

Principal Natural Therapy for Tinnitus: Interactions with Pharmaceuticals		
Natural Therapy	Pharmaceutical	Interaction
Ginkgo	Anticoagulant and antiplatelet agents	Possible increased risk of bleeding complications

Pharmaceuticals Used for Tinnitus: Possible Harmful Interactions with Natural Therapies		
Pharmaceutical	**Natural Therapy**	**Interaction**
Potassium-sparing diuretics	Arginine	Possible increased risk of hyperkalemia
	Licorice	Antagonism of drug action
	Magnesium	Risk of hypermagnesemia
	White willow	Salicylate content might interfere with spironolactone action
	Zinc	Excessive zinc levels with spironolactone
Thiazide diuretics	Calcium	Potential risk of hypercalcemia
	Dong quai, St. John's wort	Possible increased risk of photosensivitiy
	Licorice	Potentiation of hypokalemic action of drug

Pharmaceuticals Used for Tinnitus: Natural Therapies with Potential Supportive Interactions		
Pharmaceutical	**Natural Therapy**	**Interaction**
Potassium-sparing diuretics	Folate	Correction of possible drug-induced depletion
Thiazide diuretics	Magnesium, potassium, zinc	Correction of possible drug-induced depletion

ULCERATIVE COLITIS

Principal Proposed
Natural Therapies

Probiotics   [+3]

Essential fatty acids   [+2X]

(Higher numbers indicate stronger evidence; X modifier indicates contradictory results. See page xviii of the Introduction for details of the rating scale.)

Approach to the Patient

Individuals with ulcerative colitis are well known to develop deficiencies in numerous nutrients. Chronic bleeding leads to iron deficiency; malabsorption, decreased appetite, drug side effects, and increased nutrient loss through the stool may also lead to mild or profound deficiencies of protein; vitamins A, B_{12}, C, D, E, and K; folate; calcium; copper; magnesium; selenium; and zinc.[1-10] Supplementation to restore normal nutriture is advisable; recommendations to this effect will be particularly well received by many patients interested in alternative medicine.

Preliminary evidence suggests that probiotics might have benefit for ulcerative colitis as well as pouchitis following ileal pouch–anal anastomosis. Essential fatty acids might also be helpful.

Other natural treatments the patient may be using include boswellia, bromelain, glutamine, and glycosaminoglycans (GAGs). For potential safety risks with the more common of these substances, see the full herb/supplement articles.

Probiotics   + 3

A 12-week, double-blind study of 120 individuals in remission found that a nonpathogenic strain of *Escherichia coli* prevented acute attacks of ulcerative colitis as effectively as mesalazine.[11] However, due to the low rate of acute attacks reported in each group, a larger sample size is necessary to truly establish equivalence.

Probiotics may also be helpful for recurrent pouchitis after ileal pouch–anal anastomosis. A 9-month, double-blind, placebo-controlled trial of 40 individuals found that a probiotic combination could significantly reduce the risk of a pouchitis flare-up.[12] The probiotic, given at 3 or 6 g daily, was a highly concentrated formulation containing 5×10^{11} viable organisms per gram and included four strains of lactobacilli (*Lactobacillus casei*, *L. plantarum*, *L. acidophilus*, and *L. delbruekii* ssp *bulgaricus*), three strains of bifidobacteria (*Bifidobacterium longum*, *B. breve*, and *B. infantis*) and one strain of *Streptococcus salivarius* (ssp *thermophilus*). The results showed that treated individuals were much less likely to have relapses of pouchitis during the study period.

For more information, including dosage and safety issues, see the **Probiotics** article.

Essential Fatty Acids   + 2 X

The results of several small double-blind trials suggest that fish oil might be helpful for reducing symptoms of ulcerative colitis.[13-16] However, one small double-blind, placebo-controlled trial failed to find benefit.[17] Regular use of fish oil does not appear to help prevent disease flare-ups.[16,18] Evening primrose oil (*Oenothera biennis*, a source of the omega-6 fatty acid GLA) has been found beneficial in a small trial.[17]

For more information, including dosage and safety issues, see the **Fish Oil** and **Gamma-Linolenic Acid** articles.

Other Proposed Natural Therapies

Boswellia,[19] **bromelain,**[20] **glutamine,**[21-24] **blue-green algae,**[25] and **glycosaminoglycans** have been suggested for the treatment of ulcerative colitis, but the evidence for them is highly preliminary at best.

Drug Interactions

See the article on each individual supplement for a full description of the interactions summarized here.

Principal Natural Therapy for Ulcerative Colitis: Interactions with Pharmaceuticals		
Natural Therapy	Pharmaceutical	Interaction
Fish oil	Anticoagulant and antiplatelet agents	Possible increased risk of bleeding complications

Pharmaceuticals Used for Ulcerative Colitis: Possible Harmful Interactions with Natural Therapies

Pharmaceutical	Natural Therapy	Interaction
Azulfidine, sulfasalazine	Dong quai, St. John's wort	Possible increased risk of photosensitivity
	Feverfew	Possible increased risk of gastritis
	Garlic, ginkgo, high-dose vitamin E, policosanol, others	Possible increased risk of bleeding complications
	Potassium citrate	Possible decreased serum levels of drug
	White willow	Additional salicylates in herb may increase risk of all side effects
Corticosteroids	Licorice	Increased potentiation of action

Pharmaceuticals Used for Ulcerative Colitis: Natural Therapies with Potential Supportive Interactions

Pharmaceutical	Natural Therapy	Interaction
Azulfidine, sulfasalazine	Cayenne, colostrum, licorice	Possible cytoprotection
	Folate, vitamin C	Correction of possible drug-induced deficiency
Corticosteroids	Combined high-dose calcium and vitamin D, ipriflavone	Counter corticosteroid-induced osteoporosis
	Chromium	Counter corticosteroid-induced diabetes

UROLITHIASIS

Principal Proposed
Natural Therapies

Citrate [+3]

(Higher numbers indicate stronger evidence; X modifier indicates contradictory results. See page xviii of the Introduction for details of the rating scale.)

Approach to the Patient

Citrate supplements may help prevent both oxalate and uric acid stones. However, there are safety issues to consider (see Drug Interactions).

Individuals interested in natural medicine will also appreciate hearing about dietary changes that might help prevent urinary stone recurrence. Low fluid intake greatly increases the risk of developing virtually all types of stones.[1-3] However, although there is evidence that coffee, tea, beer, and wine can decrease risk of kidney stone development, apple juice and grapefruit juice may increase the risk.[4,5] Oxalate-containing foods such as spinach and cocoa, as well as sodium[2,3] and protein (particularly animal protein), may increase the risk of calcium oxalate stones,[1,3] although some studies have found that protein has no such effect.[2]

Other natural treatments your patient may be using include goldenrod and other diuretic herbs; vitamins A, B_6, and C; fish oil; GLA (gamma-linolenic acid); calcium; and magnesium. For potential safety risks with the more common of these substances, see the full herb/supplement articles.

Caution: Regular use of cranberry concentrates have been found to increase excretion of oxalate, calcium, phosphate, sodium, magnesium and potassium.[6] Because some of these ions are lithogenic and others antilithogenic, the overall effect is not clear. Nonetheless, caution is warranted.

Citrate   +3

Citrate binds with calcium in the urine, reducing the amount of calcium available to form calcium oxalate stones. Citrate also chemically inhibits calcium oxalate crystallization and alkalinizes the urine, inhibiting the development of both calcium oxalate and uric acid stones.

In a 3-year, double-blind study of 57 individuals with a history of calcium stones and low urinary citrate levels, those given potassium citrate developed fewer kidney stones than they had previously.[7] In comparison, those given placebo had no change in their rate of stone formation.

Potassium-magnesium citrate was studied in a 3-year trial involving 64 participants with a history of calcium oxalate stones.[8] During the study period, new stones formed in only 12.9% of those taking the supplement compared to 63.6% of those given placebo. Citrate is also available as calcium citrate, a popular and highly absorbable calcium supplement. However, calcium citrate has not yet been studied as a preventive for kidney stones.

Citrus juices raise urinary citrate levels as well. Lemon juice is a concentrated source of citrate.[9] Orange juice also provides citrate but significantly raises urinary oxalate.[10] Grapefruit juice is *not* advisable as a citrate source; in one large-scale study, 8 ounces of grapefruit juice daily was associated with a significant increase in stone formation.[5]

Initially it was thought that citrate supplements were only helpful for individuals whose urinary citrate excretion rate was subnormal.[10] However, citrate treatment may also be useful for those at risk for stones whose citrate excretion is normal.[8]

The proper dose of citrate depends on the chemical form: see label instructions for FDA-approved citrate salts. Caution must be exercised in individuals with severe renal disease. Standard precautions apply to the caution involved, most commonly potassium or sodium.

Other Proposed Natural Therapies

Magnesium, in the form of magnesium oxide or magnesium hydroxide, may help to prevent calcium oxalate stone development. In vitro, magnesium inhibits the growth of oxalate crystals,[11] and animal studies suggest that it decreases stone formation.[3] However, human studies have found mixed results.[12-14] In a 2-year open study, 56 participants taking magnesium hydroxide had fewer recurrences of kidney stones than 34 participants not given magnesium.[12] However, a double-blind trial of 124 participants found magnesium hydroxide not significantly more effective than placebo.[14]

Vitamin B_6 might also help prevent calcium oxalate stones. Vitamin B_6 deficiency increases the amount of oxalate in the urine of animals and humans,[3] and a small uncontrolled study found that supplementation decreased oxalate excretion in individuals with a history of urolithiasis.[15] In addition, an observational trial of 85,000 women found an inverse association between B_6 intake and urolithiasis.[16] However, an observational trial of 45,000 men found no link between B_6 and urolithiasis.[17]

Germany's Commission E recommends the following herbs for the prevention or treatment of kidney stones based on their apparent diuretic or natriuretic properties: asparagus, birch leaf, bishop's weed fruit, couch grass, goldenrod, horsetail, lovage, parsley, butterbur, and stinging nettle herb and root combination.[18] However, there is little to no evidence that they are really effective.

Several other supplements including fish oil, GLA, glycosaminoglycans (GAGs), and vitamin A[19-22] are also sometimes recommended for kidney stones, but again, there is no real evidence that they work.

Although concerns have been raised that long-term **vitamin C** treatment might increase risk of calcium oxalate stone formation, the physiological basis for this hypothesis has been challenged.[23] In addition, observational studies have found either no association or decreased risk with higher vitamin C intake.[16,17,23,24]

Nonetheless, certain individuals may be particularly at risk for vitamin C–induced kidney stones.[25] Individuals with a history of stone formation, with renal failure, or with a known defect in vitamin C or oxalate metabolism should probably restrict vitamin C intake to approximately 100 mg daily. High-dose vitamin C is also contraindicated in patients with glucose-6-phosphate dehydrogenase deficiency, iron overload, or a history of intestinal surgery.

A 5-year intervention trial of 120 men with recurrent calcium oxalate stones found that a diet with normal calcium intake but low in animal protein and salt reduced stone formation more effectively than a low calcium diet with no other changes.[28] Observational studies suggest that **calcium** *supplements* might slightly increase kidney stone risk,[26] while increased *dietary intake* of calcium reduces the risk of kidney stones.[26,27] The reason for this apparent distinction is not clear.

Drug Interactions

See the article on each individual supplement for a full description of the interactions summarized here.

Principal Natural Therapies for Urolithiasis: Interactions with Pharmaceuticals		
Natural Therapy	**Pharmaceutical**	**Interaction**
Citrate	Ephedra, flecainide, mecamylamine, methamphetamine	Increased serum levels due to decreased urinary elimination
	Lithium, methotrexate, salicylates, sulfonylureas, tetracyclines	Decreased serum levels due to increased urinary elimination
	ACE inhibitors, potassium-sparing diuretics	Hyperkalemia
Potassium citrate	Flecainide, lithium, methotrexate, salicylates, sympathomimetics, tetracyclines	Possible interactions identical to those of potassium
Sodium citrate	Lithium, methotrexate, salicylates, sulfonylureas, tetracyclines	Possible interactions identical to those of sodium

URTICARIA

Principal Proposed Natural Therapies

There are no evidence-based herbs or supplements for urticaria.

Approach to the Patient

Although there is little real evidence to support their use, patients may be using natural therapies, such as vitamins B_{12} and C and bioflavonoids, such as quercetin. For potential safety risks with the more common of these substances, see the full herb/supplement articles.

Some patients interested in alternative medicine may believe that urticaria is caused by "adrenal exhaustion." Treatments for this purported condition include various herbs and supplements, including ginseng and B vitamins; most are, at least, relatively benign.

In addition, many patients interested in alternative medicine believe that accumulated toxins are the cause of urticaria and that this can be corrected through "detoxification." The latter may involve dietary changes, "colon cleansing," and supplementation with specific herbs and supplements. Malnutrition can occur in the more extreme forms of this approach.

Other Proposed Natural Therapies

Based on poorly documented antiallergy effects, vitamins C and B_{12} and the flavonoid quercetin are sometimes suggested for urticaria in the popular literature, but there is no clinical evidence that these approaches are effective.

Drug Interactions

See the article on each individual supplement for a full description of the interactions summarized here.

Pharmaceuticals Used for Urticaria: Possible Harmful Interactions with Natural Therapies		
Pharmaceutical	Natural Therapy	Interaction
Antihistamines	Kava, valerian, other sedative herbs	Possible potentiation of sedation

VAGINAL INFECTION

Principal Proposed Natural Therapies

Probiotics [+2]

(Higher numbers indicate stronger evidence; X modifier indicates contradictory results. See page xviii of the Introduction for details of the rating scale.)

Approach to the Patient

Although there is a good rationale for the use of oral or topical probiotics (especially *Lactobacilli* and *Bifidobacteria*) to prevent or treat vaginal infections, the evidence to support this use is weak.

Other topical natural treatments the patient may be using include tea tree oil, boric acid, *Solanum nigrescens*, *Tabeuia avellanedae*, garlic, goldenseal, barberry, Oregon grape, and essential oils of cinnamon, eucalyptus, lemongrass, palmarosa, or peppermint. Be aware that these treatments can cause local inflammation and that some (such as boric acid) present toxic risk.

Probiotics +2

A review of the many studies on the use of oral and topical acidophilus to prevent vaginal yeast infections concluded that it may be effective but that more study is needed.[1-3]

In several clinical trials involving a total of 99 women with recurrent vaginitis over 7 days to 6 months, subjects using *Lactobacillus acidophilus* (taken orally, as a vaginal douche, or as a vaginal suppository) experienced improvement in symptoms as well as a decreased incidence of vaginal infections.[4-6] However, the reliability of all of these studies is questionable due to poor design.

For more information, including dosage and safety issues, see the **Probiotics** article.

Other Proposed Natural Therapies

Tea tree oil possesses antibacterial and antifungal properties[7] but appears to lack activity against Lactobacilli.[8] Tea tree oil has been tried for various types of vaginal infection, but there are no double-blind trials to support this use. Tea tree oil can cause local irritation.[9]

Boric acid suppositories and douches are also popular for vaginal infection. A double-blind comparison study of 108 women with candidal vaginitis found boric acid suppositories superior to nystatin suppositories.[10] However, there are serious safety concerns with boric acid.[11] It is toxic if absorbed internally. It should not be applied to open wounds, used by pregnant women, or applied to the skin of infants.

Various tropical plants appear to possess antifungal properties and have been tested as possible treatments for candidal yeast infections. For example, *Solanum nigrescens* has been tested in a single-blind comparison trial against the standard drug nystatin and found equally effective.[12] However, this plant has toxic constituents. Other herbs with known antifungal properties in vitro include *Tabeuia avellanedae*,[13] garlic extracts,[14-16] berberine (found in goldenseal, barberry, and Oregon grape),[17] and essential oils of various plants including cinnamon, eucalyptus, lemongrass, palmarosa, and peppermint.[18-20] Many of these may be too harsh, however, to use intravaginally.

Drug Interactions

None known.

VENOUS INSUFFICIENCY (CHRONIC)

Principal Proposed Natural Therapies

Horse chestnut [+3]

Oxerutins [+3]

Diosmin/ hesperidin [+3X]

Butcher's broom [+3]

Grape leaf [+3]

OPCs (oligomeric proanthocyanidin complexes) [+2]

Gotu kola [+2]

(Higher numbers indicate stronger evidence; X modifier indicates contradictory results. See page xviii of the Introduction for details of the rating scale.)

Approach to the Patient

Several herbs and supplements have moderately well-documented efficacy in chronic venous insufficiency (CVI) and related conditions (such as varicose veins). The best evidence is for horse chestnut and the semisynthetic bioflavonoids called oxerutins. A lesser degree of evidence supports the use of the citrus bioflavonoid combination diosmin/hesperidin, grape leaf, OPCs (oligomeric proanthocyanidin complexes), and gotu kola.

These treatments are all thought to increase venous tone and reduce capillary leakage. Improvements can be expected in pain, edema, and sensation of fatigue. Improved rate of healing of venous stasis ulcers has also been observed in some trials. Some European physicians believe that early use of these treatments will help prevent cosmetically unpleasant varicosities, but this has not been tested.

Other natural treatments the patient may be using include buckwheat tea, mesoglycans, and butcher's broom. For potential safety risks with the more common of these substances, see the full herb/supplement articles.

Caution: Many of these treatments are also advocated for phlebitis; patients should be cautioned that in Europe, physician supervision of herbal therapies is standard and that phlebitis is a situation in which self-treatment is not appropriate.

Horse Chestnut   +3

Although the research record is not complete, the balance of existing evidence indicates that horse chestnut extract (HCSE), either alone or in combination with leg compression stockings, is a useful treatment at least for the beginning stages of chronic venous insufficiency.

Four scientifically acceptable studies were published in 1986.[1-4] In general, subjective complaints of pain, itching, leg fatigue, and feelings of tension in the legs improved significantly in these studies.

One of the best was a partially blinded study of 240 patients treated for 12 weeks with placebo, compression stockings (unblinded), or HCSE (1 capsule of delayed-release horse chestnut twice daily, blinded).[5] The results showed the two therapies to be statistically equivalent and superior to placebo.

For more information, including dosage and safety issues, see the **Horse Chestnut** article.

Oxerutins   +3

At least 17 double-blind, placebo-controlled studies, enrolling a total of more than 2000 participants, have examined oxerutins in chronic venous insufficiency. All but one found oxerutins significantly more effective than placebo, providing substantial improvements in signs and symptoms.[6-18]

One of the best designed trials was a 12-week, double-blind, placebo-controlled study that enrolled 133 women with moderate chronic venous insufficiency.[8] Half received 1000 mg oxerutins daily, and the rest received matching placebo. All participants were also fitted with standard compression stockings and wore them for the duration of the study. The results showed that oxerutins significantly reduced lower leg edema compared to placebo; furthermore, these results lasted through a 6-week follow-up, even though participants were no longer taking oxerutins.

Oxerutins have also been found effective in treating impaired venous return in pregnancy.[19] There have been mixed results in treating venous stasis ulcers.[6,20,21]

For more information, including dosage and safety issues, see the **Oxerutins** article.

Diosmin/Hesperidin   +3X

A fixed micronized combination of the citrus bioflavonoids diosmin and hesperidin is used widely in Europe for the treatment of various venous conditions, and there is meaningful (if not altogether consistent) supporting evidence for this use.

For example, a 2-month, double-blind, placebo-controlled trial of 200 individuals with severe chronic venous insufficiency found that treatment with diosmin/hesperidin significantly improved symptoms compared to placebo.[43]

Another double-blind, placebo-controlled trial of diosmin/hesperidin enrolled 101 individuals with mild chronic venous insufficiency.[44] The results showed little difference between the two groups; the authors theorize that diosmin/hesperidin might be generally more effective in more severe forms of the condition.

Finally, a 2-month, double-blind, placebo-controlled trial involving 107 individuals with nonhealing venous stasis ulcers, found that diosmin/hesperidin significantly improved rate of healing.[22]

For more information, including dosage and safety issues, see the **Diosmin/Hesperidin** article.

Butcher's Broom   + 3

A 12-week, double-blind, placebo-controlled trial of 148 women found that an extract of the herb butcher's broom significantly improved symptoms of venous insufficiency.[24] The dose used supplied 10 mg of ruscogenines daily. Similar results were seen in a 12-week, double-blind, placebo-controlled trial of 141 individuals using a combination of ruscus extract and trimethyl-hesperidin chalcone.[25] However, a smaller trial using a ruscus and hesperidin combination showed only marginal results.[26]

Grape Leaf   + 3

A 12-week, double-blind, placebo-controlled study of grape leaf (red vine leaf) followed 219 individuals with CVI and found dose-dependent improvement in measurements and symptoms.[23]

Oligomeric Proanthocyanidin Complexes (OPCs)   + 2

Placebo-controlled trials involving a total of about 400 participants suggest that OPCs provide significant benefit in chronic venous insufficiency.[27-32]

For example, a 28-day, double-blind, placebo-controlled study of OPCs enrolled 92 patients with CVI and found relative improvement in subjective symptoms.[30]

For more information, including dosage and safety issues, see the **Oligomeric Proanthocyanidin Complexes** article.

Gotu Kola   + 2

Double-blind, placebo-controlled studies and other controlled trials have found a dose-dependent improvement with gotu kola in subjective and objective symptoms of CVI.[33-37]

For more information, including dosage and safety issues, see the **Gotu Kola** article.

Other Proposed Natural Therapies

Two small double-blind, placebo-controlled trials suggest that **buckwheat tea** might be effective in chronic venous insufficiency, presumably because of its content of the citrus bioflavonoid rutin (closely related to oxerutins).[38,39]

Mesoglycans (glycosaminoglycans extracted from pig intestines) have been tried for venous stasis ulcers, with some apparent benefit.[40-42,45] For example, in a double-blind, placebo-controlled trial, 183 individuals with venous stasis ulcers were treated with placebo or mesoglycans (first IM, then orally) for 24 weeks.[45] Use of mesoglyans improved the rate of ulcer healing to a statistically and clinically significant extent compared to placebo.

Other natural treatments considered for CVI include bilberry fruit, bromelain, calendula cream, and collinsonia; however, no real evidence supports these treatments at this time.

Drug Interactions

See the article on each individual supplement for a full description of the interactions summarized here.

Principal Natural Therapies for Chronic Venous Insufficiency: Interactions with Pharmaceuticals		
Natural Therapy	**Pharmaceutical**	**Interaction**
Horse chestnut, OPCs	Anticoagulant or antiplatelet agents	Possible increased risk of bleeding complications

WEIGHT LOSS

Principal Proposed
Natural Therapies

Fiber [+3X]

Chromium [+3X]

Pyruvate [+2]

5-HTP [+2]

Hydroxycitric acid (HCA) [+2X]

Caffeine-ephedrine [+3]

(Higher numbers indicate stronger evidence; X modifier indicates contradictory results. See page xviii of the Introduction for details of the rating scale.)

Approach to the Patient

There is some evidence that the supplements chromium, pyruvate, 5-HTP (5-hydroxytryptophan), and fiber might be helpful for reducing weight and/or improving body composition, but results of studies are conflicting.

Like other stimulants, a combination of caffeine and ephedra may have short-term benefit, although there are significant safety concerns with this combination. The popular diet herb *Garcinia cambogia* (a source of HCA) does not appear to be effective.

Other natural treatments the patient may be using (based on widespread marketing that varies from overly optimistic to outright deceptive) are too numerous to mention here.

Fiber   +3X

When combined with a low-calorie diet, fiber supplements may aid weight loss.[1-4] The presumed mechanism of action is appetite reduction due to mechanical filling of the stomach.

For example, in a double-blind, placebo-controlled study of 97 mildly overweight women on a hypoenergetic diet, those who took 7 g of a proprietary insoluble fiber mixture daily for 11 weeks lost 10.8 pounds compared to 7.3 pounds in the placebo group.[1] Participants were then placed on an isoenergetic diet for 16 weeks. Those taking the fiber supplement showed a decreased amount of regained weight.

Similar benefits with insoluble fiber supplements were seen in three other studies.[2,4] In these trials, insoluble fiber supplements were given 20 to 30 minutes prior to each meal at a dose of about 2.3 g, along with 8 oz of water. However, a 24-week study of 53 moderately overweight individuals found no benefit with 4 g of a proprietary insoluble fiber mixture taken daily.[5]

The crustacean-derived fiber chitosan has also been studied, with conflicting results. An 8-week, double-blind, placebo-controlled trial of 59 overweight individuals evaluated the effects 1.5 g taken prior to each of the two largest meals of the day.[6] Over the course of the study, participants in the placebo group gained a mean of 1.5 kg, while those in the chitosan group lost an average of 1.0 kg, a statistically significant difference. However, an 8-week, double-blind, placebo-controlled trial of 51 women failed to find any weight loss benefit with use of chitosan at a dose of 1200 mg twice daily.[60] Similarly, in a 28-day, double-blind trial of 30 overweight individuals, a different chitosan product taken at a dose of 1 g twice daily failed to induce weight loss compared to placebo.[7]

Benefits have also been seen with the soluble fiber glucomannan in adults,[3,8] but not in children.[9]

Chromium   + 3 X

The theory behind using chromium for weight loss invokes its apparent effects on insulin resistance. Chromium is thought to improve insulin sensitivity, causing insulin levels to fall. With reduced circulating insulin, adipose tissue may begin to initiate lipolysis. In addition, there is some evidence that chromium directly blocks insulin's effects on fat cells, interfering with its lipogenic effect.[61]

However, there are serious flaws in these arguments. For example, it has been found that even very low levels of circulating insulin are sufficient to suppress lipolysis.[62-66]

Chromium reduces insulin levels only slightly at most, probably not enough to make a significant impact.

Furthermore, the state of insulin resistance appears to affect adipose tissue as well.[67-70] Chromium supplements might therefore have the unintended effect of increasing lipolysis by reducing adipose insulin resistance.

Theory aside, the clinical evidence regarding whether chromium is an effective aid in weight loss is mixed. The largest study did find benefit, but other studies did not, possibly due to insufficient statistical power.

In a double-blind trial, 154 individuals were given either placebo or 200 or 400 μg of chromium picolinate daily.[10] Over a period of 72 days, individuals taking chromium demonstrated increase in lean body mass and loss of fat mass, resulting in a net overall weight loss versus placebo. However, in a slightly smaller double-blind study by the same researcher, no statistically significant intergroup differences were seen.[11] Researchers resorted to addititional statistical analyis in an attempt to show benefit. Smaller studies have also yielded generally negative results.[12-16]

For more information, including dosage and safety issues, see the **Chromium** article.

Pyruvate   +2

Based on its role in the Kreb's cycle, pyruvate supplements have been promoted as a treatment to enhance fat metabolism. However, the evidence that pyruvate works is limited to a number of small studies. Pyruvate also is marketed as an ergogenic aid, based on even weaker evidence.

Pyruvate is often sold in combination with dihydroxyacetone as dihydroxyacetone pyruvate (DHAP).

In a 6-week, double-blind, placebo-controlled trial, 51 individuals were given either pyruvate (6 g/day), placebo, or no treatment.[17] All participated in an exercise program. Significant decreases in fat mass (2.1 kg) and percent body fat (2.6%) were seen, along with a significant increase in lean mass (1.5 kg). No significant changes were seen in the placebo or control groups.

In a placebo-controlled study (blinding not stated), 34 modestly overweight individuals were put on a mildy low-energy diet for 4 weeks.[18] Subsequently, all participants were given a liquid supplement containing pyruvate (22 to 44 g depending on total calorie intake) or an isocaloric equivalent. Over the course of 6 weeks, individuals in the pyruvate group lost 0.7 kg versus no significant loss in the placebo group.

Other small studies using pyruvate or DHAP found similar results.[19-22]

For more information, including dosage and safety issues, see the **Pyruvate** article.

5-HTP   +2

Four small double-blind, placebo-controlled trials suggest that the serotonin precursor 5-HTP may be helpful as an aid to weight loss.[23-26]

For more information, including dosage and safety issues, see the **5-Hydroxytryptophan** article.

Hydroxycitric Acid (HCA)   +2X

Hydroxycitric acid (HCA), a derivative of citric acid, is found primarily in the small, sweet, purple fruit of the Malabar tamarind.

In vitro and animal studies, as well as one human trial, suggest that HCA might have use for weight loss.[27-36]

For example, in an 8-week, double-blind, placebo-controlled trial of 60 overweight individuals, use of HCA at a dose of 440 mg three times daily produced significant weight loss compared with placebo.[27]

However, a 12-week, double-blind, placebo-controlled trial of 135 overweight individuals given either placebo or 500 mg of HCA (*Garcinia cambogia* extract standardized to contain 50% HCA) three times daily found no effect on body weight or fat mass.[37] This study has been criticized for using a high fiber diet, which might impair HCA absorption.[38]

Negative results were seen in other small trials as well.[39-41]

For more information, including dosage and safety issues, see the **Hydroxycitric Acid** article.

Caffeine-Ephedrine   +3

Several studies suggest that a caffeine-ephedrine combination can promote short- and long-term weight loss.[42-47]

For example, a 6-month, double-blind trial with 180 obese individuals found that 20 mg of ephedrine and 200 mg of caffeine three times daily produced significant weight loss, compared with placebo or either ephedrine or caffeine given alone.[42] Tolerance did not develop over the course of the trial. However, there are real safety concerns regarding this combination.[48]

Note that these studies used the drug *ephedrine* rather than the herb *ephedra*. Ephedra presents additional safety concerns, such as unpredictable ephedrine content and the possible presence of other toxic ingredients. For more information, including dosage and safety issues, see the **Ephedra** article.

Other Proposed Natural Therapies

Results of two small double-blind, placebo-controlled studies suggest that **vitamin C** supplements might be helpful for weight loss.[49,50]

A double-blind study that enrolled 100 women found that **evening primrose oil** failed to produce any weight loss compared to placebo; however, another investigation that restricted treatment to 47 individuals with a family history of obesity found some benefit.[51]

Conjugated linoleic acid (CLA) supplements might help reduce fat mass, although the evidence is contradictory.[52-55,71] There is some evidence that **calcium** supplements might facilitate weight loss for reasons that aren't clear.[56]

Preliminary evidence suggests that the lipid **diacylglycerol** may help individuals lose fat around the abdomen.[57] Another double-blind, placebo-controlled trial investigated the possible weight-loss effects of **spirulina** but failed to find a significant difference between groups.[58]

MCTs have been used in combination with very low carbohydrate diets to promote ketosis. One study suggests that MCTs may enhance the weight loss effects of such diets, but only in the very short-term (2 weeks).[72]

Some evidence suggests that MCT consumption short of ketosis might enhance thermogenesis.[73-75] However, a 12-week, double-blind trial of 78 individuals that evaluated the effects of substituting MCTs for LCTs in otherwise equivalent low-energy diets found no significant intergroup differences regarding loss of weight or body fat; post-hoc subgroup analysis found some benefit in individuals with higher BMIs.[76] Negative results were also seen in a similar, smaller trial.[77]

A double-blind, placebo-controlled trial of 150 overweight individuals compared a low- and high-dose of a combination tablet containing **chitosan, chromium,** and ***Garcinia cambogia.***[78] The results showed dose-related weight loss and hypolipidemic effects. Benefits were also seen in a 45-day, double-blind, placebo-controlled trial of 44 overweight individuals that tested a combination product containing **yerba maté, guarana,** and **damiana.**[79]

One small double-blind study suggests that use of **colostrum** by healthy men and women undergoing exercising training may improve body composition compared to whey protein.[80]

A double-blind, placebo-controlled trial that enrolled 158 moderately overweight volunteers tested a mixture of **chromium, cayenne, inulin** (a nondigestible carbohydrate), and **phenylalanine,** as well as other herbs and nutrients.[81] All participants lost weight over the 4-week trial, but the intergroup difference was not significant.

An enormous variety of other supplements are marketed for weight loss. Most have little to no evidence behind them, and some have been found ineffective in preliminary studies.

One group of supplements, so called lipotrophics, are said to enhance lipolysis or interfere with lipogenesis, although there is no real supporting evidence. These include vitamins B_5 and B_6, biotin, choline, inositol, lecithin, and lipoic acid.

Legumes contain constituents that impair the action of amylase. Based on this fact, products containing the French white bean *Phaseolus vulgaris* are widely marketed as carbohydrate blockers.

However, there is no clinical evidence that this treatment (or any other legume) can actually aid weight loss.

A number of amino acids are claimed to reduce hunger, including phenylalanine, tyrosine, methionine, and glutamine. Because the herb kava appears to be helpful for anxiety, it has been proposed as a treatment for mood-related overeating. The antidepressant herb St. John's wort has been recommended with much the same reasoning.

Seaweeds such as kelp, bladderwrack, and sargassi are often added to diet formulas, under the unfounded presumption that they will enhance thyroid action by providing iodine. The herb guggul *(Commiphora mukul)* is also often claimed to enhance thyroid function. However there is no meaningful evidence that it actually has any thyroid-enhancing effects, and a small double-blind trial found it no more effective than placebo for weight loss.[59] Numerous herbs and supplements with potential or known effects on insulin are widely added to weight loss formulas, again, without any evidence that they are effective. These include alfalfa, *Anemarrhena asphodeloides*, arginine, *Azadirachta indica* (neem), bilberry leaf, bitter melon *(Momordica charantia)*, *Catharanthus roseus*, *Coccinia indica*, *Cucumis sativus*, *Cucurbita ficifolia*, *Cuminum cyminum* (cumin), *Euphorbia prostrata*, garlic, glucomannan, *Guaiacum coulteri*, *Guazuma ulmifolia*, guggul, holy basil *(Ocimum sanctum)*, *Lepechinia caulescens*, *Musa sapientum L.* (banana), nopal cactus *(Opuntia streptacantha)*, onion, *Psacalium peltatum*, pterocarpus, *Rhizophora mangle*, salt bush, *Spinacea oleracea*, *Tournefortia hirsutissima*, *Turnera diffusa*, and vanadium.

Herbs with laxative or diuretic reputations are also popular in weight-loss formulas, although they are unlikely to produce anything beyond a slight temporary effect. These include barberry, buchu, cascara sagrada bark, cassia powder, cleavers, corn silk, couch grass, dandelion root, fig, goldenrod, hydrangea root, juniper berry, peppermint, prune, senna leaf, tamarind, turkey rhubarb root, and uva ursi.

Herbs supposed to "strengthen" the body in general are found in many diet formulas, including ashwagandha, *Cordyceps*, *Eleutherococcus*, fo-ti, ginseng, maitake, reishi, schisandra, and suma.

Other herbs and supplements sometimes recommended for weight loss for reasons that are unclear include buckthorn, cayenne, chickweed, coenzyme Q_{10}, cranberry, fennel, flax, ginger, ginkgo, gotu kola, grape seed extract, hawthorn, licorice, milk thistle, parsley, passionflower, plantain, white willow, yellow dock, yucca, and zinc. One small double-blind trial found the supplement L-carnitine ineffective for weight loss.[82]

DHEA has been proposed as a weight loss aid, but the little evidence that is available appears more negative than positive.[83]

Drug Interactions

See the article on each individual supplement for a full description of the interactions summarized here.

Principal Natural Therapies for Weight Loss: Interactions with Pharmaceuticals		
Natural Therapy	Pharmaceutical	Interaction
5-HTP	Levodopa-carbidopa	Possible increased risk of scleroderma-like syndrome
	SSRIs, other serotonergic drugs	Possible risk of serotonin syndrome
Caffeine-Ephedra	CNS stimulants	Potentiation of stimulant side effects
Chromium	Hypoglycemic agents	Possible potentiation of drug, increasing risk of hypoglycemia

Pharmaceuticals Used for Weight Loss: Possible Harmful Interactions with Natural Therapies		
Pharmaceutical	Natural Therapy	Interaction
CNS stimulants	Stimulant herbs, such as ephedra, guarana, green tea	Potentiation of stimulant side effects
Sibutramine	5-HTP, SAMe, St. John's wort	Possible risk of serotonin syndrome

HERBS AND
SUPPLEMENTS

5-HYDROXYTRYPTOPHAN (5-HTP)

Common Uses

Depression [+2]

Anxiety [+2]

Fibromyalgia [+2]

Obesity [+2]

Tension headache (prophylaxis) [+2]

Migraine headache (prophylaxis) [+2X]

(Higher numbers indicate stronger evidence; X modifier indicates contradictory results. See page xviii of the Introduction for details of the rating scale.)

Approach to the Patient

The serotonin precursor 5-HTP has been tried for several conditions in which SSRIs might be used. Weak evidence suggests benefits of 5-HTP in depression, anxiety, fibromyalgia, and obesity, as well as tension headache and migraine prophylaxis.

Although 5-HTP is usually free of obvious side effects, there are some safety concerns (see Safety Issues and Drug Interactions).

Depression   +2

Several small studies have compared 5-HTP to standard antidepressants.[1] The best was a 6-week, double-blind trial of 63 individuals given either 5-HTP (100 mg three times daily) or fluvoxamine (50 mg three times daily).[2] The results showed equivalent improvements in depressive symptomatology.[1]

Anxiety   +2

The serotonin precursor 5-HTP is best known as a proposed treatment for depression. However, an 8-week, double-blind, placebo-controlled study compared 5-HTP and clomipramine in 45 individuals suffering from anxiety disorders.[3] The results showed that clomipramine was more effective than 5-HTP, but 5-HTP was more effective than placebo.

Fibromyalgia   +2

A 1-month, double-blind, placebo-controlled study of 50 fibromyalgia patients found significant improvement in all symptom categories with 5-HTP treatment.[4]

Obesity   +2

Four small double-blind, placebo-controlled, clinical trials, one in type 2 diabetics, suggest that 5-HTP at a dose of 750 to 900 mg daily can aid in weight loss.[5-8]

Tension Headache (Prophylaxis)   +2

An 8-week, double-blind, placebo-controlled trial of 65 individuals (mostly women) with tension headaches found that 5-HTP (100 mg three times daily) did not significantly reduce the number of headaches experienced; however, it did reduce participants' analgesic use.[9] Benefits were seen in other studies of mixed or poorly defined headache types including tension headache.[10-12]

Migraine Headache (Prophylaxis)   +2X

5-HTP may be effective for migraine prophylaxis if taken in sufficient doses. In a 6-month trial that evaluated 85 individuals, prophylactic 5-HTP (600 mg/day) proved equally effective to methysergide in reducing the intensity and duration of migraine attacks.[13] Equal benefits were also seen in a double-blind trial of 66 individuals comparing 5-HTP (400 mg/day) to pizotifen.[14]

However, in a double-blind trial that enrolled 39 individuals, 5-HTP (up to 300 mg/day) was less effective than propranolol.[15] In addition, a double-blind, placebo-controlled crossover trial of 27 children with migraines failed to demonstrate any benefit.[16]

Other studies that are sometimes quoted as evidence that 5-HTP is effective for migraines actually enrolled adults or children with many different types of headaches, including migraines.[10-12]

Other Proposed Uses

5-HTP has been recommended for all conditions in which SSRIs might be tried, including insomnia and chronic pain. However, clinical research is lacking.

Mechanism of Action

As a physiologic precursor of serotonin, 5-HTP supplements presumably alter cerebral and peripheral serotonin concentrations.

Dosage

A typical dosage of 5-HTP is 100 to 300 mg three times daily. In some clinical trials, lower maintenance doses were used after an initial response was achieved.

Safety Issues

No significant adverse effects have been reported in clinical trials of 5-HTP. Side effects appear to be limited to mild and often transient nonspecific symptoms.

In 1998 the U.S. Food and Drug Administration reported detecting low levels of the chemical contaminant known as "peak X" in one batch of 5-HTP products. Peak X is the same contaminant previously found in some L-tryptophan products, which was associated with eosinophilic myalgia and subsequently caused all L-tryptophan products to be taken off of the dietary supplement market. The FDA has yet to take action against 5-HTP products; case reports of eosinophilic myalgia with 5-HTP are rare and show weak causality.

Maximum safe dosages in individuals with severe hepatic or renal disease are not known.

Safety in Young Children and Pregnant or Lactating Women

Maximum safe dosages for young children or pregnant or lactating women have not been established. In some studies, children have been given 5-HTP without any apparent harmful effects.

Drug Interactions

Combining 5-HTP with **carbidopa** might increase the risk of a scleroderma-like syndrome in susceptible individuals.[17-19]

There are theoretical concerns (but no case reports) that 5-HTP may cause serotonin syndrome if combined with **SSRIs** or other serotonergic drugs. Because SSRIs have been associated with increased hallucinations in individuals taking zolpidem,[20] combined treatment with 5-HTP and zolpidem might present similar risk.

ALOE

(Aloe vera)

Common Uses

Genital herpes
(topical)   [+2]

Psoriasis (topical)   [+2]

Seborrhea (topical)   [+2]

Diabetes (oral)   [+1]

Wound healing
(oral and topical)   [−1X]

Burns (topical)   [−1]

(Higher numbers indicate stronger evidence; X modifier indicates contradictory results. See page xviii of the Introduction for details of the rating scale.)

Approach to the Patient

In this article, the term *aloe* refers primarily to *aloe gel*, the gelatinous substance found within the leaf of the *Aloe vera* cactus. The leaf skin contains glands that secrete laxative anthraquinones; an extract of those glands called *drug aloe* has a violent cathartic effect and is not used today. Aloe gel is not supposed to contain any leaf skin or its glands. However, a small amount of anthraquinones and other leaf skin substances may contaminate aloe gel products due to inadequate quality control during the manufacturing process, and it is has been suggested that these contaminants and not the gel itself are responsible for the effects seen in some studies. This presents the paradoxical possibility that higher purity aloe gel products may be less effective than impure ones.

Despite near-universal acceptance of the "fact" that aloe promotes burn healing, there is no evidence that this is the case. You may wish to inform your patients that aloe may actually *impair* healing of second degree burns.

Some preliminary evidence does support the use of topical aloe for genital herpes, psoriasis, and seborrhea. Weak evidence supports the use of aloe gel for improving blood sugar control. No real clinical evidence supports other medicinal uses of aloe.

Warnings that aloe can cause hypokalemia refer to drug aloe rather than aloe gel (see Safety Issues).

Genital Herpes   +2

A 2-week, double-blind, placebo-controlled trial enrolled 60 men with active genital herpes (mean 4.1 days after lesion onset).[1] Participants applied aloe cream or placebo cream three times daily for 5 days. Use of aloe cream resulted in a reduced mean time to healing and increased total number of healed patients. A previous double-blind, placebo-controlled study by the same author enrolled 120 men with genital herpes and compared aloe cream and aloe gel with placebo.[2] Aloe cream proved most effective.

Psoriasis   +2

One double-blind, placebo-controlled study of 60 patients with mild to moderate psoriasis looked at the effects of topical aloe extract (0.5%) or placebo cream applied three times daily for 4 weeks.[3] The study found that aloe cream produced significant improvement compared to placebo.

Seborrhea   +2

One recent double-blind, placebo-controlled study of 44 individuals found that 4 to 6 weeks of treatment with aloe ointment could significantly reduce symptoms of seborrhea.[4]

Diabetes   +1

A single-blind, placebo-controlled trial evaluated the potential benefits of aloe in either 72 or 40 diabetics (the study report appears to contradict itself on number of participants).[5] The re-

sults showed significantly greater improvements in blood glucose levels among those given aloe over the 2-week treatment
period. Another single-blind, placebo-controlled trial evaluated
the benefits of aloe in individuals whose blood glucose levels had
not responded to glibenclamide.[6] Of the 36 individuals who
completed the study, those taking glibenclamide and aloe
showed improvements in blood glucose levels over the 6-week
study period compared to those taking glibenclamide and
placebo.

Wound Healing   − 1X

One study evaluated the effects of aloe gel on the time interval
required for secondary intention wound healing in 21 women
who had wound complications following gynecologic surgery.[7]
The results showed a significant *delay* in wound healing in the
group receiving standard wound care and aloe gel compared to
the group receiving standard wound care alone. However, animal studies suggests that oral administration as well as topical
aloe gel application may improve healing of various forms of
wounds.[8-10]

Burns   − 1

Despite its popularity, aloe appears to be ineffective for treating
sunburn and may actually be detrimental for the healing of second degree burns.[11,12]

One double-blind trial found aloe ineffective for protecting the
skin during radiation therapy,[13] but a placebo-controlled, ob-
server-blinded trial found evidence of some benefit at higher
doses.[19]

Other Proposed Uses

Oral aloe is sometimes recommended to treat AIDS, asthma,
gastric ulcers, and general immune weakness. Although the evidence for aloe's benefit in these conditions is slight to nonexis-

tent, one of the constituents of aloe, acemannan, has been found to stimulate **immune response** and **inhibit viral replication** in animal and in vitro studies.[14-16]

Mechanism of Action

The mannan polysaccharide acemannan derived from aloe has immunomodulatory and antiviral actions. It is an FDA-approved treatment for fibrosarcoma in cats and dogs and also is used against feline leukemia virus and feline immunodeficiency virus.

Dosage

Topical aloe preparations are typically applied three to four times daily. Studies of aloe for diabetes treatment have used aloe juice at a dose of 1 tablespoon twice daily.

Safety Issues

Other than occasional allergic reactions, no serious problems have been reported with topical or oral aloe gel. However, comprehensive safety studies of aloe are lacking.

Maximum safe dosages in individuals with severe hepatic or renal disease are not known.

Drug aloe, a potent anthraquinone laxative produced from the glands in the skin of the aloe plant, can lead to hypokalemia and other toxic effects.[17] As noted above, aloe gel products may contain small amounts of drug aloe, but not in sufficient quantities to present these risks. Aloe gel does not present the same risks.

Safety in Young Children and Pregnant or Lactating Women

Maximum safe dosages for young children or pregnant or lactating women have not been established.

Drug Interactions

None are known. However, it is conceivable that the known immunomodulatory effects of acemannan could interfere with the action of immune suppressant drugs. If aloe gel does indeed possess significant hypoglycemic effects, interactions with oral hypoglycemic or insulin might be a possibility.

Aloe gel may be a useful adjuvant therapy when combined with **hydrocortisone acetate** cream.[18]

ANDROGRAPHIS
(Androgentaphis paniculata)

Common Uses

Common cold (symptom reduction) [+3]

Common cold (prophylaxis) [+3]

(Higher numbers indicate stronger evidence; X modifier indicates contradictory results. See page xviii of the Introduction for details of the rating scale.)

Approach to the Patient

Andrographis (*Andrographis paniculata*) is widely used in Scandanavia, but is not yet well known in the United States. However, this is changing due to ongoing efforts by manufacturers of andrographis to publicize the positive results seen with andrographis in scientific trials. A growing body of evidence suggests that andrographis can reduce the severity of symptoms in minor respiratory infections. The herb might also offer prophylactic effects.

Animal studies have raised concerns, however, that andrographis may have antifertility actions.

Common Cold
(Symptom Reduction) +3

The herb andrographis may offer symptomatic and prophylactic benefits in minor respiratory infections. Three double-blind, placebo-controlled studies enrolling a total of about 250 participants found that andrographis significantly reduces the duration and severity of cold symptoms.[1-3] In one of these trials, 158 adults with colds received 1200 mg daily of an andrographis extract (standardized to contain 5% andrographolide) or placebo for 4 days.[1] By day 2 of treatment, and even more by day 4, individuals given andrographis extract experienced significant improvements in symptoms compared to participants in the placebo group. The greatest response was seen in earache, sleeplessness, nasal drainage, and sore throat, but other cold symptoms improved as well.

Similar effects were seen in two double-blind, placebo-controlled studies of an herbal combination treatment containing both andrographis and eleutherococcus, enrolling a total of more than 200 individuals.[4]

In a double-blind comparative study, 6 g—but not 3 g—of andrographis proved equally effective to acetaminophen in controlling cold symptoms.[5]

Common Cold (Prophylaxis)   + 3

A 3-month, double-blind, placebo-controlled study of 107 participants found that prophylactic treatment with andrographis at the low dose of 200 mg/day significantly reduced the risk of infection.[6]

Other Proposed Uses

Preliminary animal studies suggest that andrographis may offer benefits in preventing heart disease,[7-9] providing hepatic protection against toxic insult,[10-12] and increasing CD4+ counts in HIV patients.[13]

Mechanism of Action

Some evidence suggests that andrographis may act as an immunostimulant.[14] Although the component andrographolide routinely is used for standardization purposes, it does not appear to affect immune response as much as the whole plant extract. Andrographis does not appear to possess antibacterial effects.[15]

Dosage

A typical dosage of andrographis for the treatment of minor respiratory infections is 400 mg three times a day. Doses as high as 1000 to 2000 mg three times daily have been used in some studies. Andrographis usually is standardized to its content of andrographolide, typically 4% to 6%.

Safety Issues

In human studies, andrographis has not been associated with any serious adverse effects. In one study, no changes in hepatic function, blood counts, renal function, or other laboratory measures of toxicity were found.[3]

Some studies in male and female rodents have raised concerns that andrographis may impair fertility.[16,17] However, at least one study in male rodents has contradicted these findings.[18] Because a definitive answer is lacking, these results are worrisome and suggest the need for more research.

Andrographis may stimulate gallbladder contraction; for this reason, caution should be exercised by individuals with gallbladder disease.[19]

Maximum safe dosages in individuals with severe hepatic or renal disease are not known.

Safety in Young Children and Pregnant or Lactating Women

Maximum safe dosages for young children or pregnant or lactating women have not been established.

Drug Interactions

None are known.

ANDROSTENEDIONE

Common Uses

Athletic performance enhancement   [−1]

(Higher numbers indicate stronger evidence; X modifier indicates contradictory results. See page xviii of the Introduction for details of the rating scale.)

Approach to the Patient

Androstenedione is a precursor to testosterone and estrogen. In the athletic community, androstenedione supplements are used widely in the belief that they increase testosterone production, build muscle, and enhance athletic performance and strength. However, the balance of evidence suggests that this supplement increases estrogen levels more than it increases testosterone levels and that it does not enhance athletic performance.

Explaining that androstenedione raises estrogen more than testosterone will generally discourage use of supplemental androstenedione by male athletes.

In addition, a common contaminant in androstenedione supplements (19-norandrostenedione) may cause positive urine tests for the banned steroid nandrolone.[1]

Athletic Performance Enhancement   −1

All double-blind studies of androstenedione have found that it does not alter total testosterone levels or improve sports performance, strength, or lean body mass.[2-6] In addition, all of these trials were consistent in finding that androstenedione significantly increases estrogen levels.

Only one study, an open trial of 42 healthy men taking 300 mg of androstenedione daily for 7 days, found that androstenedione significantly increased total testosterone levels.[7] However, a 3-month study found that initial increases in total testosterone were overcome by downregulation of synthesis.[6]

Mechanism of Action

Androstenedione is the physiologic precursor of testosterone and is converted to estrogen in the circulation.

Dosage

The typical recommended dose of androstenedione is 100 mg twice daily with food.

Safety Issues

Like other androgens, androstenedione may adversely affect lipid levels,[5,6] as well as cause alopecia and hirsutism.[8]

There has been one case report of priapism lasting for more than 30 hours, requiring a visit to the emergency room.[9] Although it is not certain that androstenedione was the cause in this report, it appears to be the most likely possibility.

There are theoretical concerns that androstenedione might increase the risk of liver and hormone-sensitive cancers.

Maximum safe dosages in individuals with severe hepatic or renal disease are not known.

Safety in Young Children and Pregnant or Lactating Women

No dangers are known. However, given the estrogenic effects, use of androstenedione during pregnancy and lactation is not advisable.

Drug Interactions

None are known. It seems plausible that androstenedione supplementation might alter the effects of other **hormonal therapies.**

ARGININE

Alternate Names/Supplement Forms:
Arginine Hydrochloride, L-Arginine

Common Uses

Congestive heart failure [+2]	**Interstitial cystitis** [−1]
Erectile dysfunction [+2]	**Chronic renal failure** [−1]
Peripheral vascular disease [+2]	**Asthma** [−1]
Angina [+2]	

(Higher numbers indicate stronger evidence; X modifier indicates contradictory results. See page xviii of the Introduction for details of the rating scale.)

Approach to the Patient

Arginine is an essential dibasic amino acid that promotes the formation of nitric oxide, a substance implicated in vasodilation and other aspects of smooth muscle relaxation. This action is the basis of most of the clinical purposes for which arginine has been tried.

Small randomized, double-blind, placebo-controlled trials suggest that arginine may be helpful as adjunct treatment for congestive heart failure. **Note:** Patients may need to be advised that arginine should not be used as a *substitute* for conventional therapy.

Some evidence also suggests potential utility in erectile dysfunction, peripheral arterial disease, and angina pectoris.

Because the net effect of arginine's influence on the insulin/glucagon balance may be hyperglycemia, periodic monitoring of fasting plasma glucose readings may be warranted in prediabetic or diabetic conditions or in patients taking higher doses of arginine.

Congestive Heart Failure (CHF)   + 2

Two double-blind, placebo-controlled studies enrolling a total of 55 patients with CHF found that arginine given for 4 to 6 weeks in doses of 5.6 to 8 g/day ameliorated signs and symptoms of heart failure compared to placebo.[1,2] Significant improvements were seen in arterial compliance, circulating plasma endothelin levels, and forearm blood flow during exercise, as well as walking distance and patient symptom scores.

Another double-blind, placebo-controlled trial of 17 subjects with chronic CHF found that arginine might have favorable effects on renal function over the short term.[3] Patients who received 15 g of arginine orally per day for 5 days showed improvements in glomerular filtration rate (GFR), natriuresis, and plasma endothelin levels.

Erectile Dysfunction (ED)   + 2

One double-blind, placebo-controlled trial of 50 patients with ED found subjective improvement in sexual function after 6 weeks with 5 g/day of arginine compared to placebo.[4] Those men who improved initially had low urinary nitrate levels, which doubled by the end of the study.

However, a double-blind crossover trial of 32 men using a much lower dose of arginine (1.5 mg/day) for 17 days found no effect.[26] Animal studies lend some support for this use as well.[27]

Peripheral
Vascular Disease (PVD)   + 2

Two double-blind, placebo-controlled studies involving a total of 80 patients with symptomatic PVD have found arginine effective. One study of 39 patients with intermittent claudication treated for 3 weeks with 8 g/day of arginine, 40 µg prostaglandin E_1 (PGE_1) twice a day, or placebo found improved pain-free and absolute walking distance, patient symptom scores, and endothelium-dependent vasodilation in the arginine-treated group.[5] Another study with 41 patients reported that 8 g/day of arginine combined with antioxidants, niacin, and isoflavonoids also improved pain-free and total walking distance compared to placebo or low-dose arginine.[6]

Angina   + 2

A double-blind study of 25 individuals with angina pectoris found that treatment with arginine at a dose of 6 g per day had no effect on EKG changes but significantly improved exercise tolerance.[10] The authors propose that peripheral vasodilation was involved.

A double-blind, placebo-controlled crossover trial of 36 individuals with angina found that use of arginine at a daily dose of 6.6 g daily (along with antioxidant vitamins and minerals in a food bar) reduced symptoms of angina.[28]

In an uncontrolled pilot study, 7 of 10 men with severe angina improved from functional class 4 to class 2 while taking arginine at a dose of 9 g/day.[11]

Interstitial Cystitis (IC)   − 1

In a 3-month, double-blind trial of 53 individuals with IC, 27 were given 1500 mg of arginine daily and 26 were given placebo; 21 completed the arginine arm of the study, and 25 completed the placebo arm.[7] Although consistent trends toward superior symptomatic results were seen in the verum group compared to the placebo group intention-to-treat, (ITT) analysis showed no statistically significant difference in primary outcome measures. One very small double-blind trial also found no symptomatic benefit,[8] and another study found no change in bladder NO.[9]

Note that these small studies most likely lacked statistical power to show arginine ineffective; they simply fail to provide evidence of benefit.

Chronic Renal Failure   − 1

A double-blind, placebo-controlled trial of patients with chronic renal failure found no benefit with oral L-arginine given at a dose of 0.2 g/kg body weight/day for 6 months.[12]

Asthma   − 1

A double-blind, crossover study of 14 asthmatics found L-arginine at 50 mg/kg had no effect on airway responsiveness to histamine challenge.[13]

Other Proposed Uses

A double-blind study of 40 children with recurrent **upper respiratory infections** found arginine given for 60 days at a dose of 2 to 4 g reduced the rate of infection.[14]

One small double-blind study found evidence that arginine (3 g three times daily) improved insulin sensitivity in people with type 2 **diabetes.**[15]

A double-blind, placebo-controlled, crossover trial of 10 individuals with Raynaud's phenomenon failed to find arginine at 8 g daily effective for reducing symptoms.[29]

Although arginine is sometimes proposed for enhancement of immune function in AIDS patients, there is no real evidence to support this use. Arginine has been investigated as a treatment for **male infertility,**[16-20] but the best study performed to date returned negative results.[21] Investigational uses of arginine include treatment of **hematologic disorders** such as beta-hemoglobinopathies, sickle cell disease, and beta-thalassemia.[22]

Mechanism of Action

Arginine promotes formation of the vasodilator nitric oxide (NO).[4,5,23,24] Effects on NO are the basis for the study of arginine in cardiovascular disease as well as in erectile dysfunction, female sexual dysfunction, asthma, and interstitial cystitis.

Dosage

The typical supplemental dose of arginine is 2 to 3 g daily. Doses of 6 to 15 g/day have been tried for congestive heart failure.

Safety Issues

Arginine is usually well tolerated, though minor gastrointestinal distress has been reported. Evidence from experience with intravenous use of arginine suggests that gastrin stimulation may occur, which could cause or aggravate gastritis, reflux esophagitis, and peptic ulcer disease.[31] Furthermore, a double-blind, placebo-controlled, crossover study found that an 8-day course of treatment of arginine at a dose of 30 g/day reduced pressure in the lower esophageal sphincter[29]; however, in another trial, continuous intraveneous infusion of arginine did not affect LES motility.[30]

Reports suggest that intravenous arginine might elevate BUN and potassium[31]; whether oral arginine presents the same risk remains unknown.

Given arginine's potential effects on insulin and glucagons (noted earlier), blood glucose levels should be monitored in diabetics who take arginine; however, one study suggests that arginine is safe for use by individuals with stable type 2 diabetes.[25]

Maximum safe dosages in individuals with severe hepatic disease are not known.

Safety in Young Children and Pregnant or Lactating Women

Maximum safe dosages for young children or pregnant or lactating women have not been established.

Drug Interactions

Due to arginine's effects on gastrin release when used in higher doses, patients taking the following drugs may be at increased risk of gastric irritation when taking arginine: **NSAIDs,** including aspirin; other **platelet inhibitors** such as clopidogrel or ticlodipine; **alendronate; theophylline products;** or oral or injectable **corticosteroids.**[22] Individuals who use **alcohol** excessively should avoid arginine for the same reason.

Severe, potentially fatal hyperkalemia has been reported in patients given intravenous arginine for metabolic alkalosis associated with severe liver disease and use of spironolactone. Although it is not clear whether this condition could occur with oral arginine or in individuals without severe hepatic disease, caution is warranted in patients receiving any **potassium-sparing diuretic** or **ACE inhibitors.**

ARTICHOKE LEAF
(Cynara scolymus)

Common Uses

Hyperlipidemia [+3]   **Hepatoprotection** [+1]

**Non-ulcer
dyspepsia** [+1]

*(Higher numbers indicate stronger evidence; X modifier indicates contradic-
tory results. See page xviii of the Introduction for details of the rating scale.)*

Approach to the Patient

Based on one relatively large double-blind trial, artichoke leaf
(Cynara scolymus) has received considerable publicity as a cholesterol-lowering agent. It is probably safe enough to try, but
independent confirmation of effectiveness is lacking.

The other major proposed use of artichoke leaf is non-ulcer dyspepsia. It is authorized for this purpose by Germany's Commission E, but clinical trials involved herbal combinations rather
than artichoke leaf alone.

Hyperlipidemia   +3

In a 6-week, double-blind, placebo-controlled study of 143 individuals with hyperlipidemia, artichoke leaf extract significantly improved lipid profiles.[1] Total cholesterol fell by 18.5%
compared to 8.6% in the placebo group, LDL cholesterol fell
by 23% versus 6%, and LDL/HDL ratio decreased by 20%
versus 7%.

An earlier double-blind, placebo-controlled study of 44 healthy individuals failed to find any improvement in cholesterol levels attributable to artichoke leaf.[2] Researchers noted, however, that at baseline the average cholesterol levels of the study participants were lower than normal; improvement, therefore, could not be expected.

Non-Ulcer Dyspepsia   +1

Germany's Commission E has authorized artichoke leaf for non-ulcer dyspepsia. In Europe, dyspepsia is commonly attributed to inadequate flow of bile from the gallbladder. This assumption is the basis for the use of artichoke leaf, which has been found to possess choleretic properties.[3-5] However, there is no proof that gallbladder dysfunction is actually the cause of dyspepsia, nor direct evidence that artichoke leaf improves dyspepsia symptoms. The only evidence we do have comes from open studies and a trial of a combination herbal treatment containing artichoke leaf.[4]

Hepatoprotection   +1

Highly preliminary evidence suggests that artichoke may have hepatoprotective effects.[6]

Mechanism of Action

Artichoke leaf, perhaps due to its components cynarin and luteolin, appears to interfere with cholesterol synthesis.[2,6]

Dosage

Germany's Commission E recommends 6 g of the dried herb or its equivalent per day, usually divided into three doses.

Safety Issues

Artichoke leaf has not been associated with significant side effects in studies so far, but full safety testing has not been completed.

Individuals with known allergies to artichokes or related plants in the Asteraceae family, such as arnica or chrysanthemums, should avoid using artichoke or cynarin preparations.

Because of its choleretic effects, artichoke leaf should be used with caution in individuals with gallstones or other forms of gallbladder disease.

Maximum safe dosages in individuals with severe hepatic or renal disease are not known.

Safety in Young Children and Pregnant or Lactating Women

Maximum safe dosages for young children or pregnant or lactating women have not been established.

Drug Interactions

None are known.

ASTRAGALUS
(Astragalus membranaceus)

Common Uses

Immune stimulant [+1]

(Higher numbers indicate stronger evidence; X modifier indicates contradictory results. See page xviii of the Introduction for details of the rating scale.)

Approach to the Patient

The Chinese herb astragalus *(Astragalus membranaceus)* is widely marketed as a general immune strengthener and as a treatment for the common cold.

However, a patient may be interested to hear that in traditional Chinese medicine, astragalus is not supposed to be used once an infection has begun; doing so is likened to "locking the chicken coop with the fox inside." Rather, it is supposed to be taken while well to prevent illness. (There is no meaningful evidence to support this traditional belief or any use of astragalus.)

Immune Stimulant   +1

Human, animal, and in vitro studies of astragalus, most of them performed in China, provide weak evidence that astragalus has immunomodulatory effects, increases interferon production, and T-cell, macrophage, and natural killer cell activity.[1-3,5-7,14]

Increased survival time in mice infected with NDV or Sendai virus has been reported with astragalus as well.[1]

Other Proposed
Uses of Astragalus

Weak evidence, again mostly from studies performed in China, has been used to claim that astragalus can reduce ischemia reperfusion injury.[8-12]

It has also been suggested that astragalus may have inhibitory effects on the hepatitis B virus.[13]

Mechanism of Action

Not known.

Dosage

Various standardized and unstandardized extracts of astragalus are available, each with its own recommended dosage.

Safety Issues

There have not been any reports of serious adverse effects associated with use of astragalus.

According to Chinese studies, the LD_{50} for raw astragalus delivered by intraperitoneal injection in rats is about 40 g/kg.[4] A dose of 0.5 g/kg for 30 days produced no toxic symptoms.

Maximum safe dosages in individuals with severe hepatic or renal disease are not known.

Safety in Young Children
and Pregnant or Lactating Women

Maximum safe dosages for young children or pregnant or lactating women have not been established.

Drug Interactions

None are known.

BETA-CAROTENE

Common Uses

Prevention of sunburn and photosensitivity

Reactions [+2X]

Cancer prevention [−2]

Heart disease prevention [−2]

(Higher numbers indicate stronger evidence; X modifier indicates contradictory results. See page xviii of the Introduction for details of the rating scale.)

Approach to the Patient

Beta-carotene is a member of the carotenoid family, one of the groups of chemicals responsible for giving color to fruits, vegetables, and other plants. Considerable evidence from observational studies suggests that high dietary intake of beta-carotene is associated with decreased risk of numerous illnesses, including cancer, heart disease, cataracts, and osteoarthritis.[1-8] However, dietary sources contain many types of carotenes, and there is no real evidence that isolated beta-carotene supplements offer any health benefits. Indeed, some intervention trials have found that beta-carotene supplementation may actually increase the risk of heart disease and some forms of cancer.

Thus, rather than taking beta-carotene supplements, patients might do better by increasing fruit and vegetable intake.

Trials of beta-carotene for prevention of sunburn and photosensitivity reactions have returned mixed results.

Prevention of Sunburn and Photosensitivity Reactions +2X

Results with beta-carotene for sunburn have been mixed.

In a double-blind trial, 20 young women were given 30 mg daily of beta-carotene or placebo for 10 weeks before a 13-day stretch of controlled sun exposure at a sea-level vacation spot.[9] Those who had taken the beta-carotene before and during the sun exposure experienced less skin redness than those taking placebo, even when both groups used sunscreen.

Another 10-week study found that high doses of beta-carotene produced only very minor (though statistically significant) protection against sunburn among 30 men exposed to natural sunshine compared to placebo.[10]

Mild benefits were seen in other studies as well,[11,12] although in one double-blind trial of 16 older women, beta-carotene taken for 23 days didn't provide any more protection than placebo against simulated sun exposure.[13]

Studies on the use of beta-carotene for prevention of erythropoietic protoporphyria, polymorphous light eruptions and other photosensitivity reactions have returned contradictory results.[14-20]

Cancer Prevention   − 2

Two large double-blind, placebo-controlled trials following about 50,000 subjects for up to 8 years found increased risk and incidence of lung and other cancers in individuals taking beta-carotene supplements (20 to 30 mg daily) compared to placebo.[21,22] A similar 12-year, double-blind, placebo-controlled trial of 22,000 subjects found no effect of beta-carotene on the incidence of cancer, including cancers of the lung and skin.[23,24]

Reduced lung cancer risk may be more closely associated with high intake of two carotenes other than beta-carotene: alpha-carotene and lycopene.[25,26]

Heart Disease Prevention   −2

A double-blind, placebo-controlled trial involving about 50,000 subjects found increased rates of heart disease and stroke associated with beta-carotene supplementation at a dose of 20 to 30 mg/day.[22,27-29]

Other Proposed Uses

One preliminary study found evidence that beta-carotene might be helpful for reducing pulmonary exacerbations in **cystic fibrosis.**[30]

In a 2-year, double-blind, placebo-controlled study of 141 women with early **cervical dysplasia (CIN),** 30 mg beta-carotene combined with 500 mg vitamin C per day did not make a significant impact.[31] A 9-month, double-blind, placebo-controlled study of 98 women with moderate CIN found no benefit with beta-carotene alone.[39] Absence of benefit with beta-carotene was also seen in a 2-year, double-blind, placebo-controlled trial of 103 women with high-grade CIN[40] and in a 12-month, double-blind, placebo-controlled trial of 117 women with abnormal cervical morphology of various types.[41]

A double-blind, placebo-controlled trial of 1484 individuals with **intermittent claudication** found no benefit from beta-carotene (20 mg/day), vitamin E (50 mg/day), or a combination of the two.[32]

Although mixed carotenes found in food seem to slow the progression of **cataracts** and help prevent **macular degeneration,** beta-carotene appears to be ineffective.[33-37] Beta-carotene has also been tried as a treatment for **hypertension,** but the results have not been promising.[38] Beta-carotene has been proposed as a treatment for AIDS, alcoholism, asthma, depression, epilepsy, headaches, heartburn, male and female infertility, Parkinson's disease, psoriasis, rheumatoid arthritis, and schizophrenia, but there is little to no real evidence that it works in any of these conditions.

Mechanism of Action

Beta-carotene is a known antioxidant and vitamin A precursor.

Dosage

At the present time, it is not possible to recommend any dosage of beta-carotene except as a source of supplemental vitamin A.

Safety Issues

At nutritional dosages, beta-carotene is thought to be safe. The only side effects reported from beta-carotene overdose are diarrhea and a yellowish tinge to the hands and feet. These symptoms resolve once beta-carotene ingestion is stopped or the dose reduced. However, as mentioned above, beta-carotene at a daily dosage of 20 mg or more may slightly increase the risk of heart disease and lung cancer.

Maximum safe dosages in individuals with severe hepatic or renal disease are not known.

Safety in Young Children and Pregnant or Lactating Women

Maximum safe dosages for young children or pregnant or lactating women have not been established. However, nutritional doses obtained through food sources are most likely safe.

Drug Interactions

None are known.

BETA-SITOSTEROL

Alternate Names/Supplement Forms: Sitosterols, Sitosterolins

Common Uses

Benign prostatic hyperplasia [+3]

Immunomodulation [+2]

(Higher numbers indicate stronger evidence; X modifier indicates contradictory results. See page xviii of the Introduction for details of the rating scale.)

Approach to the Patient

Beta-sitosterol, a mixture of phytosterols and sterol glucosides (sitosterolins), is a widely used European treatment for benign prostatic hyperplasia (BPH) with meaningful scientific support. Although it has not been shown to decrease prostate volume, beta-sitosterol does appear to improve subjective and objective measures of BPH severity. Much weaker evidence suggests that beta-sitosterol might have useful immunomodulatory functions.

Many products marketed for BPH contain several supplements combined, each at an inadequate dose. Patients may do better using a single-substance product that provides the dose found effective in double-blind trials. (See the article on **BPH** for several reasonably well-documented options.)

Benign Prostatic Hyperplasia +3

Three of four randomized, double-blind, placebo-controlled studies enrolling a total of 519 men with benign prostatic hyperplasia found significant benefits with beta-sitosterol.[1-4] The largest, enrolling 200 men with BPH for a period of 6 months, showed significant improvements in IPSS (International Prostate Symptom Score) and modified Boyarsky score in the treatment group compared to the placebo group, beginning at 4 weeks.[4] Significant relative improvements were also seen in peak flow and mean residual urinary volume. Reduction in prostatic volume was not observed. Similar results were seen in the second largest study, a 6-month double-blind trial of 177 individuals with BPH.[2]

Immunomodulation   +2

A small double-blind, placebo-controlled study found that sitosterol prevented the temporary immune deficiency found in ultramarathon runners, increasing CD3+ and CD4+ cell counts, and decreasing IL-6 and cortisol/DHEA ratio.[5] However, clinical parameters such as infection rate were not measured.

Other Proposed Uses

It has been suggested that beta-sitosterol and other naturally occurring sterols may, like carotenes and flavonoids, offer **general health benefits.**[6]

Mechanism of Action

Not known.

Dosage

The daily dosage of beta-sitosterol for BPH is 60 to 135 mg. In clinical trials, benefits required several weeks to develop.

Safety Issues

Although detailed safety studies have not been performed, beta-sitosterol has been well tolerated in human trials.[1,4] Maximum safe dosages in individuals with severe hepatic or renal disease are not known.

Safety in Young Children and Pregnant or Lactating Women

Maximum safe dosages for young children or pregnant or lactating women have not been established.

Drug Interactions

None are known.

BILBERRY FRUIT

(Vaccinium myrtillus)

Common Uses

Night vision improvement   [−1X]

(Higher numbers indicate stronger evidence; X modifier indicates contradictory results. See page xviii of the Introduction for details of the rating scale.)

Approach to the Patient

This article refers to the fruit of the bilberry plant *(Vaccinium myrtillus)* except where otherwise mentioned.

Bilberry became famous in World War II as an aid to night vision, but clinical studies have generally failed to support this use.

Patients may also have heard that bilberry is helpful for diabetic retinopathy, but this potential use rests on virtually no evidence.

Bilberry possesses antiplatelet effects; for this reason, caution should be exercised when combining it with anticoagulant or antiplatelet agents drugs.

Bilberry *leaf* has been proposed as a treatment for diabetes; however, this herb has far different constituents from bilberry fruit and presents toxic risks.

Night Vision Improvement   −1X

A double-blind crossover trial of 15 individuals found no improvement in night vision attributable to bilberry extract (25% anthocyanosides) taken at a dose of 160 mg twice daily, either immediately or over a period of 3 weeks.[1] Similarly negative results were seen in a double-blind, placebo-controlled crossover trial of 18 subjects[2] and another of 16 subjects.[3]

However, short-term benefits were noted in one double-blind, placebo-controlled study that found improved pupillary photomotor response for 2 hours with a single dose of bilberry extract.[4]

Other Proposed Uses

A double-blind, placebo-controlled trial of bilberry extract in 14 patients with diabetic and/or hypertensive **retinopathy** reported significant improvements in ophthalmoscopic and angiographic examination.[5]

In a single-blind, placebo-controlled study of **venous insufficiency,** bilberry extract resulted in a significant decrease in signs and symptoms over a period of 30 days.[6]

Mechanism of Action

Bilberries contain 5% to 10% catechins, 30% invertose, and relatively small amounts of anthocyanosides and flavone glycosides.[7] Anthocyanosides have received the most attention because of their antioxidant properties, influences on collagen metabolism, and apparent vasoprotective effects.[8]

Like the procyanadolic oligomers (see the **Oligomeric Proanthocyanidin Complexes**), these bioflavonoids appear to increase cross-linkage of collagen fibers, possibly increasing their stability. They also have been reported to normalize capillary permeability, inhibit collagen degradation, promote collagen biosynthesis, reduce inflammatory activity, and scavenge free radicals.[8-13] Like horse chestnut, bilberry extracts appear to reduce capillary leakage in venous insufficiency.[8] Finally, in a well-regarded animal model of ischemia reperfusion injury, 2- to 4-week pretreatment with bilberry extracts effectively decreased several measures of microvascular functional impairment.[14]

Bilberry anthocyanosides have numerous effects in the retina, including enhancing recovery of rhodopsin and altering a variety of enzymatic reactions.[15,16]

Like other flavonoids, at very high doses anthocyanosides inhibit platelet aggregation in vitro and in vivo.[8,17-19]

Dosage

The typical dose of bilberry is 160 mg twice daily of an extract standardized to contain 25% bilberry anthocyanosides.

Safety Issues

Large quantities of bilberry fruit have been administered to rats without toxic effects.[20,21] One open study of 2295 patients showed no serious side effects and only a 4% incidence of mild reactions such as gastrointestinal distress, skin rashes, and drowsiness.[22]

Maximum safe dosages in individuals with severe hepatic or renal disease are not known. The safety of bilberry leaf (as opposed to fruit) has not been well evaluated.

Safety in Young Children and Pregnant or Lactating Women

Maximum safe dosages for young children or pregnant or lactating women have not been established. However, there are no known or suspected problems with such uses, and pregnant women have been given bilberry fruit in clinical trials.[23]

Drug Interactions

Bilberry fruit may be contraindicated in patients taking **anticoagulants** or **antiplatelet agents** or in patients with bleeding disorders, because bilberry anthocyanosides mildly inhibit platelet aggregation.[8,17-19]

BIOTIN

Alternate Names/Supplement Forms:
Biocytin (Brewer's Yeast–Biotin Complex)

Common Uses

Diabetes [+1]

Brittle nails [+1]

(Higher numbers indicate stronger evidence; X modifier indicates contradictory results. See page xviii of the Introduction for details of the rating scale.)

Approach to the Patient

If the patient takes biotin, it is most likely in the belief that high doses of this supplement will promote healthy fingernails. However, there is no meaningful evidence to support this use.

High doses of biotin have also been suggested for improving blood sugar control in diabetes.

Some evidence suggests that biotin supplementation at adequate intake levels (see Dosage) may be warranted under certain circumstances. For example, marginal biotin deficiency may occur during normal pregnancy,[11] possibly increasing risks of congenital defects.[12]

Malabsorption conditions, such as inflammatory bowel disease and short bowel syndrome, may also cause biotin deficiency. Other situations that may warrant biotin supplementation include use of anticonvulsant therapy, alcohol abuse, and long-term treatment with trimethoprim-sulfamethoxazole.[9,10,13-15]

Long-term use of any antibiotic, in fact, may reduce biotin levels by killing biotin-producing colonic bacteria.

Diabetes   + 1

Highly preliminary studies suggest that supplemental biotin may help reduce blood glucose levels in individuals with either type 1 or type 2 diabetes.[1,2]

Biotin also may reduce the symptoms of diabetic neuropathy.[3]

Brittle Nails   + 1

Highly preliminary evidence in humans and animals suggests that biotin supplements may promote healthy nails.[4-6]

Other Proposed Uses

Although biotin has been suggested as a therapy for "cradle cap," there is no real evidence to support claims of efficacy in this condition.

Mechanism of Action

Biotin is a water-soluble B vitamin that is essential for fat and carbohydrate metabolism.

It has been suggested that increased expression of hepatocyte glucokinase may mediate the therapeutic activity of high-dose biotin in type 2 diabetes.[7]

Dosage

For diabetics, the usual recommended dosage of biotin is 7000 to 15,000 μg/day.

A lower dosage of 3000 μg/day has been used to treat brittle fingernails and toenails. For treating cradle cap, the usual dosage of biotin is 6000 μg/day, given to the lactating mother (not the child).

Note that the official Adequate Intake for biotin is far lower. The AI for males and females 19 and older is 30 μg.[15]

Safety Issues

Biotin is thought not to present significant toxic risk. Maximum safe dosages for individuals with severe hepatic or renal disease are not known.

Safety in Young Children and Pregnant or Lactating Women

Maximum safe dosages for young children or pregnant or lactating women have not been established.

Drug Interactions

Individuals taking **anticonvulsants** or **trimethoprim-sulfamethoxazole** might benefit from biotin supplementation at nutritional doses.[9,10,13,14]

BITTER MELON
(Momordica charantia)

Common Uses

Diabetes   [+1]

(Higher numbers indicate stronger evidence; X modifier indicates contradictory results. See page xviii of the Introduction for details of the rating scale.)

Approach to the Patient

Based on highly preliminary evidence, bitter melon *(Momordica charantia)* has been marketed as a treatment for diabetes. Patients can be advised that bitter melon is not likely successfully to replace oral hypoglycemics; at the same time, if the herb does, in fact, successfully augment the effectiveness of standard therapy, hypoglycemic reactions might occur.

Diabetes   +1

Animal studies and open human trials suggest that bitter melon may improve glucose control in type 2 diabetes.[1-4]

Other Proposed Uses

Bitter melon also has been suggested as a treatment for AIDS and cancer, but there is no evidence to support these claims.

Mechanism of Action

The aqueous extract of bitter melon appears to stimulate pancreatic insulin release through some mechanism unlike that of glucose-stimulated insulin release.[2] The constituents responsible for these hypoglycemic effects are not known.

Dosage

The usual dosage of bitter melon is one small, unripe, raw melon or about 50 to 100 ml of fresh juice divided into two or three doses over the course of the day. However, bitter melon tastes *extremely* bitter. Tinctures of bitter melon are now available and may make the herb a bit easier to swallow.

Safety Issues

As a widely eaten food in Asia, bitter melon generally is regarded as safe; however, it can cause diarrhea and stomach pain if taken in excessive amounts. In addition, if bitter melon does prove effective, hypoglycemia could result. Maximum safe dosages in individuals with severe hepatic or renal disease are not known.

Safety in Young Children and Pregnant or Lactating Women

Maximum safe dosages for young children pregnant or lactating women have not been established.

Drug Interactions

Bitter melon may potentiate the effect of oral **hypoglycemics.**[4,5]

BLACK COHOSH
(Cimicifuga racemosa)

Common Uses

Menopausal symptoms   [+2X]

(Higher numbers indicate stronger evidence; X modifier indicates contradictory results. See page xviii of the Introduction for details of the rating scale.)

Approach to the Patient

An herb native to North America, black cohosh *(Cimicifuga racemosa)* has become a staple European treatment for menopausal symptoms. However, the evidence that it is effective for this purpose rests entirely on open trials and one double-blind study the results of which are somewhat questionable.

Although the patient has probably heard that black cohosh is a phytoestrogen, the preponderance of the evidence suggests that black cohosh is not estrogenic.

No meaningful clinical evidence supports the use of black cohosh for premenstrual syndrome or dysmenorrhea.

Menopausal Symptoms   +2X

Only one double-blind, placebo-controlled study of black cohosh in menopause has been reported.[1] This trial of 80 patients at one gynecological practice compared the effects of black cohosh, conjugated estrogens (0.625 mg), and placebo over a period of 12 weeks. Black cohosh produced significantly greater improvements than placebo in the Kupperman index, the

Hamilton Anxiety scale, and the degree of proliferation of the vaginal epithelium. Estrogen proved equivalent to placebo, a result that is somewhat hard to believe.

However, a double-blind, dose-comparison study conducted by the manufacturer of Remifemin (an extract of black cohosh) found no changes in vaginal cytology nor indeed any hormonal effects of black cohosh.[2] Lack of estrogenicity also has been seen in another human trial[3] as well as in animal and in vitro studies of the herb,[4-6] although some evidence suggests possible selective estrogen receptor action.[7-9]

Based on increasing evidence that black cohosh is not estrogenic and does not affect vaginal epithelium, the results of the one positive double-blind, placebo-controlled trial is now cast in doubt. In addition, a 2-month, double-blind trial of 85 breast cancer survivors found that use of black cohosh did not reduce menopausal symptoms.[10]

Several open studies found that when black cohosh was given to women, their menopausal symptoms decreased.[11-14] These studies are widely cited in favor of black cohosh as a treatment for menopause; however, considering that hot flashes have been reported to improve by an average of 50% in the placebo arm of numerous placebo controlled trials,[15] they indicate little.

Thus on balance the evidence for black cohosh as a treatment for menopausal symptoms is very weak.

Mechanism of Action

Black cohosh contains a variety of triterpene glycosides including actein, deoxyactein, cimigoside, cimicifugoside, and racemoside, as well as phytosterins, isoflavones, isoferulic acid, and miscellaneous volatile oils. Much of the apparent vasomotor and endocrine effects of black cohosh are believed to reside in its triterpene glycoside constituents, although the phytosterin and flavone derivatives have also been investigated.[5,16,17]

Some but not all studies suggest that black cohosh may reduce luteinizing hormone (LH) levels.[2,3,5,16,18] However, in view of negative data regarding black cohosh's presumed estrogenic effect, its mechanism of action must be regarded as unknown at this time. The authors of one animal study suggest that black cohosh may act through antiestrogenic effects or even by affecting neurotransmitters.[4] Another potential explanation invokes evidence that constituents of black cohosh might lack estrogenic activity in the uterus but exert estrogenic actions elsewhere, giving the herb functional similarity to pharmaceutical selective estrogen receptor modulators.[7-9]

Dosage

The usual dosage of black cohosh is 1 or 2 tablets twice daily of a standardized extract manufactured to contain 1 mg of 27-deoxyacteine per tablet. See the Appendix for U.S. brand names of clinically tested products.

Germany's Commission E recommends the use of black cohosh for no more than 6 months due to the lack of long-term safety data in humans.

Safety Issues

In human trials, black cohosh has been well tolerated, producing only nonspecific symptoms such as occasional mild gastrointestinal distress.

Studies in rats showed no significant toxicity when black cohosh was given at 90 times the therapeutic dose for a period of 6 months.[14] Ames tests have shown no evidence of mutagenicity.[14]

Studies of breast cancer cells have found that black cohosh does not exhibit any stimulatory effect in vitro.[6,19,20] However, safety of black cohosh for those with previous breast cancer is not known, because the herb has not yet been subjected to large-scale retrospective studies.

Maximum safe dosages in individuals with severe hepatic or renal disease are not known.

Safety in Young Children
and Pregnant or Lactating Women

Because of its apparent endocrine activity, black cohosh is not
recommended for adolescents or pregnant or lactating females.

Maximum safe dosages in young children have not been established.

Drug Interactions

There are weak indications of potential interactions with **antihypertensive medications.**[4,13]

BLUE COHOSH

(Caulophyllum thalictroides)

Alternate Names/Related Species:
Beechdrops, Blue or Yellow Ginseng, Blueberry Root,
Papoose Root, Squawroot

Common Uses

Labor induction   [+1X]

(Higher numbers indicate stronger evidence; X modifier indicates contradictory results. See page xviii of the Introduction for details of the rating scale.)

Approach to the Patient

Due to serious safety concerns, patients should be advised to avoid blue cohosh *(Caulophyllum thalictroides)* entirely. A survey published in the *Journal of Nurse-Midwifery* found, rather alarmingly, that 64% of certified nurse-midwives who prescribe herbal medicines use blue cohosh to induce labor, apparently unaware of its toxicity.[1]

The herb is also often used for regulating the menstrual cycle and to induce abortion. In addition, blue cohosh is sometimes recommended for the treatment of arthritis, cramps, epilepsy, inflammation of the uterus, hiccups, colic, and sore throat.

Labor Induction   +1X

There is no evidence that blue cohosh can induce labor in humans.

Other Proposed Uses

There is no evidence that blue cohosh is effective for any of the other purposes for which it is commonly used.

Mechanism of Action

Not known.

Dosage

Blue cohosh is usually used as a tincture. Label instructions typically recommend 5 to 10 drops taken every 2 to 4 hours.

Safety Issues

Many serious safety concerns exist with blue cohosh, especially in regard to its use during pregnancy and labor (see Safety in Young Children and Pregnant or Lactating Women).

In addition, caulophyllosaponin and caulosaponin glycosides present in blue cohosh have been found to constrict coronary vessels by as much as 26% and cause substantial negative inotropic effect in animal studies.[2]

Blue cohosh also contains methylcysticine, a substance similar to nicotine.

Maximum safe dosages in individuals with severe hepatic and renal disease are not known. However, given the lack of studies to document the herb's efficacy and safety, use of blue cohosh is not recommended for use.

Safety in Young Children and Pregnant or Lactating Women

Constituents of blue cohosh such as anagyrine, N-methylcytisine, and taspine are known to interfere with implantation, produce histologic changes in uterus and thyroid tissue, and cause severe birth defects in cattle and laboratory rats.[2-4]

In addition, one case report documents profound congestive heart failure in a newborn whose mother used blue cohosh to induce labor.[2] Severe neonatal complications were seen in another case as well.[5]

Given these reports and the availability of safe alternatives for inducing labor, blue cohosh is not recommended for use in pregnancy, labor, and lactation.

Drug Interactions

None are known.

BOLDO
(Peumus boldus)

Alternate Names/Related Species: Boldu, Boldus

Common Uses

Dyspepsia [+1]

(Higher numbers indicate stronger evidence; X modifier indicates contradictory results. See page xviii of the Introduction for details of the rating scale.)

Approach to the Patient

Boldo *(Peumus boldus)* is an evergreen shrub native to South America. Although boldo has a long history of use as a culinary spice and medicinal herb, and is still one of the most common medicinal plants used in Chile, it has only recently become the subject of scientific research. It has also come to the attention of popular alternative medicine magazines, and an increasing number of patients have begun to use it for digestive problems.

Germany's Commission E has approved boldo for "spastic gastrointestinal complaints and dyspepsia."[1] This indication is primarily based on evidence that boldo stimulates gallbladder contraction.[2-4] In Europe, dyspepsia is commonly attributed to inadequate flow of bile from the gallbladder.

Boldo is also sometimes recommended as a hepatoprotectant, laxative, and antiinflammatory, but there is negligible evidence for these or any other uses.

Dyspepsia   +1

Boldo taken alone has not been clinically evaluated as a treatment for dyspepsia; however, one study evaluated the effectiveness of an herbal combination treatment containing boldo and other herbs thought to stimulate the gallbladder. In a double-blind trial, 60 individuals given either an artichoke leaf–boldo–celandine combination or placebo found improvements in symptoms of indigestion after 14 days of treatment.[5]

Celandine may be hepatotoxic.[6-8]

Other Proposed Uses

Animal studies of boldo have found some evidence of **hepatoprotectant** properties.[3,4,9] The herb also appears to have some level of **antiinflammatory** effect[3,4,10] and in addition may act as a **laxative**.[2] However, human clinical trials of boldo have not been performed.

Mechanism of Action

Not known. Boldine, a substance with antioxidant properties, is thought to be one of the active ingredients in boldo.[4,9,11]

Dosage

Germany's Commission E recommends 3 g of the dried leaf or its equivalent per day for digestive complaints.

Safety Issues

Comprehensive safety studies of boldo have not been reported. The plant's essential oils can cause kidney damage if taken alone or if large amounts of the leaf are ingested.[12] In rats, boldo extracts caused changes in bilirubin, cholesterol, alanine aminotransferase, aspartate aminotranferase, and urea levels.[12] For this reason, its use should be avoided by individuals with hepatic or renal disease.

In addition, because of its ability to stimulate gallbladder contraction, boldo use in individuals with gallbladder disease should be approached with caution.

Safety in Young Children
and Pregnant or Lactating Women

In rats, hydro-alcohol extract of boldo, as well as isolated boldine, exhibited abortive and teratogenic actions.[12] Over a period of 90-day usage, histologic transformations were not seen. In addition, the plant's essential oils can cause kidney damage if taken alone or if large amounts of the leaf are ingested.[12]

These findings contraindicate boldo use by pregnant or lactating women.

Drug Interactions

None are known; however, concomitant use with **hepatotoxic medications** should be avoided. One case report suggests that a combination of the herbs boldo and fenugreek may potentiate the effects of warfarin.[13]

BORON

Alternate Names/Supplement Forms:
Boron Chelate, Sodium Borate

Common Uses

Osteoarthritis   [+2]

Prostate cancer chemoprevention   [+1]

(Higher numbers indicate stronger evidence; X modifier indicates contradictory results. See page xviii of the Introduction for details of the rating scale.)

Approach to the Patient

Minimal evidence suggests that boron may be helpful for osteoarthritis and osteoporosis, and it is often included in supplement products marketed for those purposes. However, because supplemental boron appears to raise estrogen levels, this use may present risks in women.

Boron is found in grains, nuts, raisins, prunes, noncitrus fruits, and leafy vegetables; women interested in taking boron might do better by increasing their intake of these healthy foods than by taking boron supplements.

There is some evidence that adequate intake of boron might reduce prostate cancer risk.

Osteoarthritis   +2

In a pilot study of 20 patients with severe disease, individuals receiving boron supplementation experienced significant improvement in joint condition and less pain on passive movement compared to the placebo group.[1]

Prostate Cancer Chemoprevention   +1

Data from NHANES III found an inverse association between dietary intake of boron and risk of prostate cancer.[2] However, trials of boron supplements for chemoprevention have not been conducted.

Other Proposed Uses

Weak and contradictory evidence suggests that boron might have some utility in the treatment of **osteoporosis.**[3,4]

Boron is sometimes recommended as a treatment for rheumatoid arthritis, but there is no real evidence that it works for this condition.

Mechanism of Action

Some evidence suggests that boron may have a role in facilitating the absorption of calcium, magnesium, and phosphorus from dietary sources and in decreasing the urinary excretion of these minerals.

Dosage

No dietary or nutritional requirement for boron has been established, and boron deficiency is not known to cause any disease.

When used as a treatment for rheumatoid arthritis or osteoporosis, boron is often recommended at a dosage of 3 mg per day, an amount similar to the average daily intake from food.

Safety Issues

Because the therapeutic boron dosage is equivalent to average dietary intake of the mineral, it is probably fairly safe. Unpleasant side effects, including nausea and vomiting, are only reported at about 50 times the highest recommended dose of boron.

However, in at least two small studies, boron was found to increase estrogen levels, especially in women on estrogen replacement therapy.[3,5] Because of this finding, potential increased risk of breast and uterine cancer in postmenopausal women may be a concern with supplemental boron.

Maximum safe dosages in individuals with severe hepatic or renal disease are not known.

Safety in Young Children and Pregnant or Lactating Women

Maximum safe dosages for young children or pregnant or lactating women have not been established.

Drug Interactions

Use of boron may not be advisable for women taking **HRT (hormone replacement therapy)** due to the risk of elevating estrogen levels excessively (see Safety Issues).

BOSWELLIA
(Boswellia serrata)

Common Uses

Asthma [+2]

Rheumatoid arthritis [+2X]

(Higher numbers indicate stronger evidence; X modifier indicates contradictory results. See page xviii of the Introduction for details of the rating scale.)

Approach to the Patient

Boswellia *(Boswellia serrata)* has become increasingly popular as a treatment for bursitis, osteoarthritis, rheumatoid arthritis, and tendonitis, but the supporting evidence is weak. Better evidence, in fact, supports the use of boswellia for mild asthma, but few patients will have heard of this use.

Asthma   +2

A 6-week, double-blind, placebo-controlled study of 80 individuals with relatively mild asthma found that treatment with boswellia at a dose of 300 mg three times daily reduced the frequency of asthma attacks and improved objective measurements of pulmonary function.[1]

Rheumatoid Arthritis   +2X

According to a review of unpublished studies, preliminary double-blind trials have found boswellia effective in relieving the symptoms of rheumatoid arthritis.[2] Unfortunately, the information given in this review was insufficient to evaluate the quality of the primary research.

A double-blind, placebo-controlled study that enrolled 78 patients found no benefit of boswellia treatment.[3] However, about half of the participants dropped out, reducing the meaningfulness of the result.

Other preliminary research has suggested that boswellia may protect cartilage from damage.[4]

Other Proposed Uses

Preliminary evidence suggests that boswellia may also be helpful for **inflammatory bowel disease.**[5,10,11] Boswellic acids have been investigated as a palliative treatment for **malignant glioma.**[12-14]

Mechanism of Action

Investigations of boswellia have found that its constituents, including substances known as boswellic acids, possess antiinflammatory properties.[6-9]

Dosage

A typical dose of boswellia for asthma is 400 mg three times a day of an extract standardized to contain 37.5% boswellic acids. The full effect is said to take 4 to 8 weeks to develop.

Safety Issues

In human trials, use of boswellia has not been associated with any serious adverse effects. Maximum safe dosages in individuals with severe hepatic or renal disease are not known.

Safety in Young Children and Pregnant or Lactating Women

Maximum safe dosages for young children or pregnant or lactating women have not been established.

Drug Interactions

None are known.

BRANCHED-CHAIN AMINO ACIDS (BCAAs)

Alternate Names/Supplement Forms:
Branched-Chain Amino Acids (Combined);
or Leucine, Isoleucine, or Valine (Separately)

Common Uses

Anorexia of chronic disease [+2]

Amyotrophic lateral sclerosis [+2X]

Muscular dystrophy [−1]

Athletic performance enhancement [−1]

(Higher numbers indicate stronger evidence; X modifier indicates contradictory results. See page xviii of the Introduction for details of the rating scale.)

Approach to the Patient

Preliminary evidence suggests that branched-chain amino acid (BCAA) supplementation may be helpful for anorexia caused by chronic disease, as well as for symptoms of ALS. However patients are more likely to express interest in BCAAs as a sports supplement, a use for which the evidence is more negative than positive.

Anorexia of Chronic Disease   +2

One double-blind, placebo-controlled study looked at the effects of a daily supplement of 4.8 g BCAAs in 28 cancer patients with poor appetite due to either the disease itself or its treatment.[1]

The results showed that appetite significantly improved in individuals taking BCAAs compared to those taking placebo. Similar results were seen in a study of elderly hemodialysis patients.[2]

Amyotrophic Lateral Sclerosis + 2 X

BCAAs have been tried as a treatment for amyotrophic lateral sclerosis (ALS, Lou Gehrig's disease) based on their role in glutamate metabolism. However, study results have been mixed.[3-8] For example, one double-blind, placebo-controlled study of 18 individuals with ALS found that participants treated with BCAAs for 1 year maintained muscle strength and the ability to walk longer than those on placebo.[5] However, other controlled trials found no effect,[3] and one actually found a slight increase in deaths during the study period compared to placebo.[7]

Muscular Dystrophy − 1

A 1-year, double-blind, placebo-controlled study of 96 patients found leucine ineffective for muscular dystrophy.[9]

Athletic Performance Enhancement − 1

BCAAs are most notably used by athletes for building muscle; however, evidence suggests that these supplements do not improve performance or enhance the muscle/fat ratio in the body.[10-17]

Other Proposed Uses

Preliminary evidence suggests that BCAAs might decrease symptoms of **tardive dyskinesia**.[18]

Reports suggest that BCAAs may reduce muscle loss during recovery from surgery, but there is little real evidence of this effect.

Mechanism of Action

BCAAs (leucine, isoleucine, and valine) have a low hepatic uptake and are primarily metabolized by the peripheral skeletal muscles. BCAA metabolism in muscle has been postulated to have a regulatory function on the carbon flux in the tricarboxylic acid (TCA) cycle and to aid in the production of the amino acid glutamine.

Because both strength training and endurance exercise consume greater amounts of BCAAs than normal daily activities,[19] it has been postulated that an athlete's need for dietary intake of these amino acids is increased.

Dosage

The typical dosage of BCAAs is 1 to 5 g daily.

Safety Issues

BCAAs are believed to be safe; when taken in excess, they are simply converted into other amino acids.

Safety in Young Children and Pregnant or Lactating Women

Maximum safe dosages for young children or pregnant or lactating women have not been established.

Drug Interactions

Like other amino acids, BCAAs may interfere with **levodopa** and other antiParkinsonian medications.[20]

BROMELAIN

Alternate Names/Supplement Forms: Proteolytic Enzymes

Common Uses

Surgery [+3X]

Sports injuries [+2]

Sinusitis [+2]

Antibiotic potentiation [+2]

(Higher numbers indicate stronger evidence; X modifier indicates contradictory results. See page xviii of the Introduction for details of the rating scale.)

Approach to the Patient

Since first being manufactured on an industrial scale from the pineapple plant *(Ananas comosus)*, the proteolytic enzyme bromelain has been investigated as a treatment for various medical conditions.[1] Its most obvious use is as a digestive enzyme; however, like other proteolytic enzymes, bromelain appears to be absorbed whole to a significant extent[41,42] and may have systemic antiinflammatory, immunomodulatory, and fibrinolytic effects.

Patients are most likely to be using bromelain as a component of the various products marketed for the treatment of sports injuries. Some evidence suggests that bromelain and related enzymes can, in fact, aid recovery from injuries and surgery.

In addition, bromelain has been tried as a treatment for acute and chronic sinusitis and thrombophlebitis and as an agent for increasing antibiotic absorption.

Surgery   +3X

The evidence regarding bromelain's effectiveness in recovery from surgery is mixed.

In a double-blind, placebo-controlled study, 160 patients with mediolateral episiotomy were given 40 mg of bromelain four times daily for 3 days, beginning 4 hours after delivery.[2] The bromelain-treated group experienced a statistically significant decrease in edema, inflammation, pain, and narcotic use compared to the placebo group.

However, a randomized, unblinded, placebo-controlled study of 158 primigravidae with mediolateral episiotomies found no statistically significant differences between patients treated with bromelain (40 mg four times daily for 3 days, beginning after parturition) and those receiving placebo.[3]

Fifty-three patients undergoing rhinoplasty were randomized to receive either placebo or one of two bromelain dosing schedules.[4] In patients receiving placebo only, swelling and ecchymoses persisted for about 7 days compared to 2 days in both bromelain groups. No difference was demonstrated between the two bromelain groups.

In a double-blind, placebo-controlled trial, 95 patients undergoing iridectomy and lens extraction were randomized to take bromelain (40 mg four times daily, pre- and postoperatively) in conjunction with standard anesthetic, antiinflammatory, antibiotic, and sedative pharmaceuticals.[5] By day 7, lid edema, conjunctival hyperemia and edema, and vitreous reactions in the treated group demonstrated a statistically significant improvement compared with the placebo group.

Benefits were also seen in a small double-blind, placebo-controlled crossover study of patients undergoing dental surgery (primarily third molar extractions).[6]

However, a randomized study of 154 patients undergoing facial plastic surgery and receiving placebo or bromelain (400 mg daily, 1 day before and 4 days after the procedure) found no significant difference in edema between the control and bromelain groups.[7]

Sports Injuries   +2

A controlled study of 146 boxers (blinding not stated) with bruises on the face and hematomas on the orbits, lips, ears, chest, and arms found complete clearing of bruises in 78% of the treatment group compared to 3% of the placebo group after supplementation with 40 mg bromelain taken four times daily for 4 days.[8]

Sinusitis   +2

In a double-blind, placebo-controlled trial, 48 patients with severe to moderately severe sinusitis were randomized to receive two tablets of placebo or bromelain (dose not reported) four times daily for 6 days.[9] All patients were given standard therapy concurrently for sinusitis, which included antihistamines, analgesics, and antibiotics. On completion of the study, inflammation was reduced and breathing difficulty was relieved in greater percentages among those receiving bromelain compared to the placebo group.

Benefits were also seen in two other studies enrolling a total of more than 100 individuals with sinusitis.[10,11]

Antibiotic Potentiation   +2

In human and animal models, bromelain has been found to increase the absorption and penetration of concomitantly administered medications.

In one double-blind, placebo-controlled trial, 42 surgery patients were randomized to receive 1000 mg of amoxicillin with 160 mg of bromelain or with matching placebo.[12] Investigators found that bromelain significantly increased tissue penetration of amoxicillin in the gallbladder, bile, and skin compared to placebo. Other human and animal studies have found evidence of potentiation of amoxicillin, tetracycline, chloramphenicol, and penicillin.[13,14]

Other Proposed Uses

An 8-day, double-blind, placebo-controlled study of 73 individuals with **thrombophlebitis** evaluated bromelain as adjunct therapy, but despite a consistent trend for more rapid improvement in the bromelain group, the results achieved statistical significance only in one measure (redness).[15]

Preliminary evidence suggests that bromelain may be helpful in treating **familial amyloidotic polyneuropathy**[16] and **ulcerative colitis**.[17]

In a variety of animal models, topically applied bromelain has been found to exert a necrolytic effect on **third-degree burns**.[18-21] However, in simulated third-degree frostbite injuries conducted on swine, topical bromelain only debrided the superficial layers of the eschar.[22]

Bromelain has also been proposed as a treatment for food allergies, chronic venous insufficiency, hemorrhoids, osteoarthritis, rheumatoid arthritis, gout, and dysmenorrhea; however, there is no real evidence as yet that it is effective for any of these conditions.

Mechanism of Action

Bromelain's apparent antiinflammatory and antiedema effects may be due in part to its dose-dependent partial inhibition of the pro-inflammatory prostaglandin PGE_2, its activation of plasmin, and its antagonism or inhibition of bradykinin production.[23-25]

By depolymerizing fibrin and possibly by digesting other proteins, bromelain may increase tissue permeability, restore drainage, and re-establish circulation.[26,27] In a rat model, 10 mg/kg of intravenous bromelain reduced total plasma kininogen by

50%.[28] The mechanism by which bromelain affects hematoma resolution may be increased serum fibrinolytic activity and inhibition of plasma exudation through inhibition of bradykinin generation.[29] Bromelain may also have immunomodulatory effects.[30,43]

Dosage

Assessing the proper dose of bromelain may be difficult due to the various designations used to indicate its activity. Rohrer units (RU), gelatin dissolving units (GDU), Federation International nationale Pharmaceutique units (FIP), and milk clotting units (MCU) have been frequently used. One gram of bromelain standardized to 2000 MCU would be approximately equal to 1 g with 1200 GDU.[31]

For inflammation, studies have used 20 to 40 mg three or four times daily for 3 to 7 days. For surgical patients the recommended adult dose is 500 mg three or four times daily beginning 72 hours prior to surgery (if possible) and continuing at least 72 hours postoperatively.

Safety Issues

Bromelain appears to be essentially nontoxic. In rat studies, no toxic effects were seen at oral doses as high as 10 g/kg.[32] A 6-month study conducted in dogs with increasing daily levels of bromelain up to 750 mg/kg showed no toxic effects.[23] Rat studies have found no carcinogenicity with bromelain in doses up to 1.5 g/kg/day.[23]

Within the recommended dosage, bromelain is generally well tolerated. Patients may complain of mild gastrointestinal upset or diarrhea. Constipation has been reported in patients taking bromelain for enzyme supplementation and may be relieved by reducing the dose.

However, bromelain has been reported to cause both immediate-type and late-phase IgE-mediated reactions.[33-35] Sensitization usually occurs by inhalation and may be occupationally acquired. Symptoms may occur hours after exposure and may not be refractory to antihistamine and steroid treatments. Cross-allergenicity with bromelain has been reported for wheat flour, rye flour, kiwi fruit, perennial ryegrass, grass pollen, and birch pollen.[33,36-38]

In addition, one study that investigated the effects of bromelain in 19 hypertensive patients found a concentration-dependent increase in heart rate but not in blood pressure.[39]

One study of 47 patients with various disorders leading to edema and inflammation found no significant effects of oral bromelain (40 mg four times daily for 1 week) on bleeding, coagulation, and prothrombin time.[40]

Maximum safe dosages in individuals with severe hepatic or renal disease are not known.

Safety in Young Children and Pregnant or Lactating Women

Rat studies have found no teratogenic effects with bromelain in doses up to 1.5 g/kg/day.[23] However, due to insufficient human data, bromelain should be avoided in pregnant or lactating women. Maximum safe dosages for young children have not been established.

Drug Interactions

Though not reported to date, there are theoretical concerns regarding the concomitant use of bromelain with **anticoagulants** or **antiplatelet agents.**

As noted previously, bromelain may increase tissue levels of various **antibiotics.**

In an animal study, bromelain was found to increase pentobarbital sleeping time, suggesting the potential for interaction with other **sedatives** as well.[32]

BUGLEWEED
(Lycopus virginicus)

Alternate Names/Related Species:
Gypsyweed, Gypsywort, Sweet Bugle, Virginia Water
Horehound, Water Bugle, *Lycopus europaeus*

Common Uses

Hyperthyroidism   [+1]

Cyclic mastalgia   [+1]

(Higher numbers indicate stronger evidence; X modifier indicates contradictory results. See page xviii of the Introduction for details of the rating scale.)

Approach to the Patient

Bugleweed *(Lycopus virginicus)* has become popular as a self-treatment for hyperthyroidism. While there is some evidence bugleweed may have antithyroid effects, this is clearly not a condition in which self-treatment is advisable.

Based on weak evidence that bugleweed suppresses prolactin, it has been promoted as a treatment for cyclic mastalgia. However, there is much better evidence supporting the use of chasteberry for this condition.

Hyperthyroidism   +1

In vitro and animal studies suggest that bugleweed may reduce thyroid hormone levels in two ways: decreasing TSH release and impairing thyroid hormone synthesis.[1-5] In addition, bugleweed may block the action of the thyroid-stimulating antibodies found in Grave's disease.[2]

Cyclic Mastalgia   +1

Highly preliminary evidence suggests that bugleweed may reduce prolactin secretion.[4] Based on this effect, bugleweed has been suggested as a treatment for cyclic mastalgia. The same argument is used to support the use of the herb chasteberry; however, chasteberry actually has supporting evidence for efficacy in treating cyclic mastalgia.

Mechanism of Action

Not known.

Dosage

The dosage of bugleweed is adjusted by measuring T_4 levels; a standard starting dose is 1 to 2 g daily of the whole herb, or the equivalent dosage in extract form.

Safety Issues

The safety of bugleweed has not been established.

Long-term or high-dose use of bugleweed may cause thyroid enlargment. The herb should not be given to individuals with hypothyroidism. Sudden discontinuation of bugleweed may cause rebound hyperthyroidism.

Maximum safe dosages in individuals with severe hepatic or renal disease are not known.

Safety in Young Children and Pregnant or Lactating Women

Bugleweed should not be used by pregnant or lactating women. Maximum safe dosages for young children have not been established.

Drug Interactions

Bugleweed may interact unpredictably with **thyroid replacement therapy** and **thyroid imaging**. Due to its apparent effects on prolactin, combination treatment with **bromocriptine** or related agents might also result in unpredictable effects.

BUTTERBUR

(Petasites spp., including *Petasites hybridus,
P. albus,* and *P. vulgaris)*

Alternate Names/Related Species:
Blatterdock, Bog Rhubarb, Bogshorns, Butterfly Dock,
Capdockin, Flapperdock, Langwort, Umbrella Leaves

Common Uses

Migraines (prophylaxis) [+2]

Seasonal allergic rhinitis [+2]

(Higher numbers indicate stronger evidence; X modifier indicates contradictory results. See page xviii of the Introduction for details of the rating scale.)

Approach to the Patient

The manufacturer of standardized butterbur extract is aggressively promoting this herb for migraine headache prophylaxis and one double-blind, placebo-controlled trial supports this use. Butterbur might also be helpful for allergic rhinitis.

Based on its apparent smooth-muscle relaxant effects and possible antiinflammatory properties, butterbur has also been proposed as a treatment for asthma, irritable bowel syndrome, and tension headaches. However, the evidence for any of these uses remains indirect.

Raw butterbur contains toxic pyrrolizidine alkaloids; these are removed in the process used to manufacture the tested standardized butterbur extract.

Migraines (Prophylaxis)   + 2

A double-blind, placebo-controlled study involving 60 men and women with a history of at least three migraines per month evaluated the effectiveness of butterbur as a migraine prophylactic.[1] After a 4-week washout period, participants were given either 50 mg of butterbur extract or placebo twice daily for 3 months. The results were positive: both the number of migraine attacks and the total number of days of migraine pain were significantly reduced in the treatment group compared to the placebo group. Three of four individuals taking butterbur reported improvement compared to only one of four in the placebo group. No significant side effects were noted.

Seasonal Allergic Rhinitis   + 2

A 2-week, double-blind study of 125 individuals with seasonal allergic rhinitis compared a standardized butterbur extract against cetirizine (10 mg daily).[14] Treatment effectiveness according to the primary outcome measure, Medical Outcome Health Survey Questionnaire (SF-36), indicated that both treatments were equally effective. Equivalent effectiveness was also seen on the Physician's Clinical Global Impression score.

Other Proposed Uses

Butterbur has been investigated for use in **asthma, abdominal pain, tension headaches, back pain, bladder spasms,** and **gallbladder pain,**[2-6] but there is no real evidence as yet that it is effective in these conditions.

Mechanism of Action

Butterbur is thought to have antiinflammatory, antispasmodic, antihistaminic, and antidopaminergic effects, due to its petasin and isopetasin constituents.[2,6-9] It appears to affect peptido-leukotrienes but not prostaglandins, and the particular pattern of its actions may actually provide some gastroprotection.[10,11]

Dosage

The recommended dosage of the tested butterbur product is 50 mg twice daily. See the Appendix for U.S. brand names of clinically tested products.

Safety Issues

In clinical trials using standardized butterbur extract, no serious adverse reactions were reported. Note, however, that un-processed butterbur contains hepatotoxic and possibly carcino-genic pyrrolizidine alkaloids.[12] These must be removed during the manufacturing process to create a safe product.[13]

Maximum safe dosages in individuals with severe hepatic or re-nal disease are not known.

Safety in Young Children and Pregnant or Lactating Women

Maximum safe dosages for young children or pregnant or lac-tating women have not been established.

Drug Interactions

None are known.

CALCIUM

Alternate Names/Supplement Forms:
Bonemeal, Calcium Aspartate, Calcium Carbonate,
Calcium Chelate, Calcium Citrate, Calcium Citrate Malate,
Calcium Gluconate, Calcium Lactate, Calcium Orotate,
Dolomite, Oyster Shell Calcium, Tricalcium Phosphate

Common Uses

Osteoporosis [+4]

Premenstrual syndrome [+3]

Colon polyps [+3] **and colon cancer prevention** [+2X]

Preeclampsia [+3X]

(Higher numbers indicate stronger evidence; X modifier indicates contradictory results. See page xviii of the Introduction for details of the rating scale.)

Approach to the Patient

Good evidence indicates that calcium supplements significantly reduce osteoporosis progression, ease PMS symptoms, and reduce the incidence of colorectal polyps.

Because calcium deficiency is common, it is probably reasonable to advise most patients to consider taking calcium supplements.[1]

Patients may have heard that calcium citrate is the best absorbed form of calcium; although this is not as clear as many people believe, calcium citrate or calcium citrate malate may indeed be more effective for osteoporosis than the much cheaper calcium carbonate form (whether due to better absorption or specific effects of the anion has not been elucidated).

Osteoporosis   +4

Numerous well-designed studies indicate that calcium supplementation at recommended dosages has been found to help prevent and slow nonvertebral bone loss in postmenopausal women.[2,3] The combination of vitamin D and calcium may not only slow but also reverse both vertebral and nonvertebral bone loss.[4] Supplemental calcium also appears to enhance the effects of estrogen replacement therapy.[5] However, calcium and vitamin D use must be continued because improvements in bone rapidly disappear once the supplements are stopped.[6]

Calcium supplementation appears to be useful for increasing bone density in children and adolescent girls,[7,8] but some studies suggest that exercise may be even more important.[9]

One study found that in calcium-deficient pregnant women, calcium supplementation increases fetal bone mineralization.[10]

Use of calcium may be enhanced by other nutrients. One study found that calcium citrate malate is more effective in individuals who have a relatively high intake of protein.[76] Adding various trace minerals (15 mg zinc, 2.5 mg copper, and 5 mg manganese) along with calcium and vitamin D may also improve the outcome.[81,82] Similarly, essential fatty acids may enhance the effectiveness of calcium for osteoporosis. In one study, 65 postmenopausal women were given calcium along with either placebo or a combination of omega-6 fatty acids (from evening primrose oil) and omega-3 fatty acids (from fish oil) for a period of 18 months. At the end of the study period, the group receiving essential fatty acids had higher bone density and fewer fractures than the placebo group.[11] However, in a 12-month, double-blind trial of 85 women no benefits were seen.[12] The explanation for the discrepancy may lie in the differences between the women studied. The first study involved women living in nursing homes, the second, healthier women living on their own. The second group of women may have been better nourished and already receiving enough essential fatty acids in their diet.

Corticosteroids accelerate osteoporosis by decreasing intestinal absorption of calcium as well as through other mechanisms. Supplementation with calcium and vitamin D may help prevent the loss of bone density associated with long-term corticosteroid therapy.[13-15] A review of five studies covering a total of 274 participants reported that calcium and vitamin D supplementation significantly prevented bone loss in corticosteroid-treated individuals.[15] For example, in a 2-year, double-blind, placebo-controlled study of 130 individuals, daily supplementation with 1000 mg of calcium and 500 IU of vitamin D actually reversed steroid-induced bone loss, resulting in a net bone gain.[13]

Premenstrual Syndrome   + 3

A double-blind, placebo-controlled study of 497 women found that 1200 mg daily of calcium carbonate reduced PMS symptoms by half over a period of three menstrual cycles.[16] Improved symptoms included mood swings, headaches, food cravings, and bloating. These results corroborate earlier, smaller studies.[17,18]

Colon Polyps   + 3 and
Colon Cancer Prevention   + 2 X

A 4-year, double-blind, placebo-controlled study that followed 832 individuals with a history of polyps found that use of calcium carbonate resulted in 24% fewer polyps compared to placebo.[19]

There is also evidence from observational studies that a high calcium intake is associated with a reduced incidence of colon cancer,[20] but not all studies have found this association.[21]

Preeclampsia   + 3 X

A metaanalysis of 10 studies involving more than 6000 women found evidence that calcium may have a role in preventing pregnancy-induced hypertension, or preeclampsia, particularly in women at high risk for hypertension and/or those with low calcium intake.[22,23] However, the largest study in the

metaanalysis found no benefits. In this double-blind trial, researchers gave either 2 g of calcium or placebo daily to 4589
women from weeks 13 to 21 of their pregnancy onward. In the
end, researchers found no significant decreases in rates of hypertension or preeclampsia, not even among women with the
lowest calcium intake.[23]

Other Proposed Uses

Calcium deficiency may play a role in the development of
hypertension.[24,25] However, taking extra calcium does not appear to reduce blood pressure significantly.[26] Calcium supplements might slightly improve **lipid profile.**[26,27,77]

One preliminary study suggests that supplementation with calcium and vitamin D may be helpful for women with **polycystic
ovary syndrome.**[28]

Calcium is also sometimes recommended for attention deficit
disorder, migraine headaches, and periodontal disease, but
there is as yet little to no evidence that it is effective for these
conditions.

Mechanism of Action

Calcium is an essential component of the bony matrix and plays
a critical role in a large number of physiologic processes. Its
mechanism of action in PMS and polyp prevention is not clear
but may relate to its role as an intracellular messenger.

Dosage

Dosage recommendations for calcium vary by age. Adequate Intakes by age group are as follows: 9 to 18 years, 1300 mg; 19 to
50 years, 1000 mg; and 51 years and older, 1200 mg.

Studies suggest that no more than 500 mg of calcium is absorbed at one time, indicating that daily dosages should be di-

vided for maximal efficacy.[29] In addition, adequate levels of vitamin D are required for optimal calcium absorption.

The most clinically relevant forms of supplemental calcium are naturally derived, refined, and chelated. Naturally derived forms of calcium include bonemeal, oyster shell, and dolomite. Although they are economical and typically contain 500 to 600 mg of calcium per tablet, concerns have been raised that some of these natural forms may contain significant amounts of lead (less than 2 ppm is recommended).[30] Refined calcium carbonate is the most common commercial calcium supplement and one of the least expensive forms of calcium, but it can cause constipation and bloating and may not be well absorbed by individuals with a history of reduced gastric acid secretion. Certain forms of chelated calcium (calcium citrate and calcium citrate malate) may be more absorbable and/or more effective for osteoporosis treatment than calcium carbonate, but not all studies agree.[3,31-34,78,79] The discrepancy may be due to the particular calcium product used: some calcium carbonate formulations may dissolve better than others. It has been suggested that the citrate anion plays a positive role in osteoporosis treatment.[31-34,80]

Calcium may interfere with absorption of chromium,[35-37] manganese,[35-37] magnesium,[38,39] iron,[40-45] and zinc.[43,46-48]

A soy constituent called phytic acid can interfere with the absorption of calcium, so it may be advisable to keep soy consumption and calcium supplements 2 hours apart.

Safety Issues

Tolerable upper intake levels for calcium in adults have been set at 2500 mg daily.[49]

Though calcium *supplements* might increase kidney stone risk,[50] studies have found that increased *dietary intake* of calcium reduces the risk of kidney stones.[50,51] Maximum safe dosages in individuals with severe renal or hepatic disease are not known.

Large observational studies have found that higher intakes of calcium are associated with a greatly increased risk of prostate cancer.[52-54]

Hyperparathyroidism, sarcoidosis, and some cancers may be complicated by calcium supplementation.

Safety in Young Children and Pregnant or Lactating Women

The tolerable upper intake level of calcium for children above 1 year old and women who are pregnant or lactating has been set at 2500 mg daily.[49]

Drug Interactions

The action of **calcium channel blockers** may be affected by taking a combination of calcium supplements and high-dose vitamin D.[55]

Calcium supplements may decrease blood levels of the beta-blocker atenolol and possibly other **beta-blockers,** though the clinical effects appear to be minimal after several doses.[56]

Calcium may interfere with the absorption of antibiotics in the **tetracycline** and **fluoroquinolone** families. Individuals taking any of these medications should take calcium supplements at least 2 hours after antibiotic dosing.[57-61]

Long-term use of **thiazide diuretics** tends to increase serum calcium levels by decreasing calcium excretion.[62-65]

Weak evidence also suggests that **digoxin** may increase calcium excretion, potentially leading to depletion of the mineral.[66] The clinical significance of this finding is not known.

Corticosteroids and **anticonvulsants** such as phenytoin, carbamazepine, phenobarbital, and primidone interfere with the absorption of calcium. Though supplementation with calcium may be warranted, doses should be taken at least 2 hours apart from any of these pharmaceuticals.

Concerns have been raised that the **aluminum** content of some antacids may be harmful.[67-72] It is therefore recommended that patients take calcium citrate separately from aluminum-containing antacids, use other forms of calcium, or avoid antacids containing aluminum.

Calcium supplements may interfere with the absorption of **levothyroxine.**[73-75]

CALENDULA
(Calendula officinalis)

Common Uses

Skin injuries and lesions (topical)   [+1]

(Higher numbers indicate stronger evidence; X modifier indicates contradictory results. See page xviii of the Introduction for details of the rating scale.)

Approach to the Patient

Calendula is a common constituent of topical creams intended for the treatment of skin conditions. Although supporting evidence for effectiveness remains minimal, this is at least a harmless treatment.

Skin Injuries and Lesions (Topical)   +1

In vitro and animal studies weakly suggest that calendula cream may possess wound-healing and antiinflammatory properties.[1-5]

Based on these findings, topical calendula products are widely marketed for the treatment of skin conditions such as eczema and minor wounds. However, double-blind human trials have not been reported.

Mechanism of Action

The triterpenoid esters in calendula have been the primary focus of most research, although little is known definitively about mechanism of action (if indeed triterpenoid esters, or calendula as a whole, are clinically active).

Dosage

Calendula cream is typically applied two or three times daily to the affected area.

Safety Issues

Topical calendula is generally regarded as safe.

Safety in Young Children
and Pregnant or Lactating Women

No safety issues have been raised regarding the use of topical calendula by young children or pregnant or lactating women.

CARNITINE

Alternate Names/Supplement Forms:
Acetyl-L-Carnitine (ALC), L-Carnitine,
Propionyl-L-Carnitine (PLC), L-Propionylcarnitine (LPT),
L-Acetyl-Carnitine (LAT)

Common Uses

Post–myocardial infarction recovery [+3]

Intermittent claudication [+3]

Angina [+2]

Congestive heart failure [+2]

Dysthymia [+2]

HIV support [+1]

Dementia [−2X]

Anticonvulsant-induced carnitine deficiency [−1X]

Athletic performance enhancement [−1X]

(Higher numbers indicate stronger evidence; X modifier indicates contradictory results. See page xviii of the Introduction for details of the rating scale.)

Approach to the Patient

Medical interest in carnitine in the United States has been almost entirely restricted to its use for rare inborn errors of amino acid metabolism. However, in Europe, physicians have used various forms of carnitine for the adjunct treatment of angina, intermittent claudication, congestive heart failure, post-MI cardioprotection, dementia, and dysthymia. Supplemental carnitine has also been suggested as a treatment to correct the carnitine depletion possibly caused by various antiseizure drugs as well as counter the cardiotoxic effects of zidovudine. Carnitine has also been tried in hyperthyroidism.

It is important to caution patients that carnitine has not been suggested as an *alternative* to standard care for cardiovascular disease, but rather as an adjunct treatment.

Post-MI Recovery   +3

Two double-blind, placebo-controlled studies that followed a total of 632 individuals status post-MI found that over a 1-year period adjunct use of L-carnitine caused significant decreases in ventricular hypertrophy,[1] anginal attacks, and mortality,[2] as well as improvement in some hemodynamic parameters.[2] The dosage in the larger of the two studies was 9 g daily intravenously for 5 days followed by 6 g daily orally; the other used 4 g daily orally.

Another double-blind, placebo-controlled study that followed 101 postinfarct patients for 1 month found that use of L-carnitine reduced mean infarct size and reductions of other postinfarct complications compared to placebo.[3]

However, a double-blind, placebo-controlled study of 60 individuals status post–acute anterior MI found no relative improvement in left ventricular function after 3 months of treatment with carnitine.[85]

Intermittent Claudication   +3

A 12-month, double-blind, placebo-controlled trial of 485 patients with intermittent claudication found that propionyl-L-carnitine at a dose of 1 g twice daily produced a significant (44%) improvement in maximal walking distance in those with initial maximal walking distance less than or equal to 250 m; however, no response was seen in those with milder disease.[4] Quality of life improvements were also noted. Benefits were seen in most but not all other studies using L-carnitine or L-propionylcarnitine.[5-15]

Angina   + 2

A controlled (but not blinded) study of 200 patients taking conventional medical therapy for exercise-induced angina found significant reduction of ST-segment depression during maximal effort and improvement of hemodynamic parameters in the group receiving L-carnitine supplementation over 6 months compared to no treatment.[16] In addition, patient needs for primary medications were reduced, as were plasma cholesterol and triglyceride levels. Smaller double-blind, placebo-controlled trials using L-carnitine or L-propionylcarnitine also found positive effects.[17-21] For example, a double-blind trial of 74 individuals found that use of L-propionylcarnitine improved some, but not all, measures of angina severity compared to placebo.[86] However, a double-blind comparative trial found that L-propionyl-carnitine appeared to be less effective than diltiazem.[87]

Congestive Heart Failure (CHF)   + 2

Acute infusion of L-propionylcarnitine improves myocardial contractility and relaxation and cardiac pump function in patients with ventricular dysfunction.[22-24]

A double-blind, placebo-controlled trial that followed 50 patients with NYHA class II CHF for a period of 6 months reported that use of L-propionlylcarnitine increased exercise duration and improved hemodynamic parameters.[25] Similar results were seen in other studies.[16,26,27]

Dysthymia   + 2

One double-blind, placebo-controlled study of 60 geriatric patients with dysthymia found that treatment with 3 g/day of acetyl-L-carnitine over a 2-month period significantly improved symptoms compared to placebo.[28]

HIV Support   + 1

Preliminary evidence suggests that L-carnitine may diminish the mitochondrial toxicity associated with zidovudine (AZT) and other nucleoside analogs, exert independent positive effects on HIV infection parameters, and complement traditional chemotherapeutic regimens in HIV-infected patients.

Zidovudine therapy causes a mitochondrial myopathy characterized by depletion of mitochondrial DNA and other destructive changes that have been associated with a reduction of muscle carnitine levels.[29] Based on the observation that L-carnitine plays a major role in long-chain fatty acid transport and facilitates the beta-oxidation of fatty acids, it has been proposed as a treatment for these side effects.[30]

Other preliminary evidence suggests that L-carnitine may also enhance immune function in HIV infected individuals.[31-33]

Dementia   − 2 X

Numerous double- or single-blind studies involving a total of more than 1400 patients have evaluated acetyl-L-carnitine in the treatment of Alzheimer's disease and other forms of dementia.[34-44] Though some reported positive results in some measures of mental function, the balance of the evidence is negative. One of the largest double-blind, placebo-controlled studies, following 431 patients with mild to moderate probable Alzheimer's for 1 year, found no significant improvement with supplemental carnitine.[45] Based on benefits seen in subgroup analysis, the same researcher performed a subsequent study to evaluate whether acetyl-L-carnitine was useful in young-onset Alzheimer's disease.[14] In this 1-year, double-blind, placebo-controlled trial of 229 patients, no benefits were seen.

Anticonvulsant-Induced Carnitine Deficiency   −1X

Despite evidence that antiseizure drugs may reduce serum carnitine levels and cause carnitine-dependent metabolic dysfunction,[46-51] one double-blind, crossover study of 47 children taking anticonvulsants found no measurable benefit with carnitine supplementation.[52]

Athletic Performance Enhancement   −1X

Several small double-blind studies of L-carnitine supplementation for athletic performance enhancement in both healthy and impaired individuals have yielded contradictory results, and even the most positive studies show only slight gains.[53-60] A 1996 review article concluded that there was no scientific evidence that carnitine supplementation enhances exercise performance.[61]

Other Proposed Uses

In a large double-blind trial (n=625) in Brazil, carnitine supplementation at a dose of 100 mg/kg/day in two divided doses for 4 days reduced the incidence and mortality of **myocarditis** in cases of childhood diphtheria.[62]

A 6-month, double-blind trial evaluated the effects of L-carnitine in 50 healthy women who were taking exogenous T_4 for suppression of benign goiter.[63] The results showed that a dose of 2 or 4 g daily had bone-sparing effect and reduced other standard symptoms of **hyperthyroidism.** Previous evidence suggests that carnitine may inhibit thyroid hormone action.[64]

A 1-year, double-blind, placebo-controlled crossover trial of 24 individuals with various forms of **cerebellar ataxia** found that acetyl-L-carnitine at a dose of 1000 mg twice daily improved coordination and muscle tone.[65]

Mixed evidence suggests that intravenous L-carnitine or propionyl-L-carnitine may offer **cardioprotective effects** in cardiac surgery and improve heart function in cardiogenic shock.[22,66-69]

A 52-week, double-blind, placebo-controlled trial of 19 diabetics found that treatment with acetyl-L-carnitine at a dose of 1500 or 3000 mg daily might help prevent **diabetic cardiac autonomic neuropathy.**[70]

Evidence from three small double-blind, placebo-controlled studies enrolling a total of about 50 individuals suggests that L-carnitine can improve exercise tolerance in **COPD,** presumably by improving muscular efficiency in the lungs and other muscles.[71-73]

Carnitine may be helpful for individuals with **high levels of Lp(a) lipoprotein.**[74]

Uncontrolled studies suggest that L-carnitine or acetyl-L-carnitine may be helpful for improving sperm function.[88-96]

One study failed to find carnitine effective as a weight loss–enhancing agent.[97]

Weak to nonexistent evidence has been used to suggest that carnitine may be useful for the following conditions: arrhythmias, Down syndrome, muscular dystrophies, and alcoholic fatty liver disease.

Mechanism of Action

Carnitine is an essential factor for the transport of long-chain fatty acids into the mitochondria. Necropsy has shown decreased L-carnitine concentrations in the infarct area of patients who have suffered fatal MIs.[75] This is attributed to diffusion of L-carnitine away from ischemic tissue.[16]

Free fatty acids and acetylene–CoA in long chains accumulate under ischemic conditions. These substances degrade cellular membranes and also inhibit adenine nucleotide translocase, which catalyzes the movement of ADP from cytoplasm to mitochondria and of ATP in the reverse direction. Repletion with L-carnitine may protect the failing heart by stimulating oxidative metabolism of fatty acids and acetylene-CoA.[16,76-78]

In patients with acute MI, controlled studies have shown that oral or IV administration of carnitine reduced the levels of the MB fraction of creatine kinase.[79] Furthermore, intravenous administration of L-carnitine in patients with moderately impaired left ventricular function produced a positive inotropic effect.[76] In healthy individuals, infusion of L-propionylcarnitine increased heart rate and the effective and functional refractory period of the AV node.[80]

Acetyl-L-carnitine has been postulated to mimic some of the CNS effects of acetylcholine.[37-39,41,43,45,81,98] It may also exert a neuroprotective effect.[35]

The apparent benefits of carnitine in intermittent claudication are presumed to be due to improved muscle function rather than to normalized circulation.[5,82]

Dosage

The daily dosage usually ranges from 1500 to 6000 mg, given in three divided doses, for all forms of carnitine.

Carnitine is used in its L-form, as L-carnitine, L-propionylcarnitine (LPT), and acetyl-L-carnitine (ALC). The D- and DL-forms of carnitine should not be used (see Safety Issues).

Safety Issues

The three L-forms of carnitine appear to be safe.

In a 12-month drug-monitoring study involving more than 4000 patients with cardiovascular disease, the most common adverse effects of L-carnitine were stomach discomfort (6%), nausea (4%), and diarrhea (2%).[89]

L-Carnitine might have antithyroid actions, possibly contraindicating its use in individuals with hypothyroidism.[63,64]

One study found that hemodialysis may cause a transient carnitine deficiency, suggesting the need for supplementation in this patient group.[83] However, an earlier report suggests that patients undergoing hemodialysis might require reduced doses of carnitine.[84]

D-Carnitine is known to cause numerous problems by competitively inhibiting L-carnitine,[60] and DL-carnitine has caused a myasthenia gravis–like syndrome in hemodialysis patients.[76]

Maximum safe dosages in individuals with severe hepatic or renal disease are not known.

Safety in Young Children and Pregnant or Lactating Women

Maximum safe dosages for young children or pregnant or lactating women have not been established.

Drug Interactions

None are known.

CARTILAGE

Alternate Names/Supplement Forms:
Shark Cartilage, Bovine Cartilage

Common Uses

Cancer treatment [+2]

(Higher numbers indicate stronger evidence; X modifier indicates contradictory results. See page xviii of the Introduction for details of the rating scale.)

Approach to the Patient

Phase III studies are evaluating certain liquid shark cartilage extracts as adjunct treatment to standard chemotherapy. Individuals interested in using over-the-counter shark cartilage products for self-treatment of cancer can be advised that such products have not been shown to be effective and that, in any case, shark cartilage has not been advocated as a sole treatment for cancer.

Patients who are interested in using cartilage for osteoarthritis should be directed toward other treatments supported by stronger evidence such as glucosamine and chondroitin.

Cancer Treatment   +2

A number of in vitro studies have found that shark cartilage extract inhibits angiogenesis in chick embryos and other test systems.[1-6] These findings have led to in vitro, animal, and phase II clinical trials to investigate the possible anticancer effects of shark cartilage. The results suggest that a particular liquid shark cartilage extract called Neovastat might be useful in the treatment of various cancers, including lung, prostate, and breast cancer.[7-12] However, not all of these studies have been positive.[13,14]

Phase III trials are now under way in the United States and Canada.

Other Proposed Uses

Although meaningful evidence tells us that constituents of cartilage (glucosamine and chondroitin) benefit osteoarthritis, no studies have evaluated the effects of whole cartilage for osteoarthritis. Weak evidence suggests that shark cartilage treatment might benefit **psoriasis.**[1]

Dosage

Bovine and shark cartilage supplements are available in pill and powdered forms. Various doses of cartilage have been used in different studies, ranging from 2.5 mg to 60 g daily.

Mechanism of Action

Cartilage of all types contains angiogenesis inhibitors used to prevent excessive vascularization. In addition, shark cartilage inhibits matrix metalloproteases (MMPs), enzymes that break down the extracellular matrix.[15] Damage to the matrix is thought to facilitate tumor spread.

Safety Issues

Because cartilage is nothing more than common dietary gristle, it is presumably safe to consume. However, for reasons that are not at all clear at this time, there is a case report of hepatitis occurring with shark cartilage supplementation.[16] Full recovery occurred with discontinuation of the supplement.

Maximum safe dosages in individuals with severe hepatic or renal disease are not known.

Safety in Young Children and Pregnant or Lactating Women

Maximum safe dosages for young children or pregnant or lactating women have not been established.

Drug Interactions

None are known. The drug interactions mentioned for glucosamine could theoretically occur with whole cartilage as well.

CAT'S CLAW
(Uncaria tomentosa)

Alternate Names/Related Species: Una de gato

Common Uses

Osteoarthritis [+2]

Approach to the Patient

Cat's claw *(Uncaria tomentosa)* is a popular herb among the indigenous people of Peru, where it is used to treat cancer, diabetes, ulcers, arthritis, and infections, as well as to assist in recovery from childbirth and as a contraceptive.

Although scientific studies of cat's claw conducted in South America and Europe have yielded several interesting findings, there is no meaningful evidence for any therapeutic benefit at this time.

Patients who are interested in using cat's claw for any of the conditions or situations mentioned above should be directed toward other treatments supported by stronger evidence.

Osteoarthritis   +2

A poorly designed 4-week, double-blind, placebo-controlled trial found suggestive evidence that cat's claw might reduce osteoarthritis symptoms.[2]

Other Proposed Uses

Weak evidence suggests that cat's claw may have **chemopreventive**,[3-6] **immunomodulatory**,[7,8] and **antiviral** effects.[9]

Mechanism of Action

Not applicable.

Dosage

The optimum dosage of cat's claw is not clear. Because of the wide variation in the forms and preparations sold, patients should be instructed to follow the directions on the product label.

Safety Issues

Use of cat's claw has not generally been associated with severe adverse effects. Animal studies suggest a low order of toxicity.[6,10,11] However, there is one case report of acute renal failure in an SLE patient who began to use cat's claw.[12]

Full safety studies of the herb have not been completed.

Maximum safe dosages in individuals with severe hepatic or renal disease are not known.

Safety in Young Children and Pregnant or Lactating Women

Maximum safe dosages for young children or pregnant or lactating women have not been established.

Drug Interactions

None are known. However, evidence suggests that cat's claw might inhibit CYP3A4.[2]

CAYENNE
(Capsicum frutescens, Capsicum annuum)

Alternate Names/Related Species:
Capsicum, Grains of Paradise, African Pepper,
Bird Pepper, Chili Pepper

Common Uses

Analgesia (topical) [+4]

NSAID-induced gastritis [+1]

(Higher numbers indicate stronger evidence; X modifier indicates contradictory results. See page xviii of the Introduction for details of the rating scale.)

Approach to the Patient

Capsaicin the "hot" constituent of cayenne, has an established medicinal use in topical pain-relieving creams. However, medicinal use of oral whole cayenne is based on speculative evidence at best.

Analgesia +4

Under the brand name Zostrix, a cream containing concentrated capsaicin has been approved by the FDA for the treatment of postherpetic neuralgia.

There is also some evidence that capsaicin creams may be helpful for relieving various types of arthritis[1,2] as well as other forms of pain, such as fibromyalgia and various forms of neuropathy.[3,4]

NSAID-Induced Gastritis   +1

Limited preliminary evidence in humans and animals suggests that oral use of cayenne may provide gastric protection against nonsteroidal antiinflammatory medications.[5-7]

Other Proposed Uses

One uncontrolled study suggests that topical cayenne might be helpful for prurigo nodularis.[8]

Contrary to some reports, cayenne does not appear to be effective for treatment of *Helicobacter pylori* infection.[9]

Capsaicin is sometimes recommended for **indigestion;** however, results from a small placebo-controlled crossover study of 11 individuals suggest that 5 mg of capsaicin taken before a high-fat meal did not affect gastric function or dyspepsia symptoms.[10]

Cayenne pepper taken internally has been informally reported as a treatment for **heart disease,** but there is no scientific evidence of any such effect at this time.

Mechanism of Action

Capsaicin depletes substance P, thereby diminishing nociceptive impulses.

Dosage

Capsaicin creams are approved over-the-counter drugs and should be used as directed. For internal use, cayenne is typically taken at a dosage of 1 to 2 standard 00 gelatin capsules one to three times daily.

Safety Issues

Cayenne is generally recognized as safe. Contrary to some reports, cayenne does not appear to aggravate stomach ulcers.[11]

Maximum safe dosages in individuals with severe hepatic or renal disease are not known.

Safety in Young Children and Pregnant or Lactating Women

Maximum safe dosages for young children or pregnant or lactating women have not been established. However, use as a condiment is most likely safe.

Though it has not been proved, spicy foods are traditionally thought to stimulate colicky reactions in breast-feeding infants.

Drug Interactions

Cayenne may increase absorption of **theophylline,** possibly leading to toxic levels.[12]

Cayenne may provide a gastroprotective effect if taken with **NSAIDs.**[6,7,13]

CHAMOMILE
(German) *(Matricaria recutita)*

Common Uses

Skin inflammation and minor wounds   [+1X]

(Higher numbers indicate stronger evidence; X modifier indicates contradictory results. See page xviii of the Introduction for details of the rating scale.)

Approach to the Patient

Germany's Commission E has approved external use of chamomile for the treatment of inflammation of the skin and mucous membranes and bacterial infections of the skin and mouth. The Commission has also approved the use of inhaled chamomile oil (in steam) for symptomatic relief of respiratory tract infections and the internal use of chamomile for "spasms and inflammation of the digestive tract." However, there is, at best, scant supporting evidence for any of these uses.

Topical chamomile preparations are widely marketed as "natural hydrocortisone" and are used for skin conditions such as eczema. Although there is only minimal supporting evidence for this use, it at least a harmless treatment.

Widespread reports that chamomile is dangerously allergenic are probably baseless.

Skin Inflammation and Minor Wounds   +1X

The evidence supporting the use of chamomile cream in eczema and minor wounds is limited to case reports and controlled studies of poor quality.[1,2,9]

A placebo-controlled trial of chamomile cream for the treatment of radiation-induced skin damage in 50 women receiving radiation therapy for breast cancer found no benefit compared to placebo.[3]

Other Proposed Uses

A double-blind, placebo-controlled trial of 164 individuals found that chamomile mouthwash was not effective for treating **aphthous ulcers** induced by chemotherapy (5-FU).[4] Weak evidence suggests that oral chamomile might protect against **gastric damage** caused by alcohol or antiinflammatory drugs.[5]

A controlled study suggests that steam inhalation of chamomile essential oil produces dose-related improvements in common cold symptoms.[10]

Animal research suggests that chamomile extracts taken orally may have **anxiolytic, antispasmodic,** and **antiinflammatory** actions,[6,7] and this is the basis on which Germany's Commission E approved internal use of chamomile for "gastrointestinal spasms and inflammatory diseases of the digestive tract." However, there have been no human trials to evaluate these potential uses.

Mechanism of Action

The flavonoids apigenin, chamaxulene, and bisabolol may have antiinflammatory and antispasmodic effects.[6,7]

Dosage

Chamomile cream is applied to the affected area one to four times daily. Chamomile tea is typically made by pouring boiling water over 2 to 3 heaping teaspoons of chamomile flowers and steeping for 10 minutes. Chamomile tinctures and pills should be taken according to the directions on the label. Alcoholic tincture may be the most potent form for internal use of the herb.

Safety Issues

Chamomile is listed on the FDA's GRAS (generally recognized as safe) list. Although reports that chamomile products can cause severe reactions in individuals allergic to ragweed have received significant media attention, when all the evidence is examined, it does not appear that chamomile is particularly allergenic.[7] Some products may have been contaminated with "dog chamomile," a highly allergenic and bad-tasting plant of similar appearance.

Maximum safe dosages in individuals with severe hepatic or renal disease are not known.

Safety in Young Children and Pregnant or Lactating Women

Maximum safe dosages for young children or pregnant or lactating women have not been established. However, there have not been any credible reports of toxicity caused by this common beverage tea.

Drug Interactions

Chamomile contains coumarin compounds that might potentiate anticoagulant or antiplatelet agents, although there are no specific reports of such interactions. A general survey of plant constituents suggests that chamomile might inhibit CYP3A4.[8]

CHASTEBERRY
(Vitex agnus-castus)

Alternate Names/Related Species: Chaste Tree

Common Uses

Cyclic Mastalgia   [+3]

PMS symptoms   [+3]

Menstrual irregularities   [+2]

Menopausal symptoms, including hot flashes   [0]

(Higher numbers indicate stronger evidence; X modifier indicates contradictory results. See page xviii of the Introduction for details of the rating scale.)

Approach to the Patient

Chasteberry *(Vitex agnus-castus)* is a shrub in the verbena family that appears to inhibit prolactin secretion. The strongest evidence for its medicinal use regards cyclic mastalgia, for which several double-blind trials have found it beneficial. It also appears to be helpful for general PMS symptoms and luteal phase defect.

Note: Some Internet sources have begun promoting chasteberry as a substitute for bromocriptine, a potentially dangerous suggestion.

Cyclic Mastalgia   +3

Several double-blind trials have found chasteberry effective for cyclic mastalgia. Most used Mastodynon, a proprietary formula containing chasteberry primarily but also other herbs in homeopathic dilutions; chasteberry is the presumed active ingredient.

A double-blind, placebo-controlled trial of 97 women with symptoms of cyclic mastalgia found that treatment with chasteberry extract (as Mastodynon) significantly reduced pain intensity at the end of the first and the second menstrual cycle compared to placebo.[1] However, in the third cycle, benefits of chasteberry treatment reached a plateau, while improvements continued in the placebo group. This effect reduced the still existing difference between the groups to a point where it was no longer statistically significant.

Benefits were also seen in a double-blind trial that enrolled 160 women with cyclic mastodynia, given either chasteberry (as Mastodynon), a progestin (lynestrenol), or placebo, and followed for at least four menstrual cycles.[2] The results in patients who could be evaluated (38 placebo, 28 progestin, 55 chasteberry) showed that both chasteberry and progestin were superior to placebo.

In addition, a double-blind, placebo-controlled trial of 104 patients with mastalgia compared two forms of chasteberry over three cycles; both were more effective than placebo.[3]

Finally, a small controlled study of 56 women with cyclic breast pain found that a chasteberry combination product significantly reduced serum prolactin levels as compared to placebo.[4]

PMS Symptoms   +3

A double-blind, placebo-controlled study of 178 women found that treatment with chasteberry over three menstrual cycles significantly reduced PMS symptoms.[5] The dose used was one tablet three times daily of the chasteberry dry extract ZE 440. Women in the treatment group experienced significant improvements in symptoms, including irritability, depression, headache, and breast tenderness.

Widely cited surveys of physicians' practices involving a total of more than 3000 women suggest that chasteberry is a useful treatment for PMS.[6-8] However, because of the high level of placebo response in PMS,[9] these reported effects on premenstrual symptoms mean little.

Finally, in a 3-month, double-blind study of 175 women with PMS, chasteberry use was associated with slightly better results than vitamin B_6.[9] Unfortunately, because there was no placebo group and because the effectiveness of B_6 in PMS is controversial and modest at best,[10] this study offers no proof of chasteberry's efficacy.

Menstrual Irregularities   +2

One double-blind study evaluated 52 women with luteal phase defect due to latent hyperprolactinemia after 3 months of treatment with chasteberry.[11] The results showed reduction in prolactin release, normalization of luteal phase length, and improvements in secondary progesterone synthesis in the treated group, but not in the control group. In addition, one small uncontrolled study of secondary amenorrhea reported positive results with chasteberry.[12] However, considering that many cases of amenorrhea spontaneously remit, the predictive value of this study is questionable.

Menopausal Symptoms, Including Hot Flashes   0

There have been anecdotal reports of improvement in menopausal symptoms (primarily hot flashes) with chasteberry, but no published studies document this possible effect.

Other Proposed Uses

Based on its antiprolactive effects, chasteberry has also been tried as a **fertility drug**.[8] However, the two double-blind studies performed to evaluate this possible use failed to return statistically significant results on primary endpoints.[13,14]

Mechanism of Action

The mechanism of action of chasteberry is not yet determined. Early research into chasteberry suggested that it increased LH production and inhibited the release of FSH, causing a decrease in estrogen and an increase in progesterone.[15,16] However, subsequent investigation has focused on a reduction in prolactin secretion as the primary effect of the herb.[4,11,17-20]

Chasteberry's effect on prolactin has been attributed to dopaminergic stimulation of D_2-type receptor cells in the pituitary.[4,21]

A double-blind, placebo-controlled study of 20 normal men found greater reductions in prolactin release with a low dose of chasteberry than with a higher dose.[22]

Dosage

The usual dosage of chasteberry extract is 20 to 40 mg given in one daily dose. However, more concentrated extracts that require a different dosing schedule are also available. See the Appendix for U.S. brand names of clinically tested products.

Safety Issues

Widespread use of chasteberry in Europe has not led to any reports of significant adverse effects, other than one case of mild ovarian hyperstimulation possibly caused by chasteberry.[9,24] Drug-monitoring studies enrolling more than 3000 participants found the rate of minor side effects with chasteberry (primarily nausea, headaches, and allergy) was less than 2.5%.[6,23] A clinical study using high doses of chasteberry extract produced only mild nonspecific side effects, such as gastrointestinal disturbances.[22]

Maximum safe dosages in individuals with severe hepatic or renal disease are not known.

Safety in Young Children
and Pregnant or Lactating Women

Chasteberry presents safety concerns in pregnancy and lactation because of its prolactin-lowering effects. However, chasteberry has been tried as a galactagogue in two large unblinded controlled trials, without apparent harm.[25] (At the time of this research, chasteberry was thought to primarily affect progesterone.)

Safety of the herb in young children has not been established.

Drug Interactions

Chasteberry could conceivably interact with **bromocriptine** or other drugs intended to affect prolactin levels. For similar reasons, the herb is usually not given along with exogenous **estrogen** or **progesterone** or other treatments with endocrine activity. Its safety in combination with other herbal products commonly used for menstrual and menopausal symptoms is not known.

CHONDROITIN SULFATE

Alternate Names/Supplement Forms: Chondroitin

Common Uses

Osteoarthritis [+3]

(Higher numbers indicate stronger evidence; X modifier indicates contradictory results. See page xviii of the Introduction for details of the rating scale.)

Approach to the Patient

Chondroitin sulfate is a major component of the proteoglycans found in articular cartilage. Preliminary double-blind studies suggest that supplemental chondroitin produces a slow-acting but persistent improvement in symptoms of osteoarthritis. In addition, it may retard progression of the disease.

There are large differences in molecular weight and sulfation among chondroitin products, which lead to differences in absorption and effectiveness. The products most commonly used in double-blind trials are proprietary, and it is not clear which among the competing products are comparably effective.[1]

For retail sale, chondroitin is often combined with glucosamine. Combined glucosamine/chondroitin therapy might be superior to either treatment alone,[2,3] but this has not been solidly established. Patients may be advised to first try therapy with either treatment alone to save money.

Osteoarthritis +3

Double-blind, placebo-controlled studies, following a total of several hundred osteoarthritis (OA) patients for a duration of 3 months to 1 year, found significant improvement in subjective pain and variables related to locomotion within 3 to 6 months.[4-8] However, one double-blind, placebo-controlled trial failed to find statistically significant evidence of benefit.[9]

A double-blind comparative study of 146 individuals evaluated the effects of chondroitin versus diclofenac sodium.[10] The results suggested that chondroitin acted less rapidly, but its effects continued for at least 3 months after cessation of treatment.

Three double-blind, placebo-controlled studies of a total of about 250 patients with OA found radiologic evidence that chondroitin may slow disease progression.[6,7,11] One animal study evaluating the effects of oral and injected chondroitin found significantly more healthy cartilage remaining in the damaged joint of those treated than untreated.[12] Giving chondroitin orally was as effective as giving it by injection.

A 16-week, double-blind, placebo-controlled crossover study of 34 patients with degenerative joint disease of the knee or low back evaluated chondroitin sulfate (1200 mg per day), glucosamine HCl (1500 mg per day), and manganese ascorbate (228 mg per day).[13] The results showed statistically significant improvement in most measures of arthritis severity.

Preliminary information from one animal study suggests that combined glucosamine/chondroitin therapy may be superior to treatment with either supplement as monotherapy.[2,3] Many other positive reports with similar combination treatments can be found in the veterinary literature.[14-17] In addition, a 6-month, double-blind, placebo-controlled study using combined glucosamine, chondroitin, and manganese found evidence of significant improvement in the treated group.[18]

Other Proposed Uses

Scant evidence suggests that chondroitin may be helpful in **atherosclerosis, high cholesterol,** and **nephrolithiasis.**[19-21]

Mechanism of Action

Osteoarthritis is characterized by damage to articular cartilage, which is apparently caused by increased action of proteolytic enzymes (e.g., collagenase, elastase, and proteoglycanase). Chondroitin may help retard this damage in several ways: by blocking the action of these enzymes, by enhancing repair mechanisms by stimulating proteoglycan synthesis, and by increasing levels of protective hyaluronic acid.[22-24] Furthermore, chondroitin also appears to exert a mild direct antiinflammatory effect.[24]

Dosage

The usual dosage of chondroitin is 400 mg taken three times daily, although 1200 mg once daily appears to be equally effective.[5] Clinical trials suggest that 3 months is required for full therapeutic effect. Low molecular weight chondroitin (less than 16,900 daltons) is better absorbed orally than higher molecular weight products.[1] See Appendix for U.S. brand names of clinically tested brands.

Safety Issues

Chondroitin sulfate has not been associated with any significant side effects in clinical trials. Mild digestive disturbances and allergic reactions have been reported.[1,4-6,23] Hematologic, renal, and hepatic assessments have shown no significant difference between chondroitin treatment and placebo groups.

Chronic administration of 100 mg/kg was not associated with any significant toxicity, and intake of 1.5 g/kg caused no mortality in rats or mice.[23] Mutagenicity studies and tests for alteration of blood coagulation have been negative to date.

Maximum safe dosages in individuals with severe hepatic or renal disease are not known.

Safety in Young Children
and Pregnant or Lactating Women

Teratogenicity studies in rats and rabbits have reported no malformation of fetuses. However, newborns of gravid animals treated with chondroitin weighed 10% to 20% less than those of untreated controls.[23] For this reason, chondroitin cannot be recommended for pregnant women at this time.

Maximum safe dosages for young children or lactating women have not been established.

Drug Interactions

None are known.

CHROMIUM

Alternate Names/Supplement Forms:
Chromium Picolinate, Chromium Polynicotinate,
Chromium Chloride, High-Chromium Brewer's Yeast

Common Uses

Diabetes [+3]

Body composition (weight loss and bodybuilding) [+3X]

Insulin resistance and asymptomatic glucose intolerance [+2X]

Hyperlipidemia [+2X]

Atherosclerosis prevention [+1]

(Higher numbers indicate stronger evidence; X modifier indicates contradictory results. See page xviii of the Introduction for details of the rating scale.)

Approach to the Patient

Patients may have read that chromium deficiency is widespread and is responsible for the prevalence of adult-onset diabetes. However, the evidence that chromium is commonly deficient in the diet remains unconvincing.[1-7,54]

Nonetheless, chromium supplements may be useful for impaired glucose tolerance as well as overt diabetes. Chromium is also marketed as a weight loss aid, but the body of current evidence remains inconclusive.

Diabetics should be counseled that chromium has been advocated as adjunct, not sole, treatment for their condition.

Diabetes   + 3

Evidence from a double-blind trial enrolling 180 individuals suggests that high doses of chromium (1000 μg daily) may improve glucose control in type 2 diabetes.[8] Another double-blind trial compared placebo with chromium from brewer's yeast (23.3 μg chromium daily) and chromium chloride (200 μg chromium daily) in 78 individuals with type 2 diabetes.[9] This rather complex crossover study consisted of four 8-week intervals of treatment in random order. The results in the 67 completers showed that both active treatments significantly improved glycemic control.

A study of 243 type 1 or type 2 diabetics found that chromium supplementation decreased insulin or oral hypoglycemic medication requirements in a significant percentage of cases.[10] However, although this study is commonly reported as a controlled trial, only 10 individuals were enrolled in a double-blind protocol. The remainder of the study was open label and, as such, has little validity. Two small studies found no benefits.[11,12]

One double-blind, placebo-controlled trial of 30 pregnant women found evidence for benefit in gestational diabetes.[13]

Body Composition (Weight Loss and Bodybuilding)   + 3 X

The theory behind using chromium for weight loss rests on chromium's apparent effects on insulin resistance. (See the article on **Weight Loss** for more information.) Theory aside, the clinical evidence whether chromium is an effective aid in weight loss is mixed. The largest study did find benefit, but other studies did not, possibly due to insufficient statistical power.

In a double-blind trial, 154 individuals were given either placebo or 200 or 400 μg of chromium picolinate daily.[14] Over a period of 72 days, individuals taking chromium demonstrated increase in lean body mass and loss of fat mass, resulting in a net overall weight loss versus placebo. However, in a slightly smaller double-blind study by the same researcher, no statistically significant intergroup differences were seen.[15] Researchers resorted to ad-ditional statistical analysis in an attempt to show benefit.

Smaller studies have yielded generally negative results.[16-20]

Insulin Resistance and Asymptomatic Glucose Intolerance   +2X

Mixed evidence suggests that chromium supplementation may be beneficial for insulin resistance and mildly impaired glucose tolerance.[21-25,55]

Hyperlipidemia   +2X

Two double-blind, placebo-controlled studies following a total of 104 participants reported significant improvements in various aspects of lipid profiles with chromium supplementation at 200 to 250 µg/day.[26,27] Other studies have also found some benefit,[8,28,29] but there have been negative results as well.[21,30] One small double-blind trial study found chromium alone ineffective, but combined therapy with grapeseed extract led to statistically significant reductions in total and LDL cholesterol.[31]

Atherosclerosis Prevention   +1

Insulin resistance and mildy impaired glucose tolerance have been strongly associated with increased risk of cardiovascular disease.[32-39] Based on chromium's influence on insulin resistance, as well as its potential effects on weight and lipid variables, chromium has been evaluated for possible association with heart disease risk. An observational trial using measurements of toe-nail chromium found associations between higher chromium intake and reduced risk of myocardial infarction.[40]

Other Proposed Uses

Chromium has been suggested as an **ergogenic aid** said to improve utilization of carbohydrates. However, results of small trials have been generally negative.[41,56-64]

Mechanism of Action

For decades, it was believed that dietary chromium formed the metallic nucleus of a large molecular weight nicotinate complex called glucose tolerance factor (GTF). GTF was said to be found whole in foods such as brewer's yeast and, for this reason, such foods were described as a superior source of chromium.

However, it is now known that the hypothetical GTF molecule was actually an artifact of the analytic process rather than an actual molecule present in the body.[65-67] Current evidence indicates that an oligopeptide, named low molecular weight chromium-binding substance (LMWCr), binds to chromium and facilitates the action of insulin receptor kinase. LMWCr is not stable and is not found in foods.

Dosage

Chromium is an essential trace nutrient, but its precise daily allowance has not been determined. The estimated safe and adequate intake for individuals over 7 years of age is 50 to 200 μg.

Although one study found best results in diabetes with 1000 μg of chromium daily, the safety of such supranutritional doses has not been established (see Safety Issues). Some manufacturers claim to provide chromium in an especially bioactive form called GTF; however, current evidence indicates that GTF doesn't exist. (See Mechanism of Action).

Simultaneous intake of calcium carbonate may impair chromium absorption.[46]

Safety Issues

Trivalent chromium is generally well tolerated, and dosages within the recommendations given above are believed to be safe. Animal studies have reported no toxicity even at a 100 mg/kg dose of chromium chloride or chromium tripicolinate over a period of 24 weeks.[47] However, there have been two case reports of possible heavy metal toxicity associated with dosages of chromium picolinate in the range of 600 to 2400 μg daily for 4 to 5 months. In one, anemia, thrombocytopenia, hemolysis, weight loss, and liver and renal toxicity occurred in a woman taking 1200 to 2400 μg of chromium picolinate daily for 4 to 5 months.[48] Another found interstitial nephritis in a woman taking only 600 μg of chromium daily for 6 weeks.[49,53] The risk of chromium toxicity may be increased in individuals with pre-existing hepatic or renal disease. There has also been one report of acute generalized exanthematous pustulosis caused by a dosage of 1000 mg of chromium picolinate.[50] Although these may be idiosyncratic reactions, caution should be exercised when recommending chromium doses above nutritional needs.

It has been suggested that chromium picolinate might have unpredictable effects in psychiatric disorders, because picolinic acids may alter neurotransmitter levels or actions.[51,42]

In addition, there are also concerns that chromium picolinate could adversely affect DNA, although current evidence is incomplete and somewhat inconsistent.[52,43-45]

Maximum safe dosages in individuals with severe hepatic or renal disease are not known.

Safety in Young Children and Pregnant or Lactating Women

The official U.S. adequate intake (AI) level for pregnant women is 30 μg (29 μg if under 19 years old); the AI for lactating women is 45 μg (44 μg if under 19 years old).[53]

Drug Interactions

Chromium supplementation may be useful for correcting the reduction of HDL levels that can occur in individuals taking **beta-blockers.**[29]

COENZYME Q$_{10}$

Common Uses

Congestive heart failure   [+3]

Hypertension   [+2]

Cardiac reperfusion injury (postoperative)   [+2X]

Correction of drug-induced relative depletion   [+2]

Cardiomyopathy   [+2X]

Cardioprotective effect in doxorubicin chemotherapy   [+1]

Athletic performance enhancement   [−1]

(Higher numbers indicate stronger evidence; X modifier indicates contradictory results. See page xviii of the Introduction for details of the rating scale.)

Approach to the Patient

Some evidence indicates that various pharmaceutical treatments may deplete CoQ$_{10}$ or interfere with its action (see discussion under Correction of Drug-Induced Relative Depletion). These rather preliminary findings have been extensively popularized as a prime example of "nutrient depletion caused by drugs." Many patients believe that if they take the medications listed below (see Correction of Drug-Induced Relative Depletion), they must also take CoQ$_{10}$ supplements or run the risk of developing heart problems.

In fact, there is little meaningful evidence that CoQ$_{10}$ supplementation is necessary or beneficial for individuals using the listed medications. However, other than the cost, such supplementation is probably harmless, and the theoretical argument for supplementation is a reasonable one (see Mechanism of Action).

Better evidence supports the use of CoQ_{10} as an adjunct treatment for congestive heart failure (CHF). Supplementation with CoQ_{10} may reduce CHF symptoms and decrease the incidence of hospitalization. However, patients with heart failure who are taking CoQ_{10} should be counseled about the possibility of rebound CHF before discontinuing this therapy.

Limited evidence indicates that CoQ_{10} may be helpful for hypertension. Data supporting its usefulness in conditions such as cardiomyopathy and postoperative cardiac reperfusion injury are mixed at best. CoQ_{10} does not appear to be effective for another popular use: as a sports supplement.

Congestive Heart Failure (CHF)   + 3

A double-blind, multicenter study followed 641 patients with NYHA class III or IV failure for 1 year.[1] Half were given 2 mg/kg of CoQ_{10} orally, and the rest, placebo. Conventional therapy was continued. In the verum group, there was a progressive and statistically significant reduction in CHF class over the course of the study. No improvement in functional status was seen in the placebo group. There was also a statistically and clinically significant reduction in incidence of acute pulmonary edema, cardiac asthma, and hospitalizations for worsening heart failure in the treated group. Additionally, there was a statistically significant reduction in the percentage of patients who required one or more hospitalizations during the trial period, from 40% in the control group to about 20% in the verum group.

A double-blind study of 197 patients with heart failure from valvular disease found that 30 mg/day of CoQ_{10} significantly reduced overall symptoms.[2] A Scandinavian double-blind crossover study followed 80 patients with CHF for 6 months and found similar benefits.[3] Finally, a double-blind, placebo-controlled trial of 22 individuals with NYHA class II–III heart failure used invasive testing (right heart catheterization) and documented a significant improvement in LV performance.[4]

However, a 6-month, double-blind study of 45 individuals with CHF found no benefit.[5]

Hypertension   + 2

An 8-week, double-blind, placebo-controlled study of 59 hypertensive men receiving conventional treatment found that 120 mg of CoQ$_{10}$ daily reduced the average systolic blood pressure by 10% and diastolic blood pressure by about 9%, whereas insignificant changes were seen in the placebo group.[6]

In addition, a 12-week, double-blind study of 83 individuals with isolated systolic hypertension found improvements in the CoQ$_{10}$ group (60 mg daily) compared to the placebo group.[52] Significant improvements in systolic and diastolic blood pressure were seen in a small ($n=18$), double-blind crossover study of CoQ$_{10}$ with 10-week treatment periods.[7]

Cardiac Reperfusion Injury (Postoperative)   + 2 X

Animal studies of CoQ$_{10}$ for reducing reperfusion injury have yielded contradictory results.[8-11]

The results of human trials are similarly mixed. A double-blind trial of 20 patients with well-preserved myocardial function that evaluated the effects of two 300-mg doses of CoQ$_{10}$ in the 12 hours prior to bypass surgery showed no result.[12] However, a controlled study of 40 patients undergoing elective coronary artery bypass found that 7-day pretreatment with 150 mg of CoQ$_{10}$ significantly reduced ventricular arrhythmias; necessary dopamine dosage; and serum levels of malondialdehyde, conjugated dienes, and creatine kinase.[13] The study authors concluded that CoQ$_{10}$ might be useful in reducing peroxidative damage during routine bypass grafting. It is possible that the better result seen in this study was due to a longer period of CoQ$_{10}$ repletion.

A controlled study of 10 high-risk patients undergoing heart surgery found notable protective effects attributable to 14-day pretreatment with 100 mg/day CoQ$_{10}$.[14] Serum CoQ$_{10}$ levels were low prior to surgery in both the treated and control groups. In the treated group, significant improvements were noted in myocardial ATP, cardiac function, and the postoperative recovery time and course.

A double-blind, placebo-controlled trial of 22 patients undergoing hypothermic cardioplegic arrest found that preoperative treatment with CoQ$_{10}$ (150 to 200 mg of CoQ$_{10}$ orally per day for 5 to 7 days) resulted in lower left atrial pressure, a reduced incidence of lowered cardiac output, a wider pulse pressure, and a better preserved right and left ventricular myocardial ultrastructure.[15]

Correction of Drug-Induced Relative Depletion   +2

Some evidence suggests that a variety of pharmaceuticals might cause depletion of CoQ$_{10}$ or interfere with its action. It has been suggested (but not proved) that this CoQ$_{10}$ deficiency or inhibition may play a role in the known side effects of these treatments and that CoQ$_{10}$ supplementation may be beneficial.

The best evidence regards agents in the statin family. HMG-CoA reductase is necessary for the synthesis of both cholesterol and CoQ$_{10}$; for this reason, statin drugs would be expected to reduce CoQ$_{10}$ levels.

A randomized, double-blind, placebo-controlled trial involving 45 hypercholesterolemic patients taking either lovastatin or pravastatin over an 18-week period found a significant dose-related decline of total serum CoQ$_{10}$ levels associated with both drugs.[16] Similarly, a 3-month, double-blind, placebo-controlled study found that treatment with simvastatin or pravastatin, 20 mg/day, lowered CoQ$_{10}$ plasma levels in 30 hypercholesterolemic patients as well as 10 normal volunteers.[17]

These reductions (in the neighborhood of 30% to 50%) may be clinically significant.[18] Five hospitalized patients (43 to 72 years old) with cardiomyopathy who were treated with lovastatin showed decreased CoQ$_{10}$ blood levels and deterioration of cardiac function, including a worsening of the ejection fraction. Subsequent oral supplementation with CoQ$_{10}$ (100 to 200 mg/day) led to increased CoQ$_{10}$ blood levels and a reversal of the cardiac deterioration.

Another study found that supplemental CoQ$_{10}$ could prevent both plasma and platelet CoQ$_{10}$ reduction without affecting the therapeutic effect of simvastatin.[19]

For several other categories of drugs, the evidence is more indirect, revolving primarily around data finding inhibition of enzymes related to the production or action of CoQ$_{10}$. These proposed drug-induced depletions or interferences with CoQ$_{10}$ include sulfonylureas (Dymelor, glyburide, phenformin, and tolazamide; tolbutamide, glipizide, and chlorpropamide may be relatively noninhibitory), beta-blockers (propranolol, metoprolol, and alprenolol; timolol was relatively noninhibitory), phenothiazines, tricyclic antidepressants (supplemental CoQ$_{10}$ may be protective against cardiac side effects), diazoxide, methyldopa, hydrochlorothiazide, clonidine, and hydralazine.[20-24]

Cardiomyopathy   + 2 X

The evidence base for the use of CoQ$_{10}$ consists primarily of low-quality trials. Most were not blinded.[25-27] One double-blind trial followed patients with various cardiomyopathies over a period of 3 years.[28] In the 80 patients treated with 100 mg/day of CoQ$_{10}$, 89% of patients improved as measured by ejection fraction and subjective complaints. When the treatment was stopped, cardiac function deteriorated. However, the involvement of participants with mixed diagnoses detracts from the meaningfulness of the results. In addition, a double-blind, placebo-controlled crossover study that followed 25 patients with idiopathic dilated cardiomyopathy for a total of 8 months found no benefit with CoQ_{10} at a dose of 100 mg/day.[29]

Cardioprotective Effect in Doxorubicin Chemotherapy   +1

Animal and preliminary human trials suggest that CoQ_{10} might protect against doxorubicin cardiotoxicity.[30-32] The cardiotoxicity of doxorubicin results from its affinity to cardiolipin, a cardiac mitochondrial lipid. Because its antitumor activity is due to an entirely different mechanism (inhibiting topoisomerase II in the nucleus and producing oxygen-free radicals while the drug is bound to DNA), it is possible that CoQ_{10} may not interfere with the activity of doxorubicin.

Athletic Performance Enhancement   −1

Although most studies evaluating the use of CoQ_{10} for exercise performance improvement have found mainly negative results,[33-38] one double-blind study of 25 highly trained cross-country skiers did find some benefit.[39]

Other Proposed Uses

A 6-week, double-blind, placebo-controlled trial of 21 individuals with chronic renal failure found that use of CoQ_{10} improved creatine clearance and urine output.[53] A significant reduction in the need for dialysis was also observed in the treatment group. A double-blind, placebo-controlled trial of 21 individuals found that 2 weeks pretreatment with CoQ_{10} increased the antibody response to **hepatitis B vaccine**.[40]

On the basis of contradictory and weak evidence, respectively, CoQ_{10} has also been proposed as an aid in the treatment of **periodontal disease**[41-43] as well as **muscular dystrophy** and **neurogenic atrophy**.[44]

CoQ$_{10}$ has been tried but found ineffective for the treatment of **Huntington's disease.**[45]

Mechanism of Action

Low levels of CoQ$_{10}$ have been noted in patients with CHF.[46,47] Thus the most obvious explanation for the effectiveness of CoQ$_{10}$ in CHF is that exogenous supplementation corrects a local CoQ$_{10}$ deficiency caused by excessive myocardial exertion and that repletion should increase myocardial aerobic energy production. This explanation, although reasonable, remains unproven.

Evidence that adequate CoQ$_{10}$ is necessary for healthy heart function has been used to support the use of supplemental CoQ$_{10}$ in individuals taking medications that interfere with its action or absorption. Many of these medications are used by individuals at risk of heart disease; relative depletion of CoQ$_{10}$ can thus be seen as counterproductive in such circumstances. However, this plausible hypothesis remains unproven.

In reperfusion after ischemia, CoQ$_{10}$ may function by preventing oxidative damage to creatine kinase and other substances[13]; other authors have concluded that CoQ$_{10}$ does not scavenge the free radicals produced in reperfusion but rather enhances the recovery of high-energy phosphates, thereby preventing Ca^{2+} overload.[9]

Dosage

The typical dosage of CoQ$_{10}$ ranges from 30 to 150 mg/day, given in two or three divided doses at the higher levels. This fat-soluble substance is thought to be better absorbed when taken in oil-based soft-gel form.[48]

Safety Issues

In human trials, use of CoQ$_{10}$ has only been associated with mild, nonspecific side effects such as gastrointestinal distress.

Several studies of CoQ_{10} from 1 to 6 years in duration have reported no serious side effects, intolerance, drug interactions, or toxicity.[1,25,49] However, there have been anecdotal reports of a CoQ_{10} withdrawal syndrome in CHF, leading to temporarily worsening heart failure.

Maximum safe dosages in individuals with severe hepatic or renal disease are not known.

Safety in Young Children and Pregnant or Lactating Women

Maximum safe dosages for young children or pregnant or lactating women have not been established.

Drug Interactions

Reduced fasting glucose with CoQ_{10} was observed in one study.[6] It is possible, therefore, that individuals taking **oral hypoglycemics** might need to reduce their dosage, although this has not been reported.

Several studies have found a reduction of serum CoQ_{10} levels with **statin drug therapy.**[16,17,19] In addition, weaker evidence suggests that other drugs might either interfere with CoQ_{10} synthesis or impair the activity of enzymes containing CoQ_{10}; these drugs include **beta-blockers, clonidine, hydralazine, methyldopa, diazoxide, sulfonylureas, phenothiazines, tricyclic antidepressants,** and **thiazide diuretics.**[20-24,50] On this basis, CoQ_{10} has been proposed as a useful supplement for individuals taking these medications, but as yet there is little evidence of specific benefit.

One animal study suggests that CoQ_{10} can prolong the effects of the **antihypertensives** enalapril and nitrendipine without increasing their maximum hypotensive effect.[51]

COLOSTRUM

**Infectious gastroenteritis
(prevention and treatment) [+2X]**

*(Higher numbers indicate stronger evidence; X modifier indicates contradic-
tory results. See page xviii of the Introduction for details of the rating scale.)*

Approach to the Patient

Colostrum contains antibodies, growth factors, and transfer factor (a general immune-active substance). Most commercial
colostrum preparations are bovine in origin, and it is not clear
that the substances are active cross-species. In research studies,
cows are inoculated with specific human pathogens to create
"hyperimmune colostrum." This form of colostrum is not available over the counter; however, manufacturers who sell ordinary
colostrum sometimes use data from studies of hyperimmune
colostrum as support for their products.

Meaningful evidence suggests possible benefits of hyperimmune
colostrum supplements for some gastrointestinal infections.
Much weaker evidence suggests that ordinary bovine colostrum
might be helpful for improving body composition and protecting the stomach lining against NSAID damage.

Infectious Gastroenteritis
(Prevention and Treatment)   +2X

Preliminary evidence suggests that hyperimmune colostrum
might help prevent or possibly treat certain gastrointestinal infectious diseases.

A controlled, but not blinded, trial of 20 infants with rotaviral illness who were given hyperimmune colostrum found that the preparation could help prevent diarrhea.[1] However, once diarrhea started, treatment with colostrum was not helpful.

In contrast, a double-blind, placebo-controlled trial of 80 children with rotaviral diarrhea did find that similarly prepared colostrum could reduce symptoms and shorten recovery time.[2] Similar results were seen in another double-blind trial of about the same size.[3] However, in a double-blind trial of 135 children, colostrum prepared by immunizing cows with a simian rotavirus was found ineffective for treating rotavirus.[4] The difference among these results may lie in the level and type of antibodies found in the colostrum preparations.

A highly preliminary study suggests that hyperimmune colostrum may help prevent infection with *Cryptosporidium*.[5] Both hyperimmune and normal colostrum may also be helpful for treatment of cryptosporidial infection in individuals with AIDS.[6,7]

Other studies suggest that hyperimmune colostrum might help prevent *Shigella flexneri*[8] and *Escherichia coli* infections,[9,10] but studies have not found it effective for treating *Shigella* or *E. coli* diarrhea.[12,16]

However, a study of Bangladeshi children infected with *Helicobacter pylori* found no benefits with hyperimmune colstrum.[11]

Other Proposed Uses

One small double-blind study suggests that use of ordinary colostrum by healthy men and women undergoing exercising training may improve body composition compared to whey protein.[17] Ordinary colostrum might help protect against **gastric damage** caused by antiinflammatory drugs, at least according to one study in rats and a small human trial.[13,14]

Colostrum might also have a potential therapeutic role in individuals with **short bowel syndrome, chemotherapy-induced mouth ulcers,** or **inflammatory bowel disease,** but as yet there is no real evidence that colostrum is effective in any of these conditions.[15]

Mechanism of Action

Growth factors found in colostrum may stimulate gastric mucosal regeneration and thereby protect against NSAID-induced damage.[13,14]

Dosage

Most commercial colostrum preparations are bovine in origin and are available as capsules that contain the immune proteins in dry form. The usual recommended dosage of colostrum is 10 g daily.

Safety Issues

Colostrum does not seem to cause any significant side effects. However, comprehensive safety studies have not been performed. Concerns have been raised over possible prion infection if unsterilized products are used. Maximum safe dosages in individuals with severe hepatic or renal disease are not known.

Safety in Young Children and Pregnant or Lactating Women

Maximum safe dosages of bovine colostrum supplementation in young children or pregnant or lactating women has not been established.

Drug Interactions

None are known.

CONJUGATED LINOLEIC ACID (CLA)

Common Uses

Weight loss/body composition   [+1]

Type 2 diabetes   [+1]

(Higher numbers indicate stronger evidence; X modifier indicates contradictory results. See page xviii of the Introduction for details of the rating scale.)

Approach to the Patient

Conjugated linoleic acid (CLA) is an essential fatty acid containing several isomeric forms of linoleic acid.

Very preliminary evidence suggests that CLA may facilitate loss of body fat. It might be worth advising patients interested in CLA for this purpose to consider pyruvate instead; although supporting evidence for pyruvate is also incomplete, it is considerably more substantial than the evidence for CLA.

CLA has also been proposed as a treatment for type 2 diabetes. Again, the evidence for another supplement—chromium—is considerably stronger.

Weight Loss/Body Composition   +1

Mixed evidence from small human trials and animal studies suggests that CLA supplements may help individuals reduce body fat while retaining muscle mass.[1-4,8-10]

Type 2 Diabetes   +1

During the course of investigations into CLA for enhancing fat metabolism, some evidence was found of functional similarities to thiazolidinedione. This led to research into the possible usefulness of CLA as an oral hypoglycemic agent. One group of researchers subsquently found some evidence of benefit in preliminary animal and human trials.[5]

Other Proposed Uses

Some animal studies and in vitro research suggest that CLA might have **chemopreventive** effects.[6,11,12] However, a case control study found no association between the CLA content of breast adipose tissue and the diagnosis of breast cancer.[7]

Mechanism of Action

Not known.

Dosage

The typical dosage of CLA ranges from 3 to 5 g daily.

Safety Issues

CLA appears to be a safe nutritional substance.

Maximum safe dosages in individuals with severe hepatic or renal disease are not known.

Safety in Young Children and Pregnant or Lactating Women

Maximum safe dosages for young children or pregnant or lactating women have not been established.

Drug Interactions

None are known.

COPPER

Alternate Names/Supplement Forms:
Copper Sulfate, Copper Picolinate, Copper Gluconate,
Copper Complexes of Various Amino Acids

Common Uses

Osteoporosis [+1X]

(Higher numbers indicate stronger evidence; X modifier indicates contradictory results. See page xviii of the Introduction for details of the rating scale.)

Approach to the Patient

Despite information found on numerous web sites recommending copper supplements for arthritis, high cholesterol, osteoporosis, and heart disease, there is no evidence for therapeutic benefit.

Copper deficiency is rare. However, excessive zinc intake can markedly impair copper absorption and retention, leading to clinical signs of deficiency; this effect may endure until body stores of zinc fall to normal levels. Keep in mind that patients interested in alternative medicine may be taking zinc in high doses (see the **Zinc** article for information on popular uses of high-dose zinc). Copper deficiency may be forestalled by simultaneous administration of copper at 1 to 3 mg daily (or by avoiding high-dose zinc therapy).

Women who concomitantly take oral contraceptives and copper supplements may be at risk for hypercupremia.

Osteoporosis   + 1 X

Copper has been proposed as a treatment for osteoporosis based primarily on studies that found benefit using mixtures of various trace minerals.[1,2] However, a double-blind, placebo-controlled crossover trial of 16 healthy young adult females found no effect of copper supplementation (either 3 or 6 g of elemental Cu per day as $CuSO_4$) on markers of bone formation or resorption over 4-week periods, despite improvement in copper status.[3]

Other Proposed Uses

Contrary to some published claims that copper deficiencies may increase the risk of **hypercholesterolemia** and **heart disease,** a double-blind clinical trial of copper supplements for reducing heart disease risk found no benefit.[4]

Similarly, copper has long been mentioned as a possible treatment for osteoarthritis and rheumatoid arthritis, but there is as yet no real evidence that it works in these conditions.

Mechanism of Action

Copper is an essential component of a number of enzyme systems, including those necessary for cellular respiration and hemoglobin synthesis.

Dosage

The U.S. Dietary Reference Intake for copper for males and females 19 years and older is 900 µg.[5]

Oysters, nuts, legumes, whole grains, sweet potatoes, and dark greens are good dietary sources of copper. Water that passes through copper plumbing is also a source of this mineral, although it may provide excessive amounts.

Excessive **zinc** intake significantly reduces copper stores in the body and may cause symptoms such as anemia, neutropenia, cardiac abnormalities (including arrythmias), increased LDL levels, decreased HDL levels, decreased glucose clearance, and impaired immune function. This can be prevented by simultaneous copper supplementation.[6] In studies of high-dose zinc for preventing macular degeneration, copper was supplemented at a dose of 2 mg daily.

Safety Issues

Copper is safe when taken at nutritional dosages, but these should not be exceeded. As little as 10 mg of copper daily produces nausea in adults, and 60 mg may cause vomiting. Maximum safe dosages in individuals with severe hepatic or renal disease are not known.

Safety in Young Children and Pregnant or Lactating Women

The tolerable upper intake level of copper for pregnant or lactating women has been established at 10,000 μg daily (8000 μg if under 19 years old).[5]

Drug Interactions

Oral contraceptives might increase levels of copper in the body.[7-9] Conversely, AZT might deplete copper stores.[10]

CRANBERRY
(Vaccinium macrocarpon)

Common Uses

Prophylaxis of acute cystitis [+3]

Chronic bacteriuria/pyuria [+2X]

(Higher numbers indicate stronger evidence; X modifier indicates contradictory results. See page xviii of the Introduction for details of the rating scale.)

Approach to the Patient

Cranberry *(Vaccinium macrocarpon)* has been used for decades to prevent or treat acute urinary tract infections. However, the first double-blind trial to meaningfully support this use was reported in 2001.

Cranberry might be worth a try in patients with chronic asymptomatic bacteruria as well.

Dry cranberry extracts are far more palatable than actual cranberry juice. (Cranberry cocktail drinks contain very little cranberry.)

Prophylaxis of Acute Cystitis +3

An unpublished trial presented at the June 2001 meeting of the American Urological Association provides the only real evidence for the use of cranberry as prophylaxis for acute UTIs. This 1-year, double-blind, placebo-controlled study of 150 sexually active women compared placebo against both cranberry juice and cranberry tablets.[1] Both forms of cranberry significantly reduced the number of episodes of symptomatic UTI; however, cranberry tablets were more cost effective.

A widely reported year-long open trial of women with recurrent UTIs found cranberry to exert superior prophylaxis compared to probiotics or no treatment; but given the reputation of cranberry, the placebo effect and observer bias cannot be excluded.[2]

Chronic Bacteriuria/Pyuria   + 2 X

A double-blind, placebo-controlled study followed 153 women with a mean age of 78.5 years for a period of 6 months.[3] It was designed to examine the effects of cranberry on bacteriuria/pyuria. Half were given a standard commercial cranberry drink and the other half a placebo drink prepared to look and taste the same. Both treatments contained the identical amount of vitamin C to eliminate the possible antibacterial influence of that supplement. Despite the weak preparation of cranberry used, the results showed a 58% decrease in bacteriuria with pyuria compared to the control group. Furthermore, in women who were initially bacteriuric-pyuric, their chance of remaining so was 73% less in the treated than in the control group. However, subsequent responses to this report called it into question on statistical and methodological grounds.[4,5]

A double-blind, placebo-controlled crossover study of 15 children with neurogenic bladder reported no reduction in bacteriuria attributable to the cranberry concentrate used.[6]

Other Proposed Uses

Evidence suggests that proanthocyanidins in cranberry interfere with the coaggregation of many bacteria implicated in dental plaque formation.[7] Based on these findings, cranberry has been proposed as a prophylactic treatment for **periodontal disease**.[7] However, the sweetening agents that are typically added to cranberry to make it palatable would be expected to exert a contrary effect.

Mechanism of Action

The primary mechanism of action of cranberry juice is believed to be reduction of bacterial adherence to the epithelial cells of the bladder by interfering with the activity of adhesins that attach to oligo- or monosaccharide receptors.[8-13] These adhesins are produced by fimbriae, proteinaceous fibers of the bacterial cell wall. Inhibition has been documented in *Escherichia coli*, *Proteus*, *Klebsiella*, *Enterobacter*, and *Pseudomonas*. Some evidence suggests that in women who experience recurrent bladder infections, bacterial adherance occurs to a greater than normal extent.[14]

Cranberry also causes a decrease in urinary pH and an increase in urinary hippuric acid. However, this effect does not appear to be clinically relevant.[11]

Dosage

The usual dose of dry cranberry juice extract is 400 mg two to four times daily. Some products, including the most popular, claim to be standardized to antiadhesion activity.

Cranberry juice (pure, not cranberry cocktail) is generally taken at a dose of 4 ounces four times daily.

Safety Issues

As a food, cranberry is believed to be safe.

Concerns have been expressed about possible lithogenic effects of cranberry. Regular use of cranberry concentrates have been found to increase excretion of oxalate, calcium, phosphate, sodium, magnesium, and potassium.[15] However, some of these ions are lithogenic and others antilithogenic; the net effect is not clear.

Maximum safe dosages in individuals with severe hepatic or renal disease are not known.

Safety in Young Children and Pregnant or Lactating Women

There are no known risks or side effects of cranberry in children or pregnant or lactating women.

Drug Interactions

Excessive use of cranberry juice can increase the excretion and thus reduce the blood levels of some drugs, including certain **antidepressants, antipsychotics,** and **morphine-based analgesics.** Based on this, use of cranberry juice has been suggested as an antidote in **phencyclidine (PCP)** overdose.[16]

There are no reported interaction of cranberry with **antibiotic** treatment, but theoretically some antibiotics could be inhibited by reduced urinary pH.

CREATINE

Alternate Names/Supplement Forms:
Creatine Monohydrate

Common Uses

Ergogenic uses   [+2X]

Congestive heart failure   [+2]

(Higher numbers indicate stronger evidence; X modifier indicates contradictory results. See page xviii of the Introduction for details of the rating scale.)

Approach to the Patient

Creatine is one of the few legal sports supplements with some supporting evidence. (Caffeine is another.)

Although the evidence is far from consistent, creatine might improve performance in short-duration, high-intensity, repetitive burst exercise, as well as in resistance training. At most, however, the benefits are slight.

Patients who are not involved in these specific forms of exercise can be advised that creatine has consistently failed to show benefits in other forms of exercise.

Preliminary evidence suggests that creatine may increase exercise tolerance in patients with CHF as well as offer therapeutic benefit for difuse atrophy as well as neuromuscular diseases involving impaired muscle strength and increased fatiguability.

Ergogenic Uses   + 2 X

High-Intensity, Repetitive Burst Exercise with Short Rest Periods

Two double-blind, placebo-controlled studies involving a total of 33 individuals demonstrated improvement in high-intensity, repetitive burst exercise with short rest periods.[2,3] Comparable results were reported in many, but not all, studies of repetitive short-burst exercise.[1-6]

Resistance Training

There is some evidence that creatine supplements might be helpful in resistance training, although results are not entirely consistent.[1,7-9,48,49] One study of 19 women demonstrated that creatine at 20 g/day for 4 days followed by a maintenance dose of 5 g/day for up to 10 weeks increased maximal muscle strength and maximal intermittent arm power output.[10] Another study of strength-trained athletes who received 28 days of creatine supplementation found a significant increase in lifting repetitions.[11]

Other Forms of Exercise

In contrast to high-intensity repetitive burst exercise with short rest periods, studies of high-intensity repetitive burst exercise with longer rest periods have found unimpressive results. For example, one study noted no significant differences within or between groups for power, time to peak power, total work, or fatigue.[12] Similarly negative results have been seen in field trials of single-burst exercise as well as in studies of performance without rapid repetition.[13,14]

Negative results have also been seen in intermediate-duration high-intensity exercise. Of 13 studies reviewed, eight double-blind, placebo-controlled studies and one single-group repeated-measure study of high-intensity, intermediate-duration (30 to 150 seconds) exercise failed to show any improvement with creatine supplementation.[1] Finally, of seven double-blind, placebo-controlled studies that evaluated the use of creatine in aerobic exercise, six failed to demonstrate improvement.[1]

Congestive Heart Failure   +2

Creatine may increase exercise tolerance in congestive heart failure (CHF).

One double-blind study of 17 patients with CHF demonstrated that creatine at 20 g/day for 10 days improved exercise capacity and muscle strength, with no improvement in ejection fraction.[15] Similarly, muscle endurance during handgrip exercises improved in a double-blind, placebo-controlled crossover study of 20 males with CHF.[16]

Other Proposed Uses

In one study of 34 **hypercholesterolemic** patients, subjects were randomly assigned to receive either 5 g of creatine monohydrate plus 1 g of glucose or 6 g of glucose placebo. After 56 days, plasma cholesterol, triacylglycerols, and VLDL cholesterol were reduced in the creatine-treated group.[17]

Creatine supplements might be useful for the treatment of **disuse atrophy** after limb immobilization.[50,51]

Creatine supplementation may alleviate some of the clinical symptoms of **Duchenne's muscular dystrophy.**[18] Cultured *mdx* skeletal muscle cells have been shown to have increased cellular phosphocreatine levels, myotubule formation, and cell survival when supplemented with 20 mmol/L creatine.[19] A double-blind, placebo-controlled trial of 36 individuals with various types of muscular dystrophy found evidence of benefit in muscle strength and daily life activities.[20]

One study of 81 individuals with a variety of **neuromuscular disorders** found that creatine monohydrate (10 g/day for 5 days followed by 5 g/day for 5 to 7 days) improved handgrip, dorsiflexion, and knee extensor strength.[21]

Preliminary evidence supports the use of high-dose creatine (60 to 150 mg/kg/day) for **McArdle disease.**[22,52]

Two small studies with a total of 11 patients with **mitochondrial defects** demonstrated improvement after creatine administration. A double-blind, placebo-controlled study of seven patients demonstrated that creatine at 2 g twice daily for 2 weeks improved isometric grip strength but had no effect on aerobic cycle ergometry or body composition.[23] A study of four patients with mitochondrial encephalomyopathies showed that creatine at 0.1 to 0.2 g/kg/day improved cycle ergometry.[24]

Two studies in animal models of **chronic neurologic diseases** have indicated that creatine may be beneficial. Transgenic mice with amyotrophic lateral sclerosis supplemented with 1% to 2% creatine in the diet had increased survival and protection from neuronal loss.[25] In another study, rats fed a diet supplemented with 1% to 2% creatine were protected from malonate- or 3-nitropropionic acid–induced neural lesions that resemble those of Huntington's disease.[26]

Two case reports of patients with **defects in creatine synthesis** have shown beneficial effects of supplementary creatine. A 22-month-old infant with guanidinoacetate methyltransferase deficiency who was given creatine at 4 g/day showed clinical improvement within 2 months, accompanied by resolution of MRI abnormalities.[27] A 4-year-old girl with creatine deficiency, developmental delay, muscular disorder, and epilepsy improved after 2 months of creatine at 400 mg/kg/day.[28]

Mechanism of Action

Increased concentrations of creatine and phosphocreatine in muscle provide a ready supply of phosphorus to recharge ATP supplies; high-intensity, repetitive-burst exercise fits the physiologic picture in which this effect would be expected to be most useful.[29-33]

The mechanism of action of creatine in treatment of muscular disorders is not as well elucidated. Diminished levels of creatine in muscle may be due to disturbances in ion homeostasis that result in decreased creatine transport into the cells.[18] Diminished creatine and phosphocreatine in muscle results in increased concentrations of lactic acid and hydrogen ions that may directly affect the contractile apparatus of the muscle by affecting calcium or myosin ATPase. Acidosis also results in more rapid depletion of phosphocreatine and inhibits the enzymes of glycolysis.[34]

Impairment of energy production due to mitochondrial defects may result in lower concentrations of phosphorylated creatine and ATP, leading ultimately to cell death. Creatine stabilizes mitochondrial creatine kinase and inhibits the opening of the mitochondrial transition pore, which is linked to cell death.

Increasing creatine concentrations may increase the cerebral energy reserve and offer neuroprotection in conditions such as Huntington's disease.[26]

Authors of one study hypothesized that creatine buffers intracellular energy stores and stimulates phosphocreatine synthesis.[25] In addition, phosphocreatine serves as an energy source for glutamate uptake into synaptic vesicles; impaired glutamate uptake has been implicated in the pathogenesis of ALS.

The mechanism whereby creatine lowers lipid concentrations is not well understood. It has been suggested that creatine increases insulin sensitivity and/or postprandial signaling.[17]

Dosage

The usual dosage for creatine supplementation is 20 to 30 g of creatine monohydrate for 5 to 7 days, taken daily in four divided doses of 5 to 6 g. Thereafter, doses of 2 g/day have maintained elevated creatine concentrations in the muscle for periods up to 1 month.[33] For the average 70-kg male, this is roughly equivalent to a loading dose of 0.3 g/kg body mass per day for 5 to 6 days followed by a maintenance dose of 0.03 g/kg body mass thereafter. Some authorities do not recommend a loading dose at all and instead recommend using lower doses over a longer time.[1]

Combining carbohydrate loading with creatine may be helpful perhaps due to insulin-augmented creatine accumulation or enhanced muscle glycogen supercompensation.[35-37]

Safety Issues

The preponderance of data documenting side effects of creatine is taken from short-term studies involving healthy and/or athletic subjects, although large, systematic, long-term safety studies have not been performed.[38] Less is known about creatine supplements for individuals of other ages or states of health.

The most common side effect of creatine supplementation is weight gain.[1,2,11] Weight gain may be due to an increase in water content or in the diameter of fast-twitch (type II) glycolytic muscle fibers.[2,3,39]

Other side effects that may be caused by creatine include muscle cramping, dehydration, and gastrointestinal distress.[1,40] However, a long-term, placebo-controlled study of 100 football players found no increase in injury or cramping during 1 year of creatine supplementation.[41] Creatine does not appear to adversely affect the body's ability to exercise under hot conditions.[42]

Because excess creatine is excreted by the kidneys, the risk of renal damage must be considered when exogenous creatine is consumed. This is especially true for individuals with renal disease,[43] as well as for healthy individuals who ingest supernormal amounts of creatine or continue creatine supplementation for extended periods. However, a double-blind, placebo-controlled study of 30 young men and women did not find any adverse effects on renal function following creatine supplementation (20 g/day for 5 days).[44] Furthermore, no long-term effects of oral creatine supplementation were noted in 8 subjects who had taken creatine for periods of 10 months to 5 years in doses of 1 to 80 g/day.[45]

Nevertheless, there is one report of impaired renal functioning in a healthy individual apparently attributable to creatine.[46]

Finally, because creatine is metabolized to formaldehyde, it is possible that supplemental creatine will raise formaldehyde production sufficiently to present toxic risk.[47] However, this risk has not yet been established.

Safety in Young Children and Pregnant or Lactating Women

Maximum safe dosages for young children or pregnant or lactating women have not been established.

Drug Interactions

No drug interactions with creatine have been reported, although most studies of the supplement have prohibited concurrent use of other drugs, supplements, or steroids.

Formal drug interaction studies have not been performed.

CURCUMIN
(Extract of Turmeric, *Curcuma longa*)

Alternate Names/Related Species: *Curcuma domestica*

Common Uses

Dyspepsia [+2]   **Hyperlipidemia** [+1]

Antiinflammatory [+2X]   **Ulcers** [−2]

(Higher numbers indicate stronger evidence; X modifier indicates contradictory results. See page xviii of the Introduction for details of the rating scale.)

Approach to the Patient

Curcumin is an extract of the bright yellow spice turmeric *(Curcuma longa)*. Turmeric's components possess antioxidant and eicosanoid-modifying properties. However, while patient may have heard that turmeric works like "herbal ibuprofen," there is actually no meaningful evidence that this is the case.

One double-blind, placebo-controlled trial suggests that curcumin may be helpful for the treatment of nonulcer dyspepsia. Otherwise, there is little clinical evidence for any therapeutic action of this agent.

Dyspepsia   +2

A double-blind study performed in Thailand compared the effects of 500 mg curcumin four times daily with placebo and a locally popular over-the-counter treatment in 116 individuals with dyspepsia.[14] The results showed statistically and clinically significant benefits in the curcumin group compared to the placebo group.

Antiinflammatory   +2X

One small double-blind study of postoperative patients reported similar antiinflammatory benefits with curcumin and phenylbutazone compared to placebo.[1] However, a small double-blind, crossover trial of patients with rheumatoid arthritis found greater benefits with phenylbutazone than curcumin.[2]

Hyperlipidemia   +1

Turmeric extracts have been found to lower LDL and total cholesterol in several animal studies and one open human trial.[3-6]

Ulcers   −2

A 2-month, double-blind, placebo-controlled trial of 118 individuals with duodenal ulcers used endoscopic evaluation to study the effects of turmeric on ulcer healing but found no difference between the verum and placebo groups.[15] Another randomized controlled trial compared turmeric to liquid antacid (magnesium and aluminum hydroxide) therapy in 60 individuals; antacids proved far more effective.[16]

Other Proposed Uses

In vitro and animal studies suggest that curcumin has **chemopreventive properties.**[17-27]

Although some researchers have found evidence that curcumin (or turmeric) has hepatoprotective properties,[28-31] other researchers have failed to confirm these findings[32] and some evidence suggests that turmeric can be hepatotoxic.[33,34]

Curcumin or turmeric has also been recommended for preventing cataracts, and treating multiple sclerosis, Alzheimer's disease, and chronic anterior uveitis,[7-10] but the evidence to support these uses remains minimal.

Mechanism of Action

Although the mechanism of action of turmeric and its constituents is not known, turmeric and/or curcumin have shown
antioxidant, chemopreventive, and antiinflammatory effects in
various models.[11] It has been suggested that the apparent
chemopreventive action of curcumin is related to its ability to
competitively inhibit cytochrome P-450 isozymes responsible
for the metabolic activation of carcinogens such as benzo-
[a]pyrene and aflatoxin B_1. Curcumin selectively inhibits the
CYP 1A1/1A2 and 2B1/2B2 isozymes in the high-nanomolar to
low-micromolar range,[12] levels that are certainly achievable,
even given the poor absorption kinetics for this agent.

Dosage

The usual dose of curcumin is 400 to 600 mg three times daily,
which is equivalent to about 20 to 90 g of turmeric daily.

Safety Issues

Turmeric is on the FDA's GRAS (generally recognized as
safe) list. No LD_{50} has been discovered for curcumin, because
2.5 g/kg doses failed to cause death in various animals.[8,13] However, curcumin doses of 100 mg/kg (but not 50 mg/kg) have
been found to be ulcerogenic in rats. In addition, subchronic
oral toxicity studies of turmeric and ethanolic turmeric extract in
rats found evidence of hepatotoxicity when higher doses were
taken over a 90-day period.[33] Mice showed hepatotoxic effects
when relatively low doses were given for 14 days.

Curcumin stimulates gallbladder contraction and so could
present risks in individuals with gallbladder disease.[7]

Maximum safe dosages in individuals with severe hepatic or
renal disease are not known.

Safety in Young Children and Pregnant or Lactating Women

Maximum safe dosages for young children or pregnant or lactating women have not been established.

Drug Interactions

There is a potential for drug interactions because curcumin inhibits cytochrome P-450 isozymes.[12]

DAMIANA
(Turnera diffusa)

Alternate Names/Related Species: Damiana Leaves

Common Uses

Male aphrodisiac   [0]

(Higher numbers indicate stronger evidence; X modifier indicates contradictory results. See page xviii of the Introduction for details of the rating scale.)

Approach to the Patient

Classic herbal literature of the nineteenth century describes damiana *(Turnera diffusa)* as a tonic, or general body strengthener. Its best-known use today is as an aphrodisiac for men, but there is no evidence to support this use, and some herb experts believe that damiana's reputation as an aphrodisiac is based on a deliberate deception perpetrated more than a century ago.[4]

Male Aphrodisiac   0

The herb damiana has supposedly been used in Mexico for some time as a male aphrodisiac.[1] No scientific trials have been reported. There is no meaningful evidence to supports claims that damiana has testosterone-like actions.

Other Proposed Uses

Damiana is sometimes said to be helpful for treating **asthma** and other **respiratory diseases, depression, digestive problems, menstrual disorders,** and various forms of **sexual dysfunction;** for example, impotence in men, and inability to achieve orgasm in women.[1-3]

Damiana contains arbutin, a urinary antiseptic, at a concentration about 10 times lower than that in uva ursi (see the **Uva Ursi** article). These low levels are probably too small to make this herb a useful treatment for urinary tract infections.

Mechanism of Action

Not applicable.

Dosage

The typical dosage of damiana is 2 to 4 g taken two to three times daily.

Safety Issues

Damiana is on the FDA's GRAS (generally recognized as safe) list and is used as a food flavoring. The only common side effect of damiana is occasional mild gastrointestinal distress. However, damiana contains low levels of cyanide-like compounds, and excessive doses could be dangerous.

Maximum safe dosages in individuals with severe hepatic or renal disease are not known.

Safety in Young Children and Pregnant or Lactating Women

Maximum safe dosages for young children or pregnant or lactating women have not been established.

Drug Interactions

None are known.

DANDELION
(Taraxacum officinale)

Common Uses

Antiinflammatory [+1]   **Diuretic** [+1X]

Choleretic [+1],
"Liver Tonic" [0]

(Higher numbers indicate stronger evidence; X modifier indicates contradictory results. See page xviii of the Introduction for details of the rating scale.)

Approach to the Patient

No clinical studies of dandelion root or leaf *(Taraxacum officinale)* in humans have been reported to date. Limited animal studies suggest possible antiinflammatory actions of dandelion root and diuretic actions of dandelion leaf (and, to a lesser extent, the root as well). Based on the latter effect, it has been suggested that patients taking lithium should avoid dandelion leaf because of the risk of dehydration.

Antiinflammatory   +1

Preliminary animal evidence suggests dandelion root may have potential use in osteoarthritis and rheumatoid arthritis, as well as other inflammatory conditions.[1,2]

Choleretic   +1,
"Liver Tonic"   0

In the folk medicine of many countries, dandelion root has also been regarded as a "liver tonic," a substance believed to benefit the liver in an unspecified way. Studies in dogs and rats suggest

507

that dandelion has a choleretic effect.[3] However, human studies of the herb are lacking.

Diuretic   +1X

One animal study investigating the effects of dandelion leaf and root found diuretic and natriuretic properties in both parts of the plant, but more prominently in the leaf.[4] However, two other animal studies found no significant diuretic or natriuretic activity with *T. officinale* administration.[1,5]

Mechanism of Action

Despite dandelion's longevity in herbal medicine, very little is known regarding its constituents and actual pharmacologic mechanisms. The herb's therapeutic effects are thought to be the result of its bitter constituents. These include *p*-hydroxyphenylacetic acid, beta-sitosterol, taraxine acid-1'-O-B-D-glucopyranoside, and 11,13-dihydrotaraxic acid-1'-O-B-D-glucopyranoside.[6] Other constituents in both the dried rhizome and the root include taraxacine, various acids (e.g., caffeic and hydroxyphenylacetic acid), and vitamins (A, B, C, D, thiamine, and nicotinic acid).[1] Tetrahydroriden-tin B has been identified as well.[7]

Dosage

A typical dose of dandelion root extract (5:1) is 250 mg three to four times daily. The crude dried herb is taken at a dose of 2 to 8 g three times daily, and a 1:5 tincture in 45% alcohol is taken at 5 to 10 ml three times daily.

Safety Issues

Dandelion has been rated generally recognized as safe (GRAS) by the FDA. Animal studies indicate a low order of toxicity.[3] Only minor digestive upset and allergic reactions have been reported as side effects. Nonetheless, due to the lack of comprehensive clinical investigation into the use of this herb, the possibility of more severe but less common side effects cannot be excluded.

Dandelion can cause contact dermatitis, a generalized eczematous eruption that may be confused with atopic eczema or photosensitivity.[8]

Studies performed in the 1950s and earlier suggest that dandelion root may have choleretic and cholekinetic activity[9]; for this reason, caution may be warranted in individuals with cholelithiasis obstruction of the bile ducts or gallbladder empyema. Similarly, because dandelion root may possess some laxative properties, its use is not advised in cases of ileus.

Although some references state that dandelion root can cause hyperacidity and exacerbate ulcer pain, this concern has been disputed.[10]

There was no evidence of carcinogenicity or hepatotoxicity in rats given the dandelion species *T. platycarpum* for up to 120 days.[11] However, it is unknown if these data can be extrapolated to the *T. officinale* species or from rats to humans. Other herbs of the family Compositae, specifically coltsfoot and butterbur, have been found to be carcinogenic in rats.[12,13]

According to a fertility study conducted in mice, plant materials derived from *T. mongolicum* and other Compositae pose no risk to fertility.[14] Fertility data specific to *T. officinale* are not available.

Maximum safe dosages in individuals with severe hepatic or renal disease are not known.

Safety in Young Children and Pregnant or Lactating Women

Maximum safe dosages for young children or pregnant or lactating women have not been established, although there are no known risks among these groups.

Drug Interactions

Coumarins have been identified in dandelion leaf extracts.[15] However, there have been no reports of anticoagulant effects of dandelion. Furthermore, there have been no reports of interactions with other drugs known to affect hemostasis (e.g., warfarin, heparin, ticlopidine, clopidogrel, and nonsteroidal antiinflammatory drugs).

One case report suggests that individuals on **lithium** therapy should avoid the use of herbs with diuretic properties, due to risk of dehydration and subsequent lithium toxicity.[16]

DEVIL'S CLAW
(Harpagophytum procumbens)

Alternate Names/Related Species:
Grapple Plant, Wood Spider

Common Uses

**Arthritis
(mixed types)   [+2]**

**Chronic muscle
pain   [−2X]**

(Higher numbers indicate stronger evidence; X modifier indicates contradictory results. See page xviii of the Introduction for details of the rating scale.)

Approach to the Patient

Devil's claw *(Harpagophytum procumbens)* has shown some promise as an analgesic. However, patients may be advised that the most recent and largest studies have shown only marginal benefits at best.

Arthritis (Mixed Types)   +2

In a 4-week, double-blind trial of 63 individuals with muscular tension in the neck, shoulder, or back, use of a standardized devil's claw extract significantly improved pain levels compared to placebo.[1] Another double-blind, placebo-controlled study of 50 individuals with various types of arthritis found that 10 days of treatment with devil's claw provided significant pain relief.[2]

A 4-month, double-blind comparative study of 122 individuals with osteoarthritis of the hip and/or knee evaluated the relative efficacy of devil's claw and the European drug diacerhein.[3] Diacerhein is a member of a drug category not recognized in the United States: the so-called slow-acting drugs for osteoarthritis (SADOAs) (glucosamine and chondroitin are putative SADOAs as well). The results showed equal efficacy.

Chronic Muscle Pain   − 2X

Results of two studies on the use of devil's claw for low back pain are not easily summarized according to the rating scale used in this book. We've chosen to use −2X rather than +3X to indicate that the results on the one large "positive" trial were clinically insignificant.

A double-blind, placebo-controlled study of 197 individuals with acute exacerbations of low back pain found statistically significant but clinically marginal results with devil's claw.[4] Results in secondary measures failed to corroborate a slight dose-dependent effect seen in the primary outcome measures.

No benefit was seen on primary outcome measures in a previous double-blind study of 118 individuals with acute back pain, although secondary measures showed marginal benefit.[5]

Other Proposed Uses

Like other intensely bitter herbs, devil's claw traditionally is used as an appetite stimulant.

Mechanism of Action

Not known. Studies have found an inconsistent antiinflammatory effect,[2,6] apparently unrelated to that of NSAIDs.[7]

Dosage

A typical dosage of devil's claw is 750 mg three times daily of a preparation standardized to contain 3% iridoid glycosides.

Safety Issues

Devil's claw appears to be quite safe with no evidence of toxicity at doses many times higher than recommended.[2] A 6-month open study of 630 individuals with arthritis showed no side effects other than occasional mild gastrointestinal distress.[2] However, because of its possible gastric-stimulating action as a bitter herb, devil's claw is not recommended for individuals with ulcers.

Maximum safe dosages in individuals with severe hepatic or renal disease are not known.

Safety in Young Children and Pregnant or Lactating Women

Maximum safe dosages for young children or pregnant or lactating women have not been established.

Drug Interactions

None are known.

Devil's claw might increase the anticoagulant effects of **warfarin,** according to one case report.[8] Although the underlying pharmacology has not been eleucidated, it may be prudent to avoid simultaneous use of devil's claw with any **anticoagulant** or **antiplatelet agents,** including natural products such as **policosanol, ginkgo, garlic,** and **high-dose vitamin E.**

DEHYDROEPIANDRO-STERONE (DHEA)

Alternate Names/Supplement Forms: DHEA Sulfate

Common Uses

Systemic lupus erythematosus [+3]

Osteoporosis [+2]

Adrenal insufficiency [+2]

Sexual dysfunction in women [+2X]

Erectile dysfunction [+1]

Athletic performance enhancement [−1X]

(Higher numbers indicate stronger evidence; X modifier indicates contradictory results. See page xviii of the Introduction for details of the rating scale.)

Approach to the Patient

The majority of evidence for DHEA involves benefits in women, including evidence that it may reduce lupus symptoms in women, improve sexual function in women over 70, and also help prevent or treat osteoporosis in women of that age group.

Given that DHEA is converted into other hormones, including estrogen, use of this supplement warrants caution in women at risk for, or with a history of, hormone-sensitive diseases such as breast cancer. Adverse effects on lipid levels have been reported as well.

The long-term safety of DHEA is entirely unknown.

Systemic Lupus
Erythematosus   + 3

Growing evidence supports the use of DHEA as adjunct therapy in SLE.[7]

For example, a 12-month, double-blind, placebo-controlled trial of 381 women with mild or moderate lupus evaluated the effects of DHEA at a dose of 200 mg daily.[1] Although participants in both groups improved, DHEA was more effective than placebo, reducing many symptoms of the disease. However, DHEA was found to adversely affect the ratio of total cholesterol to HDL and to raise levels of testosterone. The study authors recommend monitoring both serum cholesterol levels and possible adverse effects caused by increased testosterone.

Similarly positive results of DHEA in lupus were seen in earlier small studies.[2,3]

DHEA might allow for a dosage reduction in standard medical therapies, as well as directly help offset some of the side effects of corticosteroid treatment, such as accelerated osteoporosis.[3,4]

Osteoporosis   + 2

A growing body of evidence suggests that DHEA may have an antiosteoporotic effect in in women (especially those over 70), but probably not in men.[3,5,52,54]

For example, in a double-blind, placebo-controlled trial of 280 men and women ranging in age from 60 to 79 years, a dose of 50 mg of DHEA daily over a 1-year period reduced bone turnover in a predefined subgroup of women over 70. However, neither men nor younger women responded.

Adrenal Insufficiency   + 2

A double-blind, placebo-controlled crossover trial of 24 women with adrenal insufficiency found that adding DHEA to the usual hormone regimen for adrenal failure improved sexual function, feelings of overall well-being, and cholesterol levels during the 4-month treatment period.[7] Another double-blind crossover trial enrolled 39 men and women and found improvements in general feelings of well-being, mood, and energy level over a 3-month treatment period.[8]

Sexual Dysfunction in Women   +2X

A 1-year controlled trial of 280 men and women, described above in the Osteoporosis section, also looked for effects on sexual function and found that DHEA at a daily dose of 50 mg improved libido and sexual satisfaction in the predefined subgroup of women over 70.[5] Effects were not seen until the sixth month, which may explain why similar trials of DHEA that only lasted 3 months did not find any effect.[10,11]

One 4-month, double-blind, placebo-controlled study of 24 women with adrenal failure found that 50 mg per day of DHEA (along with standard replacement therapy for adrenal failure) improved libido and sexual satisfaction.[7]

Two small double-blind, placebo-controlled studies tested whether a one-time dose of DHEA at 300 mg could increase sexual arousability in pre- or postmenopausal women, respectively.[56,57] As with so many other studied uses of DHEA, effects were seen in older women but not younger women.

Erectile Dysfunction   +1

A double-blind, placebo-controlled study enrolling 40 men with erectile dysfunction as well as low measured levels of DHEA indicated that DHEA at a dose of 50 mg daily improved sexual performance; however, the authors did not undertake a statistical analysis of the data.[53]

Athletic Performance Enhancement −1X

A small double-blind study found no benefit with DHEA at a dose of 150 mg per day for men undergoing weight training.[12] In addition, a 12-week, double-blind study of 40 trained male athletes given either DHEA or androstenedione at 100 mg daily found no improvement in lean body mass or strength, nor a change in testosterone levels.[13]

However, a 12-month, double-blind, placebo-controlled cross-over trial of 16 individuals aged 50 to 65 found some evidence of fat loss and strength improvement in the male participants during the period in which they received 100 mg of DHEA daily.[14] No improvement was seen in female participants.

Other Proposed Uses

DHEA is sometimes suggested for **depression** on the basis of one small double-blind study and one observational study.[15,16]

Highly preliminary evidence suggests that DHEA might be helpful for **chronic fatigue syndrome.**[17]

One small double-blind trial suggests that DHEA (50 mg/day) may improve **mood and fatigue scores** in individuals with **HIV**[6]; another small trial found inconclusive results.[9] Preliminary evidence suggests that DHEA might improve **immune response to vaccinations**[19,20] and strengthen **immunity following burns.**[21,22]

Weak evidence suggests that DHEA might reduce **heart disease risk in men.**[25-30]

Seven studies have found that DHEA supplementation does not improve mood or mental function or general sense of health and well-being in older men or women.[18,23,24,27-29,33] DHEA has also been proposed as a treatment for **Alzheimer's disease** and as an aid in **weight loss,** but the little evidence that is available appears more negative than positive.[31,32]

Mechanism of Action

Dehydroepiandrosterone (DHEA) is an adrenal hormone that is converted into testosterone and estrogen. It has been shown to possess immunomodulatory properties in numerous studies.[34-38] These properties may be the basis of its therapeutic effect in individuals with systemic lupus erythematosus.[39]

In addition, patients with SLE have been shown to have low levels of androgens, including DHEA and DHEA sulfate.[40,41] DHEA supplementation in lupus may therefore exert some of its effects by restoring normal DHEA levels.

Athletes have used DHEA in the belief that it might limit the body's response to cortisol and thereby cause an increase in muscle tissue growth. However, because study results have been mixed, it is unclear whether DHEA affects cortisol or not.[42,43]

Dosage

A typical therapeutic dosage of DHEA is 50 to 200 mg daily, although some studies used dosages above and below this range. A cream containing 10% DHEA may also be used, and is typically applied to the skin at a dosage of 3 to 5 g daily. In some studies, DHEA levels were monitored to achieve blood levels of 20 to 30 nmol/L.

For use as a dietary supplement, DHEA is manufactured synthetically from substances found in soybeans. Contrary to popular belief, there is no DHEA in wild yam.

Safety Issues

DHEA appears to be safe when taken in therapeutic doses, at least in the short term. One study found no significant side effects in 50 women who took up to 200 mg daily for up to 1 year.[2]

However, DHEA, even at the low dose of 25 mg per day, may decrease HDL levels.[1,44] In addition, DHEA may cause acne and hirsutism.[1,45]

Animal studies have found both chemopreventive and cancer-promoting effects with DHEA.[46-49] A 15-year human observational trial looking for a connection between naturally occurring DHEA levels and breast cancer found no relationship, either positive or negative.[50] However, another study found a relationship between higher levels of DHEA and ovarian cancer.[51] Overall, the long-term safety of DHEA supplements remains unknown.

Given that DHEA is converted into other hormones, including estrogen, use of this supplement warrants caution in women at risk for, or with a history of, hormone-sensitive diseases such as breast cancer.

Maximum safe dosages in individuals with severe hepatic or renal disease are not known.

Safety in Young Children and Pregnant or Lactating Women

Use of DHEA in young children or pregnant or lactating women is probably inadvisable.

Drug Interactions

Theoretically, DHEA could interact with other **hormonal treatments.** However, no such interaction has been reported at this time.

Largely on a theoretical basis, it has been suggested that DHEA supplementation may reduce some side effects of **corticosteroid drugs.**[3,4]

DIOSMIN/ HESPERIDIN

Alternate Names/Supplement Forms: Citrus Bioflavonoids

Common Uses

Hemorrhoids   [+3]   Capillary fragility   [+2]

Chronic venous   Lymphedema   [−1]
insufficiency/stasis
ulcers   [+3X]

(Higher numbers indicate stronger evidence; X modifier indicates contradictory results. See page xviii of the Introduction for details of the rating scale.)

Approach to the Patient

A fixed micronized combination of the citrus bioflavonoids diosmin (90%) and hesperidin (10%) is widely used in Europe to treat diseases of the blood vessels and lymph system. The strongest evidence supports its use in hemorrhoids. The combination also appears to have benefit in chronic venous insufficiency and venous stasis ulcers. Extensive safety evaluations have found diosmin/hesperidin free from toxicological risk.

Patients interested in trying this treatment may have trouble finding it; at the time of publication, diosmin/hesperidin is difficult to obtain in the United States. Reportedly, this may change soon.

Hemorrhoids   +3

A 2-month, double-blind, placebo-controlled trial of 120 individuals with recurrent hemorrhoid flare-ups found that treat-

ment with combined diosmin and hesperidin significantly reduced the frequency and severity of hemorrhoidal exacerbations.[1] Another double-blind, placebo-controlled trial of 100 individuals found that the same bioflavonoid preparation relieved
symptoms once an exacerbation of hemorrhoid pain had begun.[2]

Benefits of diosmin/hesperidin were also seen in a 90-day,
double-blind trial of 100 individuals with bleeding hemorrhoids.[3] In another trial, this bioflavonoid combination was
found to compare favorably with rubber band ligation.[4] However, in a trial in which both treated and placebo groups received
soluble fiber, intergroup differences were small.[5]

Chronic Venous Insufficiency/Stasis Ulcers   + 3 X

A fixed micronized combination of the citrus bioflavonoids diosmin and hesperidin is widely used in Europe for the treatment
of various venous conditions, and there is meaningful (if not altogether consistent) supporting evidence for this use.

A 2-month, double-blind, placebo-controlled trial of 200 individuals with severe chronic venous insufficiency found that
treatment with diosmin/hesperidin significantly improved
symptoms as compared to placebo.[11] Another double-blind,
placebo-controlled trial of diosmin/hesperidin enrolled 101 individuals with relatively mild chronic venous insufficiency.[12] The
results showed little difference between the two groups; the authors theorize that diosmin/hesperidin might be generally more
effective in more severe forms of the condition.

A 2-month, double-blind, placebo-controlled trial involving
107 individuals with nonhealing venous stasis ulcers found that
diosmin/hesperidin significantly improved rate of healing.[6]

Capillary Fragility   + 2

A double-blind, placebo-controlled trial of 96 individuals with
fragile capillaries (resulting in such symptoms as easy bruising

and frequent epistaxis) found that a combination of diosmin and hesperidin decreased tendency toward capillary rupture.[7]

Lymphedema   − 1

A double-blind trial that followed 94 individuals with upper limb lymphedema following breast cancer therapy found no significant difference between groups.[8] However, clinical evidence of benefit was reported in the most severely affected subgroup.

Mechanism of Action

Like oxerutins, diosmin/hesperidin appears to increase venous tone and normalize capillary permeability.

Dosage

A typical dosage of micronized diosmin/hesperidin is 500 mg twice daily. See the Appendix for U.S. brand names of clinically tested products.

Safety Issues

Micronized diosmin/hesperidin has undergone extensive safety evaluation, and appears to be essentially free from toxicological risk.[9]

Maximum safe dosages in individuals with severe hepatic or renal disease are not known.

Safety in Young Children and Pregnant or Lactating Women

Maximum safe dosages for young children or pregnant or lactating women have not been established. However, diosmin/hesperidin has been used in clinical trials of pregnant women with no apparent harm.[10]

Drug Interactions

None are known.[9]

DONG QUAI
(Angelica sinensis)

Alternate Names/Related Species: Dang Quai, Tang Quai, Dang Kwai, Dong Kwai

Common Uses

Menstrual disorders   [+1]

Menopause   [−1]

(Higher numbers indicate stronger evidence; X modifier indicates contradictory results. See page xviii of the Introduction for details of the rating scale.)

Approach to the Patient

Dong quai *(Angelica sinensis)* is a staple in the repertoire of Chinese herbology. It has become quite popular as a "women's herb" in the United States. Based on misleading reports, many patients believe that dong quai is a phytoestrogen. In fact, evidence suggests that dong quai is not estrogenic, and one study found it ineffective for the treatment of menopausal symptoms.

Dong quai is a constituent of many prepared Chinese herb formulas. However, patients can be advised that there are serious concerns that such formulas may contain unlisted pharmaceuticals and other toxic ingredients.[1,2]

Menstrual Disorders   +1

Uncontrolled (and unconvincing) studies have reported effectiveness of herbal combinations containing dong quai in a variety of conditions, including amenorrhea and dysmenorrhea.[3,4]

Menopause   − 1

A 12-week study compared the effects of dong quai to placebo in 71 postmenopausal women.[5] The results showed no statistically significant differences between groups in endometrial thickness, vaginal maturation index, number of vasomotor flushes, or the Kupperman index.

Mechanism of Action

Dong quai root contains numerous potentially active substances, including butylidene phthalide, ferulic acid, and beta-sitosterol. Nutritionally, dong quai is a source of nicotinic acid, uracil, adenine, folinic acid, vitamin E, carotene, and a subnutritional amount of vitamin B_{12}. Dong quai does not appear to have estrogenic actions.[5,6]

Dosage

The exact dosage of dong quai used in traditional Chinese formulas is highly individualized. When used in Western herbology, the typical dose is 10 to 40 drops of dong quai tincture one to three times daily or one capsule three times daily. Standardized dong quai extracts are not available.

Safety Issues

Reported side effects of dong quai are rare and consist primarily of mild gastrointestinal distress and occasional allergic reactions (rash). According to Chinese studies, dong quai possesses a low order of toxicity in rats.[7] The furocoumarins in dong quai are known photosensitizing agents, but photosensitivity has not been reported with whole dong quai herb.

Dong quai does not appear to possess phytoestrogenic effects.[11-14]

Nevertheless one case report indicates that an herb product containing dong quai caused gynecomastia.[8] The explanation may lie in the fact that such products are known to be contaminated at times with pharmaceuticals not listed on the labels.[1,2]

One in vitro trial found that, despite an absence of estrogenic action, dong quai stimulated breast cancer cell growth.[13]

Maximum safe dosages in individuals with severe renal or hepatic disease are not known.

Safety in Young Children and Pregnant or Lactating Women

Given animal and in vitro studies suggesting that dong quai can cause both uterine contractions and uterine relaxation, its use in pregnancy is not recommended. In addition, one case report suggests that maternal dong quai usage caused hypertension in both mother and nursing child[9]; again, this may be due to a pharmaceutical contaminant.

Drug Interactions

Dong quai may interact with **warfarin.** In one case report, concurrent administration of dong quai at a dose of 565 mg once to twice daily with warfarin 5 mg daily resulted in a 2.5-fold increase in PT and INR in a previously stabilized patient.[10] However, a study in rabbits found a pharmacodynamic interaction between warfarin and donq quai leading to *decreased* PT.[15]

ECHINACEA
(Echinacea purpurea)

Alternate Names/Related Species:
Purple Coneflower, Rudbeckia; *E. angustifolia, E. pallida*

Common Uses

Reducing severity and duration of upper Respiratory infections [+3]	**Prophylaxis of upper respiratory infections** [−2]
	Prophylaxis of genital herpes [−1]

(Higher numbers indicate stronger evidence; X modifier indicates contradictory results. See page xviii of the Introduction for details of the rating scale.)

Approach to the Patient

Substantial evidence suggests that various echinacea remedies can significantly reduce the duration and severity of acute upper respiratory infections and flu. However, contrary to what your patients may believe, prophylactic use of echinacea has not been found to significantly reduce the incidence of such infections. Echinacea has also failed to prove effective for herpes prophylaxis.

Goldenseal is frequently combined with echinacea in cold preparations to be taken at the onset of symptoms. However, there is no evidence that oral goldenseal is helpful in colds, nor did traditional herbalists use it in this way.[1]

Upper Respiratory Infections

Trials of echinacea have involved many different preparations, including three different species (*E. purpurea*, *E. angustifolia*, *E. pallida*) and differing mixtures of root and herb. However, the best evidence is for the above-ground portion of *E. purpurea*.

Reducing Severity and Duration   +3

In a double-blind trial, 246 individuals with recent onset of a respiratory infection were given either placebo or one of three *E. purpurea* preparations: two concentrations of a product made of 95% above-ground herb (leaves, stems, and flowers) and 5% root, and one made only from the roots of the plant.[2] The results showed significant benefit in the two above-ground preparations, but not with the root-only formula.

Another double-blind, placebo-controlled study using *E. pallida* root followed 160 adults with recent-onset URIs.[4] The results showed that treatment significantly reduced the length of illness as compared to placebo.

In a double-blind, placebo-controlled trial of 95 subjects with a recent-onset respiratory infection, a beverage tea containing above-ground portions of *E. purpurea* and *E. angustifolia* as well as an extract of *E. purpurea* root was also found effective at reducing duration and severity of infection.[5]

In a double-blind, placebo-controlled study of 120 patients with acute respiratory infections, use of Echinagard (juice extracted from the above-ground parts of *E. purpurea* harvested during the flowering stage, also known as Echinacin and EC3IJ0) resulted in a statistically significant decrease in progression to a "real cold" in the treated group as compared to the placebo group, as well as symptomatic benefit in individuals that did develop colds.[6] This included both reduced time to improvement and reduced total duration of cold. Benefits using the same product were also seen in a double-blind placebo-controlled trial of 80 individuals.[7]

Numerous earlier studies also found benefit, but many used a mixed formulation called Resistan that included other herbs as well as homeopathic preparations.[8]

Prophylaxis   − 2

Based on the popular impression that echinacea is an "immune strengthener," the herb has been used as a prophylactic treatment for respiratory infections. However, the results from properly designed studies have not been promising. If there is any prophylactic benefit of echinacea, it falls in the 10% to 20% reduction range. One unpublished study actually found a slight increase in infection rate.

For example, a double-blind, placebo-controlled study compared *E. purpurea* and *E. angustifolia* to placebo for a 12-week period in 302 volunteers.[9] The results failed to show a significant reduction in number of infections in either treatment group as compared to placebo.

Another double-blind, placebo-controlled study enrolled 109 individuals with a history of four or more colds in the previous year and gave them either *E. purpurea* juice or placebo for a period of 8 weeks.[10] No significant benefits were seen in frequency, duration, or severity of colds. Of interest, this paper is actually a more detailed look at a 1992 study widely misreported as providing evidence of benefit.[11]

Negative results were also seen in an unpublished double-blind, placebo-controlled study of 200 individuals followed for 6 months who were treated with either echinacea or placebo.[12] In this trial, individuals in the treated group actually became sick 20% more often.

Another double-blind, placebo-controlled trial followed 117 subjects, pretreated with echinacea for 14 days, and then inoculated with rhinovirus type 23.[13] No difference in rate or severity of infection was seen.

The only study with positive results found them in a subgroup analysis. This study (rating 57% on the Melchart criteria-based review) followed 609 university students.[14] Half were treated with a prophylactic dose of Resistan for at least 8 weeks, and the other half received placebo. Among a subgroup rated as more infection prone on the basis of the frequency of colds in the previous year, there was a statistically significant reduction of 20%. However, the reduction was not significant in the group as a whole.

Prophylaxis of Genital Herpes   − 1

In a 1-year, double-blind, placebo-controlled crossover trial of 50 individuals with frequently recurrent genital herpes, treatment with *E. purpurea* extract (Echinaforce, 800 mg twice daily) failed to impact disease recurrence.[15]

Other Proposed Uses

In a 10-week open trial, 203 women with candidal **vaginitis** were initially treated with a 6-day course of econazole cream and then subsequently received echinacea orally, IV, IM, or subcutaneously. Immune system parameters improved steadily over the course of treatment and recurrence of candidal vaginitis was reduced.[16] However, lack of a placebo group or blinding makes this widely reported trial relatively meaningless.

Mechanism of Action

Echinacea's mechanism of action is not known, but it is thought to involve immunomodulation.[17-26] However, in a trial that evaluated *E. purpurea* use for a period of 6 months, no changes in immune parameters were seen.[15]

Some researchers have theorized that the polysaccharide constituents of echinacea stimulate immune activity by virtue of their similarities to bacterial wall polysaccharides. However, other than the arabinogalactans, these polysaccharides are present in low to negligible amounts in most oral preparations of echinacea. Cichoric acid, which is present in typical oral preparations, also possesses phagocytosis-promoting properties. The same can be said of the alkylamide isobutylamide.

Some herbalists state that echinacea functions in the mouth rather than systemically and therefore recommend the use of liquid products.[27] The proposed method of action is direct contact and activation of the lymphatic tissues surrounding the entrance to the esophagus. However, there is no research evidence for this hypothesis.

Echinacea is not believed to exert any significant direct antibiotic action.[17]

Dosage

Echinacea dosages vary with the specific product and should be taken according to label instructions. Treatment is usually begun at the first sign of a cold and continued for 7 to 14 days. Products made from the above-ground portion of *E. purpurea* have the best supporting evidence. See the Appendix for U.S. brand names of clinically tested products.

Echinacea products frequently contain the herb goldenseal as well. However, there is no evidence that oral goldenseal is helpful in colds, nor did traditional herbalists use it for that purpose.[1]

Safety Issues

The oral use of echinacea is considered safe.[27] In rats, echinacea extracts have not been found to cause either acute or chronic toxicity, even when taken in very high doses.[28] However, there have been adverse drug reactions with parenteral use of echinacea.

According to clinical studies reported to date, oral echinacea causes few side effects.[26] The most common reports include bad taste and minor gastrointestinal symptoms. However, reports from Australia suggest that echinacea can at times cause severe allergic reactions.[32] Specific testing of individuals with a history of allergies to various plants, but who had never taken echinacea, indicated that as many as 20% nonetheless reacted to echinacea. The explanation is presumably cross-reactivity with other *Asteracea* plant species.

Germany's Commission E warns against using echinacea in autoimmune disorders such as multiple sclerosis, lupus, and rheumatoid arthritis, as well as tuberculosis and leukocytosis, based on theoretical concerns about inappropriately activating the immune system. One case report lends some support to these concerns; use of echinacea repeatedly triggered episodes of erythema nodosum (EN).[3] Finally, Commission E recommends not using echinacea for more than 8 weeks, based on evidence that parenteral echinacea reversibly depresses immune parameters.[29] However, oral use of echinacea for up to 6 months has not been associated with any measurable change in immune status.[15,16,26]

Maximum safe dosages in individuals with severe hepatic or renal disease are not known.

Safety in Young Children and Pregnant or Lactating Women

A case control study of 412 pregnant women found no adverse outcomes attributable to use of echinacea.[30]

Over 550 children with whooping cough ranging in age from infancy to 14 years old have been given parenteral echinacea extract in German studies conducted since the 1950s.[26] No significant adverse effects were reported other than occasional modest elevation in temperature, attributed to stimulation of phagocytes and the associated production of cytokines. Similar results were seen in a report on the treatment of over 500 children with tuberculosis.

Drug Interactions

Evidence suggests that *E. angustifolia* root might inhibit CYP3A4.[31]

ELDERBERRY FLOWER
(*Sambucus nigra*)

Alternate Names/Related Species: European Elder, Black Elder, Black-Berried Alder, Boor Tree, Elder

Common Uses

Viral infections   [+2]

(Higher numbers indicate stronger evidence; X modifier indicates contradictory results. See page xviii of the Introduction for details of the rating scale.)

Approach to the Patient

Sambucol, a product containing elderberry flower as well as small amounts of echinacea and bee propolis, has been widely marketed as a cold and flu remedy, but the evidence to support this use is scant.

The patient interested in using elderberry may be directed toward other natural remedies supported by stronger evidence, such as echinacea, topical zinc, or andrographis. (Elderberry flower tastes better, though.)

Viral Infections   +2

In a preliminary double-blind study, Sambucol reduced the recovery time from a particular strain of epidemic influenza by almost one-half.[1]

Elderberry is being studied for potential activity against other viral illnesses as well, including HIV[2] and herpes.[3]

Mechanism of Action

Weak evidence suggests that Sambucol may have immunomodulatory as well as direct antiviral actions.[4]

Dosage

Elderberry flower tea is made by steeping 3 to 5 g of dried flowers in 1 cup of boiling water for 10 to 15 minutes. A typical dosage is 1 cup three times daily. Standardized extracts should be taken according to the directions on the product's label. See the Appendix for U.S. brand names of clinically tested products.

Safety Issues

Elderberry flowers are generally regarded as safe. Side effects are rare and consist primarily of occasional mild gastrointestinal distress or allergic reactions.

Maximum safe dosages in individuals with severe hepatic or renal disease are not known.

Safety in Young Children and Pregnant or Lactating Women

Maximum safe dosages for young children or pregnant or lactating women have not been established.

Drug Interactions

None are known.

Eleutherococcus
(Eleutherococcus senticosus)

Alternate Names/Related Species:
Siberian Ginseng, Russian Ginseng

Common Uses

Genital herpes [+2]

Adaptogen [+2]

Immunomodulatory effects [+2]

Athletic performance enhancement [−1]

(Higher numbers indicate stronger evidence; X modifier indicates contradictory results. See page xviii of the Introduction for details of the rating scale.)

Approach to the Patient

Eleutherococcus senticosus (commonly but incorrectly known as Siberian or Russian ginseng) is only distantly related to the true ginseng species (*Panax ginseng* and *P. quinquefolius*) and possesses an altogether distinct pharmacological nature. Its popularity stems from the work of Russian scientist I.I. Brekhman, who considered *Eleutherococcus* to be functionally identical to ginseng and wrote extensively on its properties. *Eleutherococcus'* major advantage over true ginseng is its far lower cost.

Most patients believe that *Eleutherococcus* (as well as real ginseng) is a stimulant. However, Brekhman described it not as a stimulant but as an "adaptogen." Although the concept of adaptogens has not been adopted in the medical literature of the United States, herbal texts and some European medical treatises use the term freely. According to the definition of the term, an adaptogen should help the body adapt to stresses of various kinds,

534

whether heat, cold, exertion, trauma, sleep deprivation, toxic exposure, radiation, infection, or psychological stress; cause no side effects; be helpful in treating a wide variety of illnesses; and tend to return an organism toward homeostasis rather than alter variables in a fixed direction (e.g., an adaptogen should reduce serum glucose when it is high and raise serum glucose when it is low).

Regular exercise is probably the clearest example of an adaptogenic treatment. However, the evidence that *Eleutherococcus* (or any other herb) has adaptogenic properties is preliminary at best.

Eleutherococcus may reduce genital herpes recurrences. Like *Panax ginseng*, it is also widely used by athletes in the belief that it will enhance physical performance; however, this has not been documented.

Genital Herpes   +2

A 6-month, double-blind, placebo-controlled trial of 93 men and women with recurrent herpes infections found that treatment with *Eleutherococcus* (2 g daily) reduced the frequency of infections by approximately 50%.[1]

Adaptogen   +2

A review of Russian studies enrolling more than 4300 healthy and nonhealthy individuals suggests that *Eleutherococcus* may have adaptogenic effects.[2] Although the meaningfulness of these clinical trials is limited by poor design, results showed general improvement in physical performance and mental agility, adaptation to temperature fluctuations, resistance to hypoxemia and immune insults, and strengthening of cardiovascular parameters. Therapeutic benefit was also described in health conditions such as cardiovascular disease, diabetes, acute craniocerebral trauma, and various types of neuroses and pulmonary diseases. A review of animal studies also suggests adaptogenic effects.[2]

Immunomodulatory Effects   +2

In a 4-week, placebo-controlled human trial, *Eleutherococcus* increased the absolute number of immunocompetent cells, especially T-lymphocytes of the helper/inducer type.[3]

Athletic Performance Enhancement   −1

A double-blind, placebo-controlled study of 20 athletes over an 8-week period found no improvement in physical performance.[4] In addition, a small double-blind crossover trial found *Eleutherococcus* ineffective for improving performance in endurance exercise (i.e., prolonged cycling).[5] Finally, in a small double-blind, placebo-controlled trial of endurance athletes, use of *Eleutherococcus increased* physiological signs of stress during intensive training.[8]

Mechanism of Action

Some evidence suggests that *Eleutherococcus* may possess immunomodulatory actions and might also increase maximal oxygen intake under conditions of acute exercise.[9,10]

Dosage

The recommended daily dose of *Eleutherococcus* is 2 to 3 g of whole herb or 300 to 400 mg of extract. See the Appendix for U.S. brand names of clinically tested products.

Safety Issues

According to studies performed primarily in the former Soviet Union, *Eleutherococcus* appears to present a low order of toxicity in both the short and long term.[2] Human trials have not resulted in any significant side effects. The LD_{50} of *E. senticosus* root in mice was determined to be 31 g/kg. In rats, administration of a 33% ethanol extract at a dose of 5 ml/kg for 320 days produced no toxic manifestations. Studies of rats, mink, lamb, and rabbits have found no evidence of teratogenicity.

Maximum safe dosages in individuals with severe hepatic or renal disease are not known.

Safety in Young Children and Pregnant or Lactating Women

Eleutherococcus does not appear to possess teratogenic properties.[6]

Maximum safe dosages for young children or pregnant or lactating women have not been established.

Drug Interactions

None are known.

There has been one report of otherwise unexplained elevated **digoxin** levels in a patient taking digoxin and *Eleutherococcus*.[7] This appears to have been a case of interference with a diagnostic test, rather than actual elevation of digoxin levels.

Based on its purported immunomodulatory actions, *Eleutherococcus* might interfere with the action of **immunosuppressive drugs.**

EPHEDRA
(Ephedra sinica)

Alternate Names/Related Species:
Desert Herb, Ephedrine, Ma Huang, *E. equisetina,*
E. gerardiana, E. intermedia, E. major, E. shennungiana

Common Uses

**Asthma, sinus
congestion   [+4]**

**Weight loss (ephedrine/
caffeine)   [+3]**

*(Higher numbers indicate stronger evidence; X modifier indicates contradic-
tory results. See page xviii of the Introduction for details of the rating scale.)*

Approach to the Patient

Ephedra (ma huang) contains ephedrine and pseudoephedrine
(among other active alkaloids), and has actions comparable to
these drugs. However, such treatments present real risks. The
ephedrine content of ephedra is inconsistent, other toxic ingredients may be present, and severe adverse effects are possible.
Patients should be advised against using this herb.

Weight loss treatments containing ephedrine (rather than the
herb ephedra) combined with caffeine appear to be effective
and may be useful under close supervision. Once again, use of
the herb ephedra instead of ephedrine may present unpredictable risks.

Some patients may be swayed against ephedra by the fact that
traditional Chinese herbology recommends against long-term
use of the herb. Ma huang *(Ephedra sinica)* was originally used by
Chinese herbalists for the early stages of respiratory infections
and also for the short-term treatment of certain kinds of asthma,

eczema, hay fever, narcolepsy, and edema. However, it was considered inappropriate to take ma huang for an extended period of time, and individuals with less-than-robust constitutions were warned to use only low doses or to avoid ma huang altogether.

Asthma, Sinus Congestion   +4

Because it contains both ephedrine and pseudephedrine, ephedra is presumably effective as a short-term treatment for sinus congestion and mild asthma. However, it is not recommended. Modern conventional asthma treatments are safer and cause fewer side effects.

Weight Loss (Ephedrine/Caffeine)   +3

Although herbal ephedra has not been well studied as a weight loss agent, several studies have found that ephedrine/caffeine combinations are modestly effective for short- and long-term weight loss.[1-5]

For example, in a double-blind, placebo-controlled trial, 180 overweight individuals were placed on a low-energy diet and given either ephedrine/caffeine (20 mg, 200 mg), ephedrine alone (20 mg), caffeine alone (200 mg), or placebo three times daily for 24 weeks.[1] Individuals in the ephedrine/caffeine treatment group experienced weight loss of 36 pounds as compared to 29 pounds in the placebo group. Over the course of the trial, the treatment group maintained the same relative weight loss advantage over the placebo group, suggesting that tolerance to treatment did not develop.

Mechanism of Action

Ephedra's actions are presumably due to its ephedrine and pseudoephedrine content. Ephedrine suppresses appetite and increases energy expenditure.[6] The combination with caffeine appears to produce synergistic effects, with appetite suppression probably the most important overall factor.

Dosage

The therapeutic dosage of ephedra should be adjusted according to the amount of ephedrine the preparation provides. A typical adult dosage is 12.5 to 25 mg of ephedrine three times daily. It should not be used for more than 1 week.

However, a survey of ephedra products found widespread labeling errors, making determination of ephedrine content impossible in practice.[7] For this reason, as well as those given in the Safety Issues section, close medical supervision of any patient interested in using ephedra is highly recommended.

Safety Issues

There is significant controversy regarding the risks of ephedra-containing supplements, with rival analyses of case reports arriving at opposite conclusions.[8,9] However, there is no question that ephedrine is a potent sympathomimetic, and should not be taken by those with prostatic hyperplasia, hypertension, diabetes, coronary disease, atherosclerosis, or hyperthyroidism.[10] There may be risks in healthy individuals as well.[13]

One concern regards the significant potential for label inaccuracy of ephedrine content noted above. Another issue is the presence of additional ephedrine-related alkaloids, such as the schedule IV controlled substance (+)-norpseudoephedrine, that are not found in FDA-approved over-the-counter ephedra products.[7]

In addition, safety in individuals with severe hepatic or renal disease is not known.

Weight loss products and "natural" stimulants containing ephedrine, when used excessively and in combination with other stimulants such as caffeine, have resulted in severe overstimulation and even death in some individuals.[11] In 1997, the FDA proposed stiff limits on dietary supplements containing ephedrine, but these limits are presently under appeal by manufacturers.

The FDA's intervention stemmed from unscrupulous promotion (mostly via the Internet) of ma huang as a natural hallucinogen ("herbal ecstasy"). Dosages of ephedrine required to produce psychoactive effects are exceedingly cardiotoxic; the FDA has documented 38 deaths of otherwise healthy young individuals who reportedly used ephedrine for psychedelic purposes.

In addition, there has been one case report of acute hepatitis associated with the use of ma huang.[12] However, given the lack of reports in the literature of hepatotoxicity associated with ma huang and ephedrine use, the authors speculated that the ma huang product taken by the patient may have contained some other ingredient or contaminant or was misidentified.

Safety in Young Children and Pregnant or Lactating Women

Ephedra is not recommended for young children or pregnant lactating women.

Drug Interactions

Combining ephedra with **MAO inhibitors** such as phenelzine (Nardil) may lead to severe tachycardia or hypertension and may be fatal.

ESTRIOL

Alternate Names/Supplement Forms: Oestriol, Tri-Estrogen

Common Uses

Menopausal symptoms   [+4]

(Higher numbers indicate stronger evidence; X modifier indicates contradictory results. See page xviii of the Introduction for details of the rating scale.)

Approach to the Patient

Estriol, the weakest of the natural estrogens, has been popularized by some alternative physicians as a safer alternative to estrone and estradiol. However, such claims are misleading to your patients.

The balance of evidence suggests that, when taken in dosages high enough to be effective, estriol presents precisely the same risks as estradiol and estrone. Claims that estriol has an anticancer effect are based on exaggerated interpretations of very weak studies.[1-3]

There is some evidence that estriol might cause less breakthrough bleeding than other forms of estrogen.[4,5]

Menopausal Symptoms   +4

There is little doubt that estriol is effective for reducing menopausal symptoms such as hot flashes, night sweats, insomnia, vaginal dryness, and recurrent urinary tract infections.[4-10] In addition, some evidence indicates that it is helpful for postmenopausal osteoporosis.[11,12]

Mechanism of Action

Like other forms of estrogen, estriol binds to estrogen receptors on hormone-sensitive tissues.

Dosage

The usual dose of estriol is 2 to 8 mg taken once daily. A popular "alternative" product known as Tri-Estrogen contains estriol along with small amounts of estradiol and estrone.

Safety Issues

Unopposed oral estriol stimulates endometrial tissue, leading to increased risk of endometrial cancer. It may also increase breast cancer risk.[13]

In a placebo-controlled study of 1110 women, uterine tissue stimulation was seen among women given estriol orally (1 to 2 mg daily) as compared to those given placebo.[14] A large case-control study found that oral estriol increased the risk of uterine cancer.[15] In a study of 48 women given estriol at a dose of 1 mg twice daily, uterine tissue stimulation was seen in the majority of cases.[16]

However, a 12-month, double-blind, trial of oral estriol (2 mg daily) in 68 Japanese women found no effect on the uterus.[5] It may be that the high levels of soy isoflavones in the Japanese diet altered the outcome. One study also suggests that estriol is less likely to affect the uterus when taken in a once-daily dose rather than in divided doses.[17]

As with other forms of estrogen, vaginal estriol preparations appear to be safer than oral preparations.[15,18]

Maximum safe dosages in individuals with severe hepatic or renal disease are not known.

Safety in Young Children and Pregnant or Lactating Women

Estriol should not be used during pregnancy and lactation. Estriol is not intended for use by children.

Drug Interactions

Estriol's drug interactions would be expected to be identical to those of any other form of estrogen.

EYEBRIGHT
(Euphrasia officinale)

Alternate Names/Related Species: Euphrasia

Common Uses

Ocular infections   [0]

(Higher numbers indicate stronger evidence; X modifier indicates contradictory results. See page xviii of the Introduction for details of the rating scale.)

Approach to the Patient

Eyebright *(Euphrasia officinale)* has been traditionally used as an eyewash for ocular irritation and infections. There is no scientific evidence to support this medicinal use of eyebright.

Ocular Infections   0

Like many plants, eyebright contains astringent substances and volatile oils that are probably at least slightly antibacterial, but there is no evidence that eyebright is effective for treating ocular diseases. Germany's Commission E recommends against using it.

Other Proposed Uses

Eyebright tea is also sometimes taken internally to treat jaundice, respiratory infections, and memory loss. However, there is no evidence that it is effective for these conditions.

Mechanism of Action

Not applicable.

Dosage

Traditionally, eyebright tea is made by boiling 1 tablespoon of the herb in a cup of water. This is then used as an eyewash or taken internally up to three times daily.

Safety Issues

When applied topically, eyebright can cause tearing of the eyes, itching, and redness, probably due to direct irritation.[1] The safety of oral use has not been evaluated.

Maximum safe dosages in individuals with severe hepatic or renal disease are not known.

Safety in Young Children and Pregnant or Lactating Women

Maximum safe dosages for young children or pregnant or lactating women have not been established.

Drug Interactions

None are known.

FENUGREEK
(Trigonella foenum-graecum)

Alternate Names/Related Species:
Bird's Foot, Greek Hay Seed

Common Uses

Diabetes   [+1]   **Hyperlipidemia**   [+1]

(Higher numbers indicate stronger evidence; X modifier indicates contradictory results. See page xviii of the Introduction for details of the rating scale.)

Approach to the Patient

Scant preliminary evidence suggests that fenugreek *(Trigonella foenum-graecum)* may exert a hypoglycemic effect in both type 1 and 2 diabetes. However, contrary to what your patients may believe, there is no evidence that fenugreek can substitute for oral hypoglycemics.

Fenugreek may also have a hypolipidemic effect.

Diabetes   +1

In a 2-month, double-blind study of 25 individuals with type 2 diabetes, use of fenugreek (1 g per day of a standardized extract) significantly improved some measures of blood sugar control and insulin response as compared to placebo.[6] Levels of triglycerides decreased, and HDL cholesterol levels increased, presumably due to enhanced insulin sensitivity.

Animal studies, open trials, and one small, single-blind, controlled study have also reported improvements in overall blood sugar control, blood sugar elevations in response to a meal, and cholesterol levels.[1-3]

Hyperlipidemia   +1

Animal studies and open trials in humans suggest that fenugreek might have a direct hypolipidemic effect.[7-12]

Mechanism of Action

It has been suggested that fenugreek's dietary fiber may impair glucose and cholesterol absorption in the intestines; other mechanisms have been proposed as well.[3,4,7-10]

Dosage

The typical dosage is 5 to 30 g of defatted fenugreek seeds taken three times daily with meals. Because the seeds are somewhat bitter, they are best taken in capsule form. The one reported double-blind trial of fenugreek used 1 g per day of a water/ alcohol fenugreek extract.

Safety Issues

As a commonly eaten food, fenugreek is generally regarded as safe. Animal studies have found fenugreek essentially nontoxic.[7,13]

Safety in Young Children and Pregnant or Lactating Women

Pregnant women should not take fenugreek in dosages higher than is commonly used as a spice (perhaps 5 g daily). Extracts of fenugreek have been shown to stimulate uterine contractions in guinea pigs.[5]

Maximum safe dosages for young children or lactating women have not been established.

Drug Interactions

Fenugreek may cause acute hypoglycemia in diabetic patients who use **insulin** or other **hypoglycemic drugs.** One case report suggests that a combination of the herbs boldo and fenugreek may potentiate the effects of warfarin.[14]

FEVERFEW
(Tanacetum parthenium)

Alternate Names/Related Species:
Featherfew, Featherfoil, Midsummer Daisy

Common Uses

Migraine headaches (prophylaxis)   [+2X]

Rheumatoid arthritis   [−1]

(Higher numbers indicate stronger evidence; X modifier indicates contradictory results. See page xviii of the Introduction for details of the rating scale.)

Approach to the Patient

Feverfew *(Tanacetum parthenium)* may be a useful treatment for individuals with recurrent migraine headaches, but the evidence for its effectiveness is not yet strong.

While in general patients may be advised to use standardized extracts of herbs rather than cruder preparations, feverfew may be an exception. A standardized alcohol extract of feverfew failed to prove effective in one double-blind trial, but whole powdered feverfew leaf has shown efficacy in two double-blind trials.

Feverfew has antiprostaglandin effects that suggest possible drug interactions with NSAIDs as well as anticoagulant agents.

Migraine Headaches (Prophylaxis)   +2X

Imperfect evidence supports the use of some forms of feverfew for individuals with recurrent migraines.

One double-blind, placebo-controlled trial used feverfew leaf with a parthenolide content of 0.66%.[1] In this 8-month cross-over study of 59 patients, treatment with 82 mg feverfew daily was associated with a 24% reduction in the number of migraines and a significant decrease in nausea and vomiting during attacks.

A double-blind crossover trial of 57 migraine patients evaluated the effectivness of 50 mg twice daily of a whole feverfew leaf product containing only 0.2% parthenolide.[2] The results showed significant improvement in intensity of headache pain, nausea, vomiting, and photophobia, and light sensitivity in the treatment period as compared to the placebo period. Unfortunately, the study did not report whether there was an effect on migraine frequency.

In contrast to these positive results, a randomized, double-blind, placebo-controlled trial of 50 individuals given an alcohol extract of feverfew standardized to its parthenolide content found no benefit.[4] This negative outcome, in conjunction with the positive results of the low-parthenolide study mentioned above, suggests that the identification of parthenolide as the active principle was premature.

Finally, a double-blind, placebo-controlled study of 147 individuals found dose-related reduction of migraine incidence with a proprietary CO_2 feverfew extract called Mig-99, but only in a predefined subgroup with more severe migraines.[5]

Rheumatoid Arthritis   − 1

A double-blind, placebo-controlled study followed 41 symptomatic RA patients over 6 weeks, and reported no benefit with feverfew treatment.[6]

Mechanism of Action

Feverfew extract (50 or 150 μl/ml) has been shown to suppress 86% to 88% of prostaglandin production without an effect on cyclo-oxygenase.[7] Furthermore, lactones (parthenolide and epoxyartemorin) isolated from feverfew have been found to be inhibitory with IC_{50} values ranging from approximately 1 to 5 µg/ml, irreversibly inhibiting eicosanoid generation.[8]

Although parthenolide has long been considered the active ingredient in feverfew, this hypothesis was called into question by negative results with an extract standardized to its parthenolide concentration.[4] Tanetin, a lipophilic avonol (6-hydroxy-kaempferol 3,7,4'-trimethyl ether) has also been identified as a feverfew constituent that inhibits generation of pro-inflammatory eicosanoids.[9]

Given these findings, the mechanism of action of feverfew must be regarded as unknown.

Dosage

The daily dosage of herb used in the first study on feverfew mentioned above was 82 mg of dried leaf, containing 0.66% parthenolide. Subsequent dosage recommendations tended to concentrate on reproducing the same daily quantity of parthenolide. However, now that the primacy of parthenolide has been challenged, it is presently unknown which forms of feverfew may be most effective and what dosage should be taken.

Safety Issues

There are no reports of serious adverse effects associated with the use of feverfew. Animal studies have shown no adverse effects at 100 times the human daily dose; an LD_{50} has not been determined.[10]

Mouth ulcerations (from chewing feverfew leaf) and mild gastrointestinal distress have been reported.[3]

Feverfew inhibits platelet activity in vitro.[8,11-13] Despite these findings, no clinical evidence exists that feverfew adversely affects platelet function. In a study of 10 patients who had taken feverfew for 3.5 to 8 years, platelet aggregation induced by ADP and thrombin was indistinguishable between the six patients taking feverfew and the four patients who had discontinued feverfew 6 months prior.[14]

One report described a "postfeverfew syndrome" that consisted of withdrawal symptoms such as headache, insomnia, nervousness, and joint discomfort,[3] but this pattern was not seen in another study.[1] Feverfew was used for a longer time in the former case.

Maximum safe dosages in individuals with severe hepatic or renal disease are not known.

Safety in Young Children and Pregnant or Lactating Women

Safety is not established in pregnancy, and feverfew has a folk history of use as an abortifacient. It is also not recommended during lactation. Maximum safe dosages for young children have not been established.

Drug Interactions

Feverfew's effects on prostaglandins suggest that concomitant use of feverfew and **NSAIDs** might increase risk of gastropathy and nephropathy. Its antiplatelet activity suggests a potential interaction with **anticoagulant drugs,** as well as supplements such as **garlic, ginkgo, policosanol,** and high-dose **vitamin E.**

FISH OIL

Alternate Names/Supplement Forms:
Docosahexaenoic Acid (DHA), Eicosapentaenoic Acid (EPA),
Omega-3 Fatty Acids, Omega-3 Oil(s)

Common Uses

Rheumatoid arthritis [+3]

Cardiovascular disease prevention [+3X]

Dysmenorrhea [+2]

Bipolar disorder [+2]

Depression [+2]

(Higher numbers indicate stronger evidence; X modifier indicates contradictory results. See page xviii of the Introduction for details of the rating scale.)

Approach to the Patient

Fish oil contains essential fatty acids in the omega-3 family. Important constituents are EPA (eicosapentaenoic acid) and DHA (docosahexaenoic acid).

Meaningful evidence indicates that fish oil is an effective treatment for the early stages of rheumatoid arthritis. It appears to significantly reduce symptoms without side effects and may magnify the benefits of standard arthritis drugs. However, patients may be advised that it has not shown disease-modifying effects.

Numerous studies have evaluated the potential benefits of fish or fish oil for reducing cardiovascular risk. While the results have been mixed, on balance the evidence is more positive than negative. Promising preliminary evidence suggests that fish oil may also be helpful for dysmenorrhea, as well as psychological conditions, such as depression and bipolar disorder.

Rheumatoid Arthritis   +3

Thirteen double-blind, placebo-controlled studies involving a total of over 500 individuals found that the omega-3 fatty acids in fish oil can reduce the symptoms of rheumatoid arthritis.[1,2] However, unlike the DMARDs (disease-modifying anti-rheumatic drugs), fish oil is not thought to slow disease progression.

Cardiovascular
Disease Prevention   +3X

Although individual studies have produced mixed results, a meta-analysis of all published trials suggests that high intake of fish or fish oil can reduce overall mortality, heart disease mortality, and sudden cardiac death.[76]

According to many but not all studies, fish oil reduces serum triglycerides and may also modestly raise HDL levels.[3-6,77] A 24-week, double-blind, placebo-controlled trial found that use of fish oil enhanced the hypotriglyceridemic effects of simvastatin.[7] However, gemfibrozil appears to be more effective than fish oil.[8]

Additionally, fish oil may exert cardioprotective actions via anticoagulant effects and reduction of homocysteine levels.[9] Studies contradict one another regarding whether fish oil has antihypertensive effects.[10-16] A 6-week, double-blind, placebo-controlled study of 59 overweight men suggests that it is the DHA in fish oil, and not the EPA, which reduces BP.[17]

Evidence from some but not all observational trials suggests that higher dietary intake of omega-3 essential fatty acids may reduce incidence of cardiovascular disease.[18-25]

Intervention trials of fish[26,27] or fish oil[28,29,78-80] for improving the progression of cardiovascular disease have yielded mixed results.

There is some evidence that higher consumption of fish oil might help prevent sudden cardiac death,[26,31-34] possibly by helping prevent arrythmias. However, a double-blind trial of 300 individuals with acute MI found no clinical benefit with 4 g of concentrated omega-3 fatty acids daily for 12 to 14 months compared to corn oil, despite comparative improvements in HDL and triacylglycerol levels.[35]

Dysmenorrhea   + 2

In a 4-month crossover study of 42 young women aged 15 to 18, supplementation with 6 g of fish oil daily (providing 1080 mg of EPA and 720 mg of DHA) resulted in significantly reduced menstrual pain.[36]

Another double-blind study followed 78 women who received fish oil (2.5 g/day), seal oil (5 g/day), fish oil with vitamin B_{12} (2.5 g fish oil, including 7.5 μg B_{12}, daily) or placebo for three full menstrual periods.[37] Significant improvements were seen in all treatment groups, but the fish oil plus B_{12} proved most effective, and its benefits continued for the longest time after treatment was stopped (3 months). The researchers offered no explanation why B_{12} should be helpful for dysmenorrhea.

Bipolar Disorder   + 2

Preliminary evidence suggests that fish oil, a source of omega-3 fatty acids, may have a therapeutic benefit in bipolar disorder. In a double-blind study reported in 1999, 30 individuals with bipolar disorder were given either placebo or fish oil capsules for 4 months, in addition to their existing treatment.[38] The results showed longer symptom-free periods in the treated group.

This trial used rather high doses of fish oil: 7 capsules twice daily, each capsule containing 680 mg of omega-3 fatty acids (440 mg of EPA and 240 mg of DHA). By comparison, most fish oil capsules contain no more than 300 mg of total omega-3 fatty acids.

Depression   + 2

A 4-week, double-blind trial of 20 individuals with recurrent depression found that use of fish oil improved depression-index scores significantly compared to placebo.[81]

Schizophrenia   − 1 X

A double-blind, placebo-controlled trial of 87 individuals with schizophrenia or schizoaffective disorder found that adjunctive treatment with fish oil (3 g ethyl EPA daily) provided no additional benefits.[82] A much smaller previous trial did find some evidence of benefit with 2 g of EPA daily.[44]

Other Proposed Uses

Preliminary controlled studies suggest that fish oil may be of benefit in **Raynaud's phenomenon,**[39,40] **systemic lupus erythematosus,**[41] **sickle cell anemia,**[42] and **IgA nephropathy.**[43] Although one small double-blind, placebo-controlled study suggested that fish oil may reduce symptoms of **psoriasis,**[45] a subsequent larger and longer trial found no benefit.[46]

Evidence is also mixed on whether fish oil can help prevent exacerbations or reduce symptoms of **inflammatory bowel disease.** Some evidence suggests that fish oil may provide some therapeutic benefit in both **ulcerative colitis** and **Crohn's disease,**[47-52] but other trials have found no benefit.[51,53-56]

Interesting, but highly preliminary, evidence suggests that fish oil or its constituents might be helpful for treating **depression, preventing premature birth, improving vision in premature infants, treating renal calculi, alleviating the symptoms of chronic fatigue syndrome,** and **reducing the risk of prostate cancer.**[57-63] Fish oil has also been proposed as a treatment for many other conditions, including **diabetic neuropathy,**[64] allergies, and gout, but there has been little real scientific investigation of these uses.

A 16-week, double-blind, placebo-controlled study of 167 individuals with **recurrent migraine headaches** found that fish oil did not significantly reduce headache frequency or severity.[83]

Other preliminary studies suggest fish oil may help symptoms of **multiple sclerosis**[65-68]; however, the only reported double-blind study found no difference between fish oil and olive oil placebo.[69]

Docosahexaenoic acid (DHA) has been evaluated as a possible treatment for **male infertility,** but a double-blind trial of 28 men with impaired sperm activity found no benefit.[70]

DHA has also been tried as adjuvant therapy for **ADHD.** In a double-blind trial, 63 children with ADHD stabilized on stimulant therapy were additionally given either DHA (345 mg/day, from an algae source) or placebo for 4 months.[71] The results showed no difference between the treatment and placebo groups.

There is no consistent evidence that fish oil is effective for **asthma.**[72] Fish oil has been tried as an adjunctive therapy in the treatment of *Helicobacter pylori*, but the results were not promising.[30]

Mechanism of Action

EPA (eicosapentaenoic acid) and DHA (docosahexaenoic acid) are downstream intermediates in major prostaglandin and leukotriene synthesis pathways; when taken orally, they alter the balance of those pathways toward less inflammatory eicosanoids.

Dosage

Standard dosages of fish oil are 3 to 9 g daily, typically providing about 1.8 g of EPA and 0.9 g of DHA daily. However, much higher doses have also been used.

Cod liver oil is the most common form of fish oil; however, there are safety concerns regarding its high content of vitamins A and D (see Safety Issues). Salmon oil, mackerel oil, halibut oil, and the oils from other coldwater fish might be better choices. To prevent oxidation, the manufacturing process may involve adding vitamin E to or removing oxygen from fish oil capsules. Fish oil should be stored out of sunlight.

Flaxseed oil contains the omega-3 fatty acid alpha-linolenic acid (ALA). It has been suggested as a less odorous substitute for fish oil. However, ALA is farther upstream in the synthetic pathway from EPA and DHA, and it does not exert the same effect on eicosanoid synthesis.

Safety Issues

Overall, fish oil appears to be safe. It may temporarily raise LDL levels, but this effect seems to be short-lived, and levels return to normal with continued use.[4,5] Fish oil does not appear to raise glucose levels in diabetics.[5,73] Although fish oil has mild anticoagulant effects, it does not appear to cause increased risk of bleeding when taken on its own.[5]

Preliminary evidence suggests that EPA, but not other long-chain n-3 or n-6 polyunsaturated fatty acids, might suppress NK cell activity.[74]

One case report suggests that use of omega-3 fatty acids caused an incident of hypomania in a woman with a history of major depressive disorder.[75]

Cod liver oil is rich in the fat-soluble vitamins A and D. Patients using cod liver oil as a fish oil supplement should be cautioned not to exceed the safe maximum intake of these fat-soluble vitamins.

Maximum safe dosages in individuals with severe hepatic or renal disease are not known.

Safety in Young Children and Pregnant or Lactating Women

Maximum safe dosages for young children or pregnant or lactating women have not been established.

Pregnant women interested in fish oil supplements should not use cod liver oil, as excessive intake of vitamin A (>2667 IU vitamin A daily) is known to increase the risk of birth defects.

Drug Interactions

Although fish oil does not appear to potentiate bleeding complications caused by aspirin,[28] interactions with **anticoagulants** such as warfarin have not been ruled out.

FLAXSEED

(Linum usitatissimum)

Alternate Names/Related Species: Linseed

Common Uses

Constipation [+2]   **Chemoprevention** [+1]

Hyperlipidemia [+2]

(Higher numbers indicate stronger evidence; X modifier indicates contradictory results. See page xviii of the Introduction for details of the rating scale.)

Approach to the Patient

Although some patients may naturally confuse the two, flaxseeds are functionally an entirely different supplement from flaxseed oil. Flaxseeds supply soluble fiber, alpha-linolenic acid, and phytoestrogenic lignans. Flaxseed oil contains no appreciable amounts of lignans but it does contain alpha-linolenic acid; see the article on **Flaxseed Oil** for further discussion.

Flaxseed appears to be helpful for constipation and hyperlipidemia; it is also being investigated for possible chemopreventive actions based on its lignan content. Other proposed uses include menopausal symptoms and renal diseases.

Constipation   +2

Germany's Commission E authorizes the use of flaxseed for various digestive problems, such as chronic constipation, irritable bowel syndrome, diverticulitis, and general stomach discomfort.[1] In a double-blind comparative trial, 55 individuals with chronic constipation related to irritable bowel syndrome received either ground flaxseed or psyllium seed daily for 3 months.[2] The flaxseed group experienced fewer problems with constipation, abdominal pain, and bloating than the group taking psyllium.

Hyperlipidemia   +2

Small human trials suggest that flaxseed can improve lipid profiles.[3-5,21]

Chemoprevention   +1

Observational studies suggest that lignan-containing foods are associated with a lower incidence of breast and perhaps colon cancer.[6] In vitro and animal studies using flaxseed and its lignans offer supporting evidence for a potential chemopreventive effect in breast, colon, prostate, and skin cancer.[7-13]

Other Proposed Uses

Very preliminary research indicates potential benefits in treating menopausal symptoms, lupus nephritis, and polycystic kidneys.[11,14,15]

Mechanism of Action

The benefits of flaxseed in constipation and hyperlipidemia presumably are primarily due to its soluble fiber content, although its lignan and alpha-linolenic acid content may play a role as well. Lignans have estrogen antagonist/agonist action, as well as antioxidant properties.[11,12,16,17,22]

Dosage

In studies investigating flaxseed lignans, flaxseed has been taken at doses from 5 to 38 g daily.

The usual dose of flaxseed for constipation is 5 g of whole, cracked, or freshly crushed seeds (presoaked in water to soften them) taken with a glassful of liquid three times a day.[18] Children aged 6 to 12 are given half the adult dose.[18] In one study of constipation caused by irritable bowel syndrome, participants received 6 to 24 g per day of flaxseed for 6 months.[2]

Safety Issues

Use of flaxseed has not been associated with any significant adverse effects.

In vitro studies have found both chemopreventive and cancer-promoting actions of lignans.[22] For this reason, use of large amounts of flaxseed or lignans in individuals with a history of estrogen-sensitive cancer, or at high risk for it, should be considered with caution.

In diabetics, flaxseed (like other high-fiber foods) may delay glucose absorption[18] (see also Drug Interactions).

Raw flaxseeds contain small quantities of cyanide.[19] Although normal cooking and baking of whole flaxseeds or flour eliminates any detectable amounts of cyanide,[19] it is at least theoretically possible that eating huge amounts of raw or unprocessed flaxseed or flaxseed meal could pose a problem; this, however, is not considered likely.[18]

Maximum safe dosages in individuals with severe hepatic or renal disease are not known.

Safety in Young Children
and Pregnant or Lactating Women

Because the potential hormonal activity of its lignan constituents, flaxseed might not be safe for pregnant or lactating women. In one animal trial, pregnant rats who ate large amounts (5% or 10% of their diet) of flaxseed gave birth to offspring with altered reproductive organs and functions. Lignans were also found to be transferred to nursing rats.[20]

Additionally, a study in postmenopausal women found that use of flaxseed reduced estradiol and estrone levels and increased serum prolactin levels.[22]

Maximum safe dosages for young children have not been established.

Drug Interactions

As with other high-fiber foods, flaxseed supplementation could potentially require a reduction in **hypoglycemic** drug dosage.

FLAXSEED OIL
(Linum usitatissimum)

Alternate Names/Related Species: Linseed Oil

Common Uses

There are no well-documented medicinal uses of flaxseed oil at this time.

Approach to the Patient

Flaxseed oil contains both omega-3 and omega-6 essential fatty acids. Your patient may have heard that it provides all the benefits of fish oil without the bad odor. However, the principal omega-3 fatty acid in flaxseed oil (alpha-linolenic acid, or ALA) is metabolically upstream from the eicosapentaenoic acid (EPA) and docosahexaenoic acid (DHA) contained in fish oil. ALA supplementation may not increase EPA and DHA levels, and may produce significantly different physiological effects.

Whole flaxseeds contain putative chemopreventive substances known as lignans, but flaxseed oil has no lignans.[2]

Other Proposed Uses

There is some preliminary evidence that flaxseed oil may improve **lipid profile** and perhaps reduce **blood pressure.**[3]

Although flaxseed oil has been described as **chemopreventive** nutrient in some books on alternative medicine, the evidence that it works in this capacity is negligible.[4-6]

A very preliminary study suggests that flaxseed oil may be helpful for controlling **bipolar disorder** when combined with conventional medications.[7]

Flaxseed oil does not appear to be effective for reducing symptoms of **rheumatoid arthritis.**[1]

Mechanism of Action

Alpha-linolenic acid (ALA) is a precursor of EPA (eicosapentaenoic acid) and major prostaglandin and leukotriene synthesis pathways; when taken orally, it may alter the balance of those pathways, perhaps stimulating the production of less inflammatory eicosanoids.

Dosage

A typical dosage is 1 to 2 tablespoons of flaxseed oil daily. It is also available in capsule form.

The essential fatty acids in flax can be damaged by exposure to heat, light, and oxygen, and flaxseed oil should not be used for cooking (though it can be used in salad dressing). In addition, good flaxseed products are typically sold in an opaque container, processed at a temperature under 100° F and may be combined with vitamin E to prevent rancidity.

Safety Issues

Flaxseed oil appears to be a safe nutritional supplement when used as recommended.

Maximum safe dosages in individuals with severe hepatic or renal disease are not known.

Safety in Young Children and Pregnant or Lactating Women

Maximum safe dosages for young children or pregnant or lactating women have not been established. However, nutritional use is probably safe.

Drug Interactions

None are known.

FOLATE

Common Uses

Neural tube defect prevention [+4]

SSRI augmentation [+2]

Cardiovascular disease prevention [+2]

Prevention of congenital anomalies caused by folate antagonists [+1]

(Higher numbers indicate stronger evidence; X modifier indicates contradictory results. See page xviii of the Introduction for details of the rating scale.)

Approach to the Patient

Adequate folate intake can prevent neural tube defects and possibly other congenital defects as well. In addition, it may reduce the risk of cardiovascular disease and lessen the risk of developing certain forms of cancer. Folate supplementation may also augment the antidepressant effect of SSRIs.

Until recently, a good case could be made for recommending folate supplementation for most patients, due to the high prevalence of folate deficiency. However, in 1998, widespread fortification of cereal products began in the United States and Canada. As a result, the prevalence of folate deficiency decreased significantly in these countries.[1]

Neural Tube Defect Prevention   +4

Very strong evidence indicates that regular use of folate by pregnant women can reduce the risk of neural tube defects by 50% to 80%.[4,5]

Prevention of Congenital Anomalies Caused by Folate Antagonists   +1

See discussion in the Drug Interactions section.

SSRI Augmentation   +2

A 10-week, double-blind, placebo-controlled trial of 127 individuals with severe major depression (average HAM-D score above 26) found that folate supplements at a dose of 500 μg daily significantly improved the effectiveness of fluoxetine in female participants.[6] An intention-to-treat analysis showed a higher rate of responders as well as lower HAM-D scores in those who received fluoxetine plus folate as compared to fluoxetine alone. Improvements in male participants were not statistically significant. However, measurements of serum homocysteine in males showed no change with folate supplementation, suggesting that the dose of folate was inadequate.

Cardiovascular Disease Prevention   +2

Observational studies suggest that a high intake of folate may decrease the risk of cardiovascular disease by 50%, possibly by reducing homocysteine levels.[7-15] A dose of 800 μg daily may be necessary to achieve maximum homocysteine-lowering effects.[15]

Other Proposed Uses

Studies suggest that folate deficiency might predispose individuals to **cancer** of the cervix,[16] colon,[17] lung,[18] breast,[19] pancreas,[20] and oral cavity.[18] Large observational studies suggest that folate supplements may help prevent colon cancer, especially when taken for many years.[21-23] High-dose folate (10 mg daily) might be helpful for normalizing microscopic abnormalities in the appearance of the cervix in women taking oral contraceptives, but it does not appear to reverse pathologically confirmed cervical dysplasia.[24,25]

Use of folic acid supplements may help prevent **nitrate tolerance.**[26]

Folate deficiency may also increase the risk of **Alzheimer's disease,** although this has not yet been proven.[27]

Very high dosages of folate may be helpful for **gout,**[28] although it has been suggested that the benefit seen in some studies may actually be due to a folate contaminant.[29] Furthermore, other studies have found no benefit at all.[29,30]

Folate in various dosages has been suggested as a treatment for **bipolar disorder, depression, osteoarthritis** (in combination with vitamin B_{12}), **osteoporosis, restless legs syndrome, rheumatoid arthritis, seborrheic dermatitis,** and **vitiligo.**[31-47] Other conditions for which folate has been suggested include migraine headaches and periodontal disease. However, there is no definitive evidence for any of these uses.

Mechanism of Action

Folate, a B vitamin, plays a critical role in many biological processes including methylation reactions and mitosis. In addition, it appears to offer cardioprotective effects by altering homocysteine metabolism.

Dosage

In general, folate supplementation should follow daily value recommendations for age and sex. Higher dosages—up to 10 mg daily—have been used to treat specific diseases.

Safety Issues

Very high dosages of folate, greater than 5 mg daily, can cause digestive upset. Because folate supplementation can mask early symptoms of macrocytic anemia, vitamin B_{12} deficiency should be ruled out before recommending folate dosages of 800 μg or more daily.

Maximum safe dosages in individuals with severe hepatic or renal disease are not known.

Safety in Young Children and Pregnant or Lactating Women

The tolerable upper intake level of folate for pregnant or lactating women has been established at 1000 μg daily (800 μg if under 19 years old).[48]

Drug Interactions

According to a few reports, folate may increase seizures in individuals with epilepsy and may interfere with **phenytoin** therapy.[49,50]

Evidence suggests that individuals who are taking **methotrexate** for rheumatoid arthritis, juvenile rheumatoid arthritis, or psoriasis can safely take folate supplements at the same time, and some side effects (particularly elevated liver enzyme levels) may be reduced.[51-57]

Various drugs may impair the body's ability to absorb or utilize folate, including **antacids, bile acid sequestrants** (such as cholestyramine and colestipol), **H_2 blockers,** various anticonvulsants (carbamazepine, phenobarbital, phenytoin, primidone, or valproate), sulfasalazine and possibly other **NSAID-type drugs,** high-dose **triamterene, nitrous oxide,** and **trimethoprim-sulfamethoxazole.**[48,58-82] Some of these folate antagonists may increase risk of neural tube defects as well as congenital anomalies of the heart, palate, and urinary tract. An observational study suggests that folate supplements may counter this increased risk.[83]

Oral contraceptives may also affect folate slightly, although supplementation does not appear to be warranted.[2,84-85]

Pancreatin may interfere with the absorption of folate.[3]

A small double-blind trial suggests that high-dose folate may help prevent the development of tolerance during **nitrate** therapy.[26]

GAMMA-LINOLENIC ACID (GLA)

(Oenothera biennis)

Alternate Names/Supplement Forms:
GLA, Omega-6 Oil(s), Omega-6 Fatty Acids
Evening Primrose Oil, Borage Oil, Black Currant Oil

Common Uses

Diabetic neuropathy   [+3]

Rheumatoid arthritis   [+2]

Cyclic mastalgia   [+2]

Eczema   [−2X]

Obesity   [−2]

(Higher numbers indicate stronger evidence; X modifier indicates contradictory results. See page xviii of the Introduction for details of the rating scale.)

Approach to the Patient

Gamma-linolenic acid (GLA) is an important member of the essential omega-6 family of fatty acids. Sources of GLA include evening primrose oil (EPO), black currant oil, and borage oil.

Widely used in Europe for diabetic neuropathy, EPO may reduce symptoms after 3 to 6 months of use. Weaker evidence suggests that GLA may be helpful for rheumatoid arthritis and cyclic mastalgia. Although it is widely used for eczema as well, there are more studies with negative than positive results for this use.

Patients interested in using EPO can be advised that this is a very slow-acting treatment (if it works at all), and that considerable patience is necessary.

Diabetic Neuropathy   + 3

One randomized, double-blind, placebo-controlled study of 111 patients with mild diabetic neuropathy given 6 g of EPO daily for 1 year demonstrated improvement in neuropathy symptoms without change in serum glucose levels.[1] A small double-blind, placebo-controlled trial demonstrated improvement in symptoms, motor conduction velocity, muscle action potential amplitudes, nerve action potential amplitudes, and ankle heat and cold thresholds after 6 months of therapy.[2]

Rheumatoid Arthritis (RA)   + 2

GLA may be useful adjunctive therapy for RA.

In a double-blind study of 56 patients with RA, 16 of 21 patients treated with GLA for 1 year significantly improved compared to those in the placebo group.[3] This study utilized very high doses of purified GLA (2.8 g/day, equivalent to about 30 g of EPO daily). Benefits were also seen in other small trials.[4-8]

Cyclic Mastalgia   + 2

EPO has been used for a variety of breast disorders, but supporting evidence has been reported only regarding symptomatic relief in mastalgia when significant cysts or fibroadenomas are not present. In a randomized, double-blind, placebo-controlled crossover study, 73 patients with cyclical or noncyclical mastalgia (with or without palpable nodularity) experienced significantly less discomfort during the 3-month treatment period with 3 g/day of EPO.[9] However, according to a 1-year, double-blind study of 200 women with cysts large enough to be aspirated, EPO was not more effective than placebo.[10,11] Lack of benefit was also seen in a small 6-month, placebo-controlled study of 23 women with fibroadenomas.[12]

Although several small studies suggest that EPO is helpful in reducing PMS symptoms, all suffer from serious flaws.[13]

Eczema   — 2 X

Despite its widespread use in Europe, evidence on the use of EPO for eczema is more negative than positive. Studies with negative results include three double-blind, placebo-controlled trials: a 24-week study of 160 adults given GLA from borage oil,[14] a 16-week trial of EPO in 58 children,[15] and a 16-week study of EPO or EPO and fish oil in 102 patients.[16]

A 1989 review of the literature found significant benefit in nine double-blind, controlled studies performed to that date, with the greatest benefit in pruritus.[17] However, that review has been criticized for including poorly designed and unpublished studies and for possibly misinterpreting study results.[16]

One more recent double-blind trial of 51 children did find overall therapeutic benefit with EPO.[18]

Obesity   — 2

A 12-week, double-blind study that enrolled 100 significantly overweight women compared the effectiveness of EPO to placebo.[19] No difference was seen between the groups.

Another double-blind trial ($n=47$) tested the unusual hypothesis that EPO might only work in individuals with a family history of obesity.[20] Use of EPO produced a small but significant weight loss, especially in participants with both parents obese.

Other Proposed Uses

While one 3-month, double-blind, placebo-controlled study of 63 individuals with chronic fatigue syndrome found that a combination of essential fatty acids containing evening primrose oil and fish oil resulted in significant improvements,[21] a more precisely structured replication of this study in 1999 found no benefit.[22]

A small double-blind trial suggests that GLA may be beneficial for Raynaud's phenomenon.[23]

Evening primrose oil was found ineffective for attention deficit disorder symptoms in a small double-blind, placebo-controlled trial.[33] Also, in a small placebo-controlled comparative trial, evening primrose oil proved less effective than D-amphetamine.[34]

Mechanism of Action

The delta-6 desaturase conversion of dietary linoleic acid into GLA is a rate-limiting step that may be impaired in numerous conditions, including advanced age, diabetes, high alcohol intake, eczema, cyclic mastitis, viral infections, excessive saturated fat intake, elevated cholesterol levels, excessive dietary intake of *trans* and positional isomers of linoleic acid, and deficiencies of pyridoxine, zinc, magnesium, biotin, or calcium.[8,24-28] In these conditions, GLA may be useful as a "downstream" supplement, one that skips the rate-limiting delta-6 desaturase step.

Infants also appear to lack adequate delta-6 desaturase activity. Breast milk is high in GLA and related omega-6 fatty acids, whereas infant formula is not. This can lead to deficiency states in formula-fed infants and has been proposed as an explanation why breast-fed children have a lower incidence of eczema.[8]

Dosage

Since evening primrose oil is the most common form of GLA, dosages will be given in those terms.

For cyclic mastitis, the standard dose of EPO is 3 g daily in two or three divided doses. Rheumatoid arthritis has been treated with 5 to 10 g daily, although one study used concentrated GLA equivalent to 30 g of EPO. Diabetic neuropathy is typically treated with 4 to 6 g daily. There may be value in combining lipoic acid with EPO when treating this condition.[29,30] Children with eczema have been given 2 to 4 g daily. For all these conditions, the proposed minimum duration of treatment is several months.

Evening primrose oil should be given with food to minimize gastrointestinal distress.

Vitamin E is often recommended to be taken concurrently to prevent excessive lipid peroxidation and the creation of counterproductive substances.[31] Dietary reduction of less preferred fatty acids (e.g., saturated fats) has also been suggested.

See Appendix for U.S. brand names of clinically tested brands.

Safety Issues

Over 4000 patients have participated in trials of GLA, primarily in the form of EPO. No adverse effects or significant differences in rate of side effects between the treated group and the placebo group have been attributed to this treatment.[8] In animal studies, EPO has been found to be nontoxic, and noncarcinogenic.

Early reports suggested the possibility of exacerbation of temporal lobe epilepsy and mania by EPO ingestion, but further evidence has not been reported.[32]

Maximum safe dosages in individuals with severe hepatic or renal disease are not known.

Safety in Young Children and Pregnant or Lactating Women

Evidence from animal studies suggests that EPO is nonteratogenic. However, GLA may increase prostaglandin E levels in humans, a known teratogen and labor inducer.[35] For this reason, maximum safe dosages for pregnant or lactating women must be regarded as unknown. Maximum safe doses in children are also unknown.

Drug Interactions

None are known.

GARLIC

Alternate Names/Related Species:
(*Allium* spp., including *Allium sativum*)

Common Uses

Atherosclerosis [+3]

Hyperlipidemia [+3X]

**Upper respiratory infection
(prophylaxis)** [+3]

Hypertension [+2]

**Antithrombotic
effects** [+2]

Chemoprevention [+1]

Insect repellant [+2]

Antimicrobial [+1]

(Higher numbers indicate stronger evidence; X modifier indicates contradictory results. See page xviii of the Introduction for details of the rating scale.)

Approach to the Patient

Although garlic is widely regarded as an effective treatment for high cholesterol, the most recent and best designed studies suggest that the benefit, if any, is marginal. Garlic may, however, positively impact other atherosclerosis risk factors such as blood pressure, platelet aggregation, and perhaps other mechanisms.[59]

Garlic is also popularly regarded as an immune strengthener particularly effective against colds. Until recently there was no evidence for this belief, and there is still no evidence that garlic can cure a cold. However, a reasonably large and well-designed trial suggests that patients who catch colds frequently during winter months may benefit from prophylactic use of standardized garlic extract.

Contrary to what your patients may believe, garlic is not thought to exert systemic antimicrobial effects.

Patients can be advised that garlic appears to have clinically relevant antithrombotic effects. This suggests that it may potentiate pharmaceutical agents with similar actions. Furthermore, a newly popular natural product that is thought to have hypolipidemic effects, policosanol, has antiplatelet actions as well. Some patients may wish to combine treatment with the two agents in hopes of producing a stronger hypolipidemic effect. However, this might present risk of bleeding complications. Vitamin E, also popular among individuals at risk of heart disease, may further increase this risk. (See Safety Issues and Drug Interactions.)

Atherosclerosis   +3

In a 4-year, double-blind, placebo-controlled study that enrolled 280 individuals, standardized garlic powder at a dose of 900 mg/day significantly slowed the development of atherosclerosis as quantified by ultrasound measurement of intimal-medial thickness.[1] A high dropout rate (complete data were available on only 152 participants) and other statistically important complications make the results somewhat difficult to interpret precisely, but it appears that the rate of reduction in plaque growth fell in the range of 5% to 18%.

Evidence from an observational, cross-section case-control study also suggests that garlic has an overall atherosclerosis-retarding effect.[2]

One controlled (but not blinded) study of 432 patients who had suffered myocardial infarction showed significant reductions in reinfarction rate (35%) and mortality (45%) through the use of garlic oil extract over a period of 3 years.[3]

Hyperlipidemia   +3X

Despite extensive German literature finding garlic effective for hypercholesterolemia,[4-7] most recent trials have found no effect.[8-13] The explanation may lie in garlic's apparently modest benefit. A meta-analysis that accepted 13 trials found evidence of cholesterol reduction in the range of 5% compared to placebo.[14] Reported negative trials lacked study power to identify a benefit this small.

Upper Respiratory Infection (Prophylaxis)   + 3

The herb garlic has a long history of use for treating or preventing colds. However, meaningful scientific evidence to support this use first appeared in 2001.[60] In this 12-week, double-blind, placebo-controlled trial, 146 individuals received either placebo or a garlic extract between November and February. Participants receiving garlic were almost two-thirds less likely to develop a URI than those who received placebo. Furthermore, participants who did develop a URI recovered about one day faster in the garlic group as compared to the placebo group.

Hypertension   + 2

According to two small, double-blind, placebo-controlled trials of hypertensives, garlic may reduce blood pressure mildly, in the average range of 10 mm Hg for systolic blood pressure and 5 mm Hg for diastolic blood pressure, compared to placebo.[15,16] Blood pressure reduction has also been seen in normotensive individuals.[15]

Antithrombotic Effects   + 2

In a 4-week, double-blind, controlled trial, 64 individuals with consistently increased spontaneous platelet aggregation were treated with either placebo or 900 mg of standardized garlic powder daily.[17] A significant decrease in spontaneous platelet aggregation was seen in the treated group. Similar effects were seen in a smaller trial using aged garlic at a dose of 7.2 g daily.[18]

Garlic has also been found in human trials to increase fibrinolytic activity, either when taken in a single dose or over an extended period of time.[19]

Chemoprevention   +1

Several retrospective and prospective epidemiological studies have shown that individuals whose diet includes relatively large amounts of garlic tend to develop cancer less frequently.[20-25] Although the interpretation of epidemiological results is complex and always open to dispute, the cumulative evidence is significant.[20,22,26]

In one of the best epidemiological studies, the Iowa Women's Study, participants whose diet included significant quantities of garlic were about 30% less likely to develop colon cancer.[24]

Insect Repellant   +2

Oral garlic is a popular folk remedy for insect bite prevention. A double-blind, placebo-controlled crossover trial followed 80 Swedish soldiers and measured the number of tick bites received over each phase of the trial.[27] The results showed a modest but statistically significant reduction in tick bites attributable to daily consumption of 1200 mg of garlic daily (type not stated).

Antimicrobial   +1

Raw garlic extracts can kill a wide variety of microorganisms in vitro, including fungi, bacteria, viruses, and protozoa.[20,28-30] Thus it appears quite likely that topical application of garlic produces a local antibiotic effect. Topical effects could theoretically make it useful for intestinal infections,[31,32] as well as *Helicobacter pylori*.[33] However, in vivo studies of garlic for *H. pylori* have not been promising.[34,35]

There is no real evidence that garlic functions as a systemic antibiotic.

Other Proposed Uses

Garlic has been proposed as a natural therapy for the following: blood glucose regulation in diabetes and "hypoglycemia";

asthma and allergies; fungal infections including tinea pedis and vaginitis; cardiovascular support in conditions including congestive heart failure, intermittent claudication, and Raynaud's disease; parasites; arthritis; traveler's diarrhea; energy enhancement; and "liver detoxification." There is no evidence, however, to justify any of these claims.

Similarly, the widespread belief that garlic raises immunity and prevents colds is also independent of good evidence.

Mechanism of Action

The mechanism of garlic's therapeutic effects remains unknown.

Garlic's apparent antihypertensive, fibrinolytic, and antiplatelet effects may be mediated through activation of nitric oxide synthetase.[36]

The active ingredient of garlic is generally thought to be allicin. Allicin is an unstable breakdown product of the sulfur-containing substance alliin; the conversion enzyme allinase is released when garlic is cut or powdered.

In vitro and ex vivo experiments on animal hepatocytes have found that allicin and (to a lesser extent) ajoene, s-allylcystein, and related chemicals reduce cholesterol biosynthesis by inhibiting HMG-CoA reductase as well as 14-alpha-demethylase.[37-42]

Garlic concentrates selenium in a readily absorbable form, which may partially explain its antioxidant and apparent chemopreventive properties.[43] In addition, the sulfuric components of garlic may also directly bind and inactivate reactive genotoxic metabolites.[44]

Dosage

In most of the studies evaluating the effects of garlic, researchers used a dried, powdered form that contains 1.3% alliin, taken at a dose of 900 mg daily. This supplies a daily dose of about 10 mg of alliin, or a total "allicin potential" of 4 to 5 mg.

Significant technical difficulties arise in producing garlic of this type. The process of powdering and drying garlic releases allinase, which converts alliin to allicin, which in turn spontaneously degrades. Therefore ordinary garlic powder contains negligible levels of alliin and allicin by the time it reaches the consumer. In light of this, dietary supplement manufacturers have devised a number of proprietary methods to produce garlic products with stabilized allinase or allicin content.

However, not all manufacturers agree that allicin or alliin are at all relevant to garlic's activity. The widely available deodorized form of garlic called Kyolic lacks allicin and many other constituents of garlic. Nonetheless, such products have provided positive results in studies and appear to have fewer gastric side effects.[6,18]

Garlic is also sometimes sold as an oil extract. Such products contain no allicin or alliin but high levels of ajoene, dithiins, and other breakdown products.[45]

See the Appendix for U.S. brand names of clinically tested products.

Safety Issues

Garlic is on the FDA's GRAS (generally recognized as safe) list. However, garlic is usually cooked when taken as food. Typical standardized garlic products contain substances (such as alliin) not found in food garlic, making them more similar to raw garlic. Raw garlic taken in excessive doses can reportedly cause numerous symptoms, such as stomach upset, heartburn, nausea, vomiting, diarrhea, flatulence, facial flushing, rapid pulse, and insomnia. Topical garlic can cause skin irritation, blistering, and even third-degree burns.[46]

Rats fed up to 2000 mg/kg of aged garlic extract for 6 months showed no significant toxicity.[47] Genotoxicity and mutagenicity studies have been negative for aged garlic and fresh garlic.[48,49] In a chronic toxicity study in rats, long-term treatment (12 months) with standardized garlic powder at a dose equivalent to three times the usual dose produced no toxic effects in rats.[61] (Fish oil was administered simultaneously.)

In studies, garlic powder has not been associated with serious side effects. For example, an observational study followed 1997 patients given 300 mg of garlic powder three times daily over a 16-week period and found a 6% incidence of nausea, a 1.3% incidence of orthostasis, and a 1.1% incidence of allergic reactions attributable to garlic.[50] There were also a few reports of bloating, headache, sweating, and dizziness.

The most common problem with garlic is the odor. The use of so-called odorless products can alleviate, though not entirely eliminate, this problem: one study suggests that therapeutic levels of odorless garlic produce an offensive garlic smell in 50% of patients, perhaps because of allicin formed in the digestive tract.[51] This reduces patient compliance.

For theoretical reasons, garlic is not recommended for patients with brittle diabetes (garlic might possess a hypoglycemic effect), pemphigus (activated by sulfur-containing compounds), organ transplants (possible activation of immune rejection), or acute rheumatoid arthritis (possible increase in autoimmunity).

At least one case report associated garlic supplement use with a spontaneous spinal epidural hematoma.[52] Based on reports of increased bleeding following surgery, the European Scientific Cooperative on Phytotherapy recommends against using garlic before, during, or immediately after surgical procedures.[53-55] Maximum safe dosages in individuals with severe hepatic or renal disease are not known.

Safety in Young Children and Pregnant or Lactating Women

Cooked garlic in dietary doses is presumed to be safe in pregnancy and lactation based on its extensive food use. However, maximum safe dosage of standardized garlic extracts in these groups, as well as in young children and individuals with severe liver or renal disease, has not been established. There have not been any studies on teratogenicity or embryo toxicity of any form of garlic.[54]

Given the report of increased bleeding following a surgical procedure mentioned above, it might also be wise to avoid garlic supplementation during the period before and after labor and delivery.

Drug Interactions

Because garlic appears to possess antithrombotic activity, it should be used with caution in patients on **anticoagulants.** One report has indicated an increase in bleeding time in two patients taking both warfarin and garlic supplements.[56] It is also conceivable that garlic could interact with other natural substances with anticoagulant effects, such as **ginkgo, policosanol** (also used for hyperlipidemia), and high-dose **vitamin E.**

Garlic's antihypertensive effects are probably too weak to cause a problem in patients on **antihypertensive medication.**

Garlic has been found to reduce plasma concentrations of saquinavir.[57] In addition, two individuals with HIV experienced severe gastrointestinal toxicity from ritonavir after taking garlic supplements.[58]

GENISTEIN

Common Uses

Osteoporosis [+1]   **Hyperlipidemia** [+1]

Chemoprevention [+1]

(Higher numbers indicate stronger evidence; X modifier indicates contradictory results. See page xviii of the Introduction for details of the rating scale.)

Approach to the Patient

Genistein is one of the primary isoflavones in soy and possesses both phytoestrogenic and antioxidant effects. This article primarily discusses evidence specific to genistein. For general information, see the articles on **Isoflavones** and **Soy Protein.**

Preliminary evidence suggests that genistein may be useful for osteoporosis, hypercholesterolemia, and chemoprevention. However, it may be worth advising your patients that there is more evidence supporting the use of whole soy protein than any isolated isoflavone (or group of isoflavones).

Like other phytoestrogens, genistein may not be safe for pregnant or lactating women or for women with a history of breast cancer. Genistein might also inhibit thyroxin synthesis.

Osteoporosis   +1

Animal studies have found that oral or injected genistein can protect bone from osteoporosis following oophorectomy.[1-3] Unlike estrogen, which inhibits bone resorption, genistein may enhance new bone formation.[1]

Chemoprevention   + 1

Animal and in vitro studies suggest that genistein inhibits the growth of malignant cells, including hormone-insensitive cancers.[4-7]

Hyperlipidemia   + 1

Soy protein is well known to reduce cholesterol levels, and isoflavones such as genistein are thought to be important contributors to this effect.[7,8] Genistein may have other positive effects on atherosclerosis as well, such as inhibiting platelet aggregation.[7]

Other Proposed Uses

Soy protein and soy isoflavones appear to be helpful for menopausal symptoms; presumably, genistein contributes to these effects.

Genistein has also been investigated in murine models of ALS and stroke.[9]

Mechanism of Action

Genistein's actions are presumably due to its phytoestrogenic and antioxidant effects, although other mechanisms may play a role as well.[1,4,7,10]

One animal study suggests that genistein has a biphasic effect on bone density.[2]

Dosage

Most soy foods contain about 1 to 2 mg of genistein per gram of protein.[7] The optimum dosage of genistein is unknown. Asian diets typically provide 20 to 80 mg of genistein daily, along with other soy constituents.

Safety Issues

Studies in animals have found soy isoflavones, including genistein, to be essentially nontoxic.[11] However, because of its complex estrogen agonist/antagonist effects, there are at least theoretical concerns that genistein may not be safe for women with a history of breast cancer.

In a 12-month pilot study, 24 healthy pre- and postmenopausal with women, ages 30 to 58, ingested 38 g of soy protein isolate (containing 38 mg of genistein) daily during months 4 through 9. Study parameters included nipple aspiration of breast fluid, as well as blood and 24-hour urine samples for biochemistry. Results showed that prolonged consumption of soy protein isolate had a stimulatory effect on premenopausal breast tissue, characterized by increased secretion of breast fluid, the appearance of hyperplastic epithelial cells, and elevated levels of plasma estradiol. The authors concluded that these findings suggested an estrogenic stimulus from the isoflavones genistein and daidzein contained in the soy protein isolate.[12] Similar proliferative changes were noted in breast tissue biopsies of premenopausal women taking a 60-g soy supplement (containing 45 g of soy isoflavones) daily for 2 weeks.[13]

Genistein may inhibit thyroxin synthesis.[14]

Maximum safe dosages in individuals with severe hepatic or renal disease are not known.

Safety in Young Children and Pregnant or Lactating Women

Genistein may not be safe in pregnancy and lactation. One animal study found that maternal genistein exposure increases risk of mammary tumorigenesis in offspring.[15] Maximum safe dosages for young children have not been established.

Drug Interactions

None are known.

Although fears have been expressed that soy isoflavones might interfere with the action of **oral contraceptives,** one study of 40 women suggests that such concerns are groundless.[16] Another trial found that soy does not interfere with the action of **estrogen replacement therapy** in menopausal women.[17]

GINGER
(Zingiber officinale)

Common Uses

Motion sickness [+2X]

Nausea and vomiting of pregnancy [+2]

Postsurgical nausea [+3X]

Chemotherapy-induced nausea [+1]

Osteoarthritis [−1]

(Higher numbers indicate stronger evidence; X modifier indicates contradictory results. See page xviii of the Introduction for details of the rating scale.)

Approach to the Patient

Preliminary evidence suggests that ginger may be somewhat helpful for various forms of nausea, including nausea of pregnancy.

As a widely used food, the safety factor with ginger is presumed to be high. However, safety in pregnancy is not assured.

Motion Sickness +2X

Ginger may modestly improve symptoms of motion sickness when the nausea stimulus is not too strong.

A double-blind, placebo-controlled study of 79 Swedish naval cadets found that 1 g of ginger could decrease vomiting and cold sweating but without significantly decreasing nausea and vertigo.[1] Another double-blind study found equivalent benefit of ginger at a dose of 500 mg every 4 hours and dimenhydrinate 100 mg every 4 hours in a group of 60 passengers on a cruise through rough seas.[2] Similar results were also seen in two small double-blind studies using dimehydrinate.[3,4] Finally, a double-blind comparative study that followed 1489 individuals aboard ship found ginger equally effective as cinnarizine, cinnarizine with domperidone, cyclizine, dimehydrinate with caffeine, meclozine with caffeine, and scopolamine.[5]

However, a double-blind trial of 28 volunteers funded by NASA found no benefit with ginger (0.5 to 1 g) compared to scopolamine or placebo.[6] The primary measure of success was the number of swivels in a rotating chair that could be achieved without vomiting. Gastric function was also measured. The results showed no significant improvement with ginger compared to placebo other than a slight decrease in gastric hyperactivity. Negative results were seen in two other small comparative studies that used strong nausea stimuli.[7,8]

Nausea and Vomiting of Pregnancy   +2

A double-blind, placebo-controlled trial of 70 pregnant women evaluated the effectiveness of ginger for morning sickness.[9] Participants received either placebo or 250 mg of freshly prepared powdered ginger three times daily for a period of 4 days. The results indicated that ginger significantly reduced nausea and number of vomiting episodes.

Benefits were also seen in a double-blind crossover trial of 27 women.[10]

Postsurgical Nausea   +3X

The evidence regarding ginger's effectiveness in postsurgical nausea is almost perfectly mixed. It is possible that discrepancies may be due to the form of ginger used.

A double-blind British study ($n=60$) compared the effects of 1 g of ginger, placebo, and metoclopramide in the treatment of nausea following gynecological surgery.[11] The results showed that both treatments produced a similar and statistically significant benefit compared to placebo.

Another British study of similar design followed 120 women receiving elective laparoscopic gynecological surgery.[12] Whereas nausea and vomiting developed in 41% of patients given placebo, the ginger- and metoclopramide-treated patients developed these symptoms at rates of 21% and 27%, respectively.

However, a double-blind study of 108 patients undergoing similar surgery showed increased nausea and vomiting with 0.5 or 1 g of ginger compared to placebo.[13] No benefit at all was seen in another study.[14]

Chemotherapy-Induced Nausea   +1

A small open trial suggests that ginger may reduce nausea caused by 8-MOP.[15]

Osteoarthritis   −1

A double-blind, placebo-controlled crossover trial (3 weeks with each treatment) compared ginger extract (170 mg three times daily), ibuprofen (400 mg three times daily), and placebo in 56 individuals with osteoarthritis of the hip or knee.[16] Ibuprofen was superior to ginger, and only by using exploratory tests of differences was any evidence found that ginger might be superior to placebo.

A 6-week, double-blind, placebo-controlled trial evaluated a mixture of ginger and the Asian spice galanga (*Alpinia galanga*) in knee arthritis.[33] (This study was widely misreported—even in the study title—as a trial of ginger alone.) A total of 247 individuals were included in the ITT analysis, which found statistically significant evidence of efficacy in the primary outcome measure (pain on standing).

Other Proposed Uses

Ginger has been suggested as a treatment for numerous conditions, including migraine headaches, rheumatoid arthritis, hypercholesterolemia, burns, ulcers, depression, impotence, and liver toxicity. However, there is no real evidence that it is effective for these conditions.

Mechanism of Action

The mechanism of action of ginger in nausea is not known. Studies suggest that ginger does not influence the inner ear or oculomotor system.[17] Thus it appears that ginger acts on the stomach alone, perhaps overriding central nervous stimuli. However, ginger has been shown not to affect gastric emptying time.[18] A study in rabbits suggests that ginger stimulates and then fatigues cholinergic and histaminic receptors, thus producing a local anticholinergic and antihistaminic effect.[19]

Dosage

For most purposes, the typical dose of powdered ginger is 1 to 4 g daily taken in two to four divided doses. Standardized products should be taken according to label instructions. See the Appendix for U.S. brand names of clinically tested products.

For preventing motion sickness, it is usual to begin treatment 1 or 2 days before the trip and continue it throughout the period of travel.

For the nausea and vomiting of pregnancy, the best form of ginger is probably freshly brewed tea, made from boiled ginger root and diluted to taste. If chilled, carbonated, and sweetened, this would become the original form of ginger ale, a famous antinausea beverage. Powdered ginger can be used as well.

Safety Issues

Ginger is on the FDA's GRAS (generally recognized as safe) list.

Germany's Commission E mentions gallstones as a relative contraindication for ginger, without citing reasons.

The acute oral LD_{50} of ginger in rats exceeded 5 g of ginger oil/kg.[8] In mice, an 80% ethanolic extract was well tolerated at 2.5 mg/kg by gastric gavage.[20]

Ginger was found to possess antimutagenic activity in *Salmonella* TA98 using tryptophan pyrolysate as mutagen and S9 liver homogenate as activator.[21] Isolated 6-gingerol appears to be a potent mutagen, but the addition of whole ginger juice counteracts this effect.[22] Opposing effects have also been seen in other models of mutagenicity.[23] Ginger has not been systematically tested in mammalian cell cultures.[24]

Like onions and garlic, extracts of ginger inhibit platelet aggregation and thromboxane synthesis in vitro.[25-29] This has led to a concern that ginger might prolong bleeding time. However, European studies with actual oral ginger in normal quantities have not found any significant anticoagulant effects in vivo.[30-32]

Maximum safe doses in individuals with severe hepatic or renal disease are not known.

Safety in Young Children and Pregnant or Lactating Women

Despite its widespread use by pregnant women, ginger's safety in this population has not been formally established. The evidence of platelet aggregation inhibition, as well as equivocal mutagenic effects have raised concerns. Maximum safe doses for lactating women or young children have not been established.

Drug Interactions

No drug interactions are known. Because of its effects on platelet action, ginger should be used with care in patients using **anticoagulants** or **antiplatelet agents.**

GINKGO
(Ginkgo biloba)

Common Uses

Alzheimer's disease and non-alzheimer's dementia [+4]

Ordinary age-related memory loss [+3]

Improving memory and mental function in the young [+2X]

Intermittent claudication [+3]

Premenstrual syndrome [+3]

Altitude sickness [+2]

Vertiginous syndromes [+2]

Tinnitus [−2]

(Higher numbers indicate stronger evidence; X modifier indicates contradictory results. See page xviii of the Introduction for details of the rating scale.)

Approach to the Patient

A standardized extract of *Ginkgo biloba* leaf has become one of the primary European treatments for Alzheimer's and non-Alzheimer's dementia, on the basis of a respectable body of research evidence. Ginkgo may also be helpful for ordinary age-related memory loss, and intermittent claudication. Considerably weaker evidence suggests that it may be helpful for improving mental function in the young, as well as treating PMS, depression, and vertiginous syndromes and preventing altitude sickness. Ginkgo does not appear to be effective for tinnitus.

Ginkgo extract is safe and generally well tolerated. However, there are concerns related to its anticoagulant properties.

Patients can be advised not to harvest ginkgo themselves. All the proposed uses of ginkgo involve a highly concentrated standardized extract from which potentially toxic alkylphenols have been removed.

Ginkgo possesses anticoagulant properties, and as such might present risk if combined with other anticoagulant substances or used prior to surgery or labor and delivery.

Alzheimer's Disease and Non-Alzheimer's Dementia   +4

A well-regarded double-blind, placebo-controlled study of *Ginkgo biloba* in dementia (primarily Alzheimer's), involving 309 patients in a 52-week, parallel-group multicenter trial, found significant improvement in a performance-based test of memory and language (the cognitive subscale of the Alzheimer's Disease Assessment Scale, or ADAS-Cog) and a caregivers' evaluation (the Geriatric Evaluation by Relative's Rating Instrument, or GERRI).[1]

Other European studies have evaluated the effectiveness of ginkgo in Alzheimer's and non-Alzheimer's dementia and also found benefit.[2,3] In addition, over 40 other double-blind controlled trials had evaluated the benefits of ginkgo in "cerebral insufficiency" (dementia) prior to 1992.[4] Of these, eight were rated of good quality, involving a total of about 1000 patients, and results were positive in all but one of these studies.

A 24-week, double-blind, placebo-controlled study of 214 participants found no benefit with ginkgo extract at a dose of 160 or 240 mg daily.[5] This study enrolled both individuals with mild to moderate dementia and those with ordinary age-associated memory loss. However, it has been sharply criticized for a number of serious flaws in its design.[55]

Ordinary Age-Related Memory Loss   +3

The results of six double-blind studies suggest that ginkgo might be useful for ordinary age-related memory loss (technically, Age-Associated Memory Impairment, or AAMI).

In a double-blind, placebo-controlled trial, 241 seniors complaining of mildly impaired memory were given either placebo or low-dose or high-dose ginkgo for 24 weeks.[6] The results showed modest improvements in certain types of memory, especially in the low-dose ginkgo group. Benefits were also seen in three other double-blind, placebo-controlled trials of continuous ginkgo use[7-9] and in two double-blind trials that utilized one-time dosing.[10,11]

Set against these positive findings is the 24-week study mentioned above, which found no benefit in ordinary age-associated memory loss.[5] However, this study has been sharply criticized for a number of serious flaws in its design.[55]

Improving Memory and Mental Function in the Young   + 2 X

A 30-day, double-blind, placebo-controlled trial that enrolled 61 healthy men and women evaluated the effects of 120 mg of gingko extract daily.[56] The results of the per-protocol evaluation showed significant improvements in some measures of memory function, including Digit Span Backwards and Working Memory Speed; an ITT analysis was not performed.

In another double-blind, placebo-controlled crossover trial, 20 individuals aged 19 to 24 years received a one-time dose of either ginkgo at 120, 240, or 360 mg or placebo.[12] The results showed improvement with the two higher doses in various measures of mental performance, most markedly in one that measured ability to perform attention-related tasks rapidly. Mixed results were seen in two smaller double-blind, placebo-controlled crossover trials.[13,14] A double-blind, placebo-controlled study of 30 healthy males found no significant improvement in memory after 5 days' treatment with ginkgo at a dose of 120 mg daily.[15]

Intermittent Claudication   + 3

A 2000 meta-analysis of studies of ginkgo in intermittent claudication evaluated eight double-blind, placebo-controlled trials.[16] In aggregate, the results found a modest but statistically significant improvement in pain-free walking distance.

For example, a 24-week, double-blind, placebo-controlled study that enrolled 111 patients found a significant improvement in pain-free walking distance with ginkgo compared to placebo.[17] Similar improvements were also seen in a double-blind, placebo-controlled trial of 60 individuals who had achieved maximum benefit from physical therapy modalities.[18]

A 24-week, multicenter, double-blind, placebo-controlled dose-comparison study of 74 individuals with intermittent claudication reported that ginkgo at a dose of 120 mg twice daily was more effective than 60 mg twice daily.[19]

Premenstrual Syndrome   +3

One double-blind, placebo-controlled study evaluated the effect of *Ginkgo biloba* extract (80 mg twice daily) on fluid retention and other PMS symptoms over two menstrual cycles.[20] The study evaluated 143 women, 18 to 45 years of age, and followed them for two menstrual cycles. All women admitted to the study had experienced PMS-related symptoms for at least three consecutive cycles. When the study began, each woman received either 80 mg ginkgo extract twice daily or a placebo on day 16 of the first cycle. Treatment was continued until the fifth day of the next cycle and resumed again on day 16 of that cycle. Participants could double the dose if they felt they were experiencing inadequate relief. The results showed significant improvement in breast tenderness as well as emotional symptoms.

Altitude Sickness   +2

A double-blind, placebo-controlled study of 44 mountaineers on a Himalayan expedition found that 160 mg daily of standardized ginkgo extract prevented symptoms of altitude sickness, and also symptoms related to cold extremities.[30]

Vertiginous Syndromes   +2

A 3-month, double-blind trial of 70 individuals with a variety of vertiginous syndromes found that ginkgo extract given at a dose of 160 mg twice daily produced results superior to placebo.[28] However, a major limitation of this study was the large range of included disorders.

Tinnitus   −2

Three double-blind, placebo-controlled trials enrolling a total of about 220 individuals have evaluated oral *Ginkgo biloba* extract as a treatment for tinnitus, with generally positive results.[21-24] However, a more recent and much larger study found no benefit.

In this double-blind, placebo-controlled trial, 1121 individuals with tinnitus were given 12 weeks' treatment with standardized gingko at a dose of 50 mg three times daily.[25] The results showed no difference between the treated and the placebo groups.

Other Proposed Uses

Many studies of ginkgo in dementia have noted improvement in **affective symptoms.** In addition, two studies have directly evaluated this potential benefit.[26,27] For example, in an 8-week, double-blind, placebo-controlled trial, 40 depressed patients above the age of 50 who showed incomplete response to tricyclic or tetracyclic antidepressants were given adjuvant treatment with either placebo or ginkgo extract at 80 mg three times a day.[26] Patients in the treated group demonstrated significantly improved outcomes compared to the placebo group.

Weak evidence suggests that *Ginkgo biloba* extract might be useful in the treatment of **unilateral idiopathic sudden hearing loss.**[29,57] One small double-blind study suggests that ginkgo might be useful in macular degeneration.[31]

Numerous case reports and open trials suggest that ginkgo might help reduce the **sexual side effects of SSRIs,** including impotence in men and inability to achieve orgasm in women.[32-36] One small open trial failed to find benefit, but it used an unusual nonstandard form of ginkgo that does not closely resemble standard ginkgo extract.[58] However, in the absence of double-blind trials, it is quite possible that the reported benefits are due to the placebo and related effects.

Because sexual dysfunction is a major deterrent to patient compliance with SSRI antidepressants, this potential effect of ginkgo is being investigated more thoroughly.

Weak and sometimes contradictory evidence suggests that ginkgo extract might be helpful for **diabetic microvascular disease, asthma, cochlear deafness, organic impotence,** and **allergies.**[37,38] One open trial combined ginkgo and 5FU for the treatment of **pancreatic cancer,** with promising results.[39]

Chinese research suggests that ginkgo might improve the effectiveness and tolerability of neuroleptics in the treatment of **schizophrenia.**[40,59]

Mechanism of Action

The active ingredients in ginkgo are not known, and its mechanism of action is not completely elucidated. Ginkgo is thought to improve circulation by decreasing blood viscosity, antagonizing platelet-activating factor, and prolonging the half-life of endothelium-derived relaxing factor; it also decreases phospholipid destruction during hypoxia and scavenges free radicals.[37,41-43]

These effects on circulation are probably the basis for many of ginkgo's therapeutic effects. In the past, ginkgo's mechanism of action in dementia was also assumed to involve circulatory improvements, increasing oxygenation of the brain. However, as understanding of the mechanisms involved in dementia has improved, the current view is that ginkgo (and other nontropic drugs) stimulates nerve cell activity or protects nerve cell populations from further injury.[44,45]

One study suggests that ginkgo extract can competitively inhibit monoamine oxidase (MAO) A and B at therapeutic levels,[46] although no MAO-inhibitor–like reactions have been reported in the wide European usage of ginkgo. This in vitro finding is echoed by an earlier demonstration in mice of protection by ginkgo against MPTP, a neurotoxin that requires metabolic activation by MAO to exert its toxic effects.[47]

Regarding SSRI-induced impotence, nonginkgolide extracts of ginkgo have been shown to exert a relaxing effect on corpus cavernosum vasculature, but the concentrations required (about 1 mg/ml) are unlikely to be achieved in reality, suggesting that other mechanisms are at work.[48]

Dosage

The typical dose of ginkgo is 120 to 240 mg daily, in three divided doses, of a 50:1 extract standardized to contain 24% ginkgo-flavone glycosides and 6% terpenoids (2.8 to 3.4% ginkgolides A, B, and C and 2.6 to 3.2% bilobalide).[49] Ginkgolic acid content should be kept under 5 ppm. See the Appendix for U.S. brand names of clinically tested products.

Ginkgo's effects generally require 3 months of treatment to manifest fully. Preliminary dose-comparison data suggest that 240 mg daily may be more effective than 120 mg daily for intermittent claudication,[19] but not for memory loss.[8]

Safety Issues

In pooled clinical trials involving a total of almost 10,000 patients, the incidence of side effects produced by ginkgo extract was extremely small. There were 21 cases of gastrointestinal discomfort and even fewer cases of headache, dizziness, and allergic skin reactions.[37]

Animal studies of the long-term effects of continued ingestion of ginkgo extract report no evidence of organ damage; impairment of reproductive, renal, or hepatic function; or damage to health of offspring.[60]

In vitro evidence that ginkgo might function as an MAO inhibitor[46] has not been correlated by any reports of MAO-like reactions in humans.

There have been two case reports, in highly regarded journals, of subdural hematoma and hyphema association with ginkgo use.[47,50] In the former case, the patient was also taking 325 mg aspirin daily. Due to this potential risk, it might be advisable to avoid ginkgo during the perioperative period.

The ginkgo extracts approved for use in Germany are processed to remove alkylphenols, including ginkgolic acids, which have been found to be cytoxic.[51] The same ginkgo extracts are available in the United States. However, other ginkgo extracts and whole ginkgo leaf might contain appreciable levels of these dangerous constituents.

Another toxin, 4′-O-methylpyridoxine (ginkgotoxin) is a neurotoxic antivitamin B_6 found primarily in gingko seeds rather than leaves. However, very low (and probably harmless) levels have been found in the leaves as well.[52]

Apparently reliable case reports indicate that two individuals with previously well-controlled epilepsy experienced recurrent seizures upon starting use of ginkgo extract.[61] Seven other much less reliable case reports support these findings.[62] The cause might be contamination of ginkgo leaf products with ginkgo seeds. However, another possibility has been proposed as well. Ginkgo reportedly produces encephalographic changes similar to those produced by the drug tacrine, and tacrine has been associated with seizure.[62]

There is also one report of Stevens-Johnson syndrome connected with the use of *Ginkgo biloba* extract.[63]

One study found evidence that prolonged ginkgo administration alters insulin response to an oral glucose load in a manner that is complex and involves multiple effects.[53] The clinical significance of this finding is not clear.

Maximum safe dosages in individuals with severe hepatic or renal disease are not known.

Safety in Young Children and Pregnant or Lactating Women

Due to potential risk of abnormal bleeding, ginkgo supplementation should be avoided prior to childbirth.

Maximum safe dosages for pregnant or lactating women or for young children have not been established.

Drug Interactions

A limited human trial has shown that 400 mg/day of ginkgo extract does not alter hepatic microsomal enzyme activity as indicated by antipyrine clearance.[54]

One case report suggests a probable interaction between ginkgo and **aspirin.**[47] This would not be surprising, as ginkgo is known to inhibit platelet activation factor. For this reason, it is advisable to use caution when combining ginkgo with warfarin, heparin, aspirin, or any other drugs with **anticoagulant** or **antiplatelet effects.** In most of the double-blind studies of ginkgo, patients who used such drugs were excluded, so the true magnitude of this risk is not known.

It is also conceivable that ginkgo could interact with **garlic** (*Allium sativum*), **phosphatidylserine** (also used for improving mental function), policosanol (also used for intermittent claudication), high-dose **vitamin E,** and other natural products with relatively mild anticoagulant effects.

GINSENG
(Panax ginseng)

Alternate Names/Related Species:
True Ginseng, Asian Ginseng, Chinese Ginseng,
Korean Ginseng, American Ginseng *(P. quinquefolius)*

Common Uses

**Enhancing
immunity** [+3]

**Improving mental
activity** [+3]

Diabetes [+2]

**Athletic performance
enhancement** [+2X]

Adaptogen [+1]

(Higher numbers indicate stronger evidence; X modifier indicates contradictory results. See page xviii of the Introduction for details of the rating scale.)

Approach to the Patient

Asian ginseng *(Panax ginseng)* is a perennial herb of northern China, Korea, Japan, and Russia that has long played a major role in the Chinese herbal pharmacopoeia. American ginseng *(P. quinquefolius)*, a close relative, is cultivated in the United States. Siberian ginseng *(Eleutherococcus senticosus)* is often used interchangeably with *Panax* species in commercial ginseng products, but is a distant relative with a distinct pharmacological nature. This article pertains to the *Panax* species.

Because ginseng must be grown for 5 years before it is harvested, it commands a high price; for this reason, many ginseng products on the U.S. market actually contain very little *Panax ginseng*, and adulteration with caffeine or other substances is common. Dried, unprocessed ginseng root is called white ginseng, whereas a steamed, heat-dried root is called red ginseng.

Although your patient most likely regards ginseng as a kind of stimulant, its actual proposed use is somewhat different. Ginseng is said to be an "adaptogen," a substance that purportedly can help an organism adapt to stress of any kind.

Although the concept of adaptogens has not been adopted in the medical literature of the United States, herbal texts and some European medical treatises use the term freely. According to the standard definition of the term, an adaptogen should help the body adapt to stresses of various kinds, whether heat, cold, exertion, trauma, sleep deprivation, toxic exposure, radiation, infection, or psychological stress; cause no side effects; be helpful in treating a wide variety of illnesses; and tend to return an organism toward homeostasis rather than alter variables in a fixed direction (e.g., an adaptogen should reduce serum glucose when it is high and raise serum glucose when it is low).

Regular exercise is probably the clearest example of an adaptogenic treatment. However, the evidence that ginseng (or any other herb) has adaptogenic properties is preliminary at best.

Some evidence suggests that ginseng may improve immune function and mental activity, as well as help to reduce serum glucose in diabetics. The herb is also widely used by athletes in the belief that it will enhance physical performance, although the evidence for this use is contradictory at best. Contrary to some reports, ginseng does not appear to be estrogenic.

Enhancing Immunity   +3

A double-blind, placebo-controlled study of 227 participants evaluated the potential immune-stimulating effects of *Panax ginseng*.[1] After 4 weeks of treatment with 100 mg daily of Ginsana or placebo, all participants received influenza vaccine. The results showed a statistically significant decline in the frequency of colds and flus in the treated group, compared to the placebo group, from week 4 to 12. Antibody titers and measures of NK cell activity were also higher in the treated group.

Improving Mental Activity   +3

Several studies have found evidence that ginseng can improve mental function, but the effects seen are inconsistent between trials.

In a 22-month, double-blind, placebo-controlled study, 112 healthy, middle-aged adults were given either ginseng or placebo.[2] The results showed that ginseng improved abstract thinking ability. However, there were no significant changes in reaction time, memory, concentration, or overall subjective experience between the two groups. In contrast, a double-blind, placebo-controlled study of 120 individuals found that ginseng gradually improved reaction time over a 12-week treatment period among those 40 to 60 years old.[3]

Another double-blind, placebo-controlled trial of 60 elderly individuals found that 50 or 100 days of treatment with *Panax ginseng* produced improvements in numerous measures of mental function, including memory, attention, concentration, and ability to cope.[4] Benefits were still evident at 50-day follow-up. However, virtually no improvement was seen in the placebo group, a result that is highly unusual and raises doubts about the accuracy of the study. An 8-week, double-blind, placebo-controlled study enrolled 50 men and found that 8-week treatment with a ginseng extract improved ability in completion of a detail-oriented editing task.[5] Benefits were also seen in a double-blind trial of 16 healthy males.[6]

One study evaluated combined treatment with ginseng and ginkgo. (See the **Ginkgo** article for more information.[7])

Diabetes   +2

A double-blind, placebo-controlled study evaluated the effects of *Panax ginseng* (100 or 200 mg daily) on 36 newly diagnosed type 2 diabetics over an 8-week period.[8] The results showed reduction in fasting serum glucose and improved glycosylated hemoglobin and physical capacity in the ginseng group.

The effects of American ginseng *(P. quinquefolius)* on diabetes have also been evaluated in two double-blind trials. The first, a double-blind, placebo-controlled crossover study of 9 subjects with type 2 diabetes, found that a single 3-g dose of ginseng significantly reduced postprandial glycemia whether given simultaneously with the glucose challenge or 40 minutes before.[9] The second, an 8-week trial looking at longer-term control of glycemia, found that American ginseng decreased fasting plasma glucose compared to placebo.[10]

Interestingly, in double-blind trials enrolling 10 and 12 non-diabetic subjects, respectively, American ginseng only ameliorated postprandial hypoglycemia as compared to placebo when it was given 40 minutes prior to glucose challenge, rather than 0, 10, or 20 minutes prior.[9,11] Dose-dependency was evaluated in the second of these trials, but not found within a range of 1 to 3 g.[11]

Athletic Performance Enhancement   + 2 X

An 8-week, double-blind, placebo-controlled trial evaluated the effects of *Panax ginseng* with and without exercise in 41 individuals.[12] The results showed that ginseng improved aerobic capacity in ginseng-treated individuals who did not exercise, but offered no additional benefit in those who did exercise.

In a 9-week, double-blind, placebo-controlled trial of 30 highly trained athletes, treatment with *Panax ginseng* or *P. ginseng* plus vitamin E produced significant improvements in aerobic capacity.[13] Another double-blind, placebo-controlled trial of 37 individuals also found some benefit.[14]

However, negative results were seen with *Panax ginseng* in an 8-week, double-blind trial that followed 31 healthy men in their twenties.[15] Negative results have been seen in many other small trials of *Panax ginseng* as well.[16-21,56,63]

Adaptogen   + 1

The standard definition of an adaptogen includes the following concepts: an adaptogen should help the body adapt to stresses of various kinds, whether heat, cold, exertion, trauma, sleep deprivation, toxic exposure, radiation, infection, or psychological stress; it should cause no side effects; it should be helpful in treating a wide variety of illnesses; and it should tend to return an organism toward homeostasis rather than alter variables (such as serum glucose levels) in a fixed direction (e.g., an adaptogen should lower serum glucose when it is high and raise serum glucose when it is low). Regular exercise is probably the clearest example of an adaptogenic treatment.

In vitro and animal studies of ginsenosides and whole ginseng extracts (oral or intraperitoneal administration) report a wide variety of potentially adaptogenic effects including prolonged endurance; protective effects against radiation, infections, and toxins; reduction of biological changes produced by physical exhaustion and psychological stress; alterations toward homeostasis of glucose and lipid metabolism; increased alertness; increased RNA and protein synthesis; and stimulation of immune activity.[22-33]

However, there is little solid evidence from human studies. Preliminary human trials, many poorly reported and designed, suggest that *Panax ginseng* can improve glycogen utilization, alcohol clearance, serum lipids, and other metabolic parameters.[27,34,35] In addition, the studies described above regarding immunity, mental function, diabetes, and athletic performance are interpreted by proponents of the adaptogen theory as proof of ginseng's tendency to restore homeostasis.

Three double-blind, placebo-controlled studies attempted to evaluate the general sense of "well-being," an ill-defined parameter possibly related to adaptogenic effects. One followed 625 individuals (average age just under 40 years) for 12 weeks and found improvement in results on a standardized questionnaire.[36] Another followed 120 individuals and found improvement among women aged 30 to 60 years and men aged 40 to 60 years, but not among men aged 30 to 39 years.[3] However, a 60-day double-blind placebo-controlled trial of 83 adults in their mid-twenties found no benefit on measurements of affect and mood.[37] In addition, a double-blind, placebo-controlled trial of 30 young individuals found marginal benefits at 4 weeks and no significant benefits at 8 weeks.[57]

Other Proposed Uses

A double-blind, placebo-controlled study performed in China reported evidence that *Panax ginseng* can improve symptoms of **male sexual dysfunction**.[58]

A study using an untreated control found indications that *Panax ginseng* might improve **sperm count and motility**.[59]

A nonblinded pilot study provides weak evidence that *Panax ginseng* might be helpful in **chronic bronchitis**.[60]

A double-blind, placebo-controlled study of 384 postmenopausal women found no significant benefits for **menopausal symptoms** and no evidence of hormonal effects.[38]

Mechanism of Action

Not known. One poorly reported study suggests that ginseng might increase cerebrovascular flow.[39] Another study weakly suggests that ginsenosides may be the active hypoglycemic constituents in American ginseng,[40] although the lack of dose-dependency seen in another trial by the same researcher tends to discount this conclusion.[11]

Dosage

The usual daily dose of *Panax ginseng* is 200 mg of extract standardized to contain 4 to 7% ginsenosides, taken in two divided doses, or 1 g of crude herb.

See the Appendix for U.S. brand names of clinically tested products.

Safety Issues

Ginseng appears to present a low order of toxicity in both short-term and long-term use, according to the results of studies in mice, rats, dogs, chickens, minks, deer, lambs, and dwarf pigs.[27,41-43] Ginseng also does not appear to be teratogenic or carcinogenic. Studies of individual ginsenosides have also shown little toxicity.

Side effects from whole ginseng taken at appropriate doses are rare. Occasionally, women taking ginseng report menstrual abnormalities and breast tenderness; postmenopausal vaginal bleeding has also been reported.[44-47,61] However, large double-blind placebo-controlled trials have found no effects on sex hormones or gonadotropins.[3,38]

In an in vitro study, *Panax ginseng* stimulated the growth of a breast cancer cell line despite failing to show signs of estrogenicity.[62]

Overstimulation and insomnia have been reported with ginseng, and anecdotal evidence suggests that excessive doses may mildly elevate blood pressure. In addition, there has been one report of cerebral arteritis associated with ginseng use.[48] However, because there have been numerous reports of adulteration of ginseng with caffeine, germanium (which has multiple toxic effects), and other herbs, it is not clear if these reported side effects are actually due to ginseng itself.[41,49]

Reports in 1979 of a ginseng-abuse syndrome involving addiction, marked blood pressure elevation, agitation, severe sleeplessness, and hypersexuality have been thoroughly discredited.[30,50]

Maximum safe dosages in individuals with severe hepatic or renal disease are not known.

Safety in Young Children
and Pregnant or Lactating Women

Maximum safe dosages for pregnant or lactating women or for young children have not been established. However, no fetal abnormalities have been observed in rabbits and rats given high doses of ginseng extract during pregnancy.[27]

Drug Interactions

Formal drug interaction studies have not been performed. There have been reports of apparent interaction between ginseng and **phenelzine,** resulting in headache, tremulousness, and symptoms resembling mania.[51] Whether this generalizes into a drug interaction with other **MAO inhibitors** or drugs with MAO inhibitor–potential at high doses, such as **selegiline,** is not known. It is possible that the "ginseng" involved in these case reports may have been contaminated with caffeine.

One case report suggests that ginseng may inhibit CYP3A4.[52]

If it is effective for reducing serum glucose, ginseng might require a reduction in **insulin** or **oral hypoglycemic** dose.[8]

A case report suggests that *Panax ginseng* may reduce the effectiveness of **warfarin.**[53] However, a study in rats found no pharmacokinetic or pharmacodynamic interaction between warfarin and ginseng.[54]

One report indicates otherwise unexplained elevated digoxin levels in a patient taking **digoxin** and *Eleutherococcus.*[55] (Since *Eleutherococcus* is sometimes substituted for *Panax ginseng*, this finding is mentioned here.) However, this appears to have been a case of interference with a diagnostic test, rather than the actual elevation of digoxin.

GLUCOSAMINE

Alternate Names/Supplement Forms:
Glucosamine Sulfate, Glucosamine Hydrochloride,
N-Acetyl Glucosamine, Glucosamine Chloride

Common Uses

Osteoarthritis [+3X]

(Higher numbers indicate stronger evidence; X modifier indicates contradictory results. See page xviii of the Introduction for details of the rating scale.)

Approach to the Patient

Substantial but not consistent evidence suggests that glucosamine sulfate relieves symptoms of osteoarthritis more effectively than placebo. It appears to be slower acting but roughly comparable in effectiveness to NSAIDs. Importantly, glucosamine sulfate may alter the natural course of osteoarthritis by slowing progressive joint damage; however, the supporting evidence for this potentially important effect remains weak.

Because of the lack of immediate relief, some patients may quit taking glucosamine too soon and need encouragement to continue supplementation.

For retail sale, chondroitin is often combined with glucosamine. Combined glucosamine/chondroitin therapy might be superior to either treatment alone, but this has not been established.[32,33] Patients may be advised to first try therapy with either treatment alone in order to save money.

Glucosamine appears to be quite safe, except that it may present risks for diabetics (see Safety Issues).

Osteoarthritis   +3X

The evidence regarding glucosamine's effectiveness in osteoarthritis is mixed, but on balance the evidence appears to suggest that it is effective.[34]

For example, a double-blind study compared the effectiveness of glucosamine sulfate and placebo in 252 patients with radiologic stage I-III osteoarthritis of the knee.[1] The participants were treated three times daily with oral glucosamine sulfate 500 mg or placebo. At the end of the 4-week study period, ratings on Lequesne's index (a measure of osteoarthritic severity) significantly improved in the treated group as compared to placebo. Smaller double-blind studies performed in the early 1980s reported similar results.[2-4]

However, three studies enrolling a total of almost 300 individuals failed to find benefit.[5,6,35] For example, a 6-month, double-blind trial of 80 individuals with osteoarthritis of the knee failed to find glucosamine sulfate more effective than placebo.[35] The explanation for this discrepancy is not clear.

Comparison trials have also been reported. One double-blind study followed 200 subjects with osteoarthritis of the knee, half of whom received 1200 mg/day of ibuprofen and the other half, glucosamine sulfate.[7] Although ibuprofen produced faster results, both groups experienced comparable relief at the end of 4 weeks. In addition, although 35% of the ibuprofen-treated group complained of side effects, only 6% of the glucosamine group did so. Essentially equivalent results were seen in a similar 4-week, double-blind trial of 178 patients with knee osteoarthritis.[8] A 3-month, double-blind trial of 45 individuals with temporomandibular joint osteoarthritis found that glucosamine was at least as effective as ibuprofen (400 mg three times daily).[9]

Another double-blind study (published in abstract form only) followed 329 patients given piroxicam (20 mg daily), glucosamine, placebo, or glucosamine plus piroxicam for 3 months.[10] It found piroxicam and glucosamine to be equally effective, and combination treatment to be without significant additional benefit. Evaluation of patients postintervention showed that the benefits of piroxicam rapidly disappeared, while those of glucosamine were retained at near maximal levels up to the end of the monitoring period. However, the validity of this study has been questioned due to high dropout rates in both groups.

One double-blind, placebo-controlled study of 212 participants over 3 years found radiologic evidence of reduced cartilage loss in the treated group, suggesting that glucosamine is a disease-modifying drug in osteoarthritis.[11]

Other Proposed Uses

Although sports teams are known to use glucosamine as a prophylactic for muscle and tendon injury, evidence of this potential benefit has not yet been documented.

Mechanism of Action

Supplemental glucosamine may stimulate the synthesis of proteoglycans and collagen by cartilage cells and reduce phospholipase A2 activity, as well as inhibit enzymatic degradation of collagen.[2,8,12-16]

Glucosamine is also believed to exert a weak antiinflammatory effect unrelated to prostaglandins, but does not produce direct analgesia.[2,7,10,17,18]

Dosage

Glucosamine sulfate is typically taken as a dose of 500 mg three times daily. Twice daily dosing of 750 to 1000 mg is also sometimes recommended. For obese patients, a typical daily dose is 20 mg/kg body weight. Clinical trials suggest that full benefits take 4 to 6 weeks to develop.

Glucosamine hydrochloride and N-acetyl glucosamine (NAG) may produce less satisfactory results.

Glucosamine is often sold in combination with chondroitin sulfate. Preliminary information from one animal study suggests that this combination may be superior to either treatment alone.[19,20]

Safety Issues

Glucosamine sulfate appears to be essentially nontoxic.[15,16,21,22] A large, open Portuguese study of 1502 patients showed a 12% incidence of side effects, which were mainly mild to moderate gastrointestinal distress.[23] Double-blind studies show an incidence of side effects comparable to that of placebo.[7,10]

However, there are concerns that glucosamine might affect glucose metabolism through the hexosamine pathway because of the chemical similarity between glucosamine-6-phosphate and glucose-6-phosphate. Indeed, evidence from animal studies suggests that glucosamine may increase insulin resistance in diabetics.[24-28] While decreased insulin sensitivity has not been seen in human trials,[29] glucosamine has been found to increase plasma fasting glucose levels.[30] Glucosamine may increase the rate of glycosylation of tissues such as the lens, thereby increasing the risk of long-term diabetes side effects.[31]

Maximum safe dosages in individuals with severe hepatic or renal disease are not known.

Safety in Young Children and Pregnant or Lactating Women

Maximum safe dosages for pregnant or lactating women or for young children have not been established.

Drug Interactions

Results of one trial suggest that patients on **diuretics** might need to take higher doses of glucosamine for full effect.[23]

GLUTAMINE

Alternate Names/Supplement Forms: L-Glutamine

Common Uses

Post-exercise
infection   [+3]

Recovery from
critical illness   [+2]

Digestive disorders (food
allergies, chemotherapy-
induced diarrhea, Crohn's
disease, ulcerative colitis,
and irritable bowel
syndrome)   [0/−1]

*(Higher numbers indicate stronger evidence; X modifier indicates contradic-
tory results. See page xviii of the Introduction for details of the rating scale.)*

Approach to the Patient

Glutamine, or L-glutamine, is a nonessential amino acid derived
from another amino acid, glutamic acid. Because of glutamine's
role in a variety of physiologic functions, glutamine supplementation has been tried as a treatment for various conditions, including preventing the infections that often follow endurance
exercise, improving nutrition in critical illness, and treating digestive problems. Although there is limited evidence to support
the first two applications of glutamine, there is little evidence to
support its therapeutic use in other conditions.

Patients with inflammatory bowel syndrome should be cautioned that glutamine supplements are unlikely to control their
symptoms.

High doses of glutamine have been associated with manic
episodes.

Post-Exercise Infection   + 3

Endurance exercise produces immunosuppressive effects that may be related, in part, to reduction of plasma glutamine levels, although not all studies agree.[1-5,14] A double-blind, placebo-controlled study evaluated the effects of supplemental glutamine (5 g) taken at the end of exercise in 151 endurance athletes, and found a significant decrease in infections among the treated athletes.[6]

Recovery from Critical Illness   + 2

One small, double-blind study evaluated the impact of glutamine supplementation in 84 critically ill patients over a 6-month period.[7] The results showed decreased mortality as well as a decreased ICU and hospital stay in those receiving glutamine supplementation compared to those who did not.

Digestive Disorders   0/ − 1

Glutamine supplements have been suggested for individuals with various digestive problems, such as food allergies, chemotherapy-induced diarrhea, Crohn's disease, ulcerative colitis, and irritable bowel syndrome. The theoretical basis of this use invokes the high glutamine demand of intestinal cells, as well as a putative condition called "leaky gut syndrome."[8,9] However, there is no real evidence that glutamine works for these conditions.

A double-blind trial of 65 women with chemotherapy-induced diarrhea secondary to treatment for advanced breast cancer found no improvement with glutamine at a dose of 30 g per day.[10] Similarly, a double-blind trial of 14 individuals with Crohn's disease found no benefit with glutamine.[11] However, a double-blind, placebo-controlled trial of 70 individuals undergoing chemotherapy with 5-FU for colorectal cancer found evidence that glutamine at a dose of 18 g daily improved intestinal function and integrity (as measured by D-xylose urinary excreation and the cellobiose-mannitol test).[12] However, this study did not have the power to evaluate symptomatic improvement.

Other Proposed Uses

One preliminary double-blind trial suggests that glutamine supplements might have value as adjunctive therapy for angina.[15] Two small trials of glutamine as a sports supplement failed to find any enhancement of response to resistance training.[16,17]

Glutamine supplements have additionally been proposed as a treatment for athletic overtraining syndrome, attention deficit disorder, and ulcers and as a "brain booster." However, there is little to no scientific evidence for any of these uses.

Mechanism of Action

Glutamine appears to play an important role in maintaining the integrity of the gastrointestinal mucosa, especially during hypermetabolic states. It also appears to impact immune, other digestive, and myocyte functions.

Dosage

Therapeutic dosages of glutamine range from 1.5 to 6 g daily, divided into several separate doses.

Safety Issues

As a naturally occurring amino acid, glutamine is thought to be a safe supplement when taken at recommended dosages. However, individuals who are hypersensitive to monosodium glutamate (MSG) should use glutamine with caution, as it is metabolized into glutamate.

One case report suggests that high doses of glutamine could trigger manic episodes in susceptible individuals.[13]

Maximum safe dosages in individuals with severe hepatic or renal disease are not known.

Safety in Young Children and Pregnant or Lactating Women

Maximum safe dosages for pregnant or lactating women or for young children have not been established.

Drug Interactions

Because many **anticonvulsant drugs** work by blocking glutamate stimulation in the brain, there is at least a theoretical concern that high dosages of glutamine may overwhelm these drugs and pose a risk to individuals with seizure disorders.

GLYCINE

Common Uses

Cerebrovascular   **Schizophrenia**   [+2]
accident (CVA)   [+3]

(Higher numbers indicate stronger evidence; X modifier indicates contradictory results. See page xviii of the Introduction for details of the rating scale.)

Approach to the Patient

Glycine has been marketed as a memory and brain-function–enhancing supplement. The basis for this hypothesis involves its coagonist effects on glutamate brain pathways, specifically the N-methyl-D-aspartate (NMDA)–receptor. However, direct clinical evidence for this use is limited to one pilot trial. It may be advisable to steer patients toward ginkgo instead; ginkgo at least has some meaningful research to support this use. (See the **Ginkgo** article for more information.)

Building on evidence that NMDA antagonists cause schizophrenia-like symptoms, glycine has been tried as a treatment for the negative symptoms of schizophrenia (e.g., flat affect and withdrawal), with some success. Effects on NMDA are also the basis of studies investigating the use of glycine to reduce ischemic damage in strokes. However, it is possible that high-dose glycine could increase stroke damage. (See Safety Issues.)

Your patients may have encountered numerous other claims regarding glycine, such as that it can improve mental alertness, treat ADHD symptoms, aid sports performance, and reduce anxiety. However, there is no evidence at all that it is effective for these uses.

CVA   +3

A double-blind, placebo-controlled trial of 200 individuals within 6 hours of CVA onset evaluated the potential benefits of sublingual glycine at 0.5 g, 1 g, or 2 g daily over a 5-day period.[1] The results showed that 1 to 2 g daily significantly improved outcome.

There are potential concerns that high-dose glycine could also increase CVA damage (see Safety Issues).

Schizophrenia   +2

It is generally thought that antipsychotic drugs are most effective for the "positive" symptoms of schizophrenia, such as hallucinations and delusions, rather than the "negative" symptoms such as apathy, depression, and social withdrawal. Glycine has been proposed as a treatment for the latter category of symptoms.

In a placebo-controlled, double-blind crossover trial, 22 schizophrenics who were not well-managed by medications alone were randomly assigned to receive either 0.8 g/kg body weight of glycine or placebo for 6 weeks, along with standard antipsychotics.[2] The groups were then switched after a 2-week placebo washout period. Significant improvements in negative symptoms were seen with glycine as compared to placebo. In addition, the benefits appeared to continue for another 8 weeks after glycine was discontinued. No changes were seen in positive symptoms.

Three smaller double-blind, placebo-controlled clinical trials also found glycine to be helpful for negative symptoms of schizophrenia.[2-5]

One placebo-controlled trial of schizophrenics taking clozapine found that glycine was not beneficial and might in fact impair drug action.[6] However, other evidence suggests that glycine may augment clozapine's effects;[15] a conclusive analysis of this interaction awaits further research.

Other Proposed Uses

A pilot study suggests that glycine may improve memory.[16]

Preliminary clinical studies have found that glycine may be useful for treatment of **3-phosphoglycerate dehydrogenase deficiency** and **isovaleric acidemia.**[7-9]

Animal studies suggest that dietary glycine may protect against chemically induced **hepatic or renal damage.**[10-12] Other animal studies suggest that glycine may have **antitumor** effects.[13,14]

Manufacturers have made a number of additional claims for the benefits of glycine supplements, including prevention of epileptic seizures, enhancing mental alertness, treating ADHD, reducing muscle spasms, enhancing immune system function, and reducing anxiety. It is also proposed as a sports supplement, said to work in this capacity by increasing release of human growth hormone (HGH). As yet, there is no real scientific evidence for any of these uses.

Finally, because it has a sweet taste, glycine has been used as a **sugar substitute.**

Mechanism of Action

Impaired NMDA (*N*-methyl-D-aspartate) receptor–mediated glutamatergic neurotransmission may contribute to the negative symptoms of schizophrenia.[2,3] Glycine, an obligatory coagonist, may augment such neurotransmission.

Glycine's benefits in CVA may be related to interaction with inhibitory glycine and GABA receptors.[1]

Dosage

Dosages of oral glycine used for therapeutic purposes in clinical trials range from 2 to 60 g daily.

Safety Issues

No serious adverse effects of glycine have been reported, even at doses as high as 60 g/day. One participant in the 22-person trial described above developed gastric distress and vomiting, but these ceased when the glycine was discontinued.[2]

Theoretical concerns have been raised that glycine might increase cerebral injury in CVA by increasing levels of glutamate;[5] glycine antagonists have been investigated as treatments to limit the spread of ischemic injury.[17,18] However, the authors of the study on CVAs suggest that the potentiating action of glycine on NMDA receptors has a saturation limit, and that protective effects predominate.[1]

Maximum safe dosages in individuals with severe hepatic or renal disease are not known.

Safety in Young Children and Pregnant or Lactating Women

Maximum safe dosages for pregnant or lactating women or for young children have not been established.

Drug Interactions

There is mixed evidence regarding whether glycine impairs or enhances the effectiveness of **clozapine**.[15]

GOLDENROD
(*Solidago* spp.)

Alternate Names/Related Species: Aaron's Rod, Woundwort

Common Uses

Urinary tract infections and urolithiasis [0]

(Higher numbers indicate stronger evidence; X modifier indicates contradictory results. See page xviii of the Introduction for details of the rating scale.)

Approach to the Patient

Goldenrod (*Solidago* spp.) is often falsely accused of being an intensely allergenic plant because of its unfortunate tendency to bloom brightly at the same time and often in locations quite near to the truly allergenic ragweed (*Ambrosia* spp.). However, actual allergic reactions to goldenrod are unusual.

Goldenrod may have diuretic properties. For this reason, caution should be exercised in patients on lithium therapy.

Urinary Tract Infections and Urolithiasis   0

Germany's Commission E has authorized goldenrod as "irrigation therapy for inflammatory diseases of the lower urinary tract," as well as for the prevention and treatment of urolithiasis.[1] However, there is no direct evidence for any benefits in these conditions. Goldenrod does appear to increase urine flow, and may have antiinflammatory and antispasmodic effects.[2]

Mechanism of Action

Animal studies suggest that goldenrod and its constituent leio-carposide have diuretic properties.[2]

Dosage

A typical dosage is 3 to 4 g of dried herb in 150 ml of water, two to three times daily.

Safety Issues

Although no significant adverse reactions have been reported, the safety of goldenrod has not been substantially evaluated.[2]

Maximum safe dosages in individuals with severe hepatic or renal disease are not known.

Safety in Young Children and Pregnant or Lactating Women

Maximum safe dosages for pregnant or lactating women or for young children have not been established.

Drug Interactions

None known. However, one case report suggests that individuals on **lithium** therapy should avoid the use of herbs with diuretic properties, due to risk of dehydration and subsequent lithium toxicity.[3]

GOLDENSEAL

(Hydrastis canadensis)

Alternate Names/Related Species:
Yellow Root, Indian Dye, Indian Paint, Warnera, Indian Plant

Common Uses

Antimicrobial   [+1X]   **Expectorant**   [0]

(Higher numbers indicate stronger evidence; X modifier indicates contradic-
tory results. See page xviii of the Introduction for details of the rating scale.)

Approach to the Patient

Goldenseal is a highly popular herb sold almost entirely for the
wrong reasons. It is often combined with echinacea (*Echinacea
angustifolia* and other species) as an "immune booster" and "antibiotic" to be taken at the onset of a cold. However, there is no
real evidence that goldenseal increases immunity. In addition,
patients may be interested to hear that the widespread (and
false) belief that it can block a positive drug screen actually de-
rives from a novel published early last century. In *Stringtown on
the Pike* by John Uri Lloyd, a dead man is found to have traces of
goldenseal in his stomach. In fact, he had taken goldenseal regularly as a digestive aid, but a toxicology expert mistakes the
goldenseal for strychnine and deduces intentional murder.

This work of fiction sufficed to create a folkloric connection between goldenseal and drug testing. Although the goldenseal in
the story actually made a drug test come out falsely positive, this
has been turned around to become an unsubstantiated belief that
use of goldenseal will produce a "clean" urine drug screen.
Goldenseal was subsequently used (unsuccessfully) to disguise
doping of race horses, and today it is widely marketed for producing clean drug screens.

Like many other herbs, goldenseal may have topical antimicrobial properties.

Antimicrobial   +1X

Although the clinical effects of whole goldenseal root (whether oral or topical) have not been evaluated scientifically to any significant extent, its component chemical berberine has received considerable attention.

Berberine is known to possess antimicrobial activity against a wide variety of bacteria and fungi and may inhibit the growth of several intestinal parasites.[2-4] Like arbutin (a main constituent in uva ursi), berberine appears to be more effective in an alkaline environment.

Studies of oral purified berberine as an antimicrobial have found mixed results at best; in addition, absurdly high doses of goldenseal would be necessary to supply the equivalent dosage of berberine used in most trials.

One open study found that berberine can significantly inhibit intestinal hypersecretion induced by *Escherichia coli* as well as provide clinically minor benefits for *Vibrio choleraie* diarrhea.[5] Berberine did not have an additive effect when combined with tetracycline. Another study found no effect on hypersecretion in either *V. choleraie* diarrhea or nonspecific diarrhea.[6] Neither study found any reduction of *Vibrio* population attributable to berberine.

Other studies suggest that berberine can be useful in the treatment of *Giardia*.[7,8] However, the doses of berberine used in these studies would again require taking enormous quantities of oral goldenseal.

Preliminary evidence suggests that topical berberine may be effective against trachoma.[9,10]

Other Proposed Uses

Like other bitter herbs, goldenseal may stimulate appetite.

Goldenseal preparations also have been used for infections of the skin, oral cavity, urinary tract, and vagina, but there is no real evidence to support its use in these conditions.

According to traditional herbalists, oral goldenseal possesses an **expectorant** action that might make it useful in lingering respiratory infections, but this has not been scientifically documented.

Mechanism of Action

The mechanism of action of berberine as an antibiotic is not known. Although berberine does not seem to directly influence bacterial cell growth, it is known from in vitro studies to inhibit bacterial adhesion to epithelial tissues.[11]

Dosage

For systemic use, a typical dose of goldenseal is 250 to 500 mg three times daily.

Safety Issues

As many myths concern the risks of goldenseal as concern its uses. One widespread rumor claims that goldenseal is a sufficiently potent antibiotic to disrupt the normal intestinal flora. However, there is no evidence that this occurs.

Another widely quoted fallacy is that small overdoses of goldenseal are toxic and can cause ulcerations of the stomach and other mucous membranes. This warning can be traced back to a citation on "proving"—a homeopathic practice that uses massive overdoses of substances with the deliberate intent of documenting the toxic effects—in the 1892 reference *American Medicinal Plants*.[12] When used in normal doses, goldenseal is highly unlikely to cause gastric injury.

The toxicology of whole goldenseal root is not known. The LD$_{50}$ for berberine in mice is 300 mg/kg,[13] which translates to a dose of 10,000 mg/kg for goldenseal itself.

Side effects of oral goldenseal are uncommon, although there have been reports of gastrointestinal distress and increased nervousness in patients who take very high doses.

Maximum safe dosages in individuals with severe hepatic or renal disease are not known. Individuals with elevated bilirubin should avoid use of goldenseal.[14] (See Safety in Young Children and Pregnant or Lactating Women.)

Safety in Young Children and Pregnant or Lactating Women

Berberine displaces bilirubin from albumin, raising bilirubin levels, and also has been reported to cause uterine contractions in animals.[13,14] For these reasons, goldenseal is not recommended in pregnancy or lactation or for use by young children.

Drug Interactions

None are known. However, evidence suggests that goldenseal might inhibit CYP3A4.[1]

GOTU KOLA
(Centella asiatica)

Alternate Names/Related Species:
Hydrocotyle, Indian Pennywort, Marsh Penny,
Thick-Leaved Pennywort, White Rot

Common Uses

Venous insufficiency [+2]

(Higher numbers indicate stronger evidence; X modifier indicates contradictory results. See page xviii of the Introduction for details of the rating scale.)

Approach to the Patient

Like ginseng (*Panax ginseng* and other species), gotu kola *(Centella asiatica)* has been associated historically with an unusually large range of health claims, ranging from long life to increased sexual potency. However, its only indication with any substantial supporting evidence is chronic venous insufficiency of the lower limbs. Gotu kola is also used in Europe as a treatment for scleroderma and keloid scars. These three potential effects are hypothetically mediated through alterations in connective tissue formation and maintenance.

Patients interested in gotu kola for chronic venous insufficiency may be steered to treatments with better efficacy evidence, such as horse chestnut.

Gotu kola is commonly confused with the dried seed leaf of *Cola nitida*, the common kola nut. However, unlike kola nut, gotu kola contains no caffeine and is not a stimulant.

Venous Insufficiency   + 2

A double-blind study of 94 patients with venous insufficiency of the lower limbs evaluated the comparative benefits of *Centella asiatica* extract at 120 and 60 mg/day versus placebo.[1] The results showed a significant dose-related improvement in the treated groups in symptoms such as subjective heaviness, discomfort, and edema.

In a double-blind study of 87 patients with chronic venous hypertensive microangiopathy, patients were divided into three groups, one receiving placebo and the others 30 mg twice daily and 60 mg twice daily of *Centella asiatica* standardized extract, respectively.[2] The results showed a dose-related improvement in perimalleolar skin flux at rest and in transcutaneous PO_2 and PCO_2.

A placebo-controlled study (blinding not stated) of 52 patients with venous hypertension compared the effects of gotu kola extract at 60 mg three times daily and 30 mg three times daily against placebo.[3] Objective assessments included venous occlusion plethysmography (for capillary filtration rate) and AECT (ankle edema coin tester, for ankle edema). Assessed subjective symptoms included swelling, restless legs, pain, cramps, and tiredness. After 4 weeks of treatment, a significant dose-related improvement in treated patients in all parameters was observed; no change was observed in the placebo group. Ten normal subjects were also treated with the high-dose extract, but no changes were observed.

Similar results were seen in smaller, early studies.[4-7]

A 1992 review of the literature concluded that *Centella asiatica* extract provides a dose-related improvement in venous insufficiency, reducing foot swelling, ankle edema, capillary filtration rate, and microcirculatory parameters.[8]

Other Proposed Uses

Numerous clinical reports or uncontrolled studies of questionable reliability suggest that gotu kola extracts can be useful in burn and wound healing, anal fissures, bladder ulcers, dermatitis, fibrocystic breast disease, hemorrhoids, lupus erythematosus, mycosis fungoides, peptic ulcer, perineal lesions, periodontal disease, retinal detachment, tuberculosis, cellulite, cirrhosis, mental retardation, impaired memory, and scleroderma.[9] Although some of these studies are intriguing and make a good case for further research, none can be regarded as providing actual evidence of effectiveness.

One small double-blind, placebo-controlled trial looked at the benefits of oral gotu kola in **keloids,**[10] and others have examined its benefits in **leprosy.**[9]

Gotu kola has a reputation for improving **memory,** and a rat study performed in 1992 produced a temporary rush of public interest.[11] However, real evidence in humans is lacking.

A double-blind, placebo-controlled trial of 40 individuals found that gotu kola reduced the startle response to sudden loud noises.[12] The authors interpret these findings to suggest that gotu kola may have **anxiolytic effects.** Topical gotu kola is also sometimes used for psoriasis, burn healing (for which it is said to reduce scarring), and general wound healing. However, there are concerns about the safety of topical gotu kola (see Safety Issues).

Mechanism of Action

The mechanism of action of gotu kola is not known. However, because of its documented effects on venous disease, reports of efficacy in keloids, scleroderma, and burn healing, and the evidence of in vitro studies, it is tempting to conclude that gotu kola acts by improving the structure of connective tissue.[9] This may be mediated by changes in collagen and fibronectin production.[13] Much additional study is necessary to establish this effect. In leprosy, it has been suggested that gotu kola weakens the protective coating of *Mycobacterium leprae*.[14]

Dosage

The usual dose of gotu kola is 20 to 40 mg three times daily of a triterpenic extract, standardized to contain 40% asiaticoside, 29 to 30% asiatic acid, 29 to 30% madecassic acid, and 1 to 2% madecassoside.

Safety Issues

Gotu kola is generally well tolerated, the only reported side effect being rare allergic skin rash.

Toxicology studies suggest that oral asiaticoside at a dose of 1 g/kg is safe[9] and that 16 g/kg of fresh leaves are nontoxic.[11] However, asiaticoside has been found to possess weak tumor promotion properties in hairless mouse epidermis and dermis.[15]

Maximum safe dosages in individuals with severe hepatic or renal disease are not known.

Safety in Young Children and Pregnant or Lactating Women

Maximum safe dosages for pregnant or lactating women or for young children have not been established. However, Italian physicians have used gotu kola in pregnant individuals,[16] and rabbit studies suggest that gotu kola extracts are not harmful to fetal development.[10]

Drug Interactions

None are known.

GRASS POLLEN EXTRACT

Alternate Names/Related Species:
Rye Pollen Extract, Timothy Pollen Extract

Common Uses

Benign prostatic hyperplasia (BPH)   [+3]

(Higher numbers indicate stronger evidence; X modifier indicates contradictory results. See page xviii of the Introduction for details of the rating scale.)

Approach to the Patient

Like the more famous saw palmetto, grass pollen extract is used to treat benign prostatic hyperplasia, and preliminary evidence suggests that it is effective. The grasses used for this preparation are 92% rye, 5% timothy, and 3% corn.

Many products marketed for BPH contain several supplements combined, each at an inadequate dose. Your patients may do better using a single-substance product that provides the dose found effective in double-blind trials. (See the article on **Benign Prostatic Hyperplasia** for several reasonably well-documented options.)

Grass pollen has also been investigated for its potential to treat prostatitis, prostate cancer, and hypercholesterolemia.

Benign Prostatic Hyperplasia   +3

Two double-blind, placebo-controlled studies found that grass pollen extract can improve symptoms of BPH. The first enrolled 103 men with BPH for 12 weeks.[1] The results showed significant improvements in signs and symptoms. The second trial followed 57 men for 6 months, with similar outcome and significant decrease in prostate size.[2]

Other Proposed Uses

Highly preliminary evidence suggests that grass pollen might be useful for prostatitis and prostatodynia,[3-5] prostate cancer,[6-8] and hypercholesterolemia.[9]

Mechanism of Action

Not known. There is some evidence that grass pollen might act as an antiinflammatory agent in the prostate.[10]

Dosage

The recommended dosage for grass pollen extract in tablet form is 80 to 120 mg/day.[11] See the Appendix for U.S. brand names of clinically tested products.

Safety Issues

No adverse reactions were observed in any of the clinical trials discussed above, although one review author mentioned rare reports of stomach upset and skin rash.[11]

Although many individuals are allergic to grass pollen, the grass pollen products discussed in this article are processed to remove allergenic proteins.[2] It is therefore unlikely that grass-allergic individuals will have an allergic reaction to a properly prepared product.

Maximum safe dosages in individuals with severe hepatic or renal disease are not known.

Safety in Young Children and Pregnant or Lactating Women

Grass pollen extract has no proposed clinical use for pregnant or lactating women or for young children.

Drug Interactions

None are known.

GREEN TEA
(Camellia sinensis)

Alternate Names/Related Species: Black Tea, Chinese Tea

Common Uses

Periodontal disease [+2]   **Chemoprevention** [+1X]

(Higher numbers indicate stronger evidence; X modifier indicates contradictory results. See page xviii of the Introduction for details of the rating scale.)

Approach to the Patient

Green tea *(Camellia sinensis)* has developed a reputation as a healthful drink. However, observational studies form the core of this hypothesis, and they are by nature unreliable. Your patients may be taking supplements that contain concentrated green tea polyphenols; there is even less evidence that they provide health benefits.

A double-blind trial suggests that green tea candy may offer benefits for periodontal disease.

Periodontal Disease   +2

A double-blind, placebo-controlled trial of 47 individuals found evidence that use of a chewable candy containing green tea improves symptoms of gum inflammation in individuals with periodontal disease.[1]

Chemoprevention   +1X

A growing body of evidence, primarily from observational trials but also from animal and in vitro studies, suggests that regular consumption of green tea *(Camellia sinensis)* may reduce the incidence of a variety of cancers, including most prominently colon, pancreatic, and stomach cancers.[2,3] However, as usually happens with treatments supported primarily by observational trials, results of studies are inconsistent and subject to multiple interpretations.[4-6]

Other Proposed Uses

There is some evidence that consumption of green tea may reduce **heart disease** risk.[7-10]

Weak evidence suggests possible benefits of green tea in prevention of **liver disease**[7] and as a topical preventive for **sun damage.**[11-13]

Similarly weak evidence suggests that black tea, which is quite similar but not identical to green tea, may help protect against **osteoporosis**[14] and **atherosclerosis.**[15]

Mechanism of Action

Green tea contains high levels of polyphenols, such as epigallocatechin gallate, which exhibit antioxidant and chemopreventive properties.[16,17]

Dosage

Studies suggest that 3 cups of green tea daily provides protection against cancer. When taken in pill form, a typical dosage is 100 to 150 mg three times daily of a green tea extract standardized to contain 80% total polyphenols and 50% epigallocatechin gallate. However, it is unknown whether these extracts have the same effect as green tea itself.

Safety Issues

Green tea is generally regarded as safe. It does contain caffeine, although less than black tea or coffee, and can therefore cause insomnia, nervousness, and other symptoms of excess caffeine intake.

Maximum safe dosages in individuals with severe hepatic or renal disease are not known.

Safety in Young Children and Pregnant or Lactating Women

Maximum safe dosages for pregnant or lactating women have not been established. Green tea should not be given to infants or young children.

Drug Interactions

Green tea contains vitamin K, and large doses could potentially interfere with the effectiveness of **anticoagulants.**[18] In addition, the caffeine in green tea could cause significant interactions with **MAO inhibitors.**

Alternate Names/Related Species:
False Myrrh, Gum Guggulu, Gum Guggul, Gugulipid

Common Uses

Hyperlipidemia   [+2]

(Higher numbers indicate stronger evidence; X modifier indicates contradictory results. See page xviii of the Introduction for details of the rating scale.)

Approach to the Patient

Your patients are likely to use guggul *(Commiphora mukul)* for its possible hypolipidemic effects, and several double-blind trials support this use.

Guggul has been recommended for many entirely unsubstantiated uses as well, including treatment of acne, diabetes, and obesity. The last proposed use is based on unsubstantiated claims that guggul increases thyroid action. However, one study found guggul ineffective as a weight loss aid.

Hyperlipidemia   +2

The best double-blind, placebo-controlled study of guggul for reducing hyperlipidemia enrolled 61 individuals and followed them for 24 weeks.[1] Half the participants received placebo and the other half received guggul at a dose providing 100 mg of guggulsterones daily. The results after 24 weeks of treatment showed that the treated group experienced an 11.7% decrease in total cholesterol, a 12.7% decrease in LDL, a 12% decrease in triglycerides, and an 11.1% decrease in the total cholesterol/

HDL ratio. These improvements were significantly greater than those seen in the placebo group.

Similar results were seen in a double-blind, placebo-controlled trial of 40 individuals.[2]

In a double-blind comparative trial, equivalent hypolipidemic effects were seen in 228 individuals given either guggul or clofibrate.[3]

Other Proposed Uses

A small controlled trial (blinding not stated) compared oral gugulipid (50 mg of guggulsterones twice daily) against tetracycline for the treatment of **acne** and reported equivalent results.[4] An animal study found possible **antidiabetic effects.**[5]

A small double-blind trial evaluated guggulsterone as a **weight loss treatment.**[6] No statistically significant differences were seen between the verum and placebo groups.

Mechanism of Action

Guggul contains a family of ketonic steroid compounds called guggulsterones. Most studies have used a standardized ethyl acetate extract of the resin containing 4.09% Z- and E-guggulsterone. The mechanism of action of these substances is not known.

Dosage

Guggul is manufactured in a standardized form that provides a fixed amount of guggulsterones. The typical daily dose should provide 100 mg of guggulsterones.

Safety Issues

In clinical trials of standardized guggul extract, no significant side effects other than occasional mild gastrointestinal distress have been seen.[1,7,8] Laboratory tests conducted in the course of these trials did not reveal any alterations in hepatic or renal function, hematologic parameters, cardiac function, or blood chemistry. Animal studies conducted in India reportedly found no evidence of toxicity.[7]

Maximum safe dosages in individuals with severe hepatic or renal disease are not known.

Safety in Young Children
and Pregnant or Lactating Women

Maximum safe dosages for pregnant or lactating women or for young children have not been established.

Drug Interactions

None are known.

GYMNEMA
(Gymnema sylvestre)

Common Uses

Hyperglycemia [+2]

(Higher numbers indicate stronger evidence; X modifier indicates contradictory results. See page xviii of the Introduction for details of the rating scale.)

Approach to the Patient

Weak evidence suggests that gymnema *(Gymnema sylvestre)* may be an effective hypoglycemic agent. Patients should be cautioned not to substitute gymnema for standard therapy; nonetheless, when adding gymnema to a regimen of conventional care, close monitoring of serum glucose is essential to avoid hypoglycemic reactions.

Hyperglycemia +2

Two controlled studies examined the effects of an extract of *Gymnema sylvestre* (GS4) on 64 type 1 diabetics on insulin therapy and 47 type 2 diabetics on oral hypoglycemic therapy.[1,2] Both trials found significant reductions in blood glucose, glycosylated hemoglobin, and glycosylated plasma proteins, as well as decreased pharmaceutical requirements, in the treated groups. In addition, endogenous insulin secretion appeared to be enhanced. However, it is not clear from the study reports whether either of these studies was blinded.

Mechanism of Action

An ethanolic extract of the leaves of *Gymnema sylvestre* called GS4 is thought to contain the active constituents of the herb, but it has not been further analyzed. In animal studies, GS4 administration has resulted in reduced blood glucose levels.[3] In addition, histopathologic examination of pancreatic tissue in one study found evidence of an increase in the number of beta cells after GS4 supplementation.[4]

Dosage

Gymnema is usually taken at a dosage of 400 to 600 mg daily of an extract standardized to contain 24% gymnemic acid.

Safety Issues

Use of gymnema has not been associated with any reports of serious adverse effects. However, extensive toxicology studies have not been reported.

Maximum safe dosages in individuals with severe hepatic or renal disease are not known.

Safety in Young Children and Pregnant or Lactating Women

Maximum safe dosages for pregnant or lactating women or for young children have not been established.

Drug Interactions

It is possible that gymnema may potentiate the action of **insulin** or other **hypoglycemic medications,** leading to hypoglycemic reactions.

HAWTHORN

(Crataegus laevigata, C. monogyna, C. oxyacantha, C. pentagyna)

Common Uses

Congestive heart failure (CHF) [+3]

Angina [+2]

(Higher numbers indicate stronger evidence; X modifier indicates contradictory results. See page xviii of the Introduction for details of the rating scale.)

Approach to the Patient

Hawthorn is widely used in Europe for NYHA class I and II congestive heart failure (CHF). It appears to exert a positive inotropic effect on the myocardium while increasing the cardiac refractory period. However, patients may be informed that, unlike ACE inhibitors, hawthorn has not been shown to reduce the morbidity and mortality associated with CHF.

Hawthorn does potentially offer safety advantages over digoxin in early CHF, including apparent negative arrhythmogenic potential, a large therapeutic window, no contraindication in renal impairment, and no contraindication to coadministration with diuretics and laxatives.[1]

Hawthorn may also be helpful for angina. Patients may use it to treat benign arrhythmias, a use with some theoretical support but no clinical evidence. Hawthorn's effects in hypertension are marginal at best.

Congestive Heart Failure +3

Between 1981 and 2001, at least 15 controlled clinical studies (most of them double-blind) have been published on the therapeutic efficacy of hawthorn (WS 1442) in CHF.[1-5,25] Most of the almost 1000 patients participating in these studies had NYHA class II CHF. Significant improvement was generally (but not uniformly) noted in exercise tolerance, anaerobic threshold, ejection fraction, and subjective complaints. The doses of hawthorn used in these studies ranged from 180 to 900 mg/day taken for a period of 21 to 90 days (most studies lasted 42 or 56 days).

There is no evidence that hawthorn reduces CHF morbidity or mortality.

Angina   +2

In a double-blind study of 60 patients with angina, treatment for 3 weeks with 180 mg/day of hawthorn extract increased exercise tolerance.[6]

Other Proposed Uses

Hawthorn is often added to supplement products marketed to reduce blood pressure. However, if hawthorn has any effect on blood pressure, it appears to be marginal at best.[26,27] Animal studies suggest that hawthorn lengthens the myocardial refractory period and decreases the risk of **arrhythmias with reperfusion**.[1,7,8] In three rat studies, ventricular fibrillation after reperfusion dropped significantly.[9-11] No human studies of hawthorn in cardiac reperfusion have been performed.

Based on these findings, hawthorn is widely recommended by herbalists as a treatment for minor, benign arrhythmias, although there is no direct scientific basis for this use.

Mechanism of Action

The mechanism of action of hawthorn remains unknown. The most recent evidence suggests that hawthorn blocks repolarizing potassium currents in ventricular myocytes, giving the herb a functional similarity to class III antiarrhythmic drugs.[12] Other proposed explanations include activation of potassium channels, inhibition of cyclic AMP phosphodiesterase, and inhibition of angiotensin-converting enzyme.[13-16] One study found evidence that the inotropic effect of hawthorn is cAMP independent.[17]

Some of hawthorn's effects in reperfusion may be mediated through coronary artery dilation. Studies of isolated human coronary arteries showed a 14% relaxation in healthy arteries and 8% in atherosclerotic arteries.[18,19] Studies in animals have shown similar results.[20] However, one animal study suggests that hawthorn extract may aid reperfusion recovery of the myocardium through some mechanism other than increased blood flow.[21] An antioxidant mechanism has been proposed for reperfusion protection as well,[13] and extracts of well-characterized pharmaceutical hawthorn preparations are known to maintain this antioxidant activity.[22]

Dosage

The standard dose of hawthorn is 100 to 300 mg three times daily of an extract standardized to contain 2 to 3% flavonoids or 18 to 20% procyanidins. See the Appendix for U.S. brand names of clinically tested products.

A 4- to 8-week course of hawthorn is generally believed necessary for benefits to develop.

Safety Issues

Germany's Commission E lists no known risks or contraindications with hawthorn. Toxicity studies in animals suggest that the LD_{50} of hawthorn is about 500 to 1000 times the usual therapeutic dose in humans.[23-25] Studies in rats and dogs have shown no toxicity after 300 mg/kg of hawthorn were administered for 26 weeks.[1]

A water and alcohol extract of hawthorn has been shown to be nonmutagenic.[1] Other hawthorn extracts have shown mutagenicity in *Salmonella* cultures. This is presumed to be due to the presence of quercetin. However, because the quercetin content of typical hawthorn products is low compared to the amount of quercetin normally ingested with food, it has been suggested that use of hawthorn is unlikely to add significant additional risk.[1]

In clinical trials, hawthorn has been well tolerated, with side effects limited to mild gastrointestinal symptoms and allergic reactions.

Maximum safe dosages in individuals with severe hepatic or renal disease are not known.

Safety in Young Children and Pregnant or Lactating Women

No studies of embryonic or fetal toxicity have been conducted with hawthorn.

Maximum safe dosages for pregnant or lactating women or for young children have not been established.

Drug Interactions

Because of its cardiac effects, hawthorn may interact with or potentiate other **cardiovascular drugs,** and such combinations should be used with caution.

HOPS
(Humulus lupulus)

Common Uses

Sedative   [+1]

(Higher numbers indicate stronger evidence; X modifier indicates contradictory results. See page xviii of the Introduction for details of the rating scale.)

Approach to the Patient

Hops (the fruiting bodies of the hop plant, *Humulus lupulus*) is best known as the source of beer's bitter flavor, but it has a long history of use in herbal medicine as well. Although hops enjoys considerable use in Europe as a mild sedative for anxiety and insomnia, there is no meaningful evidence to support a therapeutic benefit in these conditions at this time. It is reasonable to steer patients toward therapies with more supporting evidence, such as valerian and melatonin, for insomnia.

Sedative   +1

Germany's Commission E authorizes the use of hops for "discomfort due to restlessness or anxiety and sleep disturbances." However, studies in animals and humans have generally failed to demonstrate any sedative action with hops extracts, even at high doses.[2] One study in mice did find that hops may potentiate the action of sedative drugs.[1]

Other Proposed Uses

Like other bitter herbs, hops is traditionally used to improve appetite and digestion. However, there have been no studies of this use to date.

Mechanism of Action

An observation of sleepiness in workers in the hop fields of Europe led to enthusiasm for using hops as a sedative. Subsequent investigation suggested that much of the sedative effect seen in hop fields is due to an oil that evaporates quickly in storage; for this reason, other mechanisms for the anecdotal sedative action of hops have been investigated. A sedating substance known as methylbutenol may develop in the dried herb over a period of time.[2] However, it, too, is volatile and probably is not present to any significant extent in hops products intended for oral use. Another possibility is that methylbutenol may also arise after ingestion as a metabolic product of other constituents of dried hops.

Dosage

The standard dosage of hops is 0.5 g taken one to three times daily. Because it is thought to possess at most a mild effect, hops is often combined with other herbs also thought to cause sedation.

Safety Issues

Hops is believed to be nontoxic. However, as with all herbs, some individuals are allergic to it. Some species of dogs, greyhounds in particular, appear to be sensitive to hops, and deaths have been reported in dogs.[3]

Hops possesses phytoestrogenic effects, due primarily to 8-prenylnaringenin.[4-7] The clinical significance of this finding isn't clear, but could raise issues regarding safety in individuals with a history of breast cancer.

Maximum safe dosages in individuals with severe hepatic or renal disease are not known.

Safety in Young Children and Pregnant or Lactating Women

Maximum safe dosages for pregnant or lactating women or for young children have not been established.

Drug Interactions

One animal study suggests that hops might potentiate the effects of **sedative drugs.**[1] It's possible that the phytoestrogenic action of hops could have an impact on **hormonal therapies.**

HORSE CHESTNUT
(Aesculus hippocastanum)

Alternate Names/Supplement Forms:
Buckeye, Spanish Chestnut

Common Uses

Chronic venous insufficiency   [+3]

(Higher numbers indicate stronger evidence; X modifier indicates contradictory results. See page xviii of the Introduction for details of the rating scale.)

Approach to the Patient

Standardized horse chestnut seed extract (HCSE) has been tested as a treatment for chronic venous insufficiency (CVI) in several double-blind, placebo-controlled trials conducted from the 1970s through the present.

Reasonably good evidence indicates that HCSE reduces objective measurements of lower leg edema and capillary leakage. Subjective complaints of pain, swelling, feelings of heaviness, fatigue, nocturnal calf spasms, and itching appear to improve as well. There is as yet no evidence that horse chestnut improves existing visible varicosities, although many patients may use horse chestnut for this purpose.

Like other treatments for venous insufficiency, such as oxerutins and diosmin/hesperidin, HCSE is thought to work by decreasing capillary leakage. HCSE appears to be safe when taken appropriately and exhibits only minor side effects.

Many products marketed for venous insufficiency contain several supplements combined, each at an inadequate dose. Your patients may do better using a single-substance product that provides the dose found effective in double-blind trials. (See the article on **Venous Insufficiency** [Chronic] for several reasonably well-documented options.)

The use of raw horse chestnut is not safe; only properly prepared, enteric-coated extracts should be used.

Use of oral HCSE in patients with renal or hepatic dysfunction should be approached with caution.

Chronic Venous Insufficiency   +3

Although the research record is not complete, the balance of existing evidence indicates that HCSE, either alone or in combination with leg compression stockings, is a useful treatment at least for the beginning stages of venous insufficiency.

Four reasonably well-designed studies were published in 1986.[1-4] In general, subjective complaints of pain, itching, leg fatigue, and feelings of tension in the legs improved significantly in these studies.

For example, a double-blind, placebo-controlled study of 40 patients found a significant reduction in extravascular volume after a 14-day treatment with 1 capsule twice daily of delayed-release horse chestnut versus placebo; however, no significant difference in venous capacity was noted.[3] Another study using venous plethysmography to measure the transcapillary filtration coefficient and intravascular volume of the lower leg 3 hours after a single dose of 600 mg HCSE standardized to 100 mg escin found that the filtration coefficient was significantly reduced in the verum group.[1] Both sets of authors concluded that HCSE does not exert a significant tonic effect on veins but that its contribution to reduced capillary permeability is probably of therapeutic significance.

Subsequent studies involving a total of 321 individuals also found HCSE to be significantly better than placebo for reducing leg volume and/or relieving subjective complaints.[5-7]

A partially blinded study of 240 patients treated for 12 weeks with placebo, compression stockings (unblinded), or HCSE (1 capsule of delayed-release horse chestnut twice daily) found the two therapies to be statistically equivalent and superior to placebo.[8]

Other Proposed Uses

Like other capillary stabilizers, horse chestnut or escin alone is sometimes used for **edema** following injuries such as sprains or surgery,[9] as well as for the treatment of **hemorrhoids.** In addition, based on its coumarin content, horse chestnut is sometimes administered along with standard therapy for **phlebitis.**

Mechanism of Action

The mechanism underlying the antiexudative actions of HCSE has been proposed to be related to reduced capillary permeability, a tonic effect on veins, inhibition of lysosomal glycosaminoglycan hydrolases involved in collagen breakdown, antiinflammatory activity, and increased activity of prostaglandins involved in venous contraction.[8,10-12]

It has been suggested that the active constituent escin inhibits the hypoxia-induced activation of endothelial cells and the subsequent increased adherence of neutrophils.[13] Escin (250 ng/mL) was shown to strongly inhibit the adherence of neutrophil-like HL60 cells to hypoxic venous endothelium but not to normoxic venous endothelium. Adherence of activated neutrophils may lead to alterations in the venous wall related to what occurs in CVI. The clinical significance of these findings and others in in vitro and animal studies is, of course, difficult to ascertain.

Dosage

The most common dosage of HCSE in reported clinical trials is 300 mg standardized to 50 mg escin, given twice daily in a delayed-release formulation. The best HCSE preparations certify that the toxic substance esculin has been removed. Enteric formulations must be used to prevent gastrointestinal upset. See the Appendix for U.S. brand names of clinically tested products.

Safety Issues

The saponins in horse chestnut extract irritate the gastrointestinal tract. This is the rationale for using controlled-release products, which reduce the incidence of irritation to below 1%, even at higher doses.[8] Calf cramps and pruritis are occasionally reported. Pulse and blood pressure are not affected, even in long-term treatment.

Whole horse chestnut is classified as an unsafe herb by the FDA. Poisoning by ingestion of the nuts or a tea made from the leaves and twigs is characterized by nausea, vomiting, diarrhea, salivation, headache, hemolysis, convulsions, and circulatory and respiratory failure possibly leading to death.[14] However, typical European standardized extract formulations remove the most toxic substances (i.e., esculin) and standardize the quantity of escin.

Acute oral toxicity of HCSE and escin has been studied in several animal species. The "no effect" dose is approximately 8 times higher than the recommended human dose. Mutagenic and carcinogenic studies have not been published.[15]

Use of oral HCSE in patients with renal or hepatic dysfunction should be approached with caution, as renal toxicity after high-dose oral escin has been reported.[16] In addition, acute renal failure has occurred in patients receiving intravenous escin at doses greater than 20 mg to prevent and treat postsurgical edema.[17] Drugs that displace escin from plasma-protein binding sites may also increase its nephrotoxic potential.[18]

Hepatotoxicity and shock were reported in a patient receiving an intramuscular injection of an HCSE product,[19] but there are no reports of such events involving oral HCSE products.

Safety in Young Children and Pregnant or Lactating Women

Two trials reported use of HCSE in pregnancy-related varicose veins, with good tolerability.[4,20] However, as no formal safety evaluations have been reported, compression stockings should be recommended for pregnant women before HCSE.

Animal studies to date have not shown embryotoxicity or teratogenicity.[15]

Maximum safe dosages for lactating women or young children have not been established.

Drug Interactions

Coumarins in HCSE could interfere with **anticoagulant** therapy; however, this has not been reported to date.

Escin is known to bind to plasma proteins and may thus compete with or displace drugs that are highly protein-bound. Drugs that displace escin from plasma-protein binding sites may also increase its nephrotoxic potential.[18]

HUPERZINE A

Common Uses

Memory loss [+3]

(Higher numbers indicate stronger evidence; X modifier indicates contradictory results. See page xviii of the Introduction for details of the rating scale.)

Approach to the Patient

Huperzine A is a purified alkaloid derived from a particular type of club moss *(Huperzia serrata)*. This highly specific acetylcholinesterase inhibitor is really more a drug than an herb, a point that may be worth explaining to patients motivated by an interest in natural therapies. Huperzine A is nonetheless sold over-the-counter as a dietary supplement for memory loss and mental impairment, for use in healthy individuals and those with dementia.

Memory Loss   +3

Many research papers report that huperzine A can improve memory skills in aged animals as well as in younger animals whose memories have been deliberately impaired.[1-18]

All human trials of huperzine have been performed in China and reported in Chinese.

A double-blind, placebo-controlled study evaluated 103 individuals with Alzheimer's disease who received either oral huperzine A or placebo twice a day for 8 weeks.[17] According to the English abstract, about 60% of the treated participants showed improvements in memory, cognition, and behavioral functions, compared to 36% of the placebo-treated group, a significant difference.

Benefits were also seen in an earlier double-blind trial using injected huperzine in 160 individuals with dementia or other memory disorders.[19] However, another double-blind trial of oral huperzine involving 60 individuals with Alzheimer's disease found no significant difference in symptoms between the treated and placebo groups.[20]

Huperzine is also reportedly helpful for improving memory in healthy individuals. A double-blind trial of 34 matching pairs of junior middle school students reported improvements in memory in the treated group.[21]

Mechanism of Action

Huperzine A is a potent and highly specific acetylcholinesterase inhibitor.[22-24]

Dosage

The recommended dose of huperzine A for memory loss is 100 to 200 μg twice a day.

Safety Issues

Perhaps because of its highly specific mechanism of action, huperzine A appears to have few side effects. However, minimal clinical safety information has been published at this time.

Individuals with hypertension or severe hepatic or renal disease should not take huperzine A except on medical advice.

Safety in Young Children and Pregnant or Lactating Women

Maximum safe dosages for pregnant or lactating women or for young children have not been established.

Drug Interactions

None are known.

HYDROXYCITRIC ACID

Alternate Names/Supplement Forms: *Garcinia cambogia,*
Gorikapuli, HCA, Hydroxycitrate, Malabar Tamarind

Common Uses

Weight loss   [+2X]

*(Higher numbers indicate stronger evidence; X modifier indicates contradic-
tory results. See page xviii of the Introduction for details of the rating scale.)*

Approach to the Patient

Hydroxycitric acid (HCA), a derivative of citric acid, is found
primarily in a small, sweet, purple fruit called the Malabar
tamarind, or most commonly known as *Garcinia cambogia.* Despite promising animal and in vitro trials suggesting that HCA
might suppress appetite and interfere with fat synthesis and storage, results of human trials are conflicting.

Weight Loss   +2X

In vitro and animal studies, as well as one human trial, suggest
that HCA might have utility for weight loss.[1-13]

In an 8-week, double-blind, placebo-controlled trial of 60 over
weight individuals, use of HCA at a dose of 440 mg three times
daily produced significant weight loss as compared to placebo.[13]

However, a 12-week, double-blind, placebo-controlled trial of
135 overweight individuals given either placebo or 500 mg of
HCA (*Garcinia cambogia* extract standardized to contain 50%
HCA) three times daily found no effect on body weight or fat
mass.[1] This study has been criticized for using a high fiber diet,
which might impair HCA absorption.[14]

Negative results were seen in other small trials as well.[2,3,15]

Mechanism of Action

Animal studies suggest that HCA may cause weight loss by suppressing appetite.[4-8] It has also been hypothesized that HCA may interfere with fat storage and production.[9-12] HCA may increase fat oxidation by inhibiting citrate lyase, an enzyme critical for energy metabolism during lipogenesis.[2]

Dosage

A typical dosage of HCA is 250 to 1000 mg three times daily. Supplements are available in many forms, including tablets, capsules, powders, and even snack bars. Products are often labeled *Garcinia cambogia* and standardized to contain a fixed percentage of HCA.

Safety Issues

No serious side effects have been reported in animal or human studies involving either fruit extracts or the concentrated chemical. However, formal safety studies have not been performed.

Maximum safe dosages in individuals with severe hepatic or renal disease are not known.

Safety in Young Children and Pregnant or Lactating Women

Maximum safe dosages for pregnant or lactating women or for young children have not been established.

Drug Interactions

None are known.

HYDROXYMETHYL BUTYRATE (HMB)

Alternate Names/Supplement Forms:
Beta-Hydroxy Beta-Methylbutyric Acid

Common Uses

Muscle building [+2X]

(Higher numbers indicate stronger evidence; X modifier indicates contradictory results. See page xviii of the Introduction for details of the rating scale.)

Approach to the Patient

Hydroxymethyl butyrate, or HMB, is a nonessential nutrient and a degradation product of the amino acid leucine.

Power athletes interested in enhancing strength and muscle mass typically use HMB. However, studies evaluating HMB's effects have shown contradictory results. In addition, the studies have all had small sample sizes, calling into question the reliability of the results. Larger studies will be necessary to establish whether HMB has any real benefit for athletic training.

Patients can be advised not to confuse HMB with the similar-sounding chemical gamma hydroxybutyrate (GHB—also known as the "date rape drug"); GHB can cause severe sedation, especially when combined with other sedating substances such as alcohol or anxiolytic medications.

Muscle Building   +2X

According to most, but not all, of the small double-blind trials in humans reported thus far, HMB may improve response to weight training.[1-7] However, all were small in size, and most were published only as abstracts, with many details missing.

For example, two controlled studies examined the effects of HMB supplementation in a total of 73 male volunteers.[2] In conjunction with a designated weight training program, participants received either placebo or up to 3 g of HMB daily over a 3- to 7-week period. The results suggested that HMB can enhance strength and muscle mass in direct proportion to intake and significantly increase bench-press strength, compared to placebo. However, there was no significant difference in body weight or fat mass by the end of one of these studies. Another double-blind placebo-controlled trial of 39 men and 36 women found similar results.[5]

Although two placebo-controlled studies in women found that 3 g of HMB had no effect on lean body mass and strength in sedentary women, they did find that HMB provided an additional benefit when combined with weight training.[3] In addition, a double-blind, placebo-controlled study of 31 men and women aged 70 years old undergoing resistance training found significant improvements in fat-free mass attributable to the use of HMB (3 g daily).[8]

However, other studies have found marginal or no benefits with HMB for enhancing body composition or strength.[4,6,9,13]

One review of the literature concluded that HMB is best documented for younger, relatively untrained individuals who are just beginning resistance exercise.[7] HMB might also help prevent muscle damage during prolonged exercise.[10]

Mechanism of Action

The amino acid leucine is found in particularly high concentrations in muscle tissue. During athletic training, muscle damage results in degradation of leucine as well as increased HMB levels. Some evidence suggests that HMB supplementation might provide a systemic signal to reduce the amount of muscle protein degraded during exercise.[7]

Dosage

A typical dosage of HMB is 3 g daily in pill or powdered form.

Safety Issues

HMB seems to be safe when taken at standard doses;[11,12] however, full safety studies have not been performed.

As with all supplements taken in very large doses, use of a quality HMB product is imperative, as an impurity present even in very small percentages could be problematic.

HMB should not be used by individuals with severe hepatic or renal disease except with medical advice.

Safety in Young Children and Pregnant or Lactating Women

HMB should not be used by pregnant or lactating women or in young children except with medical advice.

Drug Interactions

None are known.

INOSINE

Alternate Names/Supplement Forms:
Hypoxanthine Riboside (pure crystalline form)

Common Uses

Performance enhancement   [−1]

(Higher numbers indicate stronger evidence; X modifier indicates contradictory results. See page xviii of the Introduction for details of the rating scale.)

Approach to the Patient

Inosine has many biochemical functions, including a role in ATP production. Based on this, inosine supplements have been proposed as a metabolic enhancer for athletes, as well as a treatment for various heart conditions. However, patients can be advised that the evidence for inosine is more negative than positive.

Performance Enhancement   −1

Inosine is best known as a performance enhancer for athletes. However, most of the research on this use has failed to find evidence of benefit.[1-5] For example, inosine supplementation (5 g per day) was evaluated in 10 competitive male cyclists in a randomized, double-blind crossover trial over 5 days.[1] The results showed no improvement in aerobic cycling performance, power output, or time to fatigue. Another study of similar design found that 3-mile running performance did not improve after 2 days of inosine supplementation (6 g per day) in nine highly trained endurance runners.[3]

However, one small controlled study (blinding unknown) of 14 elite Romanian weightlifters found indirect evidence of benefit for athletic performance.[2]

Other Proposed Uses

Inosine has been proposed as a treatment for various forms of **cardiovascular disease** including cardiogenic shock, congestive heart failure, pericarditis, arrhythmia, and ischemia.[6] However, the evidence that it works for these conditions is highly preliminary.[7]

Inosine has also been suggested as a possible treatment for **Tourette's syndrome.**[8]

Dosage

When used as a sports supplement, a typical dosage of inosine in purified form is 5 to 6 g daily (see Safety Issues).

Mechanism of Action

Inosine, a nucleoside similar to the purines adenine and guanine, has been proposed as an ergogenic aid based on its physiologic role as a 2,3-diphosphoglycerate (2,3-DPG) precursor.[9,10] In addition, inosine may stimulate insulin release, resulting in carbohydrate uptake by cardiac tissue.[11]

Inosine also appears to increase cardiac contractility and elicit vasodilation of coronary vessels.[2,12] Its vasodilatory effects may be a result of adrenergic stimulation.[6]

Safety Issues

Use of inosine has not been associated with reports of serious adverse effects. However, a very small, preliminary, double-blind crossover study suggests that high doses of inosine (5000 to 10,000 mg per day for 5 to 10 days) may increase serum uric acid levels.[5]

As with all supplements taken in large doses, use of a reputable product is important because contaminants present in even small percentages could be problematic.

Maximum safe dosages in individuals with severe hepatic or renal disease are not known.

Safety in Young Children
and Pregnant or Lactating Women

Maximum safe dosages for pregnant or lactating women or for young children have not been established.

Drug Interactions

None are known.

INOSITOL (VITAMIN B$_8$)

Alternate Names/Supplement Forms:
Phytic Acid, Inositol Hexaphosphate, IP6, Myoinositol

Common Uses

Depression [+2]

Panic disorder [+2]

(Higher numbers indicate stronger evidence; X modifier indicates contradictory results. See page xviii of the Introduction for details of the rating scale.)

Approach to the Patient

Inositol is a naturally occurring isomer of glucose that is highly concentrated in cardiac and brain tissue. It has physiologic roles in the functioning of cell membranes and muscle and nervous tissue as well as in the hepatic processing of fats.

Inositol occurs in three forms in food: as phytic acid (inositol hexaphosphate, or IP6), myoinositol, and inositol combined with phospholipids.

Various forms of supplemental inositol have been proposed as a treatment for intermittent claudication as well as for a variety of neurological and psychological conditions. Preliminary evidence suggests that it may have some therapeutic benefit in individuals with depression and panic disorder; inositol is also sometimes recommended for Alzheimer's disease, obsessive-compulsive disorder, attention deficit disorder, bipolar disorder, and diabetic neuropathy. However, its proposed use in individuals with bipolar disorder warrants caution, as some evidence suggests that inositol may trigger manic episodes.

Inositol products in the phytic acid form (inositol hexaphosphate, or IP6) have been extensively marketed as a cure for a laundry list of conditions, including cancer, but supporting evidence remains highly preliminary.

It may be worth advising patients that phytic acid in foods is known to interfere with the absorption of numerous nutrients; for this reason, IP6 supplements should probably be taken at a different time of day than a multivitamin/multimineral supplement.

Depression   + 2

Several small, double-blind studies suggest that inositol may be helpful for depression.[1-3] For example, in a parallel-group, double-blind, placebo-controlled trial, 28 depressed individuals were given a daily dose of 12 g of inositol for 4 weeks.[3] By the fourth week, the group receiving inositol showed significant improvement compared to the placebo group. The only negative result was a double-blind, placebo-controlled study of 42 patients with severe depression not responding to SSRIs.[4] No improvement was seen when inositol was added.

A pilot study suggests that inositol may be helpful in conjunction with standard treatment for the depressive phase of bipolar disorder.[5] However, manic episodes have been reported (see Safety Issues).

Panic Disorder   + 2

A double-blind, placebo-controlled crossover study of 21 individuals with panic disorder found that those given 12 g of inositol daily had fewer and less severe panic attacks compared to the placebo group.[6]

A double-blind crossover study of 20 individuals compared inositol (up to 18 g daily) to fluvoxamine (up to 150 mg daily).[7]

The results over 4 weeks of treatment with each agent suggest that inositol was at least as effective as fluvoxamine.

Other Proposed Uses

Highly preliminary double-blind studies have evaluated high-dose inositol for **bulimia,**[8] **Alzheimer's disease,**[2] **obsessive-compulsive disorder,**[9,10] and **attention deficit disorder.**[2]

Inositol is also sometimes proposed as a treatment for **diabetic neuropathy,** but there have been no double-blind, placebo-controlled studies, and two uncontrolled studies had mixed results.[11,12]

Inositol has been extensively investigated for potential **chemo-preventive properties,** with some promising initial research results.[13-20]

Mechanism of Action

Although the mechanism of action of inositol is not known, it is a key intermediate in the phosphatidyl-inositol (PI) cycle, a second-messenger system used by several noradrenergic, serotonergic, and cholinergic receptors. In addition, cerebrospinal fluid levels of inositol are low in depression.[3]

It has been suggested that lithium's effects in bipolar disease might involve reduction of inositol levels; pharmacological doses of peripheral inositol have been found to reverse the behavioral effects of lithium in animals and the side effects of lithium in man.[3]

Dosage

Inositol dosages of up to 18 g daily have been tried experimentally for various conditions.

Note that phytic acid in food is known to interfere with the absorption of numerous nutrients, including iron and zinc. Since IP6 is phytic acid, it presumably would have the same effect.

Safety Issues

No serious side effects have been reported for inositol, even with a therapeutic dosage about 18 times the average dietary intake. However, no long-term safety studies have been performed.

Although inositol has sometimes been recommended for bipolar disorder, there is evidence to suggest inositol may trigger manic episodes in individuals with this condition.[21]

As with all supplements used in large doses, use of a quality product is critical as contaminants present in even small percentages could result in health problems.

Maximum safe dosages in individuals with severe hepatic or renal disease are not known.

Safety in Young Children and Pregnant or Lactating Women

Maximum safe dosages for pregnant or lactating women or for young children have not been established.

Drug Interactions

None are known.

IPRIFLAVONE

Alternate Names/Supplement Forms:
7-Isopropoxyisoflavone, Red Clover Isoflavones,
Soy Isoflavones

Common Uses

Osteoporosis, including
pain reduction from
fractures   [+3X]

Paget's disease   [+1]

Bodybuilding   [0]

(Higher numbers indicate stronger evidence; X modifier indicates contradictory results. See page xviii of the Introduction for details of the rating scale.)

Approach to the Patient

Ipriflavone, or 7-isopropoxyisoflavone, is chemically related to the isoflavone daidzen, a naturally occurring phytoestrogen found in soy and other plant products. The estrogen-like activity of ipriflavone itself, however, is believed to be limited to bone, where it appears to produce a significant antiosteoporotic effect.

Combined treatment with ipriflavone might make possible the use of lower estrogen dosages.

Note: Evidence of a possible lymphopenic effect has raised serious safety concerns regarding the use of ipriflavone. See Safety Issues and Drug Interactions.

Osteoporosis   +3X

Ipriflavone Compared to Placebo

In most double-blind, placebo-controlled studies of ipriflavone, involving a total of over 1700 enrolled subjects, results demonstrated either a significant bone-sparing effect or improvement in bone mineral density measured at the radius, whole body, or vertebrae.[1-12] These studies ranged in length from 6 months to 2 years and involved postmenopausal women (naturally, surgically, or GnRh-induced) and women with senile osteoporosis. In those studies that found improvement of bone mineral density in the ipriflavone groups, increases ranged from 0.7% to 7.1% over the course of the study. By comparison, placebo groups had losses as high as 5.0%.

One 2-year, multicenter, double-blind study evaluated ipriflavone's benefit in a group of 453 postmenopausal women (aged 50 to 65 years) with vertebral or radial mineral density 1 SD below age-matched controls.[6] They received 200 mg ipriflavone three times daily plus 1 g supplemental calcium or placebo plus calcium. Bone mass was maintained in the ipriflavone group, but the control group exhibited a significant loss in bone density. After 2 years, the results (calculated as a bone-sparing effect) were +1.6% at the lumbar spine ($P < 0.05$) and +3.5% at the radius ($P < 0.05$) compared with placebo.[6]

However, the most recent double-blind, placebo-controlled study of ipriflavone for osteoporosis found no benefits.[11] In this 3-year, double-blind, placebo-controlled trial, 474 postmenopausal women took 500 mg calcium plus either 600 mg ipriflavone or placebo daily. No intergroup differences were seen in spine, hip, or forearm density. The explanation for these negative results may lie in the calcium dosage used: virtually all other studies of ipriflavone used 1 g calcium daily.

Evidence suggests that ipriflavone can reduce the number of bone fractures. A 2-year, multicenter, randomized, double-blind study involving 100 women over 65 years of age found that patients treated with ipriflavone had a significant reduction in new fractures (along with an increase in bone mineral density).[8] A smaller study found a 50% reduction in the rate of new vertebral fractures in the first year of ipriflavone treatment.[9]

Several studies of osteoporosis have noted pain reduction during treatment with ipriflavone.[8,13,14]

Ipriflavone may also protect bone in hyperparathyroidism and during corticosteroid treatment.[15,16]

Other studies suggest that adjunctive use of ipriflavone may allow reduction of estrogen dosage while achieving an equivalent bone-sparing effect.[17-24] (See Drug Interactions for potential interaction between estrogens and ipriflavone.)

Paget's Disease   +1

Weak evidence from a small, randomized, controlled crossover trial suggests that ipriflavone treatment at 1200 mg/day followed by 600 mg/day may reduce biochemical parameters of disease activity and bone pain in patients with Paget's disease.[25]

Bodybuilding   0

Ipriflavone has also been included in bodybuilding supplements. However, no evidence suggests that ipriflavone can increase mass or strength in humans.

Mechanism of Action

The mechanism of action of ipriflavone has been suggested to be primarily antiresorptive,[3,26-28] although some studies also suggest a stimulatory effect on osteoblastic cells.[27,29-31] A study that examined the interaction of ipriflavone and estrogen on rat osteoblast-like cells concluded that ipriflavone modulates osteogenic cell differentiation and that the effect is estrogen-independent.[32]

Increased collagen synthesis in response to ipriflavone has also been suggested in a study utilizing human auditory organ cultures.[33]

A study of bone strength and mineral composition in male rats showed that a 1-month treatment with 400 mg/kg ipriflavone resulted in a 1.5-fold increase in the amount of energy required to produce a fracture of the femur.[34] However, a 12-week study of crystal formation at the same dose of ipriflavone did not show significant modifications of bone crystallinity by x-ray diffraction analysis.[34]

Dosage

The usual dosage of ipriflavone for osteoporosis is 200-mg tablets taken three times daily with meals along with 1 g calcium daily. A 300-mg ipriflavone capsule introduced for twice-daily dosing has produced excellent compliance without increased risk of adverse effects.[10] Studies of ipriflavone for Paget's disease and hyperparathyroidism have used 1200 mg/day dosing.[15,25]

A study evaluating the clearance of ipriflavone and its metabolites in subjects with mild or moderate renal failure versus normal subjects demonstrated that moderate to severe renal failure may require an adjustment of dosage.[35]

Safety Issues

Although ipriflavone is generally well tolerated, mild gastrointestinal distress can occur. It has been postulated that, in studies, the usual coadministration of 1 g calcium/day with ipriflavone may be the source of gastrointestinal disturbances.[10] However, a published case reported the reoccurrence of a gastric ulcer in a patient administered ipriflavone after surgery for a femoral fracture.[36] As studies have excluded subjects with possible gastrointestinal diseases, risk for increased gastrointestinal problems or increased severity due to treatment with ipriflavone in this population is unknown.

Atypical reactions reported for ipriflavone include rash, itching, erythema, headache, drowsiness, depression, asthenia, fatigue, and tachycardia.

Another potential risk came to the fore in the 3-year study of 474 postmenopausal women reported above; ipriflavone decreased average serum lymphocyte levels, and caused asymptomatic lymphopenia in 29 participants.[11] Similar effects were seen in one other, much smaller, study.[37] The clinical significance of this un-expected finding is not clear; however, at present it appears pru-dent to recommend that lymphopenic or immunosuppressed in-dividuals avoid ipriflavone and that healthy individuals taking ipriflavone should have routine blood counts performed.

In addition, some ipriflavone study subjects have exhibited altered hepatic and renal function test results as well as glucose and lipid metabolism changes.[3] None of these changes was permanent or resulted in disease states. However, these data cannot be used to rule out serious but rare adverse effects or those due to ipriflavone treatment beyond the average 2- to 3-year study period.

Current research suggests that ipriflavone does not increase the risk of breast cancer or other forms of cancer that are sensitive to estrogen receptor activity.[38-41] However, caution should be exer-cised in persons who have already had an occurrence of breast or reproductive cancer (see also Drug Interactions).

One study found a need for ipriflavone dosage adjustment in in-dividuals with moderate to severe renal disease.[35] Maximum safe dosages in individuals with severe hepatic disease are not known.

Safety in Young Children and Pregnant or Lactating Women

Maximum safe dosages for pregnant or lactating women, or young children, have not been established.

Drug Interactions

Ipriflavone may interact with numerous CYP enzymes, includ-ing CYP3A, CYP1A2, and CYP2C9.[42-44] These interactions may lead to increased serum levels of **theophylline, caffeine, theobromine,** other **polycyclic aromatic compounds, tolbu-tamide, phenytoin,** and **warfarin.** Both warfarin and pheny-toin contribute to osteoporosis, and warfarin is frequently pre-scribed for the elderly; the use of ipriflavone to treat iatrogenic osteoporosis caused by these pharmaceuticals could result in elevated serum levels of the drugs and potentially serious consequences.

Although ipriflavone by itself appears to have no effect on estrogen-sensitive tissues other than one, it may potentiate the effects of **estrogen** on reproductive tissue, specifically the uterus.[45-47] For this reason, HRT is preferable to ERT when ipriflavone-hormone combination treatment is considered. The finding that such potentiation is possible also suggests that there might be an increased risk of estrogen-dependent breast malignancies with such combination therapy, but thus far this potential risk has not been evaluated.

Possible interactions between ipriflavone and other medications known to produce gastrointestinal irritation, such as aspirin and **nonsteroidal antiinflammatory drugs,** are not well defined.

Based on the observed lymphopenic effects of ipriflavone, ipriflavone should be used with caution in individuals taking **immunosuppressant drugs.**

IRON

Alternate Names/Supplement Forms:
Chelated Iron, Iron Sulfate

Common Uses

Sports performance enhancement [+2]

Restless legs syndrome [−1]

(Higher numbers indicate stronger evidence; X modifier indicates contradictory results. See page xviii of the Introduction for details of the rating scale.)

Approach to the Patient

Iron deficiency is the most common nutrient deficiency in the world, prevalent in both developing and developed countries; worldwide, at least 700 million individuals have iron-deficiency anemia.[1] Groups at high risk are children, teenage girls, menstruating women, pregnant women, and the elderly.[1,2] However, patients may need to be reminded that more is not better: excessive iron supplementation may cause harmful effects. (See Safety Issues.)

The effectiveness of iron supplements in treating microcytic-hypochromic anemia is well established. Preliminary evidence also suggests that supplemental iron may improve sports performance and cognitive function in nonanemic individuals with marginal iron deficiency. Iron supplements may reduce the coughing side-effect of ACE inhibitors. However, although it is often recommended for the treatment of restless legs syndrome, a double-blind trial found iron supplementation ineffective in that condition.

Iron absorption may be affected by a broad array of pharmaceutical and nonpharmaceutical substances; conversely, iron may interfere with the absorption of these substances as well (see Drug Interactions).

Sports Performance Enhancement   + 2

A double-blind, placebo-controlled trial of 42 nonanemic women with evidence of slightly low iron reserves found that iron supplements significantly increased the benefits gained from exercise.[3] Participants were put on a daily aerobic training program for the latter 4 weeks of this 6-week trial. At the end of the trial, those receiving iron showed significantly greater gains in speed and endurance as compared to those given placebo. In addition, a double-blind, placebo-controlled study of 40 non-anemic, elite athletes with low serum ferritin found that 12 weeks of iron supplementation enhanced maximal aerobic capacity.[4]

Restless Legs Syndrome   − 1

Preliminary studies have linked iron deficiency to restless legs syndrome.[6-8] However, a double-blind study ($n=28$) of subjects with normal iron levels found no benefit with iron supplements.[9]

Other Proposed Uses

An observational study suggests that adolescent girls who are marginally iron deficient may experience **impaired mental function.**[3]

A small, double-blind trial found benefits with iron supplementation for women with menorrhagia.[5] This 1964 study reported an improvement in 75% of the women who took iron compared to 32.5% of those who took placebo. Women with higher baseline iron levels did not respond to treatment.

A study of 71 **HIV**-positive children noted a high rate of iron deficiency.[10] One observational study of 296 men with HIV infection linked high intake of iron to a decreased risk of AIDS 6 years later.[11]

A small, double-blind, placebo-controlled trial suggests that iron supplementation (256 mg ferrous sulfate) may inhibit **cough associated with use of ACE inhibitors.**[12] Researchers postulate that the mechanism of action is iron-induced suppression of NO synthase. However, due to mutual absorption interference, use of iron supplements and ACE inhibitors should be separated by 2 hours. (See Drug Interactions.)

Iron has been proposed as a treatment for attention deficit disorder, but there is no real evidence to support it.

Mechanism of Action

Iron is an essential element critical to a multitude of physiologic processes including hemoglobin and myoglobin function and DNA and ATP production.

Dosage

The typical short-term therapeutic dosage to correct iron deficiency is 100 to 200 mg daily. Once the body's iron stores reach normal levels, this dose should be reduced to the lowest level that can maintain iron balance.

The U.S. Dietary Reference Intake for iron varies with age and gender. The following daily doses are recommended: males 14 to 18 years, 11 mg; males 19 years of age and older, 8 mg; females 14 to 18 years, 15 mg; females 19 to 50 years old, 18 mg; and females 51 years and older, 8 mg.[13]

Iron and other nutrients such as **calcium,**[14-17] **soy,**[18] **zinc,**[19] **copper,**[20] and **manganese**[21] may mutually inhibit each other's absorption. Separating intake of the iron supplement and the implicated nutrient by at least 2 hours is likely to forestall any absorption problem.

Safety Issues

At the recommended dosages, iron is quite safe.

Mildly excessive levels of iron may have prooxidant effects, potentially increasing the risk of cancer and cardiovascular disease. However, evidence regarding asssociation of elevated iron with increased risk of CAD is mixed, with more evidence against such an association.[22-34]

There is some evidence that elevated iron levels may play a role in neuronal injury due to cerebral ischemia.[35] In addition, excess iron appears to increase complications of pregnancy (see below).[36]

Simultaneous use of iron and high-dose vitamin C can cause excessive iron absorption.[37-44]

Maximum safe dosages in individuals with severe hepatic or renal disease are not known.

Safety in Young Children and Pregnant or Lactating Women

The tolerable upper intake level of iron for pregnant or lactating women has been established at 45 mg daily.[13] One study suggests that iron excess may lead to increased risk of complications of pregnancy, such as preterm delivery and neonatal asphyxia.[36] For this reason, routine supplementation in the absence of deficiency should be avoided.

Drug Interactions

Absorption may be mutually inhibited with iron and the following medications: antibiotics in the **quinolone**[45-49] or **tetracycline**[50-52] families, **levodopa**,[51] **methyldopa**,[51,53] **carbidopa**,[51] **penicillamine**,[54] **thyroid hormone**,[55] and **captopril** (and possibly other **ACE inhibitors**).[51] Separating intake of the iron supplement and pharmaceutical by at least 2 hours is likely to forestall any absorption problem.

In addition, drugs in the **H₂ blocker** or **proton pump inhibitor** families may impair iron absorption through effects on digestive tract pH.[56]

Iron supplementation (256 mg ferrous sulfate) may inhibit cough associated with use of ACE inhibitors.[12]

ISOFLAVONES

Alternate Names/Supplement Forms:
Red Clover Isoflavones, Soy Isoflavones

Common Uses

Hyperlipidemia [+3]   **Osteoporosis** [+2X]

**Menopausal
symptoms** [+3X]

(Higher numbers indicate stronger evidence; X modifier indicates contradictory results. See page xviii of the Introduction for details of the rating scale.)

Approach to the Patient

Isoflavones are water-soluble chemicals which are found in many plants and may have phytoestrogenic properties. The most-investigated phytoestrogenic isoflavones, genistein and daidzein, are found in soy products and the herb red clover (*Trifolium pratense*).

Mixed evidence suggests that soy products containing isoflavones may reduce symptoms of menopausal syndrome. However, the causal role of isoflavones versus other soy constituents remains unclear, and no benefit has been found using red clover isoflavones.

Meaningful evidence supports the use of soy for improving lipid profiles. However, once again it is not clear that isoflavones are the sole soy constituent involved, and red clover isoflavones have failed to prove effective.

Evidence is mixed regarding the benefit of soy isoflavones for age-related bone loss. Soy isoflavones might present risks in pregnant women, individuals with thyroid disease, and women with a history of breast cancer (see Safety Issues).

Patients can be advised that in general there is better evidence for whole soy protein than for isolated isoflavones.

Hyperlipidemia   + 3

In 1995, a review of 38 controlled studies on soy and heart disease concluded that soy is definitely effective at reducing total cholesterol, LDL levels, and triglycerides.[1] One 1998 double-blind study involving 66 older women found improvements in HDL levels as well.[2] The FDA has approved a "heart healthy" label for soy products.

There is conflicting evidence regarding whether soy isoflavones are the active hypocholesterolemic ingredient in soy protein.[3-9,52,63] Inaccurate label claims for isoflavone content of soy products, as well as differences in the distribution of various isoflavones between products, may account for some of these contradictions.[10]

Red clover isoflavones were found ineffective for lowering cholesterol in a 12-week, double-blind study of 76 women.[11]

Menopausal Symptoms   + 3 X

According to most, but not all, studies soy protein (presumably due to its isoflavone content) can reduce vasomotor and other symptoms of menopause.[12,16,53,55,56]

For example, a double-blind, placebo-controlled study involving 104 women found that soy protein provided significant relief as compared to placebo (milk protein).[12] Similarly, after 3 weeks, participants taking daily doses of 60 g of soy protein were having 26% fewer hot flashes, and by week 12, the reduction was 45%.[12] Women taking placebo also experienced a big improvement by week 12 (30% fewer hot flashes), but the result with soy was significantly better.

However, one study did not find benefit. This 24-week, double-blind study of 69 women found no benefit with either isoflavone-rich or isoflavone-poor soy.[16] The high rate of placebo effect seen in studies of menopause may account for these discrepant results; another possibility is the between-product variability noted above. In another possibly relevant double-blind, placebo-controlled trial of 123 breast cancer survivors, soy failed to reduce vasomotor symptoms.[58]

In addition, isoflavones from red clover have also failed to show benefit. A 28-week, double-blind, placebo-controlled cross-over trial of 51 postmenopausal women found no reduction in hot flashes among those given 40 mg daily of red clover isoflavones,[17] nor were benefits seen in another double-blind, placebo-controlled trial involving 37 women given red clover isoflavones at a dose of either 40 mg or 160 mg daily.[18,58]

Osteoporosis   + 2 X

In one study that evaluated the benefits of soy isoflavones in osteoporosis, a total of 66 postmenopausal women took either placebo (soy protein with isoflavones removed) or soy protein containing 56 or 90 mg of soy isoflavones daily for 6 months.[19] The group that took the higher dosage of isoflavones showed significant gains in spinal bone density. There was little change in the placebo or low-dose isoflavone groups.

Another 24-week, double-blind trial of 69 postmenopausal women found that isoflavone-rich soy products can significantly reduce bone loss from the spine as well.[20]

Similar benefits have been seen in animal studies.[21-26] However, several animal studies and one human trial failed to find benefit.[27-29] Soy does not appear to have estrogenic effects on markers of bone resorption.[30]

Other Proposed Uses

A small ($n=18$), poorly reported, double-blind, placebo-controlled trial found weak evidence that red clover isoflavones might reduce symptoms of **cyclic mastalgia**.[59]

Soy isoflavones may exert preventive effects in some forms of **cancer,** primarily hormone-dependent cancers.[31-37]

One controlled trial found that isoflavones did not lower **blood pressure**.[38]

Mechanism of Action

Soy isoflavones (or their metabolic products) have estrogen agonist/antagonist activity. This is generally believed to be their primary mechanism of action. However, soy isoflavones are also antioxidant and may act in other ways as well.[22,31,39,40] In addition, unlike estrogen, which inhibits bone resorption, the soy isoflavone genistein may enhance new bone formation.[22]

Dosage

Although intake of isoflavones from soy in the diets of Japanese women has been estimated at up to 200 mg daily, the optimum dosage of isoflavones obtained from food is not known. According to one study, 62 mg of isoflavones daily is sufficient to reduce cholesterol.[4] However, as noted above, the causal role of isoflavones in the medicinal effects of soy remains unclear.

Safety Issues

Studies in animals have found soy isoflavones to be essentially nontoxic.[41] However, because of their complex estrogen agonist/antagonist effects, there are at least theoretical concerns that soy isoflavones may not be safe for women with a history of breast cancer.

Most but not all studies suggest that use of soy by menstruating women may reduce average estradiol levels, partially suppress the midcycle FSH surge, increase follicular phase estradiol, and extend the follicular phase by a day or two.[13-15,47,48,60,61]

The net effect of these changes may be to reduce breast cancer risk.

However, some evidence from animal trials suggests that genistein can stimulate the growth of estrogen-dependent tumors.[54,57,62]

Nonetheless, evidence from one highly preliminary study in humans found changes suggestive of increased breast cancer risk in women who took a commercial soy protein product.[42] In this 12-month pilot study, 24 healthy pre- and postmenopausal Caucasian women, ages 30 to 58 years, ingested 38 g of soy protein isolate (containing 38 mg of genistein) daily during months 4 through 9. Study parameters included nipple aspiration of breast fluid as well as blood and 24-hour urine samples for biochemistry. The study found that prolonged consumption of soy protein isolate had a stimulatory effect on premenopausal breast tissue, characterized by increased secretion of breast fluid, the appearance of hyperplastic epithelial cells, and elevated levels of plasma estradiol. The authors concluded that the findings suggested an estrogenic stimulus from the isoflavones genistein and daidzein contained in soy protein isolate. Similar proliferative changes were noted in breast tissue biopsies of premenopausal women taking a 60-g soy supplement (containing 45 g soy isoflavones) daily for 2 weeks.[43]

Soy products may inhibit thyroid synthesis or otherwise reduce thyroid activity, possibly due to the isoflavone genistein.[44-46]

Maximum safe dosages in individuals with severe hepatic or renal disease are not known.

Safety in Young Children
and Pregnant or Lactating Women

Preliminary studies and reports have raised concerns that intensive use of soy products by pregnant women could exert a hormonal effect upon unborn fetuses.[49,50] Red clover isoflavones presumably present similar risks.[51] In addition, soy and or its isoflavones may produce hypothyroidism in infants.[45,46]

Maximum safe dosages for pregnant or lactating women or for young children have not been established.

Drug Interactions

Although concerns have been expressed by some experts that soy isoflavones might interfere with the action of **oral contraceptives,** one study of 36 women suggests that such concerns are not warranted.[51] Soy products may impair thyroid function or reduce absorption of **thyroid medication,** at least in children.[44-46] For this reason, individuals with impaired thyroid function who add soy to their diet should be retested.

KAVA
(Piper methysticum)

Alternate Names/Related Species:
Ava, Ava Pepper, Intoxicating Pepper, Kava-Kava, Kawa

Common Uses

Anxiety   [+3]

(Higher numbers indicate stronger evidence; X modifier indicates contradictory results. See page xviii of the Introduction for details of the rating scale.)

Approach to the Patient

Kava *(Piper methysticum)* is a member of the pepper family that has long been cultivated by Pacific Islanders for use as a relaxing drink in social and ceremonial settings. A standardized extract of kava has become a popular European treatment for anxiety and insomnia.

Kava possesses numerous sedative constituents. Its antianxiety benefits appear to develop gradually over a period of 1 to 8 weeks and do not seem to be accompanied by a loss of mental acuity. Kava appears to be generally safe when used alone and at recommended doses. However, patients should be advised that use of kava has been linked to a number of cases of liver failure. For this reason alone, standard medications may be a preferable option. (See Safety Issues.)

Anxiety   + 3

Altogether, over 400 patients with various anxiety syndromes have participated in double-blind controlled studies of kava.[37] In the best of these studies, a 6-month, double-blind, placebo-controlled trial tested 300 mg/day of a 70% kavalactone extract in 101 outpatients with anxiety-related disorders meeting DSM-III-R criteria.[1] Participants were evaluated using the Hamilton Anxiety Scale (HAM-A, quantifying restlessness, nervousness, heart palpitations, stomach discomfort, dizziness, and chest pain) and the Clinical Global Impressions scale (CGI) as well as self-rating scales. The study found that HAM-A scores in the treated group showed clinically and statistically significant reduction compared to the placebo group beginning at 8 weeks, and that this relative improvement increased throughout the duration of the study. At 12 weeks, the CGI scale also showed statistically significant improvements in treated patients compared to the placebo group. Self-rating scales showed similar changes. This study, however, has been criticized for its heterogeneous treatment group (patients had more than one anxiety-related diagnosis) as well as significant differences in average HAM-A scores between centers.

Other studies of kava have found more rapid anxiolytic effects, demonstrable within 1 to 2 weeks.[2-4]

A 5-week double-blind placebo-controlled trial of 40 individuals with various anxiety disorders evaluated the effects of kava during and after tapering benzodiazepine medications.[5] Use of kava led to improvements of HAM-A scores as compared to baseline and as compared to placebo. Interestingly, only minimal deterioration was seen in the placebo group.

A 1993 double-blind, comparative study followed 174 patients with anxiety symptoms for a period of 6 weeks. Patients received 300 mg/day of a 70% kavalactone extract, 15 mg/day of oxazepam (a subtherapeutic dose), or 9 mg/day of bromazepam (a full therapeutic dose).[6] Similar improvement in HAM-A scores was seen in all groups, but no intergroup statistical analysis was reported.

Other double-blind, placebo-controlled studies have found anxiolytic effects with the single kavalactone kavain.[7-9] Furthermore, isolated kavain has also been found to produce effects comparable to those of benzodiazepines.[9] However, small controlled trials suggest that kava or kavalactones may impair mental function to a lesser extent than benzodiazepines.[10-13]

Other Proposed Uses

Preliminary human sleep studies have found that kava enhances sleep spindle density, reduces sleep latency, and increases slow-wave sleep without changes to REM sleep.[14]

One animal study suggests that kava may have potential value for the treatment of alcohol dependency.[38]

Mechanism of Action

The presumed active constituents of kava are fat-soluble lactones known as kavalactones. One of the most active is dihydrokavain, which has been found to produce sedative, anticonvulsant, and analgesic effects.[15-18] Other identified kavalactones include kavain, methysticin, and dihydromethysticin. Mixed kavalactones have been found to cause a mephenesin-like relaxation of skeletal muscles, and very high doses can cause ataxia and paralysis without loss of consciousness.[18-20] Nonhydrated kavalactones (kavain and methysticin)—and to a lesser extent, hydrated kavalactones (dihydrokavain and dihydromethysticin)—produce local anesthesia similar to that of cocaine, especially as topical anesthetics rather than as peripheral anesthetics.[21] Methysticin and dihydromethysticin exhibit neuroprotective properties in rodents, similar to memantine (a glutamate antagonist at NMDA-glutamate receptors, not marketed in the United States).

Initial reports suggested that kavalactones do not significantly interact with GABA receptors.[22] This led to further investigations of excitatory neuronal mechanisms. Two reports suggested that kavain, methysticin, or both can inhibit voltage-dependent sodium channels and suppress the release of the excitatory amino acid neurotransmitter glutamate.[23,24]

However, later research suggests that the effects of kavalactones may indeed involve GABA receptors, by increasing their prevalence, especially in the hippocampus and amygdala.[25] The study authors further suggest that earlier investigations erred by examining areas of the brain where kava is not believed to be active, specifically the frontal cortex and cerebellum.

It appears that kavalactones interact with some other site on GABA-A receptors other than the benzodiazepine binding site.[26] One study at nanomolar concentrations found a direct interaction between a kavain derivative and cortical neurons, suggesting a ligand-receptor interaction.[27]

Dosage

Kava products are standardized to 15 or 30% kavalactone content. (Products with a higher percentage of kavalactones are reportedly less effective, presumably due to their reduced content of unidentified active non-kavalactone constituents.) See the Appendix for U.S. brand names of clinically tested products.

For use as an antianxiety agent, the dose of kava extract should supply 60 to 210 mg of kavalactones per day, given in 2 or 3 divided doses. The total dose of kavalactones should not exceed 300 mg/day, and the course of treatment should not exceed 3 months.[9]

The usual dose for insomnia is 210 mg of kavalactones 1 hour before bedtime.

Safety Issues

Kava is usually well tolerated. A 4-week drug-monitoring study of 3029 patients given 800 mg/day of a 30% kavalactone extract yielded a 2.3% incidence of side effects, including mild headache, gastrointestinal distress, and allergic rashes. Another study of 4049 patients who took a much lower dose found side effects in 1.5% of cases, also limited mainly to mild gastrointestinal complaints or allergic rashes.[9]

Long-term kava use (months to years) in excess of 400 mg kavalactones per day can create a characteristic generalized dry, scaly dermopathy that appears primarily on the palms, soles, forearms, shins, and back.[28] The rash promptly disappears on cessation of kava.

Kava also possesses a low order of toxicity. The LD_{50} of kavalactones is about 300 to 400 mg/kg in test animals.[19] Dogs tolerate daily doses of 24 mg/kg and rats tolerate 20 mg/kg of 70% kava extract with no adverse effects.[9,19] Up to 320 mg/kg of this extract in rats caused only mild histopathological changes. No evidence of mutagenicity was observed.

However, a spate of case reports linking kava use to severe hepatotoxic reactions has led the German, Canadian, and U.S. governments to consider banning kava products.[30,31,39-41]

Due to the widespread and apparently harmless recreational use of kava in the South Pacific, it is thought that these case reports represent idiosyncratic reactions. Nonetheless, they clearly warrant caution in individuals with hepatic risk factors such as alcoholism or use of hepatotoxic medications. Furthermore, periodic liver enzyme testing may be warranted among individuals using kava.

One study of Australian aborigines who habitually consumed more than 100 times the normal dose of kava demonstrated numerous physiological changes, including decreased blood levels of albumin, plasma protein, urea, and bilirubin, accompanied by hematuria, decreased platelet count, and macrocytic red blood cells.[9,29] However, because this population also consumed large doses of alcohol and cigarettes, the extent of kava's contribution to their poor health status remains unknown.

When taken in usual doses, kava or synthetic kavain does not appear to impair reaction time or mental function.[9-13,32,33] However, high doses are known to cause inebriation.

Addiction has not been observed in European patients taking kava extracts, and animal studies suggest that typical kava products do not cause physiological tolerance or dependence.[9,34]

Three case reports appear to represent kava-induced dystonic reactions.[35] In one, a 28-year-old man exhibited abnormal ocular movements and neck spasms approximately 90 minutes after ingesting 100 mg of kava extract. This episode lasted about 40 minutes. Similar reactions were seen in two women, aged 22 and 63 years. In a fourth case, kava increased symptoms of Parkinson's disease. These cases suggest an antidopaminergic effect, at least in some individuals, indicating that kava should not be used by individuals with Parkinson's disease or with risk factors for dystonic reactions.

Maximum safe dosages in individuals with severe hepatic or renal disease are not known.

Safety in Young Children and Pregnant or Lactating Women

The German Commission E monograph warns against the use of kava during pregnancy and lactation. Safety in young children has also not been established.

Drug Interactions

According to the German Commission E, caution must be exercised when combining kava with other CNS depressants. At least one case report exists of hospitalization apparently resulting from the concomitant use of the **benzodiazepine alprazolam** and kava extract.[36] Furthermore, high doses of **alcohol** potentiate the effects and toxicity of kava in mice.[16]

The case reports mentioned above suggest that kava might increase risk of dystonic reactions in individuals on **phenothiazines,** and could additionally counteract the effectiveness of **L-dopa.**[35]

Just as antidepressants are often combined with conventional anxiolytics in the treatment of anxiety, combinations of **St. John's wort** and kava are recommended by many herbalists. Although no adverse effects have been reported, the safety of such combinations is not established. A similar lack of information prevails for the combination of kava and other herbs with a sedative reputation, such as **valerian, hops,** and **passionflower.**

KELP

Alternate Names/Supplement Forms:
Brown Seaweed, Kombu, *Laminaria* spp.

Common Uses

Vitamin and mineral supplement   [0]

(Higher numbers indicate stronger evidence; X modifier indicates contradictory results. See page xviii of the Introduction for details of the rating scale.)

Approach to the Patient

Kelp refers to several species of large, brown algae that can grow to enormous sizes in the ocean. Kelp is a type of seaweed, but not all seaweed is kelp: "seaweed" loosely describes any type of vegetation growing in the ocean, including many other types of algae and plants.

Kelp is a regular part of a normal human diet in many parts of the world, such as Japan, Alaska, and Hawaii. It has been incorporated into vitamin and mineral supplements because of its nutrient value. However, patients can be advised that iodine is not a cure-all for thyroid problems; in the absence of iodine deficiency, increased iodine intake may cause thyroid problems rather than alleviate them (see Safety Issues).

Supplements containing kelp can be purchased at most pharmacies and health food stores. Kelp used in food preparation is available at grocery stores that stock specialties for Asian cooking.

Vitamin and Mineral Supplement   0

Because it is a good source of folic acid, as well as many other vitamins and minerals, manufacturers of vitamin and mineral supplements may include kelp for additional nutrient value. However, because it may contain significant amounts of iodine, concerns about its impact on thyroid function are warranted (see Safety Issues).

Other Proposed Uses

Although kelp is used primarily as a vitamin and mineral supplement, results of highly preliminary animal and in vitro studies have suggested other potential uses.

For example, there is some evidence that elements in kelp might help to prevent infection with several kinds of **viruses,** including influenza,[1] herpes simplex,[2] and HIV.[3] Similarly, there is some evidence that kelp possesses **anticancer effects**[4-9] and may lower **blood pressure,**[10] but it would be premature to begin using kelp as a treatment for any of these health problems.

Additionally, kelp has been marketed as a weight loss product, but scientific studies of its efficacy and safety for this purpose have not been published.

Another unsubstantiated and misleading claim is that kelp can be used to treat various thyroid conditions. It is true that taking kelp may correct an iodine deficiency, but it is unlikely to benefit the thyroid in any other circumstance; as with iodine itself, excessive intake of kelp can cause thyroid dysfunction in healthy individuals (see Safety Issues).

Mechanism of Action

Not applicable.

Dosage

There is no appropriate "therapeutic" dosage of kelp, because it is not yet known whether kelp is truly therapeutic for any conditions. However, because of its high iodine content, patients should be cautioned about overuse of kelp supplementation. In 17 different kelp supplements studied by one group of researchers, the iodine content varied from 45 μg to 57,000 μg per tablet or capsule.[11] The recommended daily intake for iodine is 150 μg per day for individuals over the age of 4 years, and markedly exceeding this daily dose may cause thyroid dysfunction. (See also Safety Issues.)

Safety Issues

Excessive intake of kelp can result in iodine overload and, on that basis, induce symptoms of either hypo- or hyperthyroidism.[12-18]

In addition, published reports describe two cases of acne apparently caused or worsened by taking large doses of kelp,[19] an effect also believed due to the substantial amounts of iodine in the supplement.

Finally, some kelp and other seaweed supplements have been found to contain levels of arsenic high enough to be toxic.[20,21] Seawater contains highly diluted arsenic, but kelp (like other ocean life) can concentrate arsenic in its tissues, and there are reports of symptoms of arsenic poisoning in two individuals who had been consuming kelp. However, other studies suggest that this is uncommon.[22]

Maximum safe dosages in individuals with severe hepatic or renal disease are not known.

Safety in Young Children and Pregnant or Lactating Women

Maximum safe dosages for pregnant or lactating women or for young children have not been established.

Drug Interactions

None are known.

KUDZU
(Pueraria lobata)

Common Uses

Alcoholism [−1]

(Higher numbers indicate stronger evidence; X modifier indicates contradictory results. See page xviii of the Introduction for details of the rating scale.)

Approach to the Patient

Kudzu *(Pueraria lobata)* is cooked as food in China, and also is used as an herb in traditional Chinese medicine. However, in the United States, kudzu has become an invasive pest, with the nickname "mile-a-minute vine."

Based on the results of one animal study, kudzu received widespread press as a promising treatment for alcoholism. However, patients may not know that subsequent human research failed to corroborate these results.

Alcoholism   −1

A 1993 study evaluated the effects of kudzu in the Syrian golden hamster, a species that, if given a choice, prefers drinking alcohol to water.[1] In this study, administration of kudzu reversed that preference. Similar effects have been seen in studies involving rats.[3]

However, a 1-month, double-blind study of 38 alcoholics found no benefit in participants given kudzu as compared to those given placebo.[2]

Other Proposed Uses

In traditional Chinese medicine, kudzu is used for the acute treatment of respiratory infections accompanied by neck pain; however, there is no evidence to support this use.

Mechanism of Action

Not applicable.

Dosage

The optimum dosage of kudzu is not known. However, the double-blind study in humans mentioned above used 1.2 g of kudzu twice daily.

Safety Issues

Based on its extensive food use, kudzu is believed to be reasonably safe. Maximum safe dosages in individuals with severe hepatic or renal disease are not known.

Safety in Young Children and Pregnant or Lactating Women

Maximum safe dosages for pregnant or lactating women or for young children have not been established, but there are no known or suspected risks.

Drug Interactions

None are known.

LAPACHO
(Tabebuia impestiginosa)

Alternate Names/Related Species: Pau d'Arco, Taheebo

Common Uses

Cancer [+1]   **Antimicrobial** [+1]

(Higher numbers indicate stronger evidence; X modifier indicates contradictory results. See page xviii of the Introduction for details of the rating scale.)

Approach to the Patient

The inner bark of the lapacho tree *(Tabebuia impestiginosa)* is used in South America to treat cancer as well as a great variety of infectious diseases. Although some in vitro data has demonstrated antimicrobial and antitumor activity of the components lapachol and beta-lapachone, there are no in vivo studies to evaluate the efficacy or safety of lapacho.

Cancer   +1

Lapacho has been shown to have antitumor properties. However, the high dosage required to achieve this effect is associated with significant side effects. Another component of lapacho, beta-lapachone, is being extensively investigated as an anti-cancer agent with anticipation that it will have a more favorable side-effect profile.[1]

Antimicrobial   +1

One in vitro study demonstrated antibacterial and antifungal activity of lapachol and beta-lapachone.[2] These findings have been used in support of lapacho's traditional use to treat candidal infections, infections of the respiratory and urinary tracts, and infectious diarrhea. However, there is no evidence that the herb possesses antibiotic properties when taken orally.

Mechanism of Action

Beta-lapachone is a DNA topoisomerase inhibitor that has been found to induce apoptosis in various human cancer cells. It appears to exert its inhibitory effects by a direct interaction with topoisomerase I rather than DNA substrate.[1] Additional in vitro evidence suggests that generation of intracellular H_2O_2 plays a crucial role in beta-lapachone-induced cell death and differentiation.[3] The enzyme NAD(P)H:quinone oxidoreductase (NQO1) substantially enhances the toxicity of beta-lapachone and appears to be its intracellular target in tumor cells.[4]

Dosage

For treatment of minor infections, the standard dosage of capsulated powdered bark is 300 mg three times daily until symptoms resolve. Because many components of the bark are not water soluble, lapacho tea is not recommended.

The inner bark of the lapacho tree is believed to be the most effective part of the plant. Unfortunately, inferior products containing only the outer bark and the wood are sometimes misrepresented as "genuine inner-bark lapacho."

Safety Issues

Comprehensive safety studies of lapacho have not been reported. When taken in usual dosages, it does not appear to cause any significant side effects.[5] Maximum safe dosages in individuals with severe hepatic or renal disease are not known.

Safety in Young Children and Pregnant or Lactating Women

Because its constituent lapachol is somewhat toxic, lapacho is not recommended for pregnant or lactating women. Safety in young children has also not been established.

Drug Interactions

Because of its mechanism of action, there is at least a theoretical concern that lapacho may interfere with conventional **chemotherapeutic agents.**

LEMON BALM
(Melissa officinalis)

Alternate Names/Related Species:
Cure-All, Dropsy Plant, Honey Plant, Melissa,
Sweet Mary, Balm Mint

Common Uses

Oral and genital   **Insomnia**   [+2]
herpes (topical)   [+3]

(Higher numbers indicate stronger evidence; X modifier indicates contradictory results. See page xviii of the Introduction for details of the rating scale.)

Approach to the Patient

Lemon balm is widely sold in Europe as a topical cream for the treatment and prevention of genital and oral herpes, and identical products are available in the United States. Preliminary research suggests that the treatment may be effective. However, patients can be advised that it has not been shown to prevent transmission of the disease in sexually active or pregnant individuals.

Oral lemon balm is widely thought to have mild sedative properties, but this has not been proven.

Oral and Genital Herpes   +3

A double-blind trial evaluated 116 patients with genital or oral herpes given either lemon balm cream or placebo for a period of 5 days.[1] The largest intergroup differences were seen at day 2 of treatment, showing statistically significant improvements in favor of the treated group. In addition, the total number of patients who were completely recovered on day 5 was significantly higher in the treated group than in the placebo group. Physician and patient evaluation of the course of the outbreak was also strongly in favor of the treated group.

Additional evidence for effectiveness comes from a double-blind, placebo-controlled study that followed 66 individuals who were just beginning to develop oral herpes.[2] Treatment with lemon balm cream produced significant benefits on day 2, reducing intensity of discomfort, number of blisters, and size of lesions. Long-term but somewhat informal follow-up by the same researchers suggested that the lemon balm application also delayed the next herpes flare-up.

Insomnia   +2

No clinical studies of oral lemon balm alone have been reported. However, the herb is often combined with valerian for treatment of insomnia. One double-blind, placebo-controlled crossover study of 20 insomnia patients compared the effectiveness of a lemon balm and valerian combination against triazolam.[3] The results showed comparable benefit in the two treatment groups and a significant difference from placebo.

Other Proposed Uses

Lemon balm is often used as an ingredient in cosmetics claimed to improve skin and hair.

In Germany, a tea made from the leaves is sometimes taken as a home remedy for fevers, flus, menstrual problems, muscle spasms, anxiety, and nervous headaches.

Mechanism of Action

The antiviral mechanism of action of lemon balm is not known. However, the leading theory is that the herb blocks virus receptors on host cells.[1] In addition, lemon balm extract also has the ability to inhibit protein synthesis at the level of elongation factor eEF-2.[4] This mechanism is reminiscent of that of the interferons, whose antiviral activity is attributed in part to inhibition of the protein synthesis initiation factor eIF-2.

Dosage

For treatment of an active flare-up of herpes, the proper daily dose is four thick applications of a standard lemon balm 70:1 extract cream. This can be reduced to twice daily for preventive purposes. See the Appendix for U.S. brand names of clinically tested products.

The most studied lemon balm product is Lomaherpan, an extract standardized by bioassay. During its production, human or animal cell lines are grown in vitro and infected with herpes virus; standard paper disks infiltrated with lemon balm extract are then inserted; and the commercial extract is standardized so that a dose of 200 mcg/disc forms a 20- to 30-mm zone of inhibition of viral cellular lysis.[1]

When taken orally, the standard dose of lemon balm is 1.5 to 4.5 g/day of dried herb, according to Germany's Commission E.

Safety Issues

Topical lemon balm is not associated with any significant side effects, although allergic reactions are always possible.

Oral lemon balm is on the FDA's GRAS (Generally Recognized as Safe) list. The Ames test (with and without metabolic activation) has been found negative with oral lemon balm tincture.[5]

Maximum safe dosages in individuals with severe hepatic or renal disease are not known.

Safety in Young Children and Pregnant or Lactating Women

None are known. Maximum safe dosages for pregnant or lactating women have not been established.

In addition, pregnant women should not regard lemon balm as effective prevention against transmission of herpes to the newborn.

Drug Interactions

Lyophilized hydroethanolic extracts of lemon balm have been found to produce dose-dependent sedation and potentiation of pentobarbital in mice.[6]

LICORICE
(Glycyrrhiza glabra)

Alternate Names/Related Species:
Deglycyrrhizinated Licorice, DGL, Sweet Root;
Glycyrrhiza glanulifera, G. pallida, G. tyica, G. violocea

Common Uses

**Peptic ulcer
disease** [+1]

**Expectorant/
antitussive** [0]

(Higher numbers indicate stronger evidence; X modifier indicates contradictory results. See page xviii of the Introduction for details of the rating scale.)

Approach to the Patient

A member of the pea family, licorice root *(Glycyrrhiza glabra)* has been used as both food and medicine since ancient times. However, it has no well-documented clinical uses.

Licorice possesses a variety of active ingredients. The most analyzed is glycyrrhizin, which is known to induce pseudohyperaldosteronism, impede conversion of cortisol to cortisone, exert estrogenic effects, and decrease testosterone levels.[8-12,27,29,30]

Patients may be advised to avoid whole licorice and use the safer product deglycyrrhizinated licorice (DGL) instead. This chemically modified form of licorice is widely available in the United States. In Europe, a combination treatment containing DGL and antacids is sold as the drug Caved-S.

Peptic Ulcer Disease +1

A 12-week, controlled trial (blinding not stated) using endoscopic evaluation compared antacids, cimetidine (220 mg tid and

400 mg qhs), geranylferensylacetate (5 mg tid), and Caved-S in 874 individuals with duodenal ulcers.[13] No significant differences in outcome were observed. However, considering that Caved-S contains antacids, this study might not actually provide evidence that DGL alone is effective.

In a single-blind trial, 82 individuals with endoscopically healed gastric ulcer were treated for 2 years with cimetidine (400 mg qhs) or Caved-S. The results showed an equivalent rate of recurrence in the two groups.[14] Again, the effectiveness of DGL alone cannot be determined from this study.

There is no evidence that licorice or DGL eradicates *Helicobacter pylori*.

Weak evidence suggests that DGL might protect the gastric lining from NSAID-induced gastritis.[15]

Expectorant/Antitussive   0

Whole licorice, not DGL, is used as an expectorant for respiratory problems such as coughs and asthma. However, scientific support of this therapeutic use is lacking.

Other Proposed Uses

Oral licorice (primarily DGL) is used to relieve the discomfort of aphthous ulcers. Whole oral licorice has also been suggested as a treatment for numerous other conditions, including menopausal symptoms. Creams containing whole licorice (often combined with extract of chamomile) are in wide use as a purported "natural hydrocortisone cream." However, while topical licorice has been found to potentiate topical steroids,[31] there is no meaningful clinical evidence that topical licorice alone has significant antiinflammatory effects.

Whole licorice has been suggested as a treatment for **chronic fatigue syndrome** (CFS), based on the hypothesis that individuals with CFS often have some degree of adrenal insufficiency and **hypotension.** However, other treatments to raise blood pressure have proven ineffective for CFS; in one double-blind placebo-controlled study, a 6-week course of fludrocortisone and increased dietary sodium to raise blood pressure found no improvement in 25 individuals with CFS symptoms.[16]

Glycyrrhizin has been used intravenously, especially in Japan, for the treatment of hepatitis B and C.[30,32-34]

Mechanism of Action

The most studied ingredients are the terpenoids glycyrrhizin glycoside (glycyrrhizinic acid) and its hydrolysis product glycyrrhetinic acid. These terpenoids exert significant mineralocorticoid effects, suppressing aldosterone secretion and plasma renin activity and increasing blood pressure in a linear dose-responsive manner.[17-20] Glycyrrhizin glycoside and glycyrrhetinic acid bind to mineralocorticoid and glucocorticoid receptors. However, because mineralocorticoid actions are not seen in adrenalectomized animals, other mechanisms of action have been proposed. These include inhibition of 11-beta-OHSD, an enzyme that catalyzes the conversion of cortisol to inactive cortisone[21] as well as displacement of cortisol from transcortin.[22] In order to avoid these undesired actions, licorice products with glycyrrhizin removed are sold as deglycyrrhizinated licorice (DGL).

Glycerhetinic acid may also possess antiinflammatory, antiviral, estrogenic, and hepatoprotective actions.[1-12,23]

An ester derivative of glycyrrhetinic acid, carbenoxolone, has been used to treat gastric and esophageal ulcer disease. Researchers have postulated that it may exert a protective effect by increasing mucosal blood flow as well as mucous production, and by interfering with gastric prostanoid synthesis.[24,25]

Although whole licorice root and its preparations are thought to have mucolytic and secretagogic properties, the mechanism underlying its expectorant action is unknown.[26] Like other sweet substances, licorice may exert an antitussive effect by stimulating salivation and inducing a more frequent swallowing reflex.[26]

Dosage

As an adjuvant therapy to conventional medical care for treatment of ulcer pain, the recommended dose of DGL is two to four 380-mg tablets chewed before meals and at bedtime. A similar dose is used for apthous ulcers.

For eczema, psoriasis, or herpes, licorice cream is applied twice daily to the affected area.

A typical dose of whole licorice is 5-15 grams daily. However, dosages this high should not be used for more than one week. For long term consumption, one researcher has argued that 0.2 mg of glycyrrhizin/kg daily is an appropriate upper limit.[36] Based on a typical 4% glycyrrizin content of licorice root, this is equivalent to about 0.3 grams daily for a 130 pound adult.

Safety Issues

When taken in high enough doses, licorice can cause signs of pseudohyperaldosteronism in as little as 14 days.[35,36] See the Dosage section for a proposed safe upper intake limit for long-term consumption.

Licorice may reduce testosterone levels in men.[27] For this reason, it is not recommended for use in men with a history of impotence, infertility, or decreased libido. Similarly, due to potential estrogenic properties,[8] licorice use should be avoided by women with a history of estrogen-sensitive malignancies.

DGL products would not be expected to exert mineralacorticoid effects. However, it is not known to what extent other side effects of whole licorice may occur with DGL.

Maximum safe dosages in individuals with severe hepatic or renal disease are not known.

Safety in Young Children and Pregnant or Lactating Women

Licorice's estrogenic and mineralocorticoid actions, as well as reports of lower gestational age at birth due to licorice use,[12] contraindicate its use in pregnancy and lactation.

Drug Interactions

Licorice appears to potentiate topical and oral **corticosteroids.**[9,10,11]

Because of its mineralocorticoid activity, licorice should be used with caution in patients taking **thiazide or loop diuretics,** or **digitalis;** in addition, licorice would be expected to counter the desired actions of **potassium-sparing diuretics.** DGL products would not be expected to exert these effects.

Preliminary evidence suggests that licorice may inhibit CYP 3A4, but the clinical relevance of this finding remains unclear.[28]

LIGNANS

Alternate Names/Supplement Forms: Flaxseed, Linseed

Common Uses

Chemoprevention   [+1]

Hyperlipidemia and atherosclerosis   [+1]

(Higher numbers indicate stronger evidence; X modifier indicates contradictory results. See page xviii of the Introduction for details of the rating scale.)

Approach to the Patient

Lignans are naturally occurring chemicals widespread within the plant and animal kingdoms. Several lignans (such as secoiso-lariciresinol) have phytoestrogenic properties, and these lignans are especially abundant in flaxseed. Intestinal bacteria convert them into two other lignans, enterolactone and enterodiol, which also have estrogenic effects. In this article, the term "lignans" refers to enterolactone and enterodiol as well as the phytoestrogen lignans, but not to the wide variety of other lignans.

Like other phytoestrogens, lignans have estrogen agonist/antagonist activity. Due to these effects, lignans are being investigated for chemopreventive effects in hormonally sensitive cancers, particularly breast cancer. In addition, at least one in vitro study suggests that lignans may exert chemopreventive effects in ways that are unrelated to estrogen.[1]

Preliminary research suggests that lignans may have antihyperlipidemic effects.[4] The richest source of lignans is flaxseed (sometimes called linseed), which contains more than 100 times the amount found in other foods.[10] Patients may not realize that flaxseed oil, however, does not contain appreciable amounts of lignans.[10] Other food sources of lignans are pumpkin seeds, whole grains, cranberries, and black or green tea.[7]

Chemoprevention   + 1

The most promising use for lignans may be as chemopreventives. Observational studies suggest that individuals with a higher intake of lignan-containing foods have a lower incidence of breast and perhaps colon cancer[7]; however, other factors may be responsible for this result.

Animal studies also suggest potential chemopreventive and possibly chemotherapeutic effects. Several studies in animals suggest that lignan-rich foods (including the lignans present in flaxseed) can inhibit breast and colon cancer[10-12] as well as reduce metastasis of melanoma.[13] In vitro studies with human cell lines also suggest that flaxseed or one of its lignans can inhibit mammary tumor growth[7] and that the lignans enterolactone and enterodiol can inhibit growth of colon cancer cells.[1]

Although this preliminary research is promising, the array of substances contained in flaxseeds makes it difficult to determine whether lignans are responsible for any of the observed effects. Animal and human studies have begun to examine specific lignans, and results seem to confirm that at least some of the positive effects are probably due to the lignans themselves.[1,10,11] More and better designed trials are needed to clarify lignans' precise effects or proper dosage in cancer prevention or treatment.

Hyperlipidemia and Atherosclerosis   + 1

Studies in rabbits found that both flaxseed and one of its lignans, secoisolariciresinol diglucoside, were able to decrease hypercholesterolemic atherosclerosis.[5,6] Although the lignan also reduced cholesterol levels, whole flaxseed by itself did not.

In contrast, several human studies, two of them double-blind, found that flaxseed reduced both total cholesterol and LDL levels.[3,4,14] However, it is entirely possible that other flaxseed components such as fiber, oil, or proteins, rather than the lignans alone, contributed to the effect.[3,4] Again, more research is needed to determine whether lignans themselves play a role in reducing cholesterol and atherosclerosis.

Other Proposed Uses of Lignans

Weak evidence suggests that lignans may be helpful for treating menopausal symptoms[7] and improving renal function in lupus nephritis and polycystic kidneys.[8,9]

Mechanism of Action

Like the isoflavones found in soy, lignans (or their metabolic products) have estrogen agonist/antagonist activity. This may be their primary mechanism of action. In addition, it has been postulated that the lignan enterolactone may influence the pathogenesis of prostate cancer via an inhibition of several steroid metabolizing enzymes, such as aromatase, 5-alpha-reductase and 17-beta-hydroxysteroid dehydrogenase.[15]

The ability of lignans and their isolates (such as secoisolariciresinol diglucoside) to decrease hypercholesterolemic atherosclerosis appears to be mediated through antioxidant effects as well as antiplatelet activating factor (PAF) activity. For example, one animal study suggests that lignans act as platelet-activating factor-receptor antagonists that can inhibit the production of oxygen radicals by polymorphonuclear leukocytes.[6]

Dosage

Effective dosages of isolated lignans have not been determined. In studies, flaxseed has been taken at doses from 5 to 38 g daily.

Safety Issues

Use of flaxseed as a lignan source has not been associated with any significant adverse effects.

In vitro studies have found both chemopreventive and cancer-promoting actions of lignans.[7] Use of large amounts of flaxseed or lignans in individuals with a history of estrogen-sensitive cancer, or at high risk of it, should be considered with caution.

Maximum safe dosages in individuals with severe hepatic or renal disease are not known.

Safety in Young Children and Pregnant or Lactating Women

Because of their potential effects on estrogen, pregnant or breast-feeding women should be counseled to avoid ingesting large amounts of either flaxseed or its oil.

One study found that pregnant rats fed large amounts of flaxseed (5 or 10% of their diet), or the lignan precursor secoisolariciresinol diglycoside, gave birth to offspring with altered reproductive organs and functions, and that lignans were also transferred to the nursing rats.[16] Additionally, a study in postmenopausal women found that use of flaxseed reduced estradiol and estrone levels, and increased serum prolactin levels.[17] Maximum safe dosages for pregnant or lactating women or for young children have not been established.

Drug Interactions

None are known.

LIPOIC ACID

Alternate Names/Supplement Forms:
Alpha-Lipoic Acid, Thioctic Acid

Common Uses

Diabetic peripheral neuropathy (intravenous)   [+3], (oral)   [−2]

Diabetic autonomic neuropathy (oral)   [+2]

(Higher numbers indicate stronger evidence; X modifier indicates contradictory results. See page xviii of the Introduction for details of the rating scale.)

Approach to the Patient

Lipoic acid (or alpha-lipoic acid) is a vitamin-like substance with antioxidant properties, which serves as cofactor in the mitochondrial dehydrogenase reactions that lead to the formation of ATP. It has been widely used in Germany for over 30 years for the treatment of diabetic peripheral neuropathy, and this use has received a great deal of publicity. However, patients may not know that the only substantial evidence for efficacy in peripheral neuropathy regards intravenous rather than oral administration of lipoic acid. Oral lipoic acid has shown some promise for treating cardiac autonomic neuropathy.

Lipoic acid has been extensively hyped as a "superantioxidant." Lipoic acid does have antioxidant effects, but considering that the case for benefits with other antioxidants such as vitamin E has essentially dissolved, this fact indicates little.

Diabetic Peripheral Neuropathy (Intravenous)   +3, (Oral)   −2

Lipoic acid has been found effective in diabetic polyneuropathy; however, this benefit may occur only with intravenous administration. Two randomized, double-blind, placebo-controlled trials of diabetic polyneuropathy with a total of 831 patients demonstrated the efficacy of 3 weeks of daily intravenous alpha-lipoic acid.[1,2] However, during the 6-month period of oral alpha-lipoic acid administration in the larger of these studies, no improvement over placebo was seen.[1] Positive evidence for oral lipoic acid is limited to open trials or trials with small sample size.[2-5]

Diabetic Autonomic Neuropathy (Oral)   +2

One randomized, double-blind, placebo-controlled trial of 73 diabetic patients with symptoms of cardiac autonomic neuropathy demonstrated modest improvement compared to placebo in individuals treated with 800 mg/day oral alpha-lipoic acid for 4 months.[5]

Other Proposed Uses

Pharmacologic studies suggest that lipoic acid may improve **other aspects of diabetes,** including insulin responsiveness, microcirculation, and sugar and protein metabolism,[6-10] although the clinical relevance of these research findings remains unclear. In the major clinical studies of lipoic acid, changes in blood glucose levels were not noted.

Lipoic acid might retard the development of **diabetic cataracts.**[4,11]

Lipoic acid has been popularized as a "superantioxidant" said to prevent heart disease and cancer. Although there is no doubt that it acts as an antioxidant in both polar and lipid solutions, there is no direct evidence for these therapeutic claims.

Lipoic acid may also be useful in the treatment of **AIDS**[12] and in **cirrhosis**,[13] but the evidence is minimal at present.

Mechanism of Action

It has been clinically observed that patients with cirrhosis and diabetic polyneuropathy have lower-than-normal levels of tissue lipoic acid.[14] Research has also revealed that diabetic neuropathy[15] and many types of degenerative CNS disorders[16] are contributed to, at least in part, by oxidative stress. It is now presumed that lipoic acid appears to act by reducing free radical–induced injury of both peripheral and autonomic nerves,[3] and it might retard the development of cataracts through the same mechanism.[11]

Early research suggested that lipoic acid raises levels of vitamins C and E and that some of its benefits might be mediated through its effect on these essential nutrients. However, studies of vitamin E–deficient mice found that lipoic acid decreased symptoms of deficiency without raising vitamin E levels, suggesting that the antioxidant properties of lipoic acid might allow it to act as a substitute for vitamin E.[17]

Dosage

The typical oral dose of lipoic acid is 300 to 600 mg/day, taken in two to three divided doses. For diabetic cardiac autonomic neuropathy, the dose is 800 mg/day of alpha-lipoic acid administered orally.

Lipoic acid is well absorbed and can be taken without regard to meals.

There is some evidence that the combination of gamma linolenic acid, found in evening primrose and borage oils (see the **Gamma-Linolenic Acid** article), and lipoic acid might offer synergistic benefits in the treatment of diabetic neuropathy.[18,19]

Safety Issues

In a study of 509 type 2 diabetic patients, an oral lipoic acid dose of 1800 mg daily for 6 months was not associated with a greater incidence of side effects than placebo and did not affect glucose balance.[1] Maximum safe dosages in individuals with severe hepatic or renal disease are not known.

Safety in Young Children
and Pregnant or Lactating Women

Maximum safe dosages for pregnant or lactating women or for young children have not been established.

Drug Interactions

None are known.

Based on pharmacological studies, there are some concerns that lipoic acid might potentiate the effects of **insulin,** although this effect has not been seen in clinical trials.

LUTEIN

Common Uses

Cataract prevention and retardation   [+1]

(Higher numbers indicate stronger evidence; X modifier indicates contradictory results. See page xviii of the Introduction for details of the rating scale.)

Approach to the Patient

Lutein is a carotenoid antioxidant that has been suggested as a preventive and retardive agent against cataract formation and macular degeneration. This proposed usage is based primarily on basic science as well as epidemiologic evidence regarding dietary sources. There are no controlled clinical trials supporting the use of concentrated lutein supplements at this time. Patients will most likely have difficulty recognizing the distinction.

Cataract Prevention and Retardation   +1

Observational evidence suggests that individuals consuming lutein-rich diets are less likely to develop cataracts.[1-5]

For example, one prospective cohort study (beginning in 1986 with 8 years of follow-up) of 36,644 U.S. male health professionals found that high lutein intake is associated with decreased risk of cataracts severe enough to require extraction.[3] Another observational study (beginning in 1980 with 8 years of follow-up) of 50,828 female registered nurses found similar associations.[2]

Other Proposed Uses

Weak evidence suggests that lutein supplementation may protect against age-related **macular degeneration.**[5,6]

However, one observational study found little association be-tween macular degeneration and intake of lutein or zeathanthin.[7]

Preliminary evidence suggests that lutein may protect against **atherosclerosis**.[8]

Mechanism of Action

Lutein is a yellow-colored macular pigment that may physically screen the retina and lens from shorter wavelengths of light.[5] In addition, lutein supplementation appears to increase serum lutein levels with a concomitant increase in lutein concentration in the macula of the human eye.[5] Lutein also may prevent mac-ular degeneration and cataract formation through antioxidant effects.

Dosage

Therapeutic dosage for lutein is not established, but estimates range from 5 to 30 mg daily.

Safety Issues

Although lutein is a normal part of the diet, use as a concen-trated supplement has not undergone safety evaluation.

Maximum safe dosages in individuals with severe hepatic or re-nal disease are not known.

Safety in Young Children and Pregnant or Lactating Women

Maximum safe dosages for pregnant or lactating women or for young children have not been established.

Drug Interactions

None are known.

LYCOPENE

Common Uses

Chemoprevention [+1]

(Higher numbers indicate stronger evidence; X modifier indicates contradictory results. See page xviii of the Introduction for details of the rating scale.)

Approach to the Patient

Lycopene is a carotenoid antioxidant related to beta-carotene, which is found in many of the same foods. Most, but not all, observational studies suggest that lycopene is one of the important chemopreventive factors in fruits and vegetables; however, controlled clinical trials have not been reported at this time. Patients may need to have the distinction explained to them.

Tomatoes are one of the best dietary sources of lycopene. This antioxidant is also found in watermelon, guava, and grapefruit.

Chemoprevention   +1

Observational studies have found that high dietary lycopene intake is associated with a lower incidence of cancer, particularly cancer of the prostate, but also possibly cancer of the lung, colon, and breast.[1-7]

One prospective cohort study followed 47,894 men over a 4-year period.[1] Subjects with a high dietary intake of tomatoes or tomato sauce (including that on pizza) had lower rates of prostate cancer. In an evaluation comparing these foods to others that were studied, lycopene appeared to be the common denominator.[2]

Epidemiological evidence suggests that lycopene may have preventive effects against lung, colon, and breast cancer as well.[7] In one study, elderly Americans who consumed a diet high in tomatoes had 50% fewer cancers overall than those who did not.[3] Animal studies have also found some chemopreventive benefits with lycopene.[4,5]

However, other observational studies have not found lycopene to be the primary chemopreventive compound in fruits and vegetables.[8,9] A small, randomized, placebo-controlled trial (blinding not stated) tested a concentrated tomato supplement containing lycopene as adjunctive treatment for prostate cancer, with results that suggested benefit.[11] However, lack of equivalence in baseline parameters between the verum and placebo groups makes the outcome difficult to interpret. Essentially meaningless uncontrolled studies have been widely discussed in the press as providing supporting evidence that the same supplement may be helpful for the treatment of infertility[12] and for the prevention of cardiovascular disease.[13] An in vitro study of breast cancer cell lines found chemopreventive properties with a tomato extract but not with lycopene alone.[14]

Other Proposed Uses

A small case control study suggests that lycopene may reduce the risk of **cataracts** and **macular degeneration**.[10]

Mechanism of Action

Although the mechanism of action of lycopene has not been clearly defined, its effects are presumed to be due to its antioxidant properties.

Dosage

The optimum dosage for lycopene has not been established. However, one study on lycopene and prostate cancer found indirect evidence that 6.5 mg is an effective daily intake.[1]

Safety Issues

Although lycopene is a normal part of the diet, there has not been any formal evaluation of its safety when taken as a concentrated supplement.

Maximum safe dosages in individuals with severe hepatic or renal disease are not known.

Safety in Young Children and Pregnant or Lactating Women

Maximum safe dosages for pregnant or lactating women or for young children have not been established.

Drug Interactions

None are known.

LYSINE

Alternate Names/Supplement Forms:
L-Lysine, Lysine Hydrochloride

Common Uses

Herpes simplex (prevention)   [+2X]

(Higher numbers indicate stronger evidence; X modifier indicates contradictory results. See page xviii of the Introduction for details of the rating scale.)

Approach to the Patient

Lysine is an essential amino acid that has been suggested as a treatment for recurrent *Herpes simplex*. While some evidence suggests that a daily dose of 1250 mg or more daily may help *prevent* herpes recurrences, patients may be advised that there is no evidence supporting the use of lysine for the *treatment* of a herpes recurrence once it has occurred.

Herpes Simplex   +2X

L-Lysine may have a dose-dependent effect on herpes prophylaxis, with benefits seen at 1250 to 3000 mg daily.

A double-blind, placebo-controlled study followed 52 participants with a history of recurrent herpes.[1] While receiving 3 g of L-lysine daily for 6 months, the treatment group experienced an average of 2.4 fewer herpes infections than the placebo group—a significant difference. When infections did occur, those in the lysine group were significantly less severe and healed faster.

A double-blind, placebo-controlled crossover study (two 6-month treatment periods) of 41 subjects also found improvements in the frequency of infections with 1250 mg of lysine daily, but not with 624 mg daily.[2] However, another double-blind, placebo-controlled crossover study (two 3-month treatment periods) followed 65 patients and found no benefit with 1000 mg of lysine daily.[3] Negative results were also seen using 1200 mg of lysine daily in a small parallel-design trial with 21 subjects.[4]

Lysine has not been found effective for treating acute herpes attacks.[5]

Mechanism of Action

Preliminary in vitro studies suggest that supplemental lysine may compete with arginine, blocking viral replication.[6]

Dosage

A typical therapeutic dosage of lysine for herpes is 1 g three times daily, taken either as a prophylactic treatment or at the first sign of recurrent symptoms.

The average dietary requirement of lysine is about 1 g per day. The requirement may be greater for athletes and individuals recovering from major injuries, especially burns.

Safety Issues

Although lysine is an essential part of the diet, the safety of concentrated lysine supplements has not been well studied. High dosages have caused gallstones and hypercholesterolemia in animal studies.[7,8]

Maximum safe dosages in individuals with severe hepatic or renal disease are not known.

Safety in Young Children
and Pregnant or Lactating Women

Maximum safe dosages for pregnant or lactating women or for young children have not been established.

Drug Interactions

None are known.

MAGNESIUM

Alternate Names/Supplement Forms:
Magnesium Chloride, Magnesium Citrate,
Magnesium Fumarate, Magnesium Gluconate,
Magnesium Malate, Magnesium Oxide, Magnesium Sulfate

Common Uses

Noise-related
hearing loss   [+3]

Coronary artery
disease   [+2]

Dysmenorrhea   [+2]

PMS symptoms   [+2]

Migraine
headaches   [+2X]

Renal calculi   [−2X]

Atrial fibrillation   [−2]

(Higher numbers indicate stronger evidence; X modifier indicates contradictory results. See page xviii of the Introduction for details of the rating scale.)

Approach to the Patient

Contrary to what your patients may have heard, most individuals in North America are thought to consume adequate levels of magnesium in the diet.[55]

Certain conditions may, however, lead to depletion of magnesium. These include alcohol abuse, diabetes, and inflammatory bowel disease, as well as use of thiazide or loop diuretics, cisplatin, or cyclosporine.[1,2,31,55,56,69,70]

While it is sometimes said that calcium interferes with magnesium absorption, it apparently has no significant effect on overall magnesium status.[3,4]

Preliminary evidence suggests that magnesium supplementation might have value in preventing hearing loss caused by high-decibel noise. Other proposed uses with some evidence include treatment or prophylaxis of migraine headaches, PMS, dysmenorrhea, and coronary artery disease. However, magnesium may interfere with the absorption of various pharmaceuticals (see Drug Interactions).

Noise-Related Hearing Loss   +3

A 2-month, double-blind, placebo-controlled study of 300 military recruits found that 167 mg of magnesium daily can reduce the incidence and severity of hearing loss caused by exposure to high-volume noise[7]; this is a surprising result, as the dosage of magnesium used in the study is significantly lower than the recommended daily intake.

Coronary Artery Disease   +2

A double-blind, placebo-controlled trial of 50 individuals with stable coronary artery disease (CAD) found that supplementation with magnesium at 730 mg daily significantly improved exercise tolerance, apparently by improving endothelial function.[8] In addition, the same research group conducted a 3-month, double-blind, placebo-controlled trial of 42 individuals with CAD and found that magnesium supplementation at 800 to 1200 mg daily inhibited platelet-dependent thrombus formation.[9] The effect appears to be independent of platelet aggregation and activation and is additive with aspirin.

Dysmenorrhea   +2

A 6-month, double-blind, placebo-controlled study of 50 women with menstrual pain found that treatment with magnesium significantly improved symptoms.[10] The researchers reported evidence of reduced levels of prostaglandin F_2 alpha. Similarly positive results were seen in a double-blind, placebo-controlled study of 21 women.[11]

PMS Symptoms   + 2

A double-blind, placebo-controlled study of 32 women found that magnesium taken from day 15 of the menstrual cycle to the onset of menstrual flow could significantly improve premenstrual mood changes.[12] Another small, double-blind study (20 participants) found that magnesium supplementation can help prevent menstrual migraines.[13]

Preliminary evidence suggests that a combination of magnesium and vitamin B_6 might be more effective for PMS than either treatment alone.[14]

Migraine Headaches   + 2 X

A 12-week, double-blind, placebo-controlled study of 81 patients found that daily use of 600 mg magnesium significantly reduced recurrence of migraine headaches.[15] Side effects included diarrhea (in about one-fifth of the participants) and, less often, digestive irritation.

Similar results have been seen in other smaller double-blind studies.[13,16] One study found no benefit,[17] but it has been criticized on many significant points, including using an excessively strict definition of what constituted benefit.[18]

Renal Calculi   − 2 X

Evidence suggests that magnesium inhibits the growth of calcium oxalate stones in vitro[19] and decreases stone formation in rats.[20] However, human studies have had mixed results. Although one 2-year open study of 90 individuals found fewer recurrences of kidney stones in individuals taking magnesium hydroxide,[21] a double-blind study of 124 individuals found that magnesium hydroxide was essentially no more effective than placebo.[22]

Atrial Fibrillation   − 2

A 6-month, double-blind trial of 170 individuals found oral magnesium ineffective for preventing recurrence of atrial fibrillation.[23]

Other Proposed Uses

Several studies suggest that magnesium supplements can reduce blood pressure in **hypertension,**[24-27] although other studies have found no benefit.

Magnesium supplements have been suggested to reduce complications of pregnancy such as **preeclampsia,** but the results of large double-blind trials have been mixed.[28,29] It may be that magnesium is only helpful for this purpose in populations with particularly significant magnesium deficiency.

An interesting series of studies suggests that the combination of vitamin B_6 and magnesium may be helpful in **autism.**[33-42] Preliminary evidence suggests that magnesium may counteract the increased atherosclerosis risk associated with use of hydrogenated oils.[43]

Magnesium deficiency appears to be common in **diabetes.**[30-32] Supplementation may therefore be indicated. However, magnesium appears to increase absorption of oral hypoglycemics, potentially causing a risk of hypoglycemia (see Drug Interactions).

Magnesium has also been suggested as a treatment for osteoporosis, hypoglycemia, glaucoma, fibromyalgia, fatigue, cerebrovascular infarction, low HDL levels, Alzheimer's disease, angina, attention deficit disorder, periodontal disease, restless legs syndrome, rheumatoid arthritis, and various forms of heart disease including mitral valve prolapse and congestive heart failure. However, there is no real evidence that it is effective for any of these conditions.

One small, double-blind trial found magnesium ineffective in **asthma**.[44] Studies on magnesium supplements for improving **strength** or **sports performance** have returned contradictory results.[45-52]

Mechanism of Action

Magnesium is an essential nutrient utilized in a great variety of physiologic functions, including muscular relaxation, blood clotting, and ATP synthesis. Its ability to block calcium from entering muscle and cardiac cells may be the basis for magnesium's effects on migraine headaches and hypertension.

Dosage

The U.S. Dietary Reference Intake (DRI) for magnesium varies with age and gender as follows: males 19 to 30 years, 400 mg; males 31 years and older, 420 mg; females 19 to 30 years, 310 mg; and females 31 years and older, 320 mg.

Multivitamin/multimineral supplements seldom contain complete nutritional doses of magnesium and calcium. If supplementation with these macronutrient minerals is desired, they must be taken as separate supplements. While there is no problem combining calcium and magnesium in a single tablet, simultaneous intake of macronutrient minerals may impair absorption of micronutrient minerals, such as manganese and zinc. For this reason, it is often suggested that macro- and microminerals supplements should be taken at least two hours apart. The extent of this absorption interference is limited, however, and simultaneous use, while less than ideal, should still provide adequate nutrient supplementation.

Therapeutic dosages of magnesium range from nutritional doses to 1000 mg daily. For the treatment of PMS and dysmenorrhea, magnesium is typically taken at a dose of 500 to 1000 mg of magnesium daily, beginning on day 15 of the menstrual cycle and continuing until the onset of menstruation. Note that these doses exceed tolerable upper intake levels. (See Safety Issues.)

Safety Issues

In individuals with healthy kidneys, there is a wide margin of safety with magnesium intake. The most common complaint is loose stools.

Tolerable upper intake levels (a conservative level of intake presumed safe for virtually all healthy individuals) for magnesium *supplements* have been set as follows: children 1 to 3 years old, 65 mg; children 4 to 8 years old, 110 mg; all individuals 9 years and older (including pregnant or nursing women), 350 mg.

In some cases these numbers are lower than the DRIs; that is because the ULs for magnesium apply specifically to supplement intake, while the DRIs apply to total dietary intake.

Safety in Young Children and Pregnant or Lactating Women

The tolerable upper intake level of magnesium *supplements* for pregnant or lactating women has been established at 350 mg daily.[57]

There is one case report of fatality caused by excessive use of magnesium supplements in a developmentally and physically disabled child.[58]

Drug Interactions

Magnesium can mutually interfere with the absorption of antibiotics in the **tetracycline**[59] and **fluoroquinolone**[60-65] families, as well as **nitrofurantoin**,[66,67] **penicillamine**,[68] **ACE inhibitors, phenytoin,** and **H$_2$ blockers.** To obviate this problem, doses of magnesium should be taken at least 2 hours before or after the dose of these substances.

As noted above, **loop and thiazide diuretics, cisplatin,** and **cyclosporin** may increase the need for supplemental magnesium.

Magnesium deficiency caused by concomitant use of loop diuretics may increase risk of digoxin-related arrythmias.[1-3,69,70]

Magnesium might increase the effectiveness of oral hypoglycemics in the **sulfonylurea** family, potentially creating a risk of hypoglycemia.[5,6,53]

According to animal studies, the **potassium-sparing diuretic** amiloride may reduce urinary magnesium excretion[54]; therefore, caution should be exercised regarding magnesium supplementation in patients taking amiloride.

MAITAKE

(Grifola frondosa)

Common Uses

Chemopreventive   [+1]

(Higher numbers indicate stronger evidence; X modifier indicates contradictory results. See page xviii of the Introduction for details of the rating scale.)

Approach to the Patient

Maitake is a "medicinal" mushroom classified by contemporary herbalists as an adaptogen, a substance said to help the body adapt to stress and resist infection (see the Ginseng article for further information regarding adaptogens). Although highly preliminary data suggest that maitake may have various degrees of chemopreventive, immunomodulatory, hypolipidemic, and other therapeutic effects, patients may be advised that there have been no meaningful human trials of maitake for any medicinal purpose.

Chemopreventive   +1

A review noted that more than 50 mushroom species have exhibited anticancer activity in vitro or in animal models.[1] However, there is little other scientific evidence supporting the efficacy of maitake as a chemopreventive.

Other Proposed Uses

Highly preliminary studies suggest that maitake may have a potential therapeutic role in **AIDS, diabetes, hypertension,** and **hyperlipidemia.**[2-4] However, as yet, there is no real evidence that maitake is effective for these or any other illnesses.

Mechanism of Action

Not known. However, most investigation has focused on the polysaccharide constituents of maitake, a family of substances known to affect the human immune system in complex ways.

One recent in vitro study examining the potential antitumor effects of beta-glucan found cytotoxic effects on prostatic cancer cells.[5] The authors postulated that apoptosis was a result of an oxidative stress mechanism.

Dosage

A typical dosage of dried maitake in capsule or tablet form is 3 to 7 g daily. Maitake is an edible mushroom that can be eaten as food or made into tea.

Safety Issues

Maitake is widely believed to be safe, although formal safety studies have not been performed.

Maximum safe dosages in individuals with severe hepatic or renal disease are not known.

Safety in Young Children and Pregnant or Lactating Women

Maximum safe dosages for pregnant or lactating women or for young children have not been established.

Drug Interactions

None are known.

MALIC ACID

Alternate Names/Supplement Forms: Apple Acid

Common Uses

Fibromyalgia   [−1]

(Higher numbers indicate stronger evidence; X modifier indicates contradictory results. See page xviii of the Introduction for details of the rating scale.)

Approach to the Patient

The Krebs cycle intermediate malic acid has been heavily marketed (in combination with magnesium and other nutrients) as a treatment for fibromyalgia. However, patients may be advised that the only reported double-blind trial of malic acid for fibromyalgia found it ineffective.

Fibromyalgia   −1

In a double-blind trial, 20 individuals with fibromyalgia were given either placebo or malic acid (1200 mg per day) combined with magnesium (300 mg daily).[1] After 4 weeks of treatment, there was no significant difference between the placebo and malic acid groups.

The researchers then gave all participants the malic acid combination and increased the dose over a 6-month period. A significant improvement in fibromyalgia symptoms was found after the dose reached about 1600 mg of malic acid with 400 mg of magnesium. However, because this part of the trial was not blinded, observer bias and/or the placebo effect quite likely accounted for some or all of the results.

Mechanism of Action

Use of malic acid in fibromyalgia may be based on extremely preliminary evidence which suggests that individuals with fibromyalgia might have difficulty creating or utilizing malic acid.[2]

Dosage

In studies and commercial products, the usual dose of malic acid for fibromyalgia is 1200 to 2800 mg per day, generally combined with magnesium and other nutrients.

Safety Issues

Malic acid appears to be safe at recommended dosages. A few individuals reported loose stools at the higher doses in the above studies, possibly due to the magnesium in the combination.

Maximum safe dosages in individuals with severe hepatic or renal disease are not known.

Safety in Young Children and Pregnant or Lactating Women

Maximum safe dosages for pregnant or lactating women or for young children have not been established.

Drug Interactions

None are known.

MANGANESE

Alternate Names/Supplement Forms:
Manganese Chloride, Manganese Gluconate,
Manganese Picolinate, Manganese Sulfate

Common Uses

Dysmenorrhea [+1]   **Osteoporosis** [+1]

(Higher numbers indicate stronger evidence; X modifier indicates contradictory results. See page xviii of the Introduction for details of the rating scale.)

Approach to the Patient

The metal manganese is an important constituent of many key enzymes.

Minimal preliminary evidence suggests that manganese supplements may have some therapeutic benefit in dysmenorrhea and osteoporosis.

Dysmenorrhea   +1

A very small, double-blind study looked at the effects of dietary calcium and manganese on menstrual symptoms in 10 women with normal menses.[1] Women were assigned to each of four 39-day dietary periods: 1 or 5.6 mg of manganese per day with either 587 or 1336 mg of calcium per day. Results showed that 5.6 mg of dietary manganese significantly decreased premenstrual mood and pain symptoms. A lower dosage of 1 mg daily was not effective.

Osteoporosis   +1

Although manganese is known to play a role in bone metabolism, there is no direct evidence that manganese supplements can help prevent osteoporosis. However, one double-blind, placebo-controlled study suggests that a combination of minerals including manganese may be helpful.[2] Fifty-nine women received placebo, calcium (1000 mg daily), or calcium plus a daily mineral supplement consisting of 5 mg of manganese, 15 mg of zinc, and 2.5 mg of copper. After 2 years, the group receiving calcium plus the mineral supplement showed better bone density than the group receiving calcium alone.

Other Proposed Uses

Manganese has been suggested for muscle strains and sprains, rheumatoid arthritis, and **tardive dyskinesia,**[3] but the evidence that it works for these conditions is very weak.

Based on the observation that individuals with **seizure disorder** have lower-than-normal levels of manganese in their blood, manganese supplements have been suggested as a potentially beneficial therapy.[4]

A similar situation exists regarding **diabetes,** in which manganese deficiencies have been noted, but no trials using manganese supplements in diabetes have been reported.[5]

Mechanism of Action

Manganese is necessary for normal bone metabolism as well as a variety of enzymatic reactions. This includes its role as a cofactor for the antioxidant enzyme superoxide dismutase (SOD).

Dosage

The U.S. Adequate Intake (AI) for manganese varies by age and gender. The AI for males 14 to 18 years is 2.2 mg; 19 years and older is 2.3 mg. The AI for females 14 to 18 years is 1.6 mg; 19 years and older is 1.8 mg.[6]

A typical dosage used in studies on manganese is 3 to 6 mg daily. It is sometimes recommended at a much higher dose of 50 to 200 mg daily for 2 weeks following a muscle sprain or strain, but the safety of this dosage is not known.

Simultaneous consumption of antacids or calcium or iron supplements may impair manganese absorption.[1-3]

Safety Issues

The tolerable upper intake level of manganese for adults has been set at 11 mg.[1]

Safety in Young Children and Pregnant or Lactating Women

The maximum safe dosage of manganese for pregnant or lactating women has been established at 11 mg daily (9 mg if under 19 years old).[1]

Drug Interactions

Simultaneous consumption of **antacids** may reduce manganese absorption.[2,3]

MEDIUM-CHAIN TRIGLYCERIDES

Alternate Names/Supplement Forms: MCTs

Common Uses

Fat malabsorption [+2]   **Weight loss** [−1]

**Athletic performance
enhancement** [+2X]

*(Higher numbers indicate stronger evidence; X modifier indicates contradic-
tory results. See page xviii of the Introduction for details of the rating scale.)*

Approach to the Patient

Medium-chain triglycerides (MCTs) are fats with 8 to 10 carbon atoms, which are absorbed intact, transported to the liver,
and directly metabolized. Because of these differences from
other dietary fats, MCTs have been tried as fat substitutes
for individuals (especially those with AIDS) with malabsorption
issues.

MCTs are also popular among athletes as a proposed quick energy source and performance enhancer, although there is little
evidence as yet that they really work in these capacities.

Fat Malabsorption   +2

Two double-blind studies following a total of 48 men and
women with AIDS-related fat malabsorption found significantly
improved fat absorption and reduced stool fat content with
MCT treatment.[1,2]

In another study, patients with chronic pancreatitis appeared better able to absorb MCTs than ordinary fatty acids.[3] However, digestive enzyme supplements were used in conjunction with the MCTs.

Athletic Performance Enhancement   +2X

A number of small double-blind trials have tested MCT administration as an ergogenic aid (either taken immediately prior to the onset of exertion or administered for some extended period of time before); however, the results have been thoroughly inconsistent.[13-19]

Weight Loss   −1

Some evidence suggests that MCT consumption short of ketosis might enhance thermogenesis.[6,7,20] However, a 12-week, double-blind trial of 78 individuals evaluated the substitution of MCTs for LCTs in otherwise equivalent low-energy diets and found no significant intergroup differences regarding loss of weight or body fat; post hoc subgroup analysis found some benefit in individuals with higher BMI.[5] Negative results were also seen in a similar, smaller trial.[4] One double-blind trial suggests that MCTs may enhance the weight loss effects of ketogenic diets, but only in the very short term (2 weeks).[19]

Other Proposed Uses

MCTs have also been used to promote ketosis. Preliminary clinical evidence suggests that this metabolic state may have potential therapeutic effects in **refractory seizure disorder,** especially in children.[8-10]

Mechanism of Action

The biochemical structure of MCTs allows them to be digested and absorbed more easily than other dietary fats, which is the basis of their use in malabsorption syndromes.

The rationale for use of MCTs as an ergogenic aid is their potential to provide more energy per gram than carbohydrates and in a more easily metabolized form than ordinary dietary fats.[11] Some evidence suggests that acute or chronic treatment with MCTs may spare muscle glycogen.[17,18] Regarding weight loss, there are indications that MCT consumption might enhance thermogenesis.[6,7,20]

Dosage

When taken as an athletic performance enhancer, MCT dosages of 85 mg daily are common.

Available as purified supplements, MCTs can also be eaten as salad oil or used in cooking (coconut oil, palm oil, and butter contain up to 15% MCTs).

Safety Issues

Studies in animals and humans have found that MCTs are quite safe when consumed at a level of up to 50% of total dietary fat.[12] However, some individuals who consume MCTs, especially on an empty stomach, experience annoying (but not severe) abdominal cramps and bloating.

Maximum safe dosages in individuals with severe hepatic or renal disease are not known.

Safety in Young Children and Pregnant or Lactating Women

Maximum safe dosages for pregnant or lactating women or for young children have not been established.

Drug Interactions

None are known.

MELATONIN

Common Uses

Jet lag [+3X]

Other forms of insomnia [+2X]

Perioperative anxiety [+2]

Cancer treatment [+1]

(Higher numbers indicate stronger evidence; X modifier indicates contradictory results. See page xviii of the Introduction for details of the rating scale.)

Approach to the Patient

The pineal hormone melatonin influences circadian cycles, and exogenous melatonin may be an effective treatment for some types of circadian disturbance. Meaningful evidence supports the use of melatonin for jet lag and perhaps for other forms of insomnia. One potential use of melatonin that may interest your patients involves its possible utility as an aid in falling asleep at a reasonable hour on Sunday night, after staying up late the two nights before. (See Other Forms of Insomnia.)

The optimum dosing schedule and long-term safety of melatonin are not established at this time.

Jet lag   +3X

Most, but not all, studies of melatonin treatment for jet lag have returned positive results.

In a large, randomized, double-blind, placebo-controlled trial, 320 volunteers who had flights over six to eight time zones received placebo or melatonin in a 0.5-mg immediate-release formulation, 5-mg immediate-release formulation, or 2-mg controlled-release formulation, once daily at bedtime for 4 days after the flight.[1] The immediate-release doses appeared to be more effective than the controlled-release formulation. Self-rated sleep quality, sleep latency, fatigue, and daytime sleepiness were all significantly improved with the 5-mg dose of melatonin. In addition, the lower 0.5-mg dose was almost as effective as the 5.0-mg dose.

Benefits were also seen in smaller double-blind, placebo-controlled trials,[2-5,51] including one study that found melatonin more effective than placebo but less effective than zolpidem.[5]

However, one double-blind trial investigating placebo versus three regimens of immediate-release melatonin treatment (5 mg at bedtime, 0.5 mg at bedtime, or 0.5 mg taken on a shifting schedule) for jet lag in 237 physicians reported no significant differences between groups for sleep onset, time of awakening, hours slept, or hours napping.[6] A much smaller double-blind trial also found no benefit.[7]

Other Forms of Insomnia   + 2 X

Melatonin may also be helpful for other forms of insomnia, although the evidence is weak or inconsistent in some cases.

Studies of melatonin for the treatment of insomnia related to shift work have yielded relatively unimpressive results.[20-22,53-55]

Other small trials have examined the effects of melatonin in insomnia in the elderly, yielding generally positive results.[17-19,52,53,56] However, the results have been inconsistent regarding which part of the sleep cycle benefited from treatment.

A 4-week, double-blind trial evaluated melatonin as a treatment for chronic sleep-onset insomnia in children.[8] A total of 40 children who had experienced this condition for at least a year were given either placebo or melatonin at a dose of 5 mg. The results showed that use of melatonin significantly improved sleep onset and other sleep measures. In addition, a double-blind, placebo-controlled trial of 20 developmentally disabled children with sleep problems in which melatonin (5 mg) improved sleep latency.[9]

Individuals who frequently stay up late on Friday and Saturday nights may find it difficult to fall asleep at a reasonable hour on Sunday. A small, double-blind, placebo-controlled trial found that this delayed sleep pattern caused a phase-delay in endogenous melatonin secretion, and that use of supplemental melatonin 5.5 hours before the desired Sunday bedtime improved sleep latency.[10]

A double-blind, placebo-controlled study of 34 individuals who regularly used benzodiazepines for sleep found that controlled-release melatonin at a dose of 2 mg nightly aided drug discontinuation.[11] (See also Drug Interactions.)

Some individuals find it impossible to fall asleep until early morning, a condition called Delayed Sleep Phase Syndrome (DSPS). Melatonin may be beneficial for this syndrome.[15]

Small controlled studies using melatonin have found improved sleep in ICU patients[13] and schizophrenics with disturbed sleep patterns.[14]

Perioperative Anxiety   + 2

In a randomized, double-blind, placebo-controlled study of perioperative effects of premedication in 75 women, patients who received either 15 mg midazolam or 5 mg melatonin had a significant decrease in anxiety levels before and after surgery, as compared to placebo.[23] Except for greater preoperative sedation in the midazolam group, the two treatments were equally effective.

Similar results were seen in a subsequent double-blind trial conducted by the same researcher with 84 women.[24]

Cancer Treatment   + 1

Melatonin treatment in conjunction with conventional treatments may improve results as well as prevent some of the side effects of cancer therapy.[25-29] For example, a large randomized trial including 250 metastatic solid tumor patients with poor clinical status studied the effects of melatonin treatment in conjunction with chemotherapy.[29] Patients received melatonin (20 mg/day orally) plus chemotherapy, or chemotherapy alone. The 1-year survival rate and tumor regression rates were significantly higher in patients receiving melatonin treatment with chemotherapy. In addition, concomitant use of melatonin significantly reduced the frequency of side effects such as thrombocytopenia, neurotoxicity, cardiotoxicity, stomatitis, and asthenia.

Other Proposed Uses

A large body of research suggests that melatonin levels decline with age.[30-32] Based on these findings, as well as animal research, it has been suggested that melatonin supplementation might combat the effects of **aging**.[33] However, the basis of this hypothesis has been questioned in a more rigorous, tightly controlled study of healthy older subjects, in whom no significant difference in circulating plasma melatonin levels was observed when compared to healthy younger individuals.[34]

A 6-week, double-blind, placebo-controlled study of 22 individuals with schizophrenia and tardive dyskinesia found that melatonin at a dose of 10 mg/day significantly improved TD symptoms.[16] Preliminary evidence from small clinical studies suggests that melatonin might be useful in the treatment of **mood disorders** and **epilepsy**.[35-37] In addition, melatonin has been hypothesized to be a potential treatment for individuals with **Alzheimer's disease**.[38] Even less convincing research suggests that melatonin may enhance humoral and cell-mediated **immunity**.[39]

Melatonin at 2 mg per day was found ineffective for **tardive dyskinesia** in a small 4-week, double-blind trial.[40]

Mechanism

Melatonin is thought to reentrain the circadian rhythm. This "phase-shift" effect on the circadian rhythm is dependent on the time of melatonin administration. Some evidence suggests that melatonin may act on the GABA chloride channel complex, mimicking the actions of benzodiazepines.[41]

Melatonin has been found to inhibit the growth of estrogen-responsive breast cancer cells in vitro.[42] Although the exact mechanisms are not known, it is believed that melatonin acts to down-regulate estrogen-regulated genes, thereby inhibiting growth of breast tumor cells. Additional studies report that melatonin modulates immune function in cancer patients by activating the cytokine system, which exerts growth-inhibitory properties over a wide range of tumor cell types.[43]

Dosage

Studies of melatonin for insomnia have employed various doses ranging from 0.1 mg to several milligrams daily, taken at or within 2 hours of bedtime. For improving ability to fall asleep at a reasonable hour on Sunday night after staying up late Friday and Saturday, one study suggests using melatonin 5.5 hours before the desired bedtime.[10] The optimum dose is not clear, but may lie in the range of 0.5 mg to 5 mg. In some studies of jet lag, melatonin use was begun prior to return home and then continued for several days; others started only upon return; and more complex dosing schedules have been tried as well, but the optimum schedule is not known. For presurgical anxiolysis, a 5-mg dose has been tried.

Melatonin is available in two formulations: immediate-release gelatin capsules that produce a spike in blood melatonin levels followed by rapid elimination and controlled-release capsules that more closely mimic endogenous release. The relative value of each type for various uses has not been fully elucidated, as both positive and negative results have been seen with each form. However, evidence from a small, double-blind trial in children suggests that immediate-release melatonin helps in falling asleep, while controlled-release melatonin helps in staying asleep.[44]

Safety Issues

Melatonin may reduce mental attention for about 6 hours after use and may also cause sedation and impair balance.[13,45] For this reason, the usual sedative cautions regarding operating machinery, for example, apply.

A safety study found that melatonin at a dose of 10 mg/day produced no toxic effects when given to 40 healthy males for a period of 28 days.[46] A study in postmenopausal women found evidence that use of melatonin might impair insulin sensitivity and glucose tolerance.[47] A comparison of 12 healthy volunteers and 12 sleep-disorder patients who had been taking melatonin for 1 year found differences in levels of prolactin and LH between the two groups.[48] However, because this was an observational trial, no information on causality can be inferred. Long-term safety remains unknown.

A double-blind, placebo-controlled study of postmenopausal women found evidence that melatonin use at a dose of 1 mg each morning for 2 days impaired insulin sensitivity and glucose tolerance.[47] However, a longer study using the more typical qhs dosing found melatonin safe and effective in diabetes.[12]

Maximum safe dosages in individuals with severe hepatic or renal disease are not known.

Safety in Young Children
and Pregnant or Lactating Women

Maximum safe dosages for pregnant or lactating women or for young children have not been established.

Drug Interactions

Benzodiazepine drugs may impair melatonin release.[49,50] In addition, melatonin may mimic some actions of benzodiazepines.[41] For this reason, it has been suggested that melatonin may be particularly useful for individuals withdrawing from benzodiazepine drugs.[11,18]

METHYL SULFONYL METHANE (MSM)

Alternate Names/Supplement Forms:
Dimethyl Sulfone (DMSO$_2$)

Common Uses

Osteoarthritis   [+1]

(Higher numbers indicate stronger evidence; X modifier indicates contradictory results. See page xviii of the Introduction for details of the rating scale.)

Approach to the Patient

Methyl sulfonyl methane (MSM) is a sulfur-containing compound chemically related to DMSO (dimethyl sulfoxide). However, despite widespread marketing, there is no meaningful evidence that MSM is useful for any medical condition.

MSM supplies sulfur. Some manufacturers claim that sulfur deficiency is widespread and that for this reason alone MSM will improve the health of almost everybody who takes it. However, patients may be advised that due to the sulfur contained in the amino acids methionine, cysteine, and taurine, sulfur deficiency is not likely to occur in individuals with adequate protein intake.

Osteoarthritis   +1

The case for MSM as an osteoarthritis treatment rests on one small, poorly designed, double-blind trial that failed to conduct a statistical analysis of the results.[2]

Other Proposed Uses

A set of three small unpublished trials have been used to claim that MSM is effective for the treatment of **snoring,** aiding the growth of nails and hair, and assisting in recovery from sports injuries.[1,5,10] However, the design and reporting of each of these small studies were significantly substandard, and the results were not subjected to any statistical analysis.

One study in mice found positive effects of MSM for **rheumatoid arthritis.**[3]

MSM has been proposed as a treatment for **interstitial cystitis,** to be used by direct instillation.[4]

Animal studies suggest that MSM might have **chemopreventive properties.**[6,7]

MSM has also been marketed for allergies (including drug allergies), constipation, excess stomach acid, and scleroderma, but there is no real evidence to support these uses.

Mechanism of Action

Not known.

Dosage

Dosages of oral MSM used for therapeutic purposes range from 2000 mg to 10,000 mg daily. Creams and lotions containing MSM are also available; however, because MSM, unlike DMSO, is not absorbed through the skin, it is difficult to rationalize such use.[8]

Safety Issues

MSM is believed to be nontoxic.[9]

Maximum safe dosages in individuals with severe hepatic or renal disease are not known.

Safety in Young Children and Pregnant or Lactating Women

Not established, although there are no known or suspected risks. Maximum safe dosages for pregnant or lactating women or for young children have not been established.

Drug Interactions

None are known.

MILK THISTLE
(Silybum marianum)

Alternate Names/Related Species:
Holy Thistle, Marian Thistle, Mary Thistle, Wild Artichoke

Common Uses

Alcoholic liver disease   [+3X]

Cirrhosis   [+3X]

Viral hepatitis   [+2]

Tacrine hepatotoxicity   [−2]

Protection against other hepatotoxic chemicals   [+1]

(Higher numbers indicate stronger evidence; X modifier indicates contradictory results. See page xviii of the Introduction for details of the rating scale.)

Approach to the Patient

Although the clinical evidence is somewhat contradictory, milk thistle *(Silybum marianum)* appears to be useful in a variety of liver diseases, including alcoholic liver disease, cirrhosis, and viral hepatitis.

Milk thistle is also sometimes used empirically as adjunctive treatment along with potentially hepatotoxic pharmaceuticals. However, this use is not yet supported by clinical evidence, and a trial of individuals using tacrine found no benefits attributable to milk thistle.

Patients with chronic hepatitis C frequently take milk thistle in addition to their pharmaceutical regimen. Unfortunately, there are no available data to indicate whether this is helpful or harmful.

Alcoholic Liver Disease   + 3 X

A 1981 double-blind, placebo-controlled study followed 106 Finnish soldiers with alcoholic liver disease over a period of 4 weeks.[1] The treated group showed a significant decrease in liver enzyme levels and an improvement in liver histology as evaluated by biopsy in 29 subjects.

Two other double-blind studies also found benefit with milk thistle.[2,3] However, a 3-month, randomized, double-blind study of 116 patients showed little to no benefit, perhaps because most participants reduced their alcohol consumption to some extent and 46% stopped drinking entirely.[4] A similar study found no comparative improvement in 72 patients followed for 15 months.[5]

Cirrhosis   + 3 X

Studies of milk thistle for cirrhosis have returned inconsistent results.

A double-blind, placebo-controlled study of 170 individuals with alcoholic or nonalcoholic cirrhosis found that in the group treated with milk thistle, the 4-year survival rate was 58% as compared to only 38% in the placebo group.[6] This difference was statistically significant.

A double-blind, placebo-controlled trial that enrolled 172 individuals with cirrhosis and followed them for 4 years found reductions in mortality that just missed the conventional 0.5% cutoff for statistical significance.[7]

Finally, a 2-year, double-blind, placebo-controlled study of 200 individuals with alcoholic cirrhosis found no reduction in mortality attributable to the use of milk thistle.[8]

Other double-blind studies of cirrhotic individuals have found reductions in liver enzymes and serum bilirubin,[9,10] although one did not.[42]

Viral Hepatitis   + 2

Small double-blind studies of patients with *chronic* viral hepatitis have found significant improvement in symptoms and signs in the milk thistle–treated group.[11-13]

A 21-day, double-blind, placebo-controlled study of 57 patients with *acute* viral hepatitis found significant improvements in the group receiving milk thistle.[14] A 35-day study of 151 patients with acute hepatitis using a no-treatment control group found no benefit with milk thistle, but this study has been criticized for failing to document that the participants actually had acute viral hepatitis.[15]

Tacrine Hepatotoxicity   − 2

A double-blind, placebo-controlled study of 222 individuals with Alzheimer's disease found that 12 weeks of treatment with milk thistle did not prevent elevation of liver enzymes caused by tacrine treatment.[16]

Protection Against Other Hepatotoxic Chemicals   + 1

Numerous animal studies have found that milk thistle extract can protect against the hepatotoxicity of substances as diverse as toluene, xylene, thioacetamide, praseodymium, polycyclic aromatic hydrocarbons, acetaminophen, carbon tetrachloride, phalloidin, and tetrachloromethane.[17-21] Benefits have also been seen in humans exposed occupationally to such chemicals.[22,23] Two small series found that intravenous silibinin, one of the four isomers of silymarin found in milk thistle, reduced the death rate from *Amanita* (deathcap) mushroom poisoning.[24,25] Based on this evidence of hepatoprotective properties, milk thistle is sometimes proposed as adjunct therapy for hepatotoxic drugs. However, as noted above, milk thistle has not proven effective for adjunctive use with tacrine.

Other Proposed Uses

One placebo-controlled study suggests that milk thistle increases the liquidity of bile and could therefore be helpful in the prevention of **cholelithiasis**.[26]

Silibinin has been investigated as a protective agent against **nephrotoxicity** induced by chemotherapy with the antitumor agents cisplatin and ifosfamide.[27] Animal studies suggest that renal protection can be achieved without interfering with the antitumor effect of these drugs.[28]

Mechanism of Action

The fruit of the milk thistle plant contains four isomers collectively named silymarin: silibinin (or silybin), isosilybin, silydianin, and silychristin. Silymarin appears to induce liver cell regeneration by binding to a subunit of RNA polymerase in the nucleus, displacing an intrinsic cell regulator and leading to increased ribosomal RNA synthesis. In turn, this leads to increased protein synthesis.[29] Other suggested actions resulting in hepatoprotection include displacement of toxins from liver cell receptors, interference with Kupffer cell oxidative burst and cytokine release, inhibition of beta-glucuronidase, liver cell membrane stabilization, increased liver cell reproduction, immunomodulation, free radical scavenging, and inhibition of leukotrienes.[9,10,30-35]

Dosage

The standard dose of milk thistle extract containing 70% silymarin is 200 mg two or three times daily. Some evidence suggests that silymarin bound to phosphatidylcholine is better absorbed;[36,37] the dose of this form is 100 to 200 mg twice daily.

Safety Issues

Milk thistle is believed to possess a very low order of toxicity and is generally considered safe. Animal studies have not shown any adverse effects, even with long-term, high-dose administration.[38] A 1992 study of 2637 patients showed a low incidence of side effects, limited primarily to mild gastrointestinal disturbance.[39] However, there have been case reports of severe abdominal symptoms associated with the use of milk thistle.[40]

Milk thistle is believed safe in individuals with hepatic disease. Maximum safe dosage in individuals with severe renal disease is not known.

Safety in Young Children and Pregnant or Lactating Women

On the basis of its extensive food use, milk thistle is believed to be safe in pregnancy and lactation, and researchers have enrolled pregnant women in studies.[41] However, maximum safe dosages for pregnant or lactating women or for young children have not been established.

Drug Interactions

There is one report that silibinin can inhibit bacterial beta-glucuronidase activity.[35] Based on this, alterations in clearance of agents such as **oral contraceptives** whose durations of action depend upon bacterial beta-glucuronidase in the gut might occur. The herb does not appear to affect CYP enzymes at realistic concentrations.

N-ACETYL CYSTEINE (NAC)

Common Uses

Chronic bronchitis   [+3]   **Angina pectoris**   [+3X]

(Higher numbers indicate stronger evidence; X modifier indicates contradictory results. See page xviii of the Introduction for details of the rating scale.)

Approach to the Patient

N-acetyl cysteine (NAC) is a modified form of the dietary amino acid cysteine. Based on its role in the synthesis of glutathione, NAC has become popular as an antioxidant supplement.

Good evidence suggests that adjuvant treatment with NAC can reduce acute exacerbations of chronic bronchitis. It may also augment or maintain the effectiveness of nitroglycerin.

Chronic Bronchitis   +3

A meta-analysis of available research focused on eight reasonably well-designed, double-blind, placebo-controlled trials of NAC for chronic bronchitis.[1-9] The results of these studies, involving a total of about 1400 individuals, suggest that NAC taken daily at a dose of 400 to 1200 mg can reduce the number of acute exacerbations of chronic bronchitis.

Angina Pectoris   +3X

A 4-month double-blind placebo-controlled study of 200 individuals with unstable angina found that the combination of nitroglycerin and NAC was more effective than either one alone in preventing death, MI, or the need for revascularization.[10] The mechanism of action is not clear. Unfortunately, combined treatment was also associated with a high rate of severe headaches, a side effect seen in other studies as well.[11] One small study found that NAC helped prevent nitrate tolerance, although another found no such benefit.[12,13]

Other Proposed Uses

Preliminary evidence from double-blind, placebo-controlled studies suggests that NAC may reduce the severity of acute respiratory distress syndrome.[14] It may also have a role in treating **septic shock.**[15]

A small 6-month double-blind placebo-controlled trial found suggestive evidence that NAC may be helpful for slowing the progression of Alzheimer's disease.[17]

Although NAC has also been suggested as an aid for reducing chemotherapy side effects and as a treatment for Parkinson's disease, there is no solid scientific evidence that it is effective for these purposes.

Mechanism of Action

NAC plays a role in the biosynthesis of glutathione. Its effectiveness in bronchitis has traditionally been attributed to mucolytic actions, but other mechanisms that may play a role include antioxidant effects and intrabronchial bacteriostasis.[1] In angina, NAC is thought to act as a sulfhydryl donor, correcting the depletion of reduced sulfhydryl groups that may play a role in nitrate tolerance.[10]

Dosage

The dose of NAC used in studies of chronic bronchitis has varied from 400 to 1200 mg daily. There is no daily requirement for NAC, and it is not found in food.

Safety Issues

NAC appears to be a very safe supplement. However, one study in rats suggests that 60 to 100 times the normal dose can be hepatotoxic.[16] Maximum safe dosages in individuals with severe hepatic or renal disease are not known.

Safety in Young Children and Pregnant or Lactating Women

Maximum safe dosages for pregnant or lactating women or for young children have not been established.

Drug Interactions

Although NAC may enhance or maintain the effectiveness of **nitrate therapy,** it can also increase headaches.[10,11]

NEEM
(Azadirachta indica)

Alternate Names/Related Species:
Holy Tree, Indian Lilac, Nim, *Melia azedarach*

Common Uses

There are no well-documented uses for neem.

Approach to the Patient

Virtually all parts of the neem tree *(Azadirachta indica)*, and its close relative *Melia azedarach*, are used in the traditional medicine of India. However, patients may be advised that there are no scientifically documented clinical uses of neem.

Other Proposed Uses

The traditional uses of neem are remarkably diverse. In India the sap is used for treating fevers, general debilitation, digestive disturbances, and skin diseases; the bark gum for respiratory diseases and other infections; the leaves for digestive problems, intestinal parasites, and viral infections; the fruit for debilitation, malaria, skin diseases, and intestinal parasites; and the seed and kernel oil for diabetes, fevers, fungal infections, bacterial infections, inflammatory diseases, fertility prevention, and as an insecticide.[1,2] However, there is no scientific documentation for any of these uses.

Mechanism of Action

At least 100 bioactive substances have been found in neem, including nimbidin, azadiracthins, and other triterpenoids and

 honoids. However, the scientific evidence for neem's poten-
al pharmacology remains preliminary and inconclusive.

Dosage

Because of the numerous parts of the neem tree used and the
many different ways these can be prepared, no single dosage can
be quoted.

Safety Issues

There has not yet been a full scientific evaluation of the toxicity
and side effects of neem and its many constituents. Maximum
safe dosages in individuals with severe hepatic or renal disease
are not known.

Safety in Young Children
and Pregnant or Lactating Women

Murine genotoxicity has been reported.[3] At the present time,
neem is not recommended for use by pregnant or lactating
women. Maximum safe dosages for young children have not
been established.

Drug Interactions

None are known.

NETTLE
(Urtica dioica)

Alternate Names/Related Species: *Urtica urens*

Common Uses

Benign prostatic hyperplasia (nettle root) [+2]

Allergic rhinitis (nettle leaf) [+2]

(Higher numbers indicate stronger evidence; X modifier indicates contradictory results. See page xviii of the Introduction for details of the rating scale.)

Approach to the Patient

Like saw palmetto, pygeum, and beta-sitosterol, the root of stinging nettle *(Urtica dioica)* appears to improve urodynamic parameters in BPH. However, evidence for the efficacy of nettle is not as strong as for these other treatments.

Many products marketed for BPH contain several supplements combined, each at an inadequate dose. Your patients may do better using a single-substance product that provides the dose found effective in double-blind trials. (See the article on **Benign Prostatic Hyperplasia** for several reasonably well-documented options.)

Nettle leaf (not root) is widely used for allergies based on one preliminary double-blind trial.

Benign Prostatic Hyperplasia   +2

In a 4- to 6-week double-blind, placebo-controlled study of 72 men, treatment with nettle root produced a 14% improvement in urine flow and a 53% decrease in residual urine, a significant improvement as compared to placebo.[1] Another double-blind study of 40 men found a significant decrease in frequency of urination after 6 months.[2] Finally, a 9-week, double-blind study of 50 men found a significant improvement in urination volume, as well as a decrease in sex hormone binding globulin (SHBG).[3]

Allergic Rhinitis   +2

In a double-blind, placebo-controlled trial enrolling 98 individuals with allergic rhinitis, participants received gelatin capsules containing either 300 mg of freeze-dried nettle leaf or similar-appearing placebo and were instructed to take 2 capsules at the onset of symptoms.[4] Sixty-nine individuals completed the study. Assessment based on diary notes of symptoms 1 hour after taking the capsules showed a marginal difference, and a global assessment questionnaire showed benefit in the nettle group; however, analysis of statistical significance was not reported.

Combination therapy with saw palmetto has also been evaluated; see the **Saw Palmetto** article for details.

Mechanism of Action

Nettle root contains numerous biologically active chemicals that may influence the function of the prostate, interact with sex hormones, and reduce inflammation.[2,5-8] However, a clear pharmacologic or therapeutic mechanism has not been determined at this time. The mechanism of action of nettle leaf in allergic rhinitis is not known.

Dosage

The recommended dosage of nettle root for BPH is 4 to 6 g daily of the whole root or a proportional dose of concentrated extract. Nettle root's effectiveness might be enhanced when it is combined with pygeum.[9,10] See the Appendix for U.S. brand names of clinically tested combination products.

For allergies, the proper dosage of freeze-dried nettle leaf is 300 mg twice a day.

Safety Issues

Detailed toxicological studies of nettle root have not been reported. In one study of 4087 individuals given 600 to 1200 mg of nettle root and leaf extract daily for 6 months, less than 1% reported mild gastrointestinal distress and only 0.19% experienced allergic reactions (skin rash).[7]

Maximum safe dosages in individuals with severe hepatic or renal disease are not known.

Safety in Young Children and Pregnant or Lactating Women

Nettle has a traditional reputation as an abortifacient, and therefore should not be used by pregnant women.[11] In addition, animal studies have found evidence of uteroactivity.

Maximum safe dosages for lactating women or young children have not been established.

Drug Interactions

Based on animal studies, it has been suggested that nettle may interact with **hypoglycemic, antihypertensive,** or **sedative medications;** however, there are no case reports of interactions.[11]

NICOTINAMIDE ADENINE DINUCLEOTIDE (NADH)

Common Uses

Jet lag [+2]

Chronic fatigue syndrome [+2]

(Higher numbers indicate stronger evidence; X modifier indicates contradictory results. See page xviii of the Introduction for details of the rating scale.)

Approach to the Patient

Based primarily on the fact that nicotinamide adenine dinucleotide (NADH) plays a role in energy metabolism, NADH has become a popular sports supplement. However, patients may be advised that there is no meaningful evidence supporting the use of NADH supplements for this purpose.

Preliminary evidence does suggest that NADH may have some therapeutic utility in jet lag. One study found some evidence of efficacy in chronic fatigue syndrome, but it was marginal at best.

Jet lag +2

In a double-blind, placebo-controlled trial, 35 individuals taking an overnight flight across four time zones were given either 20 mg of NADH or placebo sublingually on the morning of arrival.[1] Participants were twice given tests of wakefulness and mental function: first at 90 minutes and then at 5 hours after landing. Individuals in the verum group scored significantly better than those in the placebo group.

Chronic Fatigue Syndrome   +2

A double-blind, placebo-controlled crossover trial that followed 26 individuals with CFS given 10 mg of NADH for a 4-week period found some improvement in symptoms during NADH treatment as compared to the period of placebo treatment (31% versus 8%).[2]

Other Proposed Uses

Besides athletic performance enhancement, NADH has been proposed as a treatment for Alzheimer's disease and Parkinson's disease; however, the few studies that have been performed on these uses are highly preliminary at best.[3-6]

Mechanism of Action

Although NADH is instrumental in energy metabolism and in the endogenous production of L-dopa, no pharmacological or therapeutic mechanism has been established.

Dosage

The typical dosage for supplemental NADH ranges from 5 to 50 mg daily.

Safety Issues

NADH appears to be safe when taken at a dosage of 5 mg daily or less. However, formal safety studies have not been completed. Maximum safe dosages in individuals with severe hepatic or renal disease are not known.

Safety in Young Children and Pregnant or Lactating Women

Maximum safe dosages for pregnant or lactating women or for young children have not been established.

Drug Interactions

None known. Possible interaction with other dopaminergic agents has not been reported to date.

NONI
(Morinda citrifolia)

Alternate Names/Related Species:
Indian Mulberry, *Morinda officinalis*

Common Uses

There are no well-documented uses for noni.

Approach to the Patient

Noni *(Morinda citrifolia)* is a small evergreen shrub or tree of the plant family Rubiaceae. Traditional Polynesian healers have apparently used the fruit for many purposes including bowel disorders (constipation and diarrhea), skin inflammation, infection, mouth sores, fever, contusions, and sprains. The primary indigenous use of this plant, however, appears to be application of the leaves as a topical treatment for wound healing.

Noni has been heavily promoted for an enormous range of uses, including abrasions, arthritis, atherosclerosis, bladder infections, boils, bowel disorders, burns, cancer, chronic fatigue syndrome, circulatory weakness, colds, cold sores, congestion, constipation, diabetes, drug addiction, eye inflammations, fever, fractures, gastric ulcers, gingivitis, headaches, heart disease, hypertension, improved digestion, immune weakness, intestinal parasites, kidney disease, malaria, menstrual cramps, menstrual irregularities, mouth sores, respiratory disorders, ringworm, sinusitis, skin inflammation, sprains, stroke, thrush, and wounds.[1] However, patients may be informed that no human clinical trials have been conducted, and no animal studies have been performed that would approximate human usage of the plant.

Marketers claim that the key medicinal component of noni is an alkaloid called "xeronine."[1] However, a thorough review of the chemical literature does not substantiate the existence of such a compound, and the original discoverer of xeronine, Dr. Heinicke, did not publish any of his findings. The only information on the subject is found in promotional materials for noni.

Other Proposed Uses

Animal studies from Hawaii suggest that large (approximately 300 to 750 mg/kg total) intraperitoneal doses of a polysaccharide-rich substance extracted from noni fruit juice may have **anticancer** activity in the Lewis lung carcinoma model in mice.[2-4] Other studies indicate damnacanthal (a purified anthraquinone compound from a chloroform extract of the root) may inhibit tyrosine kinase and stimulate UV-induced apoptosis.[5] Whether or not these effects are related to the activity of the fruit extract in the lung carcinoma model is unknown.

An in vitro study from Japan found that high concentrations (5 to 20 g/ml) of damnacanthal may have **immunomodulatory** action.[6] The lyophilized aqueous extract of *M. citrifolia* root was evaluated in another study for analgesic and behavioral effects in mice.[7] This extract at intraperitoneal doses of 800 and 1600 mg/kg had **analgesic** activity in standard writhing and hotplate tests, which were reversed by the narcotic antagonist naloxone. Administration of doses between 500 and 1600 mg/kg of the extract decreased all behavioral parameters, suggesting general **sedative** properties. However, the relevance of these huge doses of extract to therapeutic oral ingestion of plant material seems very doubtful.

Mechanism of Action

Not applicable.

Dosage

Commercial products containing noni juice or a juice concentrate (in preparations that eliminate the odor or alter the taste for palatability) are widely available and heavily promoted. Tablets and capsules of the fruit and of the whole plant are also available.

The usual recommendation is the equivalent of 4 ounces of noni juice one half-hour before breakfast. For liquid concentrates, the typical recommendation is 2 tablespoons daily; for powdered extracts, 500 to 1000 mg daily.

According to noni promoters, noni should be taken on an empty stomach and apart from coffee, tobacco, or alcohol.[8] However, there is no scientific basis for this recommendation.

Safety Issues

There are no known side effects of noni, but no safety studies have been performed. Due to the lack of evidence, use of noni by individuals with severe hepatic or renal disease is not recommended. Potassium content (similar to that of orange juice) may be sufficient to cause hyperkalemia in patients with chronic renal insufficiency.[9]

Safety in Young Children and Pregnant or Lactating Women

Maximum safe dosages for pregnant or lactating women or for young children have not been established. Due to the lack of safety data, noni should be avoided in these groups.

Drug Interactions

Due to its high potassium content, noni might interact with **potassium-sparing diuretics.**

OLIGOMERIC PROANTHOCYANIDIN COMPLEXES (OPCS)

Alternate Names/Supplement Forms:
Grape Seed *(Vitus vinifera)*, PCOs (Procyanidolic Oligomers),
Pine Bark *(Pinus pinaster)*

Common Uses

**Venous
insufficiency**   [+2]

**Atherosclerosis
prevention**   [+1]

**Edema following injury
or surgery**   [+2]

(Higher numbers indicate stronger evidence; X modifier indicates contradictory results. See page xviii of the Introduction for details of the rating scale.)

Approach to the Patient

OPCs (oligomeric proanthocyanidin complexes), also called PCOs (procyanidolic oligomers), are flavonoid-like molecules found in numerous plants and food sources. Sources include grape seed *(Vitus vinifera)*, the bark of maritime pine *(Pinus pinaster)*, and red wine. Related chemicals are found in bilberry *(Vaccinium myrtillis)* and hawthorn (*Crataegus* spp.).

OPCs extracted from French maritime pine bark have been heavily marketed in the United States under the name Pycnogenol. Grape seed OPCs are less expensive and better studied. However, to make matters confusing, grape seed extract either alone or mixed with pine bark extract was originally named

772

pycnogenol, and non–pine bark products using this name are returning to the market. Furthermore, early studies of OPCs involved a product called Endotelon, which at various times contained grape seed extract and pine bark extract in different proportions.

Some evidence suggests that OPCs increase collagen crosslinking, stabilize the capillary wall, and reduce capillary leakage. On this basis, they have been studied for the treatment of venous insufficiency and edema following surgery. Other proposed uses of OPCs based on this mechanism include capillary fragility in cirrhosis, sports injury–related edema, easy bruising, aging skin, and purpuric syndromes.

OPCs are widely marketed for heart disease prevention based primarily on their antioxidant activity, as well as results of some animal trials. However, considering the failure of vitamin E and beta-carotene to demonstrate cardiovascular benefits when they were tested in intervention trials, it is not possible to meaningfully conclude from this highly preliminary evidence that OPCs truly offer any such benefits.

OPCs appear to be nontoxic and are generally well tolerated.

Venous Insufficiency   + 2

A double-blind, placebo-controlled study evaluated the effects of a grape seed OPC formulation (Endotelon, 100 mg three times a day) on 92 patients with chronic venous insufficiency over 4 weeks.[1] Although improvement of subjective symptoms and edema were statistically significant in the treated group compared to the placebo group, there was no statistically significant difference in venous plethysmography scores.

A 2-month, double-blind, placebo-controlled trial of 40 individuals with chronic venous insufficiency found that 100 mg three times daily of Pycnogenol significantly reduced edema, pain, and the sensation of leg heaviness.[2]

An unpublished placebo-controlled study (blinding not stated) enrolled 364 individuals with chronic venous insufficiency and found that treatment with grape seed OPCs produced statistically significant improvements as compared to baseline.[3] There was a lesser response in the placebo group, but whether this difference in results was statistically significant was not stated.

A double-blind, placebo-controlled study of 20 individuals found OPCs from pine bark effective.[4]

A 1-month double-blind comparative study of 50 patients with venous insufficiency of the legs found that 150 mg/day of grape seed OPCs was more effective in reducing symptoms and signs than the citrus bioflavonoid diosmin.[5]

Edema Following Injury or Surgery   +2

A double-blind, placebo-controlled study of 63 postoperative breast cancer patients with lymphedema found that 600 mg of grape seed OPCs daily for 6 months reduced edema, pain, and paresthesias.[6]

In a double-blind, placebo-controlled study of 32 facial cosmetic surgery patients followed for 10 days, treatment with grape seed OPCs produced a statistically significant difference in the rate of edema disappearance.[7]

A 10-day, double-blind, placebo-controlled study of 50 individuals with sports injuries found that grape seed OPCs improved the rate of edema disappearance.[8]

Atherosclerosis   +1

Numerous animal studies suggest that OPCs may retard or reverse atherosclerosis.[9-12] One crossover study of 22 subjects found that 100 mg of Pycnogenol or 500 mg of aspirin were equally effective in countering increased platelet aggregation caused by smoking.[13]

One often-cited epidemiological study found an association between *dietary* flavonoids and decreased cardiovascular mortality.[14] However, the primary sources of flavonoids in this study were black tea and apples, which do not contain large quantities of OPCs.

Other Proposed Uses

A small double-blind, placebo-controlled crossover trial found indications that OPCs from pine bark might improve **asthma** symptoms and reduce serum leukotrienes.[27]

An 8-week, double-blind, placebo-controlled study of 20 patients with **cirrhosis** found that 300 mg daily of grape seed OPCs significantly improved scores on the capillary fragility index.[15]

A 6-week open study evaluated the ability of grape seed extract to improve **vision** in normal subjects.[16,17] In this trial of 100 healthy volunteers, those who received 200 mg/day of OPCs showed vision improvement compared to untreated subjects. Parameters studied included night vision and glare recovery. However, the study was not blinded.

One crossover study of 22 subjects found that 100 mg of Pycnogenol or 500 mg of aspirin were equally effective in reducing **platelet aggregation** caused by smoking.[13]

An 8-week, double-blind trial of 49 individuals found no benefit with grape seed extract (dose not stated) for **allergic rhinitis.**[18]

A small double-blind, placebo-controlled trial found that grape seed alone had no effect on lipid profiles, but combined treatment with chromium led to significant reductions in LDL and total **cholesterol.**[19]

Pilot trials using OPCs extracted from pine bark suggest possible benefit in **SLE, HTN,** and **vascular retinopathies.**[28-30]

Mechanism of Action

In vitro studies suggest that OPCs increase collagen cross-linking, decrease capillary permeability, and block the effects of hyaluronidase, elastase, collagenase, and other enzymes that degrade connective tissue.[10,20-24] Decreased capillary permeability and increased connective tissue strength are the presumed mechanisms of action in most proposed uses of OPCs.

In atherosclerosis, possible mechanisms of action for OPCs include scavenging free radicals, inhibiting platelet aggregation, altering prostaglandin metabolism, and inhibiting cholesterol binding to vessel walls.[12,20,25] However, the clinical relevance of these largely in vitro findings has yet to be established.

Dosage

OPCs are generally taken in a dose of 150 to 300 mg daily for therapy of specific diseases, and in a lower dose of 50 mg daily as a general antioxidant supplement. See the Appendix for U.S. brand names of clinically tested products.

Safety Issues

Extensive studies have shown OPCs to be essentially nontoxic, with an LD_{50} in rats and mice exceeding 4000 mg/kg.[26]

In the double-blind studies of OPCs, no significant adverse reactions were seen, and the side-effect profile was similar to that of placebo.

Maximum safe dosages in individuals with severe hepatic or renal disease are not known.

Safety in Young Children and Pregnant or Lactating Women

Maximum safe dosages for pregnant or lactating women or for young children have not been established. However, in animal studies, OPCs appear to be nonteratogenic and nonmutagenic.

Drug Interactions

Based on the activity of other flavonoids, OPCs might potentiate **anticoagulant** and **antiplatelet agents.**

OREGON GRAPE
(Mahonia aquifolium)

Alternate Names/Related Species:
Mountain Grape, Holly-Leaved Berberis, *Berberis aquifolium*

Common Uses

Psoriasis   [+2X]

(Higher numbers indicate stronger evidence; X modifier indicates contradictory results. See page xviii of the Introduction for details of the rating scale.)

Approach to the Patient

The roots and bark of the shrub Oregon grape *(Mahonia aquifolium)* have traditionally been used topically to treat skin problems.

There is considerable inconsistency about nomenclature. According to some authorities, *M. aquifolium* is identical to *Berberis aquifolium*, but others point to small distinctions. *Berberis vulgaris*, commonly called barberry, is a close relative but is not identical. All of these, as well as other herbs such as goldenseal *(Hydrastis canadensis)*, contain berberine, a presumed active ingredient.

One study suggests that Oregon grape may be helpful as a topical treatment for psoriasis, but patients may be advised that dithranol appears to be more effective. It has also been proposed as a treatment for other skin diseases such as fungal infections, eczema, and acne.

Psoriasis   + 2 X

A double-blind, placebo-controlled study involving 82 individuals with psoriasis tested the topical application of Oregon grape on one side of the body versus placebo ointment on the other.[1] Participant assessments rated the Oregon grape ointment as more effective, but physician assessments did not produce significant differences between the two. One possible design flaw was that the treatment salve was darker in color than the placebo, possibly allowing participants to guess which was which.

In another controlled study (blinding not stated) comparing topical dithranol to Oregon grape, 49 participants applied one treatment to their left side and the other to their right for 4 weeks.[2] Skin biopsies were then compared with samples taken at the beginning of the study. The physicians evaluating changes in skin tissue were unaware which treatments had been used on the samples. Greater improvements were seen in the dithranol group.

Other Proposed Uses

Oregon grape has been proposed as a treatment for **fungal infections, eczema,** and **acne.**[3-5] However, no human trials have been conducted.

Many studies have been performed on purified berberine, but it is not clear whether their results apply to the whole herb. For more information on potential uses of berberine, see the **Goldenseal** article.

Mechanism of Action

Not known.

Dosage

Topical ointments or creams containing 10% Oregon grape extract are generally applied three times daily to the affected areas.

Safety Issues

Oregon grape appears to be safe when used as directed. In an open trial, only 5 of the 443 participants using Oregon grape reported side effects such as burning, redness, and itching.[6]

Maximum safe dosages in individuals with severe hepatic or renal disease are not known.

Safety in Young Children
and Pregnant or Lactating Women

Maximum safe dosages for pregnant or lactating women or for young children have not been established. However, berberine has been reported to cause uterine contractions and to increase levels of bilirubin. For this reason, oral consumption of Oregon grape should be avoided by pregnant women.[7,8]

Drug Interactions

None are known.

ORNITHINE ALPHA-KETOGLUTARATE (OKG)

Common Uses

Sports supplement [+1]

(Higher numbers indicate stronger evidence; X modifier indicates contradictory results. See page xviii of the Introduction for details of the rating scale.)

Approach to the Patient

Ornithine alpha-ketoglutarate (OKG) is a combination of the conditionally essential amino acids ornithine and glutamine. During periods of severe stress, such as recovery from major trauma or severe illness, they may become essential. In addition, they may have anabolic or anticatabolic effects.[4] Evidence suggests that use of OKG (and related amino acids) may offer benefits for some hospitalized patients.[1,5-9]

Based on these findings (and a leap of logic), OKG has been extensively marketed as an anabolic sports supplement. However, there is no direct evidence that it is effective.

Sports Supplement   +1

The only reported controlled clinical trial of ornithine as an anabolic agent for athletes evaluated a combined arginine and ornithine supplement; it did find some evidence of benefit.[10] The relevance of this finding to OKG isn't clear.

Mechanism of Action

Under conditions of severe physical stress, glutamine and ornithine may become essential amino acids, and this may explain
their apparent usefulness in hospitalized patients. The mechanism
of the apparent anabolic and anticatabolic effects, however, is not
clear, but may involve direct effects on protein metabolism. In addition, when taken in doses of 12 mg a day, but not at lower doses,
OKG may increase growth hormone levels.[3,11,12] It has also been
suggested that OKG increases insulin release, which would have
anabolic effects; however, this has been disputed.[2]

Dosage

A typical dose of OKG is 5 to 25 g daily. It may be necessary to
increase dosage slowly to avoid digestive upset.

Safety Issues

Because it is simply ornithone and glutamine, OKG is presumably safe. However, high doses (over 5 to 10 g) can cause diarrhea and stomach cramps.[11]

Maximum safe dosages in individuals with severe hepatic or renal disease are not known.

Safety in Young Children
and Pregnant or Lactating Women

Maximum safe dosages for pregnant or lactating women or for
young children have not been established.

Drug Interactions

None are known.

OXERUTINS

Alternate Names/Supplement Forms:
Hydroxyethylrutosides (HERs), Troxerutin

Common Uses

Varicose veins/venous insufficiency [+3]

Hemorrhoids [+2X]

Lymphedema [+2]

Postsurgical edema [+2]

(Higher numbers indicate stronger evidence; X modifier indicates contradictory results. See page xviii of the Introduction for details of the rating scale.)

Approach to the Patient

Oxerutins are a group of synthetic bioflavonoids derived from rutin. Like the citrus bioflavonoids diosmin and hesperin, oxerutins appear to stabilize the capillary wall. They have been most studied for utility in chronic venous insufficiency, but also appear to be useful for hemorrhoids, lymphedema, and other conditions. Oxerutins appear to be essentially nontoxic and have been given to pregnant women in studies. However, at the time of publication, oxerutins are not easy to obtain in the United States.

Many products marketed for venous insufficiency contain several supplements combined, each at an inadequate dose. Your patients may do better using a single-substance product that provides the dose found effective in double-blind trials. (See the article on **Venous Insufficiency** for several reasonably well-documented options.)

Varicose Veins/Venous Insufficiency   +3

At least 17 double-blind, placebo-controlled studies, enrolling a total of more than 2000 participants, have examined oxerutins in chronic venous insufficiency. All but one found oxerutins significantly more effective than placebo, providing substantial improvements in signs and symptoms.[1-13]

One large double-blind, placebo-controlled study published in 1983 enrolled 660 individuals with symptoms of venous insufficiency.[2] Three out of four participants were randomly assigned to receive oxerutins (1000 mg daily) while one out of four was given placebo. After 4 weeks of treatment, those who took oxerutins reported less heaviness, aching, cramps, restless legs, and "pins and needles" symptoms than those who took placebo. This report has been criticized, however, for omitting key information, such as whether or not any participants also wore support hose.

A more recent, better designed trial also found positive results.[3] This 12-week, double-blind, placebo-controlled study enrolled 133 women with moderate chronic venous insufficiency. Half received 1000 mg oxerutins daily, and the rest received matching placebo. All participants were also fitted with standard compression stockings and wore them for the duration of the study. The results showed that oxerutins significantly reduced lower-leg edema as compared to placebo; furthermore, these results lasted through a 6-week follow-up, even though participants were no longer taking oxerutins.

Oxerutins have also been found effective in treating impaired venous return in pregnancy.[14] There have been mixed results in treating venous stasis ulcers.[1,15,16]

Hemorrhoids   +2X

A double-blind, placebo-controlled study enrolling 97 pregnant women found oxerutins significantly better than placebo at reducing the pain, bleeding, and inflammation of hemorrhoids.[17]

Benefits were seen in earlier double-blind trials as well, although one study did not find benefit.[1]

Lymphedema   +2

Three double-blind, placebo-controlled studies enrolling a total of just over 100 women have examined the effectiveness of oxerutins in lymphedema caused by breast cancer treatment.[18] In one trial, oxerutins were clinically and statistically more effective than placebo at reducing swelling, discomfort, immobility, and other measures of lymphedema over a 6-month treatment period.[19] The comparative benefit improved with successive months of treatment. The two other studies found oxerutins to be statistically more effective than placebo, but the effects were clinically modest.[18,20]

Postsurgical Edema   +2

In one double-blind, placebo-controlled trial, oxerutins given for 5 days to 40 patients recovering from surgery significantly reduced swelling and discomfort.[21]

Other Proposed Uses

One small double-blind study suggests oxerutins may be helpful for reducing vertigo and other symptoms of Meniere's disease.[22] Oxerutins have also been tried in **diabetic retinopathy, diabetic neuropathy, diabetic microangiopathy, Raynaud's phenomenon, central retinal venous occlusion,** and as an **adjuvant to radiation therapy,** with some promising results.[1]

Mechanism of Action

Oxerutins appear to inhibit capillary filtration by reducing microvascular permeability, leading to improved microcirculation and reduced edema.[1] Oxerutins may also facilitate lysis of insoluble fibrin complexes around capillaries and stimulate local macrophage activity.

Dosage

In CVI, oxerutins or troxerutin (another rutin derivative) are usually taken at a dosage of 500 mg twice daily. For lymphedema and postsurgical edema, the typical dosage is 1000 mg three times daily.

Safety Issues

Oxerutins appear to be safe and well tolerated. In most studies, oxerutins have produced no more side effects than placebo.[1] The most commonly observed side effects are nonspecific gastrointestinal symptoms, headaches, and dizziness.

Maximum safe dosages in individuals with severe hepatic or renal disease are not known.

Safety in Young Children and Pregnant or Lactating Women

Oxerutins have been used in clinical trials of pregnant women, with no apparent harmful effects.[14,17,23] However, maximum safe dosages for pregnant or lactating women, or young children, have not been established.

Drug Interactions

There are theoretical concerns that oxerutins might potentiate **anticoagulants.**

PANTETHINE

Common Uses

Hyperlipidemia [+2X]

(Higher numbers indicate stronger evidence; X modifier indicates contradictory results. See page xviii of the Introduction for details of the rating scale.)

Approach to the Patient

Closely related to the nutrient pantothenic acid, pantethine has been investigated as a treatment for hyperlipidemia. Although study results are inconsistent and trials have been small, some evidence suggests that pantethine may be useful for hyper-triglyceridemia.

Hyperlipidemia   +2X

Most, but not all, small controlled studies reported suggest that pantethine can reduce total triglyceride levels by about 30% and also improve cholesterol profile as well.[1-5] For example, a double-blind, placebo-controlled crossover study followed 29 individuals with high cholesterol and triglycerides for 8 weeks each of treatment with placebo or pantethine (300 mg three times daily).[1] The results showed most striking improvements in triglyceride levels, as well as smaller improvements in LDL and HDL levels. However, large trials have not been reported.

Mechanism of Action

Pantethine is a stable form of pantetheine, a precursor of coenzyme A, which in turn plays a role in lipid metabolism.

Dosage

The typical recommended dosage of pantethine is 300 mg three times daily.

Safety Issues

In controlled trials, no significant side effects have been reported for pantethine.

Maximum safe dosages in individuals with severe hepatic or renal disease are not known.

Safety in Young Children and Pregnant or Lactating Women

Maximum safe dosages for pregnant or lactating women or for young children have not been established.

Drug Interactions

None are known.

PASSIONFLOWER
(Passiflora incarnata)

Alternate Names/Related Species:
Granadilla, Maypop, Passion Vine

Common Uses

Anxiety [+2]   **Opiate withdrawal** [+1]

(Higher numbers indicate stronger evidence; X modifier indicates contradictory results. See page xviii of the Introduction for details of the rating scale.)

Approach to the Patient

Passionflower *(Passiflora incarnata)* is widely used as a component of "relaxing" beverage teas. Preliminary evidence suggests that passionflower may be helpful for the treatment of anxiety, as well as an aid in opiate withdrawal.

Anxiety   +2

Animal studies suggest that the leaves and stems of passionflower have sedative effects.[1-3,7]

A double-blind trial of 36 individuals compared a passionflower extract (45 drops per day) against oxazepam (30 mg/day) for the treatment of generalized anxiety disorder.[8] Oxazepam showed a more rapid onset of action, but by the end of the 4-week trial both treatments resulted in statistically equivalent improvements in HAM-A scores. Oxazepam use was associated with more problems relating to job performance.

Opiate Withdrawal   +1

A double-blind trial of 65 individuals addicted to opiate drugs compared the effectiveness of clonidine plus passionflower versus clonidine plus placebo.[9] The results over 14 days suggest that use of passionflower offered no additional benefit regarding physical symptoms of withdrawal, but did reduce subjective symptoms such as drug craving, anxiety, irritability, agitation, and dysphoria.

Mechanism of Action

The alkaloids harman and harmaline found in passionflower may possess MAO inhibitory activity.[5] Maltol, also found in passionflower, has sedative effects in mice.[3]

Dosage

Passionflower tinctures and extracts should be taken according to the label instructions. The dosage of dried passionflower is 1 cup three times daily of a tea made by steeping 1 teaspoon of the dried leaves for 10 to 15 minutes.

Safety Issues

Passionflower is on the FDA's GRAS (Generally Recognized as Safe) list. There are five case reports from Norway of individuals becoming temporarily mentally impaired from a combination herbal product containing passionflower;[6] however, it is not clear to what extent the passionflower constituent was responsible.

Maximum safe dosages in individuals with severe hepatic or renal disease are not known.

Safety in Young Children
and Pregnant or Lactating Women

The alkaloids harman and harmaline found in passionflower may possess uterotropic activity.[5] Based on this, passionflower should be avoided during pregnancy.

Maximum safe dosages for young children or lactating women have not been established.

Drug Interactions

Passionflower might potentiate **sedative medications.**[1-3]

PC-SPES

(Combination: *Isatis indigotica, Glycyrrhiza glabra,
Panax pseudoginseng, Ganoderma lucidium,
Scutellaria baicalensis, Dendranthema morifolium,
Robdosia rubescens,* and *Serenoa repens*)

Common Uses

Prostate cancer   [+1]

*(Higher numbers indicate stronger evidence; X modifier indicates contradic-
tory results. See page xviii of the Introduction for details of the rating scale.)*

Approach to the Patient

PC-SPES is said to be a formulation of eight ingredients: seven
are herbs and one is a fungus. The name is derived from the
common abbreviation for prostate cancer (PC) and the Latin
word *spes* meaning hope. After its commercial launch in 1996,
PC-SPES received increasing interest from the general public
and prostate cancer researchers, and preliminary research appeared to indicate genuine benefits in prostate cancer.

However, a chemical analysis reported in 2002 disclosed that
PC-SPES is not truly a purely herbal product: batches going
back to 1996 were found to contain diethylstilbestrol, indomethacin, and warfarin.[11] Samples subsequent to 1999 were
found to contain less DES, but, interestingly, they showed less
efficacy in treating prostate cancer.

Patients may not be aware of these facts, and may wish to try
PC-SPES—at least until the situation is explained to them.

Prostate Cancer   +1

In vitro studies found that PC-SPES decreases cancer cell growth and promotes apoptosis.[1-4] In a rat study, PC-SPES treatment reduced the occurrence of prostate cancer, inhibited tumor growth, and slowed the rate of lung metastasis.[5]

In one uncontrolled human study, PC-SPES produced a significant decrease in PSA levels for most of the 33 volunteers tested.[4] An uncontrolled study of eight individuals with hormone-sensitive prostate cancer showed that PC-SPES decreased blood levels not only of PSA, but also of testosterone;[6] this finding indicates significant hormonal activity and raises safety concerns (see Safety Issues). Benefits for androgen-independent prostate cancer were also seen in another study.[7]

Another uncontrolled clinical trial followed 16 individuals with hormone-insensitive prostate cancer for a period of 5 months.[8] The results showed decreased PSA levels and also a reduction in pain and use of analgesic medication. However, because this was not a controlled study, it is quite likely that the reported pain reduction was largely due to placebo effect.

The most extensive study reported to date is an ongoing clinical trial involving 60 individuals, half with hormone-insensitive and half with hormone-sensitive prostate cancer.[9] A preliminary presentation of the results indicated that all of the participants with hormone-sensitive PC and over half of those with hormone-insensitive PC showed significantly decreased PSA levels.[9] Additionally, benefits were seen in individuals for whom conventional chemotherapy had ceased to be effective.

Mechanism of Action

Presumably, DES is the active ingredient in PC-SPES.

Dosage

The standard dosage of PC-SPES is 6 to 9 capsules (320 mg each) per day, taken on an empty stomach at least 2 hours before or after meals.

Safety Issues

Not surprisingly, dose-related side effects of PC-SPES resemble those of estrogen when taken by men for the treatment of prostate cancer[10]; these include breast or nipple tenderness or swelling, loss of body hair, hot flashes, loss of libido, leg cramps, nausea and vomiting, and thrombophlebitis.[9] There was one case report of acquired bleeding diathesis associated with use of PC-SPES at twice the recommended dose, presumably due to its warfarin content.[6]

Safety in Young Children and Pregnant or Lactating Women

PC-SPES should not be used by young children or pregnant or lactating women.

Drug Interactions

PC-SPES might be expected to present all the same risks of drug interactions as estrogen, warfarin, and indomethacin.

PEPPERMINT
(Mentha piperita)

Alternate Names/Related Species: Brandy Mint, Lamb Mint

Common Uses

Irritable bowel syndrome [+3X]

Intestinal spasm during barium enema [+3]

(Higher numbers indicate stronger evidence; X modifier indicates contradictory results. See page xviii of the Introduction for details of the rating scale.)

Approach to the Patient

Mixed evidence suggests that enteric-coated oil of peppermint *(Mentha piperita)* may be useful in irritable bowel syndrome and other forms of intestinal spasm.

Patients should be advised that peppermint oil is not an entirely benign substance. If not enteric coated, it can cause severe gastric distress. It can also be toxic in infants and should not be used for the treatment of colic.

Irritable Bowel Syndrome   +3X

Clinical evidence regarding the use of peppermint in irritable bowel syndrome is mixed.

Several double-blind studies, involving a total of about 240 individuals with irritable bowel syndrome, found evidence that peppermint provides relief from crampy abdominal pain.[1-5] In the largest of these, 110 individuals with irritable bowel syndrome were given either enteric-coated peppermint oil (187 mg) or placebo three to four times daily, 15 to 30 minutes before meals, for 4 weeks.[3] The results in the 101 individuals who completed the trial showed significant improvements in abdominal pain, distension, stool frequency, borborygmi, and flatulence. However, smaller double-blind studies involving a total of more than 90 individuals failed to find significant improvement in symptoms as compared to placebo.[5-7] A meta-analysis concluded that while clinical trials suggest efficacy, the methodological quality of those trials was, on average, poor, preventing firm conclusions from being drawn.[16]

Intestinal Spasm During Barium Enema +3

A double-blind, controlled study of 141 individuals found that adding peppermint oil to the barium solution reduced the amount of intestinal spasm during barium enema.[8]

Other Proposed Uses

Limited evidence suggests that peppermint extracts might be helpful for **gallstones.**[9,10]

Peppermint is sometimes recommended for the treatment of excessive intestinal carriage of candida, but there is as yet no real evidence that it is effective. Menthol-containing products are used in vaporizers and salves as comfort treatments for respiratory infections.

Mechanism of Action

Menthol is the presumed primary ingredient in peppermint oil. Studies have found that very low dilutions of menthol relax gastrointestinal smooth muscle.[11-13]

Dosage

The studied dosage of peppermint oil for treating irritable bowel syndrome is 0.2 to 0.4 ml three times a day in enteric-coated capsules.

Safety Issues

At the normal dosage, enteric-coated peppermint oil is believed to be reasonably safe in healthy adults.[14,15] Nonenteric-coated peppermint oil can cause heartburn,[1,6] and the inhalation of menthol may cause laryngoconstriction and hypersensitivity reactions in some individuals.[15] In animal studies, excessive intake of peppermint oil has caused nephropathy and damage to the cerebellum.[15]

Maximum safe dosages in individuals with severe hepatic or renal disease are not known.

Safety in Young Children and Pregnant or Lactating Women

Maximum safe dosages for pregnant or lactating women or for young children have not been established. Peppermint can also cause jaundice in newborns.[15]

Drug Interactions

None are known.

PHENYLALANINE
(D- OR DL-)

Common Uses

Depression [+2] **Chronic pain** [−1X]

(Higher numbers indicate stronger evidence; X modifier indicates contradictory results. See page xviii of the Introduction for details of the rating scale.)

Approach to the Patient

L-phenylalanine is the nutritional form of phenylalanine. However, weak evidence indicates that D- (or DL-) phenylalanine may have antidepressant effects. D-phenylalanine has also been advocated as a treatment for chronic pain, but the evidence is more negative than positive.

Depression +2

Two 30-day, double-blind comparative studies enrolling a total of 100 patients with depression found D- or DL-phenylalanine (100 to 200 mg daily) as effective as equal doses of imipramine.[1,2]

Chronic Pain −1X

Preliminary evidence has suggested possible analgesic actions of D-phenylalanine[3,4]; however, these studies have been criticized for serious flaws in design.[5] Another small study found no benefit.[6]

Other Proposed Uses

In the 1970s, D-phenylalanine was tried as a treatment for **Parkinson's disease**,[7] but there have not been any follow-up studies (see Drug Interactions for precautions). Although it is sometimes proposed as a treatment for **attention deficit disorder,** study results have not been encouraging.[12,13]

Mechanism of Action

D-phenylalanine cannot be incorporated into protein and is instead metabolized into phenylethylamine,[2] a substance believed to exert stimulant effects.[8,9] In addition, D-phenylalanine may block enkephalinase, increasing enkephalin levels.[3]

Dosage

D- or DL-phenylalanine is usually used at a dose of 100 to 200 mg daily when taken for depression.

Safety Issues

Use of D- or DL-phenylalanine has not been associated with any serious adverse effects. However, long-term safety of high-dose supplementation has not been evaluated.

Maximum safe dosages in individuals with severe hepatic or renal disease are not known.

Safety in Young Children and Pregnant or Lactating Women

The maximum safe dose of D- or DL-phenylalanine for pregnant or lactating women or for young children has not been established.

Drug Interactions

There are some indications that the combined use of phenylalanine with **antipsychotic drugs** might increase the risk of developing tardive dyskinesia.[10,14,15]

PHOSPHATIDYLCHOLINE

Alternate Names/Supplement Forms:
Choline, Egg Lecithin, Lecithin, Soy Lecithin

Common Uses

Hepatic disease [+3X]   **Hyperlipidemia** [−1]

**Alzheimer's disease
(and other neurological
and psychological
disorders)** [−1X]

(Higher numbers indicate stronger evidence; X modifier indicates contradictory results. See page xviii of the Introduction for details of the rating scale.)

Approach to the Patient

Phosphatidylcholine is the presumed active ingredient in lecithin supplements. When taken orally, it is degraded into the essential nutrient choline. This article discusses investigations involving all three substances.

In Europe, phosphatidylcholine is used to treat hepatic diseases such as alcoholic fatty liver, alcoholic hepatitis, cirrhosis, and viral hepatitis. However, while there is some evidence from animal and human studies that it may be helpful for these conditions, other studies found no benefit.

More recently, phosphatidylcholine/lecithin has been proposed as a treatment for various psychological and neurological diseases such as Alzheimer's, tardive dyskinesia, and bipolar disorder, although there is little evidence that it is effective.

Lecithin has long been a popular treatment for hypercholes-terolemia. However, again there is little real evidence to support this therapeutic use.

Hepatic Disease   + 3 X

Numerous studies have found that diets extremely low in choline lead to impaired hepatic function.[1-6] Currently, the degree to which additional choline may benefit individuals with preexisting liver damage is an area of ongoing research.

One multicenter, randomized, double-blind, placebo-controlled trial evaluated the effects of polyunsaturated phosphatidyl-choline in combination with interferon alpha 2a or 2b in 176 patients with chronic hepatitis B or C.[7] In addition to their designated subcutaneous interferon doses, patients received either 1.8 g of phosphatidylcholine or placebo daily for 24 weeks. The study found a significant reduction in serum ALT levels in patients receiving phosphatidylcholine compared to the placebo group. In addition, phosphatidylcholine significantly increased the response rate to interferon in patients with hepatitis C, although it did not alter the response to interferon in patients with hepatitis B.

Another prospective double-blind trial of 15 patients with HBsAg-negative chronic active hepatitis evaluated the effects of polyunsaturated phosphatidylcholine therapy (3 g/day) or placebo given in conjunction with normal maintenance immunosuppressive therapy.[8] Histologic evidence of disease activity was significantly reduced in the phosphatidylcholine-treated group.

Evidence from animal and other preliminary human trials suggests that lecithin might be helpful in a variety of hepatic diseases including acute viral hepatitis, TPN-induced steatosis, and alcohol-induced fibrosis, cirrhosis, and fatty liver, although not all studies have had positive results.[2,9-15]

Alzheimer's Disease (and Other Neurological and Psychological Disorders) −1X

Lecithin, phosphatidylcholine, and choline have been studied in individuals with Alzheimer's disease and other neurological and psychological conditions. None of these supplements taken alone appears to diminish Alzheimer's symptoms,[16-20] nor do they appear to improve normal memory and cognition, or symptoms of tardive dyskinesia.[21-27]

However, a 1989 Canadian study suggests that lecithin may offer benefit for Alzheimer's disease when given in combination with tetrahydroaminoacridine (THA), a drug that effectively improves symptoms associated with Alzheimer's disease but is toxic to the liver at high doses.[19] By combining the two agents, researchers were able to use reduced doses of the drug and still achieve improvements in symptoms of Alzheimer's.

Hyperlipidemia −1

Lecithin has a considerable reputation as a cholesterol-lowering agent; the studies showing this positive effect, however, were poorly controlled and lacked a placebo group.[28,29] In contrast, small but better designed studies found no effect.[3,30] In one of these, a double-blind study of 23 men with hypercholesterolemia, lecithin supplementation did not improve total cholesterol, HDL, LDL, lipoprotein(a), or triglycerides.[30]

Other Proposed Uses

Use of lecithin or choline in unipolar **mania** or rapid-cycling **bipolar disorder** is based on highly preliminary evidence only.[23,24]

Phosphatidylcholine/lecithin might have value for treatment or prevention of **various liver diseases,** including alcoholic hepatitis, fatty liver and cirrhosis, chronic and acute viral hepatitis, and hepatic failure, although the evidence at present is preliminary and somewhat inconsistent.[2,7-15,31]

Based on choline's function as a methyl donor, there are at least theoretical reasons to suspect that it might have **chemopreventive** properties.[5,32-34]

Preliminary evidence suggests that choline—in concert with other methyl donors like folate, methionine, and vitamins B_{12} and B_6—may exert a **cardioprotective** effect by lowering homocysteine levels.[35,36]

Mechanism of Action

Not known. The proposed neurologic effects of choline supplements are based primarily on the nutrient's role as a precursor in acetylcholine synthesis.[5,20,21,27,37-41] Choline may also influence brain function by effects on phospholipid biosynthesis.[42-44]

Dosage

Lecithin generally contains 10 to 20% phosphatidylcholine. However, European trials have typically used products containing 90% phosphatidylcholine. Typical dosages of this more potent formulation are as follows: for hepatic disease, 350 to 500 mg three times daily; for psychological and neurologic conditions, 5 to 10 g three times daily; and for hyperlipidemia, 500 to 900 mg three times daily.

Choline is ubiquitous in nutritional sources, and the average diet provides about 500 to 1000 mg of choline per day.[3,45] According to U.S. and Canadian guidelines, the recommended daily intakes of choline vary with age and gender as follows: males 14 years and older, 550 mg; females 14 to 18 years, 400 mg; and females 19 years and older, 425 mg.

Most studies of choline as a treatment for disease have used from 1 to 30 g of choline or choline-containing supplements per day. This wide range is due to the existence of several different types of choline supplements, all with varying amounts of the active ingredient.

Safety Issues

Lecithin and choline are believed to be generally safe. At higher dosages, however, abdominal discomfort, diarrhea, and nausea may occur. Maximum safe dosages in individuals with severe hepatic or renal disease are not known.

Safety in Young Children and Pregnant or Lactating Women

Maximum safe dosages of lecithin and choline for pregnant or lactating women or for young children have not been established.

According to U.S. and Canadian guidelines, the recommended daily intake of choline for women who are pregnant is 450 mg. Lactating women are advised to take 550 mg daily.

Drug Interactions

None are known.

PHOSPHATIDYLSERINE

Common Uses

Dementia [+3]

Mild to moderate cognitive impairment [+3]

Depression [+2]

Athletic overtraining syndrome [+1]

(Higher numbers indicate stronger evidence; X modifier indicates contradictory results. See page xviii of the Introduction for details of the rating scale.)

Approach to the Patient

Like ginkgo *(Ginkgo biloba)*, phosphatidylserine appears to improve symptoms in dementia. (Most studies have not separated Alzheimer's and non-Alzheimer's dementia.) The supplement might also be helpful for milder cognitive impairment.

Much weaker evidence suggests that phosphatidylserine may be useful in depression, overtraining syndrome, and athletic performance enhancement.

Dementia +3

The largest double-blind study of supplemental phosphatidylserine for dementia followed 494 elderly patients (65 to 93 years old), recruited from 23 geriatric and general medicine centers in northeastern Italy, over a course of 6 months.[1] Participants suffered from moderate to severe cognitive decline based on the Mini Mental State Examination and Global Deterioration Scale. Half of the participants were given 300 mg of phosphatidylserine daily, and evaluation over the course of treatment showed statistically significant improvements in both behavior and cognition in the treated group compared to the placebo group. These results correlate well with those of smaller double-blind studies of supplemental phosphatidylserine involving a total of over 500 patients with Alzheimer's disease or other forms of dementia.[2-8]

Mild to Moderate Cognitive Impairment   +3

A double-blind, placebo-controlled trial evaluated the effect of supplemental phosphatidylserine in 149 individuals aged 50 to 75 whose degree of cognitive impairment fell short of clinical dementia.[9] The results over a 12-week period showed improvements with phosphatidylserine treatment in various measures of cognitive function, most strongly among the more impaired participants.

Depression   +2

One small double-blind, crossover study suggests that supplemental phosphatidylserine can be useful in geriatric patients with depression.[10] Improvements in affective symptoms were also seen in many of the studies of phosphatidylserine for dementia.

Athletic Overtraining Syndrome   +1

Preliminary studies suggest that supplemental phosphatidylserine can blunt the cortisol response to heavy physical exercise, possibly allowing more rapid muscle development in body building and other forms of athletic training, thus reducing symptoms of overtraining syndrome.[11-13]

Mechanism of Action

Exogenously administered phosphatidylserine stimulates acetylcholine release from the cerebral cortex of rats.[14] Dopaminergic effects have been seen as well.[15] In addition, phosphatidylserine has been implicated as a universal sign of apoptotic cell death: when the phospholipid is translocated from the inner layer of the cell membrane, its outer membrane presentation is a signal for the damaged cell to be phagocytized by macrophages.[16] Thus exogenous extracellular phosphatidylserine might serve as a decoy, preventing unnecessary tissue degradation by activated macrophages. This novel model is supported by earlier work demonstrating suppression of macrophage phagocytic function by phosphatidylserine.[17]

Dosage

The usual dose of phosphatidylserine is 100 mg three times daily; however, some studies have used 200 mg twice daily. It can be taken with or without food.

Phosphatidylserine is currently produced from soybeans. However, all of the research described above involved bovine-derived phosphatidylserine, which is no longer available, and there is controversy about whether soy-based phosphatidylserine is equally effective. Animal efficacy studies have yielded conflicting results,[18-20] but the latest trial did find equivalence between treatment with soy-based or bovine cortex–based phosphatidyl-serine in an avoidance task.

Safety Issues

Reported side effects of phosphatidylserine in clinical trials are rare and are usually limited to mild gastrointestinal distress.[1] In double-blind trials, biochemical evaluations have shown no adverse effects.[21] Oral dosages in rodent and dog studies showed no defined organ system toxicity, and LD_{50} values were either not determinable or were very high.[22] Phosphatidylserine has been found nonteratogenic in rats and rabbits. Mutagenic testing was negative.

Maximum safe dosages in individuals with severe hepatic or renal disease are not known.

Safety in Young Children and Pregnant or Lactating Women

Although there are no known or suspected risks, maximum safe dosages for pregnant or lactating women or for young children have not been established.

Drug Interactions

In vitro studies report that fatty acid esters of phosphatidylserine and phosphatidylethanolamine can synergistically stimulate the anticoagulant effect of **heparin.**[23]

PHYLLANTHUS
(Phyllanthus amarus)

Alternate Names/Related Species:
Phyllanthus niruri, P. urinaria

Common Uses

Chronic hepatitis B [−1X]   **Acute hepatitis B** [−1]

(Higher numbers indicate stronger evidence; X modifier indicates contradictory results. See page xviii of the Introduction for details of the rating scale.)

Approach to the Patient

Tropical plants in the genus *Phyllanthus* have a long history of folk use for hepatitis, kidney and bladder problems, intestinal parasites, and diabetes. The most studied species is *Phyllanthus amarus*, historically used for the treatment of jaundice. This traditional practice has led to scientific study of the herb in humans.

Preliminary research created interest in phyllanthus as a treatment for chronic hepatitis B; however, patients may be informed that the current balance of evidence suggests that the herb is not effective.

Chronic Hepatitis B   −1X

Despite numerous in vitro and animal studies showing efficacy against the hepatitis B virus,[1] phyllanthus has been found ineffective for chronic hepatits B in all but one human trial.[1-8]

Acute Hepatitis B   −1

In a double-blind, placebo-controlled trial enrolling 57 individuals with acute hepatitis B, results showed no improvement in speed of recovery with phyllanthus at 300 mg three times daily for 1 week.[9] However, the treatment duration in this study was oddly short.

Mechanism of Action

Not known.

Dosage

The usual dose of phyllanthus used in studies is 600 to 900 mg daily.

Safety Issues

There are no indications that phyllanthus is toxic when used at recommended doses, but comprehensive safety studies have not been performed.[2] No significant side effects have been reported in double-blind studies. Maximum safe dosages in individuals with severe hepatic or renal disease are not known.

Safety in Young Children and Pregnant or Lactating Women

Maximum safe dosages for pregnant or lactating women or for young children have not been established.

Drug Interactions

None are known.

POLICOSANOL

Alternate Names/Supplement Forms:
Octacosanol, 1-Octacosanol, *N*-Octacosanol,
Octacosyl Alcohol, Wheat Germ Oil

Common Uses

Hyperlipidemia   [+3]

**Intermittent
claudication**   [+2]

**Performance
enhancement**   [+1]

(Higher numbers indicate stronger evidence; X modifier indicates contradictory results. See page xviii of the Introduction for details of the rating scale.)

Approach to the Patient

Policosanol contains several higher aliphatic primary alcohols. The main component is octacosanol (60%), followed by triacontanol and hexacosanol.

Numerous double-blind, placebo-controlled trials, unfortunately all by a single research group, suggest that policosanol can reduce LDL and total cholesterol. Reported effects on HDL and triglycerides have been less consistent. Small comparative trials have found policosanol substantially as effective as statin drugs. Policosanol may also be helpful for intermittent claudication, presumably due to antiplatelet effects. Policosanol appears to be safe and well tolerated.

Octacosanol and policosanol are also widely marketed as sports supplements, but there is little evidence for any ergogenic effect. Other proposed uses with no real scientific support include Parkinson's disease and amyotrophic lateral sclerosis.

Patients may not realize the distinction between the tested form of policosanol and the policosanol product available in the United States. All meaningful clinical research on policosanol pertains to Cuban products derived from sugar cane. However, a product marketed in the United States under the name New Cholestin contains policosanol derived from beeswax. Beeswax extract is not identical to sugar cane policosanol and may have entirely different effects. A type of beeswax extract that has been studied in Cuba (D-002) contains more triacontanol rather than octacosanol; D-002 appears to lack hypolipidemic and antiplatelet actions.[1] It may offer promise as a cytoprotective agent, however.

The manufacturer of New Cholestin claims that their form of beeswax policosanol is different from D-002 and does reduce cholesterol. However, at press time no clinical trials of this product have been reported.

Hyperlipidemia   +3

Fifteen double-blind, placebo-controlled trials, involving over 1000 individuals and ranging in length from 6 weeks to 12 months, have found the sugar cane extract policosanol effective for improving total and LDL cholesterol levels, as well as LDL/HDL and TC/HDL ratios.[2-16] Effects on HDL cholesterol and triglycerides have been less consistent. All but one of these studies was conducted in Cuba by one research group.

The largest of these trials was a double-blind, placebo-controlled study that enrolled 437 individuals with type 2 hypercholesterolemia.[9] Participants were first placed on a step 1 diet for 5 weeks. Lipid profiles were taken twice within the next 2 weeks and averaged to provide a baseline value. Then participants received either placebo or policosanol at 5 mg/day for 12 weeks. At that point, the dosage was doubled to 10 mg/day in the treated group, and the study continued for an additional 12 weeks. The results showed significant improvements with both policosanol doses, but greater improvement at the end of the

higher-dose period. By the conclusion of the trial, LDL cholesterol in the treated group improved by 25.6%, total cholesterol
by 17.4%, HDL cholesterol by 28.4%, and triglycerides by
5.2%. These results were statistically significant from baseline as
well as compared to the outcome in the placebo group.

Seven other double-blind trials enrolling a total of about 400
individuals compared policosanol against pravastatin, fluvastatin,
simvastatin, and lovastatin, and found these agents to be essentially identical in effect on lipid parameters.[17-23] One of these
trials was reported by a different Cuban research group.[23]

Intermittent Claudication   +2

A 2-year, double-blind, placebo-controlled study of 56 individuals with intermittent claudication found that treatment with
policosanol (10 mg twice daily) improved walking distance by
more than 50% at 6 months, and the benefits increased over the
course of the study.[24] Similar results were seen with policosanol
in a 6-month, double-blind, placebo-controlled study of 62 individuals with intermittent claudication.[38]

Performance Enhancement   +1

A very small double-blind trial of octacosanol for exercise performance enhancement found evidence of benefit in some measures but not others.[25]

Other Proposed Uses

A trial of 10 individuals with **Parkinson's disease** found marginal benefits.[26]

A double-blind trial with 11 participants failed to produce any
significant benefits in **amyotrophic lateral sclerosis**.[27]

Mechanism of Action

Some evidence suggests that policosanol may impair cholesterol synthesis between the acetate and mevalonate production steps.[15,28] It also appears to increase receptor-dependent LDL processing, thereby reducing plasma LDL.

Policosanol also exhibits dose-dependent antiplatelet actions, comparable to 100 mg aspirin daily[17,28,29] and may reduce lipid peroxidation.[31,32]

Dosage

Studied dosages of policosanol for lowering elevated cholesterol levels range from 5 to 10 mg twice daily. Results may require 2 months to develop.[11,13]

At the time of publication, all published clinical trials of policosanol used sugar cane as the extraction source. However, the main U.S. product containing policosanol, New Cholestin, states that its source is beeswax.

Safety Issues

Policosanol and octacosanol are generally well tolerated. In a drug-monitoring study that followed 27,879 patients for 2 to 4 years, adverse effects were reported in only 0.31% of participants and were primarily weight loss, excessive urination and insomnia.[33] No signs of toxicity were observed in animals given very high doses of policosanol (as much as 620 times the maximum recommended dose).[34-37,40]

However, policosanol's antiplatelet effects (see Mechanism of Action) suggest caution in individuals with impaired coagulation homeostasis, as well as in the perioperative and perilabor and delivery period.

Evidence from one human trial suggests that policosanol does not affect hepatic function.[16] Nonetheless, safety in individuals with severe hepatic or renal disease has not been established. Two small double-blind trials suggest that policosanol is safe and effective for hyperlipidemia in individuals with type 2 diabetes.[8,15]

Safety in Young Children and Pregnant or Lactating Women

Not known, although there are no known or suspected risks. Maximum safe dosages for pregnant or lactating women or for young children have not been established.

Drug Interactions

In studies, policosanol has not interacted with **calcium-channel antagonists, diuretics,** or **beta-blockers.**[6] However, policosanol does appear to potentiate the antiplatelet effects of aspirin.[39] For this reason, caution should be exercised when combining policosanol with any **antiplatelet** or **anticoagulant agent.** It is also possible that policosanol could potentiate the anticoagulant properties of supplements such as garlic, ginkgo, and high-dose vitamin E.

According to one report, octacosanol or policosanol might potentiate the action of **levodopa,** causing increased dyskinesias.[26]

An experimental study in rats suggests that policosanol may potentiate the hypotensive effects of **nitroprusside** through antioxidant actions.[41]

PREGNENOLONE

Common Uses

Antiaging [0]

(Higher numbers indicate stronger evidence; X modifier indicates contradictory results. See page xviii of the Introduction for details of the rating scale.)

Approach to the Patient

Pregnenolone has been recommended as an antiaging hormone, but patients may be informed that there is no real evidence supporting this or any other use.

Antiaging 0

Pregnenolone levels have been shown not to decline with age,[1] and there is no evidence that use of pregnenolone has any therapeutic effects that can be interpreted as slowing aging.

Other Proposed Uses

Animal studies suggest that pregnenolone may enhance **memory**,[2,3] but there have been no human studies.

Pregnenolone has also been suggested as a treatment for an enormous list of health problems, including memory loss, Alzheimer's disease, menopausal symptoms, adrenal disease, Parkinson's disease, osteoporosis, fatigue, stress, depression, rheumatoid arthritis, and nerve injury, as well as a therapeutic support for enhancing weight loss, improving cognition, and increasing overall energy level; however, there is no real scientific evidence for any of these uses.

Mechanism of Action

Pregnenolone is endogenously biosynthesized from cholesterol and is a precursor to the biosynthesis of many steroidal hormones including testosterone, cortisone, progesterone, estrogen, DHEA, androstenedione, aldosterone, and others.

Dosage

A typical recommended dosage of pregnenolone is 30 mg daily, but dosages as high as 700 mg have been recommended by some. Supplemental pregnenolone is made synthetically from four substances found in soybeans.

Safety Issues

The safety and effectiveness of exogenous pregnenolone supplements have not been proven, and as with other steroid hormones, potential risks abound. Maximum safe dosages in individuals with severe hepatic or renal disease are not known.

Safety in Young Children and Pregnant or Lactating Women

Pregnenolone is not recommended for pregnant or lactating women. Maximum safe dosages for young children have not been established.

Drug Interactions

None are known.

PROBIOTICS

Alternate Names/Supplement Forms:
Bifidobacterium bifidum, B. lactis, Escherichia coli spp., Enterococcus faecium, Lactobacillus acidophilus, L. bulgaricus, L. casei, Lactobacillus GG, L. plantarum, L. reuteri, L. thermophilus, Saccharomyces boulardii, Streptococcus bulgaricus, S. thermophilus, S. salivarius

Common Uses

Traveler's diarrhea (prophylaxis)   [+3]

Acute infectious diarrhea in children (prevention and treatment)   [+3]

Inflammatory bowel disease   [+3]

Antibiotic-associated diarrhea   [+3X]

Irritable bowel syndrome (IBS)   [+2]

Eczema   [+3]

Respiratory infection prophylaxis in children   [+3]

Otitis media prophylaxis   [+3X]

Vaginal candidiasis   [+2]

Recurrent UTIs   [−1]

(Higher numbers indicate stronger evidence; X modifier indicates contradictory results. See page xviii of the Introduction for details of the rating scale.)

Approach to the Patient

Meaningful evidence supports the use of probiotic supplements in treating and preventing various forms of diarrhea.

Based on current evidence, it is reasonable to advise patients to use probiotic supplements during and immediately after a course of antibiotics, as well as while traveling in tropical countries.

Meaningful evidence also supports the use of probiotics in inflammatory bowel disease, preventing or treating childhood eczema, and preventing respiratory infections in children.

Traveler's Diarrhea + 3

One double-blind, placebo-controlled study followed 820 individuals traveling to southern Turkey and found that *Lactobacillus GG* significantly protected against intestinal infection.[1] Other studies using *Saccharomyces boulardii* have found similar benefits.[2-4] In a double-blind, placebo-controlled trial enrolling 3000 Australians, the greatest benefits were seen in those who visited North Africa and Turkey.[3] Benefit depended on consistent use of the product, and a dose of 1000 mg daily was more effective than 250 mg daily. Protection against intestinal infection has been seen with other probiotics as well.[5,6]

Acute Infectious Diarrhea in Children + 3

A review of the literature published in 2001 found 13 double-blind, placebo-controlled trials on the use of probiotics for acute infectious diarrhea in infants and children; 10 of these trials involved treatment, and 3 involved prophylaxis.[57] Overall, evidence suggests that probiotics exert a clinically and statistically significant benefit in reducing the duration of diarrhea. The evidence is strongest for the probiotic *Lactobacillus GG* and for infection with rotavirus. The evidence regarding prophylaxis is less clear.

For example, a double-blind, placebo-controlled trial of 269 children (aged 1 month to 3 years) with acute diarrhea found that those treated with *Lactobacillus GG* recovered more quickly than those given placebo.[7] The best results were seen among children with rotavirus infection. Similar results with *Lactobacillus GG* were seen in a double-blind study of 71 children.[8]

Other studies have found benefit in the treatment of acute diarrhea with *Lactobacillus LB*, *L. reuteri*, *Saccharomyces boulardii*, and other probiotics.[4,9-11]

A double-blind, placebo-controlled study of 81 hospitalized children found that treatment with *Lactobacillus GG* reduced the risk of nosocomial diarrhea, particularly rotavirus infection.[12] A double-blind, placebo-controlled study found that *Lactobacillus GG* helped prevent diarrhea in 204 undernourished children.[13] The probiotics *B. bifidum*, *Streptococcus thermophilus*, *L. casei*, *Lactobacillus LB*, and *S. boulardii* may also help prevent diarrhea in infants and children.[4,14,15]

Inflammatory Bowel Disease   + 3

A double-blind trial of 116 individuals with active ulcerative colitis compared a relatively low dose of mesalazine (1.2 to 2.4 g/day) against a nonpathogenic strain of *Escherichia coli*, 2 capsules twice daily (2.5×10^{10} viable bacteria per capsule).[16,17] The results suggest that probiotic treatment might be equally effective as low-dose mesalazine for inducing and maintaining remission. Evidence of benefit had been seen in previous trials using *E. coli* or other probiotics.[17]

A 9-month, double-blind trial of 40 individuals found that a combination of three probiotic bacteria could significantly reduce the risk of a pouchitis flare-up following partial colonic resection in ulcerative colitis.[18] Participants were given either a mixture of various probiotics, including four strains of *Lactobacilli*, three strains of *Bifidobacteria*, and one strain of *S. salivarius*, or placebo. The results showed that treated individuals were significantly less likely to have relapses of pouchitis during the study period.

Antibiotic-Associated Diarrhea   + 3 X

According to some, but not all, double-blind and open trials, probiotics (including *S. boulardii*, *Lactobacillus* spp., and *Bifidobacteria* spp.) may also help treat or prevent antibiotic-related diarrhea.[4,19-25,58] One study evaluated 180 individuals receiving either placebo or 1000 mg of saccharomyces daily along with their antibiotic treatment and found that the treated group developed diarrhea significantly less often.[20] A similar study of 193 individuals also found benefit with saccharomyces,[26] but a study of 302 individuals found no benefit with *Lactobacillus GG*.[23]

Irritable Bowel Syndrome (IBS)   + 2

Based on the theory that IBS results from a disturbance in normal gastrointestinal flora, probiotics have been tried as a treatment for IBS.

In a 4-week, double-blind, placebo-controlled crossover trial of 60 individuals with IBS, treatment with *L. plantarum* reduced flatulence significantly.[28] This benefit persisted for an additional year after treatment was stopped.

In another 4-week, double-blind trial, 40 individuals with IBS again received either *L. plantarum* or placebo.[59] The results showed improvements in pain as well as in overall symptom score.

A small 6-week trial using *L. acidophilus* also found indications of benefit.[24] However, in a double-blind, placebo-controlled crossover study of 24 individuals with irritable bowel syndrome, use of *Lactobacillus GG* failed to produce significant benefit as compared to placebo.[61]

Eczema   + 3

Use of probiotics during pregnancy and after childbirth may reduce risk of childhood eczema. In a double-blind, placebo-controlled trial that enrolled 159 women, participants received either placebo or *Lactobacillus GG* capsules beginning 2 to 4 weeks before expected delivery.[30] After delivery, breast-feeding mothers continued to take placebo or the probiotic for 6 months; formula-fed infants were given placebo or probiotic directly for the same period of time. The results showed that use of

Lactobacillus GG reduced risk of eczema developing in offspring by approximately 50%.

Two small double-blind trials found evidence that adding probiotics (*Lactobacillus GG* or *Bifidobacterium lactis*) to infant formula reduced eczema symptoms in infants with existing atopy.[31,32]

Respiratory Infection Prophylaxis in Children   + 3

A double-blind, placebo-controlled trial of 571 Finnish children in day care found that use of milk enhanced with *Lactobacillus GG* modestly but significantly reduced the rate and severity of respiratory infections.[33] Other studies have found evidence that probiotics exert an immunomodulatory effect.[34-36]

Otitis Media Prophylaxis   + 3 X

A double-blind, placebo-controlled study of 108 children (mean age 23 months) prone to recurrent otitis media examined the effects of recolonization with probiotic strains of alpha hemolytic streptococci (*S. mitis*, *S oralis*, and *S. sanguis*).[62] These strains were cultured from healthy children, and selected for their ability to inhibit *S. pneumoniae*, *H. influenzae*, *M. catarrhalis*, and *S. pyogenes*.

Participants received a 10-day course of antibiotic treatment and were then randomized to receive either active or placebo solution for 10 days. Sixty days later, another 10-day course was given. The results showed significantly decreased incidence of otitis media recurrence in the treatment group as compared to the placebo group over the 3-month study period. However, the rate of treatment failure was nonetheless high (58%). A smaller double-blind trial found no benefit.[63]

Vaginal Candidiasis   +2

A review of the many studies on the use of oral and topical acidophilus to prevent vaginal yeast infections concluded that it may be effective, but more study is needed.[4,37,38]

In several clinical trials involving a total of 99 women with recurrent vaginitis over 7 days to 6 months, subjects using *L. acidophilus* (taken orally, as a vaginal douche, or as a vaginal suppository) experienced improvement in symptoms as well as a decreased incidence of vaginal infections.[39-41] However, the reliability of all of these studies is questionable due to poor design, and at least one had a high participant dropout rate.

Recurrent UTIs   −1

Although probiotics are sometimes proposed for preventing bladder infections, a year-long open trial of 150 women found *Lactobacillus GG* ineffective as compared to cranberry juice or no treatment.[42]

Other Proposed Uses

A double-blind, placebo-controlled trial of 205 individuals found some evidence that the probiotic *L. rhamnosus* can reduce the severity of **diarrhea secondary to radiation therapy**.[43] Statistical significance was just missed, however, for primary study endpoints. In addition, a double-blind, placebo-controlled study of 144 individuals found that a probiotic form of *E. coli* reduced combined gastrointestinal and immunological side effects in individuals undergoing 5-FU chemotherapy.[44]

An 8-week, double-blind, placebo-controlled trial of 70 overweight individuals found that a probiotic treatment containing *S. thermophilus* and *Enterococcus faecium* could reduce **LDL cholesterol** levels by about 8%.[46] Similarly positive results were seen in other trials of the same or other probiotics.[47-50] However, a 6-month, double-blind, placebo-controlled trial found no

long-term benefit;[51] the researchers speculated that the participants stopped regular use of the product toward the later parts
of the study.

Probiotics have been found to exert an inhibitory action on
Helicobacter pylori.[60,64-67] While this action does not appear to
be strong enough to eradicate *Helicobacter*, evidence suggests that
Lactobacilli may be a useful adjunct to standard antibiotic therapy,
improving eradication rate and reducing side effects.[11,27,29,45,64-66]
Unfortunately, the reported studies suggesting benefit were not
double-blind.

There is some evidence that probiotics, when added to milk, can
help reduce symptoms of **milk allergies.**[52]

Probiotic treatment, both topical and oral, have also been proposed as a treatment for canker sores, but there is no solid evidence that it is effective for this purpose.

Mechanism of Action

Acidophilus and related probiotics are symbiotic organisms that
promote a normal balance of flora in the gastrointestinal and
vaginal tracts by competing with pathogenic bacteria and yeast.
In inflammatory bowel disease, normalizing luminal microbial
content might affect intestinal immune reactions and gut bar-
rier functions.[53,54]

Dosage

A typical daily dose of bacterial probiotics should supply about
3 to 5 billion live organisms, although some studies have used
doses an order of magnitude higher. A common dose of
S. boulardii yeast is 500 mg twice daily (standardized to provide
3×10^{10} colony-forming units per gram), taken while traveling
or at the beginning of using antibiotics and continuing for a few
days post-travel or after antibiotics are stopped. The most tested

form of *Lactobacillus, Lactobacillus GG,* is available in the United States. See the Appendix for U.S. brand names of clinically tested products.

One study found that most acidophilus capsules on the market contained no living acidophilus.[55] The container label should guarantee living organism counts at the time of purchase, not just at the time of manufacture.

Fructo-oligosaccharide supplements may promote intestinal probiotic colony counts.[56] The typical dose of fructo-oligosaccharides is between 2 and 8 g daily.

Safety Issues

There are no known safety problems with the use of acidophilus or other probiotics. Occasionally, some individuals notice a temporary increase in flatulence.

Safety in Young Children and Pregnant or Lactating Women

Not known. However, given that these organisms are heavily colonized in the gastrointestinal and vaginal tracts of healthy women, probiotics are probably safe.

Drug Interactions

None are known.

PROGESTERONE CREAM

Alternate Names/Supplement Forms:
Natural Progesterone, Micronized Progesterone

Common Uses

Menopausal
symptoms [+3]

Osteoporosis
treatment [−2]

(Higher numbers indicate stronger evidence; X modifier indicates contradictory results. See page xviii of the Introduction for details of the rating scale.)

Approach to the Patient

Because oral progesterone is poorly absorbed, during its initial development as a drug progesterone was delivered in cream form. Subsequently, orally absorbable progestins proved more acceptable to women and largely replaced topical progesterone. Progesterone creams became popular again in the 1990s, this time as an over-the-counter treatment surrounded by considerable misinformation.

Though progesterone cream products are typically touted as "natural progesterone," they are actually produced synthetically. In addition, the popularly marketed product, wild or Mexican yam (*Dioscorea* spp.), does not contain progesterone. It does contain diosgenin, a substance that has been used in the past as a chemical substrate for the industrial synthesis of various steroid hormones. However, it is thought unlikely that there is any physiological conversion of diosgenin to steroid hormones in the body.

A micronized form of progesterone that is chemically identical to human progesterone but can be absorbed orally (Prometrium) has been approved by the FDA. Oral micronized progesterone should be effective for all the same purposes as progestins. Progesterone cream is not absorbed in high enough concentrations to oppose estrogen, but it may be effective for controlling menopausal symptoms. Numerous books and articles have claimed that progesterone is effective for osteoporosis, perhaps even more effective than estrogen. However, there has never been any real evidence to support this belief, and a recent study found no benefit.

Menopausal Symptoms   +3

In one double-blind, placebo-controlled trial, 102 healthy women within 5 years of menopause were randomized to receive either transdermal progesterone cream (providing 20 mg progesterone daily) or placebo, along with calcium and multivitamins.[1] Use of progesterone cream significantly reduced vasomotor symptoms compared with placebo.

Osteoporosis   −2

In vitro studies and other preliminary evidence first suggested that progesterone or progestins stimulate osteoblast activity.[2,3] Subsequently, results from a series of case histories in one physician's practice were popularized as evidence that progesterone cream can slow or even reverse osteoporosis.[4-6]

However, the double-blind trial mentioned above found no evidence of any improvements in bone density attributable to progesterone.[1] Further, in a large 3-year, double-blind trial, combined estrogen and oral progesterone were no more effective for osteoporosis than estrogen alone.[7]

Mechanism of Action

The mechanism of action of progesterone in menopausal symptoms is not known.

Evidence suggesting that progesterone stimulates osteoblastic activity is the basis for investigation of its therapeutic utility in osteoporosis.[2]

Dosage

The usual dose of progesterone in cream form is 20 mg daily. Although this dose may decrease menopausal hot flashes,[1] even three to four times that amount does not provide enough progesterone to balance the uterine effects of estrogen.[3,8] A typical dose of oral micronized progesterone is 400 mg daily.

Safety Issues

In one small study, use of oral micronized progesterone at a dose of 400 mg per day was associated with dizziness, abdominal cramping, headache, breast pain, muscle pain, irritability, nausea, fatigue, diarrhea, and viral infections, at rates higher than seen in the placebo group.[9] Risks associated with progestins presumably apply as well.

Use in individuals with severe hepatic disease is contraindicated. Caution should be used in individuals with renal insufficiency.

Safety in Young Children and Pregnant or Lactating Women

Progesterone should not be used by pregnant women; safety in lactating women has not been determined. Progesterone is not intended for use in children.

Drug Interactions

A potential exists for CYP enzyme system interactions.

PROTEOLYTIC ENZYMES

Alternate Names/Supplement Forms: Bromelain, Papain, Trypsin, Chymotrypsin, Pancreatin, Digestive Enzymes

Common Uses

Surgery [+3X]

Minor injuries [+2]

Herpes zoster [+2]

Osteoarthritis/ chronic pain [+2]

(Higher numbers indicate stronger evidence; X modifier indicates contradictory results. See page xviii of the Introduction for details of the rating scale.)

Approach to the Patient

Although best known as replacement therapy in pancreatic insufficiency, pancreatic extracts and other proteolytic enzymes such as papain and bromelain also appear to have systemic effects.

Proteolytic enzymes are found in various products marketed for the treatment of sports injuries, and that is the most likely reason your patients may be using them. Evidence supports this use, although there is better evidence for using proteolytic enzymes as an aid in recovering from surgery.

Other potential uses with some supporting evidence include reducing the pain of acute herpes zoster and chronic musculoskeletal conditions.

Surgery   +3X

Studies of proteolytic enzymes following surgery have returned mixed results.

A double-blind, placebo-controlled study evaluated recovery from episiotomy in 160 women.[1] Participants given 40 mg of bromelain four times daily for 3 days, beginning 4 hours after delivery, showed statistically and clinically significant decreases in edema, inflammation, and pain. However, a similar double-blind study of 158 women failed to find significant benefit.[2]

A double-blind, placebo-controlled study that used the proteolytic enzyme product Chymoral in 204 episiotomy patients found evidence of benefit.[3] Chymoral was also found effective for reducing inflammation in a double-blind, placebo-controlled trial involving 102 surgical removals of impacted wisdom teeth[4] and in a double-blind, placebo-controlled trial of 86 individuals undergoing podiatric surgery.[32]

A controlled study of 53 individuals undergoing nasal surgery found bromelain effective at reducing bruising.[5] Benefits were also seen in a small, double-blind, placebo-controlled, crossover study of individuals undergoing dental surgery[6]; however, no significant benefits were seen in a double-blind, placebo-controlled trial of 154 individuals undergoing facial plastic surgery.[7]

In another double-blind, controlled trial, 95 patients undergoing treatment for cataracts were given 40 mg of bromelain or placebo (along with other treatments) four times daily for 2 days before surgery and for 5 days postoperatively.[8] The results showed reduced pain and inflammation in the bromelain group as compared with the placebo group.

In a double-blind, placebo-controlled trial of 80 individuals, treatment with Wobenzym (a proprietary enzyme mixture containing pancreatin, papain, bromelain, trypsin, and chymotrypsin, as well as lipase, amylase, and rutin) after knee surgery significantly improved the rate of recovery, as measured by mobility and swelling.[9] Another double-blind, placebo-controlled trial with 80 participants found benefit of the same enzyme combination in oral surgery.[10]

Minor Injuries   + 2

A double-blind, placebo-controlled study of 44 individuals with sports-related ankle injuries found that treatment with Woben-zym (described above) resulted in faster healing and reduced the time away from training by about 50%.[11] Three other small double-blind studies involving a total of about 80 athletes found that treatment with various proteolytic enzyme combinations significantly improved the rate of healing of bruises and other mild athletic injuries as compared with placebo.[12-14]

In addition, a double-blind trial of 100 individuals given a sub-cutaneous injection of their own blood to simulate bruising found that treatment with a proteolytic enzyme combination significantly speeded hematoma resolution.[15]

A double-blind, placebo-controlled trial involving 71 individuals with finger fractures found that treatment with a trypsin-chy-motrypsin combination produced a significant improvement in recovery rate.[16]

In a controlled study, 74 boxers with facial and/or upper body bruises were given bromelain until all signs of bruising had dis-appeared; another 72 boxers were given placebo.[17] Fifty-eight of the group taking bromelain lost all signs of bruising within 4 days, compared to only 10 of the group taking placebo.

Herpes Zoster   + 2

Proteolytic enzymes appear to be as effective as acyclovir for acute herpes zoster, but placebo-controlled trials have not been performed.

A double-blind trial of 192 individuals with acute herpes zoster compared the effect of a proprietary proteolytic enzyme mixture with that of acyclovir.[18] Each enzyme capsule contained 30 mg trypsin, 30 mg chymotrypsin, and 75 mg papain, as well as 30 mg thymus extract (a purported immune stimulant); the acyclovir tablets contained 200 mg of the drug. Participants were given four capsules five times daily until the disappearance of symptoms (maximum 14 days), and their pain was assessed at intervals. Statistically equivalent pain relief was demonstrated in both groups, but the acyclovir group had more side effects (primarily mild gastrointestinal disturbance). Equivalent benefits were also seen in another double-blind trial.[15]

Osteoarthritis/Chronic Pain   +2

Proteolytic enzyme combinations may be helpful for osteoarthritis and other forms of chronic musculoskeletal pain.

A 3-week, double-blind, placebo-controlled trial of 30 individuals with neck pain found that use of Wobenzym (described above) caused small but statistically significant improvements in pain.[33]

A 28-day, double-blind trial of 80 individuals with osteoarthritis of the knee compared Wobenzym (seven tablets qid) to diclofenac (50 mg bid) in a double-dummy design.[34] The results showed equivalent improvement in symptoms between the two groups.

Three double-blind trials presented in abstract form evaluated proteolytic enzymes in, respectively, 73 individuals with knee arthritis, 40 individuals with shoulder arthritis, and 120 individuals with spinal pain.[35]

These trials compared the proprietary product Phlogenzym at a dose of two tabs tid (90 mg bromelain, 48 mg trypsin, and 100 mg of the flavonoid rutoside per tablet) with diclofenac (50 mg bid in the shoulder and spine pain trials; 50 mg tid in the the knee pain trial, using a double-dummy design). Each one found statistically equivalent improvements with the enzyme combination and the drug.

A double-blind, placebo-controlled study of the oral proteolytic combination Chymroal for treatment of lumbar disk prolapse found only clinically insignificant benefits.[19]

Other Proposed Uses

Although proteolytic enzymes have been proposed as a treatment for food allergies, rheumatoid arthritis, and other autoimmune diseases, there is no real evidence as yet to substantiate these uses.

Mechanism of Action

Proteolytic enzymes appear to be absorbed whole to a certain extent[36] and to produce antiinflammatory, antiedema, immunomodulatory, and fibrinolytic effects.[10,11,13,20-29,37-39]

Dosage

Recommended dosages vary with the form of proteolytic enzymes used. See the Appendix for U.S. brand names of clinically tested products.

Safety Issues

In clinical trials, use of oral proteolytic enzyme combinations has been associated with relatively few and mild side effects, consisting primarily of gastrointestinal distress and allergic exanthema.

Bromelain is the best-studied proteolytic enzyme. In rat studies, no toxic effects were seen at oral doses as high as 10 g/kg.[40] A 6-month study conducted in dogs with increasing daily levels of bromelain up to 750 mg/kg showed no toxic effects.[41] Rat studies have found no carcinogenicity with bromelain in doses up to 1.5 g/kg/day.[41]

However, bromelain has been reported to cause both immediate-type and late-phase immunoglobulin E (IgE)–mediated reactions.[42-44]

Sensitization usually occurs by inhalation and may be occupationally acquired. Symptoms may occur hours after exposure and may not be refractory to antihistamine and steroid treatments. Cross-allergenicity with bromelain has been reported for wheat flour, rye flour, kiwi fruit, perennial ryegrass, grass pollen, and birch pollen.[42,45-47]

In addition, one study that investigated the effects of bromelain in 20 hypertensive patients found a concentration-dependent increase in both heart rate and systolic blood pressure.[48] Caution may be warranted with high doses of bromelain in hypertensive patients.

One study of 47 patients with various disorders leading to edema and inflammation found no significant effects of oral bromelain (40 mg four times daily for 1 week) on bleeding, coagulation, and prothrombin time.[49]

Maximum safe dosages in individuals with severe hepatic or renal disease are not known.

Safety in Young Children and Pregnant or Lactating Women

Maximum safe dosages for pregnant or lactating women or young children have not been established.

Drug Interactions

Papain might potentiate **anticoagulant** and **antiplatelet agents.**[30]

Pancreatin may interfere with **folate** absorption (see the **Folate** article).[31]

PYGEUM
(Prunus africana, Pygeum africanum)

Common Use

Benign prostatic hyperplasia [+3]

(Higher numbers indicate stronger evidence; X modifier indicates contradictory results. See page xviii of the Introduction for details of the rating scale.)

Approach to the Patient

Extracts of the bark of the African prune tree, pygeum *(Prunus africana, Pygeum africanum)*, have been used extensively in France and Italy to treat mild to moderate benign prostatic hyperplasia (BPH) for more than 30 years. Numerous clinical trials suggest that pygeum extract improves subjective and objective symptoms in most individuals with mild to moderate BPH (Vahlensieck stage I or II).

Many products marketed for BPH contain several supplements combined, each at an inadequate dose. Your patients may do better using a single-substance product that provides the dose found effective in double-blind trials. (See the article on Benign Prostatic Hyperplasia for several reasonably well-documented options.)

Pygeum is also used to treat infections of the prostate and seminal vesicles, as well as sexual dysfunction in men, although only small open-label studies suggest utility for these conditions.[1-3]

Benign Prostatic Hyperplasia +3

More than 10 double-blind, placebo-controlled studies of pygeum have been published, involving a total of more than 600 individuals studied for 6 to 12 weeks, using daily doses of pygeum extract from 75 to 200 mg.[4] In these trials, quality-of-life and objective measurements (urinary flow rate, residual volume, nocturia) are typically reported to improve by 2 months[4] and remain improved for at least 1 month after treatment.[5] There is no reliable evidence that pygeum can reduce prostate volume.

Most of these studies involved small numbers of patients (10 to 25 per group), but one double-blind, placebo-controlled trial of 263 men showed a reliable, statistically significant improvement with pygeum in urinary flow rate, voided volume, residual volume, daytime frequency, and nocturia.[6] No change in prostate weight was reported in this study.

Other Proposed Uses

Highly preliminary evidence suggests that pygeum might be useful for **prostatitis** as well as **male sexual dysfunction.**[1-3]

Mechanism of Action

Although the mechanism of action of pygeum extract is unknown, several synergistic mechanisms have been proposed. Phytosterols found in pygeum, such as beta-sitosterol, compete with cholesterol, an androgen precursor,[7] and inhibit the production of inflammatory arachidonic acid pathway metabolites.[4] Oleanolic and ursolic acid (pentacyclic triterpenoids) possibly exert an antiinflammatory action in the prostate by inhibiting glucosyl transferase, which is involved in proteoglycan metabolism in connective tissue.[8]

In vitro studies indicate pygeum extract is a potent inhibitor of rat prostatic fibroblast proliferation stimulated by various growth factors.[9] This may be relevant because development of BPH might be related to inappropriate growth factor activity.

Inhibition of steroid 5-alpha-reductase, the enzyme that cat-alyzes conversion of testosterone to dihydrotestosterone, is not a significant activity of pygeum extract. In vitro assays showed that the pygeum extract brand Tadenan possessed only 1/63,000 the inhibition activity of finasteride.[10]

Dosage

Clinical studies have used 75 to 200 mg daily in patients with BPH. One study indicates that once-daily dosing with 100 mg of the extract Tadenan proved as effective and free of adverse re-actions as 50 mg twice daily.[11] Once-daily dosing may improve patient compliance.

Some manufacturers standardize pygeum extracts to contain 14% triterpenoids and 0.5% n-docosanol.

Pygeum's effectiveness might be enhanced when it is combined with nettle.[12,13] See the Appendix for U.S. brand names of clin-ically tested combination products.

Safety Issues

Pygeum appears to be essentially nontoxic, both in the short and long term.[14] The most common side effect is mild gastrointesti-nal distress. Maximum safe dosages in individuals with severe hepatic or renal disease are not known.

Safety in Young Children and Pregnant or Lactating Women

Pygeum is intended only for use in men.

Drug Interactions

There are no known drug interactions.

PYRUVATE

Alternate Names/Supplement Forms:
Sodium Pyruvate, Calcium Pyruvate, Potassium Pyruvate,
Magnesium Pyruvate, Dihydroxyacetone Pyruvate (DHAP)

Common Uses

Weight reduction [+2]   **Ergogenic aid** [−1X]

(Higher numbers indicate stronger evidence; X modifier indicates contradictory results. See page xviii of the Introduction for details of the rating scale.)

Approach to the Patient

Based on its role in the Krebs cycle, pyruvate supplements have been promoted as a treatment to enhance fat metabolism. This use is supported by a number of small studies.

Pyruvate is also marketed as an ergogenic aid, but the evidence for this use is more negative than positive.

Pyruvate is often sold in combination with dihydroxyacetone as dihydroxyacetone pyruvate (DHAP).

Weight Reduction   +2

In a 6-week, double-blind, placebo-controlled trial, 51 individuals were given pyruvate (6 g/day), placebo, or no treatment.[1] All participated in an exercise program. Significant decreases in fat mass (2.1 kg) and percent body fat (2.6%) were seen, along with a significant increase in lean mass (1.5 kg). No significant changes were seen in the placebo or control groups.

In a placebo-controlled study (blinding not stated), 34 modestly overweight individuals were put on a mildly low energy diet for 4 weeks.[2] Subsequently, all participants were given a liquid supplement containing pyruvate (22 to 44 g depending on total calorie intake) or an isocaloric equivalent. Over the course of 6 weeks, individuals in the pyruvate group lost 0.7 kg vs. no significant loss in the placebo group.

Other small studies using pyruvate or DHAP found similar results.[3-6]

Ergogenic Aid   −1X

The evidence regarding pyruvate as an ergogenic aid is more negative than positive.[7-10]

Mechanism of Action

Pyruvate is endogenously biosynthesized and is involved in energy metabolism. It has been suggested that exogenous pyruvate might inhibit lipid synthesis.[11-14]

Dosage

A typical therapeutic dosage of pyruvate is 30 g daily, although 6 to 44 g daily have been used in studies. Dihydroxyacetone dosages in studies of DHAP (pyruvate plus dihydroxyacetone) have ranged from 12 to 75 g daily.

Safety Issues

In clinical trials, pyruvate and dihydroxyacetone have caused only few and nonspecific adverse effects. However, formal toxicologic studies have not been reported. Maximum safe dosages in individuals with severe hepatic or renal disease are not known.

As with all supplements used in multigram doses, use of a quality product is critical since contaminants present in even small percentages could result in toxic effects.

Safety in Young Children and Pregnant or Lactating Women

Maximum safe dosages for pregnant or lactating women or young children have not been established.

Drug Interactions

There are no known drug interactions.

QUERCETIN

Alternate Names/Supplement Forms: Quercetin Chalcone

Common Uses

Category III   **Allergy** [+1]
chronic prostatitis
(nonbacterial prostatitis/
prostatodynia) [+2]

(Higher numbers indicate stronger evidence; X modifier indicates contradictory results. See page xviii of the Introduction for details of the rating scale.)

Approach to the Patient

Quercetin is a bioflavonoid found in red wine as well as other foods. One study found quercetin supplementation effective in men with category III chronic prostatitis (nonbacterial prostatitis/prostatodynia), possibly because of inhibitory effects on nitric oxide (NO).

Your patients are more likely to have heard that quercetin is an effective treatment for allergies. It is said to function like cromolyn; however, this claim rests entirely on in vitro studies.

Category III
Chronic Prostatitis (Nonbacterial
Prostatitis/Prostatodynia) +2

A 1-month, double-blind, placebo-controlled trial of 30 men with category III chronic prostatitis found that 500 mg of quercetin twice daily produced a significant improvement in symptom score as compared with placebo.[1]

Allergy   +1

Two in vitro studies have found that quercetin decreases histamine release from mast cells and basophils.[2,3,22,23] One in vitro study demonstrated inhibition of arachidonate 5-lipoxygenase.[4]

Other Proposed Uses

A small, double-blind, placebo-controlled trial found that a supplement containing quercetin reduced symptoms of **interstitial cystitis.**[5]

Like other bioflavonoids, quercetin has **antioxidant** properties[6,7]; in vitro[8-11] and animal[12] research suggests that it might have **chemopreventive** properties; and in vitro studies indicate that it may have **antiviral** properties against herpes simplex, poliomyelitis, influenza, and respiratory viruses.[13,14]

One animal study found reduced progression of **atherosclerosis** in mice treated with quercetin,[15] and others found that quercetin reduced **cataract** formation.[16,24-26]

Mechanism of Action

Quercetin is thought to have antiinflammatory, nitric oxide–inhibiting, tyrosine kinase–inhibiting, and antioxidant properties.[1] Any of these may play a role in symptomatic relief of chronic prostatitis. Oral quercetin glucosides appear in the plasma as quercetin glucuronides rather than as glucoside or aglycone moieties; the physiologic site of hydrolysis and conjugation remains unclear.[17]

Dosage

A typical dosage is 200 to 400 mg three times daily. It is commonly stated that quercetin is poorly absorbed, and on this basis manufacturers have offered a number of quercetin products said to be better absorbed. However, this belief appears to rest on the general poor absorbability of bioflavonoids; quercetin may be better absorbed than other substances in this category.[27]

Safety Issues

Quercetin appears to be safe in adults. Although in vitro studies show quercetin has mutagenic properties on the Ames test, other evidence suggests that orally consumed quercetin is not carcinogenic and may in fact have chemopreventive properties.[10,18,19] Quercetin and other flavonoids synergistically inhibit platelet aggregation in vitro.[20]

Maximum safe dosages in individuals with severe hepatic or renal disease are not known.

Safety in Young Children and Pregnant or Lactating Women

Maximum safe dosages for pregnant or lactating women or young children have not been established. One highly preliminary study suggests that quercetin combined with other bioflavonoids in the diet of pregnant women might increase the risk of infant leukemia.[21]

Drug Interactions

There are no known drug interactions. However, because of quercetin's effects on platelet aggregation, interactions with **antiplatelet** and **anticoagulant drugs** could occur.

RED CLOVER

(Trifolium pratense)

Alternate Names/Related Species:
Wild Clover, Purple Clover, Trefoil

Common Uses

Chemoprevention [+1]   **Hyperlipidemia** [−1]

**Menopausal
symptoms** [−1]

*(Higher numbers indicate stronger evidence; X modifier indicates contradic-
tory results. See page xviii of the Introduction for details of the rating scale.)*

Approach to the Patient

Red clover *(Trifolium pratense)* is rich in various isoflavones, including daidzein and genistein (also found in soy), as well as
biochanin A and formononetin. Red clover isoflavones were extensively marketed as a treatment for menopausal symptoms before completion of any meaningful studies. Your patient may not
know that the results of two double-blind trials have now come
in; they were both negative. Red clover isoflavones have also
failed to prove effective for hyperlipidemia.

In the nineteenth century, red clover was popular among herbalists as an "alternative" or "blood purifier." These dated medical
terms refer to an ancient belief that hematologic toxins are the
root cause of many illnesses, including cancer. This belief is the
basis for red clover's inclusion in many alternative treatments
for cancer, including the Hoxsey cancer formula. Although there
is no clinical evidence that red clover can treat cancer, its
isoflavones may have chemopreventive effects.

Chemoprevention   + 1

Preliminary evidence suggests that the isoflavones present in red clover may possess chemopreventive activity.[1-5]

Menopausal Symptoms   − 1

On the basis of its high concentrations of phytoestrogenic isoflavones, red clover has been marketed as a treatment for menopausal symptoms. However, two double-blind, placebo-controlled trials involving a total of 88 women failed to show reduction of menopausal symptoms with red clover treatment.[6,7]

Hyperlipidemia   − 1

A 12-week, double-blind, placebo-controlled, ascending-dose study evaluated the effects of a purified extract of red clover in 66 postmenopausal women with moderate hypercholesterolemia.[8] Supplementation with red clover isoflavones did not significantly alter total plasma cholesterol, low-density lipoprotein (LDL), high-density lipoprotein (HDL), or triglyceride levels.

Other Proposed Uses

Based on archaic ideas about blood purification, red clover has been suggested as a treatment for acne, eczema, psoriasis, and other skin diseases. However, no evidence supports these uses.

Mechanism of Action

An isoflavone constituent of red clover, biochanin A, has been shown in vitro to inhibit carcinogen activation.[1] Another in vitro study of human stomach cancer cell lines suggests that biochanin A inhibits cell growth through activation of a signal transduction pathway for apoptosis.[2] Animal studies suggest that biochanin A as well as other constituents of red clover possess estrogenic properties.[9] Chemopreventive and phytoestrogenic properties have also been found for other isoflavones in red clover, including genistein.[3-5]

A double-blind trial of 30 individuals found that use of red clover isoflavones did not exert either a proliferatory or an antiproliferatory effect on the endometrium.[11]

Dosage

A typical dosage of red clover extract provides 40 to 160 mg of isoflavones daily. See the Appendix for U.S. brand names of clinically tested products.

Safety Issues

Red clover is on the FDA's GRAS (generally recognized as safe) list and is included in many beverage teas. However, detailed safety studies have not been performed.

Because red clover contains isoflavonoid constituents, its use in women with a history of hormone-sensitive cancer warrants caution.[10] In addition, given its coumarin constituents, use in women currently taking anticoagulants is questionable.[10]

Maximum safe dosages in individuals with severe hepatic or renal disease are not known.

See the full article on Isoflavones for other potential risks.

Safety in Young Children and Pregnant or Lactating Women

Because of its phytoestrogenic and anticoagulant components, red clover is not recommended for use in pregnant or lactating women. Safety in young children has not been established.

Drug Interactions

Formal drug interaction studies have not been performed. However, based on the presence of phytoestrogenic and anticoagulant constituents, red clover extracts may potentially interfere with **hormone therapy** and may potentiate the effect of **anticoagulant** pharmaceuticals.

RED YEAST RICE

Alternate Names/Supplement Forms:
Monascus purpureus, Monascus yeast species,
Cholestin, Hong Qu, Monacolin K

Common Use

Hyperlipidemia [+2]

(Higher numbers indicate stronger evidence; X modifier indicates contradictory results. See page xviii of the Introduction for details of the rating scale.)

Approach to the Patient

Red yeast rice (a preparation of *Monascus purpureus* yeast fermented over rice) contains several naturally occurring substances in the statin drug family (including mevinolin, identical to lovastatin). The evidence from preliminary studies suggests that red yeast rice can reduce levels of total cholesterol, low-density lipoprotein (LDL), and triglycerides in subjects with hyperlipidemia.

Like standard statin drugs, red yeast rice presumably inhibits cholesterol synthesis by impairing the action of 3-hydroxy-3-methylglutaryl coenzyme A (HMG-CoA) reductase, as well as by increasing LDL receptor prevalence.

However, your patients may not be able to get red yeast rice: because it contains lovastatin, the major brand has been taken off the market. At the time of publication, it is not clear whether any form of red yeast rice will be available.

Hyperlipidemia   + 2

An 8-week, double-blind, placebo-controlled trial of 83 subjects with hyperlipidemia evaluated red yeast rice.[1] At the end of the study after 8 weeks of administration, total cholesterol in the red yeast rice group decreased significantly compared with the placebo group: 208 mg/dL vs. 254 mg/dL. At follow-up 4 weeks later, LDL was 135 mg/dL for the treated group vs. 175 for the placebo group, and triglycerides were 124 mg/dL vs. 146 mg/dL, respectively. However, no significant differences were noted in high-density lipoprotein (HDL) levels from baseline or between groups.

Benefits with red yeast rice were also seen in U.S. and Chinese open trials.[2,3]

Mechanism of Action

The statins in red yeast rice inhibit HMG-CoA reductase. This enzyme converts HMG-CoA to mevalonate, a key step in the biosynthesis of cholesterol.

It has been suggested that the quantity of statins found in red yeast rice is insufficient to explain the hypolipidemic effect seen.[1] The overall effect may be due to the action of all the related statinlike substances found in red yeast rice, perhaps augmented by sterols, isoflavones, isoflavone glycosides, and mono-unsaturated fatty acids.

Dosage

The dosage used in most studies is 1.2 to 2.4 g of red yeast rice powder daily. The clinically tested brand (Cholestin) has been taken off the market and replaced with a policosanol product (New Cholestin).

Safety Issues

In clinical trials, use of red yeast rice has not been associated with any significant side effects. No toxic effects have been reported in studies in rats and mice given doses 125 times greater than human doses, according to unpublished results on file with one of the manufacturers of a red yeast rice product.[4] However, many red yeast rice products have been found to contain detectable levels of citrinin, a nephrotoxic mycotoxin that can form under inappropriate fermentation conditions.[5]

In addition, it is likely that red yeast rice could produce the same side effects as statin drugs. Elevations of serum aminotransferases caused by statins are usually mild, but elevations greater than three times normal have been reported. In rare cases, myopathy has developed with creatine phosphokinase levels more than 10 times the normal limit. This is more likely to occur if statin drugs are taken with gemfibrozil, high-dose niacin, or cyclosporine (see Drug Interactions).

Persons with hepatic disease or a history of alcohol abuse may develop elevated aminotransferase activity.

Maximum safe dosages in individuals with severe hepatic or renal disease are not known.

Safety in Young Children and Pregnant or Lactating Women

Red yeast rice is not recommended for pregnant or lactating women, women likely to become pregnant, or children.

Drug Interactions

The drug interactions of red yeast rice are presumably similar to those of other statin drugs: it is reasonable to assume that the incidence of myopathy or rhabdomyolysis may increase in patients also receiving **cyclosporine, fibric acid derivatives, erythromycin, azole antifungals,** and high doses of **niacin.** In addition, concomitant use of **warfarin** may increase the risk of bleeding.

Grapefruit juice reduces the activity of cytochrome P-450 3A4 enzymes, resulting in increased levels of lovastatin; presumably, consumption of grapefruit juice with red yeast rice could increase the risk of side effects.

It would not make sense to combine red yeast rice with standard **statin drugs.**

Statin drugs are known to reduce serum levels of CoQ_{10}, for which supplementation might be helpful.[6-9] Red yeast rice could do the same, but this has not been studied.

REISHI
(Ganoderma lucidum)

Common Use

Antiviral   [+1]

(Higher numbers indicate stronger evidence; X modifier indicates contradictory results. See page xviii of the Introduction for details of the rating scale.)

Approach to the Patient

Reishi *(Ganoderma lucidum)* is a "medicinal" mushroom classified by contemporary herbalists as an "adaptogen," a substance said to help the body adapt to stress and resist infection (see the article on **Ginseng** for further information regarding adaptogens). Highly preliminary data suggest that reishi may have antiviral effects. However, there have not been any meaningful clinical trials of reishi.

Antiviral   +1

In vitro studies suggest that several protein-bound polysaccharides of reishi have antiviral activities against multiple agents, including herpes simplex viruses (HSV-1, HSV-2), influenza A virus, and vesicular stomatitis virus (VSV) Indiana and New Jersey strains.[1,2] However, no clinical evidence supports the efficacy of reishi as an antiviral.

Other Proposed Uses

Reishi has been marketed for a wide variety of therapeutic benefits including chemoprevention, strengthening immunity against infection, restoring normal immune function in autoimmune diseases such as myasthenia gravis, improving symptoms of asthma and bronchitis, enhancing recovery from viral hepatitis, preventing and treating cardiovascular disease, improving mental function, healing ulcers, and preventing altitude sickness. However, there is no real evidence that reishi is effective for any of these uses.

Mechanism of Action

The mechanism of action of reishi is not known. However, most investigations have focused on its polysaccharide constituents, which may have immunomodulatory actions.

Dosage

The standard dosage of reishi is 2 to 6 g per day of raw fungus, or an equivalent dosage of concentrated extract, taken with meals. Reishi is often combined with related fungi such as shiitake, hoelen, or *Polyporus* species.

Safety Issues

Reishi is widely believed to be safe, although formal safety studies have not been performed. Occasional side effects include mild digestive upset, dry mouth, and rash.

One study in mice found no evidence of genotoxic chromosomal breakage or cytotoxic effects by *Ganoderma*.[3]

Maximum safe dosages in individuals with severe hepatic or renal disease are not known.

Safety in Young Children and Pregnant or Lactating Women

Maximum safe dosages for pregnant or lactating women or young children have not been established.

Drug Interactions

There are no known drug interactions.

RIBOSE

Coronary artery disease [+2]

Performance enhancement [−1]

(Higher numbers indicate stronger evidence; X modifier indicates contradictory results. See page xviii of the Introduction for details of the rating scale.)

Approach to the Patient

Ribose has become a popular sports supplement based on its role in adenosine triphosphate (ATP) synthesis. However, there is no evidence that oral ribose supplements produce any ergogenic effect. Weak evidence does support the use of ribose in coronary artery disease. In addition, case reports suggest potential benefit in myoadenylate deaminase deficiency.

Coronary Artery Disease   +2

One small, controlled study with 20 participants found that 3 days of ribose treatment improved before- and after-treadmill exercise tolerance in individuals with significant coronary artery disease.[1]

Performance Enhancement   −1

In a double-blind, placebo-controlled study of 20 male physical education students, use of ribose at a dose of 4 g four times daily for 6 days produced no increase in repeated maximal exercise capacity.[7] Biopsy results in a subset of participants found no change in muscle ATP resynthesis attributable to ribose.

Other Proposed Uses

In a few case reports, ribose supplements have apparently increased exercise ability in **myoadenylate deaminase (AMPD) deficiency**[3,4]; however, no double-blind studies of ribose in AMPD deficiency have been conducted. Small, double-blind studies have failed to find ribose effective in **McArdle's disease** or **Duchenne's muscular dystrophy.**[5,6]

Mechanism of Action

Exogenous ribose is thought to bypass rate-limiting steps in the oxidative pentose phosphate pathway that creates 5-phosphoribosyl-1-pyrophosphate, a necessary precursor for ATP synthesis. The net result is thought to be enhanced ATP synthesis, both in smooth and skeletal muscle.[1,2]

Dosage

Typical doses of ribose recommended by sports supplement manufacturers are 1 to 10 g per day. In the coronary artery disease study described above, participants received 60 g of ribose in water, in four divided doses.[1] In the AMPD deficiency case reports, 3 to 4 g was used every 10 to 30 minutes during exercise, sometimes totaling 50 to 60 g per day.[3,4]

Ribose is typically provided in liquid form or as a powder to be dissolved in water, but it is also available commercially in capsules. The dissolved powder has a semisweet taste that some individuals find unpleasant.[5]

Safety Issues

There are no reports of significant side effects from ribose, but formal safety studies have not yet been conducted. Reported minor side effects include diarrhea, gastrointestinal discomfort, nausea, headache, and hypoglycemia.[1]

Maximum safe dosages in individuals with severe hepatic or renal disease are not known.

As with all supplements used in multigram doses, use of a quality product is critical, since contaminants present in even small percentages could result in toxic effects.

Safety in Young Children and Pregnant or Lactating Women

Maximum safe dosages for pregnant or lactating women or young children have not been established.

Drug Interactions

There are no known drug interactions.

S-ADENOSYLMETHIONINE (SAMe)

Common Uses

Osteoarthritis [+3]   **Depression** [+2X]

Fibromyalgia [+2]   **Hepatic disease** [+1]

(Higher numbers indicate stronger evidence; X modifier indicates contradictory results. See page xviii of the Introduction for details of the rating scale.)

Approach to the Patient

Formed by the combination of the amino acid methionine and adenosine triphosphate (ATP), S-adenosylmethionine (SAMe) functions as a ubiquitous methyl donor in methyl-transferase reactions involving proteins, phospholipids, deoxyribonucleic acid (DNA), neurotransmitters, and numerous other essential biochemicals.[1] SAMe is also central to the manufacture of many sulfur-containing compounds, such as glutathione and proteoglycans.[2]

In osteoarthritis, reasonable evidence suggests that 1200 mg/day of SAMe is as effective as 750 mg of naproxen and possesses a superior side-effects profile. Preliminary evidence including one large trial suggests that oral SAMe may also be effective for depression; additional proposed uses with some evidence include fibromyalgia and various hepatic diseases.

The supplement is widely available in the United States. However, your patients may be interested to know that the label instructions advise a dose that is four times too low. This hides the high cost of SAMe; a typical full monthly dose might cost $200.

You may wish to steer your patients to glucosamine or chondroitin as less expensive and better established treatments for osteoarthritis. Similarly, St. John's wort *(Hypericum perforatum)* is better established as a treatment for depression, although it does present some significant safety risks.

Osteoarthritis   + 3

A 4-week, double-blind study investigated the effects of 1200 mg/day of SAMe (oral dose), 750 mg/day of naproxen, or placebo in 732 individuals with osteoarthritis treated at 33 centers.[3] The results showed similar benefits in the SAMe and naproxen groups.

In other double-blind studies, oral SAMe has also shown equivalent benefits to indomethacin (150 mg/day), low-dose ibuprofen (400 mg twice daily), naproxen (initially 250 mg three times daily, then twice daily), and full-dose piroxicam (20 mg daily).[4-6]

Fibromyalgia   + 2

A 6-week, double-blind study of 44 patients with fibromyalgia found improvements in disease activity, pain at rest, fatigue, and morning stiffness and in one measurement of mood in the SAMe-treated group (800 mg orally per day).[7] Similar results were found in a small, earlier study.[8] However, it is not clear whether these benefits resulted from direct improvement of fibromyalgia or, secondarily, through SAMe's probable antidepressant action.

Depression   + 2 X

The research record for SAMe in depression is modest, contradictory, and marked by numerous flaws; further, many studies involved IV or IM administration.[9]

Three double-blind, placebo-controlled studies observing a total of 135 patients with major, postmenopausal, or postpartum depression found significant improvements in depressive symptoms in those treated with oral SAMe as compared with placebo.[10-12] However, one double-blind, placebo-controlled study of 32 patients found no significant difference between treatment and control groups.[13] These studies were generally marred by poor reporting and unusually wide variation in the placebo group response (0 to 65%).

In a double-blind, placebo-controlled study of 133 depressed patients, the effects of 800 mg/day of intravenous SAMe failed to achieve significance over placebo, unless subgroup analysis or secondary outcome measures were employed.[14]

Oral SAMe has also been compared with standard agents. A 6-week, double-blind trial of 281 depressed individuals evaluated the relative effects of oral SAMe (1600 mg/day) and imipramine (150 mg/day).[15] Intention-to-treat analysis showed no differences in outcome. However, the average severity of depression in this trial was low (21-item HAM-D average score of 18); nonspecific effects could have been the primary source of the improvement seen.

Other small studies have also compared the benefits of oral or parenteral SAMe with those of tricyclic antidepressants, finding generally equivalent results.[16-19] However, marked inadequacies of study design and reporting diminish the meaningfulness of the outcomes.

In addition, SAMe might have specific utility in the depression associated with Parkinson's disease. L-Dopa depletes brain levels of SAMe.[20,21] It has been hypothesized that Parkinson's depression is related to this depletion. In a double-blind, placebo-controlled trial with 21 individuals taking L-dopa for Parkinson's disease, participants received either placebo or a combination of oral and injected SAMe for 30 days and were then crossed over.[22] The results showed improvements in symptoms of depression without loss of L-dopa efficacy.

However, there are concerns regarding long-term use of SAMe supplements in Parkinson's disease (see Drug Interactions).

Hepatic Disease   +1

A 2-year, double-blind, placebo-controlled study of 123 individuals with alcoholic cirrhosis found a statistically insignificant trend toward improvement in the verum group as compared with the placebo group; post-hoc analysis found significant differences in the subgroup with less advanced disease.[23] Small trials, some of which were double-blind, found possible value in oral contraceptive hepatotoxicity, intrahepatic cholestasis of pregnancy, and Gilbert's syndrome.[2,24-27]

Other Proposed Uses

One open study suggests that SAMe might be beneficial in **migraine headaches**.[28]

Mechanism of Action

SAMe is believed to assist metabolically in the manufacture and repair of cartilage[29,30] and to protect cartilage from damage.[31,32]

In depression, supplementation with SAMe may increase the concentration or action of dopamine and other neurotransmitters.[21,33-37] The presumed mechanism of action involves facilitated methylation of precursors as well as effects on brain cell membrane fluidity and receptor binding of neurotransmitters.

Supplementation with preformed SAMe would be expected to bypass one major need for folate (as 5-methyl-tetrahydrofolate). Because folate deficiency is linked to depression in the older population,[38] this might be one mechanism by which SAMe provides antidepressant benefits.

Dosage

To minimize possible gastrointestinal distress, SAMe is often started at an initial dose of 200 mg twice daily and then rapidly titrated upward over 1 or 2 weeks, depending on response. For osteoarthritis, 1200 mg/day in three divided doses is generally regarded as optimum for initial treatment. After symptomatic relief develops, a maintenance dose as low as 200 mg twice daily may suffice. For fibromyalgia, 800 mg orally per day was found effective in one study.[7] Although dosages of 1600 mg/day may be necessary to achieve initial response to SAMe in depression, a maintenance dose of 200 mg twice daily might suffice.

Some forms of oral SAMe may not be stable,[39] although a newly developed manufacturing technique offers promise of a more stable product.[40]

Safety Issues

In general, SAMe is very well-tolerated. In a limited study in rats and rabbits, SAMe was found to have very low toxicity in adult animals or their offspring, with the exception of an unrealistically high subcutaneous dose of 400 mg/kg.[41] SAMe does not appear to be mutagenic.[42]

Large long-term drug-monitoring studies have found that SAMe is well-tolerated.[30,43] However, the doses of SAMe used in these trials were significantly lower than the maximum amounts recommended. In a 4-week, double-blind study that involved more than 200 patients who took SAMe, 1200 mg/day, the treated group showed no more side effects than the matching placebo group.[3]

In patients with bipolar disorder, SAMe in oral doses has caused transition from a depressed to an elevated state (hypomania, mania, or euphoria).[44,45] At least one case has been reported of a manic episode induced by SAMe in a patient with no previous history of bipolar illness.[12]

Maximum safe dosages in individuals with severe hepatic or renal disease are not known.

Safety in Young Children and Pregnant or Lactating Women

Although SAMe has been used in studies of pregnant women with no apparent adverse effects,[25,27,46] maximum safe dosages for pregnant or lactating women or young children have not been established.

Drug Interactions

L-dopa is an avid acceptor of methyl groups, and its use leads to decreased levels of brain SAMe.[20,21] It has also been suggested that SAMe depletion may contribute to L-dopa side effects and gradual loss of efficacy of the drug.[21] One short-term, double-blind study did find that Parkinson's patients on L-dopa could be given SAMe without loss of L-dopa efficacy.[22] However, in the long term, SAMe supplementation might increase methylation and inactivation of L-dopa.[20]

SAMe can increase the metabolism of certain drugs by facilitating their conjugation.[47] However, the clinical significance of this observation is not known.

There has been one report of apparent serotonergic syndrome in a 71-year-old woman simultaneously taking **clomipramine** and intramuscular SAMe (100 mg/day).[48] Symptoms included hyperthermia, delirium, and myoclonic muscular rigidity.

SAW PALMETTO
(Sabal serrulata, Serenoa repens)

Alternate Names/Related Species: Permixon, Strogen Forte

Common Uses

Benign prostatic hyperplasia [+3]

Lower urinary tract symptoms in men [+2]

(Higher numbers indicate stronger evidence; X modifier indicates contradictory results. See page xviii of the Introduction for details of the rating scale.)

Approach to the Patient

Saw palmetto *(Sabal serrulata, Serenoa repens)* appears to be an effective treatment for symptoms accompanying mild to moderate benign prostatic hyperplasia (BPH) (Vahlensieck stage I or II). It is not appropriate for advanced BPH with severe urinary retention, nor should it be used without first ruling out prostate cancer.

Studies suggest that saw palmetto is approximately as effective as finasteride as well as alpha blockers. Benefits are typically reported by about 4 to 6 weeks, and about two thirds of men respond well. Unlike finasteride, which causes a greater reduction in prostate size, saw palmetto has not been shown to reduce the ultimate need for surgery. However, because finasteride lowers prostate-specific antigen (PSA) levels, it might mask prostate cancer; saw palmetto does not alter PSA levels. In addition, saw palmetto has no negative effect on sexual function.

Many products marketed for BPH contain several supplements combined, each at an inadequate dose. Your patients may do better using a single-substance product that provides the dose found effective in double-blind trials. (See the article on **Benign**

Prostatic Hyperplasia for several reasonably well-documented options.)

Saw palmetto might also be effective for nonspecific lower urinary tract symptoms (LUTS) in men.

Benign Prostatic Hyperplasia   +3

Seven double-blind, placebo-controlled trials have evaluated the effectiveness of saw palmetto in BPH.[1-10] These trials have ranged in length from 1 to 3 months and have involved a total of about 500 men. In all but one of these studies,[6] treatment with saw palmetto significantly improved urinary flow rate and most other measures of prostate disease.

Double-blind, comparative trials have also been reported. A 6-month, double-blind study of 1098 men compared finasteride with saw palmetto and found equivalent reductions in symptoms.[11] Prosate size reduction was superior with finasteride (18% vs. 6% reduction). However, this study has been criticized on the basis that its inclusion criteria regarding prostate volume and its limited duration may have precluded maximal efficacy of finasteride.[12,13] Both treatments were well-tolerated; however, sexual function scores were better in the saw palmetto group.

A 48-week, double-blind trial of 543 patients with early BPH compared combined saw palmetto and nettle root against finasteride and found equal benefits.[14] Analysis of a 431-patient subgroup with larger prostate volume (> 40 mL), for which finasteride might be more effective, found similar results.

A 52-week, double-blind study of 811 men compared saw palmetto with the alpha-blocker tamsulosin and found equivalent efficacy in subjective and objective scores of BPH severity.[15] The saw palmetto arm, however, experienced a decrease in prostate volume while a slight increase occurred among participants given tamsulosin. Both treatments were well-tolerated; however, tamsulosin caused a higher incidence of ejaculation dysfunction.

A 6-month, double-blind, placebo-controlled trial of 44 men given a saw palmetto herbal blend also containing nettle root and pumpkin seed oil found significant reduction in prostate size.[16] No significant improvement in symptoms was seen, but the study size did not have the power to detect such improvement.

Lower Urinary Tract Symptoms in Men   +2

In a 6-month, double-blind, placebo-controlled study of 81 men with moderate to severe lower urinary tract symptoms (LUTS), use of saw palmetto led to a statistically significant improvement in urinary symptoms as compared with placebo.[17] However, there was no significant improvement in measures of urinary flow or sexual function.

Other Proposed Uses

An open trial that compared saw palmetto to finasteride for the treatment of **chronic nonbacterial prostatititis** found that, while the herb produced no improvement in symptoms, the drug did prove effective.[18]

Saw palmetto is rarely used for other genitourinary complaints or for breast disorders. Its old reputation as a mild aphrodisiac has lately been resurrected in some herbal combination formulas, but there is no evidence to support this use.

Mechanism of Action

The mechanism of action of saw palmetto is not fully understood. Possible and mutually compatible explanations include prostate volume reduction, inhibition of 5-alpha-reductase, direct antiandrogen effects, interference with prostate estrogen receptors, leukotriene inhibition, and muscular relaxation.[11,16,19-29]

In rodents, saw palmetto has been found not to exhibit estrogenic or progestational properties or produce hypophyseal inhibition.[30] In humans, therapeutic doses of saw palmetto extracts do not cause alpha-1-adrenoreceptor inhibition.[31]

Dosage

The standard dose of saw palmetto is 160 mg twice per day of a lipophilic extract standardized to contain 85% to 95% fatty acids and sterols. Some evidence suggests that a once-daily dose of 320 mg is equally effective.[32,33] In a 6-month dose-determination trial, 480 mg daily was not found to be any more effective than 320 mg.[10] The most studied saw palmetto product, Permixon, uses an extraction process based on hexane. Other products use ethanol, methanol, or liquid carbon dioxide as solvents. Teas and other preparations of saw palmetto are not effective because the active constituents are lipophilic. See the Appendix for U.S. brand names of clinically tested products.

Safety Issues

Saw palmetto is well-tolerated; in clinical trials, only nonspecific side effects have been reported. In rats and dogs, saw palmetto extract administered at a dose of 2 g/kg daily for 6 months produced no toxic, mutagenic, or teratogenic effects.[30]

No clinically relevant changes in laboratory parameters have been seen in human clinical trials.[10] However, in one case report, use of saw palmetto was associated with significantly increased bleeding time and intraoperative hemorrage.[34] This report is not consistent with any known actions of saw palmetto or its constituents and awaits future elucidation.

Maximum safe dosages in individuals with severe hepatic or renal disease are not known.

Safety in Young Children and Pregnant or Lactating Women

Maximum safe dosages for pregnant or lactating women or young children have not been established; however, saw palmetto is primarily intended for use by adult men.

In rats and dogs, saw palmetto extract has been well-tolerated orally at a dose of 2 g/kg daily for 6 months and has been found devoid of mutagenic or teratogenic effects.[30]

Drug Interactions

There are no known drug interactions.

SCHISANDRA
(Schisandra chinensis)

Alternate Names/Related Species:
Wu-Wei-Zi, Magnolia Vine, Gomishi, Fructus Schizandrae

Common Uses

Hepatoprotection [+1]   **Chemoprevention** [+1]

**Athletic performance
enhancement** [+1]

(Higher numbers indicate stronger evidence; X modifier indicates contradictory results. See page xviii of the Introduction for details of the rating scale.)

Approach to the Patient

Schisandra *(Schisandra chinensis)* has long been used in the traditional medicines of Russia and China for a wide variety of conditions, including asthma, coughs, and other respiratory ailments, diarrhea, insomnia, impotence, and kidney problems. Hunters and athletes have used schisandra in the belief that it will increase endurance and counter fatigue under physical stress. More recently, schisandra has been studied for potential hepatoprotective effects.

However, you can inform your pateints that schisandra has not been evaluated in any meaningful trials. Research on the herb is limited to studies in animals as well as human trials that are not up to modern scientific standards.

Hepatoprotection   +1

Animal studies suggest that schisandra may protect the liver from toxic damage, improve hepatic function, and stimulate hepatic cell regrowth.[1-6] These findings led to its use in human trials for treating hepatitis. In a Chinese study of 189 individuals with hepatitis B, those given schisandra reportedly improved more rapidly than those given vitamins and liver extracts[6]; however, the study design and reporting were inadequate.

Athletic Performance Enhancement   +1

Preliminary studies in animals and humans suggest that schisandra or its extracts might increase stamina and speed and improve mental concentration.[1,7-9]

Chemoprevention   +1

Animal studies of schisandra have found possible chemopreventive properties.[1,6,10]

Mechanism of Action

The mechanism of action of schisandra is not known.

Dosage

Schisandra is available in capsules, tinctures, powder, tablets, and extracts. Common dosages are 1.5 to 6 g daily.

Safety Issues

Studies in mice, rats, and pigs have found schisandra to be relatively nontoxic.[1] Noticeable side effects are apparently rare; however, in large doses, schisandra may cause gastrointestinal distress or appetite suppression.[11] Allergic reactions may also occur.

Maximum safe dosages in individuals with severe hepatic or re-nal disease have not been established.

Safety in Young Children and Pregnant or Lactating Women

Maximum safe dosages for pregnant or lactating women or young children have not been established.

Drug Interactions

There are no known drug interactions.

SELENIUM

Alternate Names/Supplement Forms:
Selenite, Selenomethionine, Selenized Yeast,
Selenium Dioxide

Common Uses

Chemoprevention [+3]

Rheumatoid arthritis [−1X]

Cardiovascular disease (prevention) [−1]

(Higher numbers indicate stronger evidence; X modifier indicates contradictory results. See page xviii of the Introduction for details of the rating scale.)

Approach to the Patient

Selenium is an essential dietary mineral whose exact recommended daily intake has not been defined. Low tissue levels of selenium and inadequate dietary intake of the mineral have been associated with numerous illnesses, but an actual benefit of taking selenium supplements has not been found for any disease other than cancer—and even for cancer the evidence is incomplete.

Overt selenium deficiency has been primarily observed in parts of China where selenium soil levels are extremely low. Symptoms include heart disorders, joint damage, muscle weakness, and an increased incidence of liver cancer. The incidence of other cancers also appears to be abnormally high in areas of low soil selenium.[1,2]

Excessive doses of selenium can be toxic. See Safety Issues for tolerable upper intake levels.

Chemoprevention   +3

One multicenter, double-blind, placebo-controlled randomized trial evaluated the effects of oral selenium, 200 μg/day, against skin cancer in 1312 seniors for an average of about 6 years.[3] Average initial serum selenium levels of participants fell in the low-normal range. Although no effect was seen on that primary end-point illness, the reduction in overall cancer mortality and total cancer incidence was so significant that the blinded phase of the trial was concluded prematurely. The selenium-treated group experienced statistically significant reductions in prostate (66% relative risk [RR]), colorectal (50% RR), and lung (40% RR) cancer; they also experienced a statistically significant reduction in overall mortality (17% RR), lung cancer deaths (greater than 50% RR), and total cancer deaths (nearly 50% RR). No cases of selenium toxicity were reported. However, this study has been criticized for its reliance on secondary end points.

In an 8-year intervention trial (blinding unknown) among a population of 130,471 in the Qidong region of China,[4] the average age-adjusted incidence of liver cancer in the group given table salt fortified with 15 ppm of sodium selenite was reduced by 35.1%, with no change observed in the control group. On withdrawal of the selenium-supplemented salt, liver cancer rates returned to pretreatment levels.

Three very large observational studies report mixed evidence about the possible role of selenium deficiency in various cancers.[5-7] In one study of 120,852 men and women aged 55 to 69 years, those with selenium levels in the highest quintile (assessed by toenail selenium measurement) developed lung cancer at one half the rate of those in the lowest quintile, over the 3.3-year study period.[5] However, in a retrospective analysis of the Nurses' Health Study cohort, no correlation between dietary selenium intake and cancer in general was found.[6] Similarly, a 3.3-year prospective Dutch study of 62,573 women found no associations between dietary selenium and breast cancer.[7]

Rheumatoid Arthritis   − 1 X

Lower-than-average selenium levels have been found in individuals with rheumatoid arthritis,[8,9] and low selenium status appears to be a risk factor for Rh factor–negative rheumatoid arthritis (RA).[10] However, no improvement was seen in a double-blind study in which 40 patients with severe RA were given placebo or 256 μg of selenium in enriched yeast for 6 months.[8,9] Another double-blind study observed 55 individuals for 90 days and again found no significant improvement.[32] Similarly negative results were seen in two other small trials.[33,34] Some benefit was seen in a very small, double-blind study of mild RA.[11]

Cardiovascular Disease   − 1

The evidence for benefits of selenium supplementation in heart disease remains inconclusive.[12]

Positive associations were seen in an observational study examining the relationship between selenium status (assessed by toenail selenium measurement) and risk of acute myocardial infarction in Europe and Israel.[13] The results showed that those with the highest selenium levels had 0.63 times the chance of developing an MI as those with the lowest. On closer examination, the benefit was observed only in former cigarette smokers; those who continued to smoke or who never smoked at all showed no association. Other studies have shown a weak correlation between selenium levels and cardiovascular risk.[14-16]

A double-blind intervention trial observed 81 post-MI patients, randomizing them to receive either placebo or selenium (from selenium-rich yeast), 100 μg/day. At 6 months, the control group had experienced four fatal heart attacks and two nonfatal heart attacks, compared with no fatal heart attacks and only one nonfatal heart attack in the treated group, but the differences were not statistically significant.[17]

Other Proposed Uses

Selenium has also been proposed as a treatment for cataracts, acquired immunodeficiency syndrome (AIDS), acne, multiple sclerosis, cervical dysplasia, asthma, and osteoarthritis. However, the evidence for a beneficial effect in these conditions is indirect and is based primarily on basic science regarding antioxidants as well as observations that patients with these conditions often have lower-than-normal tissue levels of selenium.

Mechanism of Action

The antioxidant enzyme glutathione peroxidase incorporates selenium at the active sites of its chemical structure. When dietary intake of selenium is low, glutathione levels drop, potentially resulting in increased oxidative damage to a wide variety of tissues. Selenium also protects the liver, kidney, and other tissues by enhancing the detoxification of metabolically activated carcinogens. Although selenium does not appear to alter the activity of the cytochrome P-450 isozymes responsible for carcinogen-activating phase I reactions, it does induce phase II detoxification enzymes such as glutathione-S-transferase and UDP-glucuronyltransferase.[18] In addition, one study that examined the effects of 200 μg of supplemental selenium in patients who were *not* selenium deficient found a significant increase in cytotoxic lymphocyte-mediated tumor cytotoxicity and natural killer cell activity.[19]

Potential chemopreventive effects might also be related to immune status, altering viral infections that raise cancer risk.[20,21] Selenium may also enhance premalignant apoptosis.[22-24]

In addition, selenium may antagonize the absorption of lead, mercury, aluminum, and cadmium and may play a role in the production of thyroid hormone.[25,26]

Dosage

The U.S. Dietary Reference Intake for selenium for males and females 14 years and older is 55 μg.[27] In children, this is reduced to 1.5 μg/lb body weight.

Safety Issues

The tolerable upper intake levels for selenium have been set as follows: children 1 to 3 years, 90 μg; 4 to 8 years, 150 μg; 9 to 13 years, 280 μg; males and females 14 years and older, 400 μg.[27]

Toxic effects begin to be seen at levels of 750 to 1000 μg/day, including gastrointestinal distress, central nervous system (CNS) changes, garliclike breath odor, and loss of hair and fingernails.[20,28] In excessive doses, selenium can form dangerous superoxide compounds.

Maximum safe dosages in individuals with severe hepatic or renal disease are not known.

Safety in Young Children and Pregnant or Lactating Women

Needs for selenium appear to increase during pregnancy, and infants given formula alone can become selenium deficient.[28,29]

The tolerable upper intake level of selenium for pregnant or lactating women has been set at 400 μg daily.[27]

Drug Interactions

Weak evidence suggests that selenium supplementation is beneficial in preventing the nephrotoxicity and leukopenia of cancer **chemotherapy.**[30]

Treatment with **corticosteroids** may induce selenium deficiency.[31]

Proton pump inhibitors and **H$_2$ blockers** may impair absorption of selenium.

SOY PROTEIN

Alternate Names/Supplement Forms:
Hydrolyzed Soy Protein, Soy Protein Extract

Common Uses

Hyperlipidemia [+3]   **Osteoporosis** [+2X]

Menopausal   **Chemoprevention** [+1]
symptoms [+3X]

(Higher numbers indicate stronger evidence; X modifier indicates contradictory results. See page xviii of the Introduction for details of the rating scale.)

Approach to the Patient

A growing body of evidence suggests that soy foods can improve lipid profiles and reduce menopausal symptoms. Weaker evidence suggests a bone-sparing and chemopreventive role.

Your patients may be interested to know that there is better evidence for soy protein than for supplements containing isolated soy isoflavones. (For more information on the latter, see the **Isoflavone** article.)

Hyperlipidemia   +3

A metaanalysis of 38 controlled studies on soy and heart disease concluded that soy is effective at reducing total cholesterol, low-density lipoprotein (LDL), and triglyceride levels.[1] The average dosage of 47 g daily lowered total cholesterol 9%, LDL 13%, and triglycerides 10%. The effect on high-density lipoprotein (HDL) levels was less clear. Benefits have been seen in more recent studies as well,[2] and the U.S. Food and Drug Administration (FDA) has approved a "heart-healthy" label for soy products. However, one double-blind, placebo-controlled trial of men and women found evidence that use of soy protein caused a decline in endothelial function in men only, and an increase in Lp(a) overall.[3] These are potentially adverse effects.

There is conflicting evidence regarding whether soy isoflavones are the active hypocholesterolemic ingredients in soy protein.[4,32-38,57] Inaccurate label claims for isoflavone content of soy products, as well as differences in the distribution of various isoflavones among products, may account for some of these contradictions.[58]

Menopausal Symptoms   + 3 X

According to most but not all studies, soy protein can reduce vasomotor and other symptoms of menopause.[52-56]

However, in a double-blind, placebo-controlled trial of 123 breast cancer survivors, soy failed to reduce vasomotor symptoms.[51]

Osteoporosis   + 2 X

Two controlled studies with a total of 135 postmenopausal women found that isoflavone-rich soy products have a beneficial effect on bone density.[9,10] For example, a 24-week, double-blind study of 69 postmenopausal women found that soy isoflavones reduced spinal bone loss.[10]

Similar benefits have been seen in several animal studies.[11-17] However, other animal studies and one human trial failed to find benefit.[18-20] Soy does not appear to have estrogenic effects on markers of bone resorption.[21]

Chemoprevention   + 1

Observational studies, along with in vitro and limited in vivo data, suggest that soy consumption may reduce risk of hormone-sensitive cancers such as uterine, breast, and prostate cancer, as well as colon cancer.[22-29]

Mechanism of Action

Soy isoflavones are the presumed active ingredient in soy. However, although there is some evidence to support this assumption, results have been inconsistent.[20,30-38]

Soy isoflavones (or their metabolic products) have estrogen agonist/antagonist activity. This is generally believed to be their primary mechanism of action. However, soy isoflavones are also antioxidants and may act in other ways as well.[12,23,39,40] In addition, unlike estrogen, which inhibits bone resorption, the soy isoflavone genistein may enhance new bone formation.[12]

Dosage

Soy products may improve lipid levels at a dose of 25 g/day of soy protein or more.

Soy protein may decrease absorption of **zinc, iron,** or **calcium** supplements.[41-43] To avoid absorption problems, patients should be counseled to take these vitamins at least 2 hours apart from eating soy.

Safety Issues

As a widely consumed food, soy is presumed to have a high safety margin. However, because of their complex estrogen agonist/antagonist effects, there are at least theoretic concerns that soy isoflavones may not be safe for women with a history of breast cancer. See the **Isoflavone** article for more information.

Soy and the soy isoflavone genistein may impair thyroid function.[44-46]

Most but not all studies suggest that use of soy by menstruating women may reduce average estradiol levels, partially suppress the midcycle follicle-stimulating hormone (FSH) surge, increase follicular phase estradiol, and extend the follicular phase by 1 or 2 days.[3,5-8,47,50]

The net effect of these actions may be to reduce breast cancer risk.

Soy contains relatively high levels of oxalates, possibly contraindicating high intake in individuals with a tendency to form oxalate stones.[48]

Maximum safe dosages in individuals with severe hepatic or renal disease are not known.

Safety in Young Children and Pregnant or Lactating Women

Concerns have been raised about the hormonal impact that intensive use of soy products by pregnant women might have on unborn fetuses.[44,45] Soy may produce hypothyroidism in infants.[45]

Maximum safe dosages for pregnant or lactating women or young children have not been established.

Drug Interactions

Soy protein may decrease absorption and perhaps impair the action of **thyroid hormone**.[44-46] Soy does not, however, appear to interact with **oral contraceptives**.[49]

SPIRULINA AND OTHER BLUE-GREEN ALGAE PRODUCTS

Common Uses

Nutritional support   **Fibromyalgia**   [+2]
[no rating applicable]

(Higher numbers indicate stronger evidence; X modifier indicates contradictory results. See page xviii of the Introduction for details of the rating scale.)

Approach to the Patient

The supplement called spirulina consists of one or more members of a family of blue-green algae. Spirulina is currently cultivated and processed on an industrial scale in several countries, for sale in the health food market. Related products such as *Chlorella pyrenoidosa* are also discussed here.

Spirulina has been marketed for a wide range of applications, but other than being a nutritious (and expensive) food for general nutritional support, there are no well-documented uses for it. One small double-blind trial found *Chlorella pyrenoidosa* helpful for fibromyalgia.

However, patients should be informed that there are some contamination concerns regarding blue-green algae products. See Safety Issues.

Nutritional Support (No Rating Applicable)

Dried spirulina contains up to 70% protein by weight, along with relatively high levels of various B vitamins, beta-carotene, and other carotenoids; minerals including calcium, iron, magnesium, manganese, potassium, and zinc; and gamma-linolenic acid (GLA).[1] Spirulina also contains vitamin B_{12}, but it is not in an absorbable form.[1]

Fibromyalgia   +2

A double-blind, placebo-controlled, crossover trial of 37 individuals found evidence that *Chlorella pyrenoidosa* supplements might reduce symptoms of fibromyalgia.[2]

Other Proposed Uses

Evidence from animal studies and one small controlled (but not blinded) study in humans suggests that spirulina might help lower **cholesterol**.[3-5]

Preliminary evidence suggests that spirulina, like other plant foods, might have **chemopreventive** effects.[6-8]

In vitro and animal studies have found highly preliminary evidence that spirulina might have some activity against **HIV**.[9,10] Other evidence suggests that selenium deficiency may increase the infectiousness of women with HIV-1.[11]

Similarly weak evidence suggests that spirulina may have **immunomodulatory**,[12-14] **antiallergic**,[15,16] and **hepatoprotective** properties.[17,18]

A double-blind, placebo-controlled trial investigated the possible **weight-loss** effects of spirulina.[19] Although individuals taking 8.4 g of spirulina daily lost weight, the difference between the spirulina group and the placebo group was not statistically significant.

Mechanism of Action

The mechanism of action of spirulina is not known.

Dosage

Typical doses of spirulina range from 1 to 8.4 g daily.

Safety Issues

Spirulina appears to be essentially nontoxic.[1,20,21] Nevertheless, there are areas of potential concern. When spirulina is grown with the use of fermented animal waste fertilizers, contamination with pathogenic bacteria could occur.[22] Spirulina might also concentrate heavy metals such as lead and mercury,[23] but this concern has been challenged by researchers suggesting that an individual would have to consume more than 77 g daily of the most heavily contaminated spirulina to reach unsafe levels of mercury and lead consumption.[24] Other forms of blue-green algae may at times secrete hepatotoxic and/or neurotoxic substances[25,26] or harbor *Vibrio cholerae* bacteria.[27]

Because of the high nucleic acid content of spirulina, excessive consumption might increase uric acid levels. One source recommends a maximum daily intake of 50 g.[24]

Maximum safe dosages in individuals with severe hepatic or renal disease are not known.

Safety in Young Children and Pregnant or Lactating Women

Maximum safe dosages for pregnant or lactating women or young children have not been determined.

Drug Interactions

There are no known drug interactions.

Alternate Names/Related Species:
Amber, Goatweed, Hardhay, Klamath Weed, Tipton Weed

Common Uses

**Major depression
of mild to moderate
severity   [+3X]**

Polyneuropathy   [−1]

(Higher numbers indicate stronger evidence; X modifier indicates contradictory results. See page xviii of the Introduction for details of the rating scale.)

Approach to the Patient

Contrary to widespread misperception, St. John's wort has primarily been tested as a treatment for major depression, not for less severe forms of depression. However, major depression itself comes in varying levels of severity; most studies of St. John's wort evaluated the herb for major depression of mild to moderate severity. (Pharmaceutical antidepressants have primarily been evaluated for the treatment of major depression of moderate severity. There are significant ethical and safety issues involved in enrolling individuals with severe major depression in a placebo-controlled study.) Evidence from all but two trials suggests that St. John's wort is more effective than placebo and approximately as effective as standard pharmaceutical therapies.

In addition to depression, St. John's wort has been proposed for numerous other conditions that might suggest the use of a standard antidepressant, such as premenstrual syndrome (PMS), anxiety, insomnia, and menopausal symptoms. However, there have been no meaningful double-blind trials of St. John's wort for these conditions.

St. John's wort is generally well-tolerated when taken alone. However, this herb is a broad-spectrum inducer of drug-metabolizing enzymes and appears to interact with a wide variety of pharmaceuticals. Perhaps most worrisome is its ability to reduce serum levels of protease inhibitors, and nonnucleoside reverse transcriptase inhibitors, because some individuals with HIV infection take St. John's wort in the discredited belief that it has anti–human immunodeficiency virus (HIV) properties. There are many other safety concerns with St. John's wort as well (see Safety Issues).

Major Depression of Mild to Moderate Severity   +3X

Until 1998, most trials of St. John's wort for depression used LI160, a 0.3%-hypericin water and alcohol extract (the extraction process is conducted in darkness at controlled temperatures). Some subsequent studies have used either WS 5573, standardized to hyperforin-content, or ZE 117, a low-hyperforin product.

St. John's wort has primarily been evaluated as a treament for major depression of mild to moderate severity, as determined by HAM-D scores and other measures. Numerous double-blind comparative or placebo-controlled trials in this population have been reported, enrolling a total of more than 2000 individuals.[1-11,62,63] Only two of the placebo-controlled trials failed to find St. John's wort effective.[11,62] It is worth noting that 35% of all double-blind studies comparing pharmaceutical antidepressants with placebo have failed to find the active agent significantly more effective; in the more recent of the two negative trials of St. John's wort, sertraline also failed to demonstrate more effectiveness than placebo on any primary outcome measure. (The presumed causes of this relatively high rate of negative outcomes in studies of drugs known to be effective include the high rate of placebo effect in depression and the relative imprecision of the HAM-D rating scale.)

Comparative trials using appropriate doses of the pharmacologic agent found St. John's wort equally as effective as conventional antidepressants.[3-7,64] For example, an 8-week, double-blind trial of 263 individuals compared a St. John's wort product standardized to hyperforin content against placebo and imipramine.[6] Participants were diagnosed with major depression by ICD-10 criteria and had average baseline 17-item HAM-D scores of 22.6, representing a moderate level of disease severity. The results showed St. John's wort more effective at reducing HAM-D scores than placebo and as effective as imipramine, 100 mg/day.

St. John's wort has also been compared to selective serotonin reuptake inhibitors (SSRIs). A 6-week, double-blind trial of 240 individuals with mild to moderate depression compared St. John's wort with fluoxetine, 20 mg daily.[3] The results showed that St. John's wort was equally effective on the HAM-D scale, more effective on the CGI, and significantly superior in type and number of adverse events. Another 6-week, double-blind study of 149 seniors with mild to moderate depression (HAM-D average about 19) also found St. John's wort equally effective to 20 mg of fluoxetine.[4] A small trial found it equally effective as sertraline.[5] In addition, St. John's wort has been found equivalent to imipramine for mild to moderate depression[6,7] but not for severe depression.[12]

Polyneuropathy   − 1

A double-blind, placebo-controlled trial of 54 individuals found St. John's wort ineffective for polyneuropathy.[13]

Other Proposed Uses

Small double-blind trials have suggested effectiveness of St. John's wort in **seasonal affective disorder,**[14] **reactive depression,**[15] and **depression with somatic symptoms.**[16] Open trials have found it helpful in **PMS** and **menopausal symptoms.**[17,18] However, because of the typically high rate of placebo response in these conditions, such studies cannot be taken as meaningful.

Based on analogous use to standard antidepressants, St. John's wort is sometimes tried for the treatment of **insomnia**. A double-blind trial of 12 healthy volunteers found no sleep-promoting benefit, but this says little about the effectiveness of St. John's wort's in individuals with sleep problems.[19]

Neither St. John's wort nor hypericin have been shown useful in the treatment of **HIV**; in order to produce any antiviral effects, hypericin must be taken in doses high enough to cause significant toxicity.[20] In addition, as mentioned above, concerns have been raised about the ability of St. John's wort to reduce serum levels of protease inhibitors (see Drug Interactions).

Mechanism of Action

The mechanism of action of St. John's wort remains unknown. Early research suggested that extracts of St. John's wort can inhibit the enzyme monoamine oxidase in vitro.[21] However, later investigation found that the dosages of St. John's wort taken orally in actual practice were too low to inhibit monoamine oxidase.[22,23] MAO inhibitor–type reactions have never been observed with St. John's wort.

A subsequent study noted a 50% inhibition of synaptosomal uptake of serotonin, dopamine, and norepinephrine in mouse brain preparations at realistic concentrations of standard St. John's wort extracts.[24] This effect was found to correlate closely with hyperforin concentration.[25] In another study, St. John's wort extract caused down-regulation of serotonin receptors in cultured rat neuroblastoma cells.[26] Subchronic treatment in rodents has shown up-regulation of 5-HT2–receptors in the frontal cortex.[27] Administration of St. John's wort extract or imipramine for 8 weeks increased 5-HT levels in rat hypothalamus.[28]

Besides hyperforin, it appears that there are other active constituents in St. John's wort.[29] Two double-blind trials found a form of St. John's wort with low hyperforin content to be effective.[2,3] One constituent of the herb, amentoflavone, possesses high-affinity binding (IC50 about 15 nanomolar) for the benzodiazepine site of GABA-A receptors.[30] Although this effect occurs at clinically achievable concentrations, the contribution of this effect to antidepressant activity is not yet clear.[31] Various other constituents of St. John's wort, including flavonoids, may also be active.[32,33]

Hypericin is not thought to be an active ingredient causing the clinical effect of St. John's wort, although it does appear to be the primary photosensitizing constituent.

Dosage

The usual dosage of St. John's wort is 300 mg three times daily of an extract standardized to contain 0.3% hypericin or 2% to 3% hyperforin. However, some tested formulations have alternate dosing schedules, and label instructions should be followed.

See the Appendix for U.S. brand names of clinically tested products.

Safety Issues

A drug-monitoring study of 3250 patients taking St. John's wort extract for 4 weeks revealed a 2.4% overall incidence of side effects.[34] The most common were mild stomach discomfort (0.6%); allergic reactions, primarily rash (0.5%); tiredness (0.4%); and restlessness (0.3%). Only 1.5% of the patients dropped out of the study because of adverse reactions. A 1-year drug monitoring study of 313 patients found a similarly low incidence of adverse effects; further, a battery of diagnostic tests uncovered no significant posttreatment changes attributable to St. John's wort.[35]

No LD_{50} (median lethal dose) of standard St. John's wort extract was identified in studies of mice, rats, and dogs treated for 26 weeks, even at dosages of 5000 mg/kg.[36] Intolerance reactions appeared at 900 mg/kg/day. No genotoxic or mutagenic effects were noted in these studies.

St. John's wort extract has also been shown to be antimutagenic in *Escherichia coli*.[37] However, it has been recognized that hypericin can accumulate in the nucleus of cells exposed to the compound and can directly bind to deoxyribonucleic acid (DNA).[38] The relevance of these findings is unclear, and no long-term carcinogenicity testing has been conducted with St. John's wort.

Like other antidepressants, St. John's wort can cause episodes of mania.[39,40]

Hypericin is a known photosensitizing agent. Severe phototoxicity has occurred in animals that graze on St. John's wort; however, it has been estimated that these events occur at a dose of 30 to 50 times higher than the equivalent recommended dose in humans.[65] One study of sun-sensitive patients given twice the normal dose of the herb for 2 weeks showed only minimally decreased time to erythema on exposure to ultraviolet (UV) radiation.[41] Another trial found one-time dosing with two or six times the typical daily dose did not cause an increased tendency to burn in response to UVA, UVB, visible like light, or solar-simulated radiation; nor did 7 days' treatment at the normal dose.[66]

However, there is a case report of severe phototoxicity in an individual taking oral St. John's wort and subsequently receiving intensive UVB therapy.[42] In addition, there are two case reports of severe reactions to sun exposure in individuals using topical St. John's wort.[42] Based on these findings, individuals receiving UVB treatment should avoid St. John's wort entirely; sun-sensitive individuals using oral St. John's wort should take enhanced precautions against sunburn; and topical St. John's wort should be avoided. Patients who have taken a massive overdose of St. John's wort should probably be kept away from UV sources for several days.

Evidence for a potentially more worrisome effect of hypericin photosensitization was presented at a 1999 meeting of the American Society for Photobiology: photoactivation of hypericin in the lens of the eye might lead to increased risk of cataracts.[43]

One small study suggests that high doses of St. John's wort might slightly impair the performance of certain cognitive tasks.[44]

One case report associates use of St. John's wort with symptoms similar to serotonin syndrome in an individual who had previously experienced reactions to serotonergic medications.[67] Another case reported in the same communication associates use of St. John's wort with hair loss. The authors note that tricyclic antidepressants and selective serotonin reuptake inhibitors (SSRIs) have also been associated with hair loss.

A case report suggests that the herb St. John's wort may not be safe for individuals with Alzheimer's disease. Use of St. John's wort was associated with acute delirium with psychotic features in a 76-year-old woman with Alzheimer's disease.[68]

Maximum safe dosages in individuals with severe renal or hepatic disease are not known.

Safety in Young Children and Pregnant or Lactating Women

Maternal administration of St. John's wort extract (180 mg/kg—a dose calculated to mimic human dosing) in rats before and during gestation produced no effects on offspring.[45] In a study of 101 children under the age of 12 years given standardized St. John's wort extract at a dose ranging from 300 to 1800 mg, no adverse effects were seen.[69] However, maximum safe dosages for pregnant or lactating women or young children have not been established.

Drug Interactions

St. John's wort has been found to affect the activity of multiple cytochromes as well as the transport protein p-glycoprotein, and these effects are clinically relevant.[46-57,70-77]

Meaningful, and in some cases compelling, evidence indicates that the herb can reduce serum concentrations of **protease**

inhibitors, nonnucleoside reverse transcriptase inhibitors such as **nevirapine, cyclosporine, digoxin, warfarin, tricyclic antidepressants, simvastatin** (but not pravastatin), and **theophylline.**

Numerous cases of transplant rejection (heart, kidney, liver) have been reported in individuals using **cyclosporine** and St. John's wort concurrently.

A growing body of evidence suggests that the herb decreases the effectiveness of **oral contraceptives** and has caused unwanted pregnancies.[47,71,77] Interactions with numerous other drugs, such as **etoposide, teniposide, mitoxantrone, doxorubicin, cloza-pine,** and **olanzapine,** are also suspected; further, dosage adjustment to accommodate the effects of St. John's wort might lead to rebound toxicity.

Several case reports suggest that combined use of St. John's wort and other **serotonergic drugs** may result in serotonin syndrome.[58-60]

Based on its photosensitizing effects, there may be an increased risk of photosensitivity if St. John's wort is combined with **known photosensitizing agents.** In addition, **proton pump inhibitors** may potentiate the phototoxic effects of hypericin.[61]

Although it is probably advisable to discontinue all herbs and supplements before surgery and anesthesia, there does not appear to be any specific foundation to publicized claims that St. John's wort interacts with **anesthetics.**

TAURINE

Alternate Name/Supplement Form: L-Taurine

Common Uses

Congestive heart failure [+2]

Viral hepatitis [+2]

(Higher numbers indicate stronger evidence; X modifier indicates contradictory results. See page xviii of the Introduction for details of the rating scale.)

Approach to the Patient

Taurine is a nonessential amino acid synthesized from vitamin B_6 and the amino acids methionine and cysteine. Deficiencies occasionally occur in vegetarians, whose diets may not provide adequate sources for taurine synthesis.

Taurine at pharmaceutical doses offers promise as an adjuvant therapy in congestive heart failure. It may also be useful for acute viral hepatitis.

Diabetics have been found to have lower-than-average blood levels of taurine, but whether taurine supplementation is warranted in diabetes is unclear.

Your patient may have heard that taurine "calms the brain," making it a useful treatment for attention deficit hyperactivity disorder (ADHD) and epilepsy. However, no evidence supports this belief.

Congestive Heart Failure   +2

Several studies (primarily by one research group) suggest that taurine may be a useful adjuvant therapy in class II, III, and IV congestive heart failure (CHF). One 4-week, double-blind, placebo-controlled, crossover trial evaluated the effects of 2 g of taurine three times daily in 62 individuals with CHF.[1] The results showed that taurine produced significant improvement in signs and symptoms as compared with placebo. Other small blinded or open studies in humans, as well as studies in animals, have also found positive effects on CHF with taurine supplementation.[2-6]

One very small, comparative study of taurine and coenzyme Q_{10} in CHF found taurine more effective.[7] (See the article on **Coenzyme Q_{10}** for more information.)

Viral Hepatitis   +2

A double-blind, placebo-controlled study of 63 individuals with *acute* viral hepatitis (type not specified) evaluated the effects of 12 g of taurine daily or placebo.[8] The results showed significant improvements in liver function tests in the treatment group compared with the placebo group. However, a small, double-blind, placebo-controlled study found no effect of taurine therapy on liver function tests (LFTs) in individuals with *chronic* hepatitis.[9]

Other Proposed Uses

Taurine has been proposed as a treatment for numerous other conditions, including **alcoholism, cataracts, diabetes, epilepsy, gallbladder disease, hypertension, multiple sclerosis, psoriasis,** and **stroke,** but the evidence for these uses is weak and, in some cases, contradictory.[9-13]

Taurine is also sometimes combined in an "amino acid cocktail" with other amino acids for treatment of attention deficit disorder, but there is no evidence that this works.

Mechanism of Action

Found in neurologic and muscular tissue, taurine is one of the most abundant amino acids in the body. Its physiologic roles are thought to include regulation of cardiac rhythm, cellular membrane maintenance, and neurotransmitter release. It is also present in bile as taurocholic acid.

Dosage

A typical therapeutic dosage of taurine is 2 g three times daily.

Safety Issues

Because taurine is an amino acid found in dietary sources, taurine supplements are thought to be safe. However, maximum safe dosages in individuals with severe hepatic or renal disease are not known.

As with any supplement taken in multigram doses, use of a quality product is imperative; contaminants present even in small percentages may present health risks.

Safety in Young Children and Pregnant or Lactating Women

Maximum safe dosages for pregnant or lactating women or young children have not been established.

Drug Interactions

There are no known drug interactions.

TEA TREE OIL
(Melaleuca alternifolia)

Common Uses

Antifungal [+2]   **Acne** [+1]

(Higher numbers indicate stronger evidence; X modifier indicates contradictory results. See page xviii of the Introduction for details of the rating scale.)

Approach to the Patient

Tea tree oil *(Melaleuca alternifolia)* appears to be an effective topical antiseptic, active against many bacteria (including multiple-resistant strains) and fungi.[1,2] Although tea tree oil is used in mouthwashes and toothpaste, its safety for internal use has not been established.

Antifungal   +2

A double-blind, placebo-controlled trial observed 104 individuals with tinea pedis who were given a 10% tea tree oil cream, the standard drug tolnaftate, or placebo.[2] The results showed a significant reduction in clinical symptoms with either tea tree oil or tolnaftate, as compared with placebo. However, significantly more tolnaftate-treated patients than tea tree oil– or placebo-treated patients showed conversion to negative culture at the end of therapy.

Acne   +1

A single-blind comparative clinical trial of 124 patients with mild to moderate acne evaluated the efficacy and skin tolerance of 5% tea tree oil gel compared with 5% benzoyl peroxide lotion.[3] This study found that both treatments had a significant

TEA TREE OIL 895

effect in ameliorating acne by reducing the number of inflamed and noninflamed lesions (open and closed comedones), although the onset of action in the case of tea tree oil was slower. Patients treated with tea tree oil experienced fewer side effects.

Other Proposed Uses

Preliminary studies suggest that tea tree oil could be useful for treating **vaginal infections** caused by *Candida* or other organisms.[4] Tea tree oil has also been suggested as a treatment for **oral candidiasis** in human immunodeficiency virus (HIV)–infected patients.[5] A small study using tea tree oil for oral herpes found statistically insignificant trends toward benefit.[7] Australian dentists frequently administer tea tree oil mouthwash before dental procedures and recommend it as a daily preventive against periodontal disease.

Tea tree oil also appears to possess deodorant properties, probably through suppressing odor-causing bacteria.

Mechanism of Action

Terpinen-4-ol is believed to be the main antimicrobial component in tea tree oil, and species variants with higher concentrations of this ingredient are considered to be superior.[1] Its mode of action is not well-defined but may involve autolysis in the exponential growth phase.

Dosage

Tea tree preparations contain various percentages of tea tree oil. For treating fungal infections, 70% to 100% is usually used; for acne, the typical strength is 5% to 15%; and for use as a vaginal douche, 1% to 40% concentrations have been used. These products are usually applied two or three times daily until symptoms resolve. However, tea tree oil can irritate the skin, so use of lower initial concentrations is recommended.

Quality tea tree products contain oil from the *alternifolia* species of *Melaleuca* only, standardized to contain at least 30% terpinen-4-ol. Until recently, it was thought that 1,8-cineole was an undesirable ingredient responsible for local irritation and hypersensitivity reactions, but that does not appear to be correct.[1]

Safety Issues

Tea tree oil is only recommended for topical use. Although it is generally well-tolerated, an increasing number of cases of skin inflammation caused by allergy to tea tree oil have been reported.[6]

Safety in individuals with severe hepatic or renal disease is not known.

Safety in Young Children and Pregnant or Lactating Women

Safety in pregnant or lactating women or young children has not been established.

Drug Interactions

There are no known drug interactions.

THYMUS EXTRACT

Alternate Names/Supplement Forms:
Thymus Gland, Calf Thymus Extract,
Thymic Extract, Thymomodulin

Common Uses

Respiratory   **Viral hepatitis**   [−1]
infections   [−1X]

(Higher numbers indicate stronger evidence; X modifier indicates contradictory results. See page xviii of the Introduction for details of the rating scale.)

Approach to the Patient

Various extracts of bovine thymus have been tried for potential immunostimulatory properties. However, there is as yet no real evidence that thymus extracts are effective for any clinical condition; in addition, there are serious concerns regarding possible contamination with slow viruses.

Respiratory Infections   −1X

A 1-year, double-blind, placebo-controlled trial of 16 children with frequent respiratory infections found that treatment with thymus extract could reduce the rate of infection.[1]

However, results of a double-blind, placebo-controlled trial evaluating the effects of 3-month treatment with thymomodulin (a calf thymus acid lysate) in 60 athletes showed some positive trends toward benefit but no statistically significant findings.[2] The athletes were engaging in intensive training of a type thought to decrease immunity and increase risk of respiratory infections.

Viral Hepatitis   − 1

Thymus extract has been tried as a treatment for acute and chronic hepatitis B and C. However, the results of small double-blind trials have not been positive.[3-6]

Other Proposed Uses

Highly preliminary evidence suggests that thymus extracts may be helpful for **food allergies**[7] and **asthma.**[8]

Injectable forms of whole thymus extract or specific constituents have been studied as a treatment for numerous conditions including **cancer, cold sores, dermatomyositis, eczema, genital warts, hepatitis, human immunodeficiency virus (HIV) infection, leukopenia, multiple sclerosis, psoriasis, rheumatoid arthritis, scleroderma,** and **herpes zoster.**[9-16] The results of these studies have mixed. In any case, the results of trials involving injected thymus extracts cannot be considered applicable to oral thymus products.

Mechanism of Action

Presumably, thymus extracts such as thymomodulin might have the capacity to stimulate T-cell differentiation and action, with subsequent effects on B cells, macrophages, and neutrophils.[17]

Dosage

The dosage of thymus extract used in studies has varied widely, depending on the particular thymus product used.

Safety Issues

Thymus extracts have not been definitely associated with any side effects. However, there are real concerns that any glandular extract might be contaminated with slow viruses.[18] Keep in mind that there is no governmental regulation of thymus products sold as dietary supplements in the United States.

Maximum safe dosages in individuals with severe hepatic or renal disease are not known.

Safety in Young Children
and Pregnant or Lactating Women

Maximum safe dosages for pregnant or lactating women or young children have not been established.

Drug Interactions

Concomitant use of thymus extracts and **immunosuppressive therapy** should be avoided for theoretic reasons.

TRIBULUS
(Tribulus terrestris)

Alternate Names/Related Species:
Puncture Vine, Thundergod Vine

Common Use

Sports performance enhancement [−2]

(Higher numbers indicate stronger evidence; X modifier indicates contradictory results. See page xviii of the Introduction for details of the rating scale.)

Approach to the Patient

Tribulus terrestris (commonly known as puncture vine) is a tropical plant with a history of traditional medicinal use for enhancing sexual function in men and fertility in both men and women. Tribulus is widely marketed today for this use as well as for enhancing sports performance. However, no meaningful evidence supports the use of tribulus for any medical purpose.

Sports Performance Enhancement −2

At the end of an 8-week, placebo-controlled trial evaluating the effects of tribulus (3.21 mg/kg) on body composition and endurance among 15 men engaged in resistance training, the only significant difference between the two groups was in favor of placebo.[3]

Other Proposed Uses of Tribulus

Bulgarian research is the primary source of most health claims regarding tribulus. According to this research, which falls considerably short of current scientific standards, tribulus increases levels of testosterone, dehydroepiandrosterone (DHEA), estrogen, follicle-stimulating hormone (FSH), and luteinizing hormone (LH), and improves sports performance, menopausal symptoms, recovery from surgery, female fertility, and sexual function in both men and women.[7-11]

Other poor-quality studies are cited by manufacturers to support various uses of tribulus. These include an uncontrolled Chinese case series claiming to find benefits for patients with angina[12]; a study in rabbits indicating a pro-erectile effect[13]; a Chinese study in mice reporting hypolipidemic and hypoglycemic effects[14]; an in vitro study finding an antispasmodic effect[15]; and studies in rats indicating potential benefits in preventing urolithiasis.[2,16]

Mechanism of Action

Bulgarian research indicates that tribulus increases levels of various steroid hormones, but this has not been confirmed.

Dosage

Tribulus terrestris is usually taken at a dose ranging from 85 to 250 mg, three times daily with meals. Some tribulus products are standardized to provide 40% furostanol saponins; these are typically taken at a dose providing 115 mg of saponins two or three times daily.

Safety Issues

No significant adverse effects have been reported in any of the clinical trials or human research studies of tribulus. Animal studies performed in Bulgaria are said to have found that tribulus is safe in both the short and long term.[9] However, it is not clear what reliance can be placed on these conclusions. Tribulus is known to have a toxic effect on sheep.[4-6]

Maximum safe dosages in individuals with severe hepatic or renal disease are not known.

Safety in Young Children and Pregnant or Lactating Women

Because of the supposed hormonal effects of tribulus, women who are pregnant or lactating should not use any tribulus product. Maximum safe dosages for young children have not been established.

Drug Interactions

There are no known drug interactions.

TYLOPHORA
(Tylophora indica)

Alternate Names/Related Species:
Tylophora asthmatica, T. cordifolia, T. flava, T. floribunda

Common Use

Asthma   [+3X]

(Higher numbers indicate stronger evidence; X modifier indicates contradictory results. See page xviii of the Introduction for details of the rating scale.)

Approach to the Patient

Tylophora indica is a climbing perennial plant indigenous to India, where it grows wild in the southern and eastern regions and has a long-standing reputation as a remedy for asthma (hence its other name *T. asthmatica*).

Although three double-blind trials reported dramatic and long-lasting benefits from short-term treatment with tylophora, a better-designed and reported trial found no benefit.

Asthma   +3X

In a 6-day, double-blind, placebo-controlled crossover study of 195 individuals with asthma, participants showed significant improvement in symptoms when given 40 mg daily of a tylophora alcohol extract, as compared with placebo treatment.[1] Reportedly, this comparative benefit was even more marked months after use of the herb was stopped. Similarly long-lasting results were seen in two other double-blind, placebo-controlled studies involving more than 200 individuals with asthma.[2,3] However, the design of most of these studies was convoluted and the reporting incomplete.

By contrast, a better-reported, double-blind, placebo-controlled study that enrolled 135 individuals and followed a more straightforward design found no benefit of tylophora.[4]

Other Proposed Uses

Tylophora is also sometimes used for the treatment of allergies, respiratory infections, dysentery, and joint pain, but no real scientific evidence supports these uses.

Mechanism of Action

Very preliminary evidence suggests that tylophora may have antiinflammatory, antiallergic, and antispasmodic actions, perhaps mediated through stimulation of the adrenal cortex.[5-8]

Dosage

The typical dosage of tylophora leaf in dried or capsule form is 200 mg twice daily.

Safety Issues

In one double-blind trial, the chewing of whole tylophora leaf was associated with nausea, vomiting, mouth soreness, and altered taste sensation in more than one half of the participants.[2] Two other double-blind trials that used encapsulated dried tylophora leaves or powdered extract found similar side effects but far less frequently.[1,4]

Preliminary studies on animals have found tylophora extracts to be toxic only in doses far higher than the equivalent therapeutic human dose.[9]

Because of the lack of comprehensive safety studies on tylophora, the herb should not be used by individuals with severe hepatic or renal disease.

Safety in Young Children and Pregnant or Lactating Women

Until further safety evaluation is completed, children and pregnant or lactating women should avoid tylophora.

Drug Interactions

There are no known drug interactions.

TYROSINE

Alternate Name/Supplement Form: L-Tyrosine

Common Uses

Sleep deprivation [+2]   **Depression** [−1]

(Higher numbers indicate stronger evidence; X modifier indicates contradictory results. See page xviii of the Introduction for details of the rating scale.)

Approach to the Patient

Tyrosine, an amino acid derived from phenylalanine, is utilized primarily in neurotransmitter synthesis. Based on this physiologic role, tyrosine supplementation at pharmacologic doses has been proposed as a treatment for various conditions in which mental function is impaired.

Limited evidence suggests that tyrosine may be helpful in sleep deprivation. Studies do not support its use for depression. Recommendations that tyrosine be combined with other amino acids for attention deficit disorder are not supported by research evidence.

Although rare in most instances, tyrosine deficiency can occur in certain forms of severe renal disease as well as in phenylketonuria (PKU).

Sleep Deprivation   +2

A placebo-controlled study of 20 U.S. Marines found that 10 to 15 g of tyrosine twice daily improved alertness during periods of sleep deprivation.[1]

Depression   − 1

One study of nine individuals is often cited as evidence that tyrosine offers therapeutic benefit in depression.[2] However, a double-blind, placebo-controlled study of 65 individuals with depression found no benefit.[3]

Other Proposed Uses

Preliminary double-blind trials suggest tyrosine may improve **cognitive function** under conditions of physical and/or social stress.[1,7]

Tyrosine may provide some temporary benefit for **attention deficit disorder,** but the effects appear to wear off in a couple weeks.[4-6] Tyrosine is widely claimed to work better in ADD when combined in an "amino acid cocktail" with gamma-aminobutyric acid (GABA), phenylalanine, and glutamine; however, no scientific evidence supports this.

Mechanism of Action

Tyrosine is an amino acid found in numerous proteins. It is a precursor for epinephrine, melanin, and thyroxine.

Dosage

The typical recommended therapeutic dosage of tyrosine is 7 to 30 g daily.

Safety Issues

Tyrosine seems to be generally safe, although nausea, diarrhea, vomiting, and nervousness have been reported at high dosages. As with any other supplement taken in multigram doses, use of a high-quality product is imperative, since contaminants present in small percentages might present health risks.

Maximum safe dosages in individuals with severe hepatic or renal disease are not known.

Safety in Young Children and Pregnant or Lactating Women

Maximum safe dosages for pregnant or lactating women or young children have not been established.

Drug Interactions

There are no known drug interactions.

UVA URSI
(Arctostaphylos uva-ursi)

Alternate Name/Related Species: Bearberry

Common Use

Urinary tract infections (prophylaxis and treatment) [+1]

(Higher numbers indicate stronger evidence; X modifier indicates contradictory results. See page xviii of the Introduction for details of the rating scale.)

Approach to the Patient

Arctostaphylos uva-ursi, or bearberry, has a long history of use in both North America and Europe as treatment for acute urinary tract infections. Its active ingredient, arbutin, was used as a urinary antiseptic for many years. However, there is little direct evidence that uva ursi is effective.

Patients should be cautioned about the potential for hepatotoxicity, mutagenicity, and carcinogenicity with prolonged use of this herb. Because of its potential toxicity, uva ursi should not be used for prophylaxis of urinary tract infections. Uva ursi should not be used by pregnant or lactating women or patients with renal or hepatic disease.

Urinary Tract Infections (Prophylaxis and Treatment)   +1

One double-blind, placebo-controlled study observed 57 women for 1 year. None of the women who received uva ursi (combined with dandelion, a diuretic herb) developed a urinary tract infection, but five of those receiving placebo did.[1] (**Note:** Long-term use of uva ursi is not recommended; see Safety Issues.)

Mechanism of Action

The major active constituents in uva ursi are arbutin and methyl-arbutin. Other important ingredients include flavonoids, tannins, organic acids, and free hydroquinone. Arbutin is poorly absorbed from the digestive tract, but its glycosidic bond is cleaved by intestinal flora to form readily absorbable aglycone hydroquinone.[2] This appears to be conjugated to glucuronides and sulfate esters in the intestinal mucosa and liver and then excreted through the kidneys, under relatively alkaline conditions.

At a pH above 8, it has been postulated that hydroquinone reforms from its conjugates and exhibits antibiotic properties.[3] However, experimental data to support this plausible concept are lacking.

Dosage

A typical daily dose of uva ursi is 3 g dried herb.[3-5] Daily intake of 800 mg arbutin should not be exceeded. Maximum treatment duration is 2 weeks, and uva ursi should not be used more than five times per year. Uva ursi is generally taken with meals to minimize gastrointestinal upset.

Safety Issues

The major risks from uva ursi result from the arbutin metabolite hydroquinone, which is a mutagen, hepatotoxin, carcinogen, and topical irritant. For this reason, long-term use of uva ursi is contraindicated, and even short-term use should be avoided in pregnant or lactating women, young children, and individuals with severe renal or hepatic disease.

Mild gastrointestinal distress is the only commonly reported short-term side effect of uva ursi.

Safety in Young Children and Pregnant or Lactating Women

Given its possible mutagenic effects, uva ursi should not be used by young children and pregnant or lacting women.

Drug Interactions

Because uva ursi is thought to be more effective in an alkaline urine, **drugs or supplements that acidify the urine,** such as vitamin C and cranberry, should be avoided when uva ursi is being used.

VALERIAN
(Valeriana officinalis)

Common Uses

Insomnia   [+3]   **Anxiety**   [+2]

(Higher numbers indicate stronger evidence; X modifier indicates contradictory results. See page xviii of the Introduction for details of the rating scale.)

Approach to the Patient

More than 200 plant species belong to the genus *Valeriana*, but the one used for insomnia is *Valeriana officinalis*. This perennial grows abundantly in moist woodlands of Europe and North America and is under extensive cultivation to meet market demands for its medicinal root.

Preliminary evidence suggests that valerian may be an effective sleep aid; however, it is unclear whether the herb is best used for occasional insomnia or taken long term to improve sleep quality.

Insomnia   + 3

In the largest trial of valerian for insomnia, 121 patients with a history of significant insomnia were enrolled in a 28-day, double-blind, placebo-controlled study.[1] Significant improvements in sleep quality were seen at 28 days but not at 14 days. The researchers interpreted the results to indicate that valerian is most appropriately used as a long-term treatment for poor sleep rather than for occasional insomnia. In sharp contrast, smaller studies found benefits with one-time or short-term valerian use.[2-6]

A 28-day, double-blind trial of 75 individuals with various forms of insomnia compared valerian (600 mg qhs) with oxazepam (10 mg qhs).[7] The results showed no differences in efficacy.

The combination of valerian and lemon balm has also been studied for its effects on sleep, but the results have not been impressive. A poorly designed, 30-day, double-blind, placebo-controlled study of 98 individuals without insomnia found marginal evidence that a valerian–lemon balm combination improved sleep quality compared with placebo.[8] A double-blind, crossover study of 20 people with insomnia compared the benefits of the sleeping drug triazolam (Halcion), 0.125 mg, against placebo and a combination of valerian and lemon balm and failed to find the herb effective.[10] The drug, however, did prove effective.

Anxiety   + 2

Valerian is sometimes suggested as a treatment for situational and other forms of anxiety. A double-blind, placebo-controlled study of 48 participants placed under "social stress" situations compared low-dose valerian extract (100 mg), propranolol (20 mg), and the two treatments combined.[11] Use of valerian improved subjective anxiety but did not alter physiologic activation.

Mechanism of Action

The mechanism of action of valerian is unknown. Valepotriates are known to suppress the anxiogenic effects of benzodiazepine withdrawal in diazepam-dependent rats.[12] However, standard valerian preparations have little to no valepotriate content.[13,14]

Other in vitro research has shown that certain valerian extracts possess weak binding affinity to gamma-aminobutyric acid (GABA) receptors, mitochondrial benzodiazepine receptors, and barbiturate receptors.[15,16] Initial reports suggested that valerian extracts increased GABA concentration in the synaptic cleft by both increasing its secretion and impairing its uptake.[17,18] However, later research concluded that this apparent effect was actually due to GABA present in valerian extract.[19,20]

Dosage

For insomnia, the standard dose of valerian is 2 to 3 g of dried root, 270 to 450 mg of an aqueous valerian extract, or 600 mg dry ethanol extract, taken 30 to 60 minutes before bedtime.[21] The recommended sources of valerian for medicinal use are aqueous products that are valepotriate-free.[22-24] See the Appendix for U.S. brand names of clinically tested products.

Whole valerian root has been given at 2 to 3 g twice daily for anxiety.

Safety Issues

Valerian is listed on the FDA's GRAS (generally recognized as safe) list and is approved for use as a food. Except for its unpleasant odor, valerian is generally well-tolerated. In one study, only 2 out of 61 participants taking valerian reported side effects, which were headache and morning grogginess.[1] Mild gastrointestinal distress is also occasionally reported, and there are informal reports that some individuals develop a paradoxic mild stimulant effect.

One case of overdose at 20 times the standard daily dosage led to no more than minor symptoms.[25] The LD_{50} (median lethal dose) of ethanolic valerian extracts by intraperitoneal injection is 3.3 g/kg in mice. Over a 45-day period, intraperitoneal administration to rats at a level of 400 mg/kg or more produced no significant changes.[26]

There have been reports of hepatotoxicity in individuals who took combination herbal remedies containing skullcap as well as valerian.[27] However, in a series of about 50 overdose cases (including long-term follow-up) with a combination preparation called Sleep-Qik containing the anticholinergic hyoscine, the serotonin antagonist cyproheptadine, and valerian,[28,29] the expected symptoms of cyproheptadine and hyoscine toxicity developed, but there were no signs of hepatotoxicity.

Valerian does not appear to impair driving ability, reaction time, or alertness or to produce morning residual sedation when taken at night.[30-32] However, it can impair vigilance for a couple of hours immediately after use. For this reason, driving a car or operating hazardous machinery immediately after taking valerian is not recommended.

Valerian withdrawal has not been observed in animal studies or controlled human trials. However, one case report suggests the possibility. A 58-year-old man who had been taking high doses of valerian root extract (about 2.5 to 10 g daily) for many years developed delirium and sinus tachycardia during a postoperative period of no valerian use.[33]

Whole valerian contains valepotriates, substances with mutagenic and cytotoxic effects. However, these are believed not to be present in typical valerian products.[13,14,22-24] Further, their toxic effects are believed due to their metabolites baldrinal and homobaldrinal, which are subjected to a strong first-pass effect in the intestines and inactivated.[21] Nonetheless, the possibility of adverse effects in the gastrointestinal tract or liver cannot be excluded on this basis.

Maximum safe dosages in individuals with severe hepatic or renal disease are not known.

Safety in Young Children and Pregnant or Lactating Women

Maximum safe dosages of valerian for pregnant or lactating women have not been established. Valerian is generally not recommended for children under 3 years of age.[13]

Drug Interactions

A human trial found no interaction between **alcohol** and valerian as measured by concentration, attentiveness, reaction time, and driving performance.[30] However, animal studies suggest that valerian potentiates **pentobarbital, hexobarbital,** and **thiopental.**[9,30,34-36]

VANADIUM

Common Uses

Diabetes [+1]   **Bodybuilding** [−1]

(Higher numbers indicate stronger evidence; X modifier indicates contradic-
tory results. See page xviii of the Introduction for details of the rating scale.)

Approach to the Patient

Animal and preliminary studies suggest that vanadium has in-
sulinomimetic and other antidiabetic properties. Evidence does
not support the use of vanadium as an aid in bodybuilding.

There are significant concerns about possible toxicity when
vanadium is taken in supraphysiologic therapeutic doses.

Diabetes   +1

Studies in rats with and without diabetes suggest that vanadium
may have an insulin-like effect, reducing blood glucose levels.[1-11]
Most studies involve vanadium (IV)—that is, oxidation state
IV vanadium—but vanadium (V) has also been found effective in
animals.[12]

Based on these findings, preliminary studies involving human
subjects have been conducted, with mostly positive results.[13-18]
However, the doses of vanadium used, 100 to 125 mg/day, may
be toxic (see Safety Issues).

Bodybuilding   −1

A 12-week, double-blind, placebo-controlled study of 31 weight-trained athletes found no benefit with oral vanadyl sulfate at 0.5 mg/kg/day (about 1000 times nutritional needs).[19]

Other Proposed Uses

Although rodent studies have found vanadium deposited in bone,[20] no evidence as yet supports its use in osteoporosis.

Mechanism of Action

Animal studies suggest vanadium may be an essential micronutrient; however, human deficiencies have not been reported. The mechanism of action of vanadium in diabetes is thought to involve insulin enhancement through inhibition of tyrosine phosphatase enzymes, acting at one or more points in the insulin-signaling mechanism.[12]

Dosage

Estimated nutritional needs for vanadium fall in the range of 10 to 30 µg/day; the average American diet provides 10 to 60 µg/day.[21] Much higher dosages have been used in studies, but their safety is questionable (see Safety Issues).

Safety Issues

Vanadium is usually well-tolerated, although gastrointestinal distress can occur.[18] The tolerable upper intake level for vanadium in adults has been set at 1.8 mg.[22]

Studies in humans and animals suggest that excess vanadium is toxic; further, vanadium accumulation may occur if relatively small excess doses are taken for a prolonged time.[18,23-25] Possible toxic effects include hepatotoxicity, nephrotoxicity, teratogenicity, and developmental/reproductive toxicity.

Maximum safe dosages in individuals with severe hepatic or renal disease are not known.

Safety in Young Children and Pregnant or Lactating Women

Maximum safe dosages for pregnant or lactating women or young children have not been established.

Drug Interactions

The possibility of hypoglycemia in patients adding vanadium to an effective antidiabetic regimen should be considered.

VINPOCETINE

Alternate Name/Supplement Form: *Periwinkle*

Common Uses

Dementia [+3]

Acute ischemic stroke [+1]

(Higher numbers indicate stronger evidence; X modifier indicates contradictory results. See page xviii of the Introduction for details of the rating scale.)

Approach to the Patient

Vinpocetine is a chemical derived from vincamine, a substance found in the leaves of common periwinkle *(Vinca minor)* as well as in the seeds of various African plants. Developed in Hungary more than 20 years ago, vinpocetine is sold in Europe as a drug under the name Cavinton and is used for dementia as well as ordinary age-related mental impairment. In the United States, it is available as a dietary supplement. However, patients interested in natural medicine may be interested by the fact that vinpocetine more closely resembles a drug than an herb. Vinpocetine does not exist to any significant extent in nature. Producing it requires significant chemical work performed in the laboratory.

A significant amount of evidence supports the idea that vinpocetine can enhance memory and mental function, especially in those with Alzheimer's disease and related conditions. It is also reportedly helpful for those with ordinary age-related memory loss, but this has not been demonstrated. Use as a protective agent in acute ischemic stroke is undergoing active research.

Dementia   +3

A review of the literature found a total of three meaningful double-blind, placebo-controlled trials of vinpocetine extract for the treatment of dementia, enrolling a total of 327 patients.[1,2,5,15] Benefits were seen in each trial. Other positive studies have been reported as well.[3,4,6,7]

The largest of these was a 16-week, double-blind, placebo-controlled trial of 203 individuals with mild to moderate dementia.[1] The results showed significant improvement in the vinpocetine-treated group as compared with placebo.[1]

Acute Ischemic Stroke   +1

Based on its vasoactive and neuroprotective properties (see Mechanism of Action), vinpocetine has been proposed as therapy following acute ischemic stroke.

In a single-blind, placebo-controlled trial, 30 individuals status post–acute ischemic stroke received either low-molecular-weight dextran alone or dextran plus vinpocetine (10 mg IV for 5 to 7 days, followed by 10 mg orally three times daily for 30 days).[8] Vinpocetine treatment was associated with reduced risk of poor outcome at 3 months' follow-up as defined by the modified Barthel index and the modified Ranking score. There is also some suggestive evidence for benefit from other preliminary trials.[9]

Mechanism of Action

Vinpocetine appears to have several pharmacologic and biochemical actions, including stimulating cerebral vasodilation, increasing tolerance of cerebral tissue to hypoxic and ischemic insults, anticonvulsant activity, inhibitory effects on phosphodiesterase (PDE), improving hematologic flow properties, and inhibiting thrombocyte aggregation.[9-11]

Vinpocetine also appears to provide direct neuroprotective effects under in vitro and in vivo conditions. These effects appear to be related to the inhibition of voltage-dependent neuronal sodium channels, indirect inhibition of some molecular cascades initiated by the rise of intracellular calcium levels, and to a lesser extent, inhibition of adenosine reuptake.[10]

These neuroprotective effects might also be enhanced by vinpocetine's selective inhibition of calcium calmodulin–dependent cGMP-PDE.[10] This inhibition may enhance intracellular cGMP (cyclic guanosine monophosphate) levels in vascular smooth muscle, leading to reduced cerebrovascular resistance and increased cerebral blood flow.

Dosage

Vinpocetine is available in 10-mg capsules, usually taken three times per day. It appears to be better absorbed with meals.[12]

Safety Issues

Vinpocetine is generally well-tolerated, and no significant adverse effects have been seen in clinical trials. However, there is one case report of vinpocetine apparently causing reversible agranulocytosis.[13]

No serious side effects have been reported. However, maximum safe dosages in individuals with severe hepatic or renal disease are not known.

Safety in Young Children and Pregnant or Lactating Women

Maximum safe dosages for pregnant or lactating women or young children have not been established.

Drug Interactions

Vinpocetine might impair the effectiveness of **warfarin.**[14]

VITAMIN A

Alternate Name/Supplement Form: Retinol

Common Uses

**Viral infections
(children in developing
countries)** [+4]

**Respiratory
syncytial virus** [−2]

Crohn's disease [−1]

(Higher numbers indicate stronger evidence; X modifier indicates contradictory results. See page xviii of the Introduction for details of the rating scale.)

Approach to the Patient

Vitamin A deficiency is common in developing countries[1] but is relatively rare in the developed world, except among teenagers and those in lower socioeconomic groups. According to some studies,[2,3] but not all,[4,5] diabetics are frequently deficient in vitamin A. Crohn's disease, ulcerative colitis, and cystic fibrosis may also impair vitamin A absorption. There are no established therapeutic uses of exogenous vitamin A besides correcting deficiency.

Viral Infections (Children in Developing Countries) +4

A metaanalysis of 12 placebo-controlled, randomized studies found that vitamin A supplementation has considerable value in reducing morbidity and mortality of infectious illness in children growing up in developing countries.[6]

Crohn's Disease   − 1

Although inadequate vitamin A nutritional levels may be common in Crohn's disease, a double-blind, placebo-controlled study of 86 individuals found that vitamin A (50,000 IU twice daily) taken for an average of 14.1 months did not help maintain remission.[7]

Respiratory Syncytial Virus   − 2

A double-blind, placebo-controlled trial of 239 children with RSV evaluated the effects of 1-month treatment with vitamin A at a dose of 50,000 IU daily for ages 1 to 5 months, 100,000 IU for ages 6 to 11 months, and 200,000 IU for ages 12 months and older.[8] The results showed no benefit; in fact, in children aged 12 months and older, hospital stays were significantly longer.

Other Proposed Uses

Vitamin A has been studied as a treatment for various skin disorders including **acne, psoriasis, rosacea, seborrhea,** and **eczema**[9-12]; however, the benefits seen have been generally modest, and in most cases vitamin A had to be taken in potentially toxic dosages to produce results.

Vitamin A is also sometimes recommended for **menorrhagia,**[13] but there is no real evidence that it is effective.

Mechanism of Action

Vitamin A is essential for normal growth and development (including tooth and skeletal development) as well as normal function and integrity of epithelial tissues.

Vitamin A supplements presumably reduce childhood infectious disease incidence in developing countries by correcting inadequate nutritional status.

Dosage

The U.S. Dietary Reference Intake (DRI) for vitamin A varies by age and gender and is 2999 IU (900 μg) for males 14 years and older, and 2333 IU (700 μg) for females 14 years and older.

Dietary sources of vitamin A or carotenes (which are converted to vitamin A) include liver and yellow, orange, and dark green fruits and vegetables.

Safety Issues

Individuals who abuse alcohol heavily may be at higher risk of vitamin A toxicity.[14]

Excessive intake of vitamin A may increase the risk of osteoporosis.[15]

Maximum safe dosages in individuals with severe hepatic or renal disease are not known.

Safety in Young Children and Pregnant or Lactating Women

Because excessive intake of vitamin A increases risk of birth defects, it is recommended that pregnant women avoid taking vitamin A supplements. Beta-carotene supplements are recommended instead.

The tolerable upper intake level of vitamin A for pregnant or lactating women has been set at 3000 μg daily or 2800 μg if under 19 years old.[16]

Pregnant women taking valproic acid may be at increased risk of vitamin A toxicity.[17]

Drug Interactions

Vitamin A may increase the anticoagulant effects of **warfarin.**[18]

As noted above, pregnant women taking **valproic acid** may be at increased risk of adverse effects from vitamin A.[17]

Concomitant use of **isotretinoin** might also increase vitamin A toxicity because of similarity of action. The older cholesterol-lowering drugs **cholestyramine** and **colestipol** can reduce vitamin A levels; however, the effect is slight and probably not significant.[19]

Vitamin A supplementation may impair the action of vitamin D.[20]

VITAMIN B₁

Alternate Name/Supplement Form: Thiamine

Common Use

Congestive heart failure [+1]

(Higher numbers indicate stronger evidence; X modifier indicates contradictory results. See page xviii of the Introduction for details of the rating scale.)

Approach to the Patient

Vitamin B₁ deficiency is uncommon in the general population. However, loop diuretics may deplete vitamin B₁; because inadequate vitamin B₁ nutriture impairs heart function, individuals with congestive heart failure who use loop diuretics may benefit from vitamin B₁ supplements.

Vitamin B₁ supplementation may also be considered in individuals with alcoholism, anorexia, Crohn's disease, or renal failure.

Congestive Heart Failure +1

Evidence suggests that individuals with congestive heart failure are commonly deficient in vitamin B₁, presumably because of the use of loop diuretics.[1] A double-blind study of 30 individuals also found that IV administration of thiamine followed by oral supplementation could improve cardiac function in CHF.[2] As inpatients, in addition to continuation of all previous medications, patients were randomized to receive either IV thiamine, 200 mg/day, or placebo for 1 week. At discharge, all 30 patients received outpatient therapy of oral thiamine, 200 mg/day for 6 weeks.

Other Proposed Uses

Although vitamin B$_1$ is sometimes suggested as a treatment for Alzheimer's disease, the research record is contradictory.[3-7]

Vitamin B$_1$ has also been proposed as a treatment for canker sores, fibromyalgia, human immunodeficiency virus (HIV), and seizure disorders, but there is no real evidence that it is effective in these conditions.

Mechanism of Action

Thiamine is a co-enzyme in cellular energy production, plays an important role in carbohydrate metabolism, and is essential for normal functioning of nervous tissue.

Dosage

The need for vitamin B$_1$ varies with age and gender. The U.S. Dietary Reference Intake (DRI) for males 14 years and older is 1.2 mg and for females 14 to 18 years is 1.0 mg. The DRI for females 19 years and older is 1.1 mg.

Brewer's yeast and nutritional yeast are the richest dietary sources of B$_1$. Peas, beans, nuts, seeds, and whole grains also provide fairly good amounts.

Certain foods may impair absorption of B$_1$, including fish, shrimp, clams, mussels, and the herb horsetail *(Equisetum arvense)*.

Safety Issues

Vitamin B$_1$ appears to be quite safe even when taken in very high doses.

Maximum safe dosages in individuals with severe hepatic or renal disease are not known.

Safety in Young Children
and Pregnant or Lactating Women

No significant safety concerns have been raised regarding use of vitamin B$_1$ in these groups.

Drug Interactions

Loop diuretics may cause depletion of vitamin B$_1$.[1]

VITAMIN B$_2$

Alternate Names/Supplement Forms:
Riboflavin, Riboflavin-5-Phosphate

Common Use

Migraine headaches   [+2]

(Higher numbers indicate stronger evidence; X modifier indicates contradictory results. See page xviii of the Introduction for details of the rating scale.)

Approach to the Patient

Although serious riboflavin deficiencies are rare, marginal deficiencies can occur in children, elderly people, and those in poverty.[1-4]

One double-blind trial suggests that supraphysiologic doses of vitamin B$_2$ might be useful for migraine headaches.

Migraine Headaches   +2

A 3-month, double-blind, placebo-controlled study of 55 patients with migraines found that vitamin B$_2$, 400 mg/day, significantly reduced attack frequency and total headache days, for which 50% responder rates in the treated group were 56% and 59%, respectively.[5] Effects began at 1 month of B$_2$ treatment but were maximal at 3 months.

Other Proposed Uses

Although riboflavin has also been proposed as a treatment for sickle cell anemia[6] and as a performance enhancer for athletes, there is no real evidence that it is effective for these uses.

Mechanism of Action

Vitamin B$_2$ is a cofactor for vitamin B$_6$ and folate and is necessary for the biosynthesis of adenosine triphosphate (ATP). Its mechanism of action in migraine headache is not known.

Dosage

The U.S. Dietary Reference Intake for riboflavin varies by age and gender and is 1.3 mg for males 14 years and older and 1.0 mg for females 14 to 18 years of age. Females 19 years and older should take in 1.1 mg/day of vitamin B$_2$.

Riboflavin is found in organ meats and in many vegetables, nuts, legumes, and leafy greens. The richest dietary sources are torula (nutritional) yeast, brewer's yeast, and calf liver. Almonds, wheat germ, wild rice, and mushrooms are good sources as well.

Safety Issues

Riboflavin appears to present no safety risks.

Maximum safe dosages in individuals with severe hepatic or renal disease are not known.

Safety in Young Children and Pregnant or Lactating Women

Maximum safe dosages for pregnant or lactating women or young children have not been established, but no significant safety concerns have been raised.

Drug Interactions

Oral contraceptives may reduce levels of riboflavin.[7-9]

VITAMIN B₃

Alternate Names/Supplement Forms:
Niacin, Niacinamide, Nicotinamide,
Inositol Hexaniacinate, Inositol Hexanicotinate

Common Uses

**Hyperlipidemia
(niacin)** [+4]

**Intermittent
claudication (inositol
hexaniacinate)** [+3]

**Osteoarthritis
(niacinamide)** [+2]

**Raynaud's
phenomenon (inositol
hexaniacinate)** [+2]

**Diabetes
(niacinamide)** [+2X]

**Acne vulgaris
(niacinamide gel)** [+2]

(Higher numbers indicate stronger evidence; X modifier indicates contradictory results. See page xviii of the Introduction for details of the rating scale.)

Approach to the Patient

Niacin supplements can significantly improve various indices of hyperlipidemia. However, unpleasant flushing reactions and the risk of liver inflammation have kept niacin from being widely used.

A special form of so-called "flushless niacin" developed in Europe, inositol hexaniacinate, reportedly produces less flushing; it appears to be effective in intermittent claudication and perhaps in Raynaud's phenomenon. Niacinamide, which does not cause flushing, is ineffective for hyperlipidemia but may have some utility in preventing diabetes and treating osteoarthritis. Topical niacinamide gel has shown promise for the treatment of acne.

Although your patient may have heard that inositol hexaniacinate or niacinamide is less likely to cause hepatic inflammation than ordinary niacin, no meaningful evidence supports this widespread assumption.

Hyperlipidemia (Niacin)   +4

According to numerous studies, niacin can lower total and low-density lipoprotein (LDL) cholesterol by 15% to 25%, lower triglycerides by 2% to 50%, raise high-density lipoprotein (HDL) by about 15% to 30%, and reduce lipoprotein(a) by about 35%.[1-4] Combined treatment with statin drugs might offer additional benefit and appears to be safe so long as liver enzymes are monitored.[5,6] Further, long-term use of niacin has been shown to significantly reduce death rates from cardiovascular disease.[7]

Contrary to some reports, niacin appears to be safe and effective for use in diabetics.[8]

Intermittent Claudication (Inositol Hexaniacinate)   +3

Double-blind studies involving a total of about 300 individuals have found inositol hexaniacinate useful for intermittent claudication.[9-12] In one such trial, 100 individuals with intermittent claudication were given either placebo or 4 g of inositol hexaniacinate daily.[9] Over the 3-month study period, the treated group showed significant improvement in both time and total steps before onset of claudication.

Osteoarthritis (Niacinamide)   +2

In a double-blind study, 72 individuals with osteoarthritis were given either 3000 mg daily of niacinamide (in five equal doses) or placebo for 12 weeks.[13] The treated participants experienced a 29% reduction in symptoms, compared with a 10% increase in symptoms in the placebo group.

Raynaud's Phenomenon (Inositol Hexaniacinate)   +2

A double-blind study of 23 patients suggests that inositol hexaniacinate (Hexopal, 4 g/day) may be helpful for Raynaud's phenomenon.[14] Patients in the treatment group felt subjectively better and had shorter and fewer attacks of vasospasm during the trial period compared with placebo.

Diabetes (Niacinamide)   +2X

Two studies found that niacinamide may delay or prevent the onset of type 1 diabetes. In a population-based study of more than 20,000 children, 7-year treatment of islet cell antibody (ICA)–positive children with niacinamide, 25 mg/kg/day, reduced the incidence of diabetes.[15] Niacinamide might also prolong the "honeymoon period" in type 1 diabetes.[16]

However, the German portion of the ongoing European Nicotinamide Diabetes Intervention Trial has failed to demonstrate prevention of diabetes by regular use of niacinamide.[17]

Acne Vulgaris (Niacinamide Gel)   +2

In a double-blind trial, 76 individuals with moderate inflammatory acne were treated with either 4% niacinamide gel or 1% clindamycin gel.[18] Both treatments produced statistically similar improvements in acne symptoms over the 8-week trial period.

Other Proposed Uses

A preliminary study suggests that niacinamide may be helpful in **polymorphous light eruption**.[19]

Mechanism of Action

Vitamin B$_3$ is a cofactor for numerous enzymes, including those involved with cellular energy production, glycolysis, and fat synthesis. When taken at supraphysiologic doses, niacin (but not niacinamide) suppresses the synthesis of very low–density lipoprotein (VLDL) cholesterol. The mechanism of action of niacin, niacinamide, and inositol hexaniacinate in the other conditions noted above has not been elucidated.

Dosage

Therapeutic dosages range from 1 to 4 g daily of niacin, niacinamide, or inositol hexaniacinate.

The U.S. Dietary Reference Intake for niacin varies by age and gender and is 16 mg for males 14 years and older and 14 mg for females 14 years and older.

Good food sources of niacin are seeds, yeast, bran, peanuts (especially with skins), wild rice, brown rice, whole wheat, barley, almonds, and peas.

For nutritional purposes, niacin and niacinamide are interchangeable.

Safety Issues

At dosages of more than 100 mg daily, niacin frequently causes annoying skin flushing, especially in the face. This reaction may be accompanied by stomach distress, itching, and headache. In studies, as many as 43% of individuals taking niacin quit because of unpleasant side effects.[20] Slow-release niacin as well as inositol hexaniacinate may cause a lower incidence of flushing. Niacinamide does not cause flushing.

A potentially dangerous effect of high-dose niacin therapy is hepatic inflammation. Although most commonly seen with slow-release niacin, it can also occur with immediate-release niacin taken at more than 500 mg daily (usually 3 g or more). Contrary to some statements in the alternative medicine literature, there is no reason to believe that high-dose niacinamide or inositol hexaniacinate is less likely to cause this side effect. Routine hepatic function tests are therefore mandatory during high-dose treatment.

High-dose niacin may also present risks in individuals with a history of peptic ulcer disease, gout, and excess alcohol consumption.[21] However, contrary to previous reports, niacin does not appear to raise serum glucose in diabetics.[8]

Maximum safe dosages in individuals with severe hepatic or renal disease are not known.

Safety in Young Children and Pregnant or Lactating Women

The tolerable upper intake level of niacin for pregnant or lactating women has been set at 35 mg daily (30 mg if under 19 years old).[22]

Drug Interactions

Niacinamide might increase serum levels of anticonvulsant medications including **carbamazepine** and **primidone,** possibly requiring reduction in drug dosage.[23]

Although there have been concerns that high-dose niacin in combination with **statin drugs** could increase risk of liver enzyme elevation and rhabdomyolysis, studies suggest that the risk may be slight, especially in those with normal renal function,[5,6,24] and the combination may further improve lipid profiles by raising HDL levels. One study found that a low dose of niacin (100 mg) may provide a similar benefit, presumably with even less risk.[27]

Supplementation may be useful for patients taking **isoniazid,** since the drug may impair biosynthesis of niacin from tryptophan.[25,26]

VITAMIN B$_6$

Alternate Names/Supplement Forms:
Pyridoxine, Pyridoxine Hydrochloride,
Pyridoxal-5-Phosphate

Common Uses

Nausea and vomiting of pregnancy [+3]	**Carpal tunnel syndrome** [+2X]
Cardiovascular disease (prevention) [+2]	**Premenstrual syndrome** [−1X]
Asthma [+2X]	**Diabetic neuropathy** [−1]

(Higher numbers indicate stronger evidence; X modifier indicates contradictory results. See page xviii of the Introduction for details of the rating scale.)

Approach to the Patient

Mild dietary deficiencies of vitamin B$_6$ are common,[1] particularly in elderly people[2] and in children.[3] For this reason, supplementation may be appropriate on general principles.

Preliminary evidence suggests possible benefit of B$_6$ in the nausea and vomiting of pregnancy and in cardiovascular disease prevention. Evidence for usefulness in asthma, carpal tunnel syndrome, and premenstrual syndrome is weak and contradictory. Vitamin B$_6$ does not appear to be beneficial in diabetic neuropathy.

Other potential uses of vitamin B$_6$ include seborrheic dermatitis, depression, gestational diabetes, photosensitivity, and urolithiasis.

Nausea and Vomiting of Pregnancy   +3

In a double-blind trial, 342 pregnant women were given placebo or 30 mg of vitamin B$_6$ daily.[4] Subjects noted the severity of their nausea and recorded the number of vomiting episodes. The B$_6$ group experienced significantly less nausea than the placebo group. However, vomiting episodes were not significantly reduced.

Cardiovascular Disease (Prevention)   +2

Observational, case cohort, and preliminary intervention trials suggest that vitamin B$_6$ supplements with or without folic acid may significantly reduce the risk of heart disease.[5-8] The mechanism of action is presumed to involve homocysteine (see Mechanism of Action). One study found that among individuals with adequate folate and B$_{12}$ levels, low-dose supplementation with B$_6$ further reduced homocysteine levels.[9]

Asthma   +2X

Although one double-blind study of 76 children with asthma found significant benefit from vitamin B$_6$ after the second month of use,[10] a more recent double-blind study of 31 adults with steroid-dependent asthma did not.[11] The dosages of B$_6$ used in these studies were in the high range (200 to 300 mg daily), which may be associated with increased risk of sensory neuropathy (see Safety Issues).

Carpal Tunnel Syndrome   +2X

Observations in the 1970s suggested that individuals with carpal tunnel syndrome (CTS) were deficient in vitamin B$_6$.[12] This led to widespread use of vitamin B$_6$ as a CTS remedy. However, more recent evidence suggests that there is no association between CTS and vitamin B$_6$ deficiency.[13] A double-blind trial of 15 individuals found no significant differences after 10 weeks among those taking vitamin B$_6$, placebo, or nothing at all.[14] Another double-blind trial of 32 individuals found only minor benefits.[15] There was no improvement in nighttime pain, numbness, tingling, or objective measurements of median nerve function. Some improvement, however, was seen in finger swelling and discomfort after repetitive motion.

Premenstrual Syndrome   −1X

Systematic reviews have found a dozen or so double-blind studies investigating the effectiveness of vitamin B$_6$ for PMS, but none were well-designed, and overall the evidence for any benefit is weak at best.[16,17] Although it is commonly stated by B$_6$ proponents that the negative results in some of these studies were due to insufficient B$_6$ dosage, in reality there was no clear link between dosage and effectiveness.

A more recent, properly designed, double-blind trial of 120 women compared three pharmaceuticals (fluoxetine, 10 mg/day; alprazolam, 0.75 mg/day; propranolol, 20 mg/day [40 mg during the menstrual period]) with vitamin B$_6$ (pyridoxine, 300 mg/day) and placebo.[18] All participants received 3 months of treatment and 3 months of placebo. The best results were seen with fluoxetine, and pyridoxine proved no more effective than placebo.

Weak evidence suggests that the combination of magnesium and B$_6$ might offer some benefit in PMS.[19]

Diabetic Neuropathy   −1

Three double-blind, placebo-controlled trials enrolling a total of 58 individuals with diabetic neuropathy found no benefit attributable to pyridoxine supplementation.[20-22]

Other Proposed Uses

Weak evidence suggests that topical vitamin B$_6$ might be useful in **seborrheic dermatitis,**[23] and that oral vitamin B$_6$ might be useful in **depression,**[24] **gestational diabetes,**[25] **tardive dyski-**

nesia,[26-29] and **photosensitivity**[30] Vitamin B$_6$ might also help prevent calcium oxalate formation and thereby reduce the risk of **kidney stones,**[31-33] although not all studies agree.[34]

In analogy to its proposed use in pregnancy and PMS, vitamin B$_6$ has been tried as a treatment to reduce **side effects of oral contraceptives.**[61] However, a 30-day, double-blind trial of 124 women taking a low-dose combined oral contraceptive failed to find any benefit with 150 mg of vitain B$_6$ daily.

A small 30-day, double-blind trial failed to find vitamin B$_6$ at a dose of 50 mg daily helpful for **eczema.**[62]

Six double-blind, placebo-controlled trials enrolling a total of about 150 children with **autism** have found significant improvement in behavior under treatment with combination vitamin B$_6$ and magnesium therapy.[35-40] However, the study design used in many of these trials was questionable, and all were performed by one research group.

Mechanism of Action

Vitamin B$_6$ plays a major role in the biosynthesis of many proteins, hormones, and neurotransmitters. Other than improvement of nutritional levels, no specific pharmacologic or therapeutic action has been established.

It has been assumed that the mechanism of action of vitamin B$_6$ in heart disease involves homocysteine levels, but one study found evidence that vitamin B$_6$ intake itself is more strongly associated with reduced heart disease risk.[6]

Dosage

Commonly recommended therapeutic dosages of vitamin B$_6$ range from 10 to 300 mg daily. However, high dosages may present risks (see Safety Issues).

Vitamin B$_6$ requirements increase with age and vary by gender. The U.S. Dietary Reference Intake for males 14 to 50 years is 1.3 mg and for males 51 years and older is 1.7 mg. The recommended dosages are 1.2 mg in females 14 to 18 years of age, 1.3 mg in females 19 to 50 years of age, and 1.5 mg in females 51 years of age and older. Evidence has been presented, however, that these dosages should be increased.[41]

Good dietary sources of B$_6$ include nutritional (torula) yeast, brewer's yeast, sunflower seeds, wheat germ, soybeans, walnuts, lentils, lima beans, buckwheat flour, bananas, and avocados.

Safety Issues

Excessive intake of vitamin B$_6$ can cause sensory neuropathy. Although most commonly seen in dosages above 2000 mg daily, neurologic symptoms have been reported at doses as low as 200 mg daily.[42] High-dose vitamin B$_6$ may also cause or worsen acne symptoms.[43,44]

Maximum safe dosages in individuals with severe hepatic or renal disease are not known.

Safety in Young Children and Pregnant or Lactating Women

The tolerable upper intake level of vitamin B$_6$ for pregnant or lactating women has been set at 100 mg daily (80 mg if under 19 years old).[45]

Drug Interactions

Doses of vitamin B$_6$ over 5 mg may interfere with the effects of **levodopa** when the drug is taken alone.[46-48] However, **levodopa-carbidopa** combinations are not susceptible to this interference.

Supplementation might be appropriate for patients taking any of the various drugs that may impair B$_6$ nutritional levels, which include **hydralazine**,[49] **penicillamine**,[50] **theophylline**,[51-55] **MAO inhibitors**,[56] and **isoniazid**.[56-59]

Preliminary evidence suggests that vitamin B$_6$ might reduce nervous system side effects, such as hand tremors, associated with the use of **theophylline**.[60]

VITAMIN B$_{12}$

Alternate Names/Supplement Forms:
Methylcobalamin, Cyanocobalamin,
Hydrocobalamin, Cobalamin

Common Use

Male infertility   [−2]

(Higher numbers indicate stronger evidence; X modifier indicates contradictory results. See page xviii of the Introduction for details of the rating scale.)

Approach to the Patient

Aside from the treatment of pernicious anemia, there are no documented medical uses of vitamin B$_{12}$ other than to correct deficiency.

Vitamin B$_{12}$ supplementation to correct deficiency is worth considering in elderly people, total vegetarians, and individuals taking H$_2$ blockers or proton pump inhibitors. Even marginal deficiency of vitamin B$_{12}$ may impair cognitive function.[1]

Male Infertility   − 2

Adequate vitamin B$_{12}$ nutritional levels are necessary for normal sperm count and activity. For this reason, B$_{12}$ has been suggested as a treatment for infertility. However, a double-blind study of 375 oligozoospermic men found that vitamin B$_{12}$ supplements produced no benefits.[2] In a questionable post-hoc analysis, B$_{12}$ appeared to be effective in a subgroup of patients who had the lowest sperm counts and motility.

Other Proposed Uses

A 2-week, double-blind trial of 60 individuals with chronic **low back pain** found that use of intramuscular vitamin B$_{12}$ at a dose of 1000 mg daily significantly improved measures of pain and disability as compared with placebo.[41]

On the basis of weak and, in some cases, contradictory evidence, vitamin B$_{12}$ has been suggested for **AIDS**,[3,4] **asthma**,[5] **diabetic neuropathy**,[6,7] **multiple sclerosis**,[8-12] **restless legs syndrome**,[13,14] **tinnitus**,[15] and **vitiligo**.[16-18] Vitamin B$_{12}$ supplements are not effective in **Alzheimer's disease** according to one uncontrolled case series and a double-blind, placebo-controlled study.[19,20]

A double-blind trial of vitamin B$_{12}$ for seasonal affective disorder found no evidence of benefit.[42]

Vitamin B$_{12}$ is also sometimes recommended for other conditions, including depression, fatigue, osteoporosis, and periodontal disease, but no real evidence supports such uses at this time.

Mechanism of Action

Vitamin B$_{12}$ is required for normal neurophysiologic function, acts as a cofactor with folate and vitamin B$_6$ to lower serum homocysteine, and participates in the biosynthesis of S-adenosyl-methionine (SAMe). Other than correction of insufficient nutritional levels, no specific pharmacologic or therapeutic mechanism has been established.

Dosage

For pernicious anemia, vitamin B$_{12}$ injections are typically used; however, studies have found that oral B$_{12}$ is also effective when taken at sufficiently high dosages (from 300 to 1000 μg daily).[21-24]

Small amounts of vitamin B$_{12}$ suffice for daily nutritional needs. The U.S. Dietary Reference Intake for males and females 14 years and older is 2.4 μg.

Inadequate vitamin B$_{12}$ nutritional levels are relatively common in older people.[25-28] Nondairy or total vegetarians can become B$_{12}$ deficient unless they take B$_{12}$ supplements or eat B$_{12}$-enriched yeast.

Vitamin B$_{12}$ is found in most animal foods. Beef, liver, clams, and lamb provide 80 to 100 μg of B$_{12}$ per 3.5-ounce serving (at least 40 times the dietary requirement). Sardines, chicken liver, beef, kidney, and calf liver are also good sources, providing from 25 to 60 μg per serving. Trout, salmon, tuna, eggs, whey, and many cheeses provide at least the recommended daily intake.

When gastric acid is reduced, B$_{12}$ absorption from foods is diminished because of an inability to separate the vitamin from proteins. However, absorption of B$_{12}$ supplements is not affected.[25,29-33]

Safety Issues

Recommended dosages of vitamin B$_{12}$ appear to be safe.

Very high doses of vitamin B$_{12}$ may cause or worsen acne symptoms.[34,35]

Maximum safe dosages in individuals with severe hepatic or renal disease are not known.

Safety in Young Children and Pregnant or Lactating Women

No significant safety concerns have been raised for the use of vitamin B$_{12}$ in pregnant or lactating women or young children.

Drug Interactions

Although absorption of vitamin B$_{12}$ from *food* is impaired by **H$_2$ blockers** and **proton pump inhibitors,**[25,29-33] absorption of vitamin B$_{12}$ *supplements* is not affected.

Vitamin B$_{12}$ status can also be impaired by **colchicine, metformin, phenformin, zidovudine (AZT),** and **nitrous oxide.**[36-40]

VITAMIN C

Alternate Names/Supplement Forms:
Ascorbic Acid, Ascorbate

Common Uses

Upper respiratory infections

Treatment   [+3]

Prophylaxis: post–endurance exercise infection   [+3]

Prophylaxis: general   [−2]

Reflex sympathetic dystrophy (prophylaxis)   [+3]

Easy bruising   [+2]

Hypertension   [+2X]

Cervical dysplasia   [−2]

(Higher numbers indicate stronger evidence; X modifier indicates contradictory results. See page xviii of the Introduction for details of the rating scale.)

Approach to the Patient

Preliminary evidence supports the use of vitamin C in reducing the severity and duration of respiratory infections. However, the effect is extremely modest at best. Your patients may do better with echinacea, topical zinc, or andrographis.

Vitamin C is not effective for preventing colds in general. (Weak evidence suggests that vitamin C may help prevent postrace infections in endurance athletes.) Some evidence suggests, however, that garlic, probiotics, ginseng, and andrographis may have prophylactic effects against minor respiratory infections.

Vitamin C has also shown some promise in preventing reflex sympathetic dystrophy and may offer mild benefit in hypertension.

Numerous observational studies have found associations between foods rich in vitamin C and reduced incidence of various diseases. However, it is not clear whether vitamin C itself or other constituents in vitamin C–rich foods are responsible; thus no conclusions can be drawn from these studies about the effects of vitamin C supplements.

Combined treatment with vitamins C and E might be helpful for preventing preeclampsia.

One study suggests that vitamin C deficiency sufficient to cause a bleeding diathesis may occur in surgical patients more often than is usually realized.[88]

Although vitamin C is commonly recommended in multigram doses, some evidence indicates that plasma levels peak at an intake of 200 mg daily.

Upper Respiratory Infections

Treatment   +3

Numerous controlled trials of varying quality, involving a total of several thousand individuals, have found that vitamin C supplements taken at a dose of 1000 mg daily or more can very modestly reduce the duration and severity of cold symptoms.[1-3] In most of these trials, participants received vitamin C supplements on a daily basis while well, throughout a prolonged study period.

A more recent study evaluated the effects of vitamin C use at the onset of infection and found no benefit.[89] This double-blind trial of 400 individuals with new-onset cold symptoms compared the effects of vitamin C at the following daily dosages: 0.03 g daily (placebo), 1 g, 3 g, or 3 g with bioflavonoids. Participants were instructed to take the medication at the onset of cold symptoms and for the following 2 days. The results showed no difference in the duration or severity of cold symptoms between the groups.

Prophylaxis: Post–Endurance Exercise Infection   +3

Vitamin C supplements might reduce the incidence of respiratory infections following acute, but not chronic, endurance exercise.

In a double-blind, placebo-controlled study of 92 runners, using 600 mg of vitamin C for 21 days before a race made a significant difference in the incidence of respiratory infection.[4] Within 2 weeks after the race, 68% of the runners taking placebo developed cold symptoms, vs. only 33% of those taking the vitamin C supplement.

Two other studies found that vitamin C could reduce the number of colds experienced by groups of individuals under acute physical stress in cold environments.[5] One study involved 139 children attending a skiing camp in the Swiss Alps; the other enrolled 56 male soldiers engaged in a training exercise in Northern Canada during the winter months. In both cases, the participants took either 1 g of vitamin C or placebo daily at the time their training program began. Cold symptoms were monitored for 1 to 2 weeks following training, and significant differences were found in favor of vitamin C.

A study of 674 Marine recruits in basic training found no benefit of vitamin C, but their training involved chronic rather than acute physical stress.[5]

Prophylaxis: General   −2

Evidence from numerous studies has shown that regular use of vitamin C does not offer any general prophylactic benefit against respiratory infections.[6] However, vitamin C supplementation might reduce cold incidence in individuals who are ascorbate-deficient.

Reflex Sympathetic Dystrophy (Prophylaxis)   +3

A double-blind trial evaluated the potential prophylactic effect of vitamin C on RSD development in 123 individuals who had sustained wrist fractures.[7] Participants were given 500 mg of vitamin C or placebo daily for 50 days. The results showed significantly fewer cases of RSD in the treated group over a 12-month, follow-up period.

Easy Bruising   +2

A 2-month, double-blind study of 94 older individuals with marginal vitamin C deficiency found that vitamin C supplementation decreased their tendency to bruise.[8]

Hypertension   +2X

A 30-day, double-blind study of 39 individuals with hypertension found that daily treatment with 500 mg of vitamin C reduced blood pressure by about 10%.[9] Smaller benefits were seen in studies that included normotensive or borderline hypertensive individuals.[10,11] Other studies have returned inconclusive results.[12,13]

Cervical Dysplasia   −2

A double-blind, placebo-controlled study of 141 women with cervical dysplasia found that 500 mg daily of vitamin C did not help to reverse the dysplasia.[14]

Other Proposed Uses

Small double-blind studies suggest that vitamin C may be able to speed recovery from **bedsores**[15] and improve the behavior of **autistic** children.[16]

Observational studies have found that diets rich in foods containing vitamin C are associated with reduced risk of **cancer** and heart disease and a slowed rate of progression of **osteoarthritis.**[17-24] However, there is no substantive evidence that vitamin C supplements provide the same benefits.

Vitamin C supplementation has been associated with decreased incidence of **cataracts, macular degeneration, gallbladder disease in women,** and **vascular dementia.**[25-32]

A double-blind, placebo-controlled study of 283 women at increased risk for **preeclampsia** found that supplementation with vitamin C (1000 mg daily) and vitamin E (400 IU daily) significantly reduced the rate of preeclamptic symptoms.[33] Combination vitamin C and E treatment has also been found effective in a small, placebo-controlled, 8-week study of acute anterior uveitis.[34] Finally, when taken orally in combination with vitamin E but not when taken alone, vitamin C may have a modest preventive effect on sunburn.[35-40]

Topical vitamin C may offer some preventive benefits as well as improve the appearance of **aging** or **sun-damaged skin.**[37,41-43]

Many studies have tried to evaluate whether vitamin C supplements are useful for treatment of **asthma** and **allergies,** but the results have been mixed at best.[44-47]

Vitamin C has been suggested as a treatment for **male infertility**[48]; however, a double-blind study of 31 individuals found no benefit.[49]

In addition, vitamin C supplements have been recommended for bipolar disorder, bladder infections, cancer treatment, diabetes, hepatitis, herpes, insomnia, menopausal symptoms, migraine headaches, nausea, Parkinson's disease, periodontal disease, restless legs syndrome, rheumatoid arthritis, and ulcers, but no scientific evidence supports any of these uses.

Mechanism of Action

Vitamin C is a water-soluble vitamin and a strong antioxidant. It plays a significant role in the formation of intracellular cement substances such as collagen, is important in wound and bony fracture healing, and facilitates the absorption of iron.

Dosage

The U.S. Dietary Reference Intake for vitamin C varies by age and gender. The DRI for males 19 years and older is 90 mg, and for females 19 years and older it is 75 mg. Smoking significantly reduces levels of vitamin C.[50] For this reason, the recommended daily intake for smokers is 35 mg higher across all age-groups.

Proposed therapeutic dosages of vitamin C typically range from 500 mg to 3000 mg daily. However, one review of the evidence suggests that there may not be any benefit to taking more than 200 mg of vitamin C daily.[51] At dosages higher than 200 mg daily, the rate of renal excretion steadily increases and gastrointestinal (GI) absorption plateaus, resulting in a stable level of serum vitamin C comparable to that achieved with 200 mg daily. This review did not determine whether tissue concentrations of vitamin C also reach maximum levels at this dose, nor did it take into account the possible effects of divided daily doses. However, a study in young women using twice-daily doses found that both plasma and tissue levels of vitamin C reach their maximum at a daily vitamin C intake of 200 to 400 mg.[52]

Red chili peppers, sweet peppers, kale, parsley, collard, and turnip greens are excellent dietary sources of vitamin C, as are broccoli, Brussels sprouts, watercress, cauliflower, cabbage, and strawberries. Oranges and other citrus fruits are good sources, too.

Safety Issues

Recommendations regarding tolerable upper intake levels for vitamin C are as follows: children 1 to 3 years, 400 mg; 4 to 8 years, 650 mg; 9 to 13 years, 1200 mg; males and females 14 to 18 years, 1800 mg; 19 years and older, 2000 mg.

Concerns have been raised that long-term vitamin C treatment might increase risk of calcium oxalate stone formation by increasing urinary oxalate levels, although this is controversial.[53,54] Observational studies have found either no association or decreased risk with higher vitamin C intake.[55-57]

Nonetheless, certain individuals may be particularly at risk for vitamin C–induced kidney stones.[58] Individuals with a history of stone formation, with renal failure, or with a known defect in vitamin C or oxalate metabolism should probably restrict vitamin C intake to approximately 100 mg daily. High-dose vitamin C is also contraindicated in patients with glucose-6-phosphate dehydrogenase deficiency, iron overload, or a history of intestinal surgery.

Maximum safe dosages in individuals with severe hepatic or renal disease are not known.

Safety in Young Children and Pregnant or Lactating Women

The tolerable upper intake level of vitamin C for pregnant or lactating women has been set at 2000 mg daily (1800 mg if under 19 years old).

Drug Interactions

Weak evidence suggests that high doses of vitamin C might reduce the effects of **warfarin** and **heparin**.[59-62]

One study suggests that very high doses of vitamin C (3 g daily) might increase serum levels of **acetaminophen.**[63] **Aspirin** and other antiinflammatory drugs as well as **oral contraceptives** might lower blood levels of vitamin C.[64-71]

Disagreement exists regarding whether it is safe or appropriate to combine vitamin C with standard **chemotherapy drugs,** since there are concerns that the antioxidant effects of vitamin C might interfere with their action. However, there is some evidence that vitamin C may help reduce the side effects of certain chemotherapy drugs without decreasing their effectiveness.[72,73]

High-dose vitamin C supplementation may cause **copper** deficiency[74-77] and excessive **iron** absorption.[78-85]

Two small double-blind trials suggest that high-dose vitamin C therapy might help delay the onset of resistance to **nitrate** therapy.[86,87]

VITAMIN D

Alternate Names/Supplement Forms:
Cholecalciferol (Vitamin D₃), Ergocalciferol (Vitamin D₂),
Calcipotriol (Topical Vitamin D₃)

Common Use

Osteoporosis (combined with calcium)   **[+4]**

(Higher numbers indicate stronger evidence; X modifier indicates contradictory results. See page xviii of the Introduction for details of the rating scale.)

Approach to the Patient

Vitamin D deficiency occurs in elderly people as well as in people who live in northern latitudes.[1,2] It has been suggested that current intake recommendations are too low in some cases. (See Dosage.)

Solid clinical evidence indicates that the combination of calcium and vitamin D supplements may slow down or reverse osteoporosis. Vitamin D supplements alone do not appear to be effective.

Osteoporosis (Combined With Calcium)   +4

Vitamin D deficiency appears to be common among individuals with osteoporosis.[3] At least two double-blind, placebo-controlled studies observing a total of over 3500 postmenopausal women for 1 to 1.5 years found that combined vitamin D and calcium supplementation significantly increased bone density and reduced incidence of fractures.[4,5] However, calcium and vitamin D use must be continued. Improvements in bone rapidly disappear once the supplements are stopped.[6] Evidence also suggests that vitamin D combined with calcium can help protect against the bone loss caused by corticosteroid drugs.[7] However, although women with severe osteoporosis have low levels of vitamin D,[8] supplementation with vitamin D alone does not appear to be helpful.[9,10]

Other Proposed Uses

Some evidence suggests that adequate vitamin D may reduce the risk of **cancer** of the breast, colon, pancreas, prostate, and skin, but the research on this subject has yielded mixed results.[11-29] Adequate vitamin D might also reduce the risk of **hypertension.**[17,30-32]

A Finnish observational trial of 12,231 children suggests that use of vitamin D supplements reduces risk of type 1 **diabetes.**[66] Similar results were seen in other observational trials.[67,69]

One preliminary study suggests that supplementation with vitamin D and calcium may be helpful for women with **polycystic ovary syndrome.**[33]

A topical formulation of vitamin D_3 known as calcipotriol has been tried for **psoriasis,** with some success.[34]

Mechanism of Action

Vitamin D is a fat-soluble vitamin instrumental in calcium homeostasis.

Dosage

For therapeutic purposes, vitamin D is taken at nutritional doses. The Adequate Intake (AI) for vitamin D is 200 IU (5 μg) for males and females 1 to 50 years, 400 IU (10 μg) for adults 51 to 70 years of age, and 600 IU (15 μg) for adults 71 years of age and older.

However, it has been suggested that these recommendations are too low, especially for individuals with inadequate sun exposure, such as nursing home residents.[35-40] A daily dose of 1000 IU may be sufficient for sun-deprived individuals, although the optimal intake has not been determined.

There is very little vitamin D in most foods. The best dietary sources are cold-water fish. In many countries, vitamin D is added to milk and other foods, contributing to average daily intake. Relatively small levels of sunlight exposures (in the range of 5 to 15 minutes three times weekly to the hands, arms, and face) appear to supply adequate, although possibly not optimal, levels of vitamin D.[35-38]

Vitamin A supplementation may impair the action of vitamin D.[68]

Safety Issues

Vitamin D supplements are not recommended for patients with sarcoidosis or hyperparathyroidism.

When consumed in considerable excess, vitamin D supplements can cause symptoms of toxicity. Although the current recommendations set 2000 IU as the maximum safe daily intake, the dosage at which vitamin D becomes toxic is a matter of dispute.[35,41]

Maximum safe dosages in individuals with severe hepatic or renal disease are not known.

Safety in Young Children and Pregnant or Lactating Women

The Adequate Intake (AI) of vitamin D for pregnant and lactating women is 200 IU (5 μg). Tolerable upper intake levels for pregnant or lactating women and children 1 year and older have been set at 2000 IU daily.[42]

Drug Interactions

Combined vitamin D and calcium supplements might interfere with **calcium channel blockers.**[43]

The combination of calcium, vitamin D, and **thiazide diuretics** can lead to hypercalcemia.[44-46]

Phenobarbital, primidone, valproic acid, phenytoin, corticosteroids, cimetidine, heparin, isoniazid, and **rifampin** may interfere with vitamin D absorption or activity.[47-65] Supplementation may be beneficial for patients taking these medications.

VITAMIN E

Alternate Names/Supplement Forms:
Alpha-Tocopherol, D-Tocopherol, DL-Tocopherol,
DL-Alpha-Tocopherol, Tocopheryl Succinate,
Tocopheryl Acetate, D-Alpha-Tocopherol, D-Delta-Tocopherol,
D-Beta-Tocopherol, D-Gamma-Tocopherol,
Mixed Tocopherols

Common Uses

Chemoprevention   [+3]

Dysmenorrhea   [+2]

Immunomodulation   [+2]

Dementia   [+2]

Cardiac autonomic
neuropathy   [+2]

Asthenozoospermia   [+2X]

Osteoarthritis   [−1]

Tardive dyskinesia   [−2X]

Atherosclerosis   [−2]

Amyotrophic lateral
sclerosis [−2]

(Higher numbers indicate stronger evidence; X modifier indicates contradictory results. See page xviii of the Introduction for details of the rating scale.)

Approach to the Patient

Vitamin E deficiency caused by inadequate diet is relatively common in the developed world.[92] For this reason, supplementation of vitamin E at nutritional doses may be a reasonable preventive health measure.

However, despite the popularity of supraphysiologic dosages of vitamin E for heart disease prevention, evidence of benefit has not been demonstrated. Other, less well-known uses of high-dose vitamin E treatment have some supporting evidence.

Although high-dose vitamin E is reasonably safe, it may lead to increased risk of bleeding, especially when combined with antiplatelet agents.

Chemoprevention   +3

In a double-blind trial that involved 29,133 male smokers, participants given 50 mg of synthetic vitamin E daily for 5 to 8 years showed a 32% reduction in incidence of prostate cancer and a 41% drop in prostate cancer deaths, as compared with the placebo group.[1] Results were seen soon after the beginning of supplementation, suggesting that vitamin E blocks the transition phase from latent to clinical cancer. Benefits were also seen in incidence of colon cancer[2]; however, results regarding vitamin E and colon cancer from other observational and intervention trials have been mixed.[3-11] One observational study suggests that gamma-tocopherol rather than alpha-tocopherol might be the most relevant form of vitamin E for prostate cancer prevention, exerting a permissive role for both alpha-tocopherol and selenium.[12]

Observational studies also suggest benefit with vitamin E for stomach, mouth, throat, laryngeal, and liver cancer.[2,13-15]

Dysmenorrhea   +2

In a double-blind, placebo-controlled trial, 100 young women with significant menstrual pain were given either 500 IU vitamin E or placebo for 5 days.[93] Treatment began 2 days before and continued for 3 days after the expected onset of menstruation. Although both groups showed significant improvement in pain over the 2 months of the study, pain reduction was significantly greater in the treatment group as compared with the placebo group.

Immunomodulation   +2

In a double-blind, placebo-controlled trial, 88 individuals over the age of 65 years were given either placebo or vitamin E

(DL-alpha-tocopherol) at 60 mg, 200 mg, or 800 mg daily for 235 days.[16] All participants were then given diphtheria-pertussis-tetanus (DPT), pneumococcal, and hepatitis B (HepB) vaccines. The results in the 200 mg/day and 800 mg/day groups showed markedly increased hepatitis antibody titers; the 200 mg/day group also showed increased tetanus antibodies. All three treated groups showed an increased reaction on the Multi-Test Merieux delayed-type hypersensitivity skin test as compared with placebo, but only in the 200 mg/day group was the difference statistically significant.

Dementia   + 2

A 2-year, double-blind, placebo-controlled trial of 341 individuals with Alzheimer's disease found evidence that high-dose vitamin E (DL-alpha-tocopherol), 2000 IU daily (and to an even greater extent, selegiline), may significantly slow the progression of the disease.[17] Time to severe disease was increased by over 200 days in the vitamin E group as compared with the placebo group. However, because of an accident of randomization, the three groups were not equivalent, and statistical adjustment was required to reach a statistically significant outcome.

Observational studies have found associations between higher vitamin E intake and decreased risk of vascular dementia.[18]

Cardiac Autonomic Neuropathy   + 2

A 4-month, double-blind, placebo-controlled trial found that vitamin E at a dose of 600 mg daily improves the ratio of cardiac sympathetic to parasympathetic tone.[19]

Asthenozoospermia   + 2 X

A double-blind, placebo-controlled study that observed 87 men with asthenozoospermia found that treatment with vitamin E, 100 IU daily for up to 6 months, resulted in improved sperm activity.[20] However, a 56-day, double-blind study of 31 infertile men that tested combined vitamin C (1000 mg) and vitamin E (800 mg) found no benefit.[21]

Osteoarthritis   − 1

A 6-month, double-blind, placebo-controlled trial of 77 individuals with osteoarthritis found that treatment with vitamin E at a dose of 500 IU daily failed to provide any benefit as compared with placebo.[94]

Tardive Dyskinesia   − 2X

A metaanalysis of the several small double-blind studies reported before 1999 found evidence that vitamin E was more effective than placebo in the treatment of tardive dyskinesia (TD), especially recent-onset TD.[22] However, a larger double-blind trial reported in 1999 found no benefit.[23] This study included 107 participants from nine different research sites, who took 1600 IU of vitamin E or placebo daily for at least 1 year.

Atherosclerosis   − 2

Despite initial promising results from observational studies,[24-27] intervention trials suggest that vitamin E supplementation may not be effective for reducing atherosclerosis-related illness.

The Heart Outcomes Prevention Evaluation (HOPE) trial enrolled a total of 2545 women and 6996 men 55 years of age or older who were at high risk for cardiovascular events because of previous cardiovascular disease or diabetes plus one other risk factor.[28] The results over an average of 4.5 years showed that natural vitamin E (D-alpha-tocopherol) at a dose of 400 IU daily did not reduce the number of heart attacks, strokes, or deaths from heart disease. Negative results in various cardiac-related outcomes were seen in other large trials as well.[2,29-31]

In a portion of the HOPE trial, 732 individuals were treated with either vitamin E or ramipril over an average follow-up period of 4 to 5 years.[32] The results showed that ramipril slowed atherosclerosis, whereas vitamin E did not.

In addition, a large open trial evaluated the effectiveness of aspirin, vitamin E, and the combination of both for the prevention of cardiovascular events.[33] Whereas aspirin treatment proved dramatically helpful, vitamin E had little to no benefit.

The Cambridge Heart Antioxidant Study (CHAOS) trial found that participants given natural vitamin E (400 IU or 800 IU daily) had substantially fewer nonfatal heart attacks compared with the placebo group after about 1.5 years.[34] However, the number of incidents in this trial was relatively small, allowing for significant statistical error. No effects on the end points in HOPE or CHAOS were seen in two other trials; the Gruppo Italiano per lo Studio della Sopravvivenza nell'Infarto Miocardico (GISSI) and Alpha-Tocopherol, Beta-Carotene Cancer Prevention (ATBC) trials.[35,36]

It has been suggested that the relatively more abundant gamma-tocopherol might be the active form of vitamin E responsible for the inverse cardiac risk relationship seen in observational trials.[95-97] However, an observational study specifically looking to see if gamma-tocopherol levels were associated with risk of heart attack found no relationship between the two.[98]

Amyotrophic Lateral Sclerosis   − 2

A 1-year, double-blind, placebo-controlled trial of 289 individuals with ALS found that treatment with alpha-tocopherol (500 mg twice daily) combined with rituzole produced no effect on primary outcome measures (change in functional status).[38] In addition, use of vitamin E failed to alter most secondary measures. Vitamin E did appear to increase the time participants remained in the milder state of the disease as measured by the ALS Health State scale, but only when researchers collapsed the two milder AHSS states into state A and the two more severe states into state B.

Other Proposed Uses

In one observational study, high intake of vitamin E was linked to decreased risk of progression to acquired immunodeficiency syndrome (AIDS) in **HIV**-infected individuals.[39] However, a double-blind study of 49 individuals with human immunodeficiency virus (HIV) who took combined vitamins C and E or placebo for 3 months did not show any significant effects on HIV titer or the frequency of opportunistic infection.[40]

Intriguing evidence suggests that vitamin E may reduce pain in and possibly help prevent **rheumatoid arthritis**[41,42]; decrease symptoms of **menstrual pain**[93]; improve symptoms of **diabetic neuropathy**[43,44]; reduce the risk of **diabetic retinopathy** and **nephropathy**[45] and improve blood sugar control in **type 2 diabetes**[46-48]; reduce the rate of **cataract** development or progression[49-52]; control symptoms of **restless legs syndrome**[53]; reduce **muscle soreness** during resistance exercise[54]; help prevent **nitrate tolerance**[100]; and reduce symptoms of **premenstrual syndrome (PMS)**.[55,56]

Vitamin E and other antioxidants are frequently recommended for asthma, on the grounds that they may protect inflamed lung tissue, but there is no scientific evidence that they work in this manner. Similarly, although vitamin E has been suggested as a treatment for acne, Dupuytren's contracture, gout, fibromyalgia, and psoriasis, there is no real supporting evidence for any of these uses.

Vitamin E does not appear to be helpful for **cyclic mastitis,**[57] **Parkinson's disease,**[58-60] **vasomotor symptoms,**[61] **intermittent claudication,**[62] **hypertension,**[63] or **endurance exercise.**[64]

Combination Treatments

A double-blind, placebo-controlled study of 283 women at increased risk for **preeclampsia** found that supplementation with vitamin E (400 IU daily of natural vitamin E) and vitamin C (1000 mg daily) significantly reduced the rate of development of preeclampsia.[65]

When combined with vitamin C, vitamin E used orally or topically may help prevent sunburn and reduce **photosensitivity.**[66-70] However, oral vitamin E taken alone appears to be ineffective.[66,71]

A 12-month, double-blind, placebo-controlled study found that combined treatment with vitamins A and E may speed recovery after **photorefractive keratectomy** and improve long-term outcome.[72]

There is also evidence that vitamin E in combination with vitamin C may be helpful for **acute anterior uveitis.**[73]

Mechanism of Action

Vitamin E is a fat-soluble vitamin that acts as an antioxidant in lipid media. This is the basis for most of its proposed uses. However, evidence suggests that vitamin E supplementation has no effect on lipid peroxidation in vivo.[74]

Dosage

The U.S. recommendation for daily intake of vitamin E in males and females 14 years and older is 15 mg of alpha-tocopherol. Vitamin E dosages are commonly stated in terms of international units (IUs), but the equivalency depends on the form. D-Alpha-tocopherol (the primary constituent of "natural" alpha-tocopherol) is more bioactive than DL-alpha-tocopherol (the primary constituent of synthetic alpha-tocopherol); 1 IU of D-alpha-tocopherol equals 0.67 mg alpha-tocopherol, whereas 1 IU of DL-alpha-tocopherol equals 0.45 mg alpha-tocopherol.

In developed countries, dietary vitamin E deficiency is relatively common.[81-83] The best food sources of vitamin E are polyunsaturated vegetable oils, seeds, nuts, and whole grains. Typical therapeutic dosages (100 to 800 mg daily) can only be obtained through the use of a supplement.

Safety Issues

Vitamin E at therapeutic dosages has been associated with few adverse effects.

The adult safe upper intake level (UL) for vitamin E is set at 1000 mg daily.[84] The equivalent dosages are 1500 IU of natural vitamin E and 1100 IU of synthetic vitamin E. (For technical reasons, the conversion factors are slightly different than for recommended daily intake.)

However, at high dosages vitamin E does have a mild anti-platelet effect. In one study of 28,519 men, vitamin E at 50 IU/day caused an increase in fatal hemorrhagic stroke.[85] (However, overall stroke incidence was not increased.) Caution is advised in individuals with bleeding disorders or those about to undergo surgery or labor and delivery.

Controversy exists regarding whether it is safe or appropriate to use high-dose vitamin E supplements during cancer chemotherapy.[86] Concerns have been raised that vitamin E might inhibit chemotherapy action by blocking free radicals necessary for therapeutic effect. However, there is also some evidence that vitamin E might help protect against the side effects of certain chemotherapy drugs without interfering with their action.[87]

Maximum safe dosages in individuals with severe hepatic or renal disease are not known.

Safety in Young Children and Pregnant or Lactating Women

The U.S. recommendation for daily intake of vitamin E in pregnant and lactating women is 19 mg. However, the recommendation for pregnant women less than 19 years of age is 15 mg.

The tolerable upper intake level of vitamin E for pregnant or lactating women has been set at 1000 mg daily (800 mg if under 19 years old).[84]

Drug Interactions

Based on its anticoagulant properties, vitamin E might potentiate **anticoagulant** or **antiplatelet** medications. A study that evaluated vitamin E plus aspirin did, in fact, find an additive effect.[88] In contrast, a 4-week study found no interaction between vitamin E and warfarin.[89] However, combined use of high-dose vitamin E and warfarin should still be approached with caution.

There is also at least a remote possibility that vitamin E could interact with herbs and supplements that possess anticoagulant or antiplatelet effects, such as **garlic, policosanol,** and **ginkgo.**

Highly preliminary evidence suggests that vitamin E might enhance insulin sensitivity in individuals with type 2 diabetes.[46,48] This could lead to risk of hypoglycemia and may warrant adjustment of **oral hypoglycemic** medications.

Vitamin E might decrease **amiodarone**-induced lung injury.[90] Numerous animal studies and small trials in humans have examined whether vitamin E's antioxidant effects might help prevent the heart toxicity associated with doxorubicin therapy. Although some animal studies have found a heart-protective effect,[99,101-105] others have not[77-80]; human trials have found little, if any, heart-protective benefits.[37,75,76]

It has been suggested that vitamin E may enhance the antiviral effects of **zidovudine (AZT),** but evidence for this is very weak.[91] A double-blind trial of 24 individuals found that vitamin E might help prevent nitrate tolerance.[100]

VITAMIN K

Alternate Names/Supplement Forms:
Vitamin K_1 (Phylloquinone), Vitamin K_2 (Menaquinone),
Vitamin K_3 (Menadione)

Common Use

Osteoporosis [+1]

(Higher numbers indicate stronger evidence; X modifier indicates contradictory results. See page xviii of the Introduction for details of the rating scale.)

Approach to the Patient

Vitamin K is used pharmacologically to reverse the effects of anticoagulant drugs. Indirect evidence suggests possible benefits for osteoporosis.

Patients with digestive diseases such as chronic diarrhea, celiac sprue, ulcerative colitis, or Crohn's disease may become deficient in vitamin K.[1-4] Alcoholism and the use of anticonvulsants can also lead to vitamin K deficiency.[5]

Although some alternative practitioners claim that the practice of giving newborns vitamin K_1 injections may increase the risk of cancer, very large observational studies (one involving more than 1 million participants) have found no connection.[6,7]

Osteoporosis   +1

Vitamin K plays a known biochemical role in the formation of new bone. A report from 12,700 participants in the Nurses' Health Study found that higher dietary intake of vitamin K is associated with significantly reduced risk of hip fracture.[8] In this study, the most common source of vitamin K was iceberg lettuce, followed by broccoli, spinach, romaine lettuce, Brussels sprouts, and dark greens. Women who ate lettuce each day had only 55% the risk of hip fracture as those who ate it only once weekly. However, among women taking estrogen, no added benefit was seen.

Other observational studies found evidence that higher vitamin K intake is associated with a reduced incidence of hip fractures.[9,22]

Additional evidence suggests that supplemental vitamin K can reduce the amount of calcium lost in the urine.[10-12]

Other Proposed Uses

Although vitamin K has been proposed as a treatment for **menorrhagia**,[13] the last study of this was more than 55 years ago.[14] Vitamin K has also been recommended for nausea, although there is as yet little evidence supporting this use.

Mechanism of Action

Vitamin K is a fat-soluble vitamin that promotes synthesis of clotting factors. Three proteins synthesized by osteoblasts are vitamin K–dependent: osteocalcin, matrix Gla protein, and protein S.

Dosage

The U.S. Dietary Reference Intake (DRI) for vitamin K varies by age and gender. DRI for males 14 to 18 years is 75 μg, and for males 19 years and older it is 120 μg. The DRI for females 14 to 18 years is 75 μg, and for females 19 years and older it is 90 μg.[15]

However, a higher intake of vitamin K, in the range of 110 μg daily for the average woman, was associated with reduced osteoporosis in the Nurses' Health Study.

Vitamin K (in the form of K_1) is found in green leafy vegetables. Kale, green tea, and turnip greens are the best food sources, providing about 10 times the daily adult requirement in a single serving. Spinach, broccoli, lettuce, and cabbage are very rich sources as well, along with foods such as oats, green peas, whole wheat, and green beans.

Safety Issues

Vitamin K is presumably safe at the recommended therapeutic dosages, because those quantities are easily obtained from food.

Maximum safe dosages in individuals with severe hepatic or renal disease are not known.

Safety in Young Children and Pregnant or Lactating Women

No significant safety concerns have been raised regarding use of vitamin K in pregnant or lactating women or young children.

Drug Interactions

As is well known, vitamin K supplementation, or intake of foods containing high levels of this vitamin, antagonizes the action of **warfarin.** Conversely, warfarin blocks the effects of vitamin K.

Children born to mothers taking **anticonvulsants** while pregnant may be significantly deficient in vitamin K, causing bleeding problems and facial bone abnormalities.[16,17] Vitamin K supplementation during pregnancy may be helpful.

Cephalosporins and other antibiotics may impair vitamin K–dependent blood clotting in patients with vitamin K–poor diets, possibly leading to bleeding complications.[18-21]

WHITE WILLOW
(Salix spp.)

Alternate Names/Related Species:
Catkins Willow, Pussywillow, Salicin Willow, Silver Willow,
Withe Withy, *Salix alba, S. fragilis, S. purpurea*

Common Use

Analgesia   [+3]

(Higher numbers indicate stronger evidence; X modifier indicates contradictory results. See page xviii of the Introduction for details of the rating scale.)

Approach to the Patient

Willow bark has been used as a treatment for pain and fever in China since 500 BC In 1828, European chemists extracted the substance salicin from white willow *(Salix alba)*, which was soon purified to salicylic acid.

White willow may still be a viable option for treating pain. For reasons that are not entirely clearly, white willow appears to provide significant analgesia at doses that provide relatively little salicylates. It seems to produce only a low incidence of gastric distress at these doses and also does not appear to significantly impair platelet aggregation.

Analgesia   +3

In a 4-week, double-blind, placebo-controlled study of 210 individuals with back pain, two doses of willow bark extract were compared with placebo.[1] The higher-dose group received extract supplying 240 mg of salicin daily; in this group, 39% were pain free for at least 5 days of the last week of the study. In the lower-dose group (120 mg salicin daily), 21% became pain free. In contrast, only 6% of those given placebo became pain free. Stomach distress did not occur in this study. The only significant side effect seen was an allergic reaction in one participant given willow.

A double-blind, placebo-controlled trial of 78 individuals with osteoarthritis of the knee or hip found that white willow at a dose providing 240 mg of salicin daily significantly improved pain levels.[2]

Other Proposed Uses

On the basis of its salicin content, white willow is also sometimes used for analgesia in conditions such as bursitis, dysmenorrhea, headaches, rheumatoid arthritis, and tendinitis. However, its effectiveness in these conditions has not been determined.

Mechanism of Action

As noted above, white willow contains the compound salicin, a pro-drug of acetylsalicylic acid. In the body, salicin is converted to a variety of salicylates but in relatively low concentrations. Evidence suggests that standard doses of willow bark are the equivalent of about 100 mg of aspirin daily rather than a full dose.[1] It is thought that other ingredients in white willow, such as a substance called tremulacin, contribute to its analgesic effects. Both salicin and tremulacin have been found to possess antiinflammatory effects in the hen's egg chorioallantoic membrane test.[3]

Dosage

Standardized willow bark extracts should provide 120 to 240 mg of salicin daily.

Safety Issues

At standard doses, white willow does not appear to impair platelet function[4] or induce gastric irritation to the same extent as aspirin.[3] However, all risks associated with aspirin use, such as iatrogenic peptic ulcer disease, should be considered as potential risks with white willow. For this reason, white willow should not be given to children because of the risk of Reye's syndrome. It is also not recommended for use in individuals with aspirin allergies, coagulation disorders, existing peptic ulcer disease, or diabetes.

Maximum safe dosages in individuals with severe hepatic or renal disease are not known.

Safety in Young Children and Pregnant or Lactating Women

Maximum safe dosages for pregnant or lactating women have not been established. White willow should not be given to children.

Drug Interactions

Given its similarity to aspirin, white willow may adversely interact with **alcohol, anticoagulant** and **antiplatelet agents,** other **antiinflammatory agents, sulfonamide drugs, methotrexate, metoclopramide, phenytoin, probenecid, spironolactone** and other **potassium-sparing diuretics,** and **valproate.**

XYLITOL

Common Uses

Dental caries   **Otitis media**   [+3]
(prevention)   [+4]

(Higher numbers indicate stronger evidence; X modifier indicates contradictory results. See page xviii of the Introduction for details of the rating scale.)

Approach to the Patient

Strong evidence suggests that xylitol in toothpaste, gum, and lozenges can reduce dental caries; gums containing xylitol as the primary sweetener are widely available at supermarkets. However, your patients will have to read labels to discover this, since health claims are not yet permitted.

Lesser but still significant evidence suggests that xylitol may be useful in preventing otitis media as well.

Dental Caries (Prevention)   +4

Double-blind trials enrolling a total of almost 4000 individuals, mostly children, have found that xylitol significantly reduces dental caries in comparison with placebo or no treatment.[1-6] These trials used xylitol-sweetened gum, candies, or toothpaste.

In a double-blind cohort study, researchers tested gum sweetened with various concentrations of xylitol and/or sorbitol against gum sweetened with sucrose and a control receiving no gum.[2] This 40-month trial was completed by 861 children. The group with the highest xylitol intake showed the most benefits, but all of the xylitol and sorbitol gum groups showed significant reductions in cavities as compared with the no-treatment group. In contrast, the children receiving sucrose-sweetened gum had a slight increase in dental caries compared with the control group.

A double-blind, placebo-controlled study of 1677 children compared a standard fluoride toothpaste with a similar toothpaste that also contained 10% xylitol.[6] Over the 3-year study period, children given the xylitol-enriched toothpaste developed significantly fewer cavities than those in the fluoride-only group. Finally, in a 5-year study involving 740 Estonian children, both xylitol candies and chewing gums proved equally effective in caries prevention.[7]

Another series of studies suggests that children acquire caries-causing bacteria from their mothers; regular use of xylitol by a mother of a newborn child may provide some protection to the child as well.[12-14] Studies in adults have also shown benefits with xylitol gum or candy.[4] In addition, xylitol appears to help reduce gingivitis in adults.

Otitis Media   +3

A 3-month, double-blind, placebo-controlled trial of 857 children investigated the prophylactic effects of xylitol in chewing gum, syrup, and lozenges on otitis media incidence.[8] The gum was most effective, reducing the risk by 40%. Xylitol syrup was also effective, but less so. The lozenges were not effective; researchers speculated that children got tired of sucking on the large candies and did not get the proper dose of xylitol. (In addition, the children were able to distinguish between the xylitol and placebo lozenges by taste, making that portion of the study single-blind.)

Similarly positive results were seen in an earlier double-blind study by the same researchers, evaluating about 300 children over 2 months.[9]

Mechanism of Action

Xylitol replaces sugars that promote caries and also appears to directly inhibit the growth of *Streptococcus mutans*.[1,10]

Xylitol inhibits the growth and attachment of *Streptococcus pneumoniae* and perhaps the attachment of *Haemophilus influenzae* as well.[8,11]

Dosage

In the studies described above, dosages for caries prophylaxis ranged from 4.3 to 10 g per day, in divided doses. Xylitol-sweetened candy, gum, and toothpaste all appear to be effective. For otitis media prophylaxis, children given xylitol-sweetened gum received 8.4 g of xylitol daily, also in divided doses. Those who took syrup received 10 g daily. Lozenges were not effective.

Safety Issues

Xylitol is believed to be safe, but doses higher than 30 g per day can cause mild gastrointestinal distress. In studies, children taking xylitol syrup tended to have more gastrointestinal side effects than those using other forms of xylitol, possibly because it reached the stomach in a more concentrated dose.

Maximum safe dosages in individuals with severe hepatic or renal disease are not known.

Safety in Young Children and Pregnant or Lactating Women

Maximum safe dosages for pregnant or lactating women or young children have not been established.

Drug Interactions

There are no known drug interactions.

YOHIMBE
(Pausinystalia yohimbe)

Alternate Name/Related Species: *Corynanthe yohimbi*

Common Use

Erectile dysfunction [+2]

(Higher numbers indicate stronger evidence; X modifier indicates contradictory results. See page xviii of the Introduction for details of the rating scale.)

Approach to the Patient

Yohimbe *(Pausinystalia yohimbe)* is a source of the drug yohimbine, an approved but marginally effective treatment for erectile dysfunction. Yohimbine presents significant toxicologic risk; the indeterminate yohimbine content in yohimbe makes use of the herb unsafe. All studies noted below involved yohimbe rather than yohimbine.

Erectile Dysfunction   +2

Several small double-blind, placebo-controlled trials have found evidence that yohimbine is modestly effective in the treatment of erectile dysfunction.[1]

Other Proposed Uses

A small, double-blind trial suggests that combination therapy with yohimbine plus arginine may have value for the treatment of sexual dysfunction in women.[12]

Although yohimbe or yohimbine is sometimes recommended for depression, no evidence supports this use.

Mechanism of Action

The proposed mechanism of action of yohimbine involves dis-inhibition of sexual arousal nerve pathways.[1]

Dosage

The dose of yohimbe should be based on yohimbine content. Unfortunately, because of the lack of standardization of dietary supplement labeling in the United States, there is no reliable way of determining yohimbine content for a given product; one study found that the yohimbine content of yohimbe products was frequently inaccurate.[13] Some yohimbe products appear to have had purified yohimbine added.

The usual dose of yohimbine is 5.4 to 10.8 mg three times daily. Single dosing before sexual activity may be effective. Because yohimbine may have a bell-shaped dose-response curve, some experts recommend reducing the dose if there is no response at the standard doses; 2 to 3 weeks are needed to assess benefit.

Safety Issues

Yohimbine can cause anxiety, insomnia, hypertension, nausea, nervousness, and urinary frequency. Dosages greater than 40 mg/day may cause hypotension, abdominal pain, fatigue, hallu-cinations, and paralysis. Long-term toxicity or carcinogenicity has not been evaluated.

Yohimbe is not recommended for individuals with hypertension or hepatic, renal, or peptic ulcer disease.

Safety in Young Children and Pregnant or Lactating Women

Yohimbe should not be used by young children and pregnant or lactating women.

Drug Interactions

Yohimbe should not be combined with **tricyclic antidepressants, phenothiazines, antihypertensive agents,** or **central nervous system stimulants.**[2-11]

ZINC

Zinc Sulfate, Zinc Gluconate, Zinc Citrate,
Zinc Picolinate, Chelated Zinc

Common Uses

**Upper respiratory
infections (topical)** [+3X]

Oral herpes (topical) [+2]

**Infection prophylaxis
(oral)** [+3]

Sickle cell anemia [+3]

**Macular
degeneration** [+3X]

Anorexia nervosa [+2]

Acne [+2X]

Male infertility [+1]

**Rheumatoid
arthritis** [−1X]

(Higher numbers indicate stronger evidence; X modifier indicates contradictory results. See page xviii of the Introduction for details of the rating scale.)

Approach to the Patient

Inadequate zinc nutritional levels are thought to be relatively common,[95-97] especially in infants, adolescents, women, and elderly people.[98-102] For this reason, zinc supplementation may be advisable in many patients as a kind of nutritional insurance.

Alcoholism, conditions causing malabsorption, renal disease, sickle cell anemia, and any severe chronic illness or major trauma may increase zinc needs.

In addition, some medications and supplements may impair zinc absorption or increase zinc excretion (see Drug Interactions).

The best-established therapeutic use of zinc involves topical treatment: the use of zinc (as acetate or gluconate) in the form of nasal spray or lozenges to reduce the duration and severity of cold symptoms as well as, possibly, oral herpes. Uses of oral zinc at therapeutic dosages may be helpful in sickle cell anemia, macular degeneration, and acne. However, dosages of zinc above nutritional levels can cause severe copper deficiency as well as other toxic effects (see Safety Issues).

Upper Respiratory Infections (Topical)   + 3 X

It is thought that Zn^{2+} ions inhibit rhinovirus activity by binding to viral surfaces.[1] Topical zinc acetate and gluconate release Zn^{2+} and have been found effective for treating upper respiratory infections in the majority of studies; other ionic forms of zinc may be ineffective because of their physical chemistry properties (specifically, release of Zn^{2+} ions).[2,3] Two trials used zinc nasal spray, whereas previous trials used oral lozenges.

In a double-blind, placebo-controlled trial, 213 individuals with recent-onset upper respiratory infections received one inhalation of zinc gluconate or placebo nasal spray per nostril every 4 hours while awake.[1] The average duration of illness in treated participants was 2.3 days, compared with 9 days in the placebo group. This represents about a 75% reduction in the duration of symptoms. Another double-blind trial found no benefit; however, it used a 50 times lower dose of zinc.[4] In addition, the zinc salt used in this trial was zinc sulfate.

Less dramatic but still significant reduction in duration or severity of symptoms has been found in most studies of zinc acetate or gluconate lozenges.[2,3,5,6] One study in children failed to find benefit.[7] Flavoring agents such as citric acid and tartaric acid may impair ion availability and effectiveness.[2,3] Sorbitol, sucrose, dextrose, and mannitol appear to be acceptable, but information on the effect of glycine as a flavoring agent is equivocal.

Oral Herpes (Topical)   +2

In a double-blind, placebo-controlled trial, 46 individuals with active facial or circumoral herpes lesions were treated with a zinc oxide cream or placebo every 2 hours until cold sores resolved.[8] The results showed a significant reduction in severity and duration of symptoms in the treated group as compared with the placebo group. Some temporary burning and irritation from the zinc treatment were observed.

As with treatment of upper respiratory infections (URIs), proper design of the zinc formulation to release zinc ions is believed to be necessary. This trial used a zinc oxide/glycine formulation.

Infection Prophylaxis (Oral)   +3

In zinc-deficient individuals, oral zinc may be useful as prophylaxis against various infections, including pneumonia and diarrhea.[9-11]

For example, one double-blind, placebo-controlled trial evaluated the effect of daily supplementation with 10 mg of elemental zinc on the incidence and prevalence of acute lower respiratory infection in 609 children ranging in age from 6 to 35 months.[12] Supplementation and morbidity surveillance were done for 6 months. The study found a significant reduction in respiratory morbidity in children taking zinc supplements.

Sickle Cell Anemia   +3

A double-blind, placebo-controlled study of 145 sickle cell patients found that 220 mg of zinc sulfate three times daily for 18 months reduced the average number of sickle cell crises from 5.3 to 2.5 but did not decrease the length of hospitalization for each crisis.[13]

A placebo-controlled, but apparently only single-blind, study of 42 children with sickle cell disease (ages 4 to 10 years) found that use of zinc supplements for a period of 1 year enhanced growth rate.[103]

Macular Degeneration   +3X

A double-blind, placebo-controlled trial evaluated the effects of antioxidant and zinc on the progression of macular degeneration in 3640 individuals with extensive small drusen, intermediate drusen, large drusen, noncentral geographic atrophy, pigment abnormalities in one or both eyes, or advanced age-related macular degeneration (ARMD) in one eye.[104] Participants were randomly assigned to receive one of the following: antioxidants (vitamin C, 500 mg; vitamin E, 400 IU; beta-carotene, 15 mg); zinc (80 mg) and copper (2 mg); antioxidants plus zinc; or placebo. (Copper was administered along with zinc to prevent zinc-induced copper deficiency.) The results suggest that antioxidants plus zinc or zinc alone can significantly slow the progression of the disease.

A double-blind study of 151 individuals observed for 1 to 2 years found that zinc supplements at a dose of 80 mg elemental zinc daily helped preserve vision in individuals with ARMD.[14] However, another 2-year, double-blind study of 112 individuals given the same dose found no reduction in development of macular degeneration in the second eye among individuals with exudative ARMD in one eye.[15]

Anorexia Nervosa   +2

Preliminary evidence from two small double-blind trials suggests that zinc supplements might be helpful in anorexia nervosa, possibly enhancing weight gain and helping to stabilize mood.[43,105,107] One frequently quoted study often used to discredit the use of zinc in anorexia[44] appears to be relatively meaningless when inspected closely.[1,107]

Acne   + 2 X

Evidence of low serum zinc in individuals with acne[16-18] led to therapeutic trials of zinc supplementation. Several small double-blind studies involving a total of more than 300 individuals have returned somewhat conflicting results, but on balance the evidence suggests a modestly positive effect.

In one of these trials, 54 individuals with acne were given either placebo or 135 mg daily of zinc as zinc sulfate for a period of 6 weeks. Zinc produced slight but measurable benefits.[19] Similar results have been seen in most but not all studies using 90 to 135 mg of zinc daily.[20-25] Zinc in the form of zinc gluconate has been found effective at the lower (and safer) dose of 30 mg daily.[26]

Two small, double-blind trials compared zinc with tetracycline for treatment of acne. One 12-week trial found that zinc (45 mg three times daily) was as effective as tetracycline (250 mg three times daily, then twice daily, then once daily),[27] but another found the antibiotic "far more effective" when taken at 500 mg daily.[28]

A 3-month, dose-determination trial found no benefit in the use of a loading dose of zinc as opposed to continuous treatment with 30 mg daily.[29]

Male Infertility   + 1

One small, uncontrolled study of hypogonadal men found that zinc supplements increased sperm count and improved fertility.[30]

Rheumatoid Arthritis   − 1 X

The results of small double-blind studies and other forms of evidence, although mixed, suggest on balance that zinc supplements are not effective in rheumatoid arthritis (RA).[31-36,108,109] It has been proposed that zinc may only be beneficial in RA for those with zinc deficiency.[35]

Other Proposed Uses

Zinc has also been proposed as a treatment for **human immuno-deficiency virus (HIV)**,[37] **Alzheimer's disease**,[38-41] **anorexia nervosa**,[42-45] **benign prostatic hyperplasia**,[46,47] **diabetes**,[48-50] **Down's syndrome**,[51-53] **gastric and duodenal ulcers**,[54,55] **in-flammatory bowel disease**,[56-59] **osteoporosis**,[60] **prostatitis**,[61] **tinnitus**,[62,63] and **wound and burn healing**.[64-66] However, there is insufficient evidence to support these uses at this time.

There is no evidence to support the use of zinc for attention deficit disorder, cataracts, eczema, periodontal disease, urinary tract infection, or psoriasis.

An 8-week, double-blind trial of zinc at the somewhat high dose of 67 mg daily failed to find any benefit for eczema symptoms.[106]

Mechanism of Action

The efficacy of topical zinc in upper respiratory infections is thought to be a direct result of inhibition of rhinovirus replication or attachment by contact with Zn^{2+} ions.[1-3] Similar mechanisms may play a role in the treatment of herpes with topical zinc.[8]

Dosage

The U.S. Dietary Reference Intake for zinc varies by age and gender and is 11 mg in males 14 years and older. The DRI for females 14 to 18 years is 9 mg, and for females 19 years and older it is 8 mg.[67]

For treatment of upper respiratory infections, the usual topical dosage of zinc is 13 to 23 mg of zinc given as zinc gluconate, or zinc acetate lozenges every 2 hours. Other salts of zinc are not effective, and citric acid, tartaric acid, and other flavorings may block the antiviral action of zinc. Carbohydrate sweeteners are acceptable. To avoid excessive zinc intake, use of lozenges should be limited to 1 to 2 weeks. Zinc nasal spray should be used according to instructions. **Note:** Patients should be advised to avoid inhaling ("sniffing") when using zinc nasal spray, since this may result in an uncomfortable burning sensation.

See the Appendix for U.S. brand names of clinically tested products.

Extended oral treatment with high doses of elemental zinc (80 mg/day or more) has been used in research studies of various conditions such as acne, macular degeneration, and sickle cell anemia but carries a risk of toxicity related to copper deficiency (see Safety Issues). Use of copper supplements at 1 to 3 mg/day may reduce this risk. Simultaneous intake of iron or calcium supplements may reduce zinc absorption.[87-91,94]

Safety Issues

Oral zinc supplementation at nutritional doses is well-tolerated. Occasional gastric upset may occur but can be reduced by administering with food.

Recommendations regarding tolerable upper intake levels for zinc are as follows: children 1 to 3 years, 7 mg; 4 to 8 years, 12 mg; 9 to 13 years, 23 mg; males and females 14 to 18 years, 34 mg; 19 years and older, 40 mg.[67]

Long-term use of zinc at doses significantly above nutritional requirements can cause numerous toxic effects. It is thought that most, if not all, are related to zinc-induced copper deficiency. Toxic signs include anemia, neutropenia, cardiac abnormalities including arrhythmias, increased low-density lipoprotein (LDL) levels, decreased high-density lipoprotein (HDL) levels, decreased glucose clearance, and impaired immune function.[73-76] Copper supplementation may reduce this risk; however, high zinc tissue stores may significantly impair copper absorption.

Maximum safe dosages in individuals with severe hepatic or renal disease are not known.

*Safety in Young Children
and Pregnant or Lactating Women*

The tolerable upper intake level of zinc for pregnant or lactating women has been set at 40 mg daily (34 mg if under 19 years old).[67]

Drug Interactions

Zinc supplements can interfere with the absorption of **tetracyclines, fluoroquinolones,** and **penicillamine.**[69-72,78,86]

Renal handling of zinc may be altered by **diuretic therapy:** amiloride reduces, thiazides increases, and triamterene does not alter urinary zinc excretion.[80-82]

The absorption of zinc supplements may be reduced by **tetracyclines, quinolones, angiotensin-converting enzyme (ACE) inhibitors, thiazide diuretics,** and **any agent that reduces stomach acidity.** *

---

*References 68, 77, 79, 80, 82, 85, 92, 93.

APPENDIX

CLINICALLY
TESTED BRANDS

As noted in the Introduction, there is a serious bioequivalence issue regarding herbal products stemming from the presence of numerous potential active constituents in variable concentrations. Clinical results regarding one manufacturer's product may not apply to the same herb or herbal extract as supplied by a different manufacturer. This remains true even if the products are standardized to contain the same percentage of one or more ingredients.

A related consideration applies to certain nonherbal natural products as well. For example, the osteoarthritis supplement chondroitin sulfate is actually a complex mixture of chondroitins of various molecular weights; some chondroitin products may be more bioactive than others. Other supplements for which significant questions of bioactivity occur include proteolytic enzymes, citrus bioflavonoids (diosmin/hesperidin), and zinc lozenges and nasal spray.

Because of this issue, a good argument can be made for prescribing precisely the same brands of herbs and selected supplements that have been studied in double-blind trials. Competing products, especially those with similar manufacturing processes, may be equally effective. However, in the absence of corroborating trials, it is difficult to know for sure.

In order to facilitate selecting such clinically evaluated products, we have compiled the table below. It focuses on products available in the United States.

Note: This table was compiled from meaningful published studies indicating the source of the tested material. It is not meant as an endorsement of any specific product, and it is undoubtedly incomplete. We encourage manufacturers of clinically tested products not listed here to contact the editorial staff at content@healthgate.com so that these products may be included in future editions of this text.

Note also that new products can come to market at any time; in addition, manufacturers may change their suppliers. Therefore the information presented here is time-sensitive and may be out-of-date subsequent to press time.

Clinically Tested Brands		
Herb/Supplement	Tested Formulations: U.S. Brand	Tested Formulations: European Brand
Black cohosh	Remifemin (PhytoPharmica/ Enzymatic Therapy)	Remifemin (Schaper and Brummer)
Butterbur	Petadolex (Weber & Weber)	Petadolex (Weber & Weber)
Chasteberry	Femaprin (Nature's Way)	Agnolyt (Madaus)
Chondroitin sulfate	Cosamin DS (Nutramax Laboratories)	Cosamin DS (Nutramax Laboratories)
Diosmin/ hesperidin	Daflon 500 (Groupe de Recherche Servier)	Daflon 500 (Groupe de Recherche Servier)
Echinacea	EchinaGuard (Nature's Way)	Echinacin (Madaus)
	Echinoforce (Bioforce AG)	Echinoforce (Bioforce AG)
Elderberry	Sambucol (JB Harris) (Nature's Way)	Sambucol (Razei Bar Industries)

Clinically Tested Brands—cont'd		
Herb/Supplement	Tested Formulations: U.S. Brand	Tested Formulations: European Brand
Eleutherococcus	Elagen (Eladon)	Elagen (Eladon)
Gamma-linolenic acid (GLA)	Efamol (Efamol Ltd.)	Efamol (Efamol Nutraceuticals)
Garlic powder (aged)	Kyolic (Wakanuga)	Kyolic (Wakanuga)
Garlic powder (standardized for alliin content)	Kwai (Lichtwer Pharma)	Kwai (Lichtwer Pharma)
Ginger	Zintona (Pharmaton)	Zintona (Dalidar Pharma)
Gingko	Ginkai (Lichtwer Pharma)	Kaveri, LI 1370 (Lichtwer Pharma)
	Ginkoba (Pharmaton), Ginkgold (Nature's Way)	Tebonin forte, Tanakan, EGb 761 (Schwabe)
Ginseng	Ginsana (Pharmaton)	Ginsana, G115 (Pharmaton)
Grass pollen extract	Cernilton Pollen Extract Cernitin (Graminex)	Cernilton Pollen Extract (Cerniton)
Hawthorn	HeartCare (Nature's Way)	Crataegutt forte, WS 1442 (Schwabe)
Horse chestnut	Venastat (Pharmaton)	Venostasin retard (Klinge Pharma)
Kava	Kavatrol (Natrol)	Kavatrol (Natrol)
Lactobacillus GG	Culturelle (ConAgra)	

Continued

Clinically Tested Brands—cont'd		
Herb/Supplement	Tested Formulations: U.S. Brand	Tested Formulations: European Brand
Lemon balm (Melissa)	Herpalieve (PhytoPharmica), Herpilyn (Enzymatic Therapy)	Lomaherpan (Lomapharm)
Nettle/Pygeum	Prostatonin (Pharmaton)	Prostatonin (Pharmaton)
Oligomeric proanthocyanidin complexes (OPCs)	Grape Seed (PCO) Extract (PhytoPharmica/ Enzymatic Therapy), Grapenol (Solaray), Grapeseed Extract (Thorne Research)	Endotelon (Sanofi/Labaz), LeucoSelect (Indena)
Policosanol	New Cholestin (Pharmanex)	New Cholestin (Pharmanex)
Proteolytic enzymes	Wobenzym (Mucos Pharma)	Wobenzym (Mucos Pharma)
Pygeum	Pygeum Extract (Solaray)	Pygenil (Synthelabo/Sanofi), PrunaSelect (Indena)
Pygeum/Nettle	Prostatonin (Pharmaton)	Prostatonin (Pharmaton)
Red clover	Promensil (Novogen)	Promensil (Novogen)
Saw palmetto	Elusan Prostate Plants and Medicines, ProstActive (Nature's Way)	Permixon (Pierre Fabre), Prostagutt, WS 1473 (Schwabe)
Saw palmetto/ nettle	ProstActive Plus (Nature's Way)	Prostagut Forte (Schwabe)

	Clinically Tested Brands—cont'd	
Herb/Supplement	Tested Formulations: U.S. Brand	Tested Formulations: European Brand
St. John's wort	Kira (Lichtwer Pharma), Perika (Nature's Way), Movana™ (Pharmaton)	Jarsin 300, LI160, LI60WS (Lichtwer Pharma); Neuroplant, WS 5572 (Schwabe)
Valerian	Sedonium (Lichtwer Pharma)	Sedonium, LI 156 (Lichtwer Pharma)
Valerian/lemon balm	Valerian Nighttime (Nature's Way)	Euvegal forte (Schwabe)
Zinc gluconate lozenges	COLD-EEZE (Quigley Corp.)	
Zinc gluconate nasal spray	Zicam Gel Tech LLC	Zicam Gel Tech LLC

REFERENCES

Conditions

Acne

1. Pohit J, Saha KC, Pal B. Zinc status of acne vulgaris patients. *J Appl Nutr.* 1985;37:18-25.
2. Amer M, Bahgat MR, Tosson Z, et al. Serum zinc in acne vulgaris. *Int J Dermatol.* 1982;21:481-484.
3. Michaelsson G, Vahlquist A, Juhlin L. Serum zinc and retinol-binding protein in acne. *Br J Dermatol.* 1977;96:283-286.
4. Goransson K, Liden S, Odsell L. Oral zinc in acne vulgaris: a clinical and methodological study. *Acta Derm Venereol.* 1978;58:443-448.
5. Verma KC, Saini AS, Dhamija SK. Oral zinc sulfate therapy in acne vulgaris: a double-blind trial. *Acta Derm Venereol.* 1980;60:337-340.
6. Weimar VM, Puhl SC, Smith WH, et al. Zinc sulfate in acne vulgaris. *Arch Dermatol.* 1978;114:1776-1778.
7. Hillstrom L, Pettersson L, Hellbe L, et al. Comparison of oral treatment with zinc sulphate and placebo in acne vulgaris. *Br J Dermatol.* 1977;97:679-684.
8. Michaelsson G, Juhlin L, Vahlquist A. Effects of oral zinc and vitamin A in acne. *Arch Dermatol.* 1977;113:31-36.
9. Weismann K, Wadskov S, Sondergaard J. Oral zinc sulphate therapy for acne vulgaris. *Acta Derm Venereol.* 1977;57:357-360.
10. Orris L, Shalita AR, Sibulkin D, et al. Oral zinc therapy of acne. Absorption and clinical effect. *Arch Dermatol.* 1978;114:1018-1020.
11. Dreno B, Amblard P, Agache P, et al. Low doses of zinc gluconate for inflammatory acne. *Acta Derm Venereol.* 1989;69:541-543.
12. Michaelsson G, Juhlin L, Ljunghall K. A double-blind study of the effects of zinc and oxytetracycline in acne vulgaris. *Br J Dermatol.* 1977;97:561-566.
13. Cunliffe WJ, Burke B, Dodman B, et al. A double-blind trial of a zinc sulphate/citrate complex and tetracycline in the treatment of acne vulgaris. *Br J Dermatol.* 1979;101:321-325.
14. Meynadier J. Efficacy and safety study of two zinc gluconate regimens in the treatment of inflammatory acne. *Eur J Dermatol.* 2000;10:269-273.
15. Shalita AR, Smith JG, Parish LC, et al. Topical nicotinamide compared with clindamycin gel in the treatment of inflammatory acne vulgaris. *Int J Dermatol.* 1995;34:434-437.
16. Bassett IB, Pannowitz DL, Barnetson RSC. A comparative study of tea-tree oil versus benzoylperoxide in the treatment of acne. *Med J Aust.* 1990;153:455-458.
17. Thappa DM, Dogra J. Nodulocystic acne: oral gugulipid versus tetracycline. *J Dermatol.* 1994;21:729-731.

Allergic Rhinitis

1. Mittman P. Randomized, double-blind study of freeze-dried Urtica dioica in the treatment of allergic rhinitis. *Planta Med.* 1990;56:44-47.
2. Middleton E Jr, Drzewiecki G, Tatum J. The effects of citrus flavonoids on human basophil and neutrophil function. *Planta Med.* 1987;53:325-328.
3. Amellal M, Bronner C, Briancon F, et al. Inhibition of mast cell histamine release by flavonoids and biflavonoids. *Planta Med.* 1985;51:16-20.
4. Gabor M. Anti-inflammatory and anti-allergic properties of flavonoids. *Prog Clin Biol Res.* 1986;213:471-480.
5. Middleton E Jr. Effect of flavonoids on basophil histamine release and other secretory systems. *Prog Clin Biol Res.* 1986;213:493-506.
6. Ogasawara H, Middleton E Jr. Effect of selected flavonoids on histamine release (HR) and hydrogen peroxide (H2O2) generation by human leukocytes [abstract]. *J Allergy Clin Immunol.* 1985;75 (suppl 1 pt 2):184.
7. Middleton E Jr, Drzewiecki G. Flavonoid inhibition of human basophil histamine release stimulated by various agents. *Biochem Pharmacol.* 1984;33:3333-3338.

8. Pearce FL, Befus AD, Bienenstock J. Mucosal mast cells: effect of quercetin and other flavonoids on antigen-induced histamine secretion from rat intestinal mast cells. *J Allergy Clin Immunol.* 1984;73:819-823.

9. Middleton E Jr, Drzewiecki G, Krishnarao D. Quercetin: an inhibitor of antigen-induced human basophil histamine release. *J Immunol.* 1981;127:546-550.

10. Yoshimoto T, Furukawa M, Yamamoto S, et al. Flavonoids: potent inhibitors of arachidonate 5-lipoxygenase. *Biochem Biophys Res Commun.* 1983;116:612-618.

11. Kim HM, Lee EH, Cho HH, et al. Inhibitory effect of mast cell-mediated immediate-type allergic reactions in rats by spirulina. *Biochem Pharmacol.* 1998;55:1071-1076.

12. Yang HN, Lee EH, Kim HM. *Spirulina platensis* inhibits anaphyalactic reaction. *Life Sci.* 1997;61:1237-1244.

13. Bucca C, Rolla G, Oliva A, et al. Effect of vitamin C on histamine bronchial responsiveness of patients with allergic rhinitis. *Ann Allergy.* 1990;65:311-314.

14. Fortner BR II, Danziger RE, Rabinowitz PS, et al. The effect of ascorbic acid on cutaneous and nasal response to histamine and allergen. *J Allergy Clin Immunol.* 1982;69:484-488.

15. Bernstein CK, Deng C, Shuklah R, et al. Double blind placebo controlled (DBPC) study of grapeseed extract in the treatment of seasonal allergic rhinitis (SAR) [abstract]. *J Allergy Clin Immunol.* 2001;107:abstr 1018.

16. Schapowal, A. Randomised controlled trial of butterbur and cetirizine for treating seasonal allergic rhinitis. *BMJ.* 2002;324:144-146.

Altitude Sickness

1. Roncin JP, Schwartz F, D'Arbigny P. EGb 761 in control of acute mountain sickness and vascular reactivity to cold exposure. *Aviat Space Environ Med.* 1996;67:445-452.

2. Bailey DM, Davies B. Acute mountain sickness; prophylactic benefits of antioxidant vitamin supplementation at high altitude. *High Alt Med Biol.* 2001;2:21-29.

Alzheimer's Disease, Non-Alzheimer's Dementia, Ordinary Age-Related Memory Loss

1. Le Bars PL, Katz MM, Berman N, et al. A placebo-controlled, double-blind, randomized trial of an extract of *Ginkgo biloba* for dementia. North American EGb Study Group. *JAMA.* 1997;278:1327-1332.

2. Hofferberth B. The efficacy of EGb 761 in patients with senile dementia of the Alzheimer type, a double-blind, placebo-controlled study on different levels of investigation. *Hum Psychopharmacol.* 1994;9:215-222.

3. Kanowski S, Herrmann WM, Stephan K, et al. Proof of efficacy of the *Ginkgo biloba* special extract Egb 761 in outpatients suffering from mild to moderate primary degenerative dementia of the Alzheimer type or multi-infarct dementia. *Pharmacopsychiatry.* 1996;29:47-56.

4. Kleijnen J, Knipschild P. *Ginkgo biloba* for cerebral insufficiency. *Br J Clin Pharmacol.* 1992;34:352-358.

5. van Dongen MC, van Rossum E, Kessels AG, et al. The efficacy of ginkgo for elderly people with dementia and age-associated memory impairment: new results of a randomized clinical trial. *J Am Geriatr Soc.* 2000;48:1183-1194.

6. Brautigam MR, Blommaert FA, Verleye G, et al. Treatment of age-related memory complaints with *Ginkgo biloba* extract: a randomized double blind placebo-controlled study. *Phytomedicine.* 1998;5:425-434.

7. Mix JA, Crews WD Jr. An examination of the efficacy of *Ginkgo biloba* extract EGb 761 on the neuropsychologic functioning of cognitively intact older adults. *J Altern Complement Med.* 2000;6:219-229.

8. Winther K, Randlov C, Rein E, et al. Effects of *Ginkgo biloba* extract on cognitive function and blood pressure in elderly subjects. *Curr Ther Res.* 1998;59:881-888.

9. Rigney U, Kimber S, Hindmarch I. The effects of acute doses of standardized *Ginkgo biloba* extract on memory and psychomotor performance in volunteers. *Phytotherapy Res.* 1999;13:408-415.

10. Rai GS, Shovlin C, Wesnes KA. A double-blind, placebo controlled study of *Ginkgo biloba* extract ('Tanakan') in elderly outpatients with mild to moderate memory impairment. *Curr Med Res Opin.* 1991;12:350-355.

11. Allain H, Raoul P, Lieury A, et al. Effect of two doses of *Ginkgo biloba* extract (EGb 761) on the dual-coding test in elderly subjects. *Clin Ther.* 1993;15:549-558.

12. Kennedy DO, Scholey AB, Wesnes KA. The dose-dependent cognitive effects of acute administration of *Ginkgo biloba* to healthy young volunteers. *Psychopharmacology (Berl).* 2000;151:416-423.

13. Hindmarch I. Activity of *Ginkgo biloba* extract on short term memory [in French; English abstract]. *Presse Med.* 1986;15:1592-1594.

14. Warot D, Lacomblez L, Danjou P, et al. Comparative effects of *Ginkgo biloba* extracts on psychomotor performances and memory in healthy subjects [in French; English abstract]. *Therapie.* 1991;46:33-36.

15. Cenacchi T, Bertoldin T, Farina C, et al. Cognitive decline in the elderly: a double-blind, placebo-controlled multicenter study on efficacy of phosphatidylserine administration. *Aging (Milano).* 1993;5:123-133.

16. Delwaide PJ, Gyselynck-Mambourg AM, Hurlet A, et al. Double-blind randomized controlled study of phosphatidylserine in senile demented patients. *Acta Neurol Scand.* 1986;73:136-140.

17. Engel RR, Satzger W, Gunther W, et al. Double-blind cross-over study of phosphatidylserine vs. placebo in patients with early dementia of the Alzheimer type. *Eur Neuropsychopharmacol.* 1992;2:149-155.

18. Nerozzi D, Aceti F, Melia E, et al. Phosphatidylserine and memory disorders in the aged [in Italian; English abstract]. *Clin Ter.* 1987;120:399-404.

19. Funfgeld EW, Baggen M, Nedwidek P, et al. Double-blind study with phosphatidylserine (PS) in Parkinsonian patients with senile dementia of Alzheimer's type (SDAT). *Prog Clin Biol Res.* 1989;317:1235-1246.

20. Crook T, Petrie W, Wells C, et al. Effects of phosphatidylserine in Alzheimer's Disease. *Psychopharmacol Bull.* 1992;28:61-66.

21. Amaducci L, and the SMID Group. Phosphatidylserine in the treatment of alzheimer's disease: results of a multicenter study. *Psychopharmacol Bull.* 1988;24:130-134.

22. Villardita C, Grioli S, Salmeri G, et al. Multicentre clinical trial of brain phosphatidylserine in elderly patients with intellectual deterioration. *Clin Trials J.* 1987;24:84-93.

23. Palmieri G, Palmieri R, Inzoli MR, et al. Double-blind controlled trial of phosphatidylserine in patients with senile mental deterioration. *Clin Trials J.* 1987;24:73-83.

24. Crook TH, Tinklenberg J, Yesavage J, et al. Effects of phosphatidylserine in age-associated memory impairment. *Neurology.* 1991;41:644-649.

25. Wang LM, Han YF, Tang XC. Huperzine A improves cognitive deficits caused by chronic cerebral hypoperfusion in rats. *Eur J Pharmacol.* 2000;398:65-72.

26. Cheng DH, Tang XC. Comparative studies of huperzine A, E2020, and tacrine on behavior and cholinesterase activities. *Pharmacol Biochem Behav.* 1998;60:377-386.

27. Cheng DH, Ren H, Tang XC. Huperzine A, a novel promising acetylcholinesterase inhibitor. *Neuroreport.* 1996;8:97-101.

28. Xiong ZQ, Tang XC. Effect of huperzine A, a novel acetylcholinesterase inhibitor, on radial maze performance in rats. *Pharmacol Biochem Behav.* 1995;51:415-419.

29. Zhi QX, Yi FH, XI CT. Huperzine A ameliorates the spatial working memory impairments induced by AF64A. *Neuroreport.* 1995;6:2221-2224.

30. Zhu XD, Giacobini E. Second generation cholinesterase inhibitors: effect of (L)-huperzine-A on cortical biogenic amines. *J Neurosci Res.* 1995;41:828-835.

31. Zhang GB, Wang MY, Zheng JQ, et al. Facilitation of cholinergic transmission by huperzine A in toad paravertebral ganglia in vitro [in Chinese, English abstract]. *Zhongguo Yao Li Xue Bao.* 1994;15:158-161.

32. Laganiere S, Corey J, Tang XC, et al. Acute and chronic studies with the anticholinesterase Huperzine A: effect on central nervous system cholinergic parameters. *Neuropharmacology.* 1991;30:763-768.

33. Tang XC, De Sarno P, Sugaya K, et al. Effect of huperzine A, a new cholinesterase inhibitor, on the central cholinergic system of the rat. *J Neurosci Res.* 1989;24:276-285.

34. Tang XC, Han YF, Chen XP, et al. Effects of huperzine A on learning and the retrieval process of discrimination performance in rats [in Chinese]. *Zhongguo Yao Li Xue Bao.* 1986;7:507-511.

35. Guan LC, Chen SS, Lu WH, et al. Effects of huperzine A on electroencephalography power spectrum in rabbits [in Chinese, English abstract]. *Zhongguo Yao Li Xue Bao.* 1989;10:496-500.

36. Lu WH, Shou J, Tang XC. Improving effect of huperzine A on discrimination performance in aged rats and adult rats with experimental cognitive impairment [in Chinese]. *Zhongguo Yao Li Xue Bao.* 1988;9:11-15.

37. Wang YE, Feng J, Lu WH. Pharmacokinetics of huperzine A in rats and mice [in Chinese]. *Zhongguo Yao Li Xue Bao.* 1988;9:193-196.

38. Wang YE, Yue DX, Tang XC. Anti-cholinesterase activity of huperzine A [in Chinese]. *Zhongguo Yao Li Xue Bao.* 1986;7:110-113.

39. Zhu XD, Tang XC. Improvement of impaired memory in mice by huperzine A and huperzine B [in Chinese]. *Zhongguo Yao Li Xue Bao.* 1988;9:492-497.

40. Zhu XD, Tang XC. Facilitatory effects of huperzine A and B on learning and memory of spatial discrimination in mice [in Chinese]. *Yao Xue Xue Bao.* 1987;22:812-817.

41. Yan XF, Lu WH, Lou WJ, et al. Effects of huperzine A and B on skeletal muscle and the electroencephalogram [in Chinese]. *Zhongguo Yao Li Xue Bao.* 1987;8:117-123.

42. Zhang RW, Tang XC, Han YY, et al. Drug evaluation of huperzine A n the treatment of senile memory disorders [in Chinese; English abstract]. *Zhongguo Yao Li Xue Bao.* 1991;12:250-252.

43. Xu SS, Cai ZY, Qu ZW, et al. Huperzine-A in capsules and tablets for treating patients with Alzheimer disease. *Zhongguo Yao Li Xue Bao.* 1999;20:486-490.

44. Sun QQ, Xu SS, Pan JL, et al. Huperzine-A capsules enhance memory and learning performance in 34 pairs of matched adolescent students. *Zhongguo Yao Li Xue Bao.* 1999;20:601-603.

45. Hindmarch I, Fuchs HH, Erzigkeit H. Efficacy and tolerance of vinpocetine in ambulant patients suffering from mild to moderate organic psychosyndromes. *Int Clin Psychopharmacol.* 1991;6:31-43.

46. Balestreri R, Fontana L, Astengo F, et al. A double-blind placebo controlled evaluation of the safety and efficacy of vinpocetine in the treatment of patients with chronic vascular senile cerebral dysfunction. *J Am Geriatr Soc.* 1987;35:425-430.

47. Dragunow M, Faull RL. Neuroprotective effects of adenosine. *Trends Pharmacol Sci.* 1988;9:193-194.

48. Fenzl E, Apecechea M, Schaltenbrand R, et al. Efficacy and tolerance of vinpocetine administered intravenously, in addition of standard therapy, to patients suffering from an apoplectic insult. In: Krieglstein J, ed. *Pharmacology of Cerebral Ischemia: Proceedings of the International Symposium on Pharmacology of Cerebral Ischemia.* New York, NY: Elsevier Science Publishers; 1986:430-434.

49. Manconi E, Binaghi F, Pitzus F. A double-blind clinical trial of vinpocetine in the treatment of cerebral insufficiency of vascular and degenerative origin. *Curr Ther Res.* 1986;40:702-709.

50. Peruzza M, DeJacobis M. A double-blind placebo controlled evaluation of the efficacy and safety of vinpocetine in the treatment of patients with chronic vascular or degenerative senile cerebral dysfunction. *Adv Ther.* 1986;3:201-209.

51. Blaha L, Erzigkeit H, Adamczyk A, et al. Clinical evidence of the effectiveness of vinpocetine in the treatment of organic psychosyndrome. *Hum Psychopharmacol.* 1989;4:103-111. Cited by: Hindmarch I, Fuchs HH, Erzigkeit H. Efficacy and tolerance of vinpocetine in ambulant patients suffering from mild to moderate organic psychosyndromes. *Int Clin Psychopharmacol.* 1991;6:31-43.

52. Sorenson H, Sonne J. A double-masked study of the effects of ginseng on cognitive functions. *Curr Ther Res.* 1996;57:959-968.

53. Forgo I, Kayasseh L, Staub JJ. Effect of a standardized ginseng extract on general well-being, reaction time, lung function and gonadal hormones [translated from German]. *Med Welt.* 1981;32:751-756.

54. Siegl C, Siegl HJ. The possible revision of impaired mental abilities in old age: a double-blind study with *Panax ginseng* [translated from German]. *Therapiewoche.* 1979;29:4206, 4209-4216.

55. Sandberg F, Dencker L. Experimental and clinical tests on ginseng. *Z Phytother.* 1994;15:38-42.

56. D'Angelo L, Grimaldi R, Caravaggi M, et al. A double-blind, placebo-controlled clinical study on the effect of a standardized ginseng extract on psychomotor performance in healthy volunteers. *J Ethnopharmacol.* 1986;16:15-22.

57. Wesnes KA, Faleni RA, Hefting NR, et al. The cognitive, subjective, and physical effects of a *Ginkgo biloba/Panax ginseng* combination in healthy volunteers with neurasthenic complaints. *Psychopharmacol Bull.* 1997;33:677-683.

58. Sano M, Ernesto C, Thomas RG, et al. A controlled trial of selegiline, alpha-tocopherol, or both as treatment for Alzheimer's disease. *N Engl J Med.* 1997;336:1216-1222.

59. Masaki KH, Losonczy KG, Izmirlian G, et al. Association of vitamin E and C supplement use with cognitive function and dementia in elderly men. *Neurology.* 2000;54:1265-1272.

60. Bonavita E. Study of the efficacy and tolerability of L-acetylcarnitine therapy in the senile brain. *Int J Clin Pharmacol Ther Toxicol.* 1986;24:511-516.

61. Calvani M, Carta A, Caruso G, et al. Action of acetyl-L-carnitine in neurodegeneration and Alzheimer's disease. *Ann N Y Acad Sci.* 1992;663:483-486.

62. Campi N, Todeschini GP, Scarzella L. Selegiline versus L-acetylcarnitine in the treatment of Alzheimer-type dementia. *Clin Ther.* 1990;12:306-314.

63. Cipolli C, Chiari G. Effects of L-acetylcarnitine on mental deterioration in the aged: initial results [in Italian; English abstract]. *Clin Ter.* 1990;132(6 suppl):479-510.

64. Garzya G, Corallo D, Fiore A, et al. Evaluation of the effects of L-acetylcarnitine on senile patients suffering from depression. *Drugs Exp Clin Res.* 1990;16:101-106.

65. Passeri M, Cucinotta D, Bonati PA, et al. Acetyl-L-carnitine in the treatment of mildly demented elderly patients. *Int J Clin Pharmacol Res.* 1990;10:75-79.

66. Rai G, Wright G, Scott L, et al. Double-blind, placebo controlled study of acetyl-L-carnitine in patients with Alzheimer's dementia. *Curr Med Res Opin.* 1990;11:638-647.

67. Salvioli G, Neri M. L-acetylcarnitine treatment of mental decline in the elderly. *Drugs Exp Clin Res.* 1994;20:169-176.

68. Sano M, Bell K, Cote L, et al. Double-blind parallel design pilot study of acetyl levocarnitine in patients with Alzheimer's disease. *Arch Neurol.* 1992;49:1137-1141.

69. Spagnoli A, Lucca U, Menasce G, et al. Long-term acetyl-L-carnitine treatment in Alzheimer's disease. *Neurology.* 1991;41:1726-1732.

70. Vecchi GP, Chiari G, Cipolli C, et al. Acetyl-l-carnitine treatment of mental impairment in the elderly: evidence from a multicentre study. *Arch Gerontol Geriatr.* 1991;(suppl 2):159-168.

71. Thal LJ, Carta A, Clarke WR, et al. A 1-year multicenter placebo-controlled study of acetyl-L-carnitine in patients with Alzheimer's disease. *Neurology.* 1996;47:705-711.

72. Thal LJ, Calvani M, Amato A, et al. A 1-year controlled trial of acetyl-L-carnitine in early-onset AD. *Neurology.* 2000;55:805-810.

73. Chandra RK. Effect of vitamin and trace-element supplementation on cognitive function in elderly subjects. *Nutrition.* 2001;17:709-712.

74. Stough C, Lloyd J, Clarke J, et al. The chronic effects of an extract of *Bacopa monniera* (Brahmi) on cognitive function in healthy human subjects. *Psychopharmacology (Berl).* 2001;156:481-484.

75. Louwman MW, van Dusseldorp M, van de Vijver FJ, et al. Signs of impaired cognitive function in adolescents with marginal cobalamin status. *Am J Clin Nutr.* 2000;72:762-769.

76. Barrett-Connor E, Edelstein SL. A prospective study of dehydroepiandrosterone sulfate and cognitive function in an older population: the Rancho Bernardo Study. *J Am Geriatr Soc.* 1994;42:420-423.

77. Laird RD, Webb. M. Psychotic episode during use of St. John's wort. *J Herbal Pharmacother.* 2001;1:81-87.

78. Stough C, Lloyd J, Clarke J, et al. Neuropsychological changes after 30-day *Ginkgo biloba* administration in healthy participants. *Int J Neuropsychopharm.* 2001;4:131-134.

79. Hindmarch I, Fuchs HH, Erzigkeit H. Efficacy and tolerance of vinpocetine in ambulant patients suffering from mild to moderate organic psychosyndromes. *Int Clin Psychopharmacol.* 1991;6:31-43.

80. Wollschlaeger B. Efficacy of vinpocetine in the management of cognitive impairment and memory loss. *J Am Nutraceutical Assoc.* 2001;4:25-30.

Amyotrophic Lateral Sclerosis

1. Testa D, Caraceni T, Fetoni V. Branched-chain amino acids in the treatment of amyotrophic lateral sclerosis. *J Neurol.* 1989;236:445-447.

2. Tandan R, Bromberg MB, Forshew D, et al. A controlled trial of amino acid therapy in amyotrophic lateral sclerosis: I. Clinical, functional, and maximum isometric torque data. *Neurology.* 1996;47:1220-1226.

3. Plaitakis A, Smith J, Mandeli J, et al. Pilot trial of branched-chain amino acids in amyotrophic lateral sclerosis. *Lancet.* 1988;1:1015-1018.

4. Plaitakis A. Branched-chain amino acids and ALS [letter]. *Neurology.* 1994;44:1982-1983.

5. [No authors listed]. Branched-chain amino acids and amyotrophic lateral sclerosis: a treatment failure? The Italian ALS Study Group. *Neurology.* 1993;43:2466-2470.

6. Gredal O, Moller SE. Effect of branched-chain amino acids on glutamate metabolism in amyotrophic lateral sclerosis. *J Neurol Sci.* 1995;129:40-43.

7. Roufs JB. L-threonine as a symptomatic treatment for amyotrophic lateral sclerosis (ALS). *Med Hypotheses.* 1991;34:20-23.

8. Blin O, Pouget J, Aubrespy G, et al. A double-blind placebo-controlled trial of L-threonine in amyotrophic lateral sclerosis. *J Neurol.* 1992;239:79-81.

9. Testa D, Caraceni T, Fetoni V, et al. Chronic treatment with L-threonine in amyotrophic lateral sclerosis: a pilot study. *Clin Neurol Neurosurg.* 1992;94:7-9.

10. Tarnopolsky M, Martin J. Creatine monohydrate increases strength in patients with neuromuscular disease. *Neurology.* 1999;52:854-857.

11. Klivenyi P, Ferrante RJ, Matthews RT, et al. Neuroprotective effects of creatine in a transgenic animal model of amyotrophic lateral sclerosis. *Nature Med.* 1999;5:347-350.

12. Wyss M, Felber S, Skladal D, et al. The therapeutic potential of oral creatine supplementation in muscle disease. *Med Hypotheses.* 1998;51:333-336.

13. Desnuelle C, Dib M, Garrel C, et al. A double-blind, placebo-controlled randomized clinical trial of alpha-tocopherol (vitamin E) in the treatment of amyotrophic lateral sclerosis. ALS riluzole-tocopherol Study Group. *Amyotroph Lateral Scler Other Motor Neuron Disord.* 2001;2:9-18.

14. Matthews RT, Yang L, Browne S, et al. Coenzyme Q10 administration increases brain mitochondrial concentrations and exerts neuroprotective effects. *Proc Natl Acad Sci USA.* 1998;95:8892-8897.

15. Trieu VN, Uckun FM. Genistein is neuroprotective in murine models of familial amyotrophic lateral sclerosis and stroke. *Biochem Biophys Res Commun.* 1999;258:685-688.

16. Kaji R, Kodama M, Imamura A, et al. Effect of ultrahigh-dose methylcobalamin on compound muscle action potentials in amyotrophic lateral sclerosis: a double-blind controlled study. *Muscle Nerve.* 1998;21:1775-1778.

17. Norris FH Jr, Calanchini PR, Fallat RJ, et al. The administration of guanidine in amyotrophic lateral sclerosis. *Neurology.* 1974;24:721-728.

18. Beal MF. Coenzyme Q10 administration and its potential for treatment of neurodegenerative diseases. *Biofactors.* 1999;9:261-266.

19. Norris FH, Denys EH. Nutritional supplements in amyotrophic lateral sclerosis. *Adv Exp Med Biol.* 1987;209:183-189.

20. Vyth A, Timmer JG, Bossuyt PM, et al. Survival in patients with amyotrophic lateral sclerosis, treated with an array of antioxidants. *J Neurol Sci.* 1996;139(suppl):99-103.

21. Apostolski S, Marinkovic Z, Nikolic A, et al. Glutathione peroxidase in amyotrophic lateral sclerosis: the effects of selenium supplementation. *J Environ Pathol Toxicol Oncol.* 1998;17:325-329.

Angina

1. Ardissino D, Merlini PA, Savonitto S, et al. Effect of transdermal nitroglycerin or N-acetylcysteine, or both, in the long-term treatment of unstable angina pectoris. *J Am Coll Cardiol.* 1997;29:941-947.

2. Iversen HK. N-acetylcysteine enhances nitroglycerin-induced headache and cranial arterial responses. *Clin Pharmacol Ther.* 1992;52:125-133.

3. Pizzulli L, Hagendorff A, Zirbes M, et al. N-acetylcysteine attenuates nitroglycerin tolerance in patients with angina pectoris and normal left ventricular function. *Am J Cardiol.* 1997;79:28-33.

4. Hogan JC, Lewis MJ, Henderson AH. Chronic administration of N-acetylcysteine fails to prevent nitrate tolerance in patients with stable angina pectoris. *Br J Clin Pharmacol.* 1990;30:573-577.

5. Hanak T, Bruckel MH. The treatment of mild stable forms of angina pectoris using Crategutt® novo [in German; English abstract]. *Therapiewoche.* 1983;33:4331-4333.

6. Cacciatore L, Cerio R, Ciarimboli M, et al. The therapeutic effect of L-carnitine in patients with exercise-induced stable angina: a controlled study. *Drugs Exp Clin Res.* 1991;17:225-235.

7. Cherchi A, Lai C, Angelino F, et al. Effects of L-carnitine on exercise tolerance in chronic stable angina: a multicenter, double-blind, randomized, placebo controlled crossover study. *Int J Clin Pharmacol Ther Toxicol.* 1985;23:569-572.

8. Bartels GL, Remme WJ, Pillay M, et al. Effects of L-propionylcarnitine on ischemia-induced myocardial dysfunction in men with angina pectoris. *Am J Cardiol.* 1994;74:125-130.

9. Bartels GL, Remme WJ, den Hartog FR, et al. Additional antiischemic effects of long-term L-Propionylcarnitine in anginal patients treated with conventional antianginal therapy. *Cardiovasc Drugs Ther.* 1995;9:749-753.

10. Bartels GL, Remme WJ, Holwerda KJ, et al. Anti-ischaemic efficacy of L-propionylcarnitine—a promising novel metabolic approach to ischaemia? *Eur Heart J.* 1996;17:414-420.

11. Lagioia R, Scrutinio D, Mangini SG, et al. Propionil-L-carnitine: a new compound in the metabolic approach to the treatment of effort angina. *Int J Cardiol.* 1992;34:167-172.

12. Shechter M, Sharir M, Labrador MJ, et al. Oral magnesium therapy improves endothelial function in patients with coronary artery disease. *Circulation.* 2000;102:2353-2358.

13. Shechter M. The role of magnesium as antithrombotic therapy. *Wien Med Wochenschr.* 2000;150:343-347.

14. Kamikawa T, Kobayashi A, Yamashita T, et al. Effects of coenzyme Q10 on exercise tolerance in chronic stable angina pectoris. *Am J Cardiol.* 1985;56:247-251.

15. Bednarz B, Wolk R, Chamiec T, et al. Effects of oral L-arginine supplementation on exercise-induced QT dispersion and exercise tolerance in stable angina pectoris. *Int J Cardiol.* 2000;75:205-210.

16. Rapola JM, Virtamo J, Haukka JK, et al. Effect of vitamin E and beta carotene on the incidence of angina pectoris. *JAMA.* 1996;275:693-698.

17. McLean RM. Magnesium and its therapeutic uses: a review. *Am J Med.* 1994;96:63-76.

18. Maxwell AJ, Zapien MP, Pearce GL, et al. Randomized trial of a medical food for the dietary management of chronic, stable angina. *J Am Coll Cardiol.* 2002;39:37-45.

Anxiety and Panic Attacks

1. Volz HP, Kieser M. Kava-kava extract WS 1490 versus placebo in anxiety disorders— a randomized placebo-controlled 25-week outpatient trial. *Pharmacopsychiatry.* 1997;30:1-5.
2. Kinzler E, Kromer J, Lehmann E. Effect of a special kava extract in patients with anxiety-, tension-, and excitation states of non-psychotic genesis. Double blind study with placebos over 4 weeks [translated from German]. *Arzneimittelforschung.* 1991;41:584-588.
3. Warnecke G, Pfaender H, Gerster G, et al. Efficacy of an extract of kava root in patients with climacteric syndrome. A double blind study with a new mono-preparation [translated from German]. *Z Phytother.* 1990;11:81-86.
4. Warnecke G. Psychosomatic disorders in the female climacterium, clinical efficacy and tolerance of kava extract WS 1490 [translated from German]. *Fortschr Med.* 1991;109:119-122.
5. Malsch U, Klement S. Randomized placebo-controlled double-blind clinical trial of a special extract of kava roots (WS 1490) in patients with anxiety disorders of non-psychotic origin [abstract]. *Eur Phytojournal* [serial online]. 2000; Issue 1. Available at: http://www.escop.com/issue_1.htm. Accessed May 10, 2001.
6. Woelk H, Kapoula O, Lehrl S, et al. The treatment of patients with anxiety. A double-blind study: kava extract WS 1490 versus benzodiazepine [translated from German]. *Z Allgemeinmed.* 1993;69:271-277.
7. Kahn RS, Westenberg HG, Verhoeven WM, et al. Effect of a serotonin precursor and uptake inhibitor in anxiety disorders; a double-blind comparison of 5-hydroxy-tryptophan, clomipramine and placebo. *Int Clin Psychopharmacol.* 1987;2:33-45.
8. Carroll D, Ring C, Suter M, et al. The effects of an oral multivitamin combination with calcium, magnesium, and zinc on psychological well-being in healthy young male volunteers: a double-blind placebo-controlled trial. *Psychopharmacology (Berl).* 2000;150:220-225.
9. Benjamin J, Levine J, Fux M, et al. Double-blind, placebo-controlled, crossover trial of inositol treatment for panic disorder. *Am J Psychiatry.* 1995;152:1084-1086.
10. Palatnik A, Frolov K, Fux M, et al. Double-blind, controlled, crossover trial of inositol versus fluvoxamine for the treatment of panic disorder. *J Clin Psychopharmacol.* 2001;21:335-339.
11. Naguib M, Samarkandi AH. Premedication with melatonin: a double-blind, placebo-controlled comparison with midazolam. *Br J Anaesth.* 1999;82:875-880.
12. Naguib M, Samarkandi AH. The comparative dose-response effects of melatonin and midazolam for premedication of adult patients: a double-blinded, placebo-controlled study. *Anesth Analg.* 2000;91:473-479.
13. Kohnen R, Oswald WD. The effects of valerian, propranolol, and their combination on activation, performance and mood of healthy volunteers under social stress conditions. *Pharmacopsychiatry.* 1988;21:447-448.
14. Bradwejn J, Zhou Y, Koszycki D, et al. A double-blind, placebo-controlled study on the effects of Gotu Kola (Centella asiatica) on acoustic startle response in healthy subjects. *J Clin Psychopharmacol.* 2000;20:680-684.
15. Akhondzadeh S, Kashani L, Mobaseri M, et al. Passionflower in the treatment of opiates withdrawal: a double-blind randomized controlled trial. *J Clin Pharm Ther.* 2001:26;369-373.

Apthous Ulcers

1. Das SK, Das V, Gulati AK, Singh VP. Deglyceriyrrhizinated liquorice in apthous ulcers. *J Assoc Physicians India.* 1989;37:647.
2. Fidler P, Loprinzi CL, O'Fallon JR, et al. Prospective evaluation of a chamomile mouthwash for prevention of 5-FU-induced oral mucositis. *Cancer.* 1996;77:522-525.

Asthma

1. Shivpuri DN, Singhal SC, Parkash D. Treatment of asthma with an alcoholic extract of *Tylophora indica:* a cross-over, double-blind study. *Ann Allergy.* 1972;30:407-412.
2. Shivpuri DN, Menon MP, Prakash D. A crossover double-blind study on *Tylophora indica* in the treatment of asthma and allergic rhinitis. *J Allergy.* 1969;43:145-150.
3. Mathew KK, Shivpuri DN. Treatment of asthma with alkaloids of *Tylophora indica:* a double-blind study. *Aspects Allergy Appl Immunol.* 1974;7:166-179.
4. Gupta S, George P, Gupta V, et al. *Tylophora indica* in bronchial asthma—a double blind study. *Indian J Med Res.* 1979;69:981-989.
5. Gupta I, Gupta V, Parihar A, et al. Effects of *Boswellia serrata* gum resin in patients with bronchial asthma: results of a double-blind, placebo-controlled, 6-week clinical study. *Eur J Med Res.* 1998;3:511-514.
6. Collipp PJ, Goldzier S III, Weiss N, et al. Pyridoxine treatment of childhood bronchial asthma. *Ann Allergy.* 1975;35:93-97.
7. Sur S, Camara M, Buchmeier A, et al. Double-blind trial of pyridoxine (vitamin B6) in the treatment of steroid-dependent asthma. *Ann Allergy.* 1993;70:147-152.
8. Dry J, Vincent D. Effect of a fish oil diet on asthma: results of a 1-year double-blind study. *Int Arch Allergy Appl Immunol.* 1991;95:156-157.
9. Stenius-Aarniala B, Aro A, Hakulinen A, et al. Evening primrose oil and fish oil are ineffective as supplementary treatment of bronchial asthma. *Ann Allergy.* 1989;62:534-537.
10. Picado C, Castillo JA, Schinca N, et al. Effects of a fish oil enriched diet on aspirin intolerant asthmatic patients: a pilot study. *Thorax.* 1988;43:93-97.
11. Arm J. The effects of dietary supplementation with fish oil on asthmatic responses to antigen [abstract]. *J Allergy Clin Immunol.* 1988;81:183.
12. Stenius-Aarniala B, Aro A, Hakulinen A, et al. Symptomatic effects of evening primrose oil, fish oil, and olive oil in patients with bronchial asthma [abstract]. *Ann Allergy.* 1985;55:330.
13. Thien FC, Woods RK, Walters EH. Oily fish and asthma—a fishy story? *Med J Aust.* 1996;164:135-136.
14. Arm JP, Thien FC, Lee TH. Leukotrienes, fish-oil, and asthma. *Allergy Proc.* 1994;15:129-134.
15. Lee TH, Arm JP. Prospects for modifying the allergic response by fish oil diets. *Clin Allergy.* 1986;16:89-100.
16. Woods RK, Thien FC, Abramson MJ. Dietary marine fatty acids (fish oil) for asthma. *Cochrane Database Syst Rev.* 2000;(4):1-12 +5 tables.
17. Kreutner W, Chapman RW, Gulbenkian A, et al. Bronchodilatory and antiallergy activity of forskolin. *Eur J Pharmacol.* 1985;111:1-8.
18. Yousif M, Thulesius O. Forskolin reverses tachyphylaxis to the bronchodilator effects of salbutamol: an in-vitro study on isolated guinea-pig trachea. *J Pharm Pharmacol.* 1999;51:181-186.
19. Bauer K, Dietersdorfer F, Sertl K, et al. Pharmacodynamic effects of inhaled dry powder formulations of fenoterol and colforsin in asthma. *Clin Pharmacol Ther.* 1993;53:76-83.

Attention Deficit Hyperactivity Disorder (ADHD)

1. Re O. 2-Dimethylaminoethanol (deanol): a brief review of its clinical efficacy and postulated mechanism of action. *Curr Ther Res.* 1974;16:1238-1242.
2. Knobel M. Approach to a combined pharmacologic therapy of childhood hyperkinesis. *Behav Neuropsychiatry.* 1974/1975;6:87-90.
3. Fisman M, Mersky H, Helmes E. Double-blind trial of 2-dimethylaminoethanol in Alzheimer's disease. *Am J Psychiatry.* 1981;138:970-972.
4. Haug BA, Holzgraefe M. Orofacial and respiratory tardive dyskinesia: potential side effects of 2-dimethylaminoethanol (deanol). *Eur Neurol.* 1991;31:423-425.
5. Sergio W. Use of DMAE (2-dimethylaminoethanol) in the induction of lucid dreams. *Med Hypothesis.* 1988;26:255-257.

6. Voigt RG, Llorente AM, Jensen CL, et al. A randomized, double-blind, placebo-controlled trial of docosahexaenoic acid supplementation in children with attention-deficit/hyperactivity disorder. *J Pediatr.* 2001;139:189-196.
7. Richardson AJ, McDaid AM, Calvin CM, et al. Reduced behavioural and learning problems in children with specific learning difficulties after supplementation with highly unsaturated fatty acids: a randomised double-blind placebo-controlled trial. Presented at: 2nd Forum of European Neuroscience Societies; July 24-28, 2000; Brighton, United Kingdom.
8. Arnold LE, Kleykamp D, Votolato NA, et al. Gamma-linolenic acid for attention-deficit hyperactivity disorder: placebo-controlled comparison to D-amphetamine. *Biol Psychiatry.* 1989;25:222-228.
9. Kleijnen J, Knipschild P. Niacin and vitamin B6 in mental functioning: a review of controlled trials in humans. *Biol Psychiatry.* 1991;29:931-941.
10. Aman MG, Mitchell EA, Turbott SH. The effects of essential fatty acid supplementation by Efamol in hyperactive children. *J Abnorm Child Psychol.* 1987;15:75-90.

Benign Prostatic Hyperplasia (BPH)

1. Boccafoschi S, Annoscia S. Comparison of *Serenoa repens* extract with placebo by controlled clinical trial in patients with prostatic adenomatosis [in Italian]. *Urolgia.* 1983;50:1257-1268.
2. Champault G, Patel JC, Bonnard AM. A double-blind trial of an extract of the plant *Serenoa repens* in benign prostatic hyperplasia [letter]. *Br J Clin Pharmacol.* 1984;18:461-462.
3. Descotes JL, Rambeaud JJ, Deschaseaux P, et al. Placebo-controlled evaluation of the efficacy and tolerability of Permixon® in benign prostatic hyperplasia after exclusion of placebo responders. *Clin Drug Invest.* 1995;9:291-297.
4. Emili E, Lo Cigno M, Petrone U. Clinical trial of a new drug for treating hypertrophy of the prostate (Permixon®) [in Italian]. *Urolgia.* 1983;50:1042-1048.
5. Mattei FM, Capone M, Acconcia A. *Serenoa repens* extract in the medical treatment of benign prostatic hypertrophy [in Italian]. *Urolgia.* 1988;55:547-552.
6. Reece Smith H, Memon A, Smart CJ, et al. The value of Permixon® in benign prostatic hypertrophy. *Br J Urol.* 1986;58:36-40.
7. Tasca A, Barulli M, Cavazzana A, et al. Treatment of obstruction in prostatic adenoma using an extract of *Serenoa repens*. Double-blind clinical test v. placebo [in Italian; English abstract]. *Minerva Urol Nefrol.* 1985;37:87-91.
8. Bach D, Schmitt M, Ebeling L. Phytopharmaceutical and synthetic agents in the treatment of benign prostatic hyperplasia (BPH). *Phytomedicine.* 1996-1997;3:309-313.
9. Bracher F. Phytotherapy in the treatment of benign proststic hyperplasia [in German; English abstract]. *Urologe A.* 1997;36:10-17.
10. Plosker GL, Brogden RN. *Serenoa repens* (Permixon®). A review of its pharmacology and therapeutic efficacy in benign prostatic hyperplasia. *Drugs Aging.* 1996; 9:379-395.
11. Carraro JC, Raynaud JP, Koch G, et al. Comparison of phytotherapy (Permixon) with finasteride in the treatment of benign prostate hyperplasia: a randomized international study of 1,098 patients. *Prostate.* 1996;29:231-240.
12. Boyle P, Gould AL, Roehrborn CG. Prostate volume predicts outcome of treatment of benign prostatic hyperplasia with finasteride: meta-analysis of randomized clinical trials. *Urology.* 1996;48:398-405.
13. Gormley GJ, Stoner E, Bruskewitz RC, et al. The effect of finasteride in men with benign prostatic hyperplasia. *N Engl J Med.* 1992;327:1185-1191.
14. Sokeland J. Combined sabal and urtica extract compared with finasteride in men with benign prostatic hyperplasia: analysis of prostate volume and therapeutic outcome. *BJU Int.* 2000;86:439-442.
15. Debruyne F. Phytotherapy (LSESR) vs an alpha-blocker for treatment of lower urinary tract symptoms secondary to benign prostate enlargement: a randomized comparative study. Presented at: American Urological Association 2001 Annual Meeting; June 2-7, 2001; Anaheim, Calif.

16. Marks LS, Partin AW, Epstein JI, et al. Effects of a saw palmetto herbal blend in men with symptomatic benign prostatic hyperplasia. *J Urol.* 2000;163:1451-1456.

17. Andro MC, Riffaud JP. *Pygeum africanum* extract for the treatment of patients with benign prostatic hyperplasia: a review of 25 years of published experience. *Curr Ther Res.* 1995;56:796-817.

18. Breza J, Dzurny O, Borowka A, et al. Efficacy and acceptability of Tadenan® (*Pygeum africanum* extract) in the treatment of benign prostatic hyperplasia (BPH): a multicentre trial in central Europe. *Curr Med Res Opin.* 1998;14:127-139.

19. Barlet A, Albrecht J, Aubert A, et al. Efficacy of *Pygeum africanum* extract in the treatment of micturitional disorders due to benign prostatic hyperplasia: evaluation of objective and subjective parameters. A multicenter, placebo-controlled double-blind trial [translated from German]. *Wien Klin Wochenschr.* 1990;102:667-673.

20. Wilt TJ, MacDonald R, Ishani A. Beta-sitosterol for the treatment of benign prostatic hyperplasia: a systematic review. *BJU Int.* 1999;83:976-983.

21. Klippel KF, Hiltl DM, Schipp B. A multicentric, placebo-controlled, double-blind clinical trial of beta-sitosterol (phytosterol) for the treatment of benign prostatic hyperplasia. German BPH-Phyto Study group. *Br J Urol.* 1997;80:427-432.

22. Kadow C, Abrams PH. A double-blind trial of the effect of beta-sitosteryl glucoside (WA184) in the treatment of benign prostatic hyperplasia. *Eur Urol.* 1986;12:187-189.

23. Berges RR, Windeler J, Trampisch HJ, et al. Randomised, placebo-controlled, double-blind clinical trial of beta-sitosterol in patients with benign prostatic hyperplasia. Beta-sitosterol Study Group. *Lancet.* 1995;345:1529-1532.

24. Becker H, Ebeling L. Conservative therapy of benign prostatic hyperplasia (BPH) with Cernilton® N [translated from German]. *Urologe B.* 1988;28:301-306.

25. Buck AC, Cox R, Rees RW, et al. Treatment of outflow tract obstruction due to benign prostatic hyperplasia with the pollen extract, Cernilton: a double-blind, placebo-controlled study. *Br J Urol.* 1990;66:398-404.

26. Dathe G, Schmid H. Phytotherapy of benign prostate hyperplasia (BPH); double-blind study with stinging nettle root extract (Extractum Radicis Urticae—ERU) [translated from German]. *Urologe B.* 1987;27:223-226.

27. European Scientific Cooperative on Phytotherapy. *Urticae radix.* Exeter, UK: ESCOP; 1996-1997. Monographs on the Medicinal Uses of Plant Drugs, Fascicule 2:4.

28. Vontobel HP, Herzog R, Rutishauser G, et al. Results of a double-blind study on the effectiveness of ERU (extractum radicis Urticae) capsules in conservative treatment of benign prostatic hyperplasia [translated from German]. *Urologe A.* 1985; 24:49-51.

Bipolar Disorder

1. Chengappa KN, Levine J, Gershon S, et al. Inositol as an add-on treatment for bipolar depression. *Bipolar Disord.* 2000;2:47-55.

2. Levine J, Witztum E, Greenberg BD, et al. Inositol-induced mania? [letter]. *Am J Psychiatry.* 1996;153:839.

3. Mebane AH. L-glutamine and mania [letter]. *Am J Psychiatry.* 1984;141:1302-1303.

4. Stoll AL, Severus WE, Freeman MP, et al. Omega 3 fatty acids in bipolar disorder: a preliminary double-blind, placebo-controlled trial. *Arch Gen Psychiatry.* 1999; 56:407-412.

5. Stoll AL, Locke CA, Marangell LB, et al. Omega-3 fatty acids and bipolar disorder: a review. *Prostaglandins Leukot Essent Fatty Acids.* 1999;60:329-337.

6. Stoll AL, Sachs GS, Cohen BM, et al. Choline in the treatment of rapid-cycling bipolar disorder: clinical and neurochemical findings in lithium-treated patients. *Biol Psychiatry.* 1996;40:382-388.

7. Cohen BM, Lipinski JF, Altesman RI. Lecithin in the treatment of mania: double-blind, placebo-controlled trials. *Am J Psychiatry.* 1982;139:1162-1164.

8. Naylor GJ, Smith AH. Vanadium: a possible aetiological factor in manic depressive illness. *Psychol Med.* 1981;11:249-256.

9. Kay DS, Naylor GJ, Smith AH, et al. The therapeutic effect of ascorbic acid and EDTA in manic-depressive psychosis: double-blind comparisons with standard treatments. *Psychol Med.* 1984;14:533-539.
10. Coppen A, Abou-Saleh MT. Plasma folate and affective morbidity during long-term lithium therapy. *Br J Psychiatry.* 1982;141:87-89.

Cervical Dysplasia

1. Butterworth CE II, Hatch KD, Soong SJ, et al. Oral folic acid supplementation for cervical dysplasia: a clinical intervention trial. *Am J Obstet Gynecol.* 1992;166:803-809.
2. Orr J, Wilson K, Bodiford C, et al. Nutritional status of patients with untreated cervical cancer I and II. *Am J Obstet Gynecol.* 1985;151:625-635.
3. Romney SL, Palan PR, Basu J, et al. Nutrient antioxidants in the pathogenesis and prevention of cervical dysplasia and cancer. *J Cell Biochem.* 1995;23:96-103.
4. Butterworth CE II. Effect of folate on cervical cancer: synergism among risk factors. *Ann N Y Acad Sci.* 1992;669:293-299.
5. Mackerras D, Irwig L, Simpson JM, et al. Randomized double-blind trial of beta-carotene and vitamin C in women with minor cervical abnormalities. *Br J Cancer.* 1999;79:1448-1453.
6. Bell MC, Crowley-Nowick P, Bradlow HL, et al. Placebo-controlled trial of indole-3-carbinol in the treatment of CIN. *Gynecol Oncol.* 2000;78:123-129.
7. Romney SL, Palan PR, Basu J, et al. Nutrient antioxidants in the pathogenesis and prevention of cervical dysplasia and cancer. *J Cell Biochem.* 1995;23:96-103.
8. Keefe KA, Schell MJ, Brewer C, et al. A randomized double blind phase III trial using oral beta-carotene supplementation for women with high-grade cervical intraepithelial neoplasia. *Cancer Epidemiol Biomarkers Prev.* 2001;10:1029-1035.
9. Fairley CK, Tabrizi SN, Chen S, et al. A randomized clinical trial of beta carotene vs placebo for the treatment of cervical HPV infection. *Int J Gynecol Cancer.* 1996; 6:225-230.

Cholelithiasis

1. Somerville KW, Ellis WR, Whitten BH, et al. Stones in the common bile duct: experience with medical dissolution therapy. *Postgrad Med J.* 1985;61:313-316.
2. Nassuato G, Iemmolo RM, Strazzabosco M, et al. Effect of Silibinin on biliary lipid composition: experimental and clinical study. *J Hepatol.* 1991;12:290-295.
3. Leitzmann MF, Willett WC, Rimm EB, et al. A prospective study of coffee consumption and the risk of symptomatic gallstone disease in men. *JAMA.* 1999;281: 2106-2112.
4. Simon JA, Hudes ES. Serum ascorbic acid and gallbladder disease prevalence among US adults: the Third National Health and Nutrition Examination Survey (NHANES III). *Arch Intern Med.* 2000;160:931-936.

Chronic Fatigue Syndrome (CFS)

1. Forsyth LM, Preuss HG, MacDowell AL, et al. Therapeutic effects of oral NADH on the symptoms of patients with chronic fatigue syndrome. *Ann Allergy Asthma Immunol.* 1999;82:185-191.
2. Behan PO, Behan WMH, Horrobin D. Effect of high doses of essential fatty acids on the postviral fatigue syndrome. *Acta Neurol Scand.* 1990;82:209-216.
3. Warren G, McKendrick M, Peet M. The role of essential fatty acids in chronic fatigue syndrome: a case-controlled study of red-cell membrane essential fatty acids (EFA) and a placebo-controlled treatment study with high dose of EFA. *Acta Neurol Scand.* 1999;99:112-116.
4. Plioplys AV, Plioplys S. Amantadine and L-carnitine treatment of Chronic Fatigue Syndrome. *Neuropsychobiology.* 1997;35:16-23.
5. Himmel PB, Seligman TM. A pilot study employing dehydroepiandrosterone (DHEA) in the treatment of chronic fatigue syndrome. *J Clin Rheumatol.* 1999;5: 56-59.
6. Cunha BA. Beta-carotene stimulation of natural killer cell activity in adult patients with chronic fatigue syndrome. *CFIDS Chron Physicians' Forum.* Fall 1993:18-19.

7. Heath M, Klein NC, Cunha BA. Dose dependent effects of beta carotene therapy in chronic fatigue syndrome [abstract]. *Clin Res.* 1994;42:345A.

8. See DM, Broumand N, Sahl L, et al. In vitro effects of echinacea and ginseng on natural killer and antibody-dependent cell cytotoxicity in healthy subjects and chronic fatigue syndrome or acquired immunodeficiency patients. *Immunopharmacology.* 1997;35:229-235.

9. Peterson PK, Pheley A, Schroeppel J, et al. A preliminary placebo-controlled crossover trial of fludrocortisone for chronic fatigue syndrome. *Arch Intern Med.* 1998;158:908-914.

10. Martin RWY, Ogston SA, Evans JR. Effects of vitamin and mineral supplementation on symptoms associated with chronic fatigue syndrome with Coxsackie B antibodies. *J Nutr Med.* 1994;4:11-23.

Chronic Obstructive Pulmonary Disease (COPD)

1. Grandjean EM, Berthet P, Ruffmann R, et al. Efficacy of oral long-term N-acetylcysteine in chronic bronchopulmonary disease: a meta-analysis of published double-blind, placebo-controlled clinical trials. *Clin Ther.* 2000;22:209-221.

2. Hansen NC, Skriver A, Brorsen-Riis L, et al. Orally administered N-acetylcysteine may improve general well-being in patients with mild chronic bronchitis. *Respir Med.* 1994;88:531-535.

3. Grassi C, Casali L, Rossi A, et al. A comparison between different methods for detecting bronchial hyperreactivity. Bronchial hyperreactivity: methods of study. *Eur J Respir Dis Suppl.* 1980;106:19-27.

4. Grassi C, Morandini GC. A controlled trial of intermittent oral acetylcysteine in the long-term treatment of chronic bronchitis. *Eur J Clin Pharmacol.* 1976;9:393-396.

5. Riise GC, Larsson S, Larsson P et al. The intrabronchial microbial flora in chronic bronchitis patients: a target for N-acetylcsteine therapy? *Eur Respir J.* 1994;7:94-101.

6. Rasmussen JB, Glennow C. Reduction in days of illness after long-term treatment with N-acetylcysteine controlled-release tablets in patients with chronic bronchitis. *Eur Respir J.* 1988;1:351-355.

7. Parr GD, Huitson A. Oral Fabrol (oral N-acetyl-cysteine) in chronic bronchitis. *Br J Dis Chest.* 1987;81:341-348.

8. Boman G, Backer U, Larsson S, et al. Oral acetylcysteine reduces exacerbation rate in chronic bronchitis: report of a trial organized by the Swedish Society for Pulmonary Diseases. *Eur J Respir Dis.* 1983;64:405-415.

9. Verstraeten JM. Mucolytic treatment in chronic obstructive pulmonary disease: double-blind comparative clinical trial with N-acetylcysteine, bromhexine and placebo. *Acta Tuberc Pneumol Belg.* 1979;70:71-80.

10. Dal Negro R, Pomari G, Zoccatelli O, et al. L-carnitine and rehabilitative respiratory physiokinesitherapy: metabolic and ventilatory response in chronic respiratory insufficiency. *Int J Clin Pharmacol Ther Toxicol.* 1986;24:453-456.

11. Dal Negro R, Turco P, Pomari C, et al. Effects of L-carnitine on physical performance in chronic respiratory insufficiency. *Int J Clin Pharmacol Ther Toxicol.* 1988; 26:269-272.

12. Dal Negro R, Zoccatelli D, Pomari C, et al. L-carnitine and physiokinesiotherapy in chronic respiratory insufficiency: preliminary results. *Clin Trials J.* 1985;22:353-360.

13. Singh RB; et al. Dietary intake and plasma levels of antioxidant vitamins in health and disease: a hospital-based case-control study. *J Nutr Environ Med.* 1995;5:235-242.

14. Schwartz J, Weiss ST. Dietary factors and their relation to respiratory symptoms: the Second National Health and Nutrition Examination Survey. *Am J Epidemiol.* 1990;132:67-76.

15. Miedema I, Feskens EJM, Heederik D, et al. Dietary determinants of long-term incidence of chronic nonspecific lung diseases. *Am J Epidemiol.* 1993;138:37-45.

16. Sridhar MK. Nutrition and lung health. *BMJ.* 1995;310:75-76.

17. Schwartz J, Weiss ST. Relationship between dietary vitamin C intake and pulmonary function in the First National Health and Nutrition Examination Survey (NHANES I). *Am J Clin Nutr.* 1994;59:110-114.
18. Shahar E, Folsom AR, Melnick SL, et al. Dietary n-3 polyunsaturated fatty acids and smoking-related chronic obstructive pulmonary disease. *N Engl J Med.* 1994; 331:228-233.
19. Rautalahti M, Virtamo J, Haukka J, et al. The effect of alpha-tocopherol and beta-carotene supplementation on COPD symptoms. *Am J Respir Crit Care Med.* 1997;156:1447-1452.
20. Fujimoto S, Kurihara N, Hirata K, et al. Effects of coenzyme Q10 administration on pulmonary function and exercise performance in patients with chronic lung diseases. *Clin Investig.* 1993;71:S162-S166.

Cirrhosis

1. Ferenci P, Dragosics B, Dittrich H, et al. Randomized controlled trial of silymarin treatment in patients with cirrhosis of the liver. *J Hepatol.* 1989;9:105-113.
2. Benda L, Dittrich H, Ferenzi P, et al. The influence of therapy with silymarin on the survival rate of patients with liver cirrhosis [translated from German]. *Wien Klin Wochenschr.* 1980;92:678-683.
3. Pares A, Planas R, Torres M, et al. Effects of silymarin in alcoholic patients with cirrhosis of the liver: results of a controlled, double-blind, randomized and multicenter trial. *J Hepatol.* 1998;28:615-621.
4. Mato JM, Camara J, Fernandez de Paz J, et al. S-adenosylmethionine in alcoholic liver cirrhosis: a randomized, placebo-controlled, double-blind, multicenter clinical trial. *J Hepatol.* 1999;30:1081-1089.
5. Bombardieri G, Milani A, Bernardi L, et al. Effects of S-adenosyl-methionine (SAMe) in the treatment of Gilbert's Syndrome. *Curr Ther Res.* 1985;37:580-585.
6. di Padova C. S-adenosylmethionine in the treatment of osteoarthritis. Review of the clinical studies. *Am J Med.* 1987;83(5A):60-65.
7. Frezza M, Pozzato G, Chiesa L, et al. Reversal of intrahepatic cholestasis of pregnancy in women after high dose S-adenosyl-L-methionine administration. *Hepatology.* 1984;4:274-278.
8. Frezza M, Pozzato G, Pison G, et al. S-adenosylmethionine counteracts oral contraceptive hepatotoxicity in women. *Am J Med Sci.* 1987;293:234-238.
9. Nicastri PL, Diaferia A, Tartagni M, et al. A randomised placebo-controlled trial of ursodeoxycholic acid and S-adenosylmethionine in the treatment of intrahepatic cholestasis of pregnancy. *Br J Obstet Gynaecol.* 1998;105:1205-1207.
10. Marchesini G, Bianchi G, Rossi B, et al. Nutritional treatment with branched-chain amino acids in advanced liver cirrhosis. *J Gastroenterol.* 2000;35(suppl):7-12.
11. Lesbre FX, Tigaud JD. Effect of Endotelon® on the capillary fragility index of a specific controlled group: cirrhosis patients [translated from French]. *Gaz Med Fr.* 1983;90:2333-2337.
12. Matsuzaki Y, Tanaka N, Osuga T. Is taurine effective for treatment of painful muscle cramps in liver cirrhosis? [letter]. *Am J Gastroenterol.* 1993;88:1466-1467.
13. Lieber CS, Robins SJ, Li J, et al. Phosphatidylcholine protects against fibrosis and cirrhosis in the baboon. *Gastroenterology.* 1994;106:152-159.
14. Lang I, Nekam K, Gonzalez-Cabello R, et al. Hepatoprotective and immunological effects of antioxidant drugs. *Tokai J Exp Clin Med.* 1990;15:123-127.
15. Lang I, Nekan K, Deak G, et al. Immunomodulatory and hepatoprotective effects of in vivo treatment with free radical scavengers. *Ital J Gastroenterol Hepatol.* 1990; 22:283-287.
16. Lucena MI, Andrade RJ, de la Cruz JP, et al. Effects of silymarin MZ-80 on oxidative stress in patients with alcoholic cirrhosis: results of a randomized, double-blind, placebo-controlled clinical study. *Int J Clin Pharmacol Ther.* 2002;40:2-8.

Colic

1. Lucassen PL, Assendelft WJ, Gubbels JW, et al. Effectiveness of treatments for infantile colic: systematic review. *BMJ.* 1998;316:1563-1569.

2. Weizman Z, Alkrinawi S, Goldfarb D, et al. Efficacy of herbal tea preparation in infantile colic. *J Pediatr.* 1993;122:650-652.

3. Illingworth C, Timmins J. Gripe water: what is it? Why is it given? *Health Visit.* 1990;63:378.

4. Oseas RS, Phelps DL, Kaplan SA. Near fatal hyperkalemia from a dangerous treatment for colic [letter]. *Pediatrics.* 1982;69:117-118.

5. Barr RG, McMullan SJ, Spiess H, et al. Carrying as colic "therapy": a randomized controlled trial. *Pediatrics.* 1991;87:623-630.

6. Parkin PC, Schwartz CJ, Manuel BA. Randomized controlled trial of three interventions in the management of persistent crying of infancy. *Pediatrics.* 1993;92:197-201.

Congestive Heart Failure (CHF)

1. Morisco C, Trimarco B, Condorelli M. Effect of coenzyme Q10 therapy in patients with congestive heart failure: a long-term multicenter randomized study. *Clin Investig.* 1993;71(suppl 8):S134-S136.

2. Hashiba K, Kuramoto K, Ishimi Z, et al. Coenzyme-Q10 [in Japanese]. *Heart (Japanese).* 1972;4:1579-1589.

3. Hofman-Bang C, Rehnqvist N, Swedberg K, et al. Coenzyme Q10 as an adjunctive treatment of congestive heart failure. *J Am Coll Cardiol.* 1992;19:216A.

4. Munkholm H, Hansen HH, Rasmussen K. Coenzyme Q10 treatment in serious heart failure. *Biofactors.* 1999;9:285-289.

5. Khatta M, Alexander BS, Krichten CM, et al. Long-term efficacy of coenzyme Q10 therapy for congestive heart failure. Presented at: 72nd Scientific Sessions of the American Heart Association; November 7-10, 1999; Atlanta, Ga.

6. Leuchtgens VH. Crataegus Special Extract WS 1442 in NYHA II heart failure: a placebo controlled randomized double-blind study [in German; English abstract]. *Fortschr Med.* 1993;111:36-38.

7. Schulz V, Hansel R, Tyler VE. *Rational Phytotherapy: a Physicians' Guide to Herbal Medicine.* 3rd ed. Berlin, Germany: Springer-Verlag; 1998:95-98.

8. Tauchert M, Siegel G, Schulz V. Hawthorn extract as plant medication for the heart; a new evaluation of its therapeutic effectiveness [translated from German]. *MMW Munch Med Wochenschr.* 1994;136(suppl 1):S3-S5.

9. Tauchert M. *Crataegi folium* cum Flore bei Herzinsuffizienz. Cited by: Loew D. *Phytopharmaka: Forschung und Klinische Anwendung.* Darmstadt, Germany: Steinkopff; 1996:37-44.

10. Zapfe jun G. Clinical efficacy of crataegus extract WS1442® in congestive heart failure NYHA class II. *Phytomedicine.* 2001;8:262-266.

11. Caponnetto S, Canale C, Masperone MA, et al. Efficacy of L-propionylcarnitine treatment in patients with left ventricular dysfunction. *Eur Heart J.* 1994;15:1267-1273.

12. Loster H, Miehe K, Punzel M, et al. Prolonged oral L-carnitine substitution increases bicycle ergometer performance in patients with severe, ischemically induced cardiac insufficiency. *Cardiovasc Drugs Ther.* 1999;13:537-546.

13. Mancini M, Rengo F, Lingetti M, et al. Controlled study on the therapeutic efficacy of propionyl-L-carnitine in patients with congestive heart failure. *Arzneimittelforschung.* 1992;42:1101-1104.

14. Pucciarelli G, Mastursi M, Latte S, et al. The clinical and hemodynamic effects of propionyl-L-carnitine in the treatment of congestive heart failure [in Italian; English abstract]. *Clin Ter.* 1992;141:379-384.

15. Cacciatore L, Cerio R, Ciarimboli M, et al. The therapeutic effect of L-carnitine in patients with exercise-induced stable angina: a controlled study. *Drugs Exp Clin Res.* 1991;17:225-235.

16. Azuma J, Sawamura A, Awata N, et al. Double-blind randomized crossover trial of taurine in congestive heart failure. *Curr Ther Res.* 1983;34:543-557.

17. Azuma J, Sawamura A, Awata N, et al. Therapeutic effect of taurine in congestive heart failure: a double-blind crossover trial. *Clin Cardiol.* 1985;8:276-282.

18. Azuma J, Takihara K, Awata N, et al. Taurine and failing heart: experimental and clinical aspects. *Prog Clin Biol Res.* 1985;179:195-213.

19. Azuma J, Hasegawa H, Sawamura A, et al. Therapy of congestive heart failure with orally administered taurine. *Clin Ther.* 1983;5:398-408.
20. Takihara K, Azuma J, Awata N, et al. Beneficial effect of taurine in rabbits with chronic congestive heart failure. *Am Heart J.* 1986;112:1278-1284.
21. Azuma J, Takihara K, Awata N, et al. Beneficial effect of taurine on congestive heart failure induced by chronic aortic regurgitation in rabbits. *Res Commun Chem Pathol Pharmacol.* 1984;45:261-270.
22. Azuma J, Sawamura A, Awata N. Usefulness of taurine in chronic congestive heart failure and its prospective application. *Jpn Circ J.* 1992;56:95-99.
23. Hambrecht R, Hilbrich L, Erbs S, et al. Correction of endothelial dysfunction in chronic heart failure: additional effects of exercise training and oral L-arginine supplementation. *J Am Coll Cardiol.* 2000;35:706-713.
24. Rector TS, Bank AJ, Mullen KA, et al. Randomized, double-blind, placebo-controlled study of supplement oral L-arginine in patients with heart failure. *Circulation.* 1996;93:2135-2141.
25. Watanabe G, Tomiyama H, Doba N. Effects of oral administration of L-arginine on renal function in patients with heart failure. *J Hypertens.* 2000;18:229-234.
26. Gordon A, Hultman E, Kaijser L, et al. Creatine supplementation in chronic heart failure increases skeletal muscle creatine phosphate and muscle performance. *Cardiovasc Res.* 1995;30:413-418.
27. Andrews R, Greenhaff P, Curtis S, et al. The effect of dietary creatine supplementation on skeletal muscle metabolism in congestive heart failure. *Eur Heart J.* 1998; 19:617-622.
28. Brady JA, Rock CL, Horneffer MR. Thiamin status, diuretic medications, and the management of congestive heart failure. *J Am Diet Assoc.* 1995;95:541-544.
29. Shimon I, Almog S, Vered Z, et al. Improved left ventricular function after thiamine supplementation in patients with congestive heart failure receiving long-term furosemide therapy. *Am J Med.* 1995;98:485-490.
30. Keith ME, Jeejeebhoy KN, Langer A, et al. A controlled clinical trial of vitamin E supplementation in patients with congestive heart failure. *Am J Clin Nutr.* 2001;73:219-224.

Crohn's Disease

1. Sturniolo GC, Mestriner C, Lecis PE, et al. Altered plasma and mucosal concentrations of trace elements and antioxidants in active ulcerative colitis. *Scand J Gastroenterol.* 1998;33:644-649.
2. Mortensen PB, Abildgaard K, Fallingborg J. Serum selenium concentration in patients with ulcerative colitis. *Dan Med Bull.* 1989;36:568-570.
3. Dronfield MW, Malone JD, Langman MJ. Zinc in ulcerative colitis: a therapeutic trial and report on plasma levels. *Gut.* 1977;18:33-36.
4. Elsborg L, Larsen L. Folate deficiency in chronic inflammatory bowel disease. *Scand J Gastroenterol.* 1979;14:1019-1024.
5. Krasinski SD, Russell RM, Furie BC, et al. The prevalence of vitamin K deficiency in chronic gastrointestinal disorders. *Am J Clin Nutr.* 1985;41:639-643.
6. Bischoff SC, Herrmann A, Goke M, et al. Altered bone metabolism in inflammatory bowel disease. *Am J Gastroenterol.* 1997;92:1157-1163.
7. Dibble JB, Sheridan P, Losowsky MS. A survey of vitamin D deficiency in gastrointestinal and liver disorders. *Q J Med.* 1984;53:119-134.
8. Mulder TP, van der Sluys Veer A, Verspaget HW, et al. Effect of oral zinc supplementation on metallothionein and superoxide dismutase concentrations in patients with inflammatory bowel disease. *J Gastroenterol Hepatol.* 1994;9:472-477.
9. Harries AD, Brown R, Heatley RV, et al. Vitamin D status in Crohn's disease: association with nutrition and disease activity. *Gut.* 1985;26:1197-1203.
10. Harries AD, Jones LA, Danis V, et al. Controlled trial of supplemented oral nutrition in Crohn's disease. *Lancet.* 1983;1:887-890.
11. Lorenz-Meyer H, Bauer P, Nicolay C, et al. Omega-3 fatty acids and low carbohydrate diet for maintenance of remission in Crohn's disease: a randomized controlled multicenter trial. *Scand J Gastroenterol.* 1996;31:778-785.

12. Lorenz R, Weber PC, Szimnau P, et al. Supplementation with n-3 fatty acids from fish oil in chronic inflammatory bowel disease: a randomized, placebo-controlled, double-blind cross-over trial. *J Intern Med Suppl.* 1989;225:225-232.

13. Belluzzi A, Brignola C, Campieri M, et al. Effect of an enteric-coated fish-oil preparation on relapses in Crohn's disease. *N Engl J Med.* 1996;334:1557-1560.

14. Akobeng AK, Miller V, Stanton J, et al. Double-blind randomized controlled trial of glutamine-enriched polymeric diet in the treatment of active Crohn's disease. *J Pediatr Gastroenterol Nutr.* 2000;30:78-84.

15. Den Hond E, Hiele M, Peeters M, et al. Effect of long-term oral glutamine supplements on small intestinal permeability in patients with Crohn's disease. *JPEN J Parenter Enteral Nutr.* 1999;23:7-11.

16. van der Hulst RR, van Kreel BK, von Meyenfeldt MF, et al. Glutamine and the preservation of gut integrity. *Lancet.* 1993;341:1363-1365.

17. Plein K, Hotz J. Therapeutic effects of *Saccharomyces boulardii* on mild residual symptoms in a stable phase of Crohn's disease with special respect to chronic diarrhea—a pilot study. *Z Gastroenterol.* 1993;31:129-134.

18. Gupta I, Parihar A, Malhotra P, et al. Effects of *Boswellia serrata* gum resin in patients with ulcerative colitis. *Eur J Med Res.* 1997;2:37-43.

19. Gerhardt H, Seifert F, Buvari P, Vogelsang H, Repges R. Therapy of active Crohn disease with Boswellia serrata extract H 15. *Z Gastroenterol.* 2001;39:11-17.

20. Krieglstein CF, Anthoni C, Rijcken EJ, et al. Acetyl-11-keto-beta-boswellic acid, a constituent of a herbal medicine from Boswellia serrata resin, attenuates experimental ileitis. *Int J Colorectal Dis.* 2001;16:88-95.

Cystitis

1. Howell AB, Vorsa N, Der Marderosian A, et al. Inhibition of the adherence of P-fimbriated *Escherichia coli* to uroepithelial-cell surfaces by proanthocyanidin extracts from cranberries [letter]. *N Engl J Med.* 1998;339:1085-1086.

2. Ofek I, Goldhar J, Zafriri D, et al. Anti-*Escherichia coli* adhesin activity of cranberry and blueberry juices [letter]. *N Engl J Med.* 1991;324:1599.

3. Schmidt DR, Sobota AE. An examination of the anti-adherence activity of cranberry juice on urinary and nonurinary bacterial isolates. *Microbios.* 1988;55:173-181.

4. Sobota AE. Inhibition of bacterial adherence by cranberry juice: potential use for the treatment of urinary tract infections. *J Urol.* 1984;131:1013-1016.

5. Zafriri D, Ofek I, Adar R, et al. Inhibitory activity of cranberry juice on adherence of type 1 and type P fimbriated *Escherichia coli* to eucaryotic cells. *Antimicrob Agents Chemother.* 1989;33:92-98.

6. Habash MB, Van der Mei HC, Busscher HJ, et al. The effect of water, ascorbic acid, and cranberry derived supplementation on human urine and uropathogen adhesion to silicone rubber. *Can J Microbiol.* 1999;45:691-694.

7. Schaeffer AJ. Pathogenesis of recurrent urinary tract infection: use of understanding as therapy. *Urology.* 1988;32(suppl):13-15.

8. Stothers L. A randomized placebo controlled trial to evaluate naturopathic cranberry products as prophylaxis against urinary tract infection in women. Presented at: American Urological Association 2001 Annual Meeting; June 2-7, 2001; Anaheim, Calif.

9. Stothers K, Stothers L. A cost effectiveness analysis of naturopathic cranberry products used as prophylaxis against urinary tract infection in women. Presented at: American Urological Association 2001 Annual Meeting; June 2-7, 2001; Anaheim, Calif.

10. Kontiokari T, Sundqvist K, Nuutinen M, et al. Randomised trial of cranberry-lingonberry juice and *Lactobacillus GG* drink for the prevention of urinary tract infections in women. *BMJ.* 2001;322:1-5.

11. Avorn J, Monane M, Gurwitz JH, et al. Reduction of bacteriuria and pyuria after ingestion of cranberry juice. *JAMA.* 1994;271:751-754.

12. Hopkins WJ, Heisey DM, Jonler M, et al. Reduction of bacteriuria and pyuria using cranberry juice [letter]. *JAMA.* 1994;272:588-589.

13. Katz LM. Reduction of bacteriuria and pyuria using cranberry juice [letter]. *JAMA*. 1994;272:589.
14. Schlager TA, Anderson S, Trudell J, et al. Effect of cranberry juice on bacteriuria in children with neurogenic bladder receiving intermittent catheterization. *J Pediatr*. 1999;135:698-702.
15. Larsson B, Jonasson A, Fianu S. Prophylactic effect of UVA-E in women with recurrent cystitis: a preliminary report. *Curr Ther Res*. 1993;53:441-443.
16. Funfstuck R, Struabe E, Schildbach O, et al. Prevention of recurrent urinary tract infection by L-methionine [in German; English abstract]. *Med Klin*. 1997;92:574-581.

Depression (Mild to Moderate)

1. Laakmann G, Schule C, Baghai T, et al. St. John's wort in mild to moderate depression: the relevance of hyperforin for the clinical efficacy. *Pharmacopsychiatry*. 1998;31(suppl 1):54-59.
2. Linde K, Ramirez G, Mulrow CD, et al. St John's wort for depression: an overview and meta-analysis of randomised clinical trials. *BMJ*. 1996;313:253-258.
3. Philipp M, Kohnen R, Hiller KO. Hypericum extract versus imipramine or placebo in patients with moderate depression: randomised multicentre study of treatment for eight weeks. *BMJ*. 1999;319:1534-1539.
4. Schrader E, Meier B, Brattstrom A. Hypericum treatment of mild-moderate depression in a placebo-controlled study: a prospective, double-blind, randomized, placebo-controlled, multicenter study. *Hum Psychopharmacol*. 1998;13:163-169.
5. Shelton RC, Keller MB, Gelenberg A, et al. Effectiveness of St. John's wort in major depression: a randomized controlled trial. *JAMA*. 2001;285:1978-1986.
6. Kalb R, Trautmann-Sponsel RD, Kieser M. Efficacy and tolerability of hypericum extract WS 5572 versus placebo in mildly to moderately depressed patients: a randomized double-blind multicenter clinical trial. *Pharmacopsychiatry*. 2001;34:96-103.
7. Harrer G, Schmidt U, Kuhn U, et al. Comparison of equivalence between the St. John's wort extract LoHyp-57 and fluoxetine. *Arzneimittelforschung*. 1999;49:289-296.
8. Schrader E. Equivalence of St John's wort extract (Ze 117) and fluoxetine: a randomized, controlled study in mild-moderate depression. *Int Clin Psychopharmacol*. 2000;15:61-68.
9. Brenner R, Azbel V, Madhusoodanan S, et al. Comparison of an extract of hypericum (LI 160) and sertraline in the treatment of depression: a double-blind, randomized pilot study. *Clin Ther*. 2000;22:411-419.
10. Woelk H. Comparison of St John's wort and imipramine for treating depression: randomised controlled trial. *BMJ*. 2000;321:536-539.
11. Salmaggi P, Bressa GM, Nicchia G, et al. Double-blind, placebo-controlled study of S-adenosyl-L-methionine in depressed postmenopausal women. *Psychother Psychosom*. 1993;59:34-40.
12. Cerutti R, Sichel MP, Perin M, et al. Psychological distress during puerperium: a novel therapeutic approach using S-adenosylmethionine. *Curr Ther Res*. 1993;53:707-716.
13. Kagan BL, Sultzer DL, Rosenlicht N, et al. Oral S-adenosylmethionine in depression: a randomized, double-blind, placebo-controlled trial. *Am J Psychiatry*. 1990;147:591-595.
14. Fava M, Rosenbaum JF, Birnbaum R, et al. The thyrotropin response to thyrotropin-releasing hormone as a predictor of response to treatment in depressed outpatients. *Acta Psychiatr Scand*. 1992;86:42-45.
15. Delle Chiaie R, Pancheri P. Combined analysis of two controlled, multicentric, double blind studies to assess efficacy and safety of Sulfo-Adenosyl-Methionine (SAMe) vs. placebo (MC1) and imipramine (MC2) in the treatment of major depression [in Italian; English abstract]. *G Ital Psicopatol*. 1999;5:1-16.
16. Delle Chiaie R, Pancheri P, Scapicchio P. MC3: multicentre, controlled efficacy and safety trial of oral S-adenosyl-methionine (SAMe) vs. oral imipramine in the treatment of depression [abstract]. *Int J Neuropsychopharmcol*. 2000;3(suppl 1):S230.

17. Delle Chiaie R, Pancheri P, Scapicchio P. MC4: multicentre, controlled efficacy and safety trial of intramuscular S-adenosyl-methionine (SAMe) vs. oral imipramine in the treatment of depression [abstract]. *Int J Neuropsychopharmcol.* 2000;3(suppl 1):S230.

18. Levine J. Controlled trials of inositol in psychiatry. *Eur Neuropsychopharmacol.* 1997;7:147-155.

19. Benjamin J, Agam G, Levine J, et al. Inositol treatment in psychiatry. *Psychopharmacol Bull.* 1995;31:167-175.

20. Echols JC, Naidoo U, Salzman C. SAMe (S-adenosylmethionine). *Harv Rev Psychiatry.* 2000;8:84-90.

21. Heller B. Pharmacological and clinical effects of D-phenylalanine in depression and Parkinson's disease. In: Mosnaim AD, Wolf ME, eds. *Noncatecholic Phenylethylamines, Part 1.* New York, NY: Marcel Dekker; 1978:397-417.

22. Beckmann H, Athen D, Olteanu M, et al. DL-phenylalanine versus imipramine: a double-blind controlled study. *Arch Psychiatr Nervenkr.* 1979;227:49-58.

23. Beckmann H. Phenylalanine in affective disorders. *Adv Psychiatry.* 1983;10:137-147.

24. Byerley WF, Judd LL, Reimherr FW, et al. 5-hydroxytryptophan: a review of its antidepressant efficacy and adverse effects. *J Clin Psychopharmacol.* 1987;7:127-137.

25. Poldinger W, Calanchini B, Schwarz W. A functional-dimensional approach to depression: serotonin deficiency as a target syndrome in a comparison of 5-hydroxytryptophan and fluvoxamine. *Psychopathology.* 1991;24:53-81.

26. Bella R, Biondi R, Raffaele R, et al. Effect of acetyl-L-carnitine on geriatric patients suffering from dysthymic disorders. *Int J Clin Pharmacol Res.* 1990;10:355-360.

27. Cipolli C, Chiari G. Effects of L-acetylcarnitine on mental deterioration in the aged: initial results [in Italian; English abstract]. *Clin Ter.* 1990;132(suppl 6):479-510.

28. Garzya G, Corallo D, Fiore A, et al. Evaluation of the effects of L-acetylcarnitine on senile patients suffering from depression. *Drugs Exp Clin Res.* 1990;16:101-106.

29. Salvioli G, Neri M. L-acetylcarnitine treatment of mental decline in the elderly. *Drugs Exp Clin Res.* 1994;20:169-176.

30. Schubert H, Halama P. Depressive episode primarily unresponsive to therapy in elderly patients: efficacy of *Ginkgo biloba* extract EGb 761 in combination with antidepressants [translated from German]. *Geriatr Forsch.* 1993;3:45-53.

31. Eckmann F. Cerebral insufficiency: treatment with *Ginkgo-biloba* extract: time of onset of effect in a double-blind study with 60 inpatients [translated from German]. *Fortschr Med.* 1990;108:557-560.

32. Maggioni M, Picotti GB, Bondiolotti GP, et al. Effects of phosphatidylserine therapy in geriatric patients with depressive disorders. *Acta Psychiatr Scand.* 1990;81: 265-270.

33. Levine J, Barak Y, Kofman O, et al. Follow-up and relapse analysis of an inositol study of depression. *Isr J Psychiatry Relat Sci.* 1995;32:14-21.

34. Nemets B, Mishory A, Levine J, et al. Inositol addition does not improve depression in SSRI treatment failures. *J Neural Transm.* 1999;106:795-798.

35. Wolkowitz OM, Reus VI, Keebler A, et al. Double-blind treatment of major depression with dehydroepiandrosterone. *Am J Psychiatry.* 1999;156:646-649.

36. Barrett-Connor E, von Muhlen D, Laughlin GA, et al. Endogenous levels of dehydroepiandrosterone sulfate, but not other sex hormones, are associated with depressed mood in older women: the Rancho Bernardo study. *J Am Geriatr Soc.* 1999; 47:685-691.

37. Passeri M, Cucinotta D, Abate G, et al. Oral 5'-methyltetrahydrofolic acid in senile organic mental disorders with depression: results of a double-blind multicenter study. *Aging (Milano).* 1993;5:63-71.

38. Godfrey PS, Toone BK, Carney MW, et al. Enhancement of recovery from psychiatric illness by methylfolate. *Lancet.* 1990;336:392-395.

39. Heseker H, Kubler W, Pudel V, et al. Psychological disorders as early symptoms of a mild-to-moderate vitamin deficiency. *Ann N Y Acad Sci.* 1992;669:352-357.

40. Crellin R, Bottiglieri T, Reynolds EH. Folates and psychiatric disorders: clinical potential. *Drugs.* 1993;45:623-636.

41. Brattstrom LE, Hultberg BL, Hardebo JE. Folic acid responsive postmenopausal homocysteinemia. *Metabolism.* 1985;34:1073-1077.
42. Botez MI. Folate deficiency and neurological disorders in adults. *Med Hypotheses.* 1976;2:135-140.
43. Coppen A, Swade C, Jones SA, et al. Depression and tetrahydrobiopterin: the folate connection. *J Affect Disord.* 1989;16:103-107.
44. Alpert JE, Fava M. Nutrition and depression: the role of folate. *Nutr Rev.* 1997;55:145-149.
45. Coppen A, Bailey J. Enhancement of the antidepressant action of fluoxetine by folic acid: a randomised, placebo controlled trial. *J Affect Disord.* 2000;60:121-130.
46. Hibbeln JR, Salem N Jr. Dietary polyunsaturated fatty acids and depression: when cholesterol does not satisfy. *Am J Clin Nutr.* 1995;62:1-9.
47. Bell IR, Edman JS, Morrow FD, et al. B complex vitamin patterns in geriatric and young adult inpatients with major depression. *J Am Geriatr Soc.* 1991;39:252-257.
48. Zucker DK, Livingston RL, Nakra R, et al. B12 deficiency and psychiatric disorders: case report and literature review. *Biol Psychiatry.* 1981;16:197-205.
49. Hansgen KS, Vesper J. Antidepressant efficacy of a high-dose Hypericum extract (translated from German). *MMW Munch Med Wochenschr.* 1996;138:29-33.
50. Hypericum Depression Trial Study Group. Effect of Hypericum perforatum (St. John's Wort) in Major Depressive Disorder: a randomized controlled trial. *JAMA.* 2002;287:1807-1814.
51. Randlov C, Thomsen C, Winther K, et al. Effects of hypericum in mild to moderately depressed outpatients: a placebo-controlled clinical trial [abstract]. *Altern Ther Health Med.* 2001;7: 108.
52. Behnke K, Jensen GS, Graubaum HJ, et al. Hypericum perforatum versus fluoxetine in the treatment of mild to moderate depression. *Adv Ther.* 2002;19:43-52.
53. Vorbach EU, Arnoldt KH, Hubner WD. Efficacy and tolerability of St. John's wort extract LI 160 vs. imipramine in patients with severe depressive episodes according to ICD-10. *Pharmacopsychiatry.* 1997;30(suppl 2):81-85.
54. Nemets B, Stahl Z, Belmaker RH. Addition of omega-3 Fatty Acid to maintenance medication treatment for recurrent unipolar depressive disorder. *Am J Psychiatry.* 2002;159:477-479.

Diabetes

1. Ajiboye R, Harding JJ. The non-enzymic glycosylation of bovine lens proteins by glucosamine and its inhibition by aspirin, ibuprofen, and glutathione. *Exp Eye Res.* 1989;49:31-41.
2. Shankar RR, Zhu JS, Baron AD. Glucosamine infusion in rats mimics the beta-cell dysfunction of non-insulin-dependant diabetes mellitus. *Metabolism.* 1998;47:573-577.
3. Patti ME, Virkamaki A, Landaker EJ, et al. Activation of the hexosamine pathway by glucosamine in vivo induces insulin resistance of early postreceptor insulin signaling events in skelatal muscle. *Diabetes.* 1999;48:1562-1571.
4. Virkamaki A, Yki-Jarvinen H. Allosteric regulation of glycogen synthase and hexokinase by glucosamine-6-phosphate during glucosamine-induced insulin resistance in skeletal muscle and heart. *Diabetes.* 1999;48:1101-1107.
5. Almada AL, Harvey PW, Platt KJ. Effect of chronic oral glucosamine sulfate upon fasting insulin resistance index (FIRI) in nondiabetic individuals [abstract]. *FASEB J.* 2000;14:A750.
6. Monauni T, Zenti MG, Cretti A, et al. Effects of glucosamine infusion on insulin secretion and insulin action in humans. *Diabetes.* 2000;49:926-935.
7. Cagnacci A, Arangino S, Renzi A, et al. Influence of melatonin administration on glucose tolerance and insulin sensitivity of postmenopausal women. *Clin Endocrinol (Oxf).* 2001;54:339-346.
8. Anderson RA, Cheng N, Bryden NA, et al. Elevated intakes of supplemental chromium improve glucose and insulin variables in individuals with type 2 diabetes. *Diabetes.* 1997;46:1786-1791.

9. Bahijiri SM, Mira SA, Mufti AM, et al. The effects of inorganic chromium and brewer's yeast supplementation on glucose tolerance, serum lipids, and drug dosage in individuals with type 2 diabetes. *Saudi Med J.* 2000;21:831-837.

10. Rabinowitz MB, Gonick HC, Levin SR, et al. Effects of chromium and yeast supplements on carbohydrate and lipid metabolism in diabetic men. *Diabetes Care.* 1983;6:319-327.

11. Trow LG, Lewis J, Greenwood RH, et al. Lack of effect of dietary chromium supplementation on glucose tolerance, plasma insulin, and lipoprotein levels in patients with type 2 diabetes. *Int J Vitam Nutr Res.* 2000;70:14-18.

12. Jovanovic L, Gutierrez M, Peterson CM. Chromium supplementation for women with gestational diabetes mellitus. *J Trace Elem Med Biol.* 1999;12:91-97.

13. Ravina A, Slezak L, Mirsky N, et al. Control of steroid-induced diabetes with supplemental chromium. *J Trace Elem Exp Med.* 1999;12:375-378.

14. Ravina A, Slezak L, Mirsky N, et al. Reversal of corticosteroid-induced diabetes mellitis with supplemental chromium. *Diabet Med.* 1999;16:164-167.

15. Wilson BE, Gondy A. Effects of chromium supplementation on fasting insulin levels and lipid parameters in healthy, non-obese young subjects. *Diabetes Res Clin Pract.* 1995;28:179-184.

16. Cefalu WT, Bell-Farrow AD, Stegner J, et al. Effect of chromium picolinate on insulin sensitivity in vivo. *J Trace Elem Exp Med.* 1999;12:71-83.

17. Anderson RA, Polansky MM, Bryden NA, et al. Chromium supplementation of human subjects: effects on glucose, insulin and lipid variables. *Metabolism.* 1983; 32:894-899.

18. Sotaniemi EA, Haapakoski E, Rautio A. Ginseng therapy in non-insulin-dependent diabetic patients. *Diabetes Care.* 1995;18:1373-1375.

19. Vuksan V, Sievenpiper JL, Koo VY, et al. American ginseng (*Panax quinquefolius* L) reduces postprandial glycemia in nondiabetic subjects and subjects with type 2 diabetes mellitus. *Arch Intern Med.* 2000;160:1009-1013.

20. Vuksan V, Xu Z, Jenkins AL, et al. American ginseng (*Panax quinquefolium* L.) improves long term glycemic control in type 2 diabetes. Presented at: 60th Scientific Sessions of the American Diabetes Association; June 9-13, 2000; San Antonio, Tex.

21. Vuksan V, Sievenpiper JL, Wong J, et al. American ginseng (*Panax quinquefolius* L.) attenuates postprandial glycemia in a time-dependent but not dose-dependent manner in healthy individuals. *Am J Clin Nutr.* 2001;73:753-758.

22. Matsumoto J. Vanadate, molybdate, and tungstate for orthomolecular medicine. *Med Hypotheses.* 1994;43:177-182.

23. Shamberger RJ. The insulin-like effects of vanadium. *J Adv Med.* 1996;9:121-131.

24. Ramanadham S, Mongold JJ, Brownsey RW, et al. Oral vanadyl sulfate in treatment of diabetes mellitus in rats. *Am J Physiol.* 1989;257:H904-H911.

25. Brichard SM, Okitolonda W, Henquin JC. Long term improvement of glucose homeostasis by vanadate treatment in diabetic rats. *Endocrinology.* 1988;123:2048-2053.

26. Kanthasamy A, Sekar N, Govindasamy S. Vanadate substitutes insulin role in chronic experimental diabetes. *Indian J Exp Biol.* 1988;26:778-780.

27. Shechter Y. Insulin-mimetic effects of vanadate: possible implications for future treatment of diabetes. *Diabetes.* 1990;39:1-5.

28. Challiss RA, Leighton B, Lozeman FJ, et al. Effects of chronic administration of vanadate to the rat on the sensitivity of glycolysis and glycogen synthesis in skeletal muscle to insulin. *Biochem Pharmacol.* 1987;36:357-361.

29. Sakurai H, Tsuchiya K, Nakatsuka M, et al. Insulin-like effect of vanadyl ion on streptozocin-induced diabetic rats. *J Endocrinol.* 1990;126:451-459.

30. Pederson RA, Ramanadham S, Buchan AM, et al. Long-term effects of vanadyl treatment on streptozocin-induced diabetes in rats. *Diabetes.* 1989;38:1390-1395.

31. Myerovitch J, Farfel A, Sack J, et al. Oral administration of vanadate normalizes blood glucose levels in streptozocin-treated rats: characterization and mode of action. *J Biol Chem.* 1987;262:6658-6662.

32. Heylinger CE, Tahiliani AG, McNeill JH. Effect of vanadate on elevated blood glucose and depressed cardiac performance of diabetic rats. *Science.* 1985;227: 1474-1477.
33. Crans DC. Chemistry and insulin-like properties of vanadium (IV) and vanadium (V) compounds. *J Inorg Biochem.* 2000;80:123-131.
34. Boden G, Chen X, Ruiz J, et al. Effects of vanadyl sulfate on carbohydrate and lipid metabolism in patients with non-insulin-dependent diabetes mellitus. *Metabolism.* 1996;45:1130-1135.
35. Cohen N, Halberstam M, Shlimovich P, et al. Oral vanadyl sulfate improves hepatic and peripheral insulin sensitivity in patients with non-insulin-dependent diabetes mellitus. *J Clin Invest.* 1995;95:2501-2509.
36. Goldfine AB, Folli F, Patti ME, et al. Effects of sodium vanadate and in vitro insulin action in diabetes [abstract]. *Clin Res.* 1994;42:116A.
37. Halberstam M, Cohen N, Shlimovich P, et al. Oral vanadyl sulfate improves insulin sensitivity in NIDDM but not in obese nondiabetic subjects. *Diabetes.* 1996;45:659-666.
38. Goldfine AB, Patti ME, Zuberi L, et al. Metabolic effects of vanadyl sulfate in humans with non-insulin-dependent diabetes mellitus: in vivo and in vitro studies. *Metabolism.* 2000;49:400-410.
39. Srivastava AK. Anti-diabetic and toxic effects of vanadium compounds. *Mol Cell Biochem.* 2000;206:177-182.
40. Ziegler D, Gries FA. Alpha-lipoic acid in the treatment of diabetic peripheral and cardiac autonomic neuropathy. *Diabetes.* 1997;46(suppl 2):S62-S66.
41. Ziegler D, Hanefeld M, Ruhnau KJ, et al. Treatment of symptomatic diabetic polyneuropathy with the antioxidant alpha-lipoic acid: a 7-month multicenter randomized controlled trial (ALADIN III Study). ALADIN III Study Group. Alpha-Lipoic Acid in Diabetic Neuropathy. *Diabetes Care.* 1999;22:1296-1301.
42. Kahler W, Kuklinski B, Ruhlmann C, et al. Diabetes mellitus—a free radical-associated disease: results of an adjuvant antioxidant supplementation [in German; English abstract]. *Z Gesamte Inn Med.* 1993;48:223-232.
43. Packer L. Antioxidant properties of lipoic acid and its therapeutic effects in prevention of diabetes complications and cataracts. *Ann N Y Acad Sci.* 1994;738:257-264.
44. Ruhnau KJ, Meissner HP, Finn JR, et al. Effects of 3-week oral treatment with the antioxidant thioctic acid (alpha-lipoic acid) in symptomatic diabetic polyneuropathy. *Diabet Med.* 1999;16:1040-1043.
45. Ziegler D, Hanefeld M, Ruhnau KJ, et al. Treatment of symptomatic diabetic peripheral neuropathy with the anti-oxidant alpha-lipoic acid: a 3-week multicentre randomized controlled trial (ALADIN Study). *Diabetologia.* 1995;38:1425-1433.
46. Keen H, Payan J, Allawi J, et al. Treatment of diabetic neuropathy with gamma-linolenic acid: the gamma-linolenic acid multicenter trial group. *Diabetes Care.* 1993;16:8-15.
47. Jamal GA, Carmichael H. The effect of gamma-linolenic acid on human diabetic peripheral neuropathy: a double-blind placebo-controlled trial. *Diabet Med.* 1990;7:319-323.
48. Manzella D, Barbieri M, Ragno E, et al. Chronic administration of pharmacologic doses of vitamin E improves the cardiac autonomic nervous system in patients with type 2 diabetes. *Am J Clin Nutr.* 2001;73:1052-1057.
49. Elamin A, Tuvemo T. Magnesium and insulin-dependent diabetes mellitus. *Diabetes Res Clin Pract.* 1990;10:203-209.
50. Tosiello L. Hypomagnesemia and diabetes mellitus: a review of clinical implications. *Arch Intern Med.* 1996;156:1143-1148.
51. Zuccaro P, Pacifici R, Pichini S, et al. Influence of antacids on the bioavailability of glibenclamide. *Drugs Exp Clin Res.* 1989;15:165-169.
52. Kivisto KT, Neuvonen PJ. Effect of magnesium hydroxide on the absorption and efficacy of tolbutamide and chlorpropamide. *Eur J Clin Pharmacol.* 1992;42: 675-679.
53. Schmidt LE, Arfken CL, Heins JM. Evaluation of nutrient intake in subjects with non-insulin-dependent diabetes mellitus. *J Am Diet Assoc.* 1994;94:773-774.

54. Blostein-Fujii A, DeSilvestro RA, Frid D, et al. Short-term zinc supplementation in women with non-insulin-dependent diabetes mellitus: effects on plasma 5'- nucleotidase activities, insulin-like growth factor I concentrations, and lipoprotein oxidation rates in vitro. *Am J Clin Nutr.* 1997;66:639-642.

55. Sjogren A, Floren CH, Nilsson A. Magnesium, potassium, and zinc deficiency in subjects with type II diabetes mellitus. *Acta Med Scand.* 1988;224:461-465.

56. Cunningham JJ, Ellis SL, McVeigh KL, et al. Reduced mononuclear leukocyte ascorbic acid content in adults with insulin-dependent diabetes mellitus consuming adequate dietary vitamin C. *Metabolism.* 1991;40:146-149.

57. Sinclair AJ, Taylor PB, Lunec J, et al. Low plasma ascorbate levels in patients with type 2 diabetes mellitus consuming adequate dietary vitamin C. *Diabet Med.* 1994; 11:893-898.

58. Will JC, Byers T. Does diabetes mellitus increase the requirement for vitamin C? *Nutr Rev.* 1996;54:193-202.

59. Franconi F, Bennardini F, Mattana A, et al. Plasma and platelet taurine are reduced in subjects with insulin-dependent diabetes mellitus: effects of taurine supplementation. *Am J Clin Nutr.* 1995;61:1115-1119.

60. Kosenko LG. The content of some trace elements in the blood of patients suffering from diabetes mellitus [in Russian; English abstract]. *Klin Med (Mosk).* 1964; 42:113-116.

61. Bauman WA, Shaw S, Jayatilleke E, et al. Increased intake of calcium reverses vitamin B_{12} malabsorption induced by metformin. *Diabetes Care.* 2000;23:1227-1231.

62. Elliott RB, Pilcher CC, Fergusson DM, et al. A population based strategy to prevent insulin-dependent diabetes using nicotinamide. *J Pediatr Endocrinol Metab.* 1996;9:501-509.

63. Pozzilli P, Visalli N, Signore A, et al. Double blind trial of nicotinamide in recent-onset IDDM (the IMDIAB III study). *Diabetologia.* 1995;38:848-852.

64. Lampeter EF, Klinghammer A, Scherbaum WA, et al. The Deutsche Nicotinamide Intervention Study: an attempt to prevent type 1 diabetes. *Diabetes.* 1998;47:980-984.

65. Ludvigsson J, Samuelsson U, Johansson C, et al. Treatment with antioxidants at onset of type 1 diabetes in children: a randomized, double-blind placebo-controlled study. *Diabetes Metab Res Rev.* 2001;17:131-136.

66. Baskaran K, Kizar Ahamath B, Radha Shanmugasundaram K, et al. Antidiabetic effect of a leaf extract from *Gymnema sylvestre* in non-insulin-dependent diabetes mellitus patients. *J Ethnopharmacol.* 1990;30:295-305.

67. Baskaran K, Kizar Ahamath B, Radha Shanmugasundaram K, et al. Antidiabetic effect of a leaf extract from *Gymnema sylvestre* in non-insulin-dependent diabetes mellitus patients. *J Ethnopharmacol.* 1990;30:295-305.

68. Indian Council of Medical Research (ICMR). Flexible dose open trial of Vijayasar in cases of newly-diagnosed non-insulin-dependent diabetes mellitus. *Indian J Med Res.* 1998;108:24-29.

69. Bunyapraphatsara N, Yongchaiyudha S, Rungpitarangsi V, et al. Antidiabetic activity of *Aloe vera* L, juice II: clinical trial in diabetes mellitus patients in combination with glibenclamide. *Phytomedicine.* 1996;3:245-248.

70. Yongchaiyudha S, Rungpitarangsi V, Bunyapraphatsara N, et al. Antidiabetic activity of *Aloe vera* L. juice, I: clinical trial in new cases of diabetes mellitus. *Phytomedicine.* 1996;3:241-243.

71. Vogler BK, Ernst E. Aloe vera: a systematic review of its clinical effectiveness. *Br J Gen Pract.* 1999;49:823-828.

72. Roman-Ramos R, Flores-Saenz JL, Partida-Hernandez G, et al. Experimental study of the hypoglycemic effect of some antidiabetic plants. *Arch Invest Med (Mex).* 1991;22:87-93.

73. Ajabnoor MA. Effect of aloes on blood glucose levels in normal and alloxan diabetic mice. *J Ethnopharmacol.* 1990;28:215-220.

74. Ghannam N, Kingston M, Al-Meshaal IA, et al. The antidiabetic activity of aloes: preliminary clinical and experimental observations. *Horm Res.* 1986;24:288-294.

75. Sharma RD, Sarkar A, Hazra DK, et al. Use of fenugreek seed powder in the management of non-insulin dependent diabetes mellitus. *Nutr Res.* 1996;16:1331-1339.

76. Madar Z, Abel R, Samish S, et al. Glucose-lowering effect of fenugreek in non-insulin dependent diabetics. *Eur J Clin Nutr.* 1988;42:51-54.

77. Sharma RD, Raghuram TC, Rao NS. Effect of fenugreek seeds on blood glucose and serum lipids in type I diabetes. *Eur J Clin Nutr.* 1990;44:301-306.

78. Subramaniam A, Stocker C, Sennitt MV, et al. Guggul lipid reduces insulin resistance and body weight gain in C57B1/6 lep/lep mice [abstract]. *Int J Obes Relat Metab Disord.* 2001;25(suppl 2):S24.

79. Yaniv Z, Dafni A, Friedman J, et al. Plants used for the treatment of diabetes in Israel. *J Ethnopharmacol.* 1987;19:145-151.

80. Teixeira CC, Pinto LP, Kessler FHP, et al. The effect of *Syzygium cumini* (L.) skeels on post-prandial blood glucose levels in non-diabetic rats and rats with streptozotocin-induced diabetes mellitus. *J Ethnopharmacol.* 1997;56:209-213.

81. Bever BO, Zahnd GR. Plants with oral hypoglycaemic action. *Q J Crude Drug Res.* 1979;17:139-196.

82. Mathew PT, Augusti KT. Hypoglycaemic effects of onion, *Allium cepa* Linn. on diabetes mellitus: a preliminary report. *Indian J Physiol Pharmacol.* 1975;19:213-217.

83. Manickam M, Ramanathan M, Jahromi MAF, et al. Antihyperglycemic activity of phenolics from *Pterocarpus marsupium*. *J Nat Prod.* 1997;60:609-610.

84. Ahmad F, Khalid P, Khan MM, et al. Insulin-like activity in (−) epicatechin. *Acta Diabetol.* 1989;26:291-300.

85. Stern E. Successful use of *Atriplex halimus* in the treatment of type II diabetic patients: a preliminary study. Unpublished study conducted at the Zamenhoff Medical Center, Tel Aviv, Israel, 1989.

86. Earon G, Stern E, Lavosky H. Successful use of *Atriplex hamilus* in the treatment of type 2 diabetic patients: controlled clinical research report on the subject of *Atriplex*. Unpublished study conducted at the Hebrew University, Jerusalem, 1989.

87. Azad Khan AK, Akhtar S, Mahtab H. Treatment of diabetes mellitus with *Coccinia indica*. *Br Med J.* 1980;280:1044.

88. Welihinda J, Karunanayake EH, Sheriff MH, et al. Effect of *Momordica charantia* on the glucose tolerance in maturity onset diabetes. *J Ethnopharmacol.* 1986;17:277-282.

89. Akhtar MS. Trial of *Momordica charantia* Linn (Karela) powder in patients with maturity-onset diabetes. *J Pak Med Assoc.* 1982;32:106-107.

90. Leatherdale BA, Panesar RK, Singh G, et al. Improvement in glucose tolerance due to *Momordica charantia* (karela). *Br Med J.* 1981;282:1823-1824.

91. Cignarella A, Nastasi M, Cavalli E, et al. Novel lipid-lowering properties of *Vaccinium myrtillus* L. leaves, a traditional antidiabetic treatment, in several models of rat dyslipidaemia: a comparison with ciprofibrate. *Thromb Res.* 1996;84:311-322.

92. Adler JH, Lazarovici G, Marton M, et al. The diabetic response of weanling sand rats (*Psammomys obesus*) to diets containing different concentrations of salt bush (*Atriplex halimus*). *Diabetes Res.* 1986;3:169-171.

93. Aharonson Z, Shani J, Sulman FG. Hypoglycemic effect of the salt bush (*Atriplex halimus*)—a feeding source of the sand rat (*Psammomys obesus*). *Diabetologia.* 1969;5:379-383.

94. Shani J, Ahronson Z, Sulman FG, et al. Insulin-potentiating effect of salt bush (*Atriplex halimus*) ashes. *Isr J Med Sci.* 1972;8:757-758.

95. Chattopadhyay RR. Hypoglycemic effect of *Ocimum sanctum* leaf extract in normal and streptozotocin diabetic rats. *Indian J Exp Biol.* 1993;31:891-893.

96. Agrawal P, Rai V, Singh RB. Randomized placebo-controlled, single blind trial of holy basil leaves in patients with noninsulin-dependent diabetes mellitus. *Int J Clin Pharmacol Ther.* 1996;34:406-409.

97. Frati AC, Gordillo BE, Altamirano P, et al. Influence of nopal intake upon fasting glycemia in type II diabetics and healthy subjects. *Arch Invest Med (Mex).* 1991;22:51-56.

98. Frati-Munari AC, Del Valle-Martinez LM, Ariza-Andraca CR, et al. Hypoglycemic action of different doses of nopal (*Opuntia streptacantha* Lemaire) in patients with type II diabetes mellitus [in Spanish; English abstract]. *Arch Invest Med (Mex).* 1989;20:197-201.

99. Frati-Munari AC, Gordillo BE, Altamirano P, et al. Hypoglycemic effect of *Opuntia streptacantha* Lemaire in NIDDM. *Diabetes Care.* 1988;11:63-66.

100. Frati-Munari AC, Fernandez-Harp JA, de la Riva H, et al. Effects of nopal (*Opuntia* sp.) on serum lipids, glycemia, and body weight. *Arch Invest Med (Mex).* 1983;14:117-125.

101. Frati-Munari AC, de Leon C, Ariza-Andraca R, et al. Effect of a dehydrated extract of nopal (*Opuntia ficus indica* Mill.) on blood glucose [in Spanish; English abstract]. *Arch Invest Med (Mex).* 1989;20:211-216.

102. Frati Munari AC, Quiroz Lazaro JL, Altamirano Bustamante P, et al. The effect of various doses of nopal (*Opuntia streptacantha* Lemaire) on the glucose tolerance test in healthy individuals [in Spanish; English abstract]. *Arch Invest Med (Mex).* 1988;19:143-148.

103. Belury MA, Mahon A, Shi L. Role of conjugated linoleic acid (CLA) in the management of type 2 diabetes: evidence from Zucker diabetic (fa/fa) rats and human subjects. Presented at: 220th ACS National Meeting; August 20-24, 2000; Washington, DC. Abstract AGFD 26.

104. Vuksan V, Jenkins DJ, Spadafora P, et al. Konjac-mannan (glucomannan) improves glycemia and other associated risk factors for coronary heart disease in type 2 diabetes: a randomized controlled metabolic trial. *Diabetes Care.* 1999;22:913-919.

105. Doi K. Effect of konjac fibre (glucomannan) on glucose and lipids. *Eur J Clin Nutr.* 1995;(suppl 3):190-197.

106. Jayasooriya AP, Sakono M, Yukizaki C, et al. Effects of *Momordica charantia* powder on serum glucose levels and various lipid parameters in rats fed with cholesterol-free and cholesterol-enriched diets. *J Ethnopharmacol.* 2000;72:331-336.

107. Piatti PM, Monti LD, Valsecchi G, et al. Long-term oral L-arginine administration improves peripheral and hepatic insulin sensitivity in type 2 diabetic patients. *Diabetes Care.* 2001;24:875-880.

108. Gupta R, Garg VK, Mathur DK, et al. Oral zinc therapy in diabetic neuropathy. *J Assoc Physicians India.* 1998;46:939-942.

109. Alarcon-Aguilara FJ, Roman-Ramos R, Perez-Gutierrez S, et al. Study of the anti-hyperglycemic effect of plants used as antidiabetics. *J Ethnopharmacol.* 1998;61:101-110.

110. Chattopadhyay RR. A comparative evaluation of some blood sugar lowering agents of plant origin. *J Ethnopharmacol.* 1999;67:367-372.

111. Pari L, Maheswari JU. Hypoglycemic effect of *Musa sapientum* L. in alloxan-induced diabetic rats. *J Ethnopharmacol.* 1999;68:321-325.

112. Roman Ramos R, Lara Lemus A, Alarcon Aguilar F, et al. Hypoglycemic activity of some antidiabetic plants. *Arch Med Res.* 1992;23:105-109.

113. Khosla P, Bhanwra S, Singh J, et al. A study of hypoglycaemic effects of *Azadirachta indica* (Neem) in normal and alloxan diabetic rabbits. *Indian J Physiol Pharmacol.* 2000;44:69-74.

114. Roman-Ramos R, Flores-Saenz JL, Alarcon-Aguilar FJ. Anti-hyperglycemic effect of some edible plants. *J Ethnopharmacol.* 1995;48:25-32.

115. Malinow MR, McLaughlin P, Stafford C. Alfalfa seeds: effects on cholesterol metabolism. *Experientia.* 1980;36:562-564.

116. Swanston-Flatt SK, Day C, Bailey CJ, et al. Traditional plant treatments for diabetes: studies in normal and streptozotocin diabetic mice. *Diabetologia.* 1990;33:462-464.

117. Ichiki H, Miura T, Kubo M, et al. New antidiabetic compounds, mangiferin and its glucoside. *Biol Pharm Bull.* 1998;21:1389-1390.

118. Turpeinen AK, Kuikka JT, Vanninen E, et al. Long-term effect of acetyl-L-carnitine on myocardial 123I-MIBG uptake in patients with diabetes. *Clin Auton Res.* 2000;10:13-16

119. Mingrone G, Greco AV, Capristo E, et al. L-carnitine improves glucose disposal in type 2 diabetic patients. *J Am Coll Nutr.* 1999;18:77-82.
120. Montori VM, Farmer A, Wollan PC, et al. Fish oil supplementation in type 2 diabetes: a quantitative systematic review. *Diabetes Care.* 2000;23:1407-1415.
121. Elam MB, Hunninghake DB, Davis KB, et al. Effect of niacin on lipid and lipoprotein levels and glycemic control in patients with diabetes and peripheral arterial disease. The ADMIT Study: a randomized trial. *JAMA.* 2000;284:1263-1270.
122. Hypponen E, Laara E, Reunanen A, et al. Intake of vitamin D and risk of type I diabetes: a birth-cohort study. *Lancet.* 2001;358:1500-1503.
123. The EURODIAB Substudy 2 Study Group. Vitamin D supplement in early childhood and risk for Type I (insulin-dependent) diabetes mellitus. *Diabetologia.* 1999;42:51-54.
124. Stene LC, Ulriksen J, Magnus P, et al. Use of cod liver oil during pregnancy associated with lower risk of Type I diabetes in the offspring. *Diabetologia.* 2000;43:1093-1098.
125. Konno S. Maitake SX-fraction: possible hypoglycemic effect on diabetes mellitus. *Altern Comp Ther.* 2001;7:366-370.
126. Gaede P, Poulsen HE, Parving HH, et al. Double-blind randomised study of the effect of combined treatment with vitamin C and E on albuminuria in Type 2 diabetic patients. *Diabet Med.* 2001;18 756-760.

Dysmenorrhea

1. Harel Z, Biro FM, Kottenhahn RK, et al. Supplementation with omega-3 polyunsaturated fatty acids in the management of dysmenorrhea in adolescents. *Am J Obstet Gynecol.* 1996;174:1335-1338.
2. Deutch B, Jorgensen EB, Hansen JC. Menstrual discomfort in Danish women reduced by dietary supplements of omega-3 PUFA and B12 (fish oil or seal oil capsules). *Nutr Res.* 2000;20:621-631.
3. Seifert B, Wagler P, Dartsch S, et al. Magnesium: an alternative in treatment of primary dysmenorrhoea [translated from German]. *Zentralbl Gynakol.* 1989;111:755-760.
4. Fontana-Klaiber H, Hogg B. Therapeutic effects of magnesium in dysmenorrhea [in German; English abstract]. *Schweiz Rundsch Med Prax.* 1990;79:491-494.
5. Ziaei S, Faghihzadeh S, Sohrabvand F, et al. A randomized placebo-controlled trial to determine the effect of vitamin E in treatment of primary dysmenorrhoea. *BJOG.* 2001;108:1181-1183.

Dyspepsia

1. Mearin F, Balboa A, Zarate N, et al. Placebo in functional dyspepsia: symptomatic, gastrointestinal motor, and gastric sensorial responses. *Am J Gastroenterol.* 1999;94:116-125.
2. Rasyid A, Lelo A. The effect of curcumin and placebo on human gall-bladder function: an ultrasound study. *Aliment Pharmacol Ther.* 1999;13:245-249.
3. Ammon HP, Wahl MA. Pharmacology of *Curcuma longa. Planta Med.* 1991;57:1-7.
4. Thamlikitkul V, Bunyapraphatsara N, Dechatiwongse T, et al. Randomized double blind study of *Curcuma domestica* Val. for dyspepsia. *J Med Assoc Thai.* 1989;72:613-620.
5. Kupke D, von Sanden H, Trinczek-Gartner H, et al. An evaluation of the choleretic activity of a plant-based cholagogue [translated from German]. *Z Allgemeinmed.* 1991;67:1046-1058.
6. Niederau C, Gopfert E. The effect of chelidonium and turmeric root extract on upper abdominal pain due to functional disorders of the biliary system: results from a placebo-controlled double-blind study [translated from German]. *Med Klin.* 1999;94:425-430.
7. Greving I, Meister V, Monnerjahn C, et al. *Chelidonium majus:* a rare reason for severe hepatotoxic reaction. *Pharmacoepidemiol Drug Safety.* 1998;7:S66-S69.
8. Benninger J, Schneider HT, Schuppan, et al. Acute hepatitis induced by greater celandine (*Chelidonium majus*). *Gastroenterology.* 1999;117:1234-1237.

9. Strahl S, Ehret V, Dahm H, et al. Necrotizing hepatitis after taking herbal remedies [translated from German]. *Dtsch Med Wochenschr.* 1998;123:1410-1414.
10. May B, Kuntz H-D, Kieser M, et al. Efficacy of a fixed peppermint oil/caraway oil combination in non-ulcer dyspepsia. *Arzneimittelforschung.* 1996;46:1149-1153.
11. Madisch A, Heydenreich CJ, Wieland V, et al. Treatment of functional dyspepsia with a fixed peppermint oil and caraway oil combination preparation as compared to cisapride: a multicenter, reference-controlled double-blind equivalence study. *Arzneimittelforschung.* 1999;49:925-932.
12. Westphal J, Horning M, Leonhardt K. Phytotherapy in functional upper abdominal complaints. Results of a clinical study with a preparation of several plants. *Phytomedicine.* 1996;2:285-291.
13. Kleveland PM, Johannessen T, Kristensen P, et al. Effect of pancreatic enzymes in non-ulcer dyspepsia: a pilot study. *Scand J Gastroenterol.* 1990;25:298-301.
14. Arora A, Sharma MP. Use of banana in non-ulcer dyspepsia. *Lancet.* 1990;335: 612-613.
15. Rodriguez-Stanley S, Collings KL, Robinson M, et al. The effects of capsaicin on reflux, gastric emptying, and dyspepsia. *Aliment Pharmacol Ther.* 2000;14:129-134.

Easy Bruising

1. Galley P, Thiollet M. A double-blind, placebo-controlled trial of a new veno-active flavonoid fraction (S 5682) in the treatment of symptomatic capillary fragility. *Int Angiol.* 1993;12:69-72.
2. Miller MJ. Injuries to athletes: evaluation of ascorbic acid and water soluble citrus bioflavonoids in the prophylaxis of injuries in athletes. *Med Times.* 1960;88:313-316.
3. Schorah CJ, Tormey WP, Brooks GH, et al. The effect of vitamin C supplements on body weight, serum proteins, and general health of an elderly population. *Am J Clin Nutr.* 1981;34:871-876.

Eczema

1. Kalliomaki M, Salminen S, Arvilommi H, et al. Probiotics in primary prevention of atopic disease: a randomized placebo-controlled trial. *Lancet.* 2001;357:1076-1079.
2. Isolauri E. Probiotics in human disease. *Am J Clin Nutr.* 2001;73(suppl):1142S-1146S.
3. Majamaa H, Isolauri E. Probiotics: a novel approach in the management of food allergy. *J Allergy Clin Immunol.* 1997;99:179-185.
4. Patzelt-Wenczler R, Ponce-Poschl E. Proof of efficacy of Kamillosan® cream in atopic eczema. *Eur J Med Res.* 2000;5:171-175.
5. Aertgeerts P, Albring M, Klaschka F, et al. Comparison of Kamillosan cream (2 g ethanolic extract from chamomile flowers in 100 g cream) versus steroid (0.25% hydrocortisone, 0.75% fluocortin butyl ester) and non-steroid (5% bufexamac) external agents in the maintenance therapy of eczema [translated from German]. *Z Hautkr.* 1985;60:270-277.
6. Morse PF, Horrobin DF, Manku MS, et al. Meta-analysis of placebo-controlled studies of the efficacy of Epogam in the treatment of atopic eczema. Relationship between plasma essential fatty acid changes and clinical response. *Br J Dermatol.* 1989;121:75-90.
7. Berth-Jones J, Graham-Brown RA. Placebo-controlled trial of essential fatty acid supplementation in atopic dermatitis. *Lancet.* 1993;341:1557-1560.
8. Hederos CA, Berg A. Epogam evening primrose oil treatment in atopic dermatitis and asthma. *Arch Dis Child.* 1996;75:494-497.
9. Henz BM, Jablonska S, van de Kerkhof PC, et al. Double-blind, multicentre analysis of the efficacy of borage oil in patients with atopic eczema. *Br J Dermatol.* 1999;140:685-688.
10. Biagi PL, Bordoni A, Hrelia S, et al. The effect of gamma-linolenic acid on clinical status, red cell fatty acid composition, and membrane microviscosity in infants with atopic dermatitis. *Drugs Exp Clin Res.* 1994;20:77-84.
11. Stander S, Luger T, Metze D. Treatment of prurigo nodularis with topical capsaicin. *J Am Acad Dermatol.* 2001;44:471-478.

12. Fung AY, Look PC, Chong LY, et al. A controlled trial of traditional Chinese herbal medicine in Chinese patients with recalcitrant atopic dermatitis. *Int J Dermatol.* 1999;38:387-392.
13. Kramer MS, Chalmers B, Hodnett E, et al. Promotion of breastfeeding intervention trial (PROBIT). *JAMA.* 2001;285:413-420.
14. Niggemann B, Binder C, Dupont C, et al. Prospective, controlled, multi-center study on the effect of an amino-acid-based formula in infants with cow's milk allergy/intolerance and atopic dermatitis. *Pediatr Allergy Immunol.* 2001;12:78-82.
15. Mabin DC, Hollis S, Lockwood J, et al. Pyridoxine in atopic dermatitis. *Br J Dermatol.* 1995;133:764-767.
16. Ewing CI, Gibbs AC, Ashcroft C, et al. Failure of oral zinc supplementation in atopic eczema. *Eur J Clin Nutr.* 1991;45:507-510.

Erectile Dysfunction

1. Armanini D, Palermo M. Reduction of serum testosterone in men by licorice [letter]. *N Engl J Med.* 1999;341:1158.
2. Reiter WJ, Pycha A, Schatzl G, et al. Dehydroepiandrosterone in the treatment of erectile dysfunction: a prospective double-blind, randomized, placebo-controlled study. *Urology.* 1999;53:590-595.
3. Chen J, Wollman Y, Chernichovsky T, et al. Effect of oral administration of high-dose nitric oxide donor L-arginine in men with organic erectile dysfunction: results of a double-blind, randomized placebo-controlled study. *BJU Int.* 1999;83:269-273.
4. Riley AJ. Yohimbine in the treatment of erectile disorder. *Br J Clin Pract.* 1994;48:133-136.
5. Cohen AJ, Bartlik B. Ginkgo biloba for antidepressant-induced sexual dysfunction. *J Sex Marital Ther.* 1998;24:139-143.
6. McCann B. Botanical could improve sex lives of patients on SSRIs. *Drug Topics.* 1997;141:33.
7. Cohen A. Treatment of antidepressant-induced sexual dysfunction with *Ginkgo biloba* extract. Presented at: 149th Annual Meeting of the American Psychiatric Association; May 5-8, 1996; New York, N.Y. Abstract #716.
8. Cohen A, Bartlik B. Treatment of sexual dysfunction with *Ginkgo biloba* extract [scientific reports]. Presented at: 150th Annual Meeting of the American Psychiatric Association; May 18-21, 1997; San Diego, Calif.
9. Cohen A. Long term safety and efficacy of *Ginkgo biloba* extract in the treatment of anti-depressant-induced sexual dysfunction (1997). Priory Lodge Education web site. Available at: http://www.priory.com/pharmol/gingko.htm. Accessed: July 1, 1997. (Please note variant spelling of "gingko.")
10. Sikora R, Sohn M, Deutz FJ, et al. *Ginkgo biloba* extract in the therapy of erectile dysfunction [abstract]. *J Urol.* 1989;142:188A.
11. Klotz T, Mathers MJ, Braun M, et al. Effectiveness of oral L-arginine in first-line treatment of erectile dysfunction in a controlled crossover study. *Urol Int.* 1999;63(4):220-223.
12. Moody JA, Vernet D, Laidlaw S, et al. Effects of long-term administration of L-arginine on the rat erectile response. *J Urol.* 1997;158:942-947.
13. Ashton AK, Ahrens K, Gupta S, et al. Antidepressant-induced sexual dysfunction and *Ginkgo biloba* [letter]. *Am J Psychiatry.* 2000;157:836-837.
14. Choi HK, et al. Clinical efficacy of Korean red ginseng for erectile dysfunction. *Int. J Impotence Res.* 1995;7:181-186.

Fibromyalgia

1. Tavoni A, Vitali C, Bombardieri S, et al. Evaluation of S-adenosylmethionine in primary fibromyalgia: a double-blind crossover study. *Am J Med.* 1987;83(5A):107-110.
2. Tavoni A, Jeracitano G, Cirigliano G. Evaluation of S-adenosylmethionine in secondary fibromyalgia: a double-blind study [letter]. *Clin Exp Rheumatol.* 1998;16:106-107.

3. Jacobsen S, Danneskiold-Samsoe B, Andersen RB. Oral S-adenosylmethionine in primary fibromyalgia: double-blind clinical evaluation. *Scand J Rheumatol.* 1991;20: 294-302.
4. Volkmann H, Norregaard J, Jacobsen S, et al. Double-blind, placebo-controlled cross-over study of intravenous S-adenosyl-L-methionine in patients with fibromyalgia. *Scand J Rheumatol.* 1997;26:206-211.
5. Caruso I, Sarzi Puttini P, Cazzola M, et al. Double-blind study of 5-hydroxytryptophan versus placebo in the treatment of primary fibromyalgia syndrome. *J Int Med Res.* 1990;18:201-209.
6. McCarty DJ, Csuka M, McCarthy G, et al. Treatment of pain due to fibromyalgia with topical capsaicin: a pilot study. *Semin Arthritis Rheum.* 1994;23(suppl 3):41-47.
7. Merchant RE, Andre CA. A review of recent clinical trials of the nutritional supplement *Chlorella pyrenoidosa* in the treatment of fibromyalgia, hypertension, and ulcerative colitis. *Altern Ther Health Med.* 2001;7:79-80, 82-91.
8. Russell IJ, Michalek JE, Flechas JD, et al. Treatment of fibromyalgia syndrome with Super Malic: a randomized, double blind, placebo controlled, crossover pilot study. *J Rheumatol.* 1995;22:953-958.

Gout

1. Lewis AS, Murphy L, McCalla C, et al. Inhibition of mammalian xanthine oxidase by folate compounds and amethopterin. *J Biol Chem.* 1984;259:12-15.
2. Flouvier B, Devulder B. Folic acid, xanthine oxidase, and uric acid [letter]. *Ann Intern Med.* 1978;88:269.
3. Boss GR, Ragsdale RA, Zettner A, et al. Failure of folic acid (pteroylglutamic acid) to affect hyperuricemia. *J Lab Clin Med.* 1980;96:783-789.
4. European Scientific Cooperative on Phytotherapy. *Harpagophyti radix.* Exeter, UK: ESCOP; 1996-1997. Monographs on the Medicinal Uses of Plant Drugs, Fascicule 2:4.
5. Murray MT, Pizzorno JE. *Encyclopedia of Natural Medicine.* 2nd ed. Rocklin, Calif: Prima Publishing; 1998:493-494.
6. Blau LW. Cherry diet control for gout and arthritis. *Tex Rep Biol Med.* 1950;8: 309-311.

Hemorrhoids

1. Godeberge P. Daflon 500 mg in the treatment of hemorrhoidal disease: a demonstrated efficacy in comparison with placebo. *Angiology.* 1994;45:574-578.
2. Cospite M. Double-blind, placebo-controlled evaluation of clinical activity and safety of Daflon 500 mg in the treatment of acute hemorrhoids. *Angiology.* 1994; 45:566-573.
3. Misra MC, Parshad R. Randomized clinical trial of micronized flavonoids in the early control of bleeding from acute internal haemorrhoids. *Br J Surg.* 2000;87:868-872.
4. Ho YH, Tan M, Seow-Choen F. Micronized purified flavonidic fraction compared favorably with rubber band ligation and fiber alone in the management of bleeding hemorrhoids: randomized controlled trial. *Dis Colon Rectum.* 2000;43:66-69.
5. Thanapongsathorn W, Vajrabukka T. Clinical trial of oral diosmin (Daflon®) in the treatment of hemorrhoids. *Dis Colon Rectum.* 1992;35:1085-1088.
6. Wijayanegara H, Mose JC, Achmad L, et al. A clinical trial of hydroxyethylrutosides in the treatment of haemorrhoids of pregnancy. *J Int Med Res.* 1992;20:54-60.
7. Wadworth AN, Faulds D. Hydroxyethylrutosides: a review of its pharmacology and therapeutic efficacy in venous insufficiency and related disorders. *Drugs.* 1992; 44:1013-1032.
8. Saggioro A, Chiozzini G, Pallini P, et al. Treatment of hemorrhoidal crisis with mesoglycan sulfate [in Italian; English abstract]. *Minerva Dietol Gastroenterol.* 1985;31:311-315.
9. Saggioro A, Chiozzini G. Mesoglycan sulfate in acute hemorrhoidal pathology [in Italian]. *Minerva Med.* 1986;77:1909.

Hepatitis (Viral)

1. Berenguer J, Carrasco D. Double-blind trial of silymarin vs. placebo in the treatment of chronic hepatitis. *MMW Munch Med Wochenschr.* 1977;119:240-260.
2. Buzzelli G, Moscarella S, Giusti A, et al. A pilot study on the liver protective effect of silybinphosphatidylcholine complex (IdB1016) in chronic active hepatitis. *Int J Clin Pharmacol Ther Toxicol.* 1993;31:456-460.
3. Lirussi F, Okolicsanyi L. Cytoprotection in the nineties: experience with ursodeoxycholic acid and silymarin in chronic liver disease. *Acta Physiol Hung.* 1992;80:363-367.
4. Magliulo E, Gagliardi B, Fiori GP. Results of a double blind study on the effect of silymarin in the treatment of acute viral hepatitis, carried out at two medical centers [translated from German]. *Med Klin.* 1978;73:1060-1065.
5. Bode JC, Schmidt U, Durr HK. Silymarin for the treatment of acute viral hepatitis? Report of a controlled trial [translated from German]. *Med Klin.* 1977;72:513-518.
6. Matsuyama Y, Morita T, Higuchi M, et al. The effect of taurine administration on patients with acute hepatitis. *Prog Clin Biol Res.* 1983;125:461-468.
7. Podda M, Ghezzi C, Battezzati PM, et al. Effects of ursodeoxycholic acid and taurine on serum liver enzymes and bile acids in chronic hepatitis. *Gastroenterology.* 1990;98:1044-1050.
8. Berk L, de Man RA, Schalm SW, et al. Beneficial effects of *Phyllanthus amarus* for chronic hepatitis B, not confirmed. *J Hepatol.* 1991;12:405-406.
9. Arase Y, Ikeda K, Murashima N, et al. The long term efficacy of glycyrrhizin in chronic hepatitis C patients. *Cancer.* 1997;79:1494-1500.
10. Liu JP, McIntosh H, Lin H. Chinese medicinal herbs for chronic hepatitis B (Cochrane Review). *Cochrane Database Syst Rev.* 2001;(1):1-27, +7 tables.
11. Civeira MP, Castilla A, Morte S, et al. A pilot study of thymus extract in chronic non-A, non-B hepatitis. *Aliment Pharmacol Ther.* 1989;3:395-401.
12. Bortolotti F, Cadrobbi P, Crivellaro C, et al. Effect of an orally administered thymic derivative, thymomodulin, in chronic type B hepatitis in children. *Curr Ther Res.* 1988;43:67-72.
13. Galli M, Crocchiolo P, Negri C, et al. Attempt to treat acute type B hepatitis with an orally administered thymic extract (thymomodulin): preliminary results. *Drugs Exp Clin Res.* 1985;11:665-669.
14. Raymond RS, Fallon MB, Abrams GA. Oral thymic extract for chronic hepatitis C in patients previously treated with interferon: a randomized, double-blind, placebo-controlled trial. *Ann Intern Med.* 1998;129:797-800.

Herpes Simplex

1. Wolbling RH, Leonhardt K. Local therapy of herpes simplex with dried extract from *Melissa officinalis. Phytomedicine.* 1994;1:25-31.
2. Koytchev R, Alken RG, Dundarov S. Balm mint extract (Lo-701) for topical treatment of recurring *Herpes labialis. Phytomedicine.* 1999;6:225-230.
3. Syed TA, Afzal M, Ashfaq Ahmad S, et al. Management of genital herpes in men with 0.5% *Aloe vera* extract in a hydrophilic cream: a placebo-controlled double-blind study. *J Dermatol Treat.* 1997;8:99-102.
4. Syed TA, Cheema KM, Ashfaq A, et al. *Aloe vera* estract 0.5% in ahydrophilic cream versus *Aloe vera* gel for the management of genital herpes in males. A placebo-controlled, double-blind, comparative study [letter]. *J Eur Acad Dermatol Venereol.* 1996;7:294-295.
5. Williams M. Immuno-protection against herpes simplex type II infection by eleutherococcus root extract. *Int J Alt Complement Med.* 1995;13:9-12.
6. Griffith RS, Walsh DE, Myrmel KH, et al. Success of L-lysine therapy in frequently recurrent herpes simplex infection: treatment and prophylaxis. *Dermatologica.* 1987;175:183-190.
7. McCune MA, Perry HO, Muller SA, et al. Treatment of recurrent herpes simplex infections with L-lysine monohydrochloride. *Cutis.* 1984;34:366-373.
8. Milman N, Scheibel J, Jessen O. Lysine prophylaxis in recurrent herpes simplex labialis: a double-blind, controlled crossover study. *Acta Derm Venereol.* 1980;60:85-87.

9. DiGiovanna JJ, Blank H. Failure of lysine in frequently recurrent herpes simplex infection: treatment and prophylaxis. *Arch Dermatol.* 1984;120:48-51.
10. Milman N, Scheibel J, Jessen O. Failure of lysine treatment in recurrent herpes simplex labialis [letter]. *Lancet.* 1978;2:942.
11. Godfrey HR, Godfrey NJ, Godfrey JC, et al. A randomized clinical trial on the treatment of oral herpes with topical zinc oxide/glycine. *Altern Ther Health Med.* 2001;7:49-54, 56.
12. Vonau B, Chard S, Mandalia S, et al. Does the extract of the plant *Echinacea purpurea* influence the clinical course of recurrent genital herpes? *Int J STD AIDS.* 2001;12:154-158.
13. Hovi T, Hirvimies A, Stenvik M, et al. Topical treatment of recurrent mucocutaneous herpes with ascorbic acid-containing solution. *Antiviral Res.* 1995;27:263-270.
14. Terezhalmy GT, Bottomley WK, Pelleu GB. The use of water-soluble bioflavonoid-ascorbic acid complex in the treatment of recurrent herpes labialis. *Oral Surg Oral Med Oral Pathol.* 1978;45:56-62.
15. Esanu V. Research in the field of antiviral chemotherapy performed in the "Stefan S. Nicolau" Institute of Virology. *Virologie.* 1984;35:281-293.
16. Carson CF, Ashton L, Dry L, et al. *Melaleuca alternifolia* (tea tree) oil gel (6%) for the treatment of recurrent *herpes labialis. J Antimicrob Chemother.* 2001;48:450-451.

Herpes Zoster

1. Billigmann P. Enzyme therapy: an alternative in treatment of herpes zoster. A controlled study of 192 patients [translated from German]. *Fortschr Med.* 1995;113:43-48.
2. Kleine MW, Stauder GM, Beese EW. The intestinal absorption of orally administered hydrolytic enzymes and their effects in the treatment of acute herpes zoster as compared with those of oral acyclovir therapy. *Phytomedicine.* 1995;2:7-15.
3. Sklar SH, Blue WT, Alexander EJ, et al. Herpes zoster: the treatment and prevention of neuralgia with adenosine monophosphate. *JAMA.* 1985;253:1427-1430.
4. Ayres S Jr, Mihan R. Post-herpes zoster neuralgia: response to vitamin E therapy [letter]. *Arch Dermatol.* 1973;108:855-856.
5. Cochrane T. Post-herpes zoster neuralgia: response to vitamin E therapy [letter]. *Arch Dermatol.* 1975;111:396.
6. [No authors listed]. Vitamin B_{12} in herpes zoster [letter]. *JAMA.* 1951;146:1338.

HIV Support

1. de Maat MM, Hoetelmans RM, Mathot RA, et al. Drug interaction between St. John's wort and nevirapine [letter]. *AIDS.* 2001;15:420-421.
2. Durant J, Chantre PH, Gonzalez G, et al. Efficacy and saftey of *Buxus sempervirens* L. preparations (SPV-30) in HIV-infected asymptomatic patients: a multicenter, randomized, double-blind, placebo-controlled trial. *Phytomedicine.* 1998;5:1-10.
3. *PDR for Herbal Medicines.* 2nd ed. Montvale, NJ: Medical Economics Company; 2000:116.
4. *PDR for Herbal Medicines.* 1st ed. Montvale, NJ: Medical Economics Company; 1998:703.
5. Dalakas MC, Leon-Monzon ME, Bernardini I, et al. Zidovudine-induced mitochondrial myopathy is associated with muscle carnitine deficiency and lipid storage. *Ann Neurol.* 1994;35:482-487.
6. Semino-Mora MC, Leon-Monzon ME, Dalakas MC. Effect of L-carnitine on the zidovudine-induced destruction of human myotubes, part I: L-carnitine prevents the myotoxicity of AZT in vitro. *Lab Invest.* 1994;71:102-112.
7. Moretti S, Alesse E, Di Marzio L, et al. Effect of L-carnitine on human immunodeficiency virus-1 infection-associated apoptosis: a pilot study. *Blood.* 1998;91:3817-3824.
8. De Simone C, Cifone MG, Alesse E, et al. Cell associated ceramide in HIV-1-infected subjects [letter]. *AIDS.* 1996;10:675-676.
9. Kroemer G, Zamzami N, Susin SA. Mitochondrial control of apoptosis. *Immunol Today.* 1997;18:44-51.

10. Craig GB, Darnell BE, Weinsier RL, et al. Decreased fat and nitrogen losses in patients with AIDS receiving medium-chain-triglyceride-enriched formula vs. those receiving long-chain-triglyceride-containing formula. *J Am Diet Assoc.* 1997; 97:605-611.

11. Wanke CA, Pleskow D, Degirolami PC, et al. A medium chain triglyceride-based diet in patients with HIV and chronic diarrhea reduces diarrhea and malabsorption: a prospective, controlled trial. *Nutrition.* 1996;12:766-771.

12. Shabert JK, Winslow C, Lacey JM, et al. Glutamine-antioxidant supplementation increases body cell mass in AIDS patients with weight loss: a randomized, double-blind controlled trial. *Nutrition.* 1999;15:860-864.

13. Clark RH, Feleke G, Din M, et al. Nutritional treatment for acquired immunodeficiency virus-associated wasting using beta-hydroxy beta-methylbutyrate, glutamine, and arginine: a randomized, double-blind, placebo-controlled study. *JPEN J Parenter Enteral Nutr.* 2000;24:133-139.

14. Bounous G, Baruchel S, Falutz J, et al. Whey proteins as a food supplement in HIV-seropositive individuals. *Clin Invest Med.* 1993;16:204-209.

15. Scevola D, Oberto L, Faggi A, et al. Fish oil in the treatment of wasting syndrome [abstract]. *Int Conf AIDS.* 1996;11:122.

16. Akerlund B, Jarstrand C, Lindeke B, et al. Effect of *N*-acetylcysteine (NAC) treatment on HIV-1 infection: a double-blind placebo-controlled trial. *Eur J Clin Pharmacol.* 1996;50:457-461.

17. Look MP, Rockstroh JK, Rao GS, et al. Sodium selenite and *N*-acetylcysteine in antiretroviral-naive HIV-1-infected patients: a randomized, controlled pilot study. *Eur J Clin Invest.* 1998;28:389-397.

18. Walker RE, Lane HC, Boenning CM, et al. The safety, pharmacokinetics, and antiviral activity of *N*-acetylcysteine in HIV-infected individuals [abstract]. *J Cell Biochem Suppl.* 1992;16:89.

19. Calabrese C, Berman SH, Babish JG, et al. A phase I trial of andrographolide in HIV positive patients and normal volunteers. *Phytother Res.* 2000;14:333-338.

20. Pichard C, Sudre P, Karsegard V, et al. A randomized double-blind controlled study of 6 months of oral nutritional supplementation with arginine and omega-3 fatty acids in HIV-infected patients. *AIDS.* 1998;12:53-63.

21. Plettenberg A, Stoehr A, Stellbrink H-J, et al. A preparation from bovine colostrum in the treatment of HIV-positive patients with chronic diarrhea. *Clin Investig.* 1993;71:42-45.

22. Greenberg PD, Cello JP. Treatment of severe diarrhea caused by *Cryptosporidium parvum* with oral bovine immunoglobulin concentrate in patients with AIDS. *J Acquir Immune Defic Syndr Hum Retrovirol.* 1996;13:348-354.

23. Okhuysen PC, Chappell CL, Crabb J, et al. Prophylactic effect of bovine anti-Cryptosporidium hyperimmune colostrum immunoglobulin in healthy volunteers challenged with *Cryptosporidium parvum. Clin Infect Dis.* 1998;26:1324-1329.

24. Vazquez JA, Vaishampayan J, Arganoza MT, et al. Use of an over-the-counter product, Breathaway (Melaleuca Oral Solution), as an alternative agent for refractory oropharyngeal candidiasis in AIDS patients [abstract]. *Int Conf AIDS.* 1996;11:109.

25. Christeff N, Melchior JC, Mammes O, et al. Correlation between increased cortisol:DHEA ratio and malnutrition in HIV-positive men. *Nutrition.* 1999;15:534-539.

26. Cruess DG, Antoni MH, Kumar M, et al. Cognitive-behavioral stress management buffers decreases in dehydroepiandrosterone sulfate (DHEA-S) and increases in the cortisol/DHEA-S ratio and reduces mood disturbance and perceived stress among HIV-seropositive men. *Psychoneuroendocrinology.* 1999;24:537-549.

27. Rabkin JG, Ferrando SJ, Wagner GJ, et al. DHEA treatment for HIV+ patients: effects on mood, androgenic and anabolic parameters. *Psychoneuroendocrinology.* 2000; 25:53-68.

28. Burack JH, Cohen MR, Hahn JA, et al. Pilot randomized controlled trial of Chinese herbal treatment for HIV-associated symptoms. *J Acquir Immune Defic Syndr Hum Retrovirol.* 1996;12:386-393.

29. Weber R, Christen L, Loy M, et al. Randomized, placebo-controlled trial of Chinese herb therapy for HIV-1-infected individuals. *J Acquir Immune Defic Syndr Hum Retrovirol*. 1999;22:56-64.

30. Baum MK, Javier JJ, Mantero-Atienza E, et al. Zidovudine-associated adverse reactions in a longitudinal study of asymptomatic HIV-1-infected homosexual males. *J Acquir Immune Defic Syndr*. 1991;4:1218-1226.

31. Herzlich BC, Ranginwala M, Nawabi I, et al. Synergy of inhibition of DNA synthesis in human bone marrow by azidothymidine plus deficiency of folate and/or B12? *Am J Hematol*. 1990;33:177-183.

32. Mocchegiani E, Rivabene R, Santini MT. Benefit of oral zinc supplementation as an adjunct to zidovudine (AZT) therapy against opportunistic infections in AIDS. *Int J Immunopharmacol*. 1995;17:719-727.

33. Richman DD, Fischl MA, Grieco MH, et al. The toxicity of azidothymidine (AZT) in the treatment of patients with AIDS and AIDS-related complex. A double-blind, placebo-controlled trial. *N Engl J Med*. 1987;317:192-197.

34. Akerlund B, Tynell E, Bratt G, et al. *N*-acetylcysteine treatment and the risk of toxic reactions to trimethoprim-sulphamethoxazole in primary *Pneumocystis carinii* prophylaxis in HIV-infected patients. *J Infect*. 1997;35:143-147.

35. Walmsley SL, Khorasheh S, Singer J, et al. A randomized trial of *N*-acetylcysteine for prevention of trimethoprim-sulfamethoxazole hypersensitivity reactions in *Pneumocystis carinii* pneumonia prophylaxis (CTN 057). Canadian HIV Trials Network 057 Study Group. *J Acquir Immune Defic Syndr Hum Retrovirol*. 1998; 19:498-505.

36. Kahn SB, Fein SA, Brodsky I. Effects of trimethoprim on folate metabolism in man. *Clin Pharmacol Ther*. 1968;9:550-560.

37. Semba RD, Graham NM, Caiaffa WT, et al. Increased mortality associated with vitamin A deficiency during human immunodeficiency virus type 1 infection. *Arch Intern Med*. 1993;153:2149-2154.

38. Bianchi-Santamaria A, Fedeli S, Santamaria L. Short communication: possible activity of beta-carotene in patients with the AIDS related complex, a pilot study. *Med Oncol Tumor Pharmacother*. 1992;9:151-153.

39. Alexander M, Newmark H, Miller RG. Oral beta-carotene can increase the number of OKT4+ cells in human blood. *Immunol Lett*. 1985;9:221-224.

40. Fryburg DA, Mark RJ, Griffith BP, et al. The effect of supplemental beta-carotene on immunologic indices in patients with AIDS: a pilot study. *Yale J Biol Med*. 1995;68:19-23.

41. Coodley GO, Nelson HD, Loveless MO, et al. Beta-carotene in HIV infection. *J Acquir Immune Defic Syndr Hum Retrovirol*. 1993;6:272-276.

42. Coodley GO, Coodley MK, Lusk R, et al. Beta-carotene in HIV infection: an extended evaluation. *AIDS*. 1996;10:967-973.

43. Constans J, Delmas-Beauvieux MC, Sergeant C, et al. One-year antioxidant supplementation with beta-carotene or selenium for patients infected with human immunodeficiency virus: a pilot study [letters]. *Clin Infect Dis*. 1996;23:654-656.

44. Tang AM, Graham NH, Kirby AJ, et al. Dietary micronutrient intake and risk of progression to acquired immunodeficiency syndrome (AIDS) in human immunodeficiency virus type 1(HIV-1)–infected homosexual men. *Am J Epidemiol*. 1993; 138:937-951.

45. Fawzi WW, Msamanga G, Hunter D, et al. Randomized trial of vitamin supplements in relation to vertical transmission of HIV-1 in Tanzania. *J Acquir Immune Defic Syndr Hum Retrovirol*. 2000;23:246-254.

46. Coutsoudis A, Pillay K, Spooner E, et al. Randomized trial testing the effect of vitamin A supplementation on pregnancy outcomes and early mother-to-child HIV-1 transmission in Durban, South Africa. South African Vitamin A Study Group. *AIDS*. 1999;13:1517-1524.

47. Tang AM, Graham NM, Saah AJ. Effects of micronutrient intake on survival in human immunodeficiency virus type 1 infection. *Am J Epidemiol*. 1996;143:1244-1256.

48. Shor-Posner G, Morgan R, Wilkie F, et al. Plasma coabalmin levels affect information processing speed in a longitudinal study of HIV-1 disease. *Arch Neurol.* 1995;52:195-198.

49. Kieburtz KD, Giang DW, Schiffer RB, et al. Abnormal vitamin B_{12} metabolism in human immunodeficiency virus infection association with neurological dysfunction. *Arch Neurol.* 1991;48:312-314.

50. Baum MK, Shor-Posner G, Lu Y, et al. Micronutrients and HIV-1 disease progression. *AIDS.* 1995;9:1051-1056.

51. Baum MK, Mantero-Atienza E, Shor-Posner G, et al. Association of vitamin B_6 status with parameters of immune function in early HIV-1 infection. *J Acquir Immune Defic Syndr.* 1991;4:1122-1132.

52. Harakeh S, Jariwalla RJ, Pauling L. Suppression of human immunodeficiency virus replication by ascorbate in chronically and acutely infected cells. *Proc Natl Acad Sci USA.* 1990;87:7245-7249.

53. Cathcart RF 3rd. Vitamin C in the treatment of acquired immune deficiency syndrome (AIDS). *Med Hypotheses.* 1984;14:423-433.

54. Abrams B, Duncan D, Hertz-Picciotto I. A prospective study of dietary intake and acquired immune deficiency syndrome in HIV-seropositive homosexual men. *J Acquir Immune Defic Syndr.* 1993;6:949-958.

55. Allard JP, Aghdassi E, Chau J, et al. Effects of vitamin E and C supplementation on oxidative stress and viral load in HIV-infected subjects. *AIDS.* 1998;12:1653-1659.

56. Gogu SR, Beckman BS, Rangan SR, et al. Increased therapeutic efficacy of zidovudine in combination with vitamin E. *Biochem Biophys Res Commun.* 1989;165:401-407.

57. Constans J, Pellegrin JL, Sergeant C, et al. Serum selenium predicts outcome in HIV infection [letter]. *J Acquir Immune Defic Syndr Hum Retrovirol.* 1995;10:392.

58. Schrauzer GN, Sacher J. Selenium in the maintenance and therapy of HIV-infected patients. *Chem Biol Interact.* 1994;91:199-205.

59. Baum MK, Shor-Posner G, Lai S, et al. High risk of HIV-related mortality is associated with selenium deficiency. *J Acquir Immune Defic Syndr Hum Retrovirol.* 1997;15:370-374.

60. Campa A, Shor-Posner G, Indacochea F, et al. Mortality risk in selenium-deficient HIV-positive children. *J Acquir Immune Defic Syndr Hum Retrovirol.* 1999;20:508-513.

61. Zazzo JF, Chalas J, Lafont A, et al. Is nonobstructive cardiomyopathy in AIDS a selenium deficiency-related disease? [letter]. *JPEN J Parenter Enteral Nutr.* 1988;12:537-538.

62. Dworkin BM. Selenium deficiency in HIV infection and the acquired immunodeficiency syndrome (AIDS). *Chem Biol Interact.* 1994;91:181-186.

63. Baeten JM, Mostad SB, Hughes MP, et al. Selenium deficiency is associated with shedding of HIV-1—infected cells in the female genital tract. *J Acquir Immune Defic Syndr.* 2001;26:360-364.

64. Fabris N, Mocchegiani E, Galli M, et al. AIDS, zinc deficiency, and thymic hormone failure [letter]. *JAMA.* 1988;259:839-840.

65. Sappey C, Leclercq P, Coudray C, et al. Vitamin, trace element and peroxide status in HIV seropositive patients: asymptomatic patients present a severe beta-carotene deficiency. *Clin Chim Acta.* 1994;230:35-42.

66. Odeh M. The role of zinc in acquired immunodeficiency syndrome. *J Intern Med.* 1992;231:463-469.

67. Periquet BA, Jammes NM, Lambert WE, et al. Micronutrient levels in HIV-1-infected children. *AIDS.* 1995;9:887-893.

68. Tomaka FL, Imoch PJ, Reiter WM, et al. Prevalance of nutritional deficiencies in patients with HIV Infection [astract]. *Int Conf AIDS.* 1994;10:221.

69. Campa AM, Lai H, Shor-Posner G, et al. Relationship between zinc deficiency and survival in HIV+ homosexual men [abstract]. *FASEB J.* 1998;12:A217.

70. Castaldo A, Tarallo L, Palomba E, et al. Iron deficiency and intestinal malabsorption in HIV disease. *J Pediatr Gastroenterol Nutr.* 1996;22:359-363.

71. Bogden JD, Kemp FW, Han S, et al. Status of selected nutrients and progression of human immunodeficiency virus type 1 infection. *Am J Clin Nutr.* 2000;72:809-815.
72. Piscitelli SC, Burstein AH, Chaitt D, et al. Indinavir concentrations and St. John's wort [letter]. *Lancet.* 2000;355:547-548.
73. Piscitelli SC. Use of complementary medicines by patients with HIV: full sail into uncharted waters. *Medscape HIV/AIDS.* 2000;6(3).
74. Piscitelli SC, Burstein AH, Welden N, et al. The effect of garlic supplements on the pharmacokinetics of saquinavir. *Clin Infect Dis.* 2002;34:234-238.
75. Agin D, Gallagher D, Wang J, et al. Effects of whey protein and resistance exercise on body cell mass, muscle strength, and quality of life in women with HIV. *AIDS.* 2001;15:2431-2440.
76. Jacobson MA, Fusaro RE, Galmarini M, et al. Decreased serum dehydroepiandrosterone is associated with an increased progression of human immunodeficiency virus infection in men with CD4 cell counts of 200-499. *J Infect Dis.* 1991;164:864-868.
77. Mulder JW, Frissen PH, Krijnen P, et al. Dehydroepiandrosterone as predictor for progression to AIDS in asymptomatic human immunodeficiency virus-infected men. *J Infect Dis.* 1992;165:413-418.
78. Piketty C, Jayle D, Leplege A, et al. Double-blind, placebo-controlled trial of oral dehydroepiandrosterone in patients with advanced HIV disease. *Clin Endocrinol (Oxf).* 2001;55: 325-330.

Hyperlipidemia

1. Illingworth DR, Stein EA, Mitchel YB, et al. Comparative effects of lovastatin and niacin in primary hypercholesterolemia: a prospective trial. *Arch Intern Med.* 1994; 154:1586-1595.
2. Guyton JR, Goldberg AC, Kreisberg RA, et al. Effectiveness of once-nightly dosing of extended-release niacin alone and in combination for hypercholesterolemia. *Am J Cardiol.* 1998;82:737-743.
3. Vega GL, Grundy SM. Lipoprotein responses to treatment with lovastatin, gemfibrozil, and nicotinic acid in normolipidemic patients with hypoalphalipoproteinemia. *Arch Intern Med.* 1994;154:73-82.
4. Lal SM, Hewett JE, Petroski GF, et al. Effects of nicotinic acid and lovastatin in renal transplant patients: a prospective, randomized, open-label crossover trial. *Am J Kidney Dis.* 1995;25:616-622.
5. Guyton JR, Blazing MA, Hagar J, et al. Extended-release niacin vs gemfibrozil for the treatment of low levels of high-density lipoprotein cholesterol. *Arch Intern Med.* 2000;160:1177-1184.
6. Glore SR, Van Treeck D, Knehans AW, et al. Soluble fiber and serum lipids: a literature review. *J Am Diet Assoc.* 1994;94:425-436.
7. Gylling H, Miettinen TA. Serum cholesterol and cholesterol and lipoprotein metabolism in hypercholesterolaemic NIDDM patients before and during sitostanol ester-margarine treatment. *Diabetologia.* 1994;37:773-780.
8. Gylling H, Miettinen TA. Cholesterol reduction by different plant stanol mixtures and with variable fat intake. *Metabolism.* 1999;48:575-580.
9. Vanhanen HT, Blomqvist S, Ehnholm C, et al. Serum cholesterol, cholesterol precursors, and plant sterols in hypercholesterolemic subjects with different apoE phenotypes during dietary sitostanol ester treatment. *J Lipid Res.* 1993;34:1535-1544.
10. Blair SN, Capuzzi DM, Gottlieb SO, et al. Incremental reduction of serum total cholesterol and low-density lipoprotein cholesterol with the addition of plant stanol ester-containing spread to statin therapy. *Am J Cardiol.* 2000;86:46-52.
11. Nguyen TT, Dale LV, von Bergmann K, et al. Cholesterol-lowering effect of stanol ester in a US population of mildly hypercholesterolemic men and women: a randomized controlled trial. *Mayo Clin Proc.* 1999;74:1198-2206.
12. Miettinen TA, Puska P, Gylling H, et al. Reduction of serum cholesterol with sitostanol-ester margarine in a mildly hypercholesterolemic population. *N Engl J Med.* 1995;333:1308-1312.

13. Hallikainen MA, Sarkkinen ES, Uusitupa MI. Effects of low-fat stanol ester enriched margarines on concentrations of serum carotenoids in subjects with elevated serum cholesterol concentrations. *Eur J Clin Nutr.* 1999;53:966-969.

14. Gylling H, Siimes MA, Miettinen TA. Sitostanol ester margarine in dietary treatment of children with familial hypercholesterolemia. *J Lipid Res.* 1995;36:1807-1812.

15. Tammi A, Ronnemaa T, Gylling H, et al. Plant stanol ester margarine lowers serum total and low-density lipoprotein cholesterol concentrations of healthy children: the STRIP project. Special Turku Coronary Risk Factors Intervention Project. *J Pediatr.* 2000;136:503-510.

16. Hallikainen MA, Uusitupa MI. Effects of 2 low-fat stanol ester-containing margarines on serum cholesterol concentrations as part of a low-fat diet in hypercholesterolemic subjects. *Am J Clin Nutr.* 1999;69:403-410.

17. Gylling H, Radhakrishnan R, Miettinen TA. Reduction of serum cholesterol in postmenopausal women with previous myocardial infarction and cholesterol malabsorption induced by dietary sitostanol ester margarine: women and dietary sitostanol. *Circulation.* 1997;96:4226-4231.

18. Jones PJ, Ntanios FY, Raeini-Sarjaz M, et al. Cholesterol-lowering efficacy of a sitostanol-containing phytosterol mixture with a prudent diet in hyperlipidemic men. *Am J Clin Nutr.* 1999;69:1144-1150.

19. Vanhanen HT, Kajander J, Lehtovirta H, et al. Serum levels, absorption efficiency, faecal elimination, and synthesis of cholesterol during increasing doses of dietary sitostanol esters in hypercholesterolaemic subjects. *Clin Sci.* 1994;87:61-67.

20. Neil HA, Meijer GW, Roe LS. Randomized controlled trial of use by hypercholesterolaemic patients of a vegetable oil sterol-enriched fat spread. *Atherosclerosis.* 2001;156:329-337.

21. Nguyen TT. The cholesterol-lowering action of plant stanol esters. *J Nutr.* 1999; 129:2109-2112.

22. Maki KC, Davidson MH, Umporowicz DM, et al. Lipid responses to plant-sterol-enriched reduced-fat spreads incorporated into a National Cholesterol Education Program Step I diet. *Am J Clin Nutr.* 2001;74:33-43.

23. Gylling H, Miettinen TA. Effects of inhibiting cholesterol absorption and synthesis on cholesterol and lipoprotein metabolism in hypercholesterolemic non-insulin-dependent diabetic men. *J Lipid Res.* 1996;37:1776-1785.

24. Moghadasian MH, Frohlich JJ. Effects of dietary phytosterols on cholesterol metabolism and atherosclerosis: clinical and experimental evidence. *Am J Med.* 1999; 107:588-594.

25. Williams CL, Bollella MC, Strobino BA, et al. Plant stanol ester and bran fiber in childhood: effects on lipids, stool weight, and stool frequency in preschool children. *J Am Coll Nutr.* 1999;18:572-581.

26. Turnbull D, Whittaker MH, Frankos VH, et al. 13-week oral toxicity study with stanol esters in rats. *Regul Toxicol Pharmacol.* 1999;29:216-226.

27. Anderson JW, Johnstone BM, Cooke-Newell ME. Meta-analysis of the effects of soy protein intake on serum lipids. *N Engl J Med.* 1995;333:276-281.

28. Wangen KE, Duncan AM, Xu X, et al. Soy isoflavones improve plasma lipids in normocholesterolemic and mildly hypercholesterolemic postmenopausal women. *Am J Clin Nutr.* 2001;73:225-231.

29. Crouse JR III, Morgan T, Terry JG, et al. A randomized trial comparing the effect of casein with that of soy protein containing varying amounts of isoflavones on plasma concentrations of lipids and lipoproteins. *Arch Intern Med.* 1999;159:2070-2076.

30. Anthony MS, Clarkson TB, Hughes CL Jr, et al. Soybean isoflavones improve cardiovascular risk factors without affecting the reproductive system of peripubertal rhesus monkeys. *J Nutr.* 1996;126:43-50.

31. Greaves KA, Parks JS, Williams JK, et al. Intact dietary soy protein, but not adding an isoflavone-rich soy extract to casein, improves plasma lipids in ovariectomized cynomolgus monkeys. *J Nutr.* 1999;129:1585-1592.

32. Simons LA, von Konigsmark M, Simons J, et al. Phytoestrogens do not influence lipoprotein levels or endothelial function in healthy, postmenopausal women. *Am J Cardiol.* 2000;85:1297-1301.

33. Mackey R, Ekangaki A, Eden JA. The effects of soy protein in women and men with elevated plasma lipids. *Biofactors.* 2000;12:251-257.

34. Sirtori CR, Gianazza E, Manzoni C, et al. Role of isoflavones in the cholesterol reduction by soy proteins in the clinic [letter]. *Am J Clin Nutr.* 1997;65:166-167.

35. Setchell KD, Brown NM, Desai P, et al. Bioavailability of pure isoflavones in healthy humans and analysis of commercial soy isoflavone supplements. *J Nutr.* 2001;131(4 suppl):1362S-1375S.

36. Howes JB, Sullivan D, Lai N, et al. The effects of dietary supplementation with isoflavones from red clover on the lipoprotein profiles of post menopausal women with mild to moderate hypercholesterolaemia. *Atherosclerosis.* 2000;152:143-147.

37. Aneiros E, Mas R, Calderon B, et al. Effect of policosanol in lowering cholesterol levels in patients with type II hypercholesterolemia. *Curr Ther Res.* 1995;56:176-182.

38. Castano G, Canetti M, Moreira M, et al. Efficacy and tolerability of policosanol in elderly patients with type II hypercholesterolemia: a 12-month study. *Curr Ther Res.* 1995;56:819-828.

39. Castano G, Tula L, Canetti M, et al. Effects of policosanol in hypertensive patients with type II hypercholesterolemia. *Curr Ther Res.* 1996;57:691-699.

40. Torres O, Agramonte AJ, Illnait J, et al. Treatment of hypercholesterolemia in NIDDM with policosanol. *Diabetes Care.* 1995;18:393-397.

41. Aneiros E, Calderon B, Mas R, et al. Effect of successive dose increases of policosanol on the lipid profile and tolerability of treatment. *Curr Ther Res.* 1993;54:304-312.

42. Castano G, Más R, Nodarse M, et al. One-year study of the efficacy and safety of policosanol (5 mg twice daily) in the treatment of type II hypercholesterolemia. *Curr Ther Res.* 1995;56:296-304.

43. Oosthuizen W, Vorster HH, Vermaak, WJ, et al. Lecithin has no effect on serum lipoprotein, plasma fibrinogen and macro molecular protein complex levels in hyperlipidaemic men in a double-blind controlled study. *Eur J Clin Nutr.* 1998;52:419-424.

44. Pons P, Rodriguez M, Mas R, et al. One-year efficacy and safety of policosanol in patients with type II hypercholesterolemia. *Curr Ther Res.* 1994;55:1084-1092.

45. Pons P, Rodriguez M, Robaina C, et al. Effects of successive dose increases of policosanol on the lipid profile of patients with type II hypercholesterolaemia and tolerability to treatment. *Int J Clin Pharm Res.* 1994;14:27-33.

46. Pons P, Mas R, Illnait J, et al. Efficacy and safety of policosanol in patients with primary hypercholesterolemia. *Curr Ther Res.* 1992;52:507-513.

47. Mas R, Castano G, Illnait J, et al. Effects of policosanol in patients with type II hypercholesterolemia and additional coronary risk factors. *Clin Pharmacol Ther.* 1999;65:439-447.

48. Crespo N, Alvarez R, Mas R, et al. Effect of policosanol on patients with non-insulin-dependent diabetes mellitus and hypercholesterolemia: a pilot study. *Curr Ther Res.* 1997;58:44-51.

49. Castano G, Mas R, Fernandez L, et al. Effects of policosanol on postmenopausal women with type II hypercholesterolemia. *Gynecol Endocrinol.* 2000;14:187-195

50. Benitez M, Romero C, Mas R, et al. A comparative study of policosanol versus pravastatin in patients with type II hypercholesterolemia. *Curr Ther Res.* 1997;58:859-867.

51. Ortensi G, Gladstein J, Valli H, et al. A comparative study of policosanol versus simvastatin in elderly patients with hypercholesterolemia. *Curr Ther Res.* 1997;58:390-401.

52. Castano G, Mas R, Arruzazabala ML, et al. Effects of policosanol and pravastatin on lipid profile, platelet aggregation, and endothelemia in older hypercholesterolemic patients. *Int J Clin Pharmacol Res.* 1999;19:105-116.

53. Alcocer L, Fernandez L, Campos E, et al. A comparative study of policosanol versus acipimox in patients with type II hypercholesterolemia. *Int J Tissue React.* 1999;21:85-92.

54. Crespo N, Illnait J, Mas R, et al. Comparative study of the efficacy and tolerability of policosanol and lovastatin in patients with hypercholesterolemia and noninsulin dependent diabetes mellitus. *Int J Clin Pharmacol Res.* 1999;19:117-127.

55. Fernandez JC, Mas R, Castano G, et al. Comparison of the efficacy, safety, and tolerability of policosanol versus fluvastatin in elderly hypercholesterolaemic women. *Clin Drug Invest.* 2001;21:103-113.

56. Warshafsky S, Kamer RS, Sivak SL. Effect of garlic on total serum cholesterol: a meta-analysis. *Ann Intern Med.* 1993;119:599-605.

57. Mader FH. Treatment of hyperlipidaemia with garlic-powder tablets: evidence from the German Association of General Practitioners' multicentric placebo-controlled double-blind study. *Arzneimittelforschung.* 1990;40:1111-1116.

58. Steiner M, Khan AH, Holbert D, et al. A double-blind crossover study in moderately hypercholesterolemic men that compared the effect of aged garlic extract and placebo administration on blood lipids. *Am J Clin Nutr.* 1996;64:866-870.

59. Holzgartner H, Schmidt U, Kuhn U. Comparison of the efficacy and tolerance of a garlic preparation vs. bezafibrate. *Arzneimittelforschung.* 1992;42:1473-1477.

60. Neil HA, Silagy CA, Lancaster T, et al. Garlic powder in the treatment of moderate hyperlipidaemia: a controlled trial and meta-analysis. *J R Coll Physicians Lond.* 1996;30:329-334.

61. Simons LA, Balasubramaniam S, von Konigsmark M, et al. On the effect of garlic on plasma lipids and lipoproteins in mild hypercholesterolaemia. *Atherosclerosis.* 1995; 113:219-225.

62. Superko HR, Krauss RM. Garlic powder, effect on plasma lipids, postprandial lipemia, low-density lipoprotein particle size, high-density lipoprotein subclass distribution, and lipoprotein (a). *J Am Coll Cardiol.* 2000;35:321-326.

63. Isaacsohn JL, Moser M, Stein EA, et al. Garlic powder and plasma lipids and lipoproteins: a multicenter, randomized, placebo-controlled trial. *Arch Intern Med.* 1998; 158:1189-1194.

64. Gardner CD, Chatterjee LM, Carlson JJ. The effect of a garlic preparation on plasma lipid levels in moderately hypercholesterolemic adults. *Atherosclerosis.* 2001; 154:213-220.

65. Kannar D, Wattanapenpaiboon N, Savige GS, et al. Hypocholesterolemic effect of an enteric-coated garlic supplement. *J Am Coll Nutr.* 2001;20:225-231.

66. Stevinson C, Pittler MH, Ernst E. Garlic for treating hypercholesterolemia: a meta-analysis of randomized clinical trials. *Ann Intern Med.* 2000;133:420-429.

67. Englisch W, Beckers C, Unkauf M, et al. Efficacy of artichoke dry extract in patients with hyperlipoproteinemia. *Arzneimittelforschung.* 2000;50:260-265.

68. Petrowicz O, Gebhardt R, Donner M, et al. Effects of artichoke leaf extract (ALE) on lipoprotein metabolism in vitro and in vivo [abstract]. *Atherosclerosis.* 1997;129:147

69. Heber D, Yip I, Ashley JM, et al. Cholesterol-lowering effects of a proprietary Chinese red-yeast-rice dietary supplement. *Am J Clin Nutr.* 1999;69:231-236.

70. Rippe J, Bonovich K, Colfer H, et al. A multi-center, self-controlled study of Cholestin™ in subjects with elevated cholesterol [abstract]. *Circulation.* 1999; 99:1123.

71. Wang J, Lu Z, Chi J, et al. Multicenter clinical trial of the serum lipid-lowering effects of a *Monascus purpureus* (red yeast) rice preparation from traditional Chinese medicine. *Curr Ther Res.* 1997;58:964-978.

72. Singh RB, Niaz MA, Ghosh S. Hypolipidemic and antioxidant effects of Commiphora mukul as an adjunct to dietary therapy in patients with hypercholesterolemia. *Cardiovasc Drugs Ther.* 1994;8:659-664.

73. Verma SK, Bordia A. Effect of *Commiphora mukul* (gum guggulu) in patients of hyperlipidemia with special reference to HDL-cholesterol. *Indian J Med Res.* 1988;87:356-360.

74. Nityanand S, Srivastava JS, Asthana OP. Clinical trials with gugulipid: a new hypolipidaemic agent. *J Assoc Physicians India.* 1989;37:323-328.

75. Colodny LR, Montgomery A, Houston M. The role of esterin processed alfalfa saponins in reducing cholesterol. *J Am Nutraceutical Assoc.* 2001;3:6-15.

76. Vecchio F, Zanchin G, Maggioni F, et al. Mesoglycan in treatment of patients with cerebral ischemia: effects on hemorrheologic and hematochemical parameters. *Acta Neurol (Napoli).* 1993;15:449-456.

77. Saba P, Galeone F, Giuntoli F, et al. Hypolipidemic effect of mesoglycan in hyper-lipidemic patients. *Curr Ther Res.* 1986;40:761-768.
78. Postiglione A, De Simone B, Rubba P, et al. Effect of oral mesoglycan on plasma lipoprotein concentration and on lipoprotein lipase activity in primary hyperlipidemia. *Pharmacol Res Commun.* 1984;16:1-8.
79. Bell L, Halstenson CE, Halstenson CJ, et al. Cholesterol-lowering effects of calcium carbonate in patients with mild to moderate hypercholesterolemia. *Arch Intern Med.* 1992;152:2441-2444.
80. Bostick RM, Fosdick L, Grandits GA, et al. Effect of calcium supplementation on serum cholesterol and blood pressure: a randomized, double-blind, placebo-controlled, clinical trial. *Arch Fam Med.* 2000;9:31-39.
81. Ho SC, Tai ES, Eng PH, et al. In the absence of dietary surveillance, chitosan does not reduce plasma lipids or obesity in hypercholesterolaemic obese Asian subjects. *Singapore Med J.* 2001;42:6-10.
82. Tai TS, Sheu WH, Lee WJ, et al. Effect of chitosan on plasma lipoprotein concentrations in type 2 diabetic subjects with hypercholesterolemia [letter]. *Diabetes Care.* 2000;23:1703-1704.
83. Maezaki Y, Tsuji K, Nakagawa Y, et al. Hypocholesterolemic effect of chitosan in adult males. *Biosci Biotechnol Biochem.* 1993;57:1439-1444.
84. Jing SB, Li L, Ji D, et al. Effect of chitosan on renal function in patients with chronic renal failure. *J Pharm Pharmacol.* 1997;49:721-723.
85. Ormrod D, Holmes CC, Miller TE. Dietary chitosan inhibits hypercholesterolaemia and atherogenesis in the apolipoprotein E-deficient mouse model of Atherosclerosis. *Atherosclerosis.* 1998;138:329-334.
86. Deuchi K, Kanauchi O, Imasato Y, et al. Decreasing effect of chitosan on the apparent fat digestibility by rats fed on a high-fat diet. *Biosci Biotechnol Biochem.* 1994;58:1613-1616.
87. Deuchi K, Kanauchi O, Imasato Y, et al. Effect of the viscosity or deacetylation degree of chitosan on fecal fat excreted from rats fed on a high-fat diet. *Biosci Biotechnol Biochem.* 1995;59:781-785.
88. Deuchi K, Kanauchi O, Shizukuishi M, et al. Continuous and massive intake of chitosan affects mineral and fat-soluble vitamin status in rats fed on a high-fat diet. *Biosci Biotechnol Biochem.* 1995;59:1211-1216.
89. Kanauchi O, Deuchi K, Imasato Y, et al. Increasing effect of a chitosan and ascorbic acid mixture on fecal dietary fat excretion. *Biosci Biotechnol Biochem.* 1994;58:1617-1620.
90. Kobayashi T, Otsuka S, Yugari Y. Effect of chitosan on serum and liver cholesterol levels in cholesterol-fed rats. *Nutr Rep Int.* 1979;19:327-334.
91. Mertz W. Chromium in human nutrition: a review. *J Nutr.* 1993;123:626-633.
92. Press RI, Geller J, Evans GW. The effect of chromium picolinate on serum cholesterol and apolipoprotein fractions in human subjects. *West J Med.* 1990;152:41-45.
93. Roeback JR, Hla KM, Chambless LE, et al. Effects of chromium supplementation on serum high-density lipoprotein cholesterol levels in men taking beta-blockers: a randomized, controlled trial. *Ann Intern Med.* 1991;115:917-924.
94. Preuss HG, Wallerstedt D, Talpur N, et al. Effects of niacin-bound chromium and grape seed proanthocyanidin extract on the lipid profile of hypercholesterolemic subjects: a pilot study. *J Med.* 2000;31:227-246.
95. Babu PS, Srinivasan K. Hypolipidemic action of curcumin, the active principle of turmeric *(Curcuma longa)* in streptozotocin induced diabetic rats. *Mol Cell Biochem.* 1997;166:169-175.
96. Rao DS, Sekhara NC, Satyanarayana MN, et al. Effect of curcumin on serum and liver cholesterol levels in the rat. *J Nutr.* 1970;100:1307-1316.
97. Srinivasan K, Sambaiah K. The effect of spices on cholesterol 7 alpha-hydroxylase activity and on serum and hepatic cholesterol levels in the rat. *Int J Vitam Nutr Res.* 1991;61:364-369.
98. Soni KB, Kuttan R. Effect of oral curcumin administration on serum peroxides and cholesterol levels in human volunteers. *Indian J Physiol Pharmacol.* 1992;36:273-275.

99. Gonzales GF, Gonez C, Villena A. Serum lipid and lipoprotein levels in post-menopausal women: short-course effect of caigua. *Menopause*. 1995;2:225-234.

100. Asgary S, Naderi GH, Sarrafzadegan N, et al. Antihypertensive and antihyperlipi-demic effects of *Achillea wilhelmsii*. *Drugs Exp Clin Res*. 2000;26:89-93.

101. Earnest CP, Almada AL, and Mitchell TL. High-performance capillary elec-trophoresis-pure creatine monohydrate reduces blood lipids in men and women. *Clin Sci (Colch)*. 1996;91:113-118.

102. Prasad K. Dietary flax seed in prevention of hypercholesterolemic Atherosclerosis. *Atherosclerosis*. 1997;132:69-76.

103. Arjmandi BH, Khan DA, Juma S, et al. Whole flaxseed consumption lowers serum LDL-cholesterol and lipoprotein(a) concentrations in postmenopausal women. *Nutr Res*. 1998;18:1203-1214.

104. Singer P, Jaeger W, Berger I, et al. Effects of dietary oleic, linoleic, and alpha-linolenic acids on blood pressure, serum lipids, lipoproteins and the formation of eicosanoid precursors in patients with mild essential hypertension. *J Hum Hypertens*. 1990;4:227-233.

105. Harris WS. N-3 fatty acids and serum lipoproteins: human studies. *Am J Clin Nutr*. 1997;65(suppl):1645S-1654S.

106. Davini P, Bigalli A, Lamanna F, et al. Controlled study on L-carnitine therapeutic efficacy in post-infarction. *Drugs Exp Clin Res*. 1992;18:355-365.

107. Agerholm-Larsen L, Raben A, Haulrik N, et al. Effect of 8 week intake of probiotic milk products on risk factors for cardiovascular diseases. *Eur J Clin Nutr*. 2000;54:288-297.

108. Agerbaek M, Gerdes LU, Richelsen B. Hypocholesterolaemic effect of a new fer-mented milk product in healthy middle-aged men. *Eur J Clin Nutr*. 1995;49: 346-352.

109. Bertolami MC, Faludi AA, Batlouni M. Evaluation of the effects of a new fermented milk product (Gaio) on primary hypercholesterolemia. *Eur J Clin Nutr*. 1999;53: 97-101.

110. Richelsen B, Kristensen K, Pedersen SB. Long-term (6 months) effect of a new fer-mented milk product on the level of plasma lipoproteins: a placebo-controlled and double blind study. *Eur J Clin Nutr*. 1996;50:811-815.

111. Anderson JW, Gilliland SE. Effect of fermented milk (yogurt) containing *Lactobacillus acidophilus* L1 on serum cholesterol in hypercholesterolemic humans. *J Am Coll Nutr*. 1999;18:43-50.

112. Agerholm-Larsen L, Bell ML, Grunwald GK, et al. The effect of a probiotic milk product on plasma cholesterol: a meta-analysis of short-term intervention studies. *Eur J Clin Nutr*. 2000;54:856-860.

113. Iwata K, Inayama T, Kato T. Effects of *Spirulina platensis* on plasma lipoprotein li-pase activity in fructose-induced hyperlipidemic rats. *J Nutr Sci Vitaminol*. 1990; 36:165-171.

114. Gonzalez de Rivera C, Miranda-Zamora R, Diaz-Zagoya JC, et al. Preventive effect of Spirulina maxima on the fatty liver induced by a fructose-rich diet in the rat, a preliminary report. *Life Sci*. 1993;53:57-61.

115. Nakaya N, Homma Y, Goto Y. Cholesterol lowering effect of spirulina. *Nutr Rep Int*. 1988;37:1329-1337.

116. Qureshi N, Qureshi AA. Tocotrienols: novel hypocholesterolemic agents with an-tioxidant properties. In: Packer L, Fuchs J, eds. *Vitamin E in Health and Disease*. New York: Dekker; 1993:247-267.

117. Qureshi AA, Sami SA, Salser WA, et al. Synergistic effect of tocotrienol-rich frac-tion (TRF 25) of rice bran and lovastatin on lipid parameters in hypercholes-terolemic humans. *J Nutr Biochem*. 2001;12:318-329.

118. Gaddi A, Descovich GC, Noseda G, et al. Controlled evaluation of pantethine, a natural hypolipidemic compound, in patients with different forms of hyper-lipoproteinemia. *Atherosclerosis*. 1984;50:73-83.

119. Rubba P, Postiglione A, DeSimone B, et al. Comparative evaluation of the lipid-lowering effects of fenofibrate and pantethine in type II hyperlipoproteinemia. *Curr Ther Res*. 1985;38:719-727.

120. Da Col PG, Cattin L, Fonda M, et al. Pantethine in the treatment of hypercholesterolemia: a randomized double-blind trial versus tiadenol. *Curr Ther Res.* 1984; 36:314-322.

121. Angelico M, Pinto G, Ciaccheri C, et al. Improvement in serum lipid profile in hyperlipoproteinaemic patients after treatment with pantethine: a crossover, double-blind trial versus placebo. *Curr Ther Res.* 1983;33:1091-1097.

122. Durrington PN, Bhatnagar D, Mackness MI, et al. An omega-3 polyunsaturated fatty acid concentrate administered for one year decreased triglycerides in simvastatin treated patients with coronary heart disease and persisting hypertriglyceridaemia. *Heart.* 2001;85:544-548.

123. van Dam M, Stalenhoef AF, Wittekoek J, et al. Efficacy of concentrated N-3 fatty acids in hypertriglyceridaemia: a comparison with gemfibrozil. *Clin Drug Invest.* 2001;21:175-181.

124. Han KK, Soares JM, Haidar MA et al. Benefits of soy isoflavone therapeutic regimen on menopausal symptoms. *Obstet Gynecol.* 2002;99(3):389-394

125. Dewell A, Hollenbeck CB, Bruce B. The effects of soy-derived phytoestrogens on serum lipids and lipoproteins in moderately hypercholesterolemic postmenopausal women. *J Clin Endocrinol Metab.* 2002;87:118-121.

126. Wojcicki J, Pawlik A, Samochowiec L, et al. Clinical evaluation of lecithin as a lipid-lowering agent. *Phytother Res.* 1995;9:597-599.

127. Kesaniemi YA, Grundy SM. Effects of dietary polyenylphosphatidylcholine on metabolism of cholesterol and triglycerides in hypertriglyceridemic patients. *Am J Clin Nutr.* 1986;43:98-107.

128. Childs MT, Bowlin JA, Ogilvie JT, et al. The contrasting effects of a dietary soya lecithin product and corn oil on lipoprotein lipids in normolipidemic and familial hypercholesterolemic subjects. *Atherosclerosis.* 198;38:217-228.

129. Greten H, Raetzer H, Schettler G, et al. The effect of polyunsaturated phosphatidylcholine on plasma lipids and fecal sterol excretion. *Atherosclerosis.* 1980; 36:81-88.

130. Knuiman JT, Beynen AC, Katan MB. Lecithin intake and serum cholesterol. *Am J Clin Nutr.* 1989;49:266-268.

131. Valette G, Sauvaire Y, Baccou JC, Ribes G. Hypocholesterolaemic effect of fenugreek seeds in dogs. *Atherosclerosis.* 1984;50:105-111.

132. Stark A, Madar Z. The effect of an ethanol extract derived from fenugreek (Trigonella foenum-graecum) on bile acid absorption and cholesterol levels in rats. *Br J Nutr.* 1993 Jan;69(1):277-287.

133. Sowmya P, Rajyalakshmi P. Hypocholesterolemic effect of germinated fenugreek seeds in human subjects. *Plant Foods Hum Nutr.* 1999;53(4):359-365.

134. Mirkin A, Mas R, Matinto M, et al Efficacy and tolerability of policosanol in hypercholesterolemic postmenopausal women. *Int. J Clin Pharm Res.* 2001;21:31-34.

135. Sauvaire Y, Ribes G, Baccou JC, et al. Implication of steroid saponins and sapogenins in the hypocholesterolemic effect of fenugreek. *Lipids.* 1991;26(3): 191-197.

136. Evans AJ, Hood RL, Oakenfull DG, et al. Relationship between structure and function of dietary fibre: a comparative study of the effects of three galactomannans on cholesterol metabolism in the rat. *Br J Nutr.* 1992;68(1):217-229.

137. Bhardwaj PK, Dasgupta DJ, Prashar BS, Kaushal SS. Control of hyperglycaemia and hyperlipidaemia by plant product. *J Assoc Physicians India.* 1994;42:333-335.

138. Pons P, Jimenez A, Rodriquez M, et al. Effects of policosanol in elderly hypercholesterolemic patients. *Curr Ther Res.* 1993;53:265-269.

139. Wuolijoki E, Hirvela T, Ylitalo P. Decrease in serum LDL cholesterol with microcrystalline chitosan. *Methods Find Exp Clin Pharmacol.* 1999;21:357-361.

140. Zardoya R, Tula L, Castano G, et al. Effects of policosanol on hypercholesterolemic patients with abnormal serum biochemical indicators of hepatic function. *Curr Ther Res.* 1996;57:568-577.

141. Tai TS, Sheu WH, Lee WJ, et al. Effect of chitosan on plasma lipoprotein concentrations in type 2 diabetic subjects with hypercholesterolemia [letter]. *Diabetes Care.* 2000;23:1703-1704.

142. Castano G, Mas R, Fernando JC, et al. Efficacy and tolerability of policosanol compared with lovastatin in patients with type II hypercholesterolemia and concomitant coronary risk factors. *Curr Ther Res.* 2000;61:137-146.

Hypertension

1. Chan P, Tomlinson B, Chen YJ, et al. A double-blind placebo-controlled study of the effectiveness and tolerability of oral stevioside in human hypertension. *Br J Clin Pharmacol.* 2000;50:215-220.
2. Kinghorn AD, Soejarto DD. Current status of stevioside as a sweetening agent for human use. *Econ Med Plant Res.* 1985;1:2-52.
3. Silagy CA, Neil HA. A meta-analysis of the effect of garlic on blood pressure. *J Hypertens.* 1994;12:463-468.
4. Auer W, Eiber A, Hertkorn E, et al. Hypertension and hyperlipidaemia: garlic helps in mild cases. *Br J Clin Pract Suppl.* 1990;69:3-6.
5. Singh R, Niaz M, Rastogi S, et al. Effect of hydrosoluble coenzyme Q10 on blood pressures and insulin resistance in hypertensive patients with coronary artery disease. *J Hum Hypertens.* 1999;13:203-208.
6. Digiesi V, Cantini F, Brodbeck B. Effect of coenzyme Q10 on essential arterial hypertension. *Curr Ther Res.* 1990;47:841-845.
7. Danysz A, Oledzka K, Bukowska-Kiliszek M. Influence of coenzyme Q-10 on the hypotensive effects of enalapril and nitrendipine in spontaneously hypertensive rats. *Pol J Pharmacol.* 1994;46:457-461.
8. Sanjuliani AF, de Abreu Fagundes VG, Francischetti EA. Effects of magnesium on blood pressure and intracellular ion levels of Brazilian hypertensive patients. *Int J Cardiol.* 1996;56:177-183.
9. Witteman JCM, Grobbee DE, Derkx FHM, et al. Reduction of blood pressure with oral magnesium supplementation in women with mild to moderate hypertension. *Am J Clin Nutr.* 1994;60:129-135.
10. Dyckner T, Wester PO. Effect of magnesium on blood pressure. *Br Med J (Clin Res Ed).* 1983;286:1847-1849.
11. Henderson DG, Schierup J, Schodt T. Effect of magnesium supplementation on blood pressure and electrolyte concentrations in hypertensive patients receiving long term diuretic treatment. *Br Med J (Clin Res Ed).* 1986;293:664-665.
12. Whelton PK, He J, Cutler JA, et al. Effects of oral potassium on blood pressure: meta-analysis of randomized controlled clinical trials. *JAMA.* 1997;277:1624-1632.
13. Gu D, He J, Wu X, et al. Effect of potassium supplementation on blood pressure in Chinese: a randomized, placebo-controlled trial. *J Hypertens.* 2001;19:1325-1331.
14. Whelton PK, Buring J, Borhani NO, et al. The effect of potassium supplementation in persons with a high-normal blood pressure: results from phase I of the Trials of Hypertension Prevention (TOHP). Trials of Hypertension Prevention (TOPH) Collaborative Research Group. *Ann Epidemiol.* 1995;5:85-95.
15. Davis BR, Oberman A, Blaufox MD, et al. Lack of effectiveness of a low-sodium/high-potassium diet in reducing antihypertensive medication requirements in overweight persons with mild hypertension. TAIM Research Group. Trial of Antihypertensive Interventions and Management. *Am J Hypertens.* 1994;7:926-932.
16. Cappuccio FP, Elliot P, Allender PS, et al. Epidemiologic association between dietary calcium intake and blood pressure: a meta-analysis of published data. *Am J Epidemiol.* 1995;142:935-945.
17. Van Leer EM, Seidell JC, Kromhout D. Dietary calcium, potassium, magnesium, and blood pressure in the Netherlands. *Int J Epidemiol.* 1995;24:1117-1123.
18. Bostick RM, Fosdick L, Grandits GA, et al. Effect of calcium supplementation on serum cholesterol and blood pressure: a randomized, double-blind, placebo-controlled, clinical trial. *Arch Fam Med.* 2000;9:31-39.
19. Lungershausen YK, Abbey M, Nestel PJ, et al. Reduction of blood pressure and plasma triglycerides by omega-3 fatty acids in treated hypertensives. *J Hypertens.* 1994;12:1041-1045.
20. Radack K, Deck C, Huster G. The effects of low doses of n-3 fatty acid supplements on blood pressure in hypertensive subjects. *Arch Intern Med.* 1991;151:1173-1180.

21. Singer P, Jaeger W, Wirth M, et al. Lipid and blood pressure-lowering effect of mackerel diet in man. *Atherosclerosis.* 1983;49:99-108.
22. Singer P, Melzer S, Goschel M, et al. Fish oil amplifies the effect of propranolol in mild essential hypertension. *Hypertension.* 1990;16:682-691.
23. Appel LJ, Miller ER III, Seidler AJ, et al. Does supplementation of diet with 'fish oil' reduce blood pressure? A meta-analysis of controlled clinical trials. *Arch Intern Med.* 1993;153:1429-1438.
24. Whelton PK, Kumanyika SK, Cook NR, et al. Efficacy of nonpharmacologic interventions in adults with high-normal blood pressure: results from phase 1 of the Trials of Hypertension Prevention. *Am J Clin Nutr.* 1997;65(suppl):S652-S660.
25. Mori TA, Bao DQ, Burke V, et al. Docosahexaenoic acid but not eicosapentaenoic acid lowers ambulatory blood pressure and heart rate in humans. *Hypertension.* 1999;34:253-260.
26. Duffy SJ, Gokce N, Holbrook M, et al. Treatment of hypertension with ascorbic acid [letter]. *Lancet.* 1999;354:2048.
27. Osilesi O, Trout DL, Ogunwole JO, et al. Blood pressure and plasma lipids during ascorbic acid supplementation in borderline hypertensive and normotensive adults. *Nutr Res.* 1991;11:405-412.
28. Fotherby MD, Williams JC, Forster LA, et al. Effect of vitamin C on ambulatory blood pressure and plasma lipids in older persons. *J Hypertens.* 2000;18:411-415.
29. Ghosh SK, Ekpo EB, Shah IU, et al. A double-blind, placebo-controlled parallel trial of vitamin C treatment in elderly patients with hypertension. *Gerontology.* 1994;40:268-272.
30. Lovat LB, Lu Y, Palmer AJ, et al. Double-blind trial of vitamin C in elderly hypertensives. *J Hum Hypertens.* 1993;7:403-405.
31. Arvill A, Bodin L. Effect of short-term ingestion of konjac glucomannan on serum cholesterol in healthy men. *Am J Clin Nutr.* 1995;61:585-589.
32. Reffo GC. Glucomannan in hypertensive outpatients: pilot clinical trial. *Curr Ther Res.* 1988;44:22-27.
33. Vuksan V, Jenkins DJ, Spadafora P, et al. Konjac-mannan (glucomannan) improves glycemia and other associated risk factors for coronary heart disease in type 2 diabetes: a randomized controlled metabolic trial. *Diabetes Care.* 1999;22:913-919.
34. Kato H, Taguchi T, Okuda H, et al. Antihypertensive effect of chitosan in rats and humans. *J Tradit Med.* 1994;11:198-205.
35. Haji Faraji M, Haji Tarkhani AH. The effect of sour tea *(Hibiscus sabdariffa)* on essential hypertension. *J Ethnopharmacol.* 1999;65:231-236.
36. Merchant RE, Andre CA. A review of recent clinical trials of the nutritional supplement *Chlorella pyrenoidosa* in the treatment of fibromyalgia, hypertension, and ulcerative colitis. *Altern Ther Health Med.* 2001;7:79-80, 82-91.
37. Chiu KW, Fung AY. The cardiovascular effects of green beans *(Phaseolus aureus)*, common rue *(Ruta graveolens)*, and kelp *(Laminaria japonica)* in rats. *Gen Pharmacol.* 1997;29:859-862.
38. Fuller KE, Casparian JM. Vitamin D: balancing cutaneous and systematic considerations. *South Med J.* 2001;94:58-64.
39. Rostand SG. Ultraviolet light may contribute to geographic and racial blood pressure differences. *Hypertension.* 1997;30(2 pt 1):150-156.
40. Krause R, Buhring M, Hopfenmuller W, et al. Ultraviolet B and blood pressure [letter]. *Lancet.* 1998;352:709-710.
41. Scragg R. Sunlight, vitamin D, and cardiovascular disease. In: Crass MF II, Avioli LV, eds. *Calcium Regulating Hormones and Cardiovascular Function.* Boca Raton, Fla: CRC Press; 1995:213-237.
42. O'Connell TD, Simpson RU. 1,25-dihydroxyvitamin D3 and cardiac muscle structure and function. In: Crass MF II, Avioli LV, eds. *Calcium-Regulating Hormones and Cardiovascular Function.* Boca Raton, Fla: CRC Press; 1995:191-211.
43. Burke BE, Neuenschwander R, Olson RD. Randomized, double-blind, placebo-controlled trial of coenzyme Q10 in isolated systolic hypertension. *South Med J.* 2001;94:1112-1117.

Infertility (Female)

1. Propping D, Katzorke T, Belkien L. Diagnosis and therapy of corpus luteum deficiency in general practice [translated from German]. *Therapiewoche.* 1988;38: 2992-3001.
2. Gerhard I, Patek A, Monga B, et al. Mastodynon® for female infertility [in German; English abstract]. *Forsch Komplementarmed.* 1998;5:272-278.
3. Czeizel A, Metnek J, Dudas I. The effect of preconceptional multivitamin supplementation on fertility. *Int J Vitam Nutr Res.* 1996;66:55-58.
4. Thys-Jacobs S, Donovan D, Papadopoulos A, et al. Vitamin D and calcium dysregulation in the polycystic ovarian syndrome. *Steroids.* 1999;64:430-435.

Infertility (Male)

1. Armanini D, Bonanni G, Palermo M. Reduction of serum testosterone in men by licorice [letter]. *N Engl J Med.* 1999;341:1158.
2. Suleiman SA, Ali EM, Zaki ZMS, et al. Lipid peroxidation and human sperm motility: protective role of vitamin E. *J Androl.* 1996;17:530-537.
3. Rolf C, Cooper T, Yeung C, et al. Antioxidant treatment of patients with asthenozoospermia of moderate oligoasthenozoospermia with high-dose vitamin C and vitamin E: a randomized, placebo-controlled, double-blind study. *Hum Reprod.* 1999; 14:1028-1033.
4. Conquer JA, Martin JB, Tummon I, et al. Effect of DHA supplementation on DHA status and sperm motility in asthenozoospermic males. *Lipids.* 2000;35:149-154.
5. Saltzman JR, Kemp JA, Golner BB, et al. Effect of hypochlorhydria due to omeprazole treatment or atrophic gastritis on protein-bound vitamin B12 absorption. *J Am Coll Nutr.* 1994;13:584-591.
6. van Goor L, Woiski MD, Lagaay AM, et al. Review: cobalamin deficiency and mental impairment in elderly people. *Age Ageing.* 1995;24:536-542.
7. Pennypacker LC, Allen RH, Kelly JP, et al. High prevalence of cobalamin deficiency in elderly outpatients. *J Am Geriatr Soc.* 1992;40:1197-1204.
8. Yao Y, Yao SL, Yao SS, et al. Prevalence of vitamin B12 deficiency among geriatric outpatients. *J Fam Pract.* 1992;35:524-528.
9. Kumamoto Y, Maruta H, Ishigami J, et al. Clinical efficacy of mecobalamin in treatment of oligozoospermia: results of double-blind comparative clinical study [in Japanese; English abstract]. *Hinyokika Kiyo.* 1988;34:1109-1132.
10. Costa M, Canale D, Filicori M, et al. L-carnitine in idiopathic asthenozoospermia: a multicenter study. Italian Study Group on Carnitine and Male Infertility. *Andrologia.* 1994;26:155-159.
11. Vitali G, Parente R, Melotti C. Carnitine supplementation in human idiopathic asthenospermia: clinical results. *Drugs Exp Clin Res.* 1995;21:157-159.
12. Dawson EB, Harris WA, Rankin WE, et al. Effect of ascorbic acid on male fertility. *Ann NY Acad Sci.* 1987;498:312-323.
13. Wong WY, Merkus HM, Thomas CM, et al. Effects of folic acid and zinc sulfate on male factor subfertility: a double-blind, randomized, placebo-controlled trial. *Fertil Steril.* 2002;77:491-498.
14. Salvati G, Genovesi G, Marcellini L, et al. Effects of Panax Ginseng C.A. Meyer saponins on male fertility. *Panminerva Med.* 1996;38;249-254.
15. Loumbakis P, Anezinis P, Evangeliou A, et al. Effect of L-carnitine in patients with asthenospermia [abstract]. *Eur Urol.* 1996;30(suppl 2):255.
16. Muller-Tyl E, Lohninger A, Fischl F, et al. The effect of carnitine on sperm count and sperm motility [translated from German]. *Fertilitat.* 1988;4:1-4.
17. Micic S, Lalic N, Nale DJ, et al. Effects of L-carnitine on sperm motility and number in infertile men [abstract]. *Fertil Steril.* 1998;70(3 suppl 1):S12.
18. Campaniello E, Petrarolo N, Meriggiola MC, et al. Carnitine administration in asthenospermia. Presented at: 4th International Congress of Andrology; May 14-18, 1989; Florence, Italy.

19. Vicari E, Cerri L, Cataldo T, et al. Effectiveness of single and combined antioxidant therapy in patients with astheno-necrozoospermia from non-bacterial epididymitis: effects after acetyl-carnitine or carnitine-acetyl-carnitine. Presented at: 12th National Conference of the Italian Andrology Assoc.; 1999.

Injuries (Minor)

1. Baumuller M. The application of hydrolytic enzymes in blunt wounds to the soft tissue and distortion of the ankle joint: a double-blind clinical trial [translated from German]. *Allgemeinmedizin.* 1990;19:178-182.
2. Zuschlag JM. *Double-blind clinical study using certain proteolytic enzyme mixtures in karate fighters.* Gerestsried, Germany: Mucos Pharma GmbH; 1988.
3. Rathgeber WF. The use of proteolytic enzymes (chymoral) in sporting injuries. *S Afr Med J.* 1971;45:181-183.
4. Deitrick RE. Oral proteolytic enzymes in the treatment of athletic injuries: a double-blind study. *Pa Med.* 1965;68:35-37.
5. Kleine MW, Pabst H. The effect of an oral enzyme therapy on experimentally produced hematomas [translated from German]. *Forum des Prakt und Allgemeinarztes.* 1988;27:42, 45-46, 48.
6. Shaw PC. The use of a trypsin-chymotrypsin formulation in fractures of the hand. *Br J Clin Pract.* 1969;23:25-26.
7. Blonstein JL. Control of swelling in boxing injuries. *Practitioner.* 1969;203:206.
8. Parienti JJ, Parienti-Amsellem J. Post traumatic edemas in sports: a controlled test of Endotelon® [translated from French]. *Gaz Med Fr.* 1983;90:231-235.
9. Calabrese C, Preston P. Report of the results of a double-blind, randomized, single-dose trial of a topical 2% escin gel versus placebo in the acute treatment of experimentally-induced hematoma in volunteers. *Planta Med.* 1993;59:394-397.
10. Miller MJ. Injuries to athletes: evaluation of ascorbic acid and water soluble citrus bioflavonoids in the prophylaxis of injuries in athletes. *Med Times.* 1960;88:313-316.

Insomnia

1. Vorbach EU, Goetelmeyer R, Bruening J. Therapy for insomniacs: effectiveness and tolerance of valerian preparations [translated from German]. *Psychopharmakotherapie.* 1996;3:109-115.
2. Leathwood PD, Chauffard F, Heck E, et al. Aqueous extract of valerian root (*Valeriana officinalis* L.) improves sleep quality in man. *Pharmacol Biochem Behav.* 1982;17:65-71.
3. Kamm-Kohl AV, Jansen W, Brockmann P. Modern valerian therapy for nervous disorders in old age [translated from German]. *Med Welt.* 1984;35:1450-1454.
4. Lindahl O, Lindwall L. Double blind study of a valerian preparation. *Pharmacol Biochem Behav.* 1989;32:1065-1066.
5. Schulz H, Stolz C, Muller J. The effect of valerian extract on sleep polygraphy in poor sleepers: a pilot study. *Pharmacopsychiatry.* 1994;27:147-151.
6. Donath F, Quispe S, Diefenbach K. Critical evaluation of the effect of valerian extract on sleep structure and sleep quality. *Pharmacopsychiatry.* 2000;33:47-53.
7. Dorn M. Efficacy and tolerability of Baldrian versus oxazepam in non-organic and non-psychiatric insomnias: a randomized, double-blind, clinical, comparative study [translated from German]. *Forsch Komplementarmed Klass Naturheilkd.* 2000;7:79-84.
8. Cerny A, Schmid K. Tolerability and efficacy of valerian/lemon balm in healthy volunteers (a double-blind, placebo-controlled, multicentre study). *Fitoterapia.* 1999;70:221-228.
9. Schmitz M, Jackel M. Comparative study for assessing quality of life of patients with exogenous sleep disorders (temporary sleep onset and sleep interruption disorders) treated with a hops-valarian preparation and a benzodiazepine drug [translated from German]. *Wien Med Wochenschr.* 1998;148:291-298.
10. Dressing H, Riemann D, Low H, et al. Insomnia: are valerian/balm combinations of equal value to benzodiazepines? [translated from German]. *Therapiewoche.* 1992; 42:726-736.

11. Suhner A, Schlagenhauf P, Johnson R, et al. Comparative study to determine the optimal melatonin dosage form for the alleviation of jet lag. *Chronobiol Int.* 1998;15:655-666.

12. Petrie K, Dawson AG, Thompson L, et al. A double-blind trial of melatonin as a treatment for jet lag in international cabin crew. *Biol Psychiatry.* 1993;33:526-530.

13. Petrie K, Conaglen JV, Thompson L, et al. Effect of melatonin on jet lag after long haul flights. *BMJ.* 1989;298:705-707.

14. Arendt J, Aldhous M. Further evaluation of the treatment of jet-lag by melatonin: a double-blind crossover study. *Annu Rev Chronopharmacol.* 1988;5:53-55.

15. Claustrat B, Brun J, David M, et al. Melatonin and jet lag: confirmatory result using a simplified protocol. *Biol Psychiatry.* 1992;32:705-711.

16. Spitzer RL, Terman M, Williams JB, et al. Jet lag: clinical features, validation of a new syndrome-specific scale, and lack of response to melatonin in a randomized, double-blind trial. *Am J Psychiatry.* 1999;156:1392-1396.

17. Edwards BJ, Atkinson G, Waterhouse J, et al. Use of melatonin in recovery from jet-lag following an eastward flight across 10 time zones. *Ergonomics.* 2000;43: 1501-1513.

18. Suhner A, Schlagenhauf P, Hofer I, et al. Effectiveness and tolerability of melatonin and zolpidem for the alleviation of jet lag. *Aviat Space Environ Med.* 2001;72:638-646.

19. Smits MG, Nagtegaal EE, van der Heijden J, et al. Melatonin for chronic sleep onset insomnia in children: a randomized placebo-controlled trial. *J Child Neurol.* 2001;16:86-92.

20. Dodge NN, Wilson GA. Melatonin for treatment of sleep disorders in children with developmental disabilities. *J Child Neurol.* 2001;16:581-584.

21. Yang CM, Spielman AJ, D'Ambrosio P, et al. A single dose of melatonin prevents the phase delay associated with a delayed weekend sleep pattern. *Sleep.* 2001;24: 272-281.

22. Garfinkel D, Zisapel N, Wainstein J, et al. Faciliation of benzodiazepine discontinuation by melatonin:a new clinical approach. *Arch Intern Med.* 1999;159:2456-2460.

23. Kayumov L, Brown G, Jindal R, et al. A randomized, double-blind, placebo-controlled crossover study of the effect of exogenous melatonin on delayed sleep phase syndrome. *Psychosom Med.* 2001;63:40-48.

24. Zhdanova IV, Wurtman RJ, Regan MM, et al. Melatonin treatment for age-related insomnia. *J Clin Endocrinol Metab.* 2001;86:4727-4730.

25. Shilo L, Dagan Y, Smorjik Y. Effect of melatonin on sleep quality of COPD intensive care patients: a pilot study. *Chronobiol Int.* 2000;17:71-76.

26. Shamir E, Laudon M, Barak Y, et al. Melatonin improves sleep quality of patients with chronic schizophrenia. *J Clin Psychiatry.* 2000;61:373-377.

27. MacFarlane JG, Cleghorn JM, Brown GM, et al. The effects of exogenous melatonin on the total sleep time and daytime alertness of chronic insomniacs: a preliminary study. *Biol Psychiatry.* 1991;30:371-376.

28. James SP, Sack DA, Rosenthal NE, et al. Melatonin administration in insomnia. *Neuropsychopharmacology.* 1990;3:19-23.

29. Garfinkel D, Laudon M, Zisapel N. Improvement of sleep quality by controlled-release melatonin in benzodiazepine-treated elderly insomniacs. *Arch Gerontol Geriatr.* 1997;24:223-231.

30. Folkard S, Arendt J, Clark M. Can melatonin improve shift workers' tolerance of the night shift? Some preliminary findings. *Chronobiol Int.* 1993;10:315-320.

31. Dawson D, Encel N, Lushington K. Improving adaptation to simulated night shift: timed exposure to bright light versus daytime melatonin administration. *Sleep.* 1995;18:11-21.

32. Wright SW, Lawrence LM, Wrenn KD, et al. Randomized clinical trial of melatonin after night-shift work: efficacy and neuropsychologic effects. *Ann Emerg Med.* 1998;32:334-340.

33. Jan JE, Hamilton D, Seward N, et al. Clinical trials of controlled-release melatonin in children with sleep-wake cycle disorders. *J Pineal Res.* 2000;29:34-39.

34. Schulz H, Jobert M. The influence of hypericum extract on the sleep EEG in older volunteers [in German; English abstract]. *Nervenheilkunde*. 1993;12:323-327.

35. Paul MA, Brown G, Buguet A, et al. Melatonin and zopiclone as pharmacologic aids to facilitate crew rest. *Aviat Space Environ Med*. 2001;72:974-984.

36. Suhner A, Schlagenhauf P, Hofer I, et al. Effectiveness and tolerability of melatonin and zolpidem for the alleviation of jet lag *Aviat Space Environ Med*. 2001;72:638-646.

37. Chase JE, Gidal BE. Melatonin: therapeutic use in sleep disorders. *Ann Pharmacother*. 1997;31:1218-1226.

38. Sharkey KM, Fogg LF, Eastman CI. Effects of melatonin administration on daytime sleep after simulated night shift work. *J Sleep Res*. 2001;10:181-192.

39. Haimov I, Lavie P, Laudon M, et al. Melatonin replacement therapy of elderly insomniacs. *Sleep*. 1995;18:598-603.

40. Hughes RJ, Sack RL, Lewy AJ. The role of melatonin and circadian phase in age-related sleep-maintenance insomnia: assessment in a clinical trial of melatonin replacement. *Sleep*. 1998;21:52-68.

41. Garfinkel D, Laudon M, Nof D, et al. Improvement of sleep quality in elderly people by controlled-release melatonin. *Lancet*. 1995;346:541-544.

Intermittent Claudication

1. Pittler MH, Ernst E. *Ginkgo biloba* extract for the treatment of intermittent claudication: a meta-analysis of randomized trials. *Am J Med*. 2000;108:276-281.

2. Peters H, Kieser M, Holscher U. Demonstration of the efficacy of *Ginkgo biloba* special extract EGb 761 on intermittent claudication: a placebo-controlled, double-blind multicenter trial. *Vasa*. 1998;27:106-110.

3. Blume J, Kieser M, Holscher U. Placebo-controlled double-blind study of the effectiveness of *Ginkgo biloba* special extract EGb 761 in trained patients with intermittent claudication [translated from German]. *Vasa*. 1996;25:265-274.

4. Schweizer J, Hautmann C. Comparison of two dosages of *Ginkgo biloba* extract EGb 761 in patients with peripheral arterial occlusive disease Fontaine's stage IIb. A randomized, double-blind, multicentric clinical trial. *Arzneimittelforschung*. 1999;49:900-904.

5. O'Hara J, Jolly PN, Nicol CG. The therapeutic efficacy of inositol nicotinate (Hexopal) in intermittent claudication: a controlled trial. *Br J Clin Pract*. 1988;42:377-383.

6. Kiff RS, Quick CR. Does inositol nicotinate (Hexopal) influence intermittent claudication? A controlled trial. *Br J Clin Pract*. 1988;42:141-145.

7. Head A. Treatment of intermittent claudication with inositol nicotinate. *Practitioner*. 1986;230:49-54.

8. Tyson VC. Treatment of intermittent claudication. *Practitioner*. 1979;223:121-126.

9. Brevetti G, Diehm C, Lambert D. European multicenter study on propionyl-L-carnitine in intermittent claudication. *J Am Coll Cardiol*. 1999;34:1618-1624.

10. Brevetti G, Perna S, Sabba C, et al. Propionyl-L-carnitine in intermittent claudication: double-blind, placebo-controlled, dose titration, multicenter study. *J Am Coll Cardiol*. 1995;26:1411-1416.

11. Thal LJ, Calvani M, Amato A, et al. A 1-year controlled trial of acetyl-L-carnitine in early-onset AD. *Neurology*. 2000;55:805-810.

12. Bolognesi M, Amodio P, Merkel C, et al. Effect of 8-day therapy with propionyl-L-carnitine on muscular and subcutaneous blood flow of the lower limbs in patients with peripheral arterial disease. *Clin Physiol*. 1995;15:417-423.

13. Brevetti G, Perna S, Sabba C, et al. Superiority of L-propionylcarnitine vs L-carnitine in improving walking capacity in patients with peripheral vascular disease: an acute, intravenous, double-blind, cross-over study. *Eur Heart J*. 1992;13:251-255.

14. Greco AV, Mingrone G, Bianchi M, et al. Effect of propionyl-L-carnitine in the treatment of diabetic angiopathy: controlled double blind trial versus placebo. *Drugs Exp Clin Res*. 1992;18:69-80.

15. Brevetti G, Chiariello M, Ferulano G, et al. Increases in walking distance in patients with peripheral vascular disease treated with L-carnitine: a double-blind, cross-over study. *Circulation*. 1988;77:767-773.

16. Deckert J. Propionyl-L-carnitine for intermittent claudication. *J Fam Pract.* 1997;44:533-534.
17. Sabba C, Berardi E, Antonica G, et al. Comparison between the effect of L-propi-onylcarnitine, L-acetylcarnitine and nitroglycerin in chronic peripheral arterial disease: a hemodynamic double blind echo-Doppler study. *Eur Heart J.* 1994;15:1348-1352.
18. Pepine CJ. The therapeutic potential of carnitine in cardiovascular disorders. *Clin Ther.* 1991;13:2-21.
19. Brevetti G, Attisano T, Perna S, et al. Effect of L-carnitine on the reactive hyperemia in patients affected by peripheral vascular disease: a double-blind, crossover study. *Angiology.* 1989;40:857-862.
20. Hiatt WR, Regensteiner JG, Creager MA, et al. Propionyl-L-carnitine improves exercise performance and functional status in patients with claudication. *Am J Med.* 2001;110:616-622.
21. Castano G, Mas Ferreiro R, Fernandez L, et al. A long-term study of policosanol in the treatment of intermittent claudication. *Angiology.* 2001;52:115-125.
22. Castano G, Mas R, Roca J, et al. A double-blind, placebo-controlled study of the effects of policosanol in patients with intermittent claudication. *Angiology.* 1999;50:123-130.
23. Maxwell A, Anderson B, Cooke JP. Improvement in walking distance and quality of life in peripheral arterial disease by a nutritional product designed to enhance nitric oxide activity [abstract]. *J Am Coll Cardiol.* 1999;33(2 suppl A):277A.
24. Tornwall ME, Virtamo J, Haukka JK, et al. The effect of alpha-tocopherol and beta-carotene supplementation on symptoms and progression of intermittent claudication in a controlled trial. *Atherosclerosis.* 1999;147:193-197.
25. Nenci GG, Gresele P, Ferrari G, et al. Treatment of intermittent claudication with mesoglycan: a placebo-controlled, double-blind study. *Thromb Haemost.* 2001;86:1181-1187.

Interstitial Cystitis

1. Boger RH, Bode-Boger SM, Thiele W, et al. Restoring vascular nitric oxide formation by L-arginine improves the symptoms of intermittent claudication in patients with peripheral arterial occlusive disease. *J Am Coll Cardiol.* 1998;32:1336-1344.
2. Chen J, Wollman Y, Chernichovsky T, et al. Effect of oral administration of high-dose nitric oxide donor L-arginine in men with organic erectile dysfunction: results of a double-blind, randomized placebo-controlled study. *BJU Int.* 1999;83:269-273.
3. Kilroy RA, et al. Acid-base disorders. In: DiPiro JT, et al, eds. *Pharmacotherapy: A Pathophysiologic Approach.* 4th ed. Stamford, Conn: Appleton and Lange; 1999:931.
4. Korting GE, Smith SD, Wheeler MA, et al. A randomized double-blind trial of oral L-arginine for treatment of interstitial cystitis. *J Urol.* 1999;161:558-565.
5. Cartledge JJ, Davies AM, Eardley I. A randomized double-blind placebo-controlled crossover trial of the efficacy of L-arginine in the treatment of interstitial cystitis. *BJU Int.* 2000;85:421-426.
6. Ehren I, Lundberg JO, Adolfsson J, et al. Effects of L-arginine treatment on symptoms and bladder nitric oxide levels in patients with interstitial cystitis. *Urology.* 1998;52:1026-1029.
7. Rodriguez LV, Janzen N, Raz S, et al. Treatment of interstitial cystitis with a quercetin containing compound: a preliminary, double-blind placebo control trial. Presented at: American Urological Association 2001 Annual Meeting; June 2-7, 2001; Anaheim, Calif.
8. Hurst RE, Roy JB, Min RW, et al. A deficit of chondroitin sulfate proteoglycans on the bladder uroepithelium in interstitial cystitis. *Urology.* 1996;48:817-821.

Irritable Bowel Syndrome (IBS)

1. Gunn JWC. The carminative action of volatile oils. *J Pharmacol Exp Ther.* 1920;16:39-47.
2. Taylor BA, Luscombe DK, Duthie HL. Inhibitory effect of peppermint oil an gastro-intestinal smooth muscle [abstract]. *Gut.* 1983;24:A992.

3. Hawthorn M, Ferrante J, Luchowski E, et al. The actions of peppermint oil and menthol on calcium channel dependent processes in intestinal, neuronal, and cardiac preparations. *Aliment Pharmacol Ther.* 1988;2:101-118.

4. Somerville KW, Ellis WR, Whitten BH, et al. Stones in the common bile duct: experience with medical dissolution therapy. *Postgrad Med J.* 1985;61:313-316.

5. Rees WD, Evans BK, Rhodes J. Treating irritable bowel syndrome with peppermint oil. *Br Med J.* 1979;2:835-836.

6. Dew MJ, Evans BK, Rhodes J. Peppermint oil for the irritable bowel syndrome: a multicentre trial. *Br J Clin Pract.* 1984;38:394,398.

7. Liu JH, Chen GH, Yeh HZ. Enteric-coated peppermint-oil capsules in the treatment of irritable bowel syndrome: a prospective, randomized trial. *J Gastroenterol.* 1997;32:765-768.

8. Nash P, Gould SR, Barnardo DE. Peppermint oil does not relieve the pain of irritable bowel syndrome. *Br J Clin Pract.* 1986;40:292-293.

9. Lawson MJ, Knight RE, Tran K, et al. Failure of enteric-coated peppermint oil in the irritable bowel syndrome: a randomized, double-blind crossover study. *J Gastroenterol Hepatol.* 1988;3:235-238.

10. Carling L, Svedberg LE, Hulten S, et al. Short-term treatment of the irritable bowel syndrome: a placebo-controlled trial of peppermint oil against hyoscyaminme. *Opusc Med.* 1989;34:55-57.

11. Kline RM, Kline JJ, Di Palma J, et al. Enteric-coated, pH-dependent peppermint oil capsules for the treatment of irritable bowel syndrome in children. *J Pediatr.* 2001;138:125-128.

12. O'Sullivan MA, et al. Bacterial supplementaion in the irritable bowel syndrome: a randomized double-blind placebo-controlled crossover study. *Digest Liver Dis.* 2000;32:294-301.

13. Nobaek S, Johansson M-L, Molin G, et al. Alteration of intestinal microflora is associated with reduction in abdominal bloating and pain in patients with irritable bowel syndrome. *Am J Gastroenterol.* 2000;95:1231-1238.

14. Halpern GM, Prindiville T, Blankenburg M, et al. Treatment of irritable bowel syndrome with Lacteol Fort®: a randomized, double-blind, cross-over trial. *Am J Gastroenterol.* 1996;91:1579-1585.

15. Smith MA, Youngs GR, Finn R. Food intolerance, atopy, and irritable bowel syndrome [letter]. *Lancet.* 1985;2:1064.

16. Pittler M H, Ernst E. Peppermint oil for irritable bowel syndrome: a critical review and meta-analysis. *Am J Gastroenterol* 1998;93:1131-1135.

17. Niedzielin K, Kordecki H, Birkenfeld B. A controlled, double-blind, randomized study on the efficacy of Lactobacillus plantarum 299V in patients with irritable bowel syndrome. *Eur J Gastroenterol Hepatol.* 2001;13:1143-1147.

Macular Degeneration

1. Newsome DA, Swartz M, Leone NC, et al. Oral zinc in macular degeneration. *Arch Ophthalmol.* 1988;106:192-198.

2. Stur M, Tittl M, Reitner A, et al. Oral zinc and the second eye in age-related macular degeneration. *Invest Ophthalmol Vis Sci.* 1996;37:1225-1235.

3. Mares-Perlman JA, Klein R, Klein BEK, et al. Relationships between age-related maculopathy and intake of vitamin and mineral supplements [abstract]. *Invest Ophthalmol Vis Sci.* 1993;34:1133.

4. Mares-Perlman JA, Klein R, Klein BEK, et al. Association of zinc and antioxidant nutrients with age-related maculopathy. *Arch Ophthalmol.* 1996;114:991-997.

5. Seddon JM, Ajani UA, Sperduto RD, et al. Dietary carotenoids, vitamins A,C, and E, and advanced age-related macular degeneration. *JAMA.* 1994;272:1413-1420.

6. Mares-Perlman JA, Brady WE, Klein R, et al. Serum antioxidants and age-related macular degeneration in a population-based case-control study. *Arch Ophthalmol.* 1995;113:1518-1523.

7. Snodderly DM. Evidence for protection against age-related macular degeneration by carotenoids and antioxidant vitamins. *Am J Clin Nutr.* 1995;62(suppl):1448S-1461S.

8. Age Related Macular Degeneration Study Group. Multicenter ophthalmic and nutritional age-related macular degeneration study, part 2: antioxidant intervention and conclusions. *J Am Optom Assoc.* 1996;67:30-49.
9. Lebuisson DA, Leroy L, Rigal G. Treatment of senile macular degeneration with *Ginkgo biloba* extract: a preliminary double-blind, drug versus placebo study [translated from French]. *Presse Med.* 1986;15:1556-1558.
10. Landrum JT, Bone RA, Kilburn MD. The macular pigment: a possible role in protection from age-related macular degeneration. *Adv Pharmacol.* 1997;38:537-556.
11. Hammond BR Jr, Wooten BR, Snodderly DM. Density of the human crystalline lens is related to the macular pigment carotenoids, lutein and zeaxanthin. *Optom Vis Sci.* 1997;74:499-504.
12. Mares-Perlman JA, Fisher AI, Klein R, et al. Lutein and zeaxanthin in the diet and serum and their relation to age-related maculopathy in the third national health and nutrition examination survey. *Am J Epidemiol.* 2001;153:424-432.
13. Age-Related Eye Disease Study Research Group. A randomized placebo-controlled clinical trial of high-dose supplementation with vitamins C and E beta carotene and zinc for age-related macular degeneration and vision loss: AREDS Report no. 8. *Arch Ophthalmol.* 2001;119:1417-1436.

Menopausal Syndrome

1. Albertazzi P, Pansini F, Bonaccorsi G, et al. The effect of dietary soy supplementation on hot flushes. *Obstet Gynecol.* 1998;91:6-11.
2. Brzezinski A, Adlercreutz H, Shaoul R, et al. Short-term effects of phytoestrogen-rich diet on postmenopausal women. *Menopause.* 1997;4:89-94.
3. Scambia G, Mango D, Signorile PG, et al. Clinical effects of a standardized soy extract in postmenopausal women: a pilot study. *Menopause.* 2000;7:105-111.
4. Washburn S, Burke GL, Morgan T, et al. Effect of soy protein supplementation on serum lipoproteins, blood pressure, and menopausal symptoms in perimenopausal women. *Menopause.* 1999;6:7-13.
5. St. Germain A, Peterson CT, Robinson JG, et al. Isoflavone-rich or isoflavone-poor soy protein does not reduce menopausal symptoms during 24 weeks of treatment. *Menopause.* 2001;8:17-26.
6. Van Patten CL, Olivotto IA, Chambers GK, et al. Effect of soy phytoestrogens on hot flashes in postmenopausal women with breast cancer: a randomized, controlled clinical trial. *J Clin Oncol.* 2002;20:1449-1455.
7. Baber RJ, Templeman C, Morton T, et al. Randomized placebo-controlled trial of an isoflavone supplement and menopausal symptoms in women. *Climacteric.* 1999; 2:85-92.
8. Knight DC, Howes JB, Eden JA. The effect of Promensil™, an isoflavone extract, on menopausal symptoms. *Climacteric.* 1999;2:79-84.
9. Leonetti HB, Longo S, Anasti JN. Transdermal progesterone cream for vasomotor symptoms and postmenopausal bone loss. *Obstet Gynecol.* 1999;94:225-228.
10. Takahashi K, Manabe A, Okada M, et al. Efficacy and safety of oral estriol for managing postmenopausal symptoms. *Maturitas.* 2000;34:169-177.
11. Minaguchi H, Uemura T, Shirasu K, et al. Effect of estriol on bone loss in postmenopausal Japanese women: a multicenter prospective open study. *J Obstet Gynaecol Res.* 1996;22:259-265.
12. Itoi H, Minakami H, Sato I. Comparison of the long-term effects of oral estriol with the effects of conjugated estrogen, 1-alpha-hydroxyvitamin D3 and calcium lactate on vertebral bone loss in early menopausal women. *Maturitas.* 1997;28:11-17.
13. Hayashi T, Ito I, Kano H, et al. Estriol (E3) replacement improves endothelial function and bone mineral density in very elderly women. *J Gerontol A Biol Sci Med Sci.* 2000;55:B183-B190.
14. Dugal R, Hesla K, Sordal T, et al. Comparison of usefulness of estradiol vaginal tablets and estriol vagitories for treatment of vaginal atrophy. *Acta Obstet Gynecol Scand.* 2000;79:293-297.
15. Raz R, Stamm WE. A controlled trial of intravaginal estriol in postmenopausal women with recurrent urinary tract infections. *N Engl J Med.* 1993;329:753-756.

16. van der Linden MC, Gerretsen G, Brandhorst MS, et al. The effect of estriol on the cytology of urethra and vagina in postmenopausal women with genito-urinary symptoms. *Eur J Obstet Gynecol Reprod Biol.* 1993;51:29-33.

17. Holland EF, Leather AT, Studd JW. Increase in bone mass of older postmenopausal women with low mineral bone density after one year of percutaneous oestradiol implants. *Br J Obstet Gynaecol.* 1995;102:238-242.

18. Nozaki M, Hashimoto K, Inoue Y, et al. Usefulness of estriol for the treatment of bone loss in postmenopausal women [in Japanese; English abstract]. *Nippon Sanka Fujinka Gakkai Zasshi.* 1996;48:83-88.

19. Granberg S, Ylostalo P, Wikland M, et al. Endometrial sonographic and histologic findings in women with and without hormonal replacement therapy suffering from postmenopausal bleeding. *Maturitas.* 1997;27:35-40.

20. Weiderpass E, Baron JA, Adami HO, et al. Low-potency estrogen and risk of endometrial cancer: a case-control study. *Lancet.* 1999;353:1824-1828.

21. Montoneri C, Zarbo G, Garofalo A, et al. Effects of estriol administration on human postmenopausal endometrium. *Clin Exp Obstet Gynecol.* 1987;14:178-181.

22. Lippman M, Monaco ME, Bolan G. Effects of estrone, estradiol, and estriol on hormone-responsive human breast cancer in long-term tissue culture. *Cancer Res.* 1977;37:1901-1907.

23. Stoll W. Phythopharmacon influences atrophic vaginal epithelium. Double-blind study: *Cimicifuga* vs. estrogenic substances [translated from German]. *Therapeutikon.* 1987;1:23-26,28,30-31.

24. Jarry H, Harnischfeger G. Studies on the endocrine effects of the contents of *Cimicifuga racemosa:* 1. Influence on the serum concentrations of pituitary hormones in ovariectomized rats [translated from German]. *Planta Med.* 1985;(1):46-49.

25. Jarry H, Harnischfeger G, Duker E. The endocrine effects of constituents of *Cimicifuga racemosa.* 2. In vitro binding of constituents to estrogen receptors [translated from German]. *Planta Med.* 1985;(4):316-319.

26. Duker EM, Kopanski L, Jarry H, et al. Effects of extracts from *Cimicifuga racemosa* on gonadotropin release in menopausal women and ovariectomized rats. *Planta Med.* 1991;57:420-424.

27. Liske E. Therapeutic efficacy and safety of *Cimicifuga racemosa* for gynecologic disorders. *Adv Ther.* 1998;15:45-53.

28. Einer-Jensen N, Zhao J, Andersen KP, et al. *Cimicifuga* and *Melbrosia* lack oestrogenic effects in mice and rats. *Maturitas.* 1996;25:149-153.

29. Jacobson JS, Troxel AB, Evans J, et al. Randomized trial of black cohosh for the treatment of hot flashes among women with a history of breast cancer. *J Clin Oncol.* 2001;19:2739-2745.

30. Warnecke G. Influencing menopausal symptoms with a phytotherapeutic agent [in German]. *Med Welt.* 1985;36:871-874.

31. Stolze H. An alternative to treat menopausal complaints [translated from German]. *Gyne.* 1982;1:14-16.

32. Lehmann-Willenbrock VE, Riedel H-H. Clinical and endocrinologic examinations about therapy of climacteric symptoms following hysterectomy with remaining ovaries [in German; English abstract]. *Zentralbl Gynakol.* 1988;110:611-618.

33. MacLennan A, Lester S, Moore V. Oral estrogen replacement therapy versus placebo for hot flushes: a systematic review. *Climacteric.* 2001;4:58-74.

34. Wiklund IK, Mattsson LA, Lindgren R, et al. Effects of a standardized ginseng extract on quality of life and physiological parameters in symptomatic postmenopausal women: a double-blind, placebo-controlled trial. *Int J Clin Pharmacol Res.* 1999; 19:89-99.

35. Barton DL, Loprinzi CL, Quella SK, et al. Prospective evaluation of vitamin E for hot flashes in breast cancer survivors. *J Clin Oncol.* 1998;16:495-500.

36. Hirata JD, Swiersz LM, Zell B, et al. Does dong quai have estrogenic effects in postmenopausal women? A double-blind, placebo controlled trial. *Fertil Steril.* 1997; 68:981-986.

37. Kotsopoulos D, Dalais FS, Liang YL, et al. The effects of soy protein containing phytoestrogens on menopausal symptoms in postmenopausal women. *Climacteric.* 2000;3:161-167.

Migraine Headaches

1. Murphy JJ, Heptinstall S, Mitchell JR. Randomized double-blind placebo-controlled trial of feverfew in migraine prevention. *Lancet.* 1988;23:189-192.
2. Palevitch DG, Earon G, Carasso R. Feverfew *(Tanacetum parthenium)* as a prophylactic treatment for migraine: a double-blind placebo-controlled study. *Phytother Res.* 1997;11:508-511.
3. Johnson ES, Kadam NP, Hylands DM, et al. Efficacy of feverfew as prophylactic treatment of migraine. *Br Med J (Clin Res Ed).* 1985;291:569-573.
4. De Weerdt CJ, Bootsma HPR, Hendriks H. Herbal medicines in migraine prevention: randomized double-blind placebo-controlled crossover trial of a feverfew preparation. *Phytomedicine.* 1996;3:225-230.
5. Willigmann I, El Amrani M. Efficacite et innocuite de *Tanacetum parthenium* (Grande Camomille) dans la prophylaxie de la migraine: une etude dose-dependante en double-aveugle randomisee contre placebo. In: Wildi E, Winkk M, eds. *Trends in Medicinal Plant Research.* Dossenheim, Germany: Romneya-Verlag; 2001.
6. Grossmann M, Schmidramsl H. An extract of *Petasites hybridus* is effective in the prophylaxis of migraine. *Int J Clin Pharmacol Ther.* 2000;38:430-435.
7. Titus F, Davalos A, Alom J, et al. 5-Hydroxytryptophan versus methysergide in the prophylaxis of migraine: randomized clinical trial. *Eur Neurol.* 1986;25:327-329.
8. Bono G, Criscuoli M, Martignoni E, et al. Serotonin precursors in migraine prophylaxis. *Adv Neurol.* 1982;33:357-363.
9. Maissen CP, Ludin HP. Comparison of the effect of 5-hydroxytryptophan and propranolol in the interval treatment of migraine [translated from German]. *Schweiz Med Wochenschr.* 1991;121:1585-1590.
10. Santucci M, Cortelli P, Giovanardi Rossi P, et al. L-5-hydroxytryptophan versus placebo in childhood migraine prophylaxis: a double-blind crossover study. *Cephalalgia.* 1986;6:155-157.
11. De Giorgis G, Miletto R, Iannuccelli M, et al. Headache in association with sleep disorders in children: a psychodiagnostic evaluation and controlled clinical study— L-5-HTP versus placebo. *Drugs Exp Clin Res.* 1987;13:425-433.
12. Longo G, Rudoi I, Iannuccelli M, et al. Treatment of essential headache in developmental age with L-5-HTP (cross over double-blind study versus placebo) [in Italian; English abstract]. *Pediatr Med Chir.* 1984;6:241-245.
13. DeBenedittis G, Massei R. Serotonin precursors in chronic primary headache: a double-blind cross-over study with L-5-hydroxytryptophan vs. placebo. *J Neurosurg Sci.* 1985;29:239-248.
14. Peikert A, Wilimzig C, Kohne-Volland R. Prophylaxis of migraine with oral magnesium: results from a prospective, multicenter, placebo-controlled and double-blind randomized study. *Cephalalgia.* 1996;16:257-263.
15. Taubert K. Magnesium in the treatment of migraine. Result of a multicenter pilot study [in German; English abstract]. *Fortschr Med.* 1994;112:328-330.
16. Facchinetti F, Sances G, Borella P, et al. Magnesium prophylaxis of menstrual migraine: effects on intracellular magnesium. *Headache.* 1991;31:298-301.
17. Pfaffenrath V, Wessely P, Meyer C, et al. Magnesium in the prophylaxis of migraine: a double-blind, placebo-controlled study. *Cephalalgia.* 1996;16:436-440.
18. Schoenen J, Jacquy J, Lenaerts M. Effectiveness of high-dose riboflavin in migraine prophylaxis: a randomized controlled trial. *Neurology.* 1998;50:466-470.
19. Glueck CJ, McCarren T, Hitzemann R, et al. Amelioration of severe migraine with omega-3 fatty acids: a double-blind, placebo-controlled clinical trial [abstract]. *Am J Clin Nutr.* 1986;43:710.
20. McCarren T, Hitzemann R, Smith R, et al. Amelioration of severe migraine by fish oil (omega-3) fatty acids [abstract]. *Am J Clin Nutr.* 1985;41:874.
21. Pfaffenrath V, Wessely P, Meyer C, et al. Magnesium in the prophylaxis of migraine: a double-blind placebo-controlled study. *Cephalalgia.* 1996;16:436-440.

22. Pradalier A, Bakouche P, Baudesson G, et al. Failure of omega-3 polyunsaturated fatty acids in prevention of migraine: a double-blind study versus placebo. *Cephalalgia.* 2001;21:818-822.

Multiple Sclerosis (MS)

1. Swank RL. Multiple sclerosis: twenty years on low fat diet. *Arch Neurol.* 1970;23: 460-474.
2. Swank RL, Dugan BB. Effect of low saturated fat diet in early and late cases of multiple sclerosis. *Lancet.* 1990;336:37-39.
3. Millar JHD, Zikha KJ, Langman MJ, et al. Double-blind trial of linoleate supplementation of the diet in multiple sclerosis. *BMJ.* 1973;1:765-768.
4. Bates D, Fawcett PR, Shaw DA, et al. Polyunsaturated fatty acids in treatment of acute remitting multiple sclerosis. *Br Med J.* 1978;2:1390-1391.
5. Paty DW, Cousin HK, Read S, et al. Linoleic acid in multiple sclerosis: failure to show any therapeutic benefit. *Ann Neurol Scand.* 1978;58:53-58.
6. Field EJ, Joyce G. Multiple sclerosis: effect of gamma linoleate administration upon membranes and the need for extended clinical trials of unsaturated fatty acids. *Eur Neurol.* 1983;22:78-83.
7. Gallai V, Sarchielli P, Trequattrini A, et al. Cytokine secretion and eicosanoid production in the peripheral blood mononuclear cells of MS patients undergoing dietary supplementation with n-3 polyunsaturated fatty acids. *J Neuroimmunol.* 1995; 56:143-153.
8. Goldberg P. Multiple sclerosis: decrease relapse rate through dietary supplementation with calcium, magnesium, and vitamin D. *Med Hypotheses.* 1986;21:193-200.
9. Horrobin DE. Multiple sclerosis: the rational basis for treatment with colchicine and evening primrose oil. *Med Hypotheses.* 1979;5:365-378.
10. Field EJ, Joyce G. Effect of prolonged ingestion of gamma-linolenate by MS patients. *Eur Neurol.* 1978;17:67-76.
11. Bates D. Dietary lipids and multiple sclerosis. *Ups J Med Sci Suppl.* 1990;48:173-187.
12. Lee A, Patterson V. A double-blind study of L-threonine in patients with spinal spasticity. *Acta Neurol Scand.* 1993;88:334-338.
13. Hauser SL, Doolittle TH, Lopez-Bresnahan M, et al. An antispasticity effect of theonine in multiple sclerosis. *Arch Neurol.* 1992;49:923-926.
14. Simpson CA, Newell DJ, Miller H. The treatment of multiple sclerosis with massive doses of hydroxycobalamin. *Neurology.* 1965;15:599-603.
15. Goldberg P. Multiple sclerosis: vitamin D and calcium as environmental determinants of prevalence (a viewpoint). Part I: sunlight, dietary factors and epidemiology. *Int J Environ Stud.* 1974;6:19-27.
16. Hayes CE, Cantorna MT, DeLuca HF. Vitamin D and multiple sclerosis. *Proc Soc Exp Biol Med.* 1997;216:21-27.
17. Vieth R. Vitamin D supplementation, 25-hydroxyvitamin D concentrations, and safety. *Am J Clin Nutr.* 1999;69:842-856.
18. Schwartz GG. Multiple sclerosis and prostate cancer: what do their similar geographies suggest? *Neuroepidemiology.* 1992;11:244-254.
19. Winter A. New treatment for multiple sclerosis. *Neurol Orthoped J Med Surg.* 1984;5:39-43.
20. Brochet B, Guinot P, Orgogozo JM, et al. Double blind placebo controlled multicentre study of ginkgolide B in treatment of acute exacerbations of multiple sclerosis. The Ginkgolide Study Group in multiple sclerosis. *J Neurol Neurosurg Psychiatry.* 1995;58:360-362.

Nausea

1. Vutyavanich T, Wongtra-ngan S, Ruangsri R. Pyridoxine for nausea and vomiting of pregnancy: a randomized, double-blind, placebo-controlled trial. *Am J Obstet Gynecol.* 1995;173:881-884.
2. Grontved A, Brask T, Kambskard J, et al. Ginger root against seasickness: a controlled trial on the open sea. *Acta Otolaryngol (Stockh).* 1988;105:45-49.

3. Riebenfeld D, Borzone L. Randomized double-blind study comparing ginger (Zintona®) and dimenhydrinate in motion sickness. *Healthnotes Rev.* 1999;6:98-101.

4. Careddu P. Motion sickness in children: results of a double-blind study with ginger (Zintona®) and dimenhydrinate. *Healthnotes Rev.* 1999;6:102-107.

5. Mowrey DB, Clayson DE. Motion sickness, ginger, and psychophysics. *Lancet.* 1982;1:655-657.

6. Schmid R, Schick T, Steffen R, et al. Comparison of seven commonly used agents for prophylaxis of seasickness. *J Travel Med.* 1994;1:203-206.

7. Stewart JJ, Wood MJ, Wood CD, et al. Effects of ginger on motion sickness susceptibility and gastric function. *Pharmacology.* 1991;42:111-120.

8. Stott JR, Hubble MP, Spencer MB. A double-blind comparative trial of powdered ginger root, hyosine hydrobromide, and cinnarizine in the prophylaxis of motion sickness induced by cross coupled stimulation. *AGARD Conf Proc.* 1985;(372):1-6.

9. Wood CD, Manno JE, Wood MJ, et al. Comparison of efficacy of ginger with various antimotion sickness drugs. *Clin Res Pract Drug Regul Aff.* 1988;6:129-136.

10. Bone ME, Wilkinson DJ, Young JR, et al. Ginger root: a new antiemetic—the effect of ginger root on postoperative nausea and vomiting after major gynaecological sugery. *Anaesthesia.* 1990;45:669-671.

11. Phillips S, Ruggier R, Hutchinson SE, et al. *Zingiber officinale* (ginger): an antiemetic for day case surgery. *Anaesthesia.* 1993;48:715-717.

12. Arfeen Z, Owen H, Plummer JL, et al. A double-blind randomized controlled trial of ginger for the prevention of postoperative nausea and vomiting. *Anaesth Intensive Care.* 1995;23:449-452.

13. Visalyaputra S, Petchpaisit N, Somcharoen K, et al. The efficacy of ginger root in the prevention of postoperative nausea and vomiting after outpatient gynaecological laparoscopy. *Anaesthesia.* 1998;53:486-510.

14. Vutyavanich T, Kraisarin T, Ruangsri R. Ginger for nausea and vomiting in pregnancy: randomized, double-masked, placebo-controlled trial. *Obstet Gynecol.* 2001; 97:577-582.

15. Fischer-Rasmussen W, Kjaer SK, Dahl C, et al. Ginger treatment of hyperemesis gravidarum. *Eur J Obstet Gynecol Reprod Biol.* 1991;38:19-24.

Osteoarthritis

1. Altman RD, Marcussen KC. Effects of a ginger extract on knee pain in patients with osteoarthritis. *Arthritis Rheum.* 2001;44:2531-2538.

2. Bliddal H, Rosetzsky A, Schlichting P, et al. A randomized placebo-controlled crossover study of ginger extracts and ibuprofen in osteoarthritis. *Osteoarthritis Cartilage.* 2000;8:9-12.

3. Noack W, Fischer M, Forster KK, et al. Glucosamine sulfate in osteoarthritis of the knee. *Osteoarthritis Cartilage.* 1994;2:51-59.

4. Crolle G, D'Este E. Glucosamine sulphate for the management of arthrosis: a controlled clinical investigation. *Curr Med Res Opin.* 1980;7:104-109.

5. D'Ambrosio E, Casa B, Bompani R, et al. Glucosamine sulphate: a controlled clinical investigation in arthrosis. *Pharmatherapeutica.* 1981;2:504-508.

6. Drovanti A, Bignamini AA, Rovati AL. Therapeutic activity of oral glucosamine sulfate in osteoarthrosis: a placebo-controlled double-blind investigation. *Clin Ther.* 1980;3:260-272.

7. Rindone JP, Hiller D, Collacott E, et al. Randomized, controlled trial of glucosamine for treating osteoarthritis of the knee. *West J Med.* 2000;172:91-94.

8. Houpt JB, McMillian R, Wein C, et al. Effect of glucosamine hydrochloride in the treatment of pain and osteoarthritis of the knee. *J Rheumatol.* 1999;26:2423-2430.

9. Muller-Fassbender H, Bach GL, Haase W, et al. Glucosamine sulfate compared to ibuprofen in osteoarthritis of the knee. *Osteoarthritis Cartilage.* 1994;2:61-69.

10. Qiu GX, Gao SN, Giacovelli G, et al. Efficacy and safety of glucosamine sulfate versus ibuprofen in patients with knee osteoarthritis. *Arzneimittelforschung.* 1998; 48:469-474.

11. Thie NM, Prasad NG, Major PW. Evaluation of glucosamine sulfate compared to ibuprofen for the treatment of temporomandibular joint osteoarthritis: a randomized double blind controlled 3 month clinical trial. *J Rheumatol.* 2001;28:1347-1355.

12. Reginster JY, Deroisy R, Rovati LC, et al. Long-term effects of glucosamine sulphate on osteoarthritis progression: a randomized, placebo-controlled clinical trial. *Lancet.* 2001;357:251-256.

13. Bucsi L, Poor G. Efficacy and tolerability of oral chondroitin sulfate as a symptomatic slow-acting drug for osteoarthritis (SYSADOA) in the treatment of knee osteoarthritis. *Osteoarthritis Cartilage.* 1998;(6 suppl A):31-36.

14. Bourgeois P, Chales G, Dehais J, et al. Efficacy and tolerability of chondroitin sulfate 1200 mg/day vs chondroitin sulfate 3 x 400 mg/day vs placebo. *Osteoarthritis Cartilage.* 1998;(6 suppl A):25-30.

15. Uebelhart D, Thonar EJ, Delmas PD, et al. Effects of oral chondroitin sulfate on the progression of knee osteoarthritis: a pilot study. *Osteoarthritis Cartilage.* 1998;(6 suppl A):39-46.

16. Mazieres B, Loyau G, Menkes CJ, et al. Chondroitin sulfate in the treatment of gonarthrosis and coxarthrosis: 5-month result of a multicenter double-blind controlled prospective study using placebo [in French; English abstract]. *Rev Rhum Mal Osteoartic.* 1992;59:466-472.

17. Conrozier T. Anti-arthrosis treatments: efficacy and tolerance of chondroitin sulfates (CS 4&6) [translated from French]. *Presse Med.* 1998;27:1862-1865.

18. Mazieres B, Combe B, Phan Van A, et al. Chondroitin sulfate in osteoarthritis of the knee: a prospective, double blind, placebo controlled multicenter clinical study. *J Rheumatol.* 2001;28:173-181.

19. Morreale P, Manopulo R, Galati M, et al. Comparison of the antiinflammatory efficacy of chondroitin sulfate and diclofenac sodium in patients with knee osteoarthritis. *J Rheumatol.* 1996;23:1385-1391.

20. Verbruggen G, Goemaere S, Veys EM. Chondroitin sulfate: S/DMOAD (structure/disease modifying anti-osteoarthritis drug) in the treatment of finger joint OA. *Osteoarthritis Cartilage.* 1998;(6 suppl. A):37-38.

21. Uebelhart D, Thonar EJMA, Zhang J, et al. Protective effect of exogenous chondroitin 4, 6-sulfate in the acute degradation of articular cartilage in the rabbit. *Osteoarthritis Cartilage.* 1998;(6 suppl A):6-13.

22. Caruso I, Pietrogrande V. Italian double-blind multicenter study comparing S-adenosylmethionine, naproxen, and placebo in the treatment of degenerative joint disease. *Am J Med.* 1987;83(5A):66-71.

23. Maccagno A, Di Giorgio EE, Caston OL, et al. Double-blind controlled clinical trial of oral S-adenosylmethionine versus piroxicam in knee osteoarthritis. *Am J Med.* 1987;83(5A):72-77.

24. Glorioso S, Todesco S, Mazzi A, et al. Double-blind multicentre study of the activity of S-adenosylmethionine in hip and knee osteoarthritis. *Int J Clin Pharmacol Res.* 1985;5:39-49.

25. Muller-Fassbender H. Double-blind clinical trial of S-adenosylmethionine versus ibuprofen in the treatment of osteoarthritis. *Am J Med.* 1987;83(5A):81-83.

26. Vetter G. Double-blind comparative clinical trial with S-adenosylmethionine and indomethacin in the treatment of osteoarthritis. *Am J Med.* 1987;83 (5A):78-80.

27. Jonas WB, Rapoza CP, Blair WF. The effect of niacinamide on osteoarthritis: a pilot study. *Inflamm Res.* 1996;45:330-334.

28. Schmid B, Ludtke R, Selbmann HK, et al. Efficacy and tolerability of a standardized willow bark extract in patients with osteoarthritis: randomized, placebo-controlled, double blind clinical trial [translated from German]. *Z Rheumatol.* 2000;59:314-320.

29. McAlindon TE, Jacques P, Zhang Y, et al. Do antioxidant micronutrients protect against the development and progression of knee osteoarthritis? *Arthritis Rheum.* 1996;39:648-656.

30. European Scientific Cooperative on Phytotherapy. *Harpagophyti radix* (devil's claw). Exeter, UK: ESCOP; 1996-1997. Monographs on the Medicinal Uses of Plant Drugs, Fascicule 2.

31. Kuhlwein A, Meyer HJ, Koehler CO. Reduced diclofenac administration by B vitamins: results of a randomized double-blind study with reduced daily doses of diclofenac (75 mg diclofenac versus 75 mg diclofenac plus B vitamins) in acute lumbar vertebral syndromes [in German; English abstract]. *Klin Wochenschr.* 1990;68:107-115.

32. Bui LM, Pawlowski K, Bierer TL. The influence of green-lipped mussel powder *(Perna canaliculus)* on alleviating arthritic signs in dogs [abstract]. *FASEB J.* 2000;14:A218.

33. Bui LM, Pawlowski K, Bierer TL. A semi-moist treat containing green-lipped mussel *(Perna canaliculus)* can help to alleviate arthritic signs in dogs [abstract]. *FASEB J.* 2000;14:A748.

34. Bui LM, Pawlowski K, Bierer TL. Reduction of arthritic signs in dogs fed a main-meal dry diet containing green-lipped mussel *(Perna canaliculus)* [abstract]. *FASEB J.* 2000;14:A748.

35. Appelboom T, Schuermans J, Verbruggen G, et al. Symptoms modifying effect of avocado/soybean unsaponifiables (ASU) in knee osteoarthritis: a double blind prospective placebo-controlled study. *Scand J Rheumatol.* 2001;30:242-247.

36. Blotman F, Maheu E, Wulwik A, et al. Mid-term efficacy and safety of avocado and soya unsaponifiables (ASUs) in the treatment of knee and hip osteoarthritis: results of a three-month prospective, randomized, double-blind, placebo-controlled parallel groups, multicenter clinical trial. *Rev Rhum Engl Ed* 1997;64:825-834.

37. Maheu E, Mazieres B, Valat JP, et al. Symptomatic efficacy of avocado/soybean unsaponifiables in the treatment of osteoarthritis of the knee and hip: a prospective, randomized, double-blind, placebo-controlled multicenter clinical trial with a six-month treatment period and a two-month followiup demonstrating a persistent effect. *Arthritis Rheum.*1998;41:81-91.

38. Lequesne M, Maheu E, Cadet C, et al. Structural effect of avocado/soybean unsaponifiables on joint space loss in osteoarthritis of the hip. *Arthritis Rheum.* 2002;47:50-58.

39. Tilscher H, Keusch R, Neumann K. Results of a double-blind randomized comparative study of Wobenzym®-placebo in patients with cervical syndrome [translated from German]. *Wien Med Wochenschr.* 1996;146:91-95.

40. Singer F, Oberleitner H. Drug therapy of activated arthrosis. On the effectiveness of an enzyme mixture versus Diclofenac® [translated from German] *Wien Med Wochenschr.* 1996;146:55-58.

41. Klein G, Kullich W. Reducing pain by oral enzyme therapy in rheumatic diseases [translated from German]. *Wien Med Wochenschr.* 1999;149:577-580.

42. Gibson T, Dilke TF, Grahame R. Chymoral in the treatment of lumbar disc prolapse. *Rheumatol Rehabil.* 1975;14:186-190.

43. Brand C, Snaddon J, Bailey M, et al. Vitamin E is ineffective for symptomatic relief of knee osteoarthritis: a six month double blind randomized placebo controlled study. *Ann Rheum Dis.* 2001;60:946-949.

Osteoporosis

1. Minaguchi H, Uemura T, Shirasu K, et al. Effect of estriol on bone loss in postmenopausal Japanese women: a multicenter prospective open study. *J Obstet Gynaecol Res.* 1996;22:259-265.

2. Itoi H, Minakami H, Sato I. Comparison of the long-term effects of oral estriol with the effects of conjugated estrogen, 1-alpha-hydroxyvitamin D3 and calcium lactate on vertebral bone loss in early menopausal women. *Maturitas.* 1997;28:11-17.

3. Hayashi T, Ito I, Kano H, et al. Estriol (E3) replacement improves endothelial function and bone mineral density in very elderly women. *J Gerontol A Biol Sci Med Sci.* 2000;55:B183-B190.

4. Holland EF, Leather AT, Studd JW. Increase in bone mass of older postmenopausal women with low mineral bone density after one year of percutaneous oestradiol implants. *Br J Obstet Gynaecol.* 1995;102:238-242.

5. Nozaki M, Hashimoto K, Inoue Y, et al. Usefulness of estriol for the treatment of bone loss in postmenopausal women [in Japanese; English abstract]. *Nippon Sanka Fujinka Gakkai Zasshi*. 1996;48:83-88.

6. Lindsay R, Hart DM, Maclean A, et al. Bone loss during oestriol therapy in postmenopausal women. *Maturitas*. 1979;1:279-285.

7. Granberg S, Ylostalo P, Wikland M, et al. Endometrial sonographic and histologic findings in women with and without hormonal replacement therapy suffering from postmenopausal bleeding. *Maturitas*. 1997;27:35-40.

8. Weiderpass E, Baron JA, Adami HO, et al. Low-potency estrogen and risk of endometrial cancer: a case-control study. *Lancet*. 1999;353:1824-1828.

9. Montoneri C, Zarbo G, Garofalo A, et al. Effects of estriol administration on human postmenopausal endometrium. *Clin Exp Obstet Gynecol*. 1987;14:178-181.

10. Takahashi K, Manabe A, Okada M, et al. Efficacy and safety of oral estriol for managing postmenopausal symptoms. *Maturitas*. 2000;34:169-177.

11. Lippman M, Monaco ME, Bolan G. Effects of estrone, estradiol and estriol on hormone-responsive human breast cancer in long-term tissue culture. *Cancer Res*. 1977;37:1901-1907.

12. Reid IR. The roles of calcium and vitamin D in the prevention of osteoporosis. *Endocrinol Metab Clin North Am*. 1998;27:389-398.

13. Cumming RG. Calcium intake and bone mass: a quantitative review of the evidence. *Calcif Tissue Int*. 1990;47:194-201.

14. Dawson-Hughes B, Dallal GE, Krall EA, et al. A controlled trial of the effect of calcium supplementation on bone density in postmenopausal women. *N Engl J Med*. 1990;323:878-883.

15. Prince RL. Diet and the prevention of osteoporotic fractures. *N Engl J Med*. 1997;337:701-702.

16. Mezquita-Raya P, Munoz-Torres M, De Dios Luna J, et al. Relation between vitamin D insufficiency, bone density, and bone metabolism in healthy postmenopausal women. *J Bone Miner Res*. 2001;16:1408-1415.

17. Dawson-Hughes B, Harris SS, Krall EA, et al. Effect of withdrawal of calcium and vitamin D supplements on bone mass in elderly men and women. *Am J Clin Nutr*. 2000;72:745-750.

18. Buckley LM, Leib ES, Cartularo KS, et al. Calcium and vitamin D3 supplementation prevents bone loss in the spine secondary to low-dose corticosteroids in patients with rheumatoid arthritis: a randomized, double-blind, placebo-controlled study. *Ann Intern Med*. 1996;125:961-968.

19. Reid IR, Ibbertson HK. Calcium supplements in the prevention of steroid-induced osteoporosis. *Am J Clin Nutr*. 1986;44:287-290.

20. Homik J, Suarez-Almazor ME, Shea B, et al. Calcium and vitamin D for corticosteroid-induced osteoporosis. *Cochrane Database Syst Rev*. 2000;(no.30):1-9.

21. Nieves JW, Komar L, Cosman F, et al. Calcium potentiates the effect of estrogen and calcitonin on bone mass: review and analysis. *Am J Clin Nutr*. 1998;67:18-24.

22. Lloyd T, Andon MB, Rollings N, et al. Calcium supplementation and bone mineral density in adolescent girls. *JAMA*. 1993;270:841-844.

23. Barr SI, Petit MA, Vigna YM, et al. Eating attitudes and habitual calcium intake in peripubertal girls are associated with initial bone mineral content and its change over 2 years. *J Bone Miner Res*. 2001;16:940-947.

24. Lloyd T, Chinchilli VM, Johnson-Rollings N, et al. Adult female hip bone density reflects teenage sports-exercise patterns but not teenage calcium intake. *Pediatrics*. 2000;106:40-44.

25. Saltman PD, Strause LG. The role of trace minerals in osteoporosis. *J Am Coll Nutr*. 1993;12:384-389.

26. Strause L, Saltman P, Smith KT, et al. Spinal bone loss in postmenopausal women supplemented with calcium and trace minerals. *J Nutr*. 1994;124:1060-1064.

27. Kruger MC, Coetzer H, de Winter R, et al. Calcium, gamma-linolenic acid and eicosapentaenoic acid supplementation in senile osteoporosis. *Aging (Milano)*. 1998;10:385-394.

28. van Papendorp DH, Coetzer H, Kruger MC. Biochemical profile of osteoporotic patients on essential fatty acid supplementation. *Nutr Res.* 1995;15:325-334.
29. Bassey EJ, Littlewood JJ, Rothwell MC, et al. Lack of effect of supplementation with essential fatty acids on bone mineral density in healthy pre- and postmenopausal women: two randomized controlled trials of Efacal® v. calcium alone. *Br J Nutr.* 2000;83:629-635.
30. Agnusdei D, Zacchei F, Bigazzi S, et al. Metabolic and clinical effects of ipriflavone in established post-menopausal osteoporosis. *Drugs Exp Clin Res.* 1989;15:97-104.
31. Agnusdei D, Camporeale A, Zacchei F, et al. Effects of ipriflavone on bone mass and bone remodeling in patients with established postmenopausal osteoporosis. *Curr Ther Res.* 1992;51:82-91.
32. Agnusdei D, Crepaldi G, Isaia G, et al. A double blind, placebo-controlled trial of ipriflavone for prevention of postmenopausal spinal bone loss. *Calcif Tissue Int.* 1997;61:142-147.
33. Gambacciani M, Spinetti A, Piaggesi L, et al. Ipriflavone prevents the bone mass reduction in premenopausal women treated with gonadotropin hormone-releasing hormone agonists. *Bone Miner.* 1994;26:19-26.
34. Gambacciani M, Cappagli B, Piaggesi L, et al. Ipriflavone prevents the loss of bone mass in pharmacological menopause induced by GnRH-agonists. *Calcif Tissue Int.* 1997;61:S15-S18.
35. Gennari C, Adami S, Agnusdei D, et al. Effect of chronic treatment with ipriflavone in postmenopausal women with low bone mass. *Calcif Tissue Int.* 1997;61:S19-S22.
36. Kovacs AB. Efficacy of ipriflavone in the prevention and treatment of post-menopausal osteoporosis. *Agents Actions.* 1994;41:86-87.
37. Maugeri D, Panebianco P, Russo MS, et al. Ipriflavone-treatment of senile osteoporosis: results of a multicenter, double-blind clinical trial of 2 years. *Arch Gerontol Geriatr.* 1994;19:253-263.
38. Passeri M, Biondi M, Costi D, et al. Effects of 2-year therapy with ipriflavone in elderly women with established osteoporosis. *Ital J Miner Electrolyte Metab.* 1995;9:137-144.
39. Valente M, Bufalino L, Castiglione GN, et al. Effects of 1-year treatment with ipriflavone on bone in postmenopausal women with low bone mass. *Calcif Tissue Int.* 1994;54:377-380.
40. Alexandersen P, Toussaint A, Reginster J, et al. Ipriflavone has no effect on bone metabolism and causes lymphopenia in osteopenic women [abstract]. *J Bone Miner Res.* 2000;15(suppl 1):S198.
41. Melis GB, Paoletti AM, Cagnacci A. Ipriflavone prevents bone loss in post-menopausal women. *Menopause.* 1996;3:27-32.
42. Mazzuoli G, Romagnoli E, Carnevale V, et al. Effects of ipriflavone on bone remodeling in primary hyperparathyroidism. *Bone Miner.* 1992;19(suppl):S27-S33.
43. Yamazaki I, Shino A, Shimizu Y, et al. Effect of ipriflavone on glucocorticoid-induced osteoporosis in rats. *Life Sci.* 1986;38:951-958.
44. Melis GB, Paoletti AM, Bartolini R, et al. Ipriflavone and low doses of estrogens in the prevention of bone mineral loss in climacterium. *Bone Miner.* 1992;19(suppl):S49-S56.
45. Nozaki M, Hashimoto K, Inoue Y, et al. Treatment of bone loss in oophorectomized women with a combination of ipriflavone and conjugated equine estrogen. *Int J Gynaecol Obstet.* 1998;62:69-75.
46. Baulieu EE, Thomas G, Legrain S, et al. Dehydroepiandrosterone (DHEA), DHEA sulfate, and aging: contribution of the DHEAge study to a sociobiomedical issue. *Proc Natl Acad Sci.* 2000;97:4279-4284.
47. Labrie F, Diamond P, Cusan L, et al. Effect of 12-month dehydroepiandrosterone replacement therapy on bone, vagina, and endometrium in postmenopausal women. *J Clin Endocrinol Metab.* 1997;82:3498-3505.
48. van Vollenhoven RF, Park JL, Genovese MC, et al. A double-blind, placebo-controlled, clinical trial of dehydroepiandrosterone in severe systemic lupus erythematosus. *Lupus.* 1999;8:181-187.

49. Potter SM, Baum JA, Teng H, et al. Soy protein and isoflavones: their effects on blood lipids and bone density in postmenopausal women. *Am J Clin Nutr.* 1998;68(6 suppl):1375S-1379S.

50. Alekel DL, Germain AS, Peterson CT, et al. Isoflavone-rich soy protein isolate attenuates bone loss in the lumbar spine of perimenopausal women. *Am J Clin Nutr.* 2000;72:844-852.

51. Harrison E, Adjei A, Ameho C, et al. The effect of soybean protein on bone loss in a rat model of postmenopausal osteoporosis. *J Nutr Sci Vitaminol.* 1998;44:257-268.

52. Fanti O, Faugere MC, Gang Z, et al. Systematic administration of genistein partially prevents bone loss in ovariectomized rats in a nonestrogen-like mechanism [abstract]. *Am J Clin Nutr.* 1998;68(suppl):1517S-1518S.

53. Arjmandi BH, Alekel L, Hollis BW, et al. Dietary soybean protein prevents bone loss in an ovariectomized rat model of osteoporosis. *J Nutr.* 1996;126:161-167.

54. Fanti P, Monier-Faugere MC, Geng Z, et al. The phytoestrogen genistein reduces bone loss in short-term ovariectomized rats. *Osteoporos Int.* 1998;8:274-281.

55. Anderson JJ, Ambrose WW, Garner SC. Biphasic effects of genistein on bone tissue in the ovariectomized, lactating rat model. *Proc Soc Exp Biol Med.* 1998;217:345-350.

56. Arjmandi BH, Birnbaum R, Goyal NV, et al. Bone-sparing effect of soy protein in ovarian hormone-deficient rats is related to its isoflavone content. *Am J Clin Nutr.* 1998;68(6 suppl):1364S-1368S.

57. Lees CJ, Ginn TA. Soy protein isolate diet does not prevent soy increased cortical bone turnover in ovariectomized macaques. *Calcif Tissue Int.* 1998;62:557-558.

58. Jayo MJ. Dietary soy isoflavones and bone loss: a study in ovariectomized monkeys [abstract]. *J Bone Miner Res.* 1996;11:S228.

59. Gallagher JC, Rafferty K, Haynatzka V, et al. The effect of soy protein on bone metabolism [abstract]. *J Nutr.* 2000;130:667S.

60. Feskanich D, Weber P, Willett WC, et al. Vitamin K intake and hip fractures in women: a prospective study. *Am J Clin Nutr.* 1999;69:74-79.

61. Booth SL, Tucker KL, Chen H, et al. Dietary vitamin K intakes are associated with hip fracture but not with bone mineral density in elderly men and women. *Am J Clin Nutr.* 2000;71:1201-1208.

62. Prior JC. Progesterone as a bone-trophic hormone. *Endocr Rev.* 1990;11:386-398.

63. Verhaar HJ, Damen CA, Duursma SA, et al. A comparison of the action of progestins and estrogen on the growth and differentiation of normal adult human osteoblast-like cells in vitro. *Bone.* 1994;15:307-311.

64. Lee JR. Is natural progesterone the missing link in osteoporosis prevention and treatment? *Med Hypotheses.* 1991;35:316-318.

65. Lee JR. Osteoporosis reversal with transdermal progesterone [letter]. *Lancet.* 1990; 336:1327.

66. Lee JR. Osteoporosis reversal, the role of progesterone. *Int Clin Nutr Rev.* 1990; 10:384-391.

67. Leonetti HB, Longo S, Anasti JN. Transdermal progesterone cream for vasomotor symptoms and postmenopausal bone loss. *Obstet Gynecol.* 1999;94:225-228.

68. Writing Group for the PEPI Trial. Effects of hormone replacement therapy on endometrial histology in postmenopausal women: the postmenopausal estrogen/progestin interventions (PEPI) trial. *JAMA.* 1996;275:370-375.

69. Nielsen FH, Hunt CD, Mullen LM, et al. Effect of dietary boron on mineral, estrogen, and testosterone metabolism in postmenopausal women. *FASEB J.* 1987; 1:394-397.

70. Beattie JH, Peace HS. The influence of a low-boron diet and boron supplementation on bone, major minerals, and sex steroid metabolism in postmenopausal women. *Br J Nutr.* 1993;69:871-884.

71. Naghii MR, Samman S. The effect of boron supplementation on its urinary excretion and selected cardiovascular risk factors in healthy male subjects. *Biol Trace Elem Res.* 1997;56:273-286.

72. Dawson-Hughes B, Harris S. Calcium intake influences the association of protein intake with rates of bone loss in elderly men and women. *Am J Clin Nutr.* 2002; 75:773-779.

Otitis Media

1. Rosenfeld RM, Vertrees JE, Carr J, et al. Clinical efficacy of antimicrobial drugs for acute otitis media: meta-analysis of 5400 children from thirty-three randomized trials. *J Pediatr.* 1994;124:355-367.
2. Little P, Gould C, Williamson I, et al. Pragmatic randomized controlled trial of two prescribing strategies for childhood acute otitis media. *BMJ.* 2001;322:336-342.
3. Kaleida PH, Casselbrant ML, Rockette HE, et al. Amoxicillin or myringotomy or both for acute otitis media: results of a randomized clinical trial. *Pediatrics.* 1991; 87:466-474.
4. Rothrock SG, Harper MB, Green SM, et al. Do oral antibiotics prevent meningitis and serious bacterial infections in children with Streptococcus pneumoniae occult bacteremia? A meta-analysis. *Pediatrics.* 1997;99:438-444.
5. Del Mar C, Glasziou P, Hayem M. Are antibiotics indicated as initial treatment for children with acute otitis media? A meta-analysis. *BMJ.* 1997;314:1526-1529.
6. Alho OP, Laara E, Oja H. What is the natural history of recurrent acute otitis media in infancy? *J Fam Pract.* 1996;43:258-264.
7. Le CT, Freeman DW, Fireman BH. Evaluation of ventilating tubes and myringotomy in the treatment of recurrent or persistent otitis media. *Pediatr Infect Dis J.* 1991;10:2-11.
8. Uhari M, Kontiokari T, Niemela M. A novel use of xylitol sugar in preventing acute otitis media. *Pediatrics.* 1998;102:879-884.
9. Kontiokari T, Uhari M, Koskela M. Antiadhesive effects of xylitol on otopathogenic bacteria. *J Antimicrob Chemother.* 1998;41:563-565.
10. Uhari M, Kontiokari T, Koskela M. Xylitol chewing gum in prevention of acute otitis media: double blind randomized trial. *BMJ.* 1996;313:1180-1184.
11. Duncan B, Ey J, Holberg CJ, et al. Exclusive breast-feeding for at least 4 months protects against otitis media. *Pediatrics.* 1993;91:867-872.
12. Sassen ML, Brand R, Grote JJ. Breast-feeding and acute otitis media. *Am J Otolaryngol.* 1994;15:351-357.
13. Aniansson G, Alm B, Andersson B, et al. A prospective cohort study on breast-feeding and otitis media in Swedish infants. *Pediatr Infect Dis J.* 1994;13:183-188.
14. Roos K, Hakansson EG, Holm S. Effect of recolonization with interfering alpha streptococci on recurrences of acute and secretory otitis media in children: randomized placebo controlled trial. *BMJ.* 2001;322:210-212.
15. Tano K, Grahn Hakansson E, Holm SE, et al. A nasal spray with alpha-hemolytic streptococci as long term prophylaxis against recurrent otitis media. *Int J Pediatr Otorhinolaryngol.* 2002;62:17-23.
16. Sarrell EM, Mandelberg A, Cohen HA. Efficacy of naturopathic extracts in the management of ear pain associated with acute otitis media. *Arch Pediatr Adolesc Med.* 2001;155:796-799.

Parkinson's Disease

1. Schelosky L, Raffauf C, Jendroska K, et al. Kava and dopamine antagonism [letter]. *J Neurol Neurosurg Psychiatry.* 1995;58:639-640.
2. Eberhardt R, Birbamer G, Gerstenbrand F, et al. Citicoline in the treatment of Parkinson's disease. *Clin Ther.* 1990;12:489-495.
3. Birbamer G, Gerstenbrand F, Rainer J, et al. CDP-choline in the treatment of Parkinson syndrome. *New Trends Clin Neuropharmacol.* 1990;4:29-34.
4. Secades JJ, Frontera G. CDP-choline: pharmacological and clinical review. *Methods Find Exp Clin Pharmacol.* 1995;17(suppl B):1-54.
5. Agnoli A, Ruggieri S, Denaro A, et al. New strategies in the management of Parkinson's disease: a biological approach using a phospholipid precursor (CDP-choline). *Neuropsychobiology.* 1982;8:289-296.
6. Ruggieri S, Zamponi A, Casacchia M, et al. Therapeutic effects of cyticholine (cytidine-diphospho-choline) in Parkinsonian syndrome [in Italian]. *Clin Ter.* 1976;78: 515-525.
7. Lozano Fernandez R. Efficacy and safety of oral CDP-choline: drug surveillance study in 2817 cases. *Arzneimittelforschung.* 1983;33:1073-1080.

8. Liu X, Lamango N, Charlton C. L-dopa depletes S-adenosylmethionine and increases S-adenosyl homocysteine: relationship to the wearing-off effects [abstract]. *Abstr Soc Neurosci.* 1998;24:1469.

9. Bottiglieri T, Hyland K, Reynolds EH. The clinical potential of ademetionine (S-Adenosylmethionine) in neurological disorders. *Drugs.* 1994;48:137-152.

10. Bressa GM. S-adenosyl-l-methionine (SAMe) as antidepressant: meta-analysis of clinical studies. *Acta Neurol Scand Suppl.* 1994;154:7-14.

11. Carrieri PB, Indaco A, Gentile S, et al. S-adenosylmethionine treatment of depression in patients with Parkinson's disease: a double-blind, crossover study versus placebo. *Curr Ther Res.* 1990;48:154-160.

12. Mayeux R, Stern Y, Sano M, et al. The relationship of serotonin to depression in Parkinson's disease. *Mov Disord.* 1988;3:237-244.

13. Sternberg EM, Van Woert MH, Young SN, et al. Development of a scleroderma-like illness during therapy with L-5-hydroxytryptophan and carbidopa. *N Engl J Med.* 1980;303:782-787.

14. Joly P, Lampert A, Thomine E, et al. Development of pseudobullous morphea and scleroderma-like illness during therapy with L-5-hydroxytryptophan and carbidopa. *J Am Acad Dermatol.* 1991;25:332-333.

15. Auffranc JC, Berbis P, Fabre JF, et al. Sclerodermiform and poikilodermal syndrome observed during treatment with carbidopa and 5-hydroxytryptophan [translated from French]. *Ann Dermatol Venereol.* 1985;112:691-692.

16. Funfgeld EW, Baggen M, Nedwidek P, et al. Double-blind study with phosphatidylserine (PS) in Parkinsonian patients with senile dementia of Alzheimer's type (SDAT). *Prog Clin Biol Res.* 1989;317:1235-1246.

17. Parkinson Study Group. Effects of tocopherol and deprenyl on the progression of disability in early Parkinson's disease. *N Engl J Med.* 1993;328:176-183.

18. Parkinson Study Group. Impact of deprenyl and tocopherol treatment on Parkinson's disease in DATATOP patients requiring levodopa. *Ann Neurol.* 1996;39: 37-45.

19. Kieburtz K, McDermott M, Como P, et al. The effect of deprenyl and tocopherol on cognitive performance in early untreated Parkinson's disease. *Neurology.* 1994;44: 1756-1759.

20. Reilly DK, Hershey L, Rivera-Calimlim L, et al. On-off effects in Parkinson's disease: a controlled investigation of ascorbic acid therapy. *Adv Neurol.* 1983;37:51-60.

21. Dizdar N, Kagedal B, Lindvall B. Treatment of Parkinson's disease with NADH. *Acta Neurol Scand.* 1994;90:345-347.

22. Kuhn W, Muller T, Winkel R, et al. Parenteral application of NADH in Parkinson's disease: clinical improvement partially due to stimulation of endogenous levodopa biosynthesis. *J Neural Transm.* 1996;103:1187-1193.

23. Birkmayer JG, Vrecko C, Volc D, et al. Nicotinamide adenine dinucleotide (NADH)—a new therapeutic approach to Parkinson's disease: comparison of oral and parenteral application. *Acta Neurol Scand Suppl.* 1993;146:32-35.

24. Sechi G, Deledda MG, Bua G, et al. Reduced intravenous glutathione in the treatment of early Parkinson's disease. *Prog Neuropsychopharmacol Biol Psychiatry.* 1996; 20:1159-1170.

25. Snider SR. Octacosanol in parkinsonism [letter]. *Ann Neurol.* 1984;16:723.

26. Heller B, Fischer E, Martin R. Therapeutic action of d-phenylalanine in Parkinson's disease. *Arzneimittelforschung.* 1976;26:577-579.

27. Smythies JR, Halsey JH. Treatment of Parkinson's disease with L-methionine. *South Med J.* 1984;77:1577.

28. Meininger V, Flamier A, Phan T, et al. L-methionine treatment of Parkinson's disease: preliminary results [in French; English abstract]. *Rev Neurol (Paris).* 1982;138: 297-303.

29. Nutt JG, Woodward WR, Hammerstad JP, et al. The "on-off" phenomenon in Parkinson's disease. Relation to levodopa absorption and transport. *N Engl J Med.* 1984;310:483-488.

Peptic Ulcer Disease

1. Kassir ZA. Endoscopic controlled trial of four drug regimens in the treatment of chronic duodenal ulceration. *Ir Med J.* 1985;78:153-156.

2. Morgan AG, Pacsoo C, McAdam WAF. Maintenance therapy: a two-year comparison between caved-S and cimetidine treatment in the prevention of symptomatic gastric ulcer recurrence. *Gut.* 1985;26:599-602.

3. Rees WD, Rhodes J, Wright JE, et al. Effect of deglycyrrhizinated liquorice on gastric mucosal damage by aspirin. *Scand J Gastroenterol.* 1979;14:605-607.

4. Sakamoto I, Igarashi M, Kimura K, et al. Suppressive effect of *Lactobacillus gasseri* OLL 2716 (LG21) on *Helicobacter pylori* infection in humans. *J Antimicrob Chemother.* 2001;47:709-710.

5. Beil W, Birkholz C, Sewing KF. Effects of flavonoids on parietal cell acid secretion, gastric mucosal prostaglandin production, and *Helicobacter pylori* growth. *Arzneimittelforschung.* 1995;45:697-700.

6. Sivam GP. Protection against *Helicobacter pylori* and other bacterial infections by garlic. *J Nutr.* 2001;131(3 suppl):1106S-1108S.

7. Armuzzi A, Cremonini F, Ojetti V, et al. Effect of *Lactobacillus GG* supplementation on antibiotic-associated gastrointestinal side effects during *Helicobacter pylori* eradication therapy: a pilot study. *Digestion.* 2001;63:1-7.

8. Playford RJ, Floyd DN, Macdonald CE, et al. Bovine colostrum is a health food supplement which prevents NSAID induced gut damage. *Gut.* 1999;44:653-658.

9. Macdonald CE, Calnan DP, Podas T, et al. Clinical trial of colostrum for protection against NSAID induced enteropathy [abstract]. *Gastroenterology.* 1998;114:G0856.

10. Abdel Salam OM, Mozsik G, Szolcsanyi J. Studies on the effect of intragastric capsaicin on gastric ulcer and on the prostacyclin-induced cytoprotection in rats. *Pharmacol Res.* 1995;32:209-215.

11. Holzer P, Pabst MA, Lippe IT. Intragastric capsaicin protects against aspirin-induced lesion formation and bleeding in the rat gastric mucosa. *Gastroenterology.* 1989;96:1425-1433.

12. Yeoh KG, Kang JY, Yap I, et al. Chili protects against aspirin-induced gastroduodenal mucosal injury in humans. *Dig Dis Sci.* 1995;40:580-583.

13. Van Dau N, Ngoc Ham N, Huy Khac D, et al. The effects of a traditional drug, tumeric *(Curcuma longa)*, and placebo on the healing of duodenal ulcer. *Phytomedicine.* 1998;5:29-34.

14. Kositchaiwat C, Kositchaiwat S, Havanondha J. *Curcuma longa* Linn. in the treatment of gastric ulcer comparison to liquid antacid: a controlled clinical trial. *J Med Assoc Thai.* 1993;76:601-605.

15. Gupta D, Kulshrestha VK, Srivastava RK, et al. Mechanisms of curcumin induced gastric ulcer in rats. *Indian J Med Res.* 1980;71:806-814.

16. Graham DY, Anderson SY, Lang T. Garlic or jalapeno peppers for treatment of *Helicobacter pylori* infection. *Am J Gastroenterol.* 1999;94:1200-1202.

17. Aydin A, Ersoz G, Tekesin O, et al. Garlic oil and *Helicobacter pylori* infection [letter]. *Am J Gastroenterol.* 2000;95:563-564.

18. Aiba Y, Suzuki N, Kabir AM, et al. Lactic acid-mediated suppression of *Helicobacter pylori* by the oral administration of Lactobacillus salivarius as a probiotic in a gnotobiotic murine model. *Am J Gastroenterol.* 1998;93:2097-2101.

19. Sakamoto I, Igarashi M, Kimura K, et al. Suppressive effect of Lactobacillus gasseri OLL 2716 (LG21) on Helicobacter pylori infection in humans. *J Antimicrob Chemother.* 2001;47:709-710.

20. Wendakoon CN, Thomson AB, Ozimek L. Lack of therapeutic effect of a specially designed yogurt for the eradication of Helicobacter pylori infection. *Digestion.* 2002;65:16-20.

21. Felley CP, Corthesy-Theulaz I, Rivero JL, et al. Favorable effect of an acidified milk (LC-1) on Helicobacter pylori gastritis in man. *Eur J Gastroenterol Hepatol.* 2001;13:25-29.

22. Michetti P, Dorta G, Wiesel PH, et al. Effect of whey-based culture supernatant of Lactobacillus acidophilus (johnsonii) La1 on Helicobacter pylori infection in humans. *Digestion.* 1999;60:203-209.
23. Armuzzi A, Cremonini F, Bartolozzi F, et al. The effect of oral administration of Lactobacillus GG on antibiotic-associated gastrointestinal side-effects during Helicobacter pylori eradication therapy. *Aliment Pharmacol Ther.* 2001;15:163-169.
24. Canducci F, Armuzzi A, Cremonini F, et al. A lyophilized and inactivated culture of Lactobacillus acidophilus increases Helicobacter pylori eradication rates. *Aliment Pharmacol Ther.* 2000;14:1625-1629.
25. De Francesco V, Stoppino V, Sgarro C, et al. Lactobacillus acidophilus administration added to omeprazole/amoxycillin-based double therapy in Helicobacter pylori eradication. *Dig Liver Dis.* 2000;32:746-747.
26. Meier R, Wettstein A, Drewe J, et al. Fish oil (Eicosapen) is less effective than metronidazole in combination with pantoprazole and clarithromycin for Helicobacter pylori eradication. *Aliment Pharmacol Ther.* 2001;15:851-855.

Photosensitivity

1. Gould JW, Mercurio MG, Elmets CA. Cutaneous photosensitivity diseases induced by exogenous agents. *J Am Acad Dermatol.* 1995;33:551-573.
2. Suhonen R, Plosila M. The effect of beta-carotene in combination with canthaxanthin, Ro 8-8427 (Phenoro), in treatment of polymorphous light eruptions. *Dermatologica.* 1981;163:172-176.
3. Corbett MF, Hawk JL, Herxheimer A, et al. Controlled therapeutic trials in polymorphic light eruption. *Br J Dermatol.* 1982;107:571-581.
4. Krook G, Haeger-Aronsen B. Beta-carotene in the treatment of erythropoietic protoporphyria. *Acta Derm Venereol Suppl (Stockh).* 1982;100:125-129.
5. Mathews-Roth MM, Pathak MA, Fitzpatrick TB, et al. Beta-carotene as an oral photoprotective agent in erythropoietic protoporphyria. *JAMA.* 1974;228:1004-1008.
6. Mathews-Roth MM. Carotenoids in erythropoietic protoporphyria and other photosensitivity diseases. *Ann NY Acad Sci.* 1993;691:127-138.
7. Corbett MF, Herxheimer A, Magnus IA, et al. The long term treatment with beta-carotene in erythropoietic protoporphyria: a controlled trial. *Br J Dermatol.* 1977;97:655-662.
8. Gollnick HP, Hopfenmuller W, Hemmes C, et al. Systemic beta carotene plus topical UV sunscreen are an optimal protection against harmful effects of natural UV-sunlight: results of the Berlin-Eilath study. *Eur J Dermatol.* 1996;6:200-205.
9. Lee J, Jiang S, Levine N, et al. Carotenoid supplementation reduces erythema in human skin after simulated solar radiation exposure. *Proc Soc Exp Biol Med.* 2000;223:170-174.
10. Stahl W, Heinrich U, Jungmann H, et al. Carotenoids and carotenoids plus vitamin E protect against ultraviolet light-induced erythema in humans. *Am J Clin Nutr.* 2000;71:795-798.
11. Mathews-Roth MM, Pathak MA, Parrish J, et al. A clinical trial of the effects of oral beta-carotene on the responses of human skin to solar radiation. *J Invest Dermatol.* 1972;59:349-353.
12. Garmyn M, Ribaya-Mercado JD, Russel RM, et al. Effect of beta-carotene supplementation on the human sunburn reaction. *Exp Dermatol.* 1995;4:104-111.
13. Wolf C, Steiner A, Honigsmann H. Do oral carotenoids protect human skin against ultraviolet erythema, psoralen phototoxicity, and ultraviolet-induced DNA damage? *J Invest Dermatol.* 1988;90:55-57.
14. Darr D, Combs S, Dunston S, et al. Topical vitamin C protects porcine skin from ultraviolet radiation-induced damage. *Br J Dermatol.* 1992;127:247-253.
15. Darr D, Dunston S, Faust H, et al. Effectiveness of antioxidants (vitamin C and E) with and without sunscreens as topical photoprotectants. *Acta Derm Venereol.* 1996;76:264-268.

16. Trevithick JR, Shum DT, Redae S, et al. Reduction of sunburn damage to skin by topical application of vitamin E acetate following exposure to ultraviolet B radiation: effect of delaying application or of reducing concentration of vitamin E acetate applied. *Scanning Microsc.* 1993;7:1269-1281.

17. Trevithick JR, Xiong H, Lee S, et al. Topical tocopherol acetate reduces post-UVB, sunburn-associated erythema, edema, and skin sensitivity in hairless mice. *Arch Biochem Biophys.* 1992;296:575-582.

18. Katiyar SK, Elmets CA, Agarwal R, et al. Protection against ultraviolet-B radiation-induced local and systemic suppression of contact hypersensitivity and edema responses in C3H/HeN mice by green tea polyphenols. *Photochem Photobiol.* 1995;62:855-861.

19. Katiyar SK, Matsui MS, Elmets CA, et al. Polyphenolic antioxidant (−)-epigallo-catechin-3-gallate from green tea reduces UVB-induced inflammatory responses and infiltration of leukocytes in human skin. *Photochem Photobiol.* 1999;69:148-153.

20. Eberlein-Konig B, Placzek M, Przybilla B. Protective effect against sunburn of combined systemic ascorbic acid (vitamin C) and d-alpha-tocopherol (vitamin E). *J Am Acad Dermatol.* 1998;38:45-48.

21. Fuchs J, Kern H. Modulation of UV-light-induced skin inflammation by D-alpha-tocopherol and L-ascorbic acid: a clinical study using solar simulated radiation. *Free Radic Biol Med.* 1998;25:1006-1012.

22. Werninghaus K, Meydani M, Bhawan J, et al. Evaluation of the photoprotective effect of oral vitamin E supplementation. *Arch Dermatol.* 1994;130:1257-1261.

23. Boffa MJ, Ead RD, Reed P, et al. A double-blind, placebo-controlled, crossover trial of oral vitamin C in erythropoietic protoporphyria. *Photodermatol Photoimmunol Photomed.* 1996;12:27-30.

24. Gajdos A. Letter: A.M.P. in porphyria cutanea tarda. *Lancet.* 1974;1:163.

25. Ross JB, Moss MA. Relief of the photosensitivity of erythropoietic protoporphyria by pyridoxine. *J Am Acad Dermatol.* 1990;22(2 pt 2):340-342.

26. Elmets CA, Singh D, Tubesing K, et al. Cutaneous photoprotection from ultraviolet injury by green tea polyphenols. *J Am Acad Dermatol.* 2001;44:425-432.

Pregnancy Support

1. Lao TT, Tam K, Chan LY. Third trimester iron status and pregnancy outcome in non-anaemic women: pregnancy unfavourably affected by maternal iron excess. *Hum Reprod.* 2000;15:1843-1848.

2. Hemminki E, Rimpela U. A randomized comparison of routine versus selective iron supplementation during pregnancy. *J Am Coll Nutr.* 1991;10:3-10.

3. Hemminki E, Merilainen J. Long-term follow-up of mothers and their infants in a randomized trial on iron prophylaxis during pregnancy. *Am J Obstet Gynecol.* 1995;173:205-209.

4. Vutyavanich T, Wongtra-ngan S, Ruangsri R. Pyridoxine for nausea and vomiting of pregnancy: a randomized, double-blind, placebo-controlled trial. *Am J Obstet Gynecol.* 1995;173:881-884.

5. Vutyavanich T, Kraisarin T, Ruangsri R. Ginger for nausea and vomiting in pregnancy: randomized, double-masked, placebo-controlled trial. *Obstet Gynecol.* 2001;97:577-582.

6. Fischer-Rasmussen W, Kjaer SK, Dahl C, et al. Ginger treatment of hyperemesis gravidarum. *Eur J Obstet Gynecol Reprod Biol.* 1991;38:19-24.

7. Merkel RL. The use of menadione bisulfite and ascorbic acid in the treatment of nausea and vomiting of pregnancy. *Am J Obstet Gynecol.* 1952;64:416-418.

8. Aikins Murphy P. Alternative therapies for nausea and vomiting of pregnancy. *Obstet Gynecol.* 1998;91:149-155.

9. Bergstein NA. Clinical study on the efficacy of O-(beta-hydroxyethyl) rutoside (HR) in varicosis of pregnancy. *J Int Med Res.* 1975;3:189-193.

10. Steiner M, Hillemanns HG. Investigation of the anti-edemic efficacy of Venostasin® retard [translated from German]. *MMW Munch Med Wochenschr.* 1986;128:551-552.

11. Basellini A, Agus GB, Antonucci E, et al. Varices in pregnancy (an up-date) [translated from Italian]. *Ann Obstet Ginecol Med Perinat.* 1985;106:337-341.

12. Wijayanegara H, Mose JC, Achmad L, et al. A clinical trial of hydroxyethylrutosides in the treatment of haemorrhoids of pregnancy. *J Int Med Res.* 1992;20:54-60.

13. Wadworth AN, Faulds D. Hydroxyethylrutosides: a review of its pharmacology, and therapeutic efficacy in venous insufficiency and related disorders. *Drugs.* 1992; 44:1013-1032.

14. Buckshee K, Takkar D, Aggarwal N. Micronized flavonoid therapy in internal hemorrhoids of pregnancy. *Int J Gynaecol Obstet.* 1997;57:145-151.

15. Atallah AN, Hofmeyr GJ, Duley L. Calcium supplementation during pregnancy for preventing hypertensive disorders and related problems. *Cochrane Database Syst Rev.* 2000;(3):1-16.

16. Levine RJ, Hauth JC, Curet LB, et al. Trial of calcium to prevent preeclampsia. *N Engl J Med.* 1997;337:69-76.

17. Chappell LC, Seed PT, Briley AL, et al. Effect of antioxidants on the occurrence of pre-eclampsia in women at increased risk: a randomized trial. *Lancet.* 1999;354:810-816.

18. Gulmezoglu AM, Hofmeyr GJ, Oosthuisen MM. Antioxidants in the treatment of severe pre-eclampsia: an explanatory randomized controlled trial. *Br J Obstet Gynaecol.* 1997;104:689-696.

19. Jonsson B, Hauge B, Larsen MF, et al. Zinc supplementation during pregnancy: a double blind randomized controlled trial. *Acta Obstet Gynecol Scand.* 1996;75: 725-729.

20. Hunt IF, Murphy NJ, Cleaver AE, et al. Zinc supplementation during pregnancy: effects on selected blood constituents and on progress and outcome of pregnancy in low-income women of Mexican descent. *Am J Clin Nutr.* 1984;40:508-521.

21. Mahomed K, James DK, Golding J, et al. Zinc supplementation during pregnancy: a double blind randomized controlled trial. *BMJ.* 1989;299:826-830.

22. Moutquin JM, Garner PR, Burrows RF, et al. Report of the Canadian Hypertension Society Consensus Conference: 2. Nonpharmacologic management and prevention of hypertensive disorders in pregnancy. *CMAJ.* 1997;157:907-919.

23. Salvig JD, Olsen SF, Secher NJ. Effects of fish oil supplementation in late pregnancy on blood pressure: a randomized controlled trial. *Br J Obstet Gynaecol.* 1996;103: 529-533.

24. Onwude JL, Lilford RJ, Hjartardottir H, et al. A randomized double blind placebo controlled trial of fish oil in high risk pregnancy. *Br J Obstet Gynaecol.* 1995;102:95-100.

25. Bulstra-Ramakers MT, Huisjes HJ, Visser GH. The effects of 3 g eicosapentaenoic acid daily on recurrence of intrauterine growth retardation and pregnancy induced hypertension. *Br J Obstet Gynaecol.* 1995;102:123-126.

26. Olsen SF, Secher NJ. A possible preventive effect of low-dose fish oil on early delivery and pre-eclampsia: indications from a 50-year-old controlled trial. *Br J Nutr.* 1990;64:599-609.

27. Sibai BM, Villar MA, Bray E. Magnesium supplementation during pregnancy: a double-blind randomized controlled clinical trial. *Am J Obstet Gynecol.* 1989;161:115-119.

28. Spatling L, Spatling G. Magnesium supplementation in pregnancy: a double-blind study. *Br J Obstet Gynaecol.* 1988;95:120-125.

29. Rudnicki M, Frolich A, Rasmussen WF, et al. The effect of magnesium on maternal blood pressure in pregnancy-induced hypertension: a randomized double-blind placebo-controlled trial. *Acta Obstet Gynecol Scand.* 1991;70:445-450.

30. Moodley J, Norman RJ. Attempts at dietary alteration of prostaglandin pathways in the management of pre-eclampsia. *Prostaglandins Leukot Essent Fatty Acids.* 1989; 37:145-147.

31. Sanchez-Ramos L, Adair CD, Kaunitz AM, et al. Calcium supplementation in mild preeclampsia remote from term: a randomized double-blind clinical trial. *Obstet Gynecol.* 1995;85:915-918.

32. Dahle LO, Berg G, Hammar M, et al. The effect of oral magnesium substitution on pregnancy-induced leg cramps. *Am J Obstet Gynecol.* 1995;173:175-180.

33. Hammar M, Berg G, Solheim F, et al. Calcium and magnesium status in pregnant women: a comparison between treatment with calcium and vitamin C in pregnant women with leg cramps. *Int J Vitam Nutr Res.* 1987;57:179-183.
34. Avsar AF, Ozmen S, Soylemez F. Vitamin B1 and B6 substitution in pregnancy for leg cramps [letter]. *Am J Obstet Gynecol.* 1996;175:233-234.
35. Pack AR, Thomson ME. Effects of topical and systemic folic acid supplementation on gingivitis in pregnancy. *J Clin Periodontol.* 1980;7:402-413.
36. Thomson ME, Pack AR. Effects of extended systemic and topical folate supplementation on gingivitis of pregnancy. *J Clin Periodontol.* 1982;9:275-280.
37. Jovanovic L, Gutierrez M, Peterson CM. Chromium supplementation for women with gestational diabetes mellitus. *J Trace Elem Exp Med.* 1999;12:91-97.
38. Bennink HJ, Schreurs WH. Improvement of oral glucose tolerance in gestational diabetes by pyridoxine. *Br Med J.* 1975;3:13-15.
39. Olsen SF, Sorensen JD, Secher NJ, et al. Randomized controlled trial of effect of fish-oil supplementation on pregnancy duration. *Lancet.* 1992;339:1003-1007.
40. Villar J, Repke JT. Calcium supplementation during pregnancy may reduce preterm delivery in high-risk populations. *Am J Obstet Gynecol.* 1990;163(4 pt 1):1124-1131.
41. Crowther CA, Hiller JE, Pridmore B, et al. Calcium supplementation in nulliparous women for the prevention of pregnancy-induced hypertension, preeclampsia and preterm birth: an Australian randomized trial. FRACOG and the ACT Study Group. *Aust N Z J Obstet Gynaecol.* 1999;39:12-18.
42. Ramakrishnan U, Manjrekar R, Rivera J, et al. Micronutrients and pregnancy outcome: a review of the literature. *Nutr Res.* 1999;19:103-159.
43. Cherry FF, Sandstead HH, Rojas P, et al. Adolescent pregnancy: associations among body weight, zinc nutriture, and pregnancy outcome. *Am J Clin Nutr.* 1989;50:945-954.
44. Goldenberg RL, Tamura T, Neggers Y, et al. The effect of zinc supplementation on pregnancy outcome. *JAMA.* 1995;274:463-468.
45. Caulfield LE, Zavaleta N, Figueroa A, et al. Maternal zinc supplementation does not affect size at birth or pregnancy duration in Peru. *J Nutr.* 1999;129:1563-1568.
46. Kovacs L, Molnar BG, Huhn E, et al. Magnesium substitution in pregnancy: a prospective, randomized double-blind study [translated from German]. *Geburtsh Frauenheilk.* 1988;48:595-600.
47. Villar J, Gulmezoglu AM, de Onis M. Nutritional and antimicrobial interventions to prevent preterm birth and overview of randomized controlled trials. *Obstet Gynecol Surv.* 1998;53:575-585.
48. Hemminki E, Rimpela U. Iron supplementation, maternal packed cell volume, and fetal growth. *Arch Dis Child.* 1991;66:422-425.
49. Simpson M, Parsons M, Greenwood J, et al. Raspberry leaf in pregnancy: its safety and efficacy in labor. *J Midwifery Womens Health.* 2001;46:51-59.
50. Gunn TR, Wright IM. The use of black and blue cohosh in labor. *NZ Med J.* 1996;109:410-411.
51. Jones TK, Lawson BM. Profound neonatal congestive heart failure caused by maternal consumption of blue cohosh herbal medication. *J Pediatr.* 1998;132:550-552.
52. Newall CA, Anderson LA, Phillipson JD. *Herbal Medicines: A Guide for Health-Care Professionals.* London: Pharmaceutical Press; 1996:15-16, 274.
53. Strandberg TE, Jarvenpaa AL, Vanhanen H, et al. Birth outcome in relation to licorice consumption during pregnancy. *Am J Epidemiol.* 2001;153:1085-1088.

Premenstrual Syndrome (PMS)

1. Thys-Jacobs S, Starkey P, Bernstein D, et al. Calcium carbonate and the premenstrual syndrome: effects on premenstrual and menstrual symptoms. Premenstrual Syndrome Study Group. *Am J Obstet Gynecol.* 1998;179:444-452.
2. Alvir JM, Thys-Jacobs S. Premenstrual and menstrual symptom clusters and response to calcium treatment. *Psychopharmacol Bull.* 1991;27:145-148.

3. Thys-Jacobs S, Ceccarelli S, Bierman A, et al. Calcium supplementation in premenstrual syndrome: a randomized crossover trial. *J Gen Intern Med.* 1989;4:183-189.

4. Schellenberg R. Treatment for the premenstrual syndrome with Agnus castus fruit extract: prospective, randomized, placebo controlled study. *BMJ.* 2001;322:134-137.

5. Halaska M, Beles P, Gorkow C, et al. Treatment of cyclical mastalgia with a solution containing a *Vitex agnus* castus extract: results of a placebo-controlled double-blind study. *Breast.* 1999;8:175-181.

6. Kubista E, Muller G, Spona J. Treatment of mastopathy associated with cyclic mastodynia: clinical results and hormone profiles [translated from German]. *Gynakol Rundsch.* 1986;26:65-79.

7. Wuttke W, Splitt G, Gorkow C, et al. Treatment of cyclical mastalgia: results of a randomized, placebo-controlled, double-blind study [translated from German]. *Geburtsh Frauenheilk.* 1997;57:569-574.

8. Tamborini A, Taurell R. Value of standardized *Ginkgo biloba* extract (Egb 761) in the management of congestive symptoms of premenstrual syndrome [translated from French]. *Rev Fr Gynecol Obstet.* 1993;88:447-457.

9. Facchinetti F, Borella P, Sances G, et al. Oral magnesium successfully relieves premenstrual mood changes. *Obstet Gynecol.* 1991;78:177-181.

10. Walker AF, De Souza MC, Vickers MF, et al. Magnesium supplementation alleviates premenstrual symptoms of fluid retention. *J Womens Health.* 1998;7:1157-1165.

11. Facchinetti F, Sances G, Borella P, et al. Magnesium prophylaxis of menstrual migraine: effects on intracellular magnesium. *Headache.* 1991;31:298-301.

12. Chakmakjian ZH, Higgins CE, Abraham GE. The effect of nutritional supplement, Optivite for Women, on premenstrual tension syndromes: II. Effect on symptomatology, using a double-blind cross-over design. *J Appl Nutr.* 1985;37:12-17.

13. Stewart A. Clinical and biochemical effects of nutritional supplementation on the premenstrual syndrome. *J Reprod Med.* 1987;32:435-441.

14. London RS, Bradley L, Chiamori NY. Effect of a nutritional supplement on premenstrual symptomatology in women with premenstrual syndrome: a double-blind longitudinal study. *J Am Coll Nutr.* 1991;10:494-499.

15. De Souza MC, Walker AF, Robinson PA, et al. A synergistic effect of a daily supplement for 1 month of 200 mg magnesium plus 50 mg vitamin B6 for the relief of anxiety-related premenstrual symptoms: a randomized, double-blind, crossover study. *J Womens Health Gend Based Med.* 2000;9:131-139.

16. Horrobin DF, Manku M, Brush M, et al. Abnormalities in plasma essential fatty acid levels in women with premenstrual syndrome and with nonmalignant breast disease. *J Nutr Med.* 1991;2:259-264.

17. Pashby NL, Mansel RE, Hughes LE, et al. A clinical trial of evening primrose oil in mastalgia [abstract]. *Br J Surg.* 1981;68:801.

18. Mansel RE, Gateley CA, Harrison BJ, et al. Effects and tolerability of n-6 essential fatty acid supplementation in patients with recurrent breast cysts: a randomized double-blind placebo-controlled trial. *J Nutr Med.* 1990;1:195-200.

19. Mansel RE, Harrison BJ, Melhuish J, et al. A randomized trial of dietary intervention with essential fatty acids in patients with categorized cysts. *Ann NY Acad Sci.* 1990; 586:288-294.

20. Kollias J, Macmillan RD, Sibbering DM, et al. Effect of evening primrose oil on clinically diagnosed fibroadenomas. *Breast.* 2000;9:35-36.

21. Budeiri D, Li Wan Po A, Dornan JC. Is evening primrose oil of value in the treatment of premenstrual syndrome? *Control Clin Trials.* 1996;17:60-68.

22. Wyatt KM, Dimmock PW, Jones PW, et al. Efficacy of vitamin B6 in the treatment of premenstrual syndrome: systematic review. *BMJ.* 1999;318:1375-1381.

23. Kleijnen J, Ter Riet G, Knipschild P. Vitamin B6 in the treatment of the premenstrual syndrome: a review. *Br J Obstet Gynaecol.* 1990;97:847-852.

24. Diegoli MS, da Fonseca AM, Diegoli CA, et al. A double-blind trial of four medications to treat severe premenstrual syndrome. *Int J Gynaecol Obstet.* 1998;62:63-67.

25. Ingram DM, Hickling C, West L, et al. A double-blind randomized controlled trial of isoflavones in the treatment of cyclical mastalgia. *Breast* 2002;11:170-174.

Psoriasis

1. Syed TA, Ahmad SA, Holt AH, et al. Management of psoriasis with *Aloe vera* extract in a hydrophilic cream: a placebo-controlled, double-blind study. *Trop Med Int Health.* 1996;1:505-509.
2. Wiesenauer M, Ludtke R. Mahonia aquifolium in patients with psoriasis vulgaris: an intraindividual study. *Phytomedicine.* 1996;3:231-235.
3. Augustin M, Andrees U, Grimme H, et al. Effects of *Mahonia aquifolium* ointment on the expression of adhesion, proliferation, and activation markers in the skin of patients with psoriasis. *Forsch Komplementarmed.* 1999;6(suppl 2):19-21.
4. Soyland E, Funk J, Rajka G, et al. Effect of dietary supplementation with very-long-chain n-3 fatty acids in patients with psoriasis. *N Engl J Med.* 1993;328:1812-1816.
5. Bittiner SB, Tucker WF, Cartwright I, et al. A double-blind, randomized, placebo-controlled trial of fish oil in psoriasis. *Lancet.* 1988;1:378-380.
6. Dupont E, Savard PE, Jourdain C, et al. Antiangiogenic properties of a novel shark cartilage extract: potential role in the treatment of psoriasis. *J Cutan Med Surg.* 1998;2:146-152.

Raynaud's Phenomenon

1. DiGiacomo RA, Kremer JM, Shah DM. Fish-oil dietary supplementation in patients with Raynaud's phenomenon: a double-blind, controlled, prospective study. *Am J Med.* 1989;86:158-164.
2. Ringer TV, Hughes GS, Spillers. Fish oil blunts the pain response to cold pressor testing in normal males [abstract]. *J Am Coll Nutr.* 1989;8:435.
3. Belch JJ, Shaw B, O'Dowd A, et al. Evening primrose oil (Efamol) in the treatment of Raynaud's phenomenon: a double blind study. *Thromb Haemost.* 1985;54:490-494.
4. Sunderland GT, Belch JJ, Sturrock RD, et al. A double blind randomized placebo controlled trial of hexopal in primary Raynaud's disease. *Clin Rheumatol.* 1988;7:46-49.
5. Jung F, Mrowietz C, Kiesewetter H, et al. Effect of *Ginkgo biloba* on fluidity of blood and peripheral microcirculation in volunteers. *Arzneimittelforschung.* 1990;40:589-593.
6. Roncin JP, Schwartz F, D'Arbigny P. EGb 761 in control of acute mountain sickness and vascular reactivity to cold exposure. *Aviat Space Environ Med.* 1996;67:445-452.

Respiratory Infections (Minor)

1. Audera C, Patulny RV, Sander BH, et al. Mega-dose vitamin C in treatment of the common cold: a randomized controlled trial. *Med J Aust.* 2001;175:359-362.
2. Brinkeborn RM, Shah DV, Degenring FH. Echinaforce and other *Echinacea* fresh plant preparations in the treatment of the common cold: a randomized, placebo controlled, double-blind clinical trial. *Phytomedicine.* 1999;6:1-5.
3. Josling P. Preventing the common cold with a garlic supplement: a double-blind, placebo-controlled survey. *Adv Ther.* 2001;18(4):189-193.
4. Dorn M, Knick E, Lewith G. Placebo-controlled double-blind study of *Echinacea pallidae* radix in upper respiratory tract infections. *Complement Ther Med.* 1997;5:40-42.
5. Lindenmuth GF, Lindenmuth EB. The efficacy of echinacea compound herbal tea preparation on the severity and duration of upper respiratory and flu symptoms: a randomized, double-blind placebo-controlled study. *J Altern Complement Med.* 2000;6:327-334.
6. Hoheisel O, Sandberg M, Bertram S, et al. Echinagard® treatment shortens the course of the common cold: a double-blind placebo-controlled clinical trial. *Eur J Clin Res.* 1997;9:261-268.
7. Schulten B, Bulitta M, Ballering-Bruhl B, et al. Efficacy of *Echinacea purpurea* in patients with a common cold. A placebo-controlled, randomized, double-blind clinical trial. *Arzneimittelforschung.* 2001;51:563-568.
8. Melchart D, Linde K, Worku F, et al. Immunomodulation with echinacea: a systematic review of controlled clinical trials. *Phytomedicine.* 1994;1:245-254.
9. Melchart D, Walther E, Linde K, et al. *Echinacea* root extracts for the prevention of upper respiratory tract infections: a double-blind, placebo-controlled randomized trial. *Arch Fam Med.* 1998;7:541-545.

10. Grimm W, Muller H. A randomized controlled trial of the effect of fluid extract of *Echinacea purpurea* on the incidence and severity of colds and respiratory infections. *Am J Med*. 1999;106:138-143.

11. Chamberlain C. Take echinacea? Bless You (April 27, 1999). ABC News web site. http://www.abcnews.go.com/sections/living/DailyNews/echinacea990427.html. Accessed July 15, 2000.

12. Turner RB, Riker DK, Gangemi JD. Ineffectiveness of echinacea for prevention of experimental rhinovirus colds. *Antimicrob Agents Chemother*. 2000;44:1708-1709.

13. Schmidt U, Albrecht M, Schenk N. Immunostimulator decreases the frequency of influenza-like syndromes: double-blind placebo-controlled trial on 646 students of the University of Cologne [in German; English abstract]. *Natur und Ganzheitsmedizin*. 1990;3:277-281.

14. Hirt M, Nobel S, Barron E. Zinc nasal gel for the treatment of common cold symptoms: a double-blind, placebo-controlled trial. *Ear Nose Throat J*. 2000;79:778-781.

15. Eby GA. Linearity in dose-response from zinc lozenges in treatment of common colds. *J Pharm Technol*. 1995;11:110-122.

16. Eby GA. Zinc ion availability: the determinant of efficacy in zinc lozenge treatment of common colds. *J Antimicrob Chemother*. 1997;40:483-493.

17. Belongia EA, Berg R, Liu K. A randomized trial of zinc nasal spray for the treatment of upper respiratory illness in adults. *Am J Med*. 2001;111:103-108.

18. Marshall S. Zinc gluconate and the common cold: review of randomized controlled trials. *Can Fam Physician*. 1998;44:1037-1042.

19. Prasad AS, Fitzgerald JT, Bao B, et al. Duration of symptoms and plasma cytokine levels in patients with the common cold treated with zinc acetate: a randomized, double-blind, placebo-controlled trial. *Ann Intern Med*. 2000;133:245-252.

20. Macknin ML. Zinc gluconate lozenges for treating the common cold in children: a randomized controlled trial. *JAMA*. 1998;279:1962-1967.

21. Hemila H. Does vitamin C alleviate the symptoms of the common cold? A review of current evidence. *Scand J Infect Dis*. 1994;26:1-6.

22. Hemila H. Vitamin C and the common cold. *Br J Nutr*. 1992;67:3-16.

23. Hemila H. Vitamin C supplementation and common cold symptoms: factors affecting the magnitude of the benefit. *Med Hypotheses*. 1999;52:171-178.

24. Hemila H. Vitamin C intake and susceptibility to the common cold. *Br J Nutr*. 1997;77:59-72.

25. Peters EM, Goetzsche JM, Grobbelaar B, et al. Vitamin C supplementation reduces the incidence of postrace symptoms of upper-respiratory-tract infection in ultramarathon runners. *Am J Clin Nutr*. 1993;57:170-174.

26. Hemila H. Vitamin C and common cold incidence: a review of studies with subjects under heavy physical stress. *Int J Sports Med*. 1996;17:379-383.

27. Caceres DD, Hancke JL, Burgos RA, et al. Use of visual analogue scale measurements (VAS) to assess the effectiveness of standardized *Andrograpahis paniculata* extract SHA-10 in reducing the symptoms of common cold: a randomized double blind placebo study. *Phytomedicine*. 1999;6:217-223.

28. Melchior J, Palm S, Wikman G. Controlled clinical study of standardized *Andrographis paniculata* extract in common cold: a pilot trial. *Phytomedicine*. 1996-1997;3:314-318.

29. Hancke J, Burgos R, Caceres D, et al. A double-blind study with a new monodrug Kan Jang: decrease of symptoms and improvements in the recovery from common colds. *Phytother Res*. 1995;9:559-562.

30. Melchior J, Spasov AA, Ostrovskij OV, et al. Double-blind, placebo-controlled pilot and phase III study of activity of standardized *Andrographis paniculata* Herba Nees extract fixed combination (Kan jang) in the treatment of uncomplicated upper-respiratory tract infection. *Phytomedicine*. 2000;7:341-350.

31. Thamlikitkul V, Theerapong S, Boonroj P et al. Efficacy of *Andrographis paniculata* (Nees) for pharyngotonsillitis in adults. *J Med Assoc Thai*. 1991;74:437-442.

32. Caceres DD, Hancke JL, Burgos RA, et al. Prevention of common colds with *Andrographis paniculata* dried extract: a pilot double blind trial. *Phytomedicine*. 1997;4:101-104.

33. Hatakka K, Savilahti E, Ponka A, et al. Effect of long term consumption of probiotic milk on infections in children attending day care centres: double blind, randomized trial. *BMJ*. 2001;322:1-5.
34. Meydani SN, Ha WK. Immunological effects of yogurt. *Am J Clin Nutr*. 2000;71: 861-872.
35. Arunachalam K, Gill HS, Chandra RK. Enhancement of natural immune function by dietary consumption of *Bifidobacterium lactis*. *Eur J Clin Nutr*. 2000;54:263-267.
36. Scaglione F, Cattaneo G, Alessandria M, et al. Efficacy and safety of the standardized ginseng extract G 115 for potentiating vaccination against common cold and/or influenza syndrome. *Drugs Exp Clin Res*. 1996;22:65-72.
37. Meydani SN, Meydani M, Blumberg JB, et al. Vitamin E supplementation and in vivo immune response in healthy elderly subjects: a randomized controlled trial. *JAMA*. 1997;277:1380-1386.
38. Zakay-Rones Z, Varsano N, Zlotnik M, et al. Inhibition of several strains of influenza virus in vitro and reduction of symptoms by an elderberry extract (*Sambucus nigra* L.) during an outbreak of influenza B Panama. *J Altern Complement Med*. 1995;1: 361-369.
39. Baligan M, Giardina A, Giovannini G, et al. L-arginine and immunity: study of pediatric subjects [translated from Italian]. *Minerva Pediatr*. 1997;49:537-542.
40. Fiocchi A, Borella E, Riva E, et al. A double-blind clinical trial for the evaluation of the therapeutical effectiveness of a calf thymus derivative (Thymomodulin) in children with recurrent respiratory infections. *Thymus*. 1986;8:331-339.
41. Castell LM, Poortmans JR, Newsholme EA. Does glutamine have a role in reducing infections in athletes? *Eur J Appl Physiol*. 1996;73:488-490.
42. Castell LM, Newsholme EA. Glutamine and the effects of exhaustive exercise upon the immune response. *Can J Physiol Pharmacol*. 1998;76:524-532.
43. Girodon F, Lombard M, Galan P, et al. Effect of micronutrient supplementation on infection in institutionalized elderly subjects: a controlled trial. *Ann Nutr Metab*. 1997;41:98-107.
44. Girodon F. Impact of trace elements and vitamin supplementation on immunity and infections in institutionalized elderly patients. *Arch Intern Med*. 1999;748-754.
45. Chandra RK. Effect of vitamin and trace-element supplementation on immune responses and infection in elderly subjects. *Lancet*. 1992;340:1124-1127.
46. Jain AL. Influence of vitamins and trace-elements on the incidence of respiratory infection in the elderly. *Nutr Res*. 2002;22:85-87.
47. Chandra RK, Puri S. Nutritional support improves antibody response to influenza virus vaccine in the elderly. *BMJ (Clin Res Ed)*. 1985;291;705-706.
48. Ender PT, DeRussy PK, Caldwell MM, et al. The effect of a multivitamin on the immunologic response to the influenza vaccine in the elderly. *Infect Dis Clin Pract*. 2001;10:81-85.

Restless Legs Syndrome

1. O'Keeffe ST. Restless legs syndrome: a review. *Arch Intern Med*. 1996;156:243-248.
2. Sun ER, Chen CA, Ho G, et al. Iron and the restless legs syndrome. *Sleep*. 1998;21: 371-377.
3. O'Keeffe ST, Gavin K, Lavan JN. Iron status and restless legs syndrome in the elderly. *Age Ageing*. 1994;23:200-203.
4. Davis BJ, Rajput A, Rajput ML, et al. A randomized, double-blind placebo-controlled trial of iron in restless legs syndrome. *Eur Neurol*. 2000;43:70-75.
5. Hornyak M, Voderholzer U, Hohagen F, et al. Magnesium therapy for periodic leg movements-related insomnia and restless legs syndrome: an open pilot study. *Sleep*. 1998;21:501-505.
6. Popoviciu L, Asgian B, Delast-Popoviciu D, et al. Clinical, EEG, electromyographic and polysomnographic studies in restless legs syndrome caused by magnesium deficiency. *Rom J Neurol Psychiatry*. 1993;31:55-61.
7. Ayres S Jr, Mihan R. "Restless legs" syndrome: response to vitamin E. *J Appl Nutr*. 1973;25:8-15.
8. Silber MH. Restless legs syndrome. *Mayo Clin Proc*. 1997;72:261-264.

Rheumatoid Arthritis

1. James MJ, Cleland LG. Dietary n-3 fatty acids and therapy for rheumatoid arthritis. *Semin Arthritis Rheum.* 1997;27:85-97.

2. Volker D, Fitzgerald P, Major G, et al. Efficacy of fish oil concentrate in the treatment of rheumatoid arthritis. *J Rheumatol.* 2000;27:2343-2346.

3. Zurier RB, Rossetti RG, Jacobson EW, et al. Gamma-linolenic acid treatment of rheumatoid arthritis: a randomized, placebo-controlled trial. *Arthritis Rheum.* 1996;39:1808-1817.

4. Leventhal LJ, Boyce EG, Zurier RB. Treatment of rheumatoid arthritis with gammalinolenic acid. *Ann Intern Med.* 1993;119:867-873.

5. Leventhal LJ, Boyce EG, Zurier RB. Treatment of rheumatoid arthritis with blackcurrant seed oil. *Br J Rheumatol.* 1994;33:847-852.

6. Rothman D, DeLuca P, Zurier RB. Botanical lipids: effects on inflammation, immune responses, and rheumatoid arthritis. *Semin Arthritis Rheum.* 1995;25:87-96.

7. Belch JJ, Ansell D, Madhok R, et al. Effects of altering dietary essential fatty acids on requirements for non-steroidal anti-inflammatory drugs in patients with rheumatoid arthritis: a double blind placebo controlled study. *Ann Rheum Dis.* 1988;47:96-104.

8. Horrobin DF. Nutritional and medical importance of gamma-linolenic acid. *Prog Lipid Res.* 1992;31:163-194.

9. European Scientific Cooperative on Phytotherapy. *Harpagophyti radix* (devil's claw). Exeter, UK: ESCOP; 1996-1997. Monographs on the Medicinal Uses of Plant Drugs, Fascicule 2:4-5.

10. Etzel R. Special extract of *Boswellia serrata* (H 15)* in the treatment of rheumatoid arthritis. *Phytomedicine.* 1996;3:91-94.

11. Sander O, Herborn G, Rau R. Is H15 (resin extract of *Boswellia serrata*, "incense") a useful supplement to established drug therapy of chronic polyarthritis? Results of a double-blind pilot study [in German; English abstract]. *Z Rheumatol.* 1998;57:11-16.

12. Reddy GK, Chandrakasan G, Dhar SC. Studies on the metabolism of glycosaminoglycans under the influence of new herbal anti-inflammatory agents. *Biochem Pharmacol.* 1989;38:3527-3534.

13. Tarp U. Selenium in rheumatoid arthritis: a review. *Analyst.* 1995;120:877-881.

14. Tarp U, Overvad K, Hansen JC, et al. Low selenium level in severe rheumatoid arthritis. *Scand J Rheumatol.* 1985;14:97-101.

15. Knekt P, Heliovaara M, Aho K, et al. Serum selenium, serum alpha-tocopherol, and the risk of rheumatoid arthritis. *Epidemiology.* 2000;11:402-405.

16. Peretz A, Neve J, Duchateau J, et al. Adjuvant treatment of recent onset rheumatoid arthritis by selenium supplementation: preliminary observations [letter]. *Br J Rheumatol.* 1992;31:281-286.

17. Peretz A, Neve J, Jeghers O, et al. Zinc distribution in blood components, inflammatory status, and clinical indexes of disease activity during zinc supplementation in inflammatory rheumatic diseases. *Am J Clin Nutr.* 1993;57:690-694.

18. Rasker JJ, Kardaun SH. Lack of beneficial effect of zinc sulphate in rheumatoid arthritis. *Scand J Rheumatol.* 1982;11:168-170.

19. Simkin PA. Treatment of rheumatoid arthritis with oral zinc sulfate. *Agents Actions Suppl.* 1981;8:587-596.

20. Edmonds SE, Winyard PG, Guo R, et al. Putative analgesic activity of repeated oral doses of vitamin E in the treatment of rheumatoid arthritis: results of a prospective placebo controlled double blind trial. *Ann Rheum Dis.* 1997;56:649-655.

21. Helmy M, Shohayeb M, Helmy MH, et al. Antioxidants as adjuvant therapy in rheumatoid disease. *Arzneimittelforschung.* 2001;51:293-298.

22. Tao X, Lipsky PE. The Chinese anti-inflammatory and immunosuppressive herbal remedy *Tripterygium wilfordii* Hook F. *Rheum Dis Clin North Am.* 2000;26:29-50.

23. Bingham R, Bellew BA, Bellew JG. Yucca plant saponin in the management of arthritis. *J Appl Nutr.* 1975;27:45-51.

24. Murav'ev IuV, Venikova MS, Pleskovskaia GN, et al. Effect of dimethyl sulfoxide and dimethyl sulfone on a destructive process in the joints of mice with spontaneous arthritis [in Russian; English abstract]. *Patol Fiziol Eksp Ter.* 1991;2:37-39.

25. Deodhar SD, Sethi R, Srimal RC. Preliminary study on antirheumatic activity of curcumin (diferuloyl methane). *Indian J Med Res.* 1980;71:632-634.

26. Huber B. Therapy of degenerative rheumatic diseases: need for additional analgesic medication with Phytodolor® N [translated from German]. *Fortschr Med.* 1991;109: 248-250.

27. Chopra A, Lavin P, Patwardhan B, et al. Randomized double blind trial of an ayurvedic plant derived formulation for treatment of rheumatoid arthritis. *J Rheumatol.* 2000; 27:1365-1372.

28. Cazzola M, Antivalle M, Sarzi-Puttini P, et al. Oral type II collagen in the treatment of rheumatoid arthritis: a six-month double blind placebo-controlled study. *Clin Exp Rheumatol.* 2000;18:571-577.

29. Peretz A, Siderova V, Neve J. Selenium supplementation in rheumatoid arthritis investigated in a double blind placebo-controlled trial. *Scand J Rheumatol.* 2001;30: 208-212.

30. Petersson I, Majberger E, Palm S, et al. Treatment of rheumatoid arthritis with selenium and vitamin E [abstract]. *Scand J Rheumatol.* 1991;20:218.

31. Jantti J, Vapaatalo H, Seppala E, et al. Treatment of rheumatoid arthritis with fish oil selenium vitamins A and E and placebo [abstract]. *Scand J Rheumatol.* 1991;20:225.

Sexual Dysfunction in Women

1. Baulieu EE, Thomas G, Legrain S, et al. Dehydroepiandrosterone (DHEA), DHEA sulfate, and aging: contribution of the DHEAge study to a sociobiomedical issue. *Proc Natl Acad Sci.* 2000;97:4279-4284.

2. Morales AJ, Nolan JJ, Nelson JC, et al. Effects of replacement dose of dehydroepiandrosterone in men and women of advancing age. *J Clin Endocrinol Metab.* 1994;78:1360-1367.

3. Flynn MA, Weaver-Osterholtz D, Sharpe-Timms KL, et al. Dehydroepiandrosterone replacement in aging humans. *J Clin Endocrinol Metab.* 1999;84:1527-1533.

4. Arlt W, Callies F, van Vlijmen JC, et al. Dehydroepiandrosterone replacement in women with adrenal insufficiency. *N Engl J Med.* 1999;341:1013-1020.

5. Cohen AJ, Bartlik B. *Ginkgo biloba* for antidepressant-induced sexual dysfunction. *J Sex Marital Ther.* 1998;24:139-143.

6. McCann B. Botanical could improve sex life of patients on SSRIs. *Drug Topics.* 1997;141:33.

7. Cohen A, Bartlik B. Treatment of sexual dysfunction with *Ginkgo biloba* extract [scientific reports]. Presented at: 150th Annual Meeting of the American Psychiatric Association; May 18-21, 1997; San Diego, Calif.

8. Cohen A. Long term safety and efficacy of *Ginkgo biloba* extract in the treatment of anti-depressant-induced sexual dysfunction (1997). Priory Lodge Education web site. http://www.priory.com/pharmol/gingko.htm. Accessed: July 1, 1997. (Please note variant spelling of "ginkgo.")

9. Ito TY, Trant AS, Polan ML. A double-blind placebo-controlled study of ArginMax, a nutritional supplement for enhancement of female sexual function. *J Sex Marital Ther.* 2001;27:541-549.

10. Meston CM, Worcel M. The effects of L-arginine and yohimbine on sexual arousal in postmenopausal women with female sexual arousal disorder. Presented at: 26th Annual Meeting of the International Academy of Sex Research; June 21-24, 2000; Paris, France.

11. Meston CM, Heiman JR. Acute dehydroepiandrosterone effects on sexual arousal in premenopausal women. *J Sex Marital Ther.* 2002;28:53-60.

12. Hackbert L, Heiman JR. Acute dehydroepiandrosterone (DHEA) effects on sexual arousal in postmenopausal women. *J Womens Health Gend Based Med.* 2002;11:155-162.

13. Ashton AK, Ahrens K, Gupta S, et al. Antidepressant-induced sexual dysfunction and *Ginkgo biloba* [letter]. *Am J Psychiatry.* 2000;157:836-837.

Sunburn

1. Trevithick JR, Xiong H, Lee S, et al. Topical tocopherol acetate reduces post-UVB, sunburn-associated erythema, edema, and skin sensitivity in hairless mice. *Arch Biochem Biophys.* 1992;296:575-582.
2. Trevithick JR, Shum DT, Redae S, et al. Reduction of sunburn damage to skin by topical application of vitamin E acetate following exposure to ultraviolet B radiation: effect of delaying application or of reducing concentration of vitamin E acetate applied. *Scanning Microsc.* 1993;7:1269-1281.
3. Darr D, Combs S, Dunston S, et al. Topical vitamin C protects porcine skin from ultraviolet radiation-induced damage. *Br J Dermatol.* 1992;127:247-253.
4. Darr D, Dunston S, Faust H, et al. Effectiveness of antioxidants (vitamin C and E) with and without sunscreens as topical photoprotectants. *Acta Derm Venereol.* 1996;76:264-268.
5. Eberlein-Konig B, Placzek M, Przybilla B. Protective effect against sunburn of combined systemic ascorbic acid (vitamin C) and d-alpha-tocopherol (vitamin E). *J Am Acad Dermatol.* 1998;38:45-48.
6. Fuchs J, Kern H. Modulation of UV-light-induced skin inflammation by D-alpha-tocopherol and L-ascorbic acid: a clinical study using solar simulated radiation. *Free Radic Biol Med.* 1998;25:1006-1012.
7. Werninghaus K, Meydani M, Bhawan J, et al. Evaluation of the photoprotective effect of oral vitamin E supplementation. *Arch Dermatol.* 1994;130:1257-1261.
8. Traikovich SS. Use of topical ascorbic acid and its effects on photodamaged skin topography. *Arch Otolaryngol Head Neck Surg.* 1999;125:1091-1098.
9. Katiyar SK, Elmets CA, Agarwal R, et al. Protection against ultraviolet-B radiation-induced local and systemic suppression of contact hypersensitivity and edema responses in C3H/HeN mice by green tea polyphenols. *Photochem Photobiol.* 1995; 62:855-861.
10. Katiyar SK, Matsui MS, Elmets CA, et al. Polyphenolic antioxidant (−)-epigallo-catechin-3-gallate from green tea reduces UVB-induced inflammatory responses and infiltration of leukocytes in human skin. *Photochem Photobiol.* 1999;69:148-153.
11. Gollnick HP, Hopfenmuller W, Hemmes C, et al. Systemic beta carotene plus topical UV sunscreen are an optimal protection against harmful effects of natural UV-sunlight: results of the Berlin-Eilath study. *Eur J Dermatol.* 1996;6:200-205.
12. Mathews-Roth MM, Pathak MA, Parrish J, et al. A clinical trial of the effects of oral beta-carotene on the responses of human skin to solar radiation. *J Invest Dermatol.* 1972;59:349-353.
13. Garmyn M, Ribaya-Mercado JD, Russel RM, et al. Effect of beta-carotene supplementation on the human sunburn reaction. *Exp Dermatol.* 1995;4:104-111.
14. Crowell J, Penneys N. The effect of *Aloe vera* on cutaneus erythema and blood-flow following ultraviolet-B (UVB) exposure [abstract]. *Clin Res.* 1987;35:A676.

Surgery Support

1. Schmidt JM, Greenspoon JS. *Aloe vera* dermal wound gel is associated with a delay in wound healing. *Obstet Gynecol.* 1991;78:115-117.
2. Zatuchni GI, Colombi DJ. Bromelains therapy for the prevention of episiotomy pain. *Obstet Gynecol.* 1967;29:275-278.
3. Howat RC, Lewis GD. The effect of bromelain therapy on episiotomy wounds-a double blind controlled clinical trial. *J Obstet Gynaecol Br Commow.* 1972;79:951-953.
4. Soule SD, Wasserman HC, Burstein R. Oral proteolytic enzyme therapy (Chymoral) in episiotomy patients. *Am J Obstet Gynecol.* 1966;95:820-823.
5. Cameron IW. An investigation into some of the factors concerned in the surgical removal of the impacted lower wisdom tooth, including a double blind trial of chymoral. *Br J Oral Surg.* 1980;18:112-124.
6. Seltzer AP. Minimizing post-operative edema and ecchymoses by the use of an oral enzyme preparation (bromelain): a controlled study of 53 rhinoplasty cases. *Eye Ear Nose Throat Mon.* 1962;41:813-817.
7. Spaeth GL. The effect of bromelains on the inflammatory response caused by cataract extraction: a double-blind study. *Eye Ear Nose Throat Mon.* 1968;47:634-639.

8. Tassman GC, Zafran JN, Zayon GM. Evaluation of a plant proteolytic enzyme for the control of inflammation and pain. *J Dent Med.* 1964;19:73-77.

9. Gylling U, Rintala A, Taipale S, et al. The effect of a proteolytic enzyme combinate (bromelain) on the postoperative edema by oral application: a clinical and experimental study. *Acta Chir Scand.* 1966;131:193-196.

10. Rahn H-D. Efficacy of hydrolytic enzymes in surgery. Presented at: Symposium on Enzyme Therapy in Sports Injuries: XXIV FIMS World Congress of Sport Medicine; May 29, 1990; Amsterdam.

11. Vinzenz K. Treatment of edema with hydrolytic enzymes in oral surgical procedures [translated from German]. *Quintessenz.* 1991;42:1053-1064.

12. Taylor HM, Rose KE, Twycross RG. A double-blind clinical trial of hydroxyethyl-rutosides in obstructive arm lymphoedema. *Phlebology.* 1993;1:22-28.

13. Mortimer PS, Badger C, Clarke I, et al. A double-blind, randomized, parallel-group, placebo-controlled trial of O-(beta-hydroxyethyl)-rutosides in chronic arm edema resulting from breast cancer treatment. *Phlebology.* 1995;10:51-55.

14. Piller NB, Morgan RG, Casley-Smith JR. A double-blind, cross-over trial of O-(beta-hydroxyethyl)-rutosides (benzo-pyrones) in the treatment of lymphoedema of the arms and legs. *Br J Plast Surg.* 1988;41:20-27.

15. Casley-Smith JR, Casley-Smith JR. Modern treatment of lymphoedema. II. The benzopyrones. *Australas J Dermatol.* 1992;33:69-74.

16. Pecking AP, Fevrier B, Wargon C, et al. Efficacy of Daflon 500 mg in the treatment of lymphedema (secondary to conventional therapy of breast cancer). *Angiology.* 1997;48:93-98.

17. Fassina A, Rubinacci A. Post-traumatic edema: a controlled study into the activity of hydroxyethyl rutoside [translated from Italian]. *Gazz Med Ital Arch Sci.* 1987;146: 103-109.

18. Pecking A, Desprez-Curely JP, Megret G. Oligomeric grape flavanols (Endotelon®) in the treatment of secondary upper limb lymphedemas [translated from French]. Paris, France: Association de Lymphologie de Lange Francaise Hopital Saint-Louis; 1989:69-73.

19. Baruch J. Effect of Endotelon in postoperative edema: results of a double-blind study versus placebo in 32 female patients [translated from French]. *Ann Chir Plast Esthet.* 1984;29:393-395.

20. Bone ME, Wilkinson DJ, Young JR, et al. Ginger root: a new antiemetic. The effect of ginger root on postoperative nausea and vomiting after major gynaecological sugery. *Anaesthesia.* 1990;45:669-671.

21. Phillips S, Ruggier R, Hutchinson SE, et al. *Zingiber officinale* (ginger): an antiemetic for day case surgery. *Anaesthesia.* 1993;48:715-717.

22. Arfeen Z, Owen H, Plummer JL, et al. A double-blind randomized controlled trial of ginger for the prevention of postoperative nausea and vomiting. *Anaesth Intensive Care.* 1995;23:449-452.

23. Visalyaputra S, Petchpaisit N, Somcharoen K, et al. The efficacy of ginger root in the prevention of postoperative nausea and vomiting after outpatient gynaecological laparoscopy. *Anaesthesia.* 1998;53:506-510.

24. Naguib M, Samarkandi AH. Premedication with melatonin: a double-blind, placebo-controlled comparison with midazolam. *Br J Anaesth.* 1999;82:875-880.

25. Naguib M, Samarkandi AH. The comparative dose-response effects of melatonin and midazolam for premedication of adult patients: a double-blinded, placebo-controlled study. *Anesth Analg.* 2000;91:473-479.

26. Tepaske R, Velthuis H, Oudemans-van Straaten HM, et al. Effect of preoperative oral immune-enhancing nutritional supplement on patients at high risk of infection after cardiac surgery: a randomized placebo-controlled trial. *Lancet.* 2001;358:696-701.

27. Magro Filho O, de Carvalho AC. Topical effect of propolis in the repair of sulcoplasties by the modified Kazanjian technique: cytological and clinical evaluation. *J Nihon Univ Sch Dent.* 1994;36:102-111.

28. Wilhelm K, Feldmeier C. Thermometric investigations about the efficacy of Beta-escin to reduce postoperative edema [in German; English abstract]. *Med Klin.* 1977;72:128-134.

29. European Scientific Cooperative on Phytotherapy. *Allii sativi bulbus* (garlic). Exeter, UK: ESCOP; 1996-1997. Monographs on the Medicinal Uses of Plant Drugs, Fascicule 3.

30. Burnham BE. Garlic as a possible risk for postoperative bleeding [letter]. *Plast Reconstr Surg.* 1995;95:213.

31. German K, Kumar U, Blackford HN. Garlic and the risk of TURP bleeding. *Br J Urol.* 1995;76:518.

32. Frank SC. Use of chymoral as an anti-inflammatory agent following surgical trauma. *J Am Podiatr Assoc.* 1966;55:706-709.

33. Cheema P, El-Mefty O, Jazieh AR. Intraoperative hemorrhage associated with the use of extract of Saw Palmetto herb: a case report and review of literature. *J Intern Med.* 2001;250:167-169.

Systemic Lupus Erythematosus

1. Mease PJ, Merrill JT, Lahita R, et al. GL701 (prasterone, dehydroepiandrosterone) improves or stabilizes disease activity in systemic lupus erythematosus. Presented at: The Endocrine Society's 82nd Annual Meeting; June 21-24, 2000; Toronto.

2. van Vollenhoven RF, Morabito LM, Engelman EG, et al. Treatment of systemic lupus erythematosus with dehydroepiandrosterone: 50 patients treated up to 12 months. *J Rheumatol.* 1998;25:285-289.

3. van Vollenhoven RF, Park JL, Genovese MC, et al. A double-blind, placebo-controlled, clinical trial of dehydroepiandrosterone in severe systemic lupus erythematosus. *Lupus.* 1999;8:181-187.

4. Hall AV, Parbtani A, Clark WF, et al. Abrogation of MRL/lpr lupus nephritis by dietary flaxseed. *Am J Kidney Dis.* 1993;22:326-332.

5. Clark WF, Parbtani A, Huff MW, et al. Flaxseed: a potential treatment for lupus nephritis. *Kidney Int.* 1995;48:475-480.

6. Clark WF, Parbtani A, Naylor CD, et al. Fish oil in lupus nephritis: clinical findings and methodological implications. *Kidney Int.* 1993;44:75-86.

7. Clark WF, Parbtani A. Omega-3 fatty acid supplementation in clinical and experimental lupus nephritis. *Am J Kidney Dis.* 1994;23:644-647.

8. Walton AJ, Snaith ML,Locniskar M. Dietary fish oil and the severity of symptoms in patients with systemic lupus erythematosus. *Ann Rheum Dis.* 1991;50:463-466.

9. Roberts JL, Hayashi JA. Exacerbation of SLE associated with alfalfa ingestion[letter]. *N Engl J Med.* 1983;308:1361.

10. Malinow MR, Bardana EJ, Pirofsky B, et al. Systemic lupus erythematosus-like syndrome in monkeys fed alfalfa sprouts: role of a nonprotein amino acid. *Science.* 1982;216:415-417.

Tardive Dyskinesia

1. Richardson MA. *Amino Acids in Psychiatric Disease.* Washington, DC: American Psychiatric Press; 1990.

2. Gardos G, Cole JO, Matthews JD, et al. The acute effects of a loading dose of phenylalanine in unipolar depressed patients with and without tardive dyskinesia. *Neuropsychopharmacology.* 1992;6:241-247.

3. Mosnik DM, Spring B, Rogers K, et al. Tardive dyskinesia exacerbated after ingestion of phenylalanine by schizophrenic patients. *Neuropsychopharmacology.* 1997;16:136-146.

4. Adler LA, Rotrosen J, Edson R, et al. Vitamin E treatment for tardive dyskinesia. *Arch Gen Psychiatry.* 1999;56:836-841.

5. Boomershine KH, Shelton PS, Boomershine JE. Vitamin E in the treatment of tardive dyskinesia. *Ann Pharmacother.* 1999;33:1195-1202.

6. Joe SH. Effect of lecithin on tardive dyskinesia. *Korea Univ Med J.* 1985;22:197-206.

7. Gelenberg AJ, Dorer DJ, Wojcik JD, et al. A crossover study of lecithin treatment of tardive dyskinesia. *J Clin Psychiatry.* 1990;51:149-153.

8. Domino EF, May WW, Demetriou S, et al. Lack of clinically significant improvement of patients with tardive dyskinesia following phosphatidylcholine therapy. *Biol Psychiatry.* 1985;20:1189-1196.
9. Growdon JH, Hirsch MJ, Wurtman RJ, et al. Oral choline administration to patients with tardive dyskinesia. *N Engl J Med.* 1977;297:524-527.
10. Nasrallah HA, Dunner FJ, Smith RE, et al. Variable clinical response to choline in tardive dyskinesia. *Psychol Med.* 1984;14:697-700.
11. Gelenberg AJ, Wojcik J, Falk WE, et al. CDP-choline for the treatment of tardive dyskinesia: a small negative series. *Compr Psychiatry.* 1989;30:1-4.
12. Alphs L, Davis JM. Noncatecholaminergic treatments of tardive dyskinesia. *J Clin Psychopharmacol.* 1982;2:380-385.
13. Richardson MA, Bevans ML, Weber JB, et al. Branched chain amino acids decrease tardive dyskinesia symptoms. *Psychopharmacology.* 1999;143:358-364.
14. Kunin RA. Manganese and niacin in the treatment of drug-induced tardive dyskinesias. *J Orthomol Psychiatry.* 1976;5:4-27.Cited by: Werbach MR. *Nutritional Influences on Illness* [book on CD-ROM]. Tarzana, Calif: Third Line Press; 1998.
15. DeVeaugh-Geiss J, Manion L. High-dose pyridoxine in tardive dyskinesia. *J Clin Psychiatry.* 1978;39:573-575.
16. Sandyk R, Pardeshi R. Pyridoxine improves drug-induced Parkinsonism and psychosis in a schizophrenic patient. *Int J Neurosci.* 1990;52:225-232.
17. Lerner V, Kaptsan A, Miodownik C, et al. Vitamin B6 in treatment of tardive dyskinesia: a preliminary case series study. *Clin Neuropharmacol.* 1999;22:241-243.
18. Lerner V, Miodownik C, Kaptsan A, et al. Vitamin B(6) in the treatment of tardive dyskinesia: a double-blind, placebo-controlled, crossover study. *Am J Psychiatry.* 2001;158:1511-1514.
19. Peet M, Laugharne JD, Mellor J, et al. Essential fatty acid deficiency in erythrocyte membranes from chronic schizophrenic patients, and the clinical effects of dietary supplementation. *Prostaglandins Leukot Essent Fatty Acids.* 1996;55:71-75.
20. Wolkin A, Jordan B, Peselow E, et al. Essential fatty acid supplementation in tardive dyskinesia. *Am J Psychiatry.* 1986;143:912-914.
21. Vaddadi KS, Courtney P, Gilleard CJ, et al. A double-blind trial of essential fatty acid supplementation in patients with tardive dyskinesia. *Psychiatry Res.* 1989;27:313-323.
22. Vaddadi K. Dyskinesias and their treatment with essential fatty acids: a review. *Prostaglandins Leukot Essent Fatty Acids.* 1996;55:89-94.
23. Hawkins DR. Successful prevention of tardive dyskinesia. *J Orthomolec Med.* 1989;4:35-36.
24. Shamir E, Barak Y, Plopsky I, et al. Is melatonin treatment effective for tardive dyskinesia? *J Clin Psychiatry.* 2000;61:556-558.
25. Shamir E, Barak Y, Shalman I, et al. Melatonin treatment for tardive dyskinesia: a double-blind, placebo-controlled, crossover study. *Arch Gen Psychiatry.* 2001;58:1049-1052.

Tinea Pedis

1. Williams LR, Home VN, Zhang X, et al. The composition and bactericidal activity of oil of *Melaleuca alternifolia* (tea tree oil). *Int J Aromather.* 1988;1:15-17.
2. May J, Chan CH, King A, et al. Time-kill studies of tea tree oils on clinical isolates. *J Antimicrob Chemother.* 2000;45:639-643.
3. Tong MM, Altman PM, Barnetson RS. Tea tree oil in the treatment of tinea pedis. *Australas J Dermatol.* 1992;33:145-149.
4. Buck DS, Nidorf DM, Addino JG. Comparison of two topical preparations for the treatment of onychomycosis: *Melaleuca alternifolia* (tea tree) oil and clotrimazole. *J Fam Pract.* 1994;38:601-605.
5. Ledezma E, Marcano K, Jorquera A, et al. Efficacy of ajoene in the treatment of tinea pedis: a double-blind and comparative study with terbinafine. *J Am Acad Dermatol.* 2000;43:829-832.
6. Ramadan W, Mourad B, Ibrahim S, et al. Oil of bitter orange: new topical antifungal agent. *Int J Dermatol.* 1996;35:448-449.

7. Pattnaik S, Subramanyam VR, Bapaji M, et al. Antibacterial and antifungal activity of aromatic constituents of essential oils. *Microbios*. 1997;89:39-46.

8. Lozoya X, Navarro V, Garcia M, et al. *Solanum chrysotrichum* (Schldl): a plant used in Mexico for the treatment of skin mycosis. *J Ethnopharmacol*. 1992;36:127-132.

9. Ali-Shtayeh MS, Abu Ghdeib SI. Antifungal activity of plant extracts against dermatophytes. *Mycoses*. 1999;42:665-672.

10. McCutcheon AR, Ellis SM, Hancock REW, et al. Antifungal screening of medicinal plants of British Columbian native peoples. *J Ethnopharmacol*. 1994;44:157-169.

11. Caceres A, Jauregui E, Herrera D, et al. Plants used in Guatemala for the treatment of dermatomucosal infections. 1: Screening of 38 plant extracts for anticandidal activity. *J Ethnopharmacol*. 1991;33:277-283.

12. Guiraud P, Steiman R, Campos-Takaki GM, et al. Comparison of antibacterial and antifungal activities of lapachol and beta-lapachone. *Planta Med*. 1994;60:373-374.

13. Chandra B, Lakshmi V, Srivastava OP, et al. In vitro antifungal activity of constituents of *Hypericum mysorense* Heyne against *Trichophyton mentagrophytes*. *Indian Drugs*. 1989;26:678-679.

14. Zehavi U, Polacheck I. Saponins as antimycotic agents: glycosides of medicagenic acid. *Adv Exp Med Biol*. 1996;404:535-546.

Tinnitus

1. Ernst E, Stevinson C. *Ginkgo biloba* for tinnitus: a review. *Clin Otolaryngol*. 1999;24:164-167.

2. Holgers KM, Axelsson A, Pringle I. *Ginkgo biloba* extract for the treatment of tinnitus. *Audiology*. 1994;33:85-92.

3. Meyer B. Multicenter randomized double-blind drug vs. placebo study of the treatment of tinnitus with *Ginkgo biloba* extract [translated from French]. *Presse Med*. 1986;15:1562-1564.

4. Morgenstern C, Biermann E. Long-term tinnitus therapy with ginkgo special extract EGb 761 [translated from German]. *Fortschr Med*. 1997;115(29):57-58.

5. Drew S, Davies E. Effectiveness of *Ginkgo biloba* in treating tinnitus: double blind, placebo controlled trial. *BMJ*. 2001;322:73-75.

6. Shemesh Z, Attias J, Ornan M, et al. Vitamin B12 deficiency in patients with chronic-tinnitus and noise-induced hearing loss. *Am J Otolaryngol*. 1993;14:94-99.

7. Romeo G, Giorgetti M. Therapeutic effects of vitamin A associated with vitamin E in perceptual hearing loss [translated from Italian]. *Acta Vitaminol Enzymol*. 1985;7:139-143.

8. Gersdorff M, Robillard T, Stein F, et al. The zinc sulfate overload test in patients suffering from tinnitus associated with low serum zinc: preliminary report [in French; English abstract]. *Acta Otorhinolaryngol Belg*. 1987;41:498-505.

9. Paaske PB, Pedersen CB, Kjems G, et al. Zinc in the management of tinnitus: placebo-controlled trial. *Ann Otol Rhinol Laryngol*. 1991;100:647-649.

10. Ehrenberger K, Brix R. Glutamic acid and glutamic acid diethylester in tinnitus treatment. *Acta Otolaryngol (Stockh)*. 1983;95:599-605.

11. Sziklai I, Komora V, Ribari O. Double-blind study on the effectiveness of a bioflavonoid in the control of tinnitus in otosclerosis. *Acta Chir Hung*. 1992-1993;33:101-107.

12. Moser M, Ranacher G, Wilmot TJ, et al. A double-blind clinical trial of hydroxy-ethylrutosides in Meniere's disease. *J Laryngol Otol*. 1984;98:265-272.

13. Dobie RA. A review of randomized clinical trials in tinnitus. *Laryngoscope*. 1999;109:1202-1211.

14. Rosenberg SI, Silverstein H, Rowan PT, et al. Effect of melatonin on tinnitus. *Laryngoscope*. 1998;108:305-310.

Ulcerative Colitis

1. Sturniolo GC, Mestriner C, Lecis PE, et al. Altered plasma and mucosal concentrations of trace elements and antioxidants in active ulcerative colitis. *Scand J Gastroenterol*. 1998;33:644-649.

2. Mortensen PB, Abildgaard K, Fallingborg J. Serum selenium concentration in patients with ulcerative colitis. *Dan Med Bull.* 1989;36:568-570.

3. Dronfield MW, Malone JD, Langman MJ. Zinc in ulcerative colitis: a therapeutic trial and report on plasma levels. *Gut.* 1977;18:33-36.

4. Elsborg L, Larsen L. Folate deficiency in chronic inflammatory bowel disease. *Scand J Gastroenterol.* 1979;14:1019-1024.

5. Krasinski SD, Russell RM, Furie BC, et al. The prevalence of vitamin K deficiency in chronic gastrointestinal disorders. *Am J Clin Nutr.* 1985;41:639-643.

6. Bischoff SC, Herrmann A, Goke M, et al. Altered bone metabolism in inflammatory bowel disease. *Am J Gastroenterol.* 1997;92:1157-1163.

7. Dibble JB, Sheridan P, Losowsky MS. A survey of vitamin D deficiency in gastrointestinal and liver disorders. *Q J Med.* 1984;53:119-134.

8. Mulder TP, van der Sluys Veer A, Verspaget HW, et al. Effect of oral zinc supplementation on metallothionein and superoxide dismutase concentrations in patients with inflammatory bowel disease. *J Gastroenterol Hepatol.* 1994;9:472-477.

9. Ainley CC, Cason J, Carlsson LK, et al. Zinc status in inflammatory bowel disease. *Clin Sci (Colch).* 1988;75:277-283.

10. Halsted CH, Ghandi G, Tamura T. Sulfasalazine inhibits the absorption of folates in ulcerative colitis. *N Engl J Med.* 1981;305:1513-1517.

11. Kruis W, Schutz E, Fric P, et al. Double-blind comparison of an oral *Escherichia coli* preparation and mesalazine in maintaining remission of ulcerative colitis. *Aliment Pharmacol Ther.* 1997;11:853-858.

12. Gionchetti P, Rizzello F, Venturi A, et al. Oral bacteriotherapy as maintenance treatment in patients with chronic pouchitis: a double-blind, placebo-controlled trial. *Gastroenterology.* 2000;119:305-309.

13. Aslan A, Triadafilopoulos G. Fish oil fatty acid supplementation in active ulcerative colitis: a double-blind, placebo-controlled, crossover study. *Am J Gastroenterol.* 1992;87:432-437.

14. Almallah YZ, El-Tahir A, Heys SD, et al. Distal procto-colitis and n-3 polyunsaturated fatty acids: the mechanism(s) of natural cytotoxicity inhibition. *Eur J Clin Invest.* 2000;30:58-65.

15. Stenson WF, Cort D, Rodgers J, et al. Dietary supplementation with fish oil in ulcerative colitis. *Ann Intern Med.* 1992;116:609-614.

16. Hawthorne AB, Daneshmend TK, Hawkey CJ, et al. Treatment of ulcerative colitis with fish oil supplementation: a prospective 12 month randomized controlled trial. *Gut.* 1992;33:922-928.

17. Greenfield SM, Green AT, Teare JP, et al. A randomized controlled study of evening primrose oil and fish oil in ulcerative colitis. *Aliment Pharmacol Ther.* 1993;7:159-166.

18. Loeschke K, Ueberschaer B, Pietsch A, et al. n-3 fatty acids only delay early relapse of ulcerative colitis in remission. *Dig Dis Sci.* 1996;41:2087-2094.

19. Gupta I, Parihar A, Malhotra P, et al. Effects of *Boswellia serrata* gum resin in patients with ulcerative colitis. *Eur J Med Res.* 1997;2:37-43.

20. Kane S, Goldberg MJ. Use of bromelain for mild ulcerative colitis [letter]. *Ann Intern Med.* 2000;132:680.

21. Alverdy JC. Effects of glutamine-supplemented diets on immunology of the gut. *JPEN J Parenter Enteral Nutr.* 1990;14(4 suppl):109S-113S.

22. Fox AD, Kripke SA, Berman JR, et al. Reduction of the severity of enterocolitis by glutamine-supplemented enteral diets. *Surg Forum.* 1987;38:43-44.

23. Fujita T, Sakurai K. Efficacy of glutamine-enriched enteral nutrition in an experimental model of mucosal ulcerative colitis. *Br J Surg.* 1995;82:749-751.

24. van der Hulst RR, van Kreel BK, von Meyenfeldt MF, et al. Glutamine and the preservation of gut integrity. *Lancet.* 1993;341:1363-1365.

25. Merchant RE, Andre CA. A review of recent clinical trials of the nutritional supplement *Chlorella pyrenoidosa* in the treatment of fibromyalgia, hypertension, and ulcerative colitis. *Altern Ther Health Med.* 2001;7:79-80, 82-91.

Urolithiasis

1. Trinchieri A, Mandressi A, Luongo P, et al. The influence of diet on urinary risk factors for stones in healthy subjects and idiopathic renal calcium stone formers. *Br J Urol.* 1991;67:230-236.

2. Ruml LA, Pearle MS, Pak CY. Medical therapy, calcium oxalate urolithiasis. *Urol Clin North Am.* 1997;24:117-133.

3. Parivar F, Low RK, Stoller ML. The influence of diet on urinary stone disease. *J Urol.* 1996;155:432-440.

4. Curhan GC, Willett WC, Rimm EB, et al. Prospective study of beverage use and the risk of kidney stones. *Am J Epidemiol.* 1996;143:240-247.

5. Curhan GC, Willett WC, Speizer FE, et al. Beverage use and risk for kidney stones in women. *Ann Intern Med.* 1998;128:534-540.

6. Terris MK, Issa MM, Tacker JR. Dietary supplementation with cranberry concentrate tablets may increase the risk of nephrolithiasis. *Urology.* 2001;57:26-29.

7. Barcelo P, Wuhl O, Servitge E, et al. Randomized double-blind study of potassium citrate in idiopathic hypocitraturic calcium nephrolithiasis. *J Urol.* 1993;150:1761-1764.

8. Ettinger B, Pak CY, Citron JT, et al. Potassium-magnesium citrate is an effective prophylaxis against recurrent calcium oxalate nephrolithiasis. *J Urol.* 1997;158:2069-2073.

9. Seltzer MA, Low RK, McDonald M, et al. Dietary manipulation with lemonade to treat hypocitraturic calcium nephrolithiasis. *J Urol.* 1996;156:907-909.

10. Pak CY. Citrate and renal calculi: an update. *Miner Electrolyte Metab.* 1994;20:371-377.

11. Li MK, Blacklock NJ, Garside J. Effects of magnesium on calcium oxalate crystallization. *J Urol.* 1985;133:123-125.

12. Johansson G, Backman U, Danielson BG, et al. Biochemical and clinical effects of the prophylactic treatment of renal calcium stones with magnesium hydroxide. *J Urol.* 1980;124:770-774.

13. Wilson DR, Strauss AL, Manuel MA. Comparison of medical treatments for the prevention of recurrent calcium nephrolithiasis [abstract]. *Urol Res.* 1984;12:39-40.

14. Ettinger B, Citron JT, Livermore B, et al. Chlorthalidone reduces calcium oxalate calculous recurrence but magnesium hydroxide does not. *J Urol.* 1988;139:679-684.

15. Murthy MS, Farooqui S, Talwar HS, et al. Effect of pyridoxine supplementation on recurrent stone formers. *Int J Clin Pharmacol Ther Toxicol.* 1982;20:434-437.

16. Curhan GC, Willett WC, Speizer FE, et al. Intake of vitamins B6 and C and the risk of kidney stones in women. *J Am Soc Nephrol.* 1999;10:840-845.

17. Curhan GC, Willett WC, Rimm EB, et al. A prospective study of the intake of vitamins C and B6, and the risk of kidney stones in men. *J Urol.* 1996;155:1847-1851.

18. Blumenthal M, ed. *The Complete German Commission E Monographs, Therapeutic Guide to Herbal Medicines.* Boston: Integrative Medicine Communications; 1998:429.

19. Baggio B, Gambaro G, Marchini F, et al. Correction of erythrocyte abnormalities in idiopathic calcium-oxalate nephrolithiasis and reduction of urinary oxalate by oral glycosaminoglycans. *Lancet.* 1991;338:403-405.

20. Buck AC, Jenkins A, Lingam K, et al. The treatment of idiopathic recurrent urolithiasis with fish oil (EPA) and evening primrose oil (GLA): a double blind study [abstract]. *J Urol.* 1993;149:253A.

21. Tulloch I, Smellie WS, Buck AC. Evening primrose oil reduces urinary calcium excretion in both normal and hypercalciuric rats. *Urol Res.* 1994;22:227-230.

22. Bichler KH, Kirchner C, Weiser H, et al. Influence of vitamin A deficiency on the excretion of uromucoid and other substances in the urine of rats. *Clin Nephrol.* 1983;20:32-39.

23. Gerster H. No contribution of ascorbic acid to renal calcium oxalate stones. *Ann Nutr Metab.* 1997;41:269-282.

24. Simon JA, Hudes ES. Relation of serum ascorbic acid to serum vitamin B12, serum ferritin, and kidney stones in US adults. *Arch Intern Med.* 1999;159:619-624.

25. Auer BL, Auer D, Rodgers AL. Relative hyperoxaluria, crystalluria, and haematuria after megadose ingestion of vitamin C. *Eur J Clin Invest.* 1998;28:695-700.

26. Curhan GC, Willett WC, Rimm EB. Comparison of dietary calcium with supple-mental calcium and other nutrients as factors affecting the risk for kidney stones in women. *Ann Intern Med.* 1997;126:497-504.

27. Curhan GC, Willett WC, Rimm EB, et al. A prospective study of dietary calcium and other nutrients and the risk of symptomatic kidney stones. *N Engl J Med.* 1993;328:833-838.

28. Borghi L, Schianchi T, Meschi T, et al. Comparison of two diets for the prevention of recurrent stones in idiopathic hypercalciuria. *N Engl J Med.* 2002;346:77-84.

Vaginal Infection

1. Elmer GW, Surawicz CM, McFarland LV. Biotherapeutic agents: a neglected modal-ity for the treatment and prevention of selected intestinal and vaginal infections. *JAMA.* 1996;275:870-876.

2. Reid G, Bruce AW, McGroarty JA, et al. Is there a role for lactobacilli in prevention of urogenital and intestinal infections. *Clin Microbiol Rev.* 1990;3:335-344.

3. McGroarty JA. Probiotic use of lactobacilli in the human female urogenital tract. *FEMS Immunol Med Microbiol.* 1993;6:251-264.

4. Hilton E, Rindos P, Isenberg HD. *Lactobacillus GG* vaginal supositories and vagini-tis [letter]. *J Clin Microbiol.* 1995;33:1433.

5. Friedlander A, Druker MM, Schachter A. *Lactobacillus acidophillus* and vitamin B com-plex in the treatment of vaginal infection. *Panminerva Med.* 1986;28:51-53.

6. Hilton E, Isenberg HD, Alperstein P, et al. Ingestion of yogurt containing *Lactobacillus acidophilus* as prophylaxis for candidal vaginitis. *Ann Intern Med.* 1992;116:353-357.

7. Williams LR, Home VN, Zhang X, et al. The composition and bactericidal activity of oil of *Melaleuca alternifolia* (tea tree oil). *Int J Aromather.* 1988;1:15-17.

8. Hammer KA, Carson CF, Riley TV. In vitro susceptibilities of lactobacilli and or-ganisms associated with bacterial vaginosis to *Melaleuca alternifolia* (tea tree) oil [letter]. *Antimicrob Agents Chemother.* 1999;43:196.

9. Lippert U, Walter A, Hausen B, et al. Increasing incidence of contact dermatitis to tea tree oil [abstract]. *J Allergy Clin Immunol.* 2000;105(1 pt 2):A127.

10. van Slyke KK, Michel VP, Rein MF. Treatment of vulvovaginal candidiasis with boric acid powder. *Am J Obstet Gynecol.* 1981;141:145-148.

11. Penna RP, ed. *Handbook of Nonprescription Drugs.* 6th ed. Washington, DC: American Pharmaceutical Association; 1979:424.

12. Giron LM, Aguilar GA, Caceres A, et al. Anticandidal activity of plants used for the treatment of vaginitis in Guatemala and clinical trial of a *Solanum nigrescens* prepa-ration. *J Ethnopharmacol.* 1988;22:307-313.

13. Guiraud P, Steiman R, Campos-Takaki GM, et al. Comparison of antibacterial and antifungal activities of lapachol and beta-lapachone. *Planta Med.* 1994;60:373-374.

14. Sandhu DK, Warraich MK, Singh S. Sensitivity of yeasts isolated from cases of vaginitis to aqueous extracts of garlic. *Mykosen.* 1980;23:691-698.

15. Ghannoum MA. Studies on the anticandidal mode of action of *Allium sativum* (garlic). *J Gen Microbiol.* 1988;134:2917-2924.

16. Hughes BG, Lawson LD. Antimicrobial effects of *Allium sativum* L. (garlic), *Allium ampeloprasum* L. (elephant garlic), and *Allium cepa* L. (onion), garlic compounds and commercial garlic supplement products. *Phytother Res.* 1991;5:154-158.

17. Kaneda Y, Torii M, Tanaka T, et al. In vitro effects of berberine sulphate on the growth and structure of *Entamoeba histolytica*, *Giardia lamblia* and *Trichomonas vagi-nalis*. *Ann Trop Med Parasitol.* 1991;85:417-425.

18. Pattnaik S, Subramanyam VR, Bapaji M, et al. Antibacterial and antifungal activity of aromatic constituents of essential oils. *Microbios.* 1997;89:39-46.

19. Quale JM, Landman D, Zaman MM, et al. In vitro activity of *Cinnamomum zeylan-icum* against azole resistant and sensitive *Candida* species and a pilot study of cinna-mon for oral candidiasis. *Am J Chin Med.* 1996;24:103-109.

20. Singh HB, Srivastava M, Singh AB, et al. Cinnamon bark oil, a potent fungitoxicant against fungi causing respiratory tract mycoses. *Allergy.* 1995;50:995-999.

Venous Insufficiency (Chronic)

1. Bisler H, Pfeifer R, Kluken N, et al. Effect of horse-chestnut seed extract on trans-capillary filtration in chronic venous insufficiency [translated from German]. *Dtsch Med Wochenschr.* 1986;111:1321-1329.

2. Lohr E, Garanin G, Jesau P, Fischer H. Anti-edemic therapy in chronic venous insufficiency with tendency to formation of edema [translated from German]. *MMW Munch Med Wochenschr.* 1986;128:579-581.

3. Rudofsky G, Neiss A, Otto K, Seibel K. Antiedematous effects and clinical effectiveness of horse chestnut seed extract in double blind studies [translated from German]. *Phlebol Proktol.* 1986;15:47-54.

4. Steiner M, Hillemanns HG. Investigation of the anti-edemic efficacy of Venostasin® retard [translated from German]. *MMW Munch Med Wochenschr.* 1986;128:551-552.

5. Diehm C. The role of edema protective drugs in the treatment of chronic venous insufficiency: a review of evidence based on placebo-controlled clinical trials with regard to efficacy and tolerance. *Phlebology.* 1996;11:23-29.

6. Wadworth AN, Faulds D. Hydroxyethylrutosides. A review of its pharmacology, and therapeutic efficacy in venous insufficiency and related disorders. *Drugs.* 1992;44:1013-1032.

7. Pulvertaft TB. General practice treatment of symptoms of venous insufficiency with oxerutins: results of a 660 patient multicentre study in the UK. *Vasa.* 1983;12:373-376.

8. Unkauf M, Rehn D, Klinger J, et al. Investigation of the efficacy of oxerutins compared to placebo in patients with chronic venous insufficiency treated with compression stockings. *Arzneimittelforschung.* 1996;46:478-482.

9. MacLennan WJ, Wilson J, Rattenhuber V, et al. Hydroxyethylrutosides in elderly patients with chronic venous insufficiency: its efficacy and tolerability. *Gerontology.* 1994;40:45-52.

10. Rehn D, Brunnauer H, Diebschlag W, et al. Investigation of the therapeutic equivalence of different galenical preparations of O-(beta-hydroxyethyl)-rutosides following multiple dose peroral administration. *Arzneimittelforschung.* 1996;46:488-492.

11. Rehn D, Unkauf M, Klein P, et al. Comparative clinical efficacy and tolerability of oxerutins and horse chestnut extract in patients with chronic venous insufficiency. *Arzneimittelforschung.* 1996;46:483-487.

12. Balmer A, Limoni C. A double blind placebo-controlled clinical trial of Venoruton on the symptoms and signs of chronic venous insufficiency: the importance of patient selection [in German; English abstract]. *Vasa.* 1980;9:76-82.

13. Bergqvist D, Hallbook T, Lindblad B, et al. A double-blind trial of O-(beta-hydroxyethyl)-Rutoside in patients with chronic venous insufficiency. *Vasa.* 1981;10:253-260.

14. Anderson JH, Geraghty JG, Wilson YT, et al. Paroven© and graduated compression hosiery for superficial venous insufficiency. *Phlebology.* 1990;5:271-276.

15. van Cauwenberge H. Double blind study of the efficacy of O-beta-hydroxyethyl)-rutosides in the treatment of venous conditions [in French]. *Med Hyg (Geneve).* 1978;36:4175-4177.

16. de Jongste AB, Jonker JJ, Huisman MV, et al. A double blind three center clinical trial on the short-term efficacy of 0-(beta-hydroxyethyl)-rutosides in patients with post-thrombotic syndrome. *Thromb Haemost.* 1989;62:826-829.

17. Prerovsky I, Roztocil K, Hlavova A, et al. The effect of hydroxyethylrutosides after acute and chronic oral administration in patients with venous diseases: a double-blind study. *Angiologica.* 1972;9:408-414.

18. Cappelli R, Pecchi S, Oberhausser V, et al. Efficacy of O-(beta-hydroxyethyl)-rutosides at high dosages in counteracting the unwanted activity of oral contraceptives on venous function. *Int J Clin Pharmacol Res.* 1987;7:291-299.

19. Bergstein NA. Clinical study on the efficacy of O-(beta-hydroxyethyl)rutoside (HR) in varicosis of pregnancy. *J Int Med Res.* 1975;3:189-193.

20. Stegmann W, Hubner K, Deichmann B, et al. The efficacy of O-(beta-hydroxyethyl)-rutosides in the treatment of venous leg ulcers [in French; English abstract]. *Phlebologie.* 1987;40:149-156.

21. Wright DD, Franks PJ, Blair SD, et al. Oxerutins in the prevention of recurrence in chronic venous ulceration: randomized controlled trial. *Br J Surg.* 1991;78: 1269-1270.

22. Guilhou JJ, Dereure O, Marzin L, et al. Efficacy of Daflon 500 mg in venous leg ulcer healing: a double-blind, randomized, controlled versus placebo trial in 107 patients. *Angiology.* 1997;48:77-85.

23. Kiesewetter H, Koscielny J, Kalus U, et al. Efficacy of orally administered extract of red vine leaf AS 195 (folia itis viniferae) in chronic venous insufficiency (stages I-II): a randomized, double-blind, placebo-controlled trial. *Arzneimittelforschung.* 2000;50:109-117.

24. Lucker P, Jost V, Wolna P, et al. Efficacy and safety of ruscus extract compared to placebo in patients suffering from chronic venous insufficiency [abstract]. *Phytomedicine.* 2000;7(suppl 2):P-155.

25. Rudofsky G, Diehm C, Gruss JD, et al. Chronic venous insufficiency: treatment with *Ruscus* extract and trimethylhesperidin chalcone [in German; English abstract]. *MMW Munch Med Wochenschr.* 1990;132:205-210.

26. Weindorf N, Schultz-Ehrenburg U. Controlled study of increasing venous tone in primary varicose veins by oral administration of *Ruscus aculeatus* and trimethylhespiridinchalcone [in German; English abstract]. *Z Hautkr.* 1987;62:28-30, 35-38.

27. Bombardelli E, Morazzoni P. *Vitis vinifera* L. *Fitoterapia.* 1995;66:291-317.

28. Henriet JP. Exemplary study for a phlebotropic substance, the EIVE Study [translated from French]. Fairfield, Conn: Primary Source; not dated.

29. Delacroix P. Double-blind study of Endotelon® in chronic venous insufficiency [translated from French]. *La Revue de Medecine.* 1981;22:1793-1802.

30. Thebaut JF, Thebaut P, Vin F. Study of Endotelon® in functional manifestations of peripheral venous insufficiency. Results of a double-blind study of 92 patients [translated from French]. *Gaz Med.* 1985;92:96-100.

31. Arcangeli P. Pycnogenol® in chronic venous insufficiency. *Fitoterapia.* 2000;71: 236-244.

32. Petrassi C, Mastromarino A, Spartera C. Pycnogenol® in chronic venous insufficiency. *Phytomedicine.* 2000;7:383-388.

33. Belcaro GV, Grimaldi R, Guidi G. Improvement of capillary permeability in patients with venous hypertension after treatment with TTFCA. *Angiology.* 1990;41:533-540.

34. Belcaro GV, Rulo A, Grimaldi R. Capillary filtration and ankle edema in patients with venous hypertension treated with TTFCA. *Angiology.* 1990;41:12-18.

35. Cesarone MR, Laurora G, De Sactis MT, et al. The microcirculatory activity of *Centella asiatica* in venous insufficiency: a double-blind study [translated from Italian]. *Minerva Cardioangiol.* 1994;42:299-304.

36. Pointel JP, Boccalon H, Cloarec M, et al. Titrated extract of *Centella asiatica* (TECA) in the treatment of venous insufficiency of the lower limbs. *Angiology.* 1987;38:46-50.

37. Cesarone MR, Laurora G, De Sanctis MT, et al. Activity of *Centella asiatica* in venous insufficiency [in Italian; English abstract]. *Minerva Cardioangiol.* 1992;40:137-143.

38. Ihme N, Kiesewetter H, Jung F, et al. Leg edema protection from a buckwheat herb tea in patients with chronic venous insufficiency: a single-center, randomized, double-blind, placebo-controlled clinical trial. *Eur J Clin Pharmacol.* 1996;50:443-447.

39. Koscielny J, Radtke H, Hoffmann KH, et al. Fagorutin buckwheat herb tea in chronic venous insufficiency [translated from German]. *Z Phytother.* 1996;17:147-150,153-156,159.

40. Petruzzellis V, Velon A. Therapeutic action of oral doses of mesoglycan in the pharmacological treatment of varicose syndrome and its complications [in Italian; English abstract]. *Minerva Med.* 1985;76:543-548.

41. Sangrigoli V, Carra G, Lazzara N, et al. Mesoglycan in acute and chronic venous insufficiency of the legs [in Italian; English abstract]. *Clin Ter.* 1989;129:207-209.

42. Oddone G, Fiscella GF, de Franceschi T. Assessment of the effects of oral mesoglycan sulphate in patients with chronic venous pathology of the lower extremities [in Italian; English abstract]. *Gazz Med Ital.* 1987;146:111-114.

43. Laurent R, Gilly R, Frileux C. Clinical evaluation of a venotropic drug in man. Example of Daflon 500 mg. *Int Angiol.* 1988;7:39-43.

44. Danielsson G, Jungbeck C, Peterson K, et al. A randomized controlled trial of micronized purified flavonoid fraction vs placebo in patients with chronic venous disease. *Eur J Vasc Endovasc Surg.* 2002;23:73-76.
45. Arosio E, Ferrari G Santoro L, et al. A placebo-controlled double-blind study of mesoglycan in the treatment of chronic venous ulcers. *Eur J Vasc Endovasc Surg.* 2001;22:365-372.

Weight Loss

1. Ryttig KR, Tellnes G, Haegh L, et al. A dietary fibre supplement and weight maintenance after weight reduction: a randomized, double-blind, placebo-controlled long-term trial. *Int J Obes.* 1989;13:165-171.
2. Rigaud D, Ryttig KR, Angel LA, et al. Overweight treated with energy restriction and a dietary fibre supplement: a 6-month randomized, double-blind, placebo-controlled trial. *Int J Obes.* 1990;14:763-769.
3. Walsh DE, Yaghoubian V, Behforooz A. Effect of glucomannan on obese patients: a clinical study. *Int J Obes.* 1984;8:289-293.
4. Rossner S, von Zweigbergk D, Ohlin A, et al. Weight reduction with dietary fibre supplements: results of two double-blind randomized studies. *Acta Med Scand.* 1987;222:83-88.
5. Birketvedt GS, Aaseth J, Florholmen JR, et al. Long-term effect of fiber supplement and reduced energy intake on body weight and blood lipids in overweight subjects. *Acta Medica (Hradec Kralove).* 2000;43:129-132.
6. Schiller RN, Barrager E, Schauss AG, et al. A randomized, double-blind, placebo-controlled study examining the effects of a rapidly soluble chitosan dietary supplement on weight loss and body composition in overweight and mildly obese individuals. *J Am Nutraceutical Assoc.* 2001;4:42-49.
7. Pittler MH, Abbot NC, Harkness EF, et al. Randomized, double-blind trial of chitosan for body weight reduction. *Eur J Clin Nutr.* 1999;53:379-381.
8. Reffo GC. Glucomannan in hypertensive outpatients: pilot clinical trial. *Curr Ther Res.* 1988;44:22-27.
9. Vido L, Facchin P, Antonello I, et al. Childhood obesity treatment: double blinded trial on dietary fibres (glucomannan) versus placebo. *Padiatr Padol.* 1993;28:133-136.
10. Kaats GR, Blum K, Fisher JA, et al. Effects of chromium picolinate supplementation on body composition: a randomized, double-masked, placebo-controlled study. *Curr Ther Res.* 1996;57:747-765.
11. Kaats GR, Blum K, Pullin D, et al. A randomized, double-masked, placebo-controlled study of the effects of chromium picolinate supplementation on body composition: a replication and extension of a previous study. *Curr Ther Res.* 1998;59:379-388.
12. McCarty MF. The case for supplemental chromium and a survey of clinical studies with chromium picolinate. *J Appl Nutr.* 1991;43:58-66.
13. Trent LK, Thieding-Cancel D. Effects of chromium picolinate on body composition. *J Sports Med Phys Fitness.* 1995;35:273-280.
14. Clancy SP, Clarkson PM, DeCheke ME, et al. Effects of chromium picolinate supplementation on body composition, strength, and urinary chromium loss in football players. *Int J Sport Nutr.* 1994;4:142-153.
15. Hallmark MA, Reynolds TH, DeSouza CA, et al. Effects of chromium and resistive training on muscle strength and body composition. *Med Sci Sports Exerc.* 1996;28:139-144.
16. Volpe SL, Huang HW, Larpadisorn K, et al. Effect of chromium supplementation and exercise on body composition, resting metabolic rate and selected biochemical parameters in moderately obese women following an exercise program. *J Am Coll Nutr.* 2001;20:293-306.
17. Kalman D, Colker CM, Stark S, et al. Effect of pyruvate supplementation on body composition and mood. *Curr Ther Res.* 1998;59:793-802.
18. Stanko RT, Reynolds HR, Hoyson R, et al. Pyruvate supplementation of a low-cholesterol, low-fat diet: Effects on plasma lipid concentrations and body composition in hyperlipidemic patients. *Am J Clin Nutr.* 1994;59:423-427.

19. Stanko RT, Tietze DL, Arch JE. Body composition, energy utilization, and nitrogen metabolism with a 4.25-MJ/d low-energy diet supplemented with pyruvate. *Am J Clin Nutr.* 1992;56:630-635.

20. Stanko RT, Arch JE. Inhibition of regain in body weight and fat with addition of 3-carbon compound to the diet with hyperenergetic refeeding after weight reduction. *Int J Obes Relat Metab Disord.* 1996;20:925-930.

21. Stanko RT, Tietze DL, Arch JE. Body composition, energy utilization, and nitrogen metabolism with a severely restricted diet supplemented with dihydroxyacetone and pyruvate. *Am J Clin Nutr.* 1992;55:771-772.

22. Kalman D, Colker CM, Wilets I, et al. The effects of pyruvate supplementation on body composition in overweight individuals. *Nutrition.* 1999;15:337-340.

23. Ceci F, Cangiano C, Cairella M, et al. The effects of oral 5-hydroxytryptophan administration on feeding behavior in obese adult female subjects. *J Neural Transm.* 1989;76:109-117.

24. Cangiano C, Ceci F, Cairella M, et al. Effects of 5-hydroxytryptophan on eating behavior and adherence to dietary prescriptions in obese adult subjects. *Adv Exp Med Biol.* 1991;294:591-593.

25. Cangiano C, Ceci F, Cascino A, et al. Eating behavior and adherence to dietary prescriptions in obese adult subjects treated with 5-hydroxytryptophan. *Am J Clin Nutr.* 1992;56:863-867.

26. Cangiano C, Laviano A, Del Ben M, et al. Effects of oral 5-hydroxy-tryptophan on energy intake and macronutrient selection in non-insulin dependent diabetic patients. *Int J Obes Relat Metab Disord.* 1998;22:648-654.

27. Thom E. Hydroxycitrate (HCA) in the treatment of obesity [abstract]. *Int J Obes Relat Metab Disord.* 1996;20(suppl 4):75.

28. Greenwood MRC, Cleary MP, Gruen R, et al. Effect of (−)-hydroxycitrate on development of obesity in the Zucker obese rat. *Am J Physiol.* 1981;240:E72-E78.

29. Sullivan C, Triscari J. Metabolic regulation as a control for lipid disorders. I. Influence of (−)-hydroxycitrate on experimentally induced obesity in the rodent. *Am J Clin Nutr.* 1977;30:767-776.

30. Sullivan AC, Triscari J, Hamilton JG, et al. Effect of (−)-hydroxycitrate upon the accumulation of lipid in the rat. I. Lipogenesis. *Lipids.* 1974;9:121-128.

31. Sullivan AC, Triscari J, Hamilton JG, et al. Effect of (−)-hydroxycitrate upon the accumulation of lipid in the rat. II. Appetite. *Lipids.* 1974;9:129-134.

32. Sergio W. A natural food, the malabar tamarind, may be effective in the treatment of obesity. *Medical Hypothesis.* 1988;27:39-40.

33. Lowenstein JM. Effect of (−)-hydroxycitrate on fatty acid synthesis by rat liver in vivo. *J Biol Chem.* 1971;246:629-632.

34. Triscari J, Sullivan AC. Comparative effects of (−)-hydroxycitrate and (+)-allo-hydroxycitrate on acetyl CoA carboxylase and fatty acid and cholesterol synthesis in vivo. *Lipids.* 1977;12:357-363.

35. Cheema-Dhadli S, Halperin ML, Leznoff CC. Inhibition of enzymes which interact with citrate by (−)-hydroxycitrate and 1,2,3,-tricarboxybenzene. *Eur J Biochem.* 1973;38:98-102.

36. Sullivan AC, Hamilton JG, Miller ON, et al. Inhibition of lipogenesis in rat liver by (−)-hydroxycitrate. *Arch Biochem Biophys.* 1972;150:183-190.

37. Heymsfield SB, Allison DB, Vasselli JR, et al. *Garcinia cambogia* (hydroxycitric acid) as a potential antiobesity agent: a randomized controlled trial. *JAMA.* 1998;280:1596-1600.

38. Badmaev V, Majeed M, Conte AA, et al. *Garcinia cambogia* for weight loss [letter]. *JAMA.* 1999;282:233-234.

39. Kovacs EM, Westerterp-Plantenga MS, Saris WH. The effects of 2-week ingestion of (−)-hydroxycitrate and (−)-hydroxycitrate combined with medium-chain triglycerides on satiety, fat oxidation, energy expenditure, and body weight. *Int J Obes Relat Metab Disord.* 2001;25:1087-1094.

40. Kriketos AD, Thompson HR, Greene H, et al. (−)-Hydroxycitric acid does not affect energy expenditure and substrate oxidation in adult males in a post-absorptive state. *Int J Obes Relat Metab Disord.* 1999;23:867-873.

41. Mattes RD, Bormann L. Effects of (−)-hydroxycitric acid on appetitive variables. *Physiol Behav.* 2000;71:87-94.

42. Astrup A, Breum L, Toubro S. Pharmacological and clinical studies of ephedrine and other thermogenic agonists. *Obes Res.* 1995;3:537S-540S.

43. Breum L, Pedersen JK, Ahlstrom F, et al. Comparison of an ephedrine/caffeine combination and dexfenfluramine in the treatment of obesity: a double-blind multicenter trial in general practice. *Int J Obes Relat Metab Disord.* 1994;18:99-103.

44. Molnar D, Torok K, Erhardt E, et al. Safety and efficacy of treatment with an ephedrine/caffeine mixture. The first double-blind placebo-controlled pilot study in adolescents. *Int J Obes Relat Metab Disord.* 2000;24:1573-1578.

45. Norregaard J, Jorgensen S, Mikkelsen KL, et al. The effect of ephedrine plus caffeine on smoking cessation and postcessation weight gain. *Clin Pharmacol Ther.* 1996;60: 679-686.

46. Astrup A, Breum L, Toubro S, et al. The effect and safety of an ephedrine/caffeine compound compared to ephedrine, caffeine, and placebo in obese subjects on an energy restricted diet: a double-blind trial. *Int J Obes Relat Metab Disord.* 1992;16: 269-277.

47. Boozer CN, Nasser JA, Heymsfield SB, et al. An herbal supplement containing Ma Huang-Guarana for weight loss: a randomized, double-blind trial. *Int J Obes Relat Metab Disord.* 2001;25:316-324.

48. Haller CA, Benowitz NL. Adverse cardiovascular and central nervous system events associated with dietary supplements containing ephedra alkaloids. *N Engl J Med.* 2000;343:1833-1838.

49. Naylor GJ, McHarg AM, Edwards L. A double blind placebo controlled trial of ascorbic acid in obesity. *IRCS J Med Sci.* 1982;10:848-849.

50. Naylor GJ, Grant L, Smith C. A double blind placebo controlled trial of ascorbic acid in obesity. *Nutr Health.* 1985;4:25-28.

51. Garcia CM, Carter J, Chou A. Gamma linolenic acid causes weight loss and lower blood pressure in overweight patients with family history of obesity. *Swed J Biol Med.* 1986;4:8-11.

52. Thom E. A pilot study with the aim of studying the efficacy and tolerability of CLA (Tonalin™) on the body composition in humans [unpublished]. July 1997.

53. West DB, Camet PM, Maddus CD, et al. Reduced body fat with conjugated linoleic acid feeding in the mouse [abstract]. *FASEB J.* 1997;11:A599.

54. Ferreira M, Kreider R, Wilson M, et al. Effects of conjugated linoleic acid (CLA) supplementation during resistance training on body composition and strength [abstract]. *J Strength Cond Res.* 1997;11:280.

55. Blankson H, Stakkestad JA, Fagertun H, et al. Conjugated linoleic acid reduces body fat mass in overweight and obese humans. *J Nutr.* 2000;130:2943-2948.

56. Davies KM, Heaney RP, Recker RR, et al. Calcium intake and body weight. *J Clin Endocrinol Metab.* 2000;85:4635-4638.

57. Nagao T, Watanabe H, Goto N, et al. Dietary diacylglycerol suppresses accumulation of body fat compared to triacylglycerol in men in a double-blind controlled trial. *J Nutr.* 2000;130:792-797.

58. Becker EW, Jakober B, Luft D, et al. Clinical and biochemical evaluations of the alga Spirulina with regard to its application in the treatment of obesity: a double-blind cross-over study. *Nutr Rep Int.* 1986;33:565-574.

59. Antonio J, Colker CM, Torina GC, et al. Effects of a standardized guggulsterone phosphate supplement on body composition in overweight adults: a pilot study. *Curr Ther Res.* 1999;60:220-227.

60. Wuolijoki E, Hirvela T, Ylitalo P. Decrease in serum LDL cholesterol with microcrystalline chitosan. *Methods Find Exp Clin Pharmacol.* 1999;21:357-361.

61. Dibling D, Zemel MB. Chromium picolinate antagonized the lipogenic and antilipolytic effects of insulin in human adipocytes [abstract]. *FASEB J.* 1998;12:A505.

62. Cheuvront SN. The zone diet and athletic performance. *Sports Med.* 1999;27: 213-228.

63. Coulston AM, Liu GC, Reaven GM. Plasma glucose insulin and lipid responses to high-carbohydrate low-fat diets in normal humans. *Metabolism.* 1983;32:52-56.

64. Lefebvre PJ, Luyckx AS. Effect of insulin on glucagon enhanced lipolysis in vitro. *Diabetologia.* 1969;5:195-197.

65. Jensen MD, Caruso M, Heiling V, et al. Insulin regulation of lipolysis in nondiabetic and IDDM subjects. *Diabetes.* 1989;38:1595-1601.

66. Howard BV, Savage PJ, Nagulesparan M, et al. Evidence for marked sensitivity to the antilipolytic action of insulin in obese maturity-onset diabetics. *Metabolism.* 1979;28:744-750.

67. Fraze E, Donner CC, Swislocki AL, et al. Ambient plasma free fatty acid concentrations in noninsulin-dependent diabetes mellitus: evidence for insulin resistance. *J Clin Endocrinol Metab.* 1985;61:807-811.

68. Sigal RJ, El-Hashimy M, Martin BC, et al. Acute postchallenge hyperinsulinemia predicts weight gain: a prospective study. *Diabetes.* 1997;46:1025-1029.

69. Olefsky JM, Nolan JJ. Insulin resistance and non-insulin-dependent diabetes mellitus: cellular and molecular mechanisms. *Am J Clin Nutr.* 1995;61(4 suppl):980S-986S.

70. Eckel RH. Insulin resistance: an adaptation for weight maintenance. *Lancet.* 1992;340:1452-1453.

71. Smedman A, Vessby B. Conjugated linoleic acid supplementation in humans: metabolic effects. *Lipids.* 2001;36:773-781.

72. Krotkiewski M Value of VLCD supplementation with medium chain triglycerides. *Int J Obes.* 2001;25:1393-1400.

73. Seaton TB, Welle SL, Warenko MK, et al. Thermic effect of medium-chain and long-chain triglycerides in man. *Am J Clin Nutr.* 1986;44:630-634.

74. Scalfi L, Coltorti A, Contaldo F. Postprandial thermogenesis in lean and obese subjects after meals supplemented with medium-chain and long-chain triglycerides. *Am J Clin Nutr.* 1991;53: 1130-1133.

75. Baba N, Bracco EF, Hashim SA. Enhanced thermogenesis and diminished deposition of fat in response to overfeeding with diet containing medium chain triglyceride. *Am J Clin Nutr.* 1982;35:678-682.

76. Tsuji H, Kasai M, Takeuchi H, et al. Dietary medium-chain triacylglycerols suppress accumulation of body fat in a double-blind controlled trial in healthy men and women. *J Nutr.* 2001;131:2853-2856.

77. Yost TJ, Eckel RH. Hypocaloric feeding in obese women: metabolic effects of medium-chain triglyceride substitution. *Am J Clin Nutr.* 1989;49:326-330.

78. Girola M, de Bernardi M, Contos S, et al. Dose effect in lipid-lowering activity of a new dietary integrator (chitosan Garcinia cambogia extract and chrome). *Acta Toxicol Ther.* 1996;17:25-40.

79. Andersen T, Fogh J. Weight loss and delayed gastric emptying following a South American herbal preparation in overweight patients. *J Hum Nutr Diet.* 2001;14:243-250.

80. Antonio J, Sanders MS, Van Gammeren D. The effects of bovine colostrum supplementation on body composition and exercise performance in active men and women. *Nutrition.* 2001;17:243-247.

81. Hoeger WWK, Harris C, Long EM, et al. Four-week supplementation with a natural dietary compound produces favorable changes in body composition. *Adv Ther.* 1998;15:305-314.

82. Villani RG, Gannon J, Self M, et al. L-Carnitine supplementation combined with aerobic training does not promote weight loss in moderately obese women. *Int J Sport Nutr Exerc Metab.* 2000;10:199-207.

83. Vogiatzi MG, Boeck MA, Vlachopapadopoulou E, et al. Dehydroepiandrosterone in morbidly obese adolescents: effects on weight, body composition, lipids, and insulin resistance. *Metabolism.* 1996;45:1011-1015.

Herbs and Supplements

5-Hydroxytryptophan (5-HTP)

1. Byerley WF, Judd LL, Reimherr FW, et al. 5-hydroxytryptophan: a review of its antidepressant efficacy and adverse effects. *J Clin Psychopharmacol.* 1987;7:127-137.
2. Poldinger W, Calanchini B, Schwarz W. A functional-dimensional approach to depression: serotonin deficiency as a target syndrome in a comparison of 5-hydroxytryptophan and fluvoxamine. *Psychopathology.* 1991;24:53-81.
3. Kahn RS, Westenberg HG, Verhoeven WM, et al. Effect of a serotonin precursor and uptake inhibitor in anxiety disorders: a double-blind comparison of 5-hydroxytryptophan, clomipramine, and placebo. *Int Clin Psychopharmacol.* 1987;2:33-45.
4. Caruso I, Sarzi Puttini P, Cazzola M, et al. Double-blind study of 5-hydroxytryptophan versus placebo in the treatment of primary fibromyalgia syndrome. *J Int Med Res.* 1990;18:201-209.
5. Ceci F, Cangiano C, Cairella M, et al. The effects of oral 5-hydroxytryptophan administration on feeding behavior in obese adult female subjects. *J Neural Transm.* 1989;76:109-117.
6. Cangiano C, Ceci F, Cairella M, et al. Effects of 5-hydroxytryptophan on eating behavior and adherence to dietary prescriptions in obese adult subjects. *Adv Exp Med Biol.* 1991;294:591-593.
7. Cangiano C, Ceci F, Cascino A, et al. Eating behavior and adherence to dietary prescriptions in obese adult subjects treated with 5-hydroxytryptophan. *Am J Clin Nutr.* 1992;56:863-867.
8. Cangiano C, Laviano A, Del Ben M, et al. Effects of oral 5-hydroxy-tryptophan on energy intake and macronutrient selection in non-insulin dependent diabetic patients. *Int J Obes Relat Metab Disord.* 1998;22:648-654.
9. Ribeiro CAF. L-5-Hydroxytryptophan in the prophylaxis of chronic tension-type headache: a double-blind, randomized, placebo-controlled study. *Headache.* 2000;40:451-456.
10. De Giorgis G, Miletto R, Iannuccelli M, et al. Headache in association with sleep disorders in children: a psychodiagnostic evaluation and controlled clinical study: L-5-HTP versus placebo. *Drugs Exp Clin Res.* 1987;13:425-433.
11. Longo G, Rudoi I, Iannuccelli M, et al. Treatment of essential headache in developmental age with L-5-HTP (cross over double-blind study versus placebo) [in Italian; English abstract]. *Pediatr Med Chir.* 1984;6:241-245.
12. DeBenedittis G, Massei R. Serotonin precursors in chronic primary headache: a double-blind cross-over study with L-5-hydroxytryptophan vs. placebo. *J Neurosurg Sci.* 1985;29:239-248.
13. Titus F, Davalos A, Alom J, et al. 5-Hydroxytryptophan versus methysergide in the prophylaxis of migraine: randomized clinical trial. *Eur Neurol.* 1986;25:327-329.
14. Bono G, Criscuoli M, Martignoni E, et al. Serotonin precursors in migraine prophylaxis. *Adv Neurol.* 1982;33:357-363.
15. Maissen CP, Ludin HP. Comparison of the effect of 5-hydroxytryptophan and propranolol in the interval treatment of migraine [translated from German]. *Schweiz Med Wochenschr.* 1991;121:1585-1590.
16. Santucci M, Cortelli P, Giovanardi Rossi P, et al. L-5-hydroxytryptophan versus placebo in childhood migraine prophylaxis: a double-blind crossover study. *Cephalalgia.* 1986;6:155-157.
17. Sternberg EM, Van Woert MH, Young SN, et al. Development of a scleroderma-like illness during therapy with L-5-hydroxytryptophan and carbidopa. *N Engl J Med.* 1980;303:782-787.
18. Joly P, Lampert A, Thomine E, et al. Development of pseudobullous morphea and scleroderma-like illness during therapy with L-5-hydroxytryptophan and carbidopa. *J Am Acad Dermatol.* 1991;25:332-333.
19. Auffranc JC, Berbis P, Fabre JF, et al. Sclerodermiform and poikilodermal syndrome observed during treatment with carbidopa and 5-hydroxytryptophan [translated from French]. *Ann Dermatol Venereol.* 1985;112:691-692.

20. Elko CJ, Burgess JL, Robertson WO. Zolpidem-associated hallucinations and serotonin reuptake inhibition: a possible interaction. *Clin Toxicol.* 1998;36:195-203.

Aloe

1. Syed TA, Afzal M, Ashfaq Ahmad S, et al. Management of genital herpes in men
with 0.5% *Aloe vera* extract in a hydrophilic cream: a placebo-controlled double-
blind study. *J Dermatol Treat.* 1997;8:99-102.

2. Syed TA, Cheema KM, Ashfaq A, et al. *Aloe vera* extract 0.5% in ahydrophilic cream
versus *Aloe vera* gel for the management of genital herpes in males: a placebo-
controlled, double-blind, comparative study [letter]. *J Eur Acad Dermatol Venereol.*
1996;7:294-295.

3. Syed TA, Ahmad SA, Holt AH, et al. Management of psoriasis with *Aloe vera* extract
in a hydrophilic cream: a placebo-controlled, double-blind study. *Trop Med Int
Health.* 1996;1:505-509.

4. Vardy DA, Cohen AD, Tchetov T, et al. A double blind, placebo-controlled trial of
an *Aloe vera* (*A. barbadensis*) emulsion in the treatment of seborrheic dermatitis.
J Dermatol Treat. 1999;10:7-11.

5. Yongchaiyudha S, Rungpitarangsi V, Bunyapraphatsara N, et al. Antidiabetic activity
of *Aloe vera* L. juice. I. Clinical trial in new cases of diabetes mellitus. *Phytomedicine.*
1996;3:241-243.

6. Bunyapraphatsara N, Yongchaiyudha S, Rungpitarangsi V, et al. Antidiabetic activity
of *Aloe vera* L. juice II. Clinical trial in diabetes mellitus patients in combination with
glibenclamide. *Phytomedicine.* 1996;3:245-248.

7. Schmidt JM, Greenspoon JS. *Aloe vera* dermal wound gel is associated with a delay
in wound healing. *Obstet Gynecol.* 1991;78:115-117.

8. Chithra P, Sajithlal GB, Chandrakasan G. Influence of *Aloe vera* on collagen characteristics in healing dermal wounds in rats. *Mol Cell Biochem.* 1998;181:71-76.

9. Fulton JE Jr. The stimulation of postdermabrasion wound healing with stabilized
Aloe vera gel-polyethylene oxide dressing. *J Dermatol Surg Oncol.* 1990;16:460-467.

10. Davis RH, Leitner MG, Russo JM, et al. Wound healing: oral and topical activity of
Aloe vera. J Am Podiatr Med Assoc. 1989;79:559-562.

11. Kaufman T, Kalderon N, Ullmann Y, et al. *Aloe vera* gel hindered wound healing of
experimental second-degree burns: a quantitative controlled study. *J Burn Care
Rehabil.* 1988;9:156-159.

12. Crowell J, Penneys N. The effect of *Aloe vera* on cutaneus erythema and blood-flow
following ultraviolet-B (UVB) exposure [abstract]. *Clin Res.* 1987;35:A676.

13. Williams MS, Burk M, Loprinzi CL, et al. Phase III double-blind evaluation of an
Aloe vera gel as a prophylactic agent for radiation-induced skin toxicity. *Int J Radiat
Oncol Biol Phys.* 1996;36:345-349.

14. 't Hart LA, Nibbering PH, van den Barselaar MT, et al. Effects of low molecular
weight constituents from aloe vera gel on oxidative metabolism and cytotoxic and
bacteriacidal activities of human neutrophlis. *Int J Immunopharmacol.* 1990;12:
427-434.

15. Sheets MA, Unger BA, Giggleman GF Jr, et al. Studies of the effect of acemannan on
retrovirus infections: clinical stabilization of feline leukemia virus-infected cats. *Mol
Biother.* 1991;3:41-45.

16. Kemp MC, Kahlon JB, Chinnah AD, et al. In-vitro evaluation of the antiviral effects of acemannan on the replication and pathogensis of HIV-1 and other enveloped
viruses: modification of the processing of glycoprotein precursors [abstract]. *Antiviral
Res.* 1990;13(suppl):83.

17. Shah AH, Qureshi S, Tariq M, et al. Toxicity studies on six plants used in the traditional Arab system of medicine. *Phytother Res.* 1989;3:25-29.

18. Davis RH, Parker WL, Murdoch DP. *Aloe vera* as a biologically active vehicle for
hydrocortisone acetate. *J Am Podiatr Assoc.* 1991;81:1-9.

19. Olsen DL, Raub W Jr., Bradley C, et al. The effect of aloe vera gel/mild soap versus
mild soap alone in preventing skin reactions in patients undergoing radiation therapy. *Oncol Nurs Forum.* 2001;28:543-547.

Andrographis

1. Caceres DD, Hancke JL, Burgos RA, et al. Use of visual analogue scale measurements (VAS) to asses the effectiveness of standardized *Andrograpahis paniculata* extract SHA-10 in reducing the symptoms of common cold: a randomized double blind placebo study. *Phytomedicine.* 1999;6:217-223.
2. Melchior J, Palm S, Wikman G. Controlled clinical study of standardized *Andrographis paniculata* extract in common cold: a pilot trial. *Phytomedicine.* 1996-1997; 3:314-318.
3. Hancke J, Burgos R, Caceres D, et al. A double-blind study with a new monodrug Kan Jang: decrease of symptoms and improvements in the recovery from common colds. *Phytother Res.* 1995;9:559-562.
4. Melchior J, Spasov AA, Ostrovskij OV, et al. Double-blind, placebo-controlled pilot and phase III study of activity of standardized *Andrographis paniculata* Herba Nees extract fixed combination (Kan jang) in the treatment of uncomplicated upper-respiratory tract infection. *Phytomedicine.* 2000;7:341-350.
5. Thamlikitkul V, Theerapong S, Boonroj P et al. Efficacy of *Andrographis paniculata* (Nees) for pharyngotonsillitis in adults. *J Med Assoc Thai.* 1991;74:437-442.
6. Caceres DD, Hancke JL, Burgos RA, et al. Prevention of common colds with *Andrographis paniculata* dried extract: a pilot double blind trial. *Phytomedicine.* 1997;4:101-104.
7. Zhao HY, Fang WY. Antithrombotic effects of *Andrographis paniculata* Nees in preventing myocardial infarction. *Chin Med J (Engl).* 1991;104:770-775.
8. Zhang CY, Tan BKH. Mechanisms of cardiovascular activity of *Andrographis paniculata* in the anaesthetized rat. *J Ethnopharmacol.* 1997;56:97-101.
9. Wang DW, Zhao HY. Prevention of atherosclerotic arterial stenosis and restenosis after angioplasty with *Andrographis paniculata* nees and fish oil: experimental studies of effects and mechanisms. *Chin Med J.* 1994;107:464-470.
10. Visen PKS, Shukla B, Patnaik GK, et al. Andrographolide protects rat hepatocytes against paracetamol-induced damage. *J Ethnopharmacol.* 1993;40:131-136.
11. Kapil A, Koul IB, Banerjee SK, et al. Antihepatotoxic effects of major diterpenoid constituents of *Andrographis paniculata*. *Biochem Pharmacol.* 1993;46:182-185.
12. Handa SS, Sharma A. Hepatoprotective efects of andrographolide from *Andrographis paniculata* against carbontetrachloride. *Indian J Med Res.* 1990;92:276-283.
13. Calabrese C, Berman SH, Babish JG, et al. A phase I trial of andrographolide in HIV positive patients and normal volunteers. *Phytother Res.* 2000;14:333-338.
14. Puri A, Saxena R, Saxena RP, et al. Immunostimulant agents from *Andrographis paniculata*. *J Nat Prod.* 1993;56:995-999.
15. Leelarasamee A, Trakulsomboon S, Sittisomwong N. Undetectable anti-bacterial activity of *Andrographis paniculata* (Burma) wall. ex ness. *J Med Assoc Thai.* 1990;73: 299-304.
16. Akbarsha MA, Manivannan B, Shahul K, et al. Antifertility effect of *Andrographis paniculata* (Nees) in male albino rat. *Indian J Exp Biol.* 1990;28:421-426.
17. Zoha MS, Hussain AHM, Choudhury SAR. Antifertility effect of *Andrographis paniculata* in mice. *Bangladesh Med Res Counc Bull.* 1989;15:34-37.
18. Burgos RA, Caballero EE, Sanchez NS, et al. Testicular toxicity assessment of *Andrographis paniculata* dried extract in rats. *J Ethnopharmacol.* 1997;58:219-224.
19. Shukla B, Visen PK, Patnaik GK, et al. Choleretic effect of andrographolide in rats and guinea pigs. *Planta Med.* 1992;58:146-149.

Androstenedione

1. Catlin DH, Leder BZ, Ahrens B, et al. Trace contamination of over-the-counter androstenedione and positive urine test results for a nandrolone metabolite. *JAMA.* 2000; 284:2618-2621.
2. King DS, et al. Effect of oral androstenedione on serum testosterone and adaptations to resistance training in young men. *JAMA.* 1999;281:2020-2028.
3. Wallace MB, Lim J, Cutler A, et al. Effects of dehydroepiandrosterone vs. androstenedione supplementation in men. *Med Sci Sports Exerc.* 1999;31:1788-1792.

4. Ballantyne CS, Phillips SM, MacDonald JR, et al. The acute effects of androstene-dione supplementation in healthy young males. *Can J Appl Physiol.* 2000;25:68-78.

5. Brown GA, Vukovich MD, Martini ER, et al. Endocrine responses to chronic an-drostenedione intake in 30- to 56-year-old men. *J Clin Endocrinol Metab.* 2000;85: 4074-4080.

6. Broeder CE, Quindry J, Brittingham K, et al. The andro project: physiological and hormonal influences of androstenedione supplementation in men 35 to 65 years old participating in a high-intensity resistance training program. *Arch Intern Med.* 2000;160:3093-3104.

7. Leder BZ, Longcope C, Catlin DH, et al. Oral androstenedione administration and serum testosterone concentrations in young men. *JAMA.* 2000;283:779-782.

8. Yesalis CE, ed. *Anabolic Steroids in Sport and Exercise.* Champaign, Ill: Human Kinetics; 1993.

9. Kachhi PN, Henderson SO. Priapism after androstenedione intake for athletic per-formance enhancement. *Ann Emerg Med.* 2000;35:391-393.

Arginine

1. Hambrecht R, Hilbrich L, Erbs S, et al. Correction of endothelial dysfunction in chronic heart failure: additional effects of exercise training and oral L-arginine sup-plementation. *J Am Coll Cardiol.* 2000;35:706-713.

2. Rector TS, Bank AJ, Mullen KA, et al. Randomized, double-blind, placebo-controlled study of supplement oral L-arginine in patients with heart failure. *Circulation.* 1996;93:2135-2141.

3. Watanabe G, Tomiyama H, Doba N. Effects of oral administration of L-arginine on renal function in patients with heart failure. *J Hypertens.* 2000;18:229-234.

4. Chen J, Wollman Y, Chernichovsky T, et al. Effect of oral administration of high-dose nitric oxide donor L-arginine in men with organic erectile dysfunction: results of a double-blind, randomized placebo-controlled study. *BJU Int.* 1999;83:269-273.

5. Boger RH, Bode-Boger SM, Thiele W, et al. Restoring vascular nitric oxide forma-tion by L-arginine improves the symptoms of intermittent claudication in patients with peripheral arterial occlusive disease. *J Am Coll Cardiol.* 1998;32:1336-1344.

6. Maxwell AJ, Anderson BE, Cooke JP. Nutritional therapy for peripheral arterial dis-ease: a double-blind, placebo-controlled, randomized trial of HeartBar. *Vasc Med.* 2000;5(1):11-9.

7. Korting GE, Smith SD, Wheeler MA, et al. A randomized double-blind trial of oral L-arginine for treatment of interstitial cystitis. *J Urol.* 1999;161:558-565.

8. Cartledge JJ, Davies AM, Eardley I. A randomized double-blind placebo-controlled crossover trial of the efficacy of L-arginine in the treatment of interstitial cystitis. *BJU Int.* 2000;85:421-426.

9. Ehren I, Lundberg JON, Adolfsson J, et al. Effects of L-arginine treatment on symp-toms and bladder nitric oxide levels in patients with interstitial cystitis. *Urology.* 1998;52:1026-1029.

10. Bednarz B, Wolk R, Chamiec T, et al. Effects of oral L-arginine supplementation on exercise-induced QT dispersion and exercise tolerance in stable angina pectoris. *Int J Cardiol.* 2000;75:205-210.

11. Blum A, Porat R, Rosenschein U, et al. Clinical and inflammatory effects of dietary L-arginine in patients with intractable angina pectoris. *Am J Cardiol.* 1999;83:1488-1490.

12. De Nicola L, Bellizzi V, Minutolo R, et al. Randomized, double-blind, placebo-controlled study of arginine supplementation in chronic renal failure. *Kidney Int.* 1999;56:674-684.

13. de Gouw HW, Verbruggen MB, Twiss IM, et al. Effect of oral L-arginine on airway hyperresponsiveness to histamine in asthma. *Thorax.* 1999;54:1033-1035.

14. Baligan M, Giardina A, Giovannini G, et al. L-Arginine and immunity: study of pe-diatric subjects [translated from Italian]. *Minerva Pediatr.* 1997;49:537-542.

15. Piatti PM, Monti LD, Valsecchi G, et al. Long-term oral L-arginine administration improves peripheral and hepatic insulin sensitivity in type 2 diabetic patients. *Diabetes Care.* 2001;24:875-880.

16. De Aloysio D, Mantuano R, Mauloni M, et al. The clinical use of arginine aspartate in male infertility. *Acta Eur Fertil.* 1982;13:133-167.
17. Mroueh A. Effect of arginine on oligospermia. *Fertil Steril.* 1970;21:217-219.
18. Schacter A, Goldman JA, Zukerman Z. Treatment of oligospermia with the amino acid arginine. *J Urol.* 1973;110:311-313.
19. Schachter A, Friedman S, Goldman JA, et al. Treatmant of oligospermia with the amino acid arginine. *Int J Gynaecol Obstet.* 1973;11:206-209.
20. Tanimura J. Studies on arginine in human semen, part II: The effects of medication with L-arginine-HCL on male infertility. *Bull Osaka Med Sch.* 1967;13:84-89.
21. Pryor JP, Blandy JP, Evans P et al. Controlled clinical trial of arginine for infertile men with oligozoospermia. *Br J Urol.* 1978;50:47-50.
22. *USP DI. Vol. III, Approved Drug Products and Legal Requirements.* 20th ed. Rockville, Md: United States Pharmacopeial Convention; 2000.
23. American Society of Health-System Pharmacists. *AHFS Drug Information.* Bethesda, Md: American Society of Health-System Pharmacists; 2000:2306-2307.
24. Kilroy RA, et al. Acid-base disorders. In: DiPiro JT, et al., eds. *Pharmacotherapy: A Pathophysiologic Approach.* 4th ed. Stamford, Conn: Appleton & Lange; 1999:931.
25. Bruinsma KA, Anderson BE, Prendergast JJ, et al. Effects of an L-arginine-enriched medical food in patients with type II diabetes [abstract]. *Diabetes.* 2001;50(suppl 2):Abst #1796-PO.
26. Klotz T, Mathers MJ, Braun M, et al. Effectiveness of oral L-arginine in first-line treatment of erectile dysfunction in a controlled crossover study. *Urol Int.* 1999;63(4):220-223.
27. Moody JA, Vernet D, Laidlaw S, et al. Effects of long-term administration of L-arginine on the rat erectile response. *J Urol* 1997;158:942-947.
28. Maxwell AJ, Zapien MP, Pearce GL, et al. Randomized trial of a medical food for the dietary management of chronic, stable angina. *J Am Coll Cardiol.* 2002;39:37-45.
29. Luiking YC, Weusten BL, Portincasa P, et al. Effects of long-term oral L-arginine on esophageal motility and gallbladder dynamics in healthy humans. *Am J Physiol.* 1998;274(6 pt 1):G984-G991.
30. Straathof JW, Adamse M, Onkenhout W, et al. Effect of L-arginine on lower oesophageal sphincter motility in man. *Eur J Gastroenterol Hepatol.* 2000;12:419-424.
31. American Society of Health-System Pharmacists. *AHFS Drug Information.* Bethesda, MD: American Society of Health-System Pharmacists; 2000:2306-2307.

Artichoke Leaf

1. Englisch W, Beckers C, Unkauf M, et al. Efficacy of Artichoke dry extract in patients with hyperlipoproteinemia. *Arzneimittelforschung.* 2000;50:260-265.
2. Petrowicz O, Gebhardt R, Donner M, et al. Effects of artichoke leaf extract (ALE) on lipoprotein metabolism in vitro and in vivo [abstract]. *Atherosclerosis.* 1997;129:147.
3. Kirchhoff R, Beckers CH, Kichhoff GM, et al. Increase in choleresis by means of artichoke extract. *Phytomedicine.* 1994;1:107-115.
4. Kupke D, von Sanden H, Trinczek-Gartner H, et al. An evaluation of the choleretic activity of a plant-based cholagogue [translated from German]. *Z Allgemeinmed.* 1991;67:1046-1058.
5. Matuschowski P, et al. Testing of *Cynara scolymus* in the isolated perfused rat liver. Presented at: 43rd Annual Congress on Medicinal Plant Research; September 3-7, 1995; Halle (Saale), Germany.
6. Kraft K. Artichoke leaf extract: recent findings reflecting effects on lipid metabolism, liver and gastrointestinal tracts. *Phytomedicine.* 1997;4:369-378.

Astragalus

1. Hou Y, Ma G, Wu S, et al. Effect of Radix *Astragali seu* Hedysari on the interferon system. *Chin Med J.* 1981;94:35-40.
2. Lau BHS, Ruckle HC, Botolazzo T, et al. Chinese medicinal herbs inhibit growth of murine renal cell carcinoma. *Cancer Biother.* 1994;9:153-161.

3. Sun Y, Hersh EM, Talpaz M, et al. Immune restoration and/or augmentation of local graft versus host reaction by traditional Chinese medicinal herbs. *Cancer.* 1983;52:70-73.
4. Bensky D, Gamble A, Kaptchuk TJ. *Chinese Herbal Medicine: Materia Medica.* Seattle, Wash: Eastland Press; 1986:457-459.
5. Chu DT, Sun Y, Hersh EM, et al. Immune restoration and/or augmentation of local graft versus host reaction by traditional Chinese medicinal herbs. *Cancer.* 1983;52:70-73.
6. Gao C, Wang R, Liu D, et al. The effects of astragalus and shenmai injections on macrophage function in burned mice. *Zhonghua Shao Shang Za Zhi.* 2000;17:163-167.
7. Jiao Y, Wen J, Yu X. Related influence of flavonoid of Astragalus membranaceus's stem and leaves on the function of cell mediated immunity in mice. *Zhongguo Zhong Xi Yi Jie He Za Zhi.* 1999;19:356-358.
8. Chen LX, Liao JZ, Guo WQ. Effects of Astragalus membranaceus on left ventricular function and oxygen free radical in acute myocardial infarction patients and mechanism of its cardiotonic action. *Zhongguo Zhong Xi Yi Jie He Za Zhi.* 1995;15:141-143.
9. Chu L, Shi X, Xi S. Experimental studies on improving heart preservation effect of Astragalus saponins. *Zhongguo Zhong Xi Yi Jie He Za Zhi.* 1999;19:481-483.
10. Li SQ, Yuan RX, Gao H. Clinical observation on the treatment of ischemic heart disease with Astragalus membranaceus. *Zhongguo Zhong Xi Yi Jie He Za Zhi.* 1995; 15:77-80.
11. Quan J, Du G. Protective effect of Astragalus membranaceus (Fisch.) Bge. and Hedysarum polybotrys Hand.-Mazz. on experimental model of cerebral ischemia in rats. *Zhongguo Zhong Xi Yi Jie He Za Zhi.* 1998;23:371-373.
12. Wang D, Wang C, Tian Y. Effect of total flavonoids of Astragalus on nitroxide in ischemia reperfusion injury. *Hongguo Zhong Xi Yi Jie He Za Zhi.* 1999;19:221-223.
13. Fan T, et al. The inhibitory effect of some Chinese herbs on hepatitis B virus replication in vitro and its mechanism. *Chin J Exper Clin Virol.* 1996;10:27-30.
14. Shon YH, Kim JH, Nam KS. Effect of Astragali radix extract on lipopolysaccharide-induced inflammation in human amnion. *Biol Pharm Bull.* 2002;25:77-80.

Beta-Carotene

1. McAlindon TE, Jacques P, Zhang Y, et al. Do antioxidant micronutrients protect against the development and progression of knee osteoarthritis? *Arthritis Rheum.* 1996;39:648-656.
2. Steinmetz KA, Potter JD. Vegetables, fruit, and cancer prevention: a review. *J Am Diet Assoc.* 1996;96:1027-1039.
3. Ziegler RG. A review of epidemiologic evidence that carotenoids reduce the risk of cancer. *J Nutr.* 1989;119:116-122.
4. Flagg EW, Coates RJ, Greenberg RS. Epidemiologic studies of antioxidants and cancer in humans. *J Am Coll Nutr.* 1995;14:419-427.
5. Vena JE, Graham S, Freudenheim J, et al. Diet in the epidemiology of bladder cancer in western New York. *Nutr Cancer.* 1992;18:255-264.
6. Rock CL, Saxe GA, Ruffin MT IV, et al. Carotenoids, vitamin A, and estrogen receptor status in breast cancer. *Nutr Cancer.* 1996;25:281-296.
7. Zheng W, Sellers TA, Doyle TJ, et al. Retinol, antioxidant vitamins, and cancers of the upper digestive tract in a prospective cohort study of postmenopausal women. *Am J Epidemiol.* 1995;142:955-960.
8. Kohlmeier L, Hastings SB. Epidemiologic evidence of a role of carotenoids in cardiovascular disease prevention. *Am J Clin Nutr.* 1995.62(suppl):1370S-1376S.
9. Gollnick HPM, Hopfenmuller W, Hemmes C, et al. Systemic beta carotene plus topical UV sunscreen are an optimal protection against harmful effects of natural UV-sunlight: results of the Berlin-Eilath study. *Eur J Dermatol.* 1996;6:200-205.
10. Mathews-Roth MM, Pathak MA, Parrish J, et al. A clinical trial of the effects of oral beta-carotene on the responses of human skin to solar radiation. *J Invest Dermatol.* 1972;59:349-353.
11. Lee J, Jiang S, Levine N, et al. Carotenoid supplementation reduces erythema in human skin after simulated solar radiation exposure. *Proc Soc Exp Biol Med.* 2000; 223:170-174.

12. Stahl W, Heinrich U, Jungmann H, et al. Carotenoids and carotenoids plus vitamin E protect against ultraviolet light-induced erythema in humans. *Am J Clin Nutr.* 2000; 71:795-798.

13. Garmyn M, Ribaya-Mercado JD, Russel RM, et al. Effect of beta-carotene supplementation on the human sunburn reaction. *Exp Dermatol.* 1995;4:104-111.

14. Krook G, Haeger-Aronsen B. Beta-carotene in the treatment of erythropoietic protoporphyria. *Acta Derm Venereol Suppl (Stockh).* 1982;100:125-129.

15. Suhonen R, Plosila M. The effect of beta-carotene in combination with canthaxanthin, Ro 8-8427 (Phenoro), in treatment of polymorphous light eruptions. *Dermatologica.* 1981;163:172-176.

16. Corbett MF, Hawk JL, Herxheimer A, et al. Controlled therapeutic trials in polymorphic light eruption. *Br J Dermatol.* 1982;107:571-581.

17. Corbett MF, Herxheimer A, Magnus IA, et al. The long term treatment with beta-carotene in erythropoietic protoporphyria: a controlled trial. *Br J Dermatol.* 1977;97: 655-662.

18. Mathews-Roth MM, Pathak MA, Fitzpatrick TB, et al. Beta-carotene as an oral photoprotective agent in erythropoietic protoporphyria. *JAMA.* 1974;228:1004-1008.

19. Mathews-Roth MM. Carotenoids in erythropoietic protoporphyria and other photosensitivity diseases. *Ann N Y Acad Sci.* 1993;691:127-138.

20. Wolf C, Steiner A, Honigsmann H. Do oral carotenoids protect human skin against ultraviolet erythema, psoralen phototoxicity, and ultraviolet-induced DNA damage? *J Invest Dermatol.* 1988;90:55-57.

21. Albanes D, Heinonen OP, Huttunen JK, et al. Effects of alpha-tocopherol and beta-carotene supplements on cancer incidence in the Alpha-Tocopherol Beta-Carotene Cancer Prevention Study. *Am J Clin Nutr.* 1995;62(suppl):1427S-1430S.

22. Omenn GS, Goodman GE, Thornquist MD, et al. Effects of a combination of beta carotene and vitamin A on lung cancer and cardiovascular disease. *N Engl J Med.* 1996;334:1150-1155.

23. Hennekens CH, Buring JE, Manson JE, et al. Lack of effect of long-term supplementation with beta carotene on the incidence of malignant neoplasms and cardiovascular disease. *N Engl J Med.* 1996;334:1145-1149.

24. Frieling UM, Schaumberg DA, Kupper TS, et al. A randomized, 12-year primary-prevention trial of beta carotene supplementation for nonmelanoma skin cancer in the physician's health study. *Arch Dermatol.* 2000;136:179-184.

25. Michaud DS, Feskanich D, Rimm EB, et al. Intake of specific carotenoids and risk of lung cancer in 2 prospective US cohorts. *Am J Clin Nutr.* 2000;72:990-997.

26. Speizer FE, Colditz GA, Hunter DJ, et al. Prospective study of smoking, antioxidant intake, and lung cancer in middle-aged women (USA). *Cancer Causes Control.* 1999;10:475-482.

27. Alpha-tocopherol, Beta Carotene Cancer Prevention Study Group. The effect of vitamin E and beta-carotene on the incidence of lung cancer and other cancers in male smokers. *N Engl J Med.* 1994;330:1029-1035.

28. Rapola JM, Virtamo J, Ripatti S, et al. Randomized trial of alpha-tocopherol and beta-carotene supplements on incidence of major coronary events in men with previous myocardial infarction. *Lancet.* 1997;349:1715-1720.

29. Rapola JM, Virtamo J, Haukka JK, et al. Effect of vitamin E and beta carotene on the incidence of angina pectoris. *JAMA.* 1996;275:693-698.

30. Renner S, Rath R, Rust P, et al. Effects of beta-carotene supplementation for six months on clinical and laboratory parameters in patients with cystic fibrosis. *Thorax.* 2001;56:48-52.

31. Mackerras D, Irwig L, Simpson JM, et al. Randomized double-blind trial of beta-carotene and vitamin C in women with minor cervical abnormalities. *Br J Cancer.* 1999;79:1448-1453.

32. Tornwall ME, Virtamo J, Haukka JK, et al. The effect of alpha-tocopherol and beta-carotene supplementation on symptoms and progression of intermittent claudication in a controlled trial. *Atherosclerosis.* 1999;147:193-197.

33. Carson C, Lee S, De Paola C, et al. Antioxidant intake and cataract in the Melbourne Visual Impairment Project [abstract]. *Am J Epidemiol.* 1994;139(11 suppl):Abst 65.

34. Vitale S, West S, Hallfrish J, et al. Plasma antioxidants and risk of cortical and nuclear cataract. *Epidemiology.* 1993;4:195-203.
35. Teikari JM, Rautalahti M, Haukka J, et al. Incidence of cataract operations in Finnish male smokers unaffected by alpha tocopherol or beta carotene supplements. *J Epidemiol Community Health.* 1998;52:468-472.
36. Seddon JM, Ajani UA, Sperduto RD, et al. Dietary carotenoids, vitamins A,C, and E, and advanced age-related macular degeneration. *JAMA.* 1994;272:1413-1420.
37. Goldberg J, Flowerdew G, Smith E, et al. Factors associated with age-related macular degeneration: an analysis of data from the first National Health and Nutrition Examination Survey. *Am J Epidemiol.* 1988;128:700-710.
38. Kostis JB, Wilson AC, Lacy CR. Hypertension and ascorbic acid [letter]. *Lancet.* 2000;355:1272.
39. Romney SL, Ho GY, Palan PR, et al. Effects of beta-carotene and other factors on outcome of cervical dysplasia and human papillomavirus infection. *Gynecol Oncol.* 1997;65:483-492.
40. Keefe KA, Schell MJ, Brewer C, et al. A randomized double blind phase III trial using oral beta-carotene supplementation for women with high-grade cervical intra-epithelial neoplasia. *Cancer Epidemiol Biomarkers Prev.* 2001;10:1029-1035.
41. Fairley CK, Tabrizi SN, Chen S, et al. A randomized clinical trial of beta carotene vs. placebo for the treatment of cervical HPV infection. *Int J Gynecol Cancer.* 1996;6:225-230.

Beta-Sitosterol

1. Wilt TJ, MacDonald R, Ishani A. Beta-sitosterol for the treatment of benign prostatic hyperplasia: a systematic review. *BJU Int.* 1999;83:976-983.
2. Klippel KF, Hiltl DM, Schipp B. A multicentric, placebo-controlled, double-blind clinical trial of beta-sitosterol (phytosterol) for the treatment of benign prostatic hyperplasia. German BPH-Phyto Study group. *Br J Urol.* 1997;80:427-432.
3. Kadow C, Abrams PH. A double-blind trial of the effect of beta-sitosteryl glucoside (WA184) in the treatment of benign prostatic hyperplasia. *Eur Urol.* 1986;12:187-189.
4. Berges RR, Windeler J, Trampisch HJ, et al. Randomized, placebo-controlled, double-blind clinical trial of beta-sitosterol in patients with benign prostatic hyperplasia. Beta-sitosterol Study Group. *Lancet.* 1995;345:1529-1532.
5. Bouic PJD, Clark A, Lamprecht J, et al. The effects of B-stitosterol (BSS) and B-Sitosterol glucoside (BSSG) mixture on selected immune parameters of marathon runners: inhibition of post marathon immune suppression and inflammatioin. *Int J Sport Nutr.* 1999;20:258-262.
6. Pegel K. The importance of sitosterol and sitosterolin in human and animal nutrition. *S Afr J Sci.* 1997;93:263-268.

Bilberry Fruit

1. Muth ER, Laurent JM, Jasper P. The effect of bilberry nutritional supplementation on night visual acuity and contrast sensitivity. *Altern Med Rev.* 2000;5:164-173.
2. Zadok D, Levy Y, Glovinsky Y. The effect of anthocyanosides in a multiple oral dose on night vision. *Eye.* 1999;13:734-736.
3. Levy Y, Glovinsky Y. The effect of anthocyanosides on night vision. *Eye.* 1998;12:967-969.
4. Vannini L, Samually R, Coffano M, et al. Pupillographic study after administration of anthocyanosides [in Italian; English abstract]. *Boll Ocul.* 1986;65:569-577.
5. Perossini M, Guidi G, Chiellini S, et al. Diabetic and hypertensive retinopathy therapy with *Vaccinium Myrtillus* anthocyanosides (tegens): double blind placebo-controlled clinical trial [in Italian; English abstract]. *Ann Ottalmol Clin Ocul.* 1987;12:1174-1190.
6. Gatta L, et al. Bilberry. *Fitoterapia.* 1988;59(suppl 1):19. Cited by: Bone K. Bilberry: the vision herb. *Mediherb Professional Rev.* 1997;59(3):1-4.
7. Schulz V, Hansel R, Tyler VE. *Rational Phytotherapy: A Physicians' Guide to Herbal Medicine.* 3rd ed. Berlin, Germany: Springer-Verlag; 1998:193.
8. Morazzoni P, Bombardelli E. Vaccinium Myrtillus L. *Fitoterapia.* 1996;67:3-29.

9. Gabor M. Pharmacologic effects of flavonoids on blood vessels. *Angiologica*. 1972; 9:355-374.

10. Havsteen B. Flavonoids, a class of natural products of high pharmacological potency. *Biochem Pharmacol*. 1983;32:1141-1148.

11. Mian E, Curri SB, Lietti A, et al. Anthocyanosides and microvessels wall: new findings on the mechanism of action of their protective effect in syndromes due to abnormal capillary fragility [in Italian; English abstract]. *Minerva Med*. 1977;68:3565-3581.

12. Monboisse JC, Braquet P, Randoux A, et al. Non-enzymatic degradation of acid-soluble calf skin collagen by superoxide ion: protective effect of flavonoids. *Biochem Pharmacol*. 1983;32:53-58.

13. Pulliero G, Montin S, Bettini R, et al. Ex vivo study of the inhibitory effects of *Vaccinium myrtillus* anthocyanosides on human platelet aggregation. *Fitoterapia*. 1989;60:69-75.

14. Bertuglia S, Malandrino S, Colantuoni A. Effect of *Vaccinium myrtillus* anthocyanosides on ischaemia reperfusion injury in hamster cheek pouch microcirculation. *Pharmacol Res*. 1995;31:183-187.

15. Cluzel C, Bastide P, Wegman R, et al. Enzymatic activities in the retina and anthocyanosides extracted from *Vaccinium myrtillus* [translated from French]. *Biochem Pharmacol*. 1970;19:2295-2302.

16. Wegmann R, et al. Effects of anthocyanosides on photo receptors. Cyto-enzymatic aspects [translated from French]. *Ann Histochim*. 1969;14:237-256.

17. Bottecchia D, Bettini V, Martino R, et al. Preliminary report on the inhibitory effect of *Vaccinium myrtillus* anthocyanosides on platelet aggregation and clot retraction. *Fitoterapia*. 1987;58:3-8.

18. Morazzoni P, Magistretti MJ. Effects of *Vaccinium myrtillus* anthocyanosides on prostacyclin-like activity in rat arterial tissue. *Fitoterapia*. 1986;57:11-14.

19. Zaragoza F, Iglesias I, Benedi J. Comparative study of the anti-aggregation effects of anthocyanosides and other agents [in Spanish; English abstract]. *Arch Farmacol Toxicol*. 1985;11:183-188.

20. Lietti A, Cristoni A, Picci M. Studies on *Vaccinium myrtillus* anthocyanosides. I. Vasoprotective and antiinflammatory activity. *Arzneimittelforschung*. 1976;26: 829-832.

21. Lietti A, Forni G. Studies on *Vaccinium myrtillus* anthocyanosides. II. Aspects of anthocyanins pharmacokinetics in the rat. *Arzneimittelforschung*. 1976;26:832-835.

22. Eandi M. Post marketing investigation on Tegens® preparation with respect to side effects. [data on file]. 1987. Cited by: Morazzoni P, Bombardelli E. *Vaccinium myrtillus* L. *Fitoterapia*. 1996;67:3-29.

23. Grismondi GL. Treatment of phlebopathies caused by stasis in pregnancy [translated from Italian]. *Minerva Ginecol*. 1981;33:221-230.

Biotin

1. Maebashi M, Makino Y, Furukawa Y, et al. Therapeutic evaluation of the effect of biotin on hyperglycemia in patients with non-insulin dependent diabetes mellitus. *J Clin Biochem Nutr*. 1993;14:211-218.

2. Coggeshall J, Heggers JP, Robson MC, et al. Biotin status and plasma glucose in diabetics. *Ann N Y Acad Sci*. 1985;447:389-392.

3. Koutsikos D, Agroyannis B, Tzanatos-Exarchou H. Biotin for diabetic peripheral neuropathy. *Biomed Pharmacother*. 1990;44:511-514.

4. Floersheim GL. Treatment of brittle fingernails with biotin [in German; English abstract]. *Z Hautkr*. 1989;64:41-48.

5. Colombo VE, Gerber F, Bronhofer M, et al. Treatment of brittle fingernails and onychoschizia with biotin: scanning electron microscopy. *J Am Acad Dermatol*. 1990;23:1127-1132.

6. Hochman LG, Scher RK, Meyerson MS. Brittle nails: response to daily biotin supplementation. *Cutis*. 1993;51:303-305.

7. McCarty MF. Toward practical prevention of type 2 diabetes. *Med Hypotheses*. 2000;54:786-793.

8. Dietary reference intakes for thiamin, riboflavin, niacin, vitamin B_6, folate, vitamin B12, pantothenic acid, biotin, and choline. (1998). Available at http://www.nap.edu. Accessed October 4, 2001.

9. Krause KH, Bonjour JP, Berlit P, et al. Biotin status of epileptics. *Ann NY Acad Sci.* 1985;447:297-313.

10. Said HM, Redha R, Nylander W. Biotin transport in the human intestine: inhibition by anticonvulsant drugs. *Am J Clin Nutr.* 1989;49:127-131.

11. Mock DM, Quirk JG, Mock NI. Marginal biotin deficiency during normal pregnancy. *Am J Clin Nutr.* 2002;75:295-299.

12. Zempleni J, Mock DM. Marginal biotin deficiency is teratogenic. *Proc Soc Exp Biol Med.* 2000;223:14-21.

13. Schulpis KH, Karikas GA, Tjamouranis J, et al. Low serum biotinidase activity in children with valproic acid monotherapy. *Epilepsia.* 2001;42:1359-1362.

14. Mock DM, Dyken ME. Biotin catabolism is accelerated in adults receiving long-term therapy with anticonvulsants. *Neurology.* 1997;49:1444-1447.

15. Groff, J. *Advanced Nutrition and Human Metabolism.* 2nd ed. St. Paul, Mn.: West Publishing Company; 1995.

Bitter Melon

1. Srivastava Y, Venkatakrishna-Bhatt H, Verma Y, et al. Antidiabetic and adaptogenic properties of *Momordica charantia* extract: an experimental and clinical evaluation. *Phytother Res.* 1993;7:285-289.

2. Welihinda J, Arvidson G, Gylfe E, et al. The insulin-releasing activity of the tropical plant *Momordica charantia. Acta Biol Med Ger.* 1982;41:1229-1240.

3. Welihinda J, Karunanayake EH, Sheriff MHR, et al. Effect of *Momordica charantia* on the glucose tolerance in maturity onset diabetes. *J Ethnopharmacol.* 1986;17:277-282.

4. Leatherdale BA, Panesar RK, Singh G, et al. Improvement in glucose tolerance due to *Momordica charantia* (karela). *Br Med J (Clin Res Ed).* 1981;282:1823-1824.

5. Aslam M, Stockley IH. Interaction between curry ingredient (karela) and drug (chlorpropamide). *Lancet.* 1979;1:607.

Black Cohosh

1. Stoll W. Phythopharmacon influences atrophic vaginal epithelium: double-blind study: *Cimicifuga* vs. estrogenic substances [translated from German]. *Therapeutikon.* 1987;1:23-26,28,30-31.

2. Liske E, Hanggi W, Henneicke-Von Zepelin HH, et al. Physiological investigation of a unique extract of black cohosh *(Cimicifugae racemosae rhizoma):* a 6-month clinical study demonstrates no systemic estrogenic effect. *J Womens Health Gend Based Med.* 2002;11:163-174.

3. Nesselhut T, Liske E. Pharmacological measures in postmenopausal women with an isopropanolic aqueous extract of *Cimicifugae racemosae* rhizoma [abstract]. *Menopause.* 1999;6:Abst. #99.012.

4. Einer-Jensen N, Zhao J, Andersen KP, et al. *Cimicifuga* and *Melbrosia* lack estrogenic effects in mice and rats. *Maturitas.* 1996;25:149-153.

5. Jarry H, Harnischfeger G. Studies on the endocrine effects of the contents of *Cimicifuga racemosa:* 1. Influence on the serum concentrations of pituitary hormones in ovariectomized rats [translated from German]. *Planta Med.* 1985;(1):46-49.

6. Zava DT, Dollbaum CM, Blen M. Estrogen and progestin bioactivity of foods, herbs, and spices. *Proc Soc Exp Biol Med.* 1998;217:369-378.

7. Seidlova-Wuttke D, Wuttke W. Selective estrogen receptor modulator activity of *Cimicifuga racemosa* extract: clinical data [abstract]. *Phytomedicine.* 2000;7(suppl 2):11.

8. Seidlova-Wuttke D, Jarry H, Heiden I, et al. Effects of *Cimicifuga racemosa* on estrogen-dependent tissues [abstract]. *Phytomedicine.* 2000;7(suppl 2):11-12.

9. Wuttke W, Jarry H, Heiden I, et al. Selective estrogen receptor modulator (SERM) activity of the *Cimicifuga racemosa* extract BNO 1055: pharmacology and mechanisms of action [abstract]. *Phytomedicine.* 2000;7(suppl 2):12.

10. Jacobson JS, Troxel AB, Evans J, et al. Randomized trial of black cohosh for the treatment of hot flashes among women with a history of breast cancer. *J Clin Oncol.* 2001;19:2739-2745.

11. Stolze H. An alternative to treat menopausal complaints [translated from German]. *Gyne.* 1982;1:14-16.

12. Warnecke G. Influencing menopausal symptoms with a phytotherapeutic agent [in German]. *Med Welt.* 1985;36:871-874.

13. Lehmann-Willenbrock VE, Riedel H-H. Clinical and endocrinologic examinations about therapy of climacteric symptoms following hysterectomy with remaining ovaries [in German; English abstract]. *Zentralbl Gynakol.* 1988;110:611-618.

14. Liske E. Therapeutic efficacy and safety of *Cimicifuga racemosa* for gynecologic disorders. *Adv Ther.* 1998;15:45-53.

15. MacLennan A, Lester S, Moore V. Oral estrogen replacement therapy versus placebo for hot flushes: a systematic review. *Climacteric.* 2001;4:58-74.

16. Jarry H, Harnischfeger G, Duker E. The endocrine effects of constituents of *Cimicifuga racemosa*. 2. In vitro binding of constituents to estrogen receptors [translated from German]. *Planta Med.* 1985;(4):316-319.

17. Schulz V, Hansel R, Tyler VE. *Rational Phytotherapy: A Physicians' Guide to Herbal Medicine.* 3rd ed. Berlin, Germany: Springer-Verlag; 1998:243.

18. Duker EM, Kopanski L, Jarry H, et al. Effects of extracts from *Cimicifuga racemosa* on gonadotropin release in menopausal women and ovariectomized rats. *Planta Med.* 1991;57:420-424.

19. Nesselhut T, Schellhase C, Dietrich R, et al. Investigations into the growth-inhibitive efficacy of phytopharmacopia with estrogen-like influences on mammary gland carcinoma cells [translated from German]. *Arch Gynecol Obstet.* 1993;254:817-818.

20. Freudenstein J, Dasenbrock C, Nisslein T. Lack of promotion of estrogen dependent mammary gland tumors in vivo by an isopropanolic black cohosh extract [abstract]. *Phytomedicine.* 2000;7(suppl 2):13.

Blue Cohosh

1. McFarlin BL, Gibson MH, O'Rear J, et al. A national survey of herbal preparation use by nurse-midwives for labor stimulation: review of the literature and recommendations for practice. *J Nurse Midwifery.* 1999;44:205-216.

2. Jones TK, Lawson BM. Profound neonatal congestive heart failure caused by maternal consumption of blue cohosh herbal medication. *J Pediatr.* 1998;132:550-552.

3. Chandrasekhar K, Vishwanath CR. Studies on the effect of *Caulophyllum* on implantation in rats [abstract]. *J Reprod Fertil.* 1974;38:245-246.

4. Chandrasekhar K, Sarma GH. Observations on the effect of low and high doses of *Caulophyllum* on the ovaries and the consequential changes in the uterus and thyroid in rats [abstract]. *J Reprod Fertil.* 1974;38:236-237.

5. Gunn TR, Wright IM. The use of black and blue cohosh in labour. *NZ Med J.* 1996;109:410-411.

Boldo

1. Blumenthal M, ed. *The Complete German Commission E Monographs, Therapeutic Guide to Herbal Medicines.* Boston, Mass: Integrative Medicine Communications; 1998.

2. Magistretti MJ. Remarks on the pharmacological examinaiton of plant extracts. *Fitoterapia.* 1980;51:67-79.

3. Lanhers MC, Joyeux M, Soulimani R, et al. Hepatoprotective and anti-inflammatory effects of a traditional medicinal plant of Chile, *Peumus boldus. Planta Med.* 1991;57:110-115.

4. Speisky H, Cassels BK. Boldo and boldine: an emerging case of natural drug development. *Pharmacol Res.* 1994;29:1-12.

5. Kupke D, von Sanden H, Trinczek-Gartner H, et al. An evaluation of the choleretic activity of a plant-based cholagogue [translated from German]. *Z Allgemeinmed.* 1991;67:1046-1058.

6. Greving I, Meister V, Monnerjahn C, et al. *Chelidonium majus:* a rare reason for severe hepatotoxic reaction. *Pharmacoepidemiol Drug Safety.* 1998;7:S66-S69.

7. Benninger J, Schneider HT, Schuppan, et al. Acute hepatitis induced by greater celandine *(Chelidonium majus). Gastroenterology.* 1999;117:1234-1237.
8. Strahl S, Ehret V, Dahm HH, et al. Necrotizing hepatitis after taking herbal remedies. *Dtsch Med Wochenschr.* 1998;123:1410-1414.
9. Jimenez I, Speisky H. Biological disposition of boldine: in vitro and in vivo studies. *Phytother Res.* 2000;14:254-260.
10. Backhouse N, Delporte C, Givernau M, et al. Anti-inflammatory and antipyretic effects of boldine. *Agents Actions.* 1994;42:114-117.
11. Jimenez I, Garrido A, Bannach R, et al. Protective effects of boldine against free radical-induced erythrocyte lysis. *Phytother Res.* 2000;14:339-343.
12. Almeida ER, Melo AM, Xavier H. Toxicological evaluation of the hydro-alcohol extract of the dry leaves of *Peumus boldus* and boldine in rats. *Phytother Res.* 2000;14:99-102.
13. Lambert JP, Cormier A. Potential interaction between warfarin and boldo-fenugreek. *Pharmacotherapy.* 2001;21:509-512.

Boron

1. Travers RL, Rennie GC, Newnham RE. Boron and arthritis: the results of a double-blind pilot study. *J Nutr Med.* 1990;1:127-132.
2. Zhang ZF, Winton MI, Rainey C, et al. Boron is associated with decreased risk of human prostate cancer. Presented at: Experimental Biology 2001; March 31-April 4, 2001; Orlando, FL.
3. Nielsen FH, Hunt CD, Mullen LM, et al. Effect of dietary boron on mineral, estrogen, and testosterone metabolism in postmenopausal women. *FASEB J.* 1987;1:394-397.
4. Beattie JH, Peace HS. The influence of a low-boron diet and boron supplementation on bone, major mineral and sex steroid metabolism in postmenopausal women. *Br J Nutr.* 1993;69:871-884.
5. Naghii MR, Samman S. The effect of boron supplementation on its urinary excretion and selected cardiovascular risk factors in healthy male subjects. *Biol Trace Elem Res.* 1997;56:273-286.

Boswellia

1. Gupta I, Gupta V, Parihar A, et al. Effects of *Boswellia serrata* gum resin in patients with bronchial asthma: results of a double-blind, placebo-controlled, 6-week clinical study. *Eur J Med Res.* 1998;3:511-514.
2. Etzel R. Special extract of *Boswellia serrata* (H 15)* in the treatment of rheumatoid arthritis. *Phytomedicine.* 1996;3:91-94.
3. Sander O, Herborn G, Rau R. Is H15 (resin extract of *Boswellia serrata*, "incense") a useful supplement to established drug therapy of chronic polyarthritis? Results of a double-blind pilot study [in German; English abstract]. *Z Rheumatol.* 1998;57:11-16.
4. Reddy GK, Chandrakasan G, Dhar SC. Studies on the metabolism of glycosaminoglycans under the influence of new herbal anti-inflammatory agents. *Biochem Pharmacol.* 1989;38:3527-3534.
5. Gupta I, Parihar A, Malhotra P, et al. Effects of *Boswellia serrata* gum resin in patients with ulcerative colitis. *Eur J Med Res.* 1997;2:37-43.
6. Safayhi H, Sailer ER, Ammon HPT. 5-lipoxygenase inhibition by acetyl-11-keto-beta-boswellic acid (AKBA) by a novel mechanism. *Phytomedicine.* 1996;3:71-72.
7. Singh GB, Atal CK. Pharmacology of an extract of salai guggal ex-*Boswellia serrata*, a new non-steroidal anti-inflammatory agent. *Agents Actions.* 1986;18:407-412.
8. Wildfeuer A, Neu IS, Safayhi H, et al. Effects of boswellic acids extracted from a herbal medicine on the biosynthesis of leukotrienes and the course of experimental autoimmune encephalomyelitis. *Arzneimittelforschung.* 1998;48:668-674.
9. Safayhi H, Boden SE, Schweizer S, et al. Concentration-dependent potentiating and inhibitory effects of *Boswellia* extracts on 5-lipoxygenase product formation in stimulated PMNL. *Planta Med.* 2000;66:110-113.
10. Gerhardt H, Seifert F, Buvari P, et al. Therapy of active Crohn disease with Boswellia serrata extract H 15. *Z Gastroenterol.* 2001;39:11-17.

11. Krieglstein CF, Anthoni C, Rijcken F,J, et al. Acetyl-11-keto-beta-boswellic acid, a constituent of a herbal medicine from Boswellia serrata resin, attenuates experimental ileitis. *Int J Colorectal Dis.* 2001;16:88-95.

12. Janssen G, Bode U, Breu H, et al. Boswellic acids in the palliative therapy of children with progressive or relapsed brain tumors. *Klin Padiatr.* 2000;212:189-195.

13. Winking M, Sarikaya S, Rahmanian A, et al. Boswellic acids inhibit glioma growth: a new treatment option? *J Neurooncol.* 2000;46:97-103.

14. Glaser T, Winter S, Groscurth P, et al. Boswellic acids and malignant glioma: induction of apoptosis but no modulation of drug sensitivity. *Br J Cancer.* 1999;80: 756-765.

Branched-Chain Amino Acids (BCAAs)

1. Cangiano C, Laviano A, Meguid MM, et al. Effects of administration of oral branched-chain amino acids on anorexia and caloric intake in cancer patients. *J Natl Cancer Inst.* 1996;88:550-551.

2. Hiroshige K, Sonta T, Suda T, et al. Oral supplementation of branched-chain amino acid improves nutritional status in elderly patients on chronic hemodialysis. *Nephrol Dial Transplant.* 2001;16:1856-1862.

3. Testa D, Caraceni T, Fetoni V. Branched-chain amino acids in the treatment of amyotrophic lateral sclerosis. *J Neurol.* 1989;236:445-447.

4. Tandan R, Bromberg MB, Forshew D, et al. A controlled trial of amino acid therapy in amyotrophic lateral sclerosis. I. Clinical, functional, and maximum isometric torque data. *Neurology.* 1996;47:1220-1226.

5. Plaitakis A, Smith J, Mandeli J, et al. Pilot trial of branched-chain aminoacids in amyotrophic lateral sclerosis. *Lancet.* 1988;1:1015-1018.

6. Plaitakis A. Branched-chain amino acids and ALS [letter]. *Neurology.* 1994;44: 1982-1983.

7. [No authors listed]. Branched-chain amino acids and amyotrophic lateral sclerosis: a treatment failure? The Italian ALS Study Group. *Neurology.* 1993;43;2466-2470.

8. Gredal O, Moller SE. Effect of branched-chain amino acids on glutamate metabolism in amyotrophic lateral sclerosis. *J Neurol Sci.* 1995;129:40-43.

9. Mendell JR, Griggs RC, Moxley RT III, et al. Clinical investigation in duchenne muscular dystrophy. IV. Double-blind controlled trial of leucine. *Muscle Nerve.* 1984;7:535-541.

10. Kelly GS. Sports nutrition: a review of selected nutritional supplements for bodybuilders and strength athletes. *Altern Med Rev.* 1997;2:184-201.

11. Bigard AX, Lavier P, Ullmann L, et al. Branced-chain amino acid supplementation during repeated prolonged skiing exercises at altitude. *Int J Sport Nutr.* 1996;6; 295-306.

12. Struder HK, Hollmann W, Platen P, et al. Influence of paroxetine, branched-chain amino acids and tyrosine on neuroendocrine system responses and fatigue in humans. *Horm Metab Res.* 1998;30:188-194.

13. Davis JM, Welsh RS, De Volve KL, et al. Effects of branched-chain amino acids and carbohydrate on fatigue during intermittent, high intensity running. *Int J Sports Med.* 1999;20:309-314.

14. Mero A. Leucine supplementation and intensive training. *Sports Med.* 1999;27: 347-358.

15. van Hall G, Raaymakers JS, Saris WH, et al. Ingestion of branched-chain amino acids and tryptophan during sustained exercise in man: failure to affect performance. *J Physiol.* 1995;486(Pt 3):789-794.

16. Williams MH. Facts and fallacies of purported ergogenic amino acid supplements. *Clin Sports Med.* 1999;18:633-649.

17. Wagenmakers AJ. Amino acid supplements to improve athletic performance. *Curr Opin Clin Nutr Metab Care.* 1999;2:539-544.

18. Richardson MA, Bevans ML, Weber JB, et al. Branched chain amino acids decrease tardive dyskinesia symptoms. *Psychopharmacology.* 1999;143:358-364.

19. Wagenmakers A. Amino acid metabolism, muscular fatigue and muscle wasting, speculations on adaptations to high altitude. *Int J Sport Med.* 1992;13:S110-S113.

20. Robertson DR, Higginson I, Macklin BS, et al. The influence of protein containing meals on the pharmacokinetics of levodopa in healthy volunteers. *Br J Clin
Pharmacol.* 1991;31:413-417.

Bromelain

1. Taussig SJ, Nieper HA. Bromelain: its use in prevention and treatment of cardiovascular disease present status. *J Int Acad Prev Med.* 1979;6:139-151.
2. Zatuchni GI, Colombi DJ. Bromelains therapy for the prevention of episiotomy
pain. *Obstet Gynecol.* 1967;29:275-278.
3. Howat RC, Lewis GD. The effect of bromelain therapy on episiotomy wounds: a
double blind controlled clinical trial. *J Obstet Gynaecol Br Commow.* 1972;79:951-953.
4. Seltzer AP. Minimizing post-operative edema and ecchymoses by the use of an oral
enzyme preparation (bromelain): a controlled study of 53 rhinoplasty cases. *Eye Ear
Nose Throat Mon.* 1962;41:813-817.
5. Spaeth GL. The effect of bromelains on the inflammatory response caused by
cataract extraction: a double-blind study. *Eye Ear Nose Throat Mon.* 1968;47:634-639.
6. Tassman GC, Zafran JN, Zayon GM. Evaluation of a plant proteolytic enzyme for
the control of inflammation and pain. *J Dent Med.* 1964;19:73-77.
7. Gylling U, Rintala A, Taipale S, et al. The effect of a proteolytic enzyme combinate
(bromelain) on the postoperative edema by oral application: a clinical and experimental study. *Acta Chir Scand.* 1966;131:193-196.
8. Blonstein JL. Control of swelling in boxing injuries. *Practitioner.* 1969;203:206.
9. Ryan RE. A double-blind clinical evaluation of bromelains in the treatment of acute
sinusitis. *Headache.* 1967;7:13-17.
10. Taub SJ. The use of ananase in sinusitis: a study of 60 patients. *Eye Ear Nose Throat
Mon.* 1966;45:96-98.
11. Seltzer AP. Adjunctive use of bromelains in sinusitis: a controlled study. *Eye Ear Nose
Throat Mon.* 1967;46:1281-1288.
12. Tinozzi S, Venegoni A. Effect of bromelain on serum and tissue levels of amoxy-
cillin. *Drugs Exp Clin Res.* 1978;4:39-44.
13. Luerti M, Vignali M. Influence of bromelain on penetration of antibiotics in uterus,
salpinx and ovary. *Drugs Exp Clin Res.* 1978;4:45-48.
14. Mori S, Ojima Y, Hirose T, et al. The clinical effect of proteolytic enzyme containing bromelain and trypsin on urinary tract infection evaluated by double blind
method. *Acta Obstet Gynaecol Jpn.* 1972;19:147-153.
15. Seligman B. Oral Bromelains as adjuncts in the treatment of acute thrombophlebitis.
Angiology. 1969;20:22-26.
16. Adachi N, Koh CS, Tsukada N, et al. In vitro degradation of amyloid material by
four proteases in tissue of a patient with familial amyloidotic polyneuropathy.
J Neurol Sci. 1988;84:295-299.
17. Kane S, Goldberg MJ. Use of bromelain for mild ulcerative colitis [letter]. *Ann Intern
Med.* 2000;132:680.
18. Levenson SM, Kan D, Gruber C, et al. Chemical debridement of burns. *Ann Surg.*
1974;180:670-704.
19. Levine N, Seifter E, Connerton C, et al. Debridement of experimental skin burns of
pigs with bromelain, a pineapple-stem enzyme. *Plast Reconstr Surg.* 1973;52:413-424.
20. Klein GK. Enzymatic debridement of third degree burns in animals with bromelains: a preliminary report. *J Maine Med Assoc.* 1964;55:169-171.
21. Klaue P, Aman G, Romaen W. Chemical debridement of the burn eschar in rats with
bromelain combined with topical antmicrobial agents. *Eur Surg Res.* 1979;11:
353-359.
22. Ahle NW, Hamlet MP. Enzymatic frostbite eschar debridement by bromelain. *Ann
Emerg Med.* 1987;16:1063-1065.
23. Taussig SJ, Yokoyama MM, Chinen A, et al. Bromelain, a proteolytic enzyme and its
clinical application: a review. *Hiroshima J Med Sci.* 1975;24:185-193.
24. Taussig SJ. The mechanism of the physiological action of bromelain. *Med Hypotheses.*
1980;6:99-104.

25. Taussig SJ, Batkin S. Bromelain, the enzyme complex of pineapple *(Ananas comosus)* and its clinical application. An update. *J Ethnopharmacol.* 1988;22:191-203.

26. Ako H, Cheung AHS, Matsuura PK. Isolation of a fibrinolysis enzyme activator from commercial bromelain (1). *Arch Int Pharmacodyn Ther.* 1981;254:157-167.

27. Martin GJ, Ehrenreich J, Asbell N. Bromelian. Pineapple protease with anti-edema-activity. *Exp Med Surg.* 1962;20:227-247.

28. Barrett AJ, Starkey PM. The interaction of alpha 2-macroglobulin with proteinases: characteristics and specificity of the reaction, and a hypothesis concerning its molecular mechanism. *Biochem J.* 1973;133:709-724.

29. Petry JJ. Surgically significant nutritional supplements. *Plast Reconstr Surg.* 1996;97:233-240.

30. Desser L, Rehberger A, Paukovits W. Proteolytic enzymes and amylase induce cytokine production in human peripheral blood mononuclear cells in vitro. *Cancer Biother.* 1994;9:253-263.

31. [No authors listed]. Bromelain. *Altern Med Rev.* 1998;3:302-305.

32. Moss JN, Frazier CV, Martin GJ. Bromelains: the pharmacology of the enzymes. *Arch Int Pharmacodyn Ther.* 1963;145:166-188.

33. Baur X. Studies on the specificity of human IgE-antibodies to the plant proteases papain and bromelain. *Clin Allergy.* 1979;9:451-457.

34. Baur X, Fruhmann G. Allergic reactions, including asthma, to the pineapple protease bromelain following occupational exposure. *Clin Allergy.* 1979;9:443-450.

35. Gailhofer G, Wilders-Truschnig M, Smolle J, et al. Asthma caused by bromelain: an occupational allergy. *Clin Allergy.* 1988;18:445-450.

36. Gall H, Kalveram KJ, Forck G, et al. Kiwi fruit allergy: a new birch pollen-associated food allergy. *J Allergy Clin Immunol.* 1994;94:70-76.

37. Pike RN, Bagarozzi D Jr, Travis J. Immunological cross-reactivity of the major allergen from perennial ryegrass (Lolium perenne), Lol p I, and the cysteine proteinase, bromelain. *Int Arch Allergy Immunol.* 1997;112:412-414.

38. Tanabe S, Tesaki S, Watanabe M, et al. Cross-reactivity between bromelain and soluble fraction from wheat flour [in Japanese; English abstract]. *Arerugi.* 1997;46:1170-1173.

39. Gutfreund AE, Taussig SJ, Morris AK. Effect of oral bromelain on blood pressure and heart rate of hypertensive patients. *Hawaii Med J.* 1978;37:143-146.

40. Cirelli MG, Smyth RD. Effects of bromelain anti-edema therapy on coagulation, bleeding, and prothrombin times. *J New Drugs.* 1963;3:37-39.

41. Kolac C, Streichhan P, Lehr CM. Oral bioavailability of proteolytic enzymes *Eur J Pharm Biopharm.* 1996;42:222-232.

42. Smyth RD, Brennan R, Martin GJ. Studies establishing the absorption of the bromelains (proteolytic enzymes) from the gastrointestinal tract. *Exp Med Surg.* 1964;22:46-59.

43. Brakebusch M, Wintergerst U, Petropoulou T, et al. Bromelain is an accelerator of phagocytosis respiratory burst and killing of Candida albicans by human granulocytes and monocytes. *Eur J Med Res.* 2001;6;193-200.

Bugleweed

1. Kohrle J, Auf'mkolk M, Winterhoff H, et al. Iodothyronine deiodinases: inhibition by plant extracts. *Acta Endocrinol.* 1981;96 (suppl):15-16.

2. Auf'mkolk M, Ingbar JC, Kubota K, et al. Extracts and auto-oxidized constituents of certain plants inhibit the receptor-binding and biological activity of Graves' disease immunoglobulins. *Endocrinology.* 1985;116:1687-1693.

3. Auf'mkolk M, Kohrle J, Gumbinger H, et al. Antihormonal effects of plant extracts: iodothyronine deiodinase of rat liver is inhibited by extracts and secondary metabolites of plants. *Horm Metab Res.* 1984;16:188-192.

4. Sourgens H, Winteroff H, Gumbinger HG, et al. Antihormonal effects of plant extracts: TSH and prolactin-suppressing properties of *Lithospermum officinale* and other plants. *Planta Med.* 1982;45:78-86.

5. Brinker F. Inhibition of endocrine function by botanical agents. I. *Boraginaceae* and *Labiatae. J Naturopath Med.* 1990;1:10-18.

Butterbur

1. Grossmann M, Schmidramsl H. An extract of *Petasites hybridus* is effective in the prophylaxis of migraine. *Int J Clin Pharmacol Ther.* 2000;38:430-435.
2. Reglin F. Butterbur root: a pain reliever with wide range application possibilities. *Praxis-Telegram.* 1998;1:13-14.
3. *PDR for Herbal Medicines.* 1st ed. Montvale, NJ: Medical Economics Co; 1998: 1020-1022.
4. Carle R. Plant-based antiphlogistics and spasmolytics [translated from German]. *Z Phytother.* 1988;9:67-76.
5. Ziolo G, Samochowiec L. Study on clinical properties and mechanisms of action of *Petasites* in bronchial asthma and chronic obstructive bronchitis. *Pharm Acta Helv.* 1998;72:378-380.
6. Scheidegger C, Dahinden C, Wiesmann U. Effects of extracts and of individual components from *Petasites* on prostaglandin synthesis in cultured skin fibroblasts and on leucotriene synthesis in isolated human peripheral leucocytes. *Pharm Acta Helv.* 1998;72:376-378.
7. Grossman W. Migraine prophylaxis with a phytopharmaceutical remedy: the results of a randomized, placebo-controlled, double-blind clinical study with Petadolex™. *Der Freie Arzt.* 1996;(3):1-7.
8. Carle R. Plant-based antiphlogistics and spasmolytics [translated from German]. *Z Phytother.* 1988;9:67-76.
9. Berger D, Burkard W, Schaffner W. Influence of *Petasites hybridus* on dopamine-D2 and histamine-H1 receptors. *Pharm Acta Helv.* 1998;72:373-375.
10. Brune K, Bickel D, Peskar BA. Gastro-protective effects by extracts of *Petasites hybridus:* the role of inhibition of peptido-leukotriene synthesis. *Planta Med.* 1993; 59:494-496.
11. Bickel D, Roder T, Bestmann HJ, et al. Identification and characterization of inhibitors of peptido-leukotriene-synthesis from *Petasites hybridus. Planta Med.* 1994; 60:318-322.
12. Luthy J, Zweifel U, Schmid P, et al. Pyrrolizidine alkaloids in *Petasites hybridus* L. and P. albus L. [in German; English abstract]. *Pharm Acta Helv.* 1983;58:98-100.
13. Mauz C, Candrian U, Luthy J, et al. Method for the reduction of pyrrolizidine alkaloids from medicinal plant extracts [in German; English abstract]. *Pharm Acta Helv.* 1985;60:256-259.
14. Schapowal, A. Randomized controlled trial of butterbur and cetirizine for treating seasonal allergic rhinitis. *BMJ.* 2002;324:144-146.

Calcium

1. McCarron DA, Hatton D. Dietary calcium and lower blood pressure: we can all benefit. *JAMA.* 1996;275:1128-1129.
2. Cumming RG. Calcium intake and bone mass: a quantitative review of the evidence. *Calcif Tissue Int.* 1990;47:194-201.
3. Dawson-Hughes B, Dallal GE, Krall EA, et al. A controlled trial of the effect of calcium supplementation on bone density in postmenopausal women. *N Engl J Med.* 1990;323:878-883.
4. Prince RL. Diet and the prevention of osteoporotic fractures. *N Engl J Med.* 1997;337:701-702.
5. Nieves JW, Komar L, Cosman F, et al. Calcium potentiates the effect of estrogen and calcitonin on bone mass: review and analysis. *Am J Clin Nutr.* 1998;67:18-24.
6. Dawson-Hughes B, Harris SS, Krall EA, et al. Effect of withdrawal of calcium and vitamin D supplements on bone mass in elderly men and women. *Am J Clin Nutr.* 2000;72:745-750.
7. Lloyd T, Andon MB, Rollings N, et al. Calcium supplementation and bone mineral density in adolescent girls. *JAMA.* 1993;270:841-844.
8. Barr SI, Petit MA, Vigna YM, et al. Eating attitudes and habitual calcium intake in peripubertal girls are associated with initial bone mineral content and its change over 2 years. *J Bone Miner Res.* 2001;16:940-947.

9. Lloyd T, Chinchilli VM, Johnson-Rollings N, et al. Adult female hip bone density reflects teenage sports-exercise patterns but not teenage calcium intake. *Pediatrics.* 2000;106:40-44.

10. Koo WW, Walters JC, Esterlitz J, et al. Maternal calcium supplementation and fetal bone mineralization. *Obstet Gynecol.* 1999;94:577-582.

11. Kruger MC, Coetzer H, de Winter R, et al. Calcium, gamma-linolenic acid and eicosapentaenoic acid supplementation in senile osteoporosis. *Aging (Milano).* 1998;10:385-394.

12. Bassey EJ, Littlewood JJ, Rothwell MC, et al. Lack of effect of supplementation with essential fatty acids on bone mineral density in healthy pre- and postmenopausal women: two randomized controlled trials of Efacal® v. calcium alone. *Br J Nutr.* 2000;83:629-635.

13. Buckley LM, Leib ES, Cartularo KS, et al. Calcium and vitamin D_3 supplementation prevents bone loss in the spine secondary to low-dose corticosteroids in patients with rheumatoid arthritis: a randomized, double-blind, placebo-controlled study. *Ann Intern Med.* 1996;125:961-968.

14. Reid IR, Ibbertson HK. Calcium supplements in the prevention of steroid-induced osteoporosis. *Am J Clin Nutr.* 1986;44:287-290.

15. Homik J, Suarez-Almazor ME, Shea B, et al. Calcium and vitamin D for corticosteroid-induced osteoporosis. *Cochrane Database Syst Rev.* 2000;(no.30):1-9.

16. Thys-Jacobs S, Starkey P, Bernstein D, et al. Calcium carbonate and the premenstrual syndrome: effects on premenstrual and menstrual symptoms. Premenstrual Syndrome Study Group. *Am J Obstet Gynecol.* 1998;179:444-452.

17. Thys-Jacobs S, Ceccarelli S, Bierman A, et al. Calcium supplementation in premenstrual syndrome: a randomized crossover trial. *J Gen Intern Med.* 1989;4:183-189.

18. Penland JG, Johnson PE. Dietary calcium and manganese effects on menstrual cycle symptoms. *Am J Obstet Gynecol.* 1993;168:1417-1423.

19. Baron JA, Beach M, Mandel JS, et al. Calcium supplements for the prevention of colorectal adenomas. *N Engl J Med.* 1999;340:101-107.

20. Hyman J, Baron JA, Dain BJ, et al. Dietary and supplemental calcium and the recurrence of colorectal adenomas. *Cancer Epidemiol Biomarkers Prev.* 1998;7:291-295.

21. Kearney J, Giovannucci E, Rimm E, et al. Calcium, vitamin D, and dairy foods and the occurrence of colon cancer in men. *Am J Epidemiol.* 1996;143:907-917.

22. Atallah AN, Hofmeyr GJ, Duley L. Calcium supplementation during pregnancy for preventing hypertensive disorders and related problems. *Cochrane Database Syst Rev.* 2000;(3):1-16.

23. Levine RJ, Hauth JC, Curet LB, et al. Trial of calcium to prevent preeclampsia. *N Engl J Med.* 1997;337:69-76.

24. Cappuccio FP, Elliott P, Allender PS, et al. Epidemiologic association between dietary calcium intake and blood pressure: a meta-analysis of published data. *Am J Epidemiol.* 1995;142:935-945.

25. Van Leer EM, Seidell JC, Kromhout D. Dietary calcium, potassium, magnesium and blood pressure in the Netherlands. *Int J Epidemiol.* 1995;24:1117-1123.

26. Bostick RM, Fosdick L, Grandits GA, et al. Effect of calcium supplementation on serum cholesterol and blood pressure: a randomized, double-blind, placebo-controlled, clinical trial. *Arch Fam Med.* 2000;9:31-38.

27. Bell L, Halstenson CE, Halstenson CJ, et al. Cholesterol-lowering effects of calcium carbonate in patients with mild to moderate hypercholesterolemia. *Arch Intern Med.* 1992;152:2441-2444.

28. Thys-Jacobs S, Donovan D, Papadopoulos A, et al. Vitamin D and calcium dysregulation in the polycystic ovarian syndrome. *Steroids.* 1999;64:430-435.

29. Harvey JA, Zobitz MM, Pak CYC. Dose dependency of calcium absorption: a comparison of calcium carbonate and calcium citrate. *J Bone Miner Res.* 1988;3(3):253-258.

30. Bourgoin BP, Evans DR, Cornett JR, et al. Lead content in 70 brands of dietary calcium supplements. *Am J Public Health.* 1993;83:1155-1160.

31. Heller HJ, Stewart A, Haynes S, et al. Pharmacokinetics of calcium absorption from two commercial calcium supplements. *J Clin Pharmacol.* 1999;39:1151-1154.

32. Sheikh MS, Santa Ana CA, Nicar MJ, et al. Gastrointestinal absorption of calcium from milk and calcium salts. *N Engl J Med.*1987;317:532-536.

33. Miller J, Smith DL, Flora L, Slemenda C, et al. Calcium absorption from calcium carbonate and a new form of calcium (CCM) in healthy male and female adolescents. *Am J Clin Nutr.* 1988;48:1291-1294.

34. Heller HJ, Greer LG, Haynes SD, et al. Pharmacokinetic and pharmacodynamic comparison of two calcium supplements in postmenopausal women. *J Clin Pharmacol.* 2000;40:1237-1244.

35. Seaborn CD, Stoecker BJ. Effects of antacid or ascorbic acid on tissue accumulation and urinary excretion of 51-chromium. *Nutr Res.* 1990;10:1401-1407.

36. Freeland-Graves JH; Lin PH. Plasma uptake of manganese as affected by oral loads of manganese, calcium, milk, phosphorous, copper, and zinc. *J Am Coll Nutr.* 1991;10:38-43.

37. Davidsson L, Cederblad A, Lonnerdal B, et al. The effect of individual dietary components on manganese absorption in humans. *Am J Clin Nutr.* 1991;54:1065-1070.

38. Lewis NM, Marcus MSK, Behling AR, et al. Calcium supplements and milk: effects on acid-base balance and on retention of calcium, magnesium, and phosphorus. *Am J Clin Nutr.* 1989;49:527-533.

39. Andon MB, Ilich JZ, Tzagournis MA, et al. Magnesium balance in adolescent females consuming a low- or high-calcium diet. *Am J Clin Nutr.* 1996;63:950-953.

40. Hallberg L. Does calcium interfere with iron absorption? *Am J Clin Nutr.* 1998;68:3-4.

41. Minihane AM, Fairweather-Tait SJ. Effect of calcium supplementation on daily non-heme-iron absorption and long-term iron status. *Am J Clin Nutr.* 1998;68:96-102.

42. Cook JD, Dassenko SA, Whittaker P. Calcium supplementation: effect on iron absorption. *Am J Clin Nutr.* 1991;53:106-111.

43. Dawson-Hughes B, Seligson FH, Hughes VA. Effects of calcium carbonate and hydroxyapatite on zinc and iron retention in postmenopausal women. *Am J Clin Nutr.* 1986;44:83-88.

44. Read MH, Medeiros D, Bendel R, et al. Mineral supplementation practices of adults in seven western states. *Nutr Res.* 1986;6:375-383.

45. Sokoll LJ, Dawson-Hughes B. Calcium supplementation and plasma ferritin concentrations in premenopausal women. *Am J Clin Nutr.* 1992;56:1045-1048.

46. Argiratos V, Samman S. The effect of calcium carbonate and calcium citrate on the absorption of zinc in healthy female subjects. *Eur J Clin Nutr.* 1994;48:198-204.

47. Spencer H, Kramer L, Norris C, et al. Effect of calcium and phosphorus on zinc metabolism in man. *Am J Clin Nutr.* 1984;40:1213-1218.

48. Spencer H, Norris C, Osis D. Further studies of the effect of zinc on intestinal absorption of calcium in man. *J Am Coll Nutr.* 1992;11:561-566.

49. Institute of Medicine. *Dietary Reference Intakes for Calcium, phosphorus, magnesium, vitamin D and fluoride.* Washington DC:National Academy Press; 2001.

50. Curhan GC, Willett WC, Rimm EB. Comparison of dietary calcium with supplemental calcium and other nutrients as factors affecting the risk for kidney stones in women. *Ann Intern Med.* 1997;126:497-504.

51. Curhan GC, Willett WC, Rimm EB, et al. A prospective study of dietary calcium and other nutrients and the risk of symptomatic kidney stones. *N Engl J Med.* 1993; 328:833-838.

52. Giovannucci E, Rimm EB, Wolk A, et al. Calcium and fructose intake in relation to risk of prostate cancer. *Cancer Res.* 1998;58:442-447.

53. Chan JM, Giovannuci E, Andersson S-O, et al. Dairy products, calcium, phosphorous, vitamin D, and risk of prostate cancer (Sweden). *Cancer Causes Control.* 1998; 9:559-566.

54. Giovannucci E. Dietary influences of 1,25(OH)2 vitamin D in relation to prostate cancer: a hypothesis. *Cancer Causes Control.* 1998;9:567-582.

55. Bar-Or D, Gasiel Y. Calcium and calciferol antagonise effect of verapamil in atrial fibrillation. *Br Med J (Clin Res Ed).* 1981;282:1585-1586.

56. Kirch W, Schafer-Korting M, Axthelm T, et al. Interaction of atenolol with furosemide and calcium and aluminum salts. *Clin Pharmacol Ther.* 1981;30:429-435.

57. Neuvonen PJ, Kivisto KT, Lehto P. Interference of dairy products with the absorption of ciprofloxacin. *Clin Pharmacol Ther.* 1991;50(5 pt 1):498-502.

58. Minami R, Inotsume N, Nakano M, et al. Effect of milk on absorption of norfloxacin in healthy volunteers. *J Clin Pharmacol.* 1993;33:1238-1240.

59. Lehto P, Kivisto KT. Different effects of products containing metal ions on the absorption of lomefloxacin. *Clin Pharmacol Ther.* 1994;56:477-482.

60. Dudley MN, Marchbanks CR, Flor SC, et al. The effect of food or milk on the absorption kinetics of ofloxacin. *Eur J Clin Pharmacol.* 1991;41:569-571.

61. Flor S, Guay DR, Opsahl JA, et al. Effects of magnesium-aluminum hydroxide and calcium carbonate antacids on bioavailability of ofloxacin. *Antimicrob Agents Chemother.* 1990;34:2436-2438.

62. Riis B, Christiansen C. Actions of thiazide on vitamin D metabolism: a controlled therapeutic trial in normal women early in the postmenopause. *Metabolism.* 1985; 34:421-424.

63. Lemann J Jr, Gray RW, Maierhofer WJ, et al. Hydrochlorothiazide inhibits bone resorption in men despite experimentally elevated serum 1,25-dihydroxyvitamin D concentrations. *Kidney Int.* 1985;28:951-958.

64. Crowe M, Wollner L, Griffiths RA. Hypercalcemia following vitamin D and thiazide therapy in the elderly. *Practitioner.* 1984;228:312-313.

65. Gora ML, Seth SK, Bay WH, et al. Milk-alkali syndrome associated with use of chlorothiazide and calcium carbonate. *Clin Pharm.* 1989;8:227-229.

66. Kupfer S, Kosovsky JD. Effects of cardiac glycosides on renal tubular transport of calcium, magnesium, inorganic phosphate, and glucose in the dog. *J Clin Invest.* 1965;44:1132-1143.

67. Gaby AR. Aluminum: the ubiquitous poison contributing to Alzheimer's and osteoporsis, with advice on avoiding exposure. *Nutr Healing.* 1997;4:3-4,11.

68. Walker JA, Sherman RA, Cody RP. The effect of oral bases on enteral aluminum absorption. *Arch Intern Med.* 1990;150:2037-2039.

69. [No authors listed]. Preliminary findings suggest calcium citrate supplements may raise aluminum levels in blood, urine. *Fam Pract News.* 1992;22:74-75.

70. Weberg R, Berstad A. Gastrointestinal absorption of aluminium from single doses of aluminium containing antacids in man. *Eur J Clin Invest.* 1986;16:428-432.

71. Nolan CR, Califano JR, Butzin CA. Influence of calcium acetate or calcium citrate on intestinal aluminum absorption. *Kidney Int.* 1990;38:937-941.

72. Slanina P, Frech W, Bernhardson A, et al. Influence of dietary factors on aluminium absorption and retention in the brain and bone of rats. *Acta Pharmacol Toxicol (Copenh).* 1985;56:331-336.

73. Butner LE, Fulco PP, Feldman G. Calcium carbonate–induced hypothyroidism [letter]. *Ann Intern Med.* 2000;132:595.

74. Schneyer CR. Calcium carbonate and reduction of levothyroxine efficacy [letter]. *JAMA.* 1998;279:750.

75. Singh N, Singh PN, Hershman JM. Effect of calcium carbonate on the absorption of levothyroxine. *JAMA.* 2000;283:2822-2825.

76. Dawson-Hughes B, Harris S. Calcium intake influences the association of protein intake with rates of bone loss in elderly men and women. *Am J Clin Nutr.* 2002;75:773-779.

77. Reid IR, Mason B, Horne A, et al. Effects of calcium supplementation on serum lipid concentrations in normal older women: a randomized controlled trial. *Am J Med.* 2002;112:343-347.

78. Heaney RP, Dowell MS, Bierman J, et al. Absorbability and cost effectiveness in calcium supplementation. *J Am Coll Nutr.* 2001;20(3):239-246.

79. Heaney RP, Dowell MS, Barger-Lux MJ. Absorption of calcium as the carbonate and citrate salts, with some observations on method. *Osteoporos Int.* 1999;9:19-23.

80. Dawson-Hughes B, Dallal GE, Krall EA, et al. A controlled trial of the effect of calcium supplementation on bone density in postmenopausal women. *N Engl J Med.* 1990;323:878-883.

81. Saltman PD, Strause LG. The role of trace minerals in osteoporosis. *J Am Coll Nutr.* 1993;12:384-389.

82. Strause L, Saltman P, Smith KT, et al. Spinal bone loss in postmenopausal women supplemented with calcium and trace minerals. *J Nutr.* 1994;124:1060-1064.

Calendula

1. Patrick KFM, Kumar S, Edwardson PAD, et al. Induction of vascularisation by an aqueous extract of the flowers of *Calendula officinalis* L: the European marigold. *Phytomedicine.* 1996;3:11-18.
2. Della Loggia R, Tubaro A, Sosa S, et al. The role of triterpenoids in the topical anti-inflammatory activity of *Calendula officinalis* flowers. *Planta Med.* 1994;60:516-520.
3. Della Loggia R, Becker H, Isaac O, et al. Topical anti-inflammatory activity of *Calendula officinalis* extracts. *Planta Med.* 1990;56:658.
4. Zitterl-Eglseer K, Sosa S, Jurenitsch J, et al. Anti-edematous activities of the main triterpendiol esters of marigold (*Calendula officinalis* L.). *J Ethnopharmacol.* 1997; 57(2):139-44.
5. Schmidgall J, Schnetz E, Hensel A. Evidence for bioadhesive effects of polysaccharides and polysaccharide-containing herbs in an ex vivo bioadhesion assay on buccal membranes. *Planta Medica.* 2000;66:48-53.

Carnitine

1. Iliceto S, Scrutinio D, Bruzzi P, et al. Effects of L-carnitine administration on left ventricular remodeling after acute anterior myocardial infarction: the L-Carnitine Ecocardiografia Digitalizzata Infarto Miocardico (CEDIM) Trial. *J Am Coll Cardiol.* 1995;26:380-387.
2. Davini P, Bigalli A, Lamanna F, et al. Controlled study on L-carnitine therapeutic efficacy in post-infarction. *Drugs Exp Clin Res.* 1992;18:355-365.
3. Singh RB, Niaz MA, Agarwal P, et al. A randomized, double-blind, placebo-controlled trial of L-carnitine in suspected acute myocardial infarction. *Postgrad Med J.* 1996;72:45-50.
4. Brevetti G, Diehm C, Lambert D. European multicenter study on propionyl-L-carnitine in intermittent claudication. *J Am Coll Cardiol.* 1999;34:1618-1624.
5. Brevetti G, Perna S, Sabba C, Martone VD, et al. Propionyl-L-carnitine in intermittent claudication: double-blind, placebo-controlled, dose titration, multicenter study. *J Am Coll Cardiol.* 1995;26:1411-1416.
6. Bolognesi M, Amodio P, Merkel C, et al. Effect of 8-day therapy with propionyl-L-carnitine on muscular and subcutaneous blood flow of the lower limbs in patients with peripheral arterial disease. *Clin Physiol.* 1995;15:417-423.
7. Brevetti G, Perna S, Sabba C, et al. Superiority of L-propionylcarnitine vs. L-carnitine in improving walking capacity in patients with peripheral vascular disease: an acute, intravenous, double-blind, cross-over study. *Eur Heart J.* 1992;13:251-255.
8. Greco AV, Mingrone G, Bianchi M, et al. Effect of propionyl-L-carnitine in the treatment of diabetic angiopathy: controlled double blind trial versus placebo. *Drugs Exp Clin Res.* 1992;18:69-80.
9. Brevetti G, Chiariello M, Ferulano G, et al. Increases in walking distance in patients with peripheral vascular disease treated with L-carnitine: a double-blind, cross-over study. *Circulation.* 1988;77:767-773.
10. Deckert J. Propionyl-L-carnitine for intermittent claudication. *J Fam Pract.* 1997;44:533-534.
11. Sabba C, Berardi E, Antonica G, et al. Comparison between the effect of L-propionylcarnitine, L-acetylcarnitine and nitroglycerin in chronic peripheral arterial disease: a hemodynamic double blind echo-Doppler study. *Eur Heart J.* 1994;15: 1348-1352.
12. Pepine CJ. The therapeutic potential of carnitine in cardiovascular disorders. *Clin Ther.* 1991;13:2-21.
13. Brevetti G, Attisano T, Perna S, et al. Effect of L-carnitine on the reactive hyperemia in patients affected by peripheral vascular disease: a double-blind, crossover study. *Angiology.* 1989;40:857-862.
14. Thal LJ, Calvani M, Amato A, et al. A 1-year controlled trial of acetyl-L-carnitine in early-onset AD. *Neurology.* 2000;55:805-810.

15. Hiatt WR, Regensteiner JG, Creager MA, et al. Propionyl-L-carnitine improves exercise performance and functional status in patients with claudication. *Am J Med.* 2001;110:616-622.

16. Cacciatore L, Cerio R, Ciarimboli M, et al. The therapeutic effect of L-carnitine in patients with exercise-induced stable angina: a controlled study. *Drugs Exp Clin Res.* 1991;17:225-235.

17. Bartels GL, Remme WJ, Pillay M, et al. Effects of L-propionylcarnitine on ischemia-induced myocardial dysfunction in men with angina pectoris. *Am J Cardiol.* 1994; 74:125-130.

18. Bartels GL, Remme WJ, den Hartog FR, et al. Additional antiischemic effects of long-term L-Propionylcarnitine in anginal patients treated with conventional antianginal therapy. *Cardiovasc Drugs Ther.* 1995;9:749-753.

19. Bartels GL, Remme WJ, Holwerda KJ, et al. Anti-ischaemic efficacy of L-propionylcarnitine: a promising novel metabolic approach to ischaemia? *Eur Heart J.* 1996;17:414-420.

20. Cherchi A, Lai C, Angelino F, et al. Effects of L-carnitine on exercise tolerance in chronic stable angina: a multicenter, double-blind, randomized, placebo controlled crossover study. *Int J Clin Pharmacol Ther Toxicol.* 1985;23:569-572.

21. Lagioia R, Scrutinio D, Mangini SG, et al. Propionil-L-carnitine: a new compound in the metabolic approach to the treatment of effort angina. *Int J Cardiol.* 1992;34:167-172.

22. Bartels GL, Remme WJ, Pillay M, et al. Acute improvement of cardiac function with intravenous L-propionylcarnitine in humans. *J Cardiovasc Pharmacol.* 1992;20: 157-164.

23. Chiddo A, Gaglione A, Musci S, et al. Hemodynamic study of intravenous propionyl-L-carnitine in patients with ischemic heart disease and normal left ventricular function. *Cardiovasc Drugs Ther.* 1991;5(suppl 1):107-111.

24. Anand I, Chandrashekhan Y, De Giuli F, et al. Acute and chronic effects of propionyl-L-carnitine on the hemodynamics, exercise capacity, and hormones in patients with congestive heart failure. *Cardiovasc Drugs Ther.* 1998;12:291-299.

25. Caponnetto S, Canale C, Masperone MA, et al. Efficacy of L-propionylcarnitine treatment in patients with left ventricular dysfunction. *Eur Heart J.* 1994;15:1267-1273.

26. Mancini M, Rengo F, Lingetti M, et al. Controlled study on the therapeutic efficacy of propionyl-L-carnitine in patients with congestive heart failure. *Arzneimittelforschung.* 1992;42:1101-1104.

27. Pucciarelli G, Mastursi M, Latte S, et al. The clinical and hemodynamic effects of propionyl-L-carnitine in the treatment of congestive heart failure. *Clin Ter.* 1992; 141:379-384.

28. Bella R, Biondi R, Raffaele R, et al. Effect of acetyl-L-carnitine on geriatric patients suffering from dysthymic disorders. *Int J Clin Pharmacol Res.* 1990;10:355-360.

29. Dalakas MC, Leon-Monzon ME, Bernardini I, et al. Zidovudine-induced mitochondrial myopathy is associated with muscle carnitine deficiency and lipid storage. *Ann Neurol.* 1994;35:482-487.

30. Semino-Mora MC, Leon-Monzon ME, Dalakas MC. Effect of L-carnitine on the zidovudine-induced destruction of human myotubes, part I: L-carnitine prevents the myotoxicity of AZT in vitro. *Lab Invest.* 1994;71:102-112.

31. Moretti S, Alesse E, Di Marzio L, et al. Effect of L-carnitine on human immunodeficiency virus-1 infection-associated apoptosis: a pilot study. *Blood.* 1998;91:3817-3824.

32. De Simone C, Cifone MG, Alesse E, et al. Cell-associated ceramide in HIV-1-infected subjects. *AIDS.* 1996;10:675-676.

33. Kroemer G, Zamzami N, Susin SA. Mitochondrial control of apoptosis. *Immunol Today.* 1997;18:44-51.

34. Bonavita E. Study of the efficacy and tolerability of L-acetylcarnitine therapy in the senile brain. *Int J Clin Pharmacol Ther Toxicol.* 1986;24:511-516.

35. Calvani M, Carta A, Caruso G, et al. Action of acetyl-L-carnitine in neurodegeneration and Alzheimer's disease. *Ann NY Acad Sci.* 1992;663:483-486.

36. Campi N, Todeschini GP, Scarzella L. Selegiline versus L-acetylcarnitine in the treatment of Alzheimer-type dementia. *Clin Ther.* 1990;12:306-314.

37. Cipolli C, Chiari G. Effects of L-acetylcarnitine on mental deterioration in the aged: initial results [in Italian; English abstract]. *Clin Ter.* 1990;132(6 suppl):479-510.

38. Garzya G, Corallo D, Fiore A, et al. Evaluation of the effects of L-acetylcarnitine on senile patients suffering from depression. *Drugs Exp Clin Res.* 1990;16:101-106.

39. Passeri M, Cucinotta D, Bonati PA, et al. Acetyl-L-carnitine in the treatment of mildly demented elderly patients. *Int J Clin Pharmacol Res.* 1990;10:75-79.

40. Rai G, Wright G, Scott L, et al. Double-blind, placebo controlled study of acetyl-L-carnitine in patients with Alzheimer's dementia. *Curr Med Res Opin.* 1990;11:638-647.

41. Salvioli G, Neri M. L-acetylcarnitine treatment of mental decline in the elderly. *Drugs Exp Clin Res.* 1994;20:169-176.

42. Sano M, Bell K, Cote L, et al. Double-blind parallel design pilot study of acetyl levocarnitine in patients with Alzheimer's disease. *Arch Neurol.* 1992;49:1137-1141.

43. Spagnoli A, Lucca U, Menasce G, et al. Long-term acetyl-L-carnitine treatment in Alzheimer's disease. *Neurology.* 1991;41:1726-1732.

44. Vecchi GP, Chiari G, Cipolli C, et al. Acetyl-L-carnitine treatment of mental impairment in the elderly: evidence from a multicenter study. *Arch Gerontol Geriatr.* 1991;(suppl 2):159-168.

45. Thal LJ, Carta A, Clarke WR, et al. A 1-year multicenter placebo-controlled study of acetyl-L-carnitine in patients with Alzheimer's disease. *Neurology.* 1996;47:705-711.

46. Matsuda I, Ohtani Y. Carnitine status in Reye and Reye-like syndromes. *Pediatr Neurol.* 1986;2:90-94.

47. Camina MF, Rozas I, Gomez M, et al. Short-term effects of administration of anticonvulsant drugs on free carnitine and acylcarnitine in mouse serum and tissues. *Br J Pharmacol.* 1991;103:1179-1183.

48. De Vivo DC, Bohan TP, Coulter DL, et al. L-Carnitine supplementation in childhood epilepsy: current perspectives. *Epilepsia.* 1998;39:1216-1225.

49. Zelnik N, Fridkis I, Gruener N. Reduced carnitine and antiepileptic drugs: cause relationship or co-existence? *Acta Paediatr.* 1995;84:93-95.

50. Rodriguez-Segade S, de la Pena CA, Tutor JC, et al. Carnitine deficiency associated with anticonvulsant therapy. *Clin Chim Acta.* 1989;181:175-181.

51. Hug C, McGraw CA, Bates SR, et al. Reduction of serum carnitine concentrations during anticonvulsant therapy with phenobarbital, valproic acid, phenytoin, and carbamazepine in children. *J Pediatr.* 1991;119:799-802.

52. Freeman JM, Vining EP, Cost S, et al. Does carnitine administration improve the symptoms attributed to anticonvulsant medications?: a double-blinded, crossover study. *Pediatrics.* 1994;93(6 pt 1):893-895.

53. Decombaz J, Deriaz O, Acheson K, et al. Effect of L-carnitine on submaximal exercise metabolism after depletion of muscle glycogen. *Med Sci Sports Exerc.* 1993;25:733-740.

54. Dragan AM, Vasilic D, Eremia NMD. Studies concerning some acute biological changes after endovenous administration of 1 g 1-carnitine in elite athletes. *Physiologie.* 1987;24:231-234.

55. Dragan GI, Wagner W, Ploesteanu E. Studies concerning the ergogenic value of protein supply and 1-carnitine in elite junior cyclists. *Physiologie.* 1988;25:129-132.

56. Greig C, Finch KM, Jones DA, et al. The effect of oral supplementation with L-carnitine on maximum and submaximum exercise capacity. *Eur J Appl Physiol Occup Physiol.* 1987;56:457-460.

57. Marconi C, Sassi G, Carpinelli A, Cerretelli P. Effects of L-carnitine loading on the aerobic and anaerobic performance of endurance athletes. *Eur J Appl Physiol.* 1985;54:131-135.

58. Soop M, Bjorkman O, Cederblad G, et al. Influence of carnitine supplementation on muscle substrate and carnitine metabolism during exercise. *J Appl Physiol.* 1988;64:2394-2399.

59. Vecchiet L, Di Lisa F, Pieralisi G, et al. Influence of L-carnitine administration on maximal physical exercise. *Eur J Appl Physiol.* 1990;61:486-490.

60. Watanabe S, Ajisaka R, Masuoka T, et al. Effects of L- and DL-carnitine on patients with impaired exercise tolerance. *Jpn Heart J.* 1995;36:319-331.

61. Heinonen OJ. Carnitine and physical exercise. *Sports Med.* 1996;22:109-132.

62. Ramos AC, Barrucand L, Elias PR, et al. Carnitine supplementation in diphtheria. *Indian Pediatr.* 1992;29:1501-1505.

63. Benvenga S, Ruggeri RM, Russo A, et al. Usefulness of L-carnitine, a naturally occurring peripheral antagonist of thyroid hormone action, in iatrogenic hyperthyroidism: a randomized, double-blind, placebo-controlled clinical trial. *J Clin Endocrinol Metab.* 2001;86:3579-3594.

64. Benvenga S, Lakshmanan M, Trimarchi F. Carnitine is a naturally occurring inhibitor of thyroid hormone nuclear uptake. *Thyroid.* 2000;10;1043-1050.

65. Sorbi S, Forleo P, Fani C, et al. Double-blind, crossover, placebo-controlled clinical trial with L-acetylcarnitine in patients with degenerative cerebellar ataxia. *Clin Neuropharmacol.* 2000;23:114-118.

66. Golba KS, Wos S, Deja MA, et al. Cardioplegia supplementation with L-carnitine enhances myocardial protection in patients with low ejection fraction. *Kardiol Pol.* 2000;51:181-184.

67. Pastoris O, Dossena M, Foppa P, et al. Effect of L-carnitine on myocardial metabolism: results of a balanced, placebo-controlled, double-blind study in patients undergoing open heart surgery. *Pharmacol Res.* 1998;37:115-122.

68. Corbucci GG, Loche F. L-Carnitine in cardiogenic shock therapy: pharmacodynamic aspects and clinical data. *Int J Clin Pharmacol Res.* 1993;13:87-91.

69. Gasparetto A, Corbucci GG, De Blasi RA, et al. Influence of acetyl-L-carnitine infusion on hemodynamic parameters and survival of circulatory-shock patients. *Int J Clin Pharmacol Res.* 1991;11:83-92.

70. Turpeinen AK, Kuikka JT, Vanninen E, et al. Long-term effect of acetyl-L-carnitine on myocardial 123I-MIBG uptake in patients with diabetes. *Clin Auton Res.* 2000; 10:13-16.

71. Dal Negro R, Pomari G, Zoccatelli O, et al. L-carnitine and rehabilitative respiratory physiokinesitherapy: metabolic and ventilatory response in chronic respiratory insufficiency. *Int J Clin Pharmacol Ther Toxicol.* 1986;24:453-456.

72. Dal Negro R, Turco P, Pomari C, et al. Effects of L-carnitine on physical performance in chronic respiratory insufficiency. *Int J Clin Pharmacol Ther Toxicol.* 1988; 26:269-272.

73. Dal Negro R, Zoccatelli D, Pomari C, et al. L-carnitine and physiokinesiotherapy in chronic respiratory insufficiency: preliminary results. *Clin Trials J.* 1985;22:353-360.

74. Sirtori CR, Calabresi L, Ferrara S, et al. L-carnitine reduces plasma lipoprotein(a) levels in patients with hyper Lp(a). *Nutr Metab Cardiovasc Dis.* 2000;10:247-251.

75. Spagnoli LG Corsi M, Villaschi S, et al. Myocardial carnitine deficiency in acute myocardial infarction. *Lancet.* 1982;1:1419-1420.

76. Goa KL, Brogden RN. L-carnitine: a preliminary review of its pharmacokinetics, and its therapeutic use in ischaemic cardiac disease and primary and secondary carnitine deficiencies in relationship to its role in fatty acid metabolism. *Drugs.* 1987; 34:1-24.

77. Opie LH. Role of carnitine in fatty acid metabolism of normal and ischemic myocardium. *Am Heart J.* 1979;97:375-388.

78. Ferrari R, Cucchini F, Di Lisa F, et al. The effect of L-carnitine (carnitene) on myocardial metabolism of patients with coronary artery disease. *Clin Trials J.* 1984; 21:40-50.

79. Rebuzzi AG, Schiavoni G, Amico CM, et al. Beneficial effects of L-carnitine in the reduction of the necrotic area in acute myocardial infarction. *Drugs Exp Clin Res.* 1984;10:219-223.

80. Di Biase M, Tritto M, Pitzalis MV, et al. Electrophysiologic evaluation of intravenous L-propionylcarnitine in man. *Int J Cardiol.* 1991;30:329-333.

81. Carta A, Calvani M, Bravi D, et al. Acetyl-L-carnitine and Alzheimer's disease: pharmacological considerations beyond the cholinergic sphere. *Ann NY Acad Sci.* 1993; 695:324-326.

82. Brevetti G, Perna S, Sabba C, et al. Effect of propionyl-L-carnitine on quality of life in intermittent claudication. *Am J Cardiol.* 1997;79:777-780.

83. Jackson, JM, Lee HA. L-Carnitine and acetyl-L-carnitine status during hemodialysis with acetate in humans: a kinetic analysis. *Am J Clin Nutr.* 1996;64:922-927.

84. Weschler A, Aviram M, Levin M, et al. High dose of L-carnitine increases platelet aggregation and plasma triglyceride levels in uremic patients on hemodialysis. *Nephron.* 1984;38:120-124.

85. Iyer R, Gupta A, Khan A, et al. Does left ventricular function improve with L-carnitine after acute myocardial infarction? *J Postgrad Med.* 1999;45:38-41.

86. Bartels GL, Remme WJ, den Hartog FR, et al. Additional antiischemic effects of long-term L-Propionylcarnitine in anginal patients treated with conventional antianginal therapy. *Cardiovasc Drugs Ther.* 1995;9:749-753.

87. Bartels GL, Remme WJ, Holwerda KJ, et al. Anti-ischaemic efficacy of L-propionylcarnitine: a promising novel metabolic approach to ischaemia? *Eur Heart J.* 1996;17:414-420.

88. Loumbakis P, Anezinis P, Evangeliou A, et al. Effect of L-carnitine in patients with asthenospermia [abstract] *Eur Urol.* 1996; 30(suppl 2):255.

89. Muller-Tyl E, Lohninger A, Fischl F, et al. The effect of carnitine on sperm count and sperm motility [translated from German]. *Fertilitat.* 1988;4:1-4.

90. Micic S, Lalic N, Nale DJ, et al. Effects of L-carnitine on sperm motility and number in infertile men [abstract]. *Fertil Steril.* 1998;70(3 suppl 1):S12.

91. Vicari E. Effectiveness of a short-term anti-oxidative high-dose therapy on IVF program outcome in infertile male patients with previous excessive sperm. Radical Oxygen Species production persistent even following antimicrobials administered for epididymitis: prelim misc. 1997;93-97.

92. Vicari E, Cerri L, Cataldo T, et al. Effectiveness of single and combined antioxidant therapy in patients with astheno-necrozoospermia from non-bacterial epididymitis: effects after acetyl-carnitine or carnitine-acetyl-carnitine. Presented at: 12th National Conference, Italian Andrology Assoc;1999.

93. Campaniello E, Petrarolo N, Meriggiola MC, et al. Carnitine administration in asthenospermia. Presented at: 4th International Congress of Andrology; May 14-18, 1989. Florence;1989.

94. Costa M, Canale D, Filicori M, et al. L-carnitine in idiopathic asthenozoospermia: a multicenter study. *Andrologia.*1994;26:155-159.

95. Vitali G, Parente R, Melotti C. Carnitine supplementation in human idiopathic asthenospermia: clinical results. *Drugs Exp Clin Res.* 1995;21:157-159.

96. Moncada ML, Vicari E, Cimino C, et al. Effect of acetylcarnitine treatment in oligoasthenospermic patients. *Acta Eur Fertil.* 1992;23:221-224.

97. Villani RG, Gannon J, Self M, et al. L-carnitine supplementation combined with aerobic training does not promote weight loss in moderately obese women. *Int J Sport Nutr Exerc Metab.* 2000;10:199-207.

98. Pettegrew JW, Levine J, McClure RJ. Acetyl-L-carnitine physical-chemical metabolic and therapeutic properties: relevance for its mode of action in Alzheimer's disease and geriatric depression. *Mol Psychiatry.* 2000;5:616-632.

Cartilage

1. Dupont E, Savard PE, Jourdain C, et al. Antiangiogenic properties of a novel shark cartilage extract: potential role in the treatment of psoriasis. *J Cutan Med Surg.* 1998;2:146-152.

2. Sheu JR, Fu CC, Tsai ML, et al. Effect of U-995, a potent shark cartilage-derived angiogenesis inhibitor, on anti-angiogenesis and anti-tumor activities. *Anticancer Res.* 1998;18:4435-4441.

3. Davis PF, He Y, Furneaux RH, et al. Inhibition of angiogenesis by oral ingestion of powdered shark cartilage in a rat model. *Microvasc Res.* 1997;54:178-182.

4. Oikawa T, Ashino-Fuse H, Shimamura M, et al. A novel angiogenic inhibitor de-rived from Japanese shark cartilage (I): extraction and estimation of inhibitory activ-ities toward tumor and embryonic angiogenesis. *Cancer Lett.* 1990;51:181-186.

5. McGuire TR, Kazakoff PW, Hoie EB, et al. Antiproliferative activity of shark carti-lage with and without tumor necrosis factor-alpha in human umbilical vein endo-thelium. *Pharmacotherapy.* 1996;16:237-244.

6. Lee A, Langer R. Shark cartilage contains inhibitors of tumor angiogenesis. *Science.* 1983;221:1185-1187.

7. Riviere M, Latreille J, Falardeau P, et al. AE-941 (Neovastat), an inhibitor of angio-genesis: phase I/II cancer clinical trial results. *Cancer Invest.* 1999;17(suppl 1):16-17.

8. Jamali M-A, Riviere M, Falardeau P, et al. Effect of AE-941 (neovastat), an angio-genesis inhibitor, in the Lewis lung carcinoma metastatic model, efficacy, toxicity prevention and survival [abstract]. *Clin Invest Med.* 1998;(suppl):S16.

9. Riviere M, Falardeau P, Latreille J, et al. Phase I/II lung cancer clinical trial results with AE-941 (neovastat), an inhibitor of angiogenesis [abstract]. *Clin Invest Med.* 1998;(suppl):S14.

10. Riviere M, Alaoui-Jamali M, Falardeau P, et al. Neovastat: an inhibitor of angiogen-esis with anti-cancer activity. Presented at: American Association for Cancer Research Annual Meeting 39; March 28-April 1, 1998; New Orleans, 1998.

11. Blasecki J, Alaoui-Jamali M, Wang T, et al. Oral administration of Neovastat inhibits tumor progression in animal models of progressive tumor growth and metastasis. *Int J Oncol.* 1997;11(suppl):934.

12. Dupont E, Alaoui-Jamali M, Wang T, et al. Angiostatic and antitumoral activity of AE-941 (Neovastat), a molecular fraction derived from shark cartilage. Presented at: American Association for Cancer Research Annual Meeting 38; April 12-16, 1997; San Diego; 1997.

13. Horsman MR, Alsner J, Overgaard J. The effect of shark cartilage extracts on the growth and metastatic spread of the SCCVII carcinoma. *Acta Oncol.* 1998;37:441-445.

14. Miller DR, Anderson GT, Stark JJ, et al. Phase I/II trial of the safety and efficacy of shark cartilage in the treatment of advanced cancer. *J Clin Oncol.* 1998;16:3649-3655.

15. Wojtowicz-Praga S. Clinical potential of matrix metalloprotease inhibitors. *Drugs R D.* 1999;1:117-129.

16. Ashar B, Vargo E. Shark cartilage-induced hepatitis [letter]. *Ann Intern Med.* 1996;125:780-781.

Cat's Claw

1. Sudzinski JW, Foster BC, Vandenhoek S, et al. An in vitro evaluation of human cy-tochrome P450 3A4 inhibition by selected commercial herbal extracts and tinctures. *Phytomedicine.* 2000;7:273-282.

2. Piscoya J, Rodriguez Z, Bustamante SA, et al. Efficacy and safety of freeze-dried cat's claw in osteoarthritis of the knee: mechanisms of action of the species Uncaria guia-nensis. *Inflamm Res.* 2001;50:442-448.

3. Sheng Y, Pero RW, Amiri A, et al. Induction of apoptosis and inhibition of prolifer-ation in human tumor cells treated with extracts of Uncaria tomentosa. *Anticancer Res.* 1998; 18:3363-3368.

4. Riva L, Coradini D, Di Fronzo G, et al. The antiproliferative effects of Uncaria to-mentosa extracts and fractions on the growth of breast cancer cell line. *Anticancer Res.* 2001;21:2457-2561.

5. Sandoval M, Charbonnet RM, Okuhama NN, et al. Cat's claw inhibits TNFalpha production and scavenges free radicals: role in cytoprotection. *Free Radic Biol Med.* 2000;29:71-78.

6. Sheng Y, Bryngelsson C, Pero RW. Enhanced DNA repair, immune function and reduced toxicity of C-MED-100, a novel aqueous extract from Uncaria tomentosa. *J Ethnopharmacol.* 2000;69:115-126.

7. Wagner H, Kreutzkamp B, Jurcic K. The alkaloids of Uncaria tomentosa and their phagocytosis stimulating action. *Planta Med.* 1985:419-423.

8. Lamm S, Sheng Y, Pero RW. Persistent response to pneumococcal vaccine in individuals supplemented with a novel water-soluble extract of Uncaria tomentosa, C-Med-100. *Phytomedicine.* 2001 Jul;8:267-274.
9. Williams JE. Review of antiviral and immunomodulating properties of plants of the Peruvian rainforest with a particular emphasis on Una de Gato and Sangre de Grade. *Altern Med Rev.* 2001;6:567-579.
10. Rizzi R, Re F, Bianci A, et al. Mutagenic and antimutagenic activities of Uncaria tomentosa and its extracts. *J Ethnopharmacology.* 1993; 38:63-77.
11. Santa Maria A, Lopez A, Diaz MM, et al. Evaluation of the toxicity of Uncaria tomentosa by bioassays in vitro. *Journal of Ethnopharmacology.* 1997; 57:183-187.
12. Hilepo JN, Bellucci AG, Mossey RT. Acute renal failure caused by "cat's claw" herbal remedy in a patient with systemic lupus erythematosus. *Nephron.* 1997;77:361.

Cayenne

1. Deal CL, Schnitzer TJ, Lipstein E, et al. Treatment of arthritis with topical capsaicin: a double blind trial. *Clin Ther.* 1991;13:383-395.
2. McCarthy GM, McCarty DJ. Effect of topical capsaicin in the therapy of painful osteoarthritis of the hands. *J Rheumatol.* 1992;19:604-607.
3. McCarty DJ, Csuka M, McCarthy, et al. Treatment of pain due to fibromyalgia with topical capsaicin: a pilot study. *Semin Arthritis Rheum.* 1994;23(suppl 3):41-47.
4. McCleane G. Topical application of doxepin hydrochloride, capsaicin and a combination of both produces analgesia in chronic human neuropathic pain: a randomized, double-blind, placebo-controlled study. *Br J Clin Pharmacol.* 2000;49:574-579.
5. Yeoh KG, Kang JY, Yap I, et al. Chili protects against aspirin-induced gastroduodenal mucosal injury in humans. *Dig Dis Sci.* 1995;40:580-583.
6. Abdel Salam OM, Moszik G, Szolcsanyi J. Studies on the effect of intragastric capsaicin on gastric ulcer and on the prostacyclin-induced cytoprotection in rats. *Pharmacol Res.* 1995;32:209-215.
7. Holzer P, Pabst MA, Lippe IT. Intragastric capsaicin protects against aspirin-induced lesion formation and bleeding in the rat gastric mucosa. *Gastroenterology.* 1989;96:1425-1433.
8. Stander S, Luger T, Metze D. Treatment of prurigo nodularis with topical capsaicin. *J Am Acad Dermatol.* 2001;44:471-478.
9. Graham DY, Anderson SY, Lang T. Garlic or jalapeno peppers for treatment of *Helicobacter pylori* infection. *Am J Gastroenterol.* 1999;94:1200-1202.
10. Rodriguez-Stanley S, Collings KL, Robinson M, et al. The effects of capsaicin on reflux, gastric emptying and dyspepsia. *Aliment Pharmacol Ther.* 2000;14:129134.
11. Graham DY, Smith JL, Opekun AR. Spicy food and the stomach. Evaluation by videoendoscopy. *JAMA.* 1988;260:3473-3475.
12. Bouraoui A, Toumi A, Mustapha HB, et al. Effects of capsicum fruit on theophylline absorption and bioavailability in rabbits. *Drug Nutr Interact.* 1998;5:345-350.
13. Yeoh KG, Kang JY, Yap I, et al. Chili protects against aspirin-induced gastroduodenal mucosal injury in humans. *Dig Dis Sci.* 1995;40:580-583.

Chamomile

1. Hormann HP, Korting HC. Evidence for the efficacy and safety of topical herbal drugs in dermatology: Part 1: anti-inflammatory agents. *Phytomedicine.* 1994;1:161-171.
2. Aertgeerts P, Albring M, Klaschka F, et al. Comparative testing of Kamillosan cream and steroidal (0.25% hydrocortisone, 0.75% fluocortin butyl ester) and non-steroidal (5% bufexamac) dermatologic agents in maintenance therapy of eczematous diseases [translated from German]. *Z Hautkr.* 1985;60:270-277.
3. Maiche AG, Grohn P, Maki-Hokkonen H. Effect of chamomile cream and almond ointment on acute radiation skin reaction. *Acta Oncol.* 1991;30:395-396.
4. Fidler P, Loprinzi CL, O'Fallon JR, et al. Prospective evaluation of a chamomile mouthwash for prevention of 5-FU-induced oral mucositis. *Cancer.* 1996;77:522-525.

5. Szelenyi I, Isaac O, Thiemer K. Pharmacological experiments with compounds of chamomile. III. Experimental studies of the ulcerprotective effect of chamomile (in German). *Planta Med.* 1979;35:218-227.

6. Viola H, Wasowski C, de Stein ML, et al. Apigenin, a component of *Matricaria recutita* flowers, is a central benzodiazepine receptors-ligand with anxiolytic effects. *Planta Med.* 1995;61:213-216.

7. Schulz V, Hansel R, Tyler VE. *Rational Phytotherapy: A Physicians' Guide to Herbal Medicine.* 3rd ed. Berlin, Germany: Springer-Verlag; 1998: 254-256.

8. Budzinski JW, Foster BC, Vandenhoek S, et al. An in vitro evaluation of human cytochrome P450 3A4 inhibition by selected commercial herbal extracts and tinctures. *Phytomedicine.* 2000;7:273-282.

9. Patzelt-Wenczler R, Ponce-Poschl E. Proof of efficacy of Kamillosan® cream in atopic eczema. *Eur J Med Res.* 2000;5:171-175.

10. Saller R, Beschorner M, Hellenbrecht D, Bühring M. Dose-dependency of symptomatic relief of complaints by chamomile steam inhalation in patients with common cold. *Eur J Pharm.* 1990;183:728.

Chasteberry

1. Halaska M, Beles P, Gorkow C, et al. Treatment of cyclical mastalgia with a solution containing a *Vitex agnus* castus extract: results of a placebo-controlled double-blind study. *Breast* 1999;8:175-181.

2. Kubista E, Muller G, Spona J. Treatment of mastopathy associated with cyclic mastodynia: clinical results and hormone profiles [translated from German]. *Gynakol Rundsch.* 1986;26:65-79.

3. Wuttke W, Splitt G, Gorkow C, et al. Treatment of cyclical mastalgia: results of a randomized, placebo-controlled, double-blind study [translated from German]. *Geburtsh Frauenheilk.* 1997;57:569-574.

4. Wuttke W, et al. Dopaminergic compounds in *Vitex agnus* castus. In: Lowe D, Rietbrock N, eds. *Phytopharmaka in Forschung und klinischer Anwendung.* Darmstadt, Germany: Steinkopff Verlag; 1995;81-91.

5. Schellenberg R. Treatment for the premenstrual syndrome with *Agnus castus* fruit extract: prospective, randomized, placebo controlled study. *BMJ.* 2001;322:134-137.

6. Dittmar FW, Bohnert KJ, Peeters M, et al. Premenstrual syndrome: treatment with a phytopharmaceutical [translated from German]. *Ther Gynakol.* 1992;5:60-68.

7. Peters-Welte C, Albrecht M. Menstrual abnormalities and PMS: *Vitex agnus* castus [translated from German]. *Therapie Woche Gynakol.* 1994;7:49-52.

8. Propping D, Katzorke T, Belkien L. Diagnosis and therapy of corpus luteum deficiency in general practice [translated from German]. *Therapiewoche.* 1988;38:2992-3001.

9. Schulz V, Hansel R, Tyler VE. *Rational Phytotherapy: A Physicians' Guide to Herbal Medicine.* 3rd ed. Berlin, Germany: Springer-Verlag; 1998:243, 246.

10. Kleijnen J, Ter Riet G, Knipschild P. Vitamin B_6 in the treatment of the premenstrual syndrome: a review. *Br J Obstet Gynaecol.* 1990;97:847-852.

11. Milewicz A, Gejdel E, Sworen H, et al. *Vitex agnus* castus extract in the treatment of luteal phase defects due to latent hyperprolactinemia: results of a randomized placebo-controlled double-blind study [translated from German]. *Arzneimittelforschung.* 1993;43:752-756.

12. Loch E-G, Kaiser E. Diagnosis and treatment of amenorrhea in practice [in German; English abstract]. *Gynakol Praxis.* 1990;14:489-495.

13. Gerhard I, Patek A, Monga B, et al. Mastodynon® for female infertility [in German; English abstract]. *Forsch Komplementarmed.* 1998;5:272-278.

14. Bergmann J, Luft B, Boehmann S, et al. The effectiveness of the complex agent, Phyto-Hypophyson® L, in female sterility of hormonal origin [translated from German]. *Forsch Komplementarmed Klass Naturheilkd.* 2000;7:190-199.

15. Amann W. Elimination of obstipation with Agnolyt® [in German]. *Ther Gegw.* 1965;104:1263-1265.

16. Weiss RF, Meuss AR. *Herbal Medicine.* Beaconsfield, United Kingdom: Beaconsfield Publishers; 1988:317-318.

17. Jarry H, Leonhardt S, Wuttke W, et al. *Agnus castus* as a dopaminergic active principle in Mastodynon® N [in German; English abstract]. *Z Phytother.* 1991;12:77-82.
18. Jarry H, Leonhardt S, Gorkow C, et al. In vitro prolactin but not LH and FSH release is inhibited by compounds in extracts of *Agnus castus:* direct evidence for a dopaminergic principle by the dopamine receptor assay. *Exp Clin Endocrinol.* 1994;102:448-454.
19. Sliutz G, Speiser P, Schultz AM, et al. *Agnus castus* extracts inhibit prolactin secretion of rat pituitary cells. *Horm Metab Res.* 1993;25:253-255.
20. Winterhoff H. Medicinal plants witwh endocrine efficacy. Effects on thyroid and ovary function [translated from German]. *Z Phytother.* 1993;14:83-94.
21. Meier B, Berger D, Hoberg E, et al. Pharmacological activities of *Vitex agnus*-castus extracts in vitro. *Phytomedicine.* 2000;7:373-381.
22. Merz PG, Gorkow C, Schrodter A, et al. The effects of a special *Agnus castus* extract (BP1095E1) on prolactin secretion in healthy male subjects. *Exp Clin Endocrinol Diabetes.* 1996;104:447-453.
23. Propping D, Bohnert KJ, Peeters M, et al. *Agnus-castus:* treatment of gynaecological syndromes [translated from German]. *Therapeutikon.* 1991;5:581-585.
24. Cahill DJ, Fox R, Wardle PG, et al. Multiple follicular development associated with herbal medicine. *Hum Reprod.* 1994;9:1469-1470.
25. Bruckner C. Use and value of common European lactation-promoting medicinal plants [translated from German]. *Padiatr Grenzgeb.* 1991;28:403-410.

Chondroitin Sulfate

1. Adebowale AO, Cox DS, Liang Z, et al. Analysis of glucosamine and chondroitin sulfate content in marketed products and the Caco-2 permeability of chondroitin sulfate raw materials. *J Am Nutraceutical Assoc.* 2000;3:37-44.
2. Lippiello L, Woodward J, Karpman R, et al. In vivo chondroprotection and metabolic synergy of glucosamine and chondroitin sulfate. *Clin Orthop.* 2000;381: 229-240.
3. Lippiello L, Karpman RR, Hammad T. Synergistic effect of glucosamine HCL and chondroitin sulfate on in vitro proteoglycan synthesis by bovine chondrocytes. Presented at: American Academy of Orthopaedic Surgeons 67th Annual Meeting; March 15-19, 2000; Orlando, Fla.
4. Bucsi L, Poor G. Efficacy and tolerability of oral chondroitin sulfate as a symptomatic slow-acting drug for osteoarthritis (SYSADOA) in the treatment of knee osteoarthritis. *Osteoarthritis Cartilage.* 1998;6 suppl A:31-36.
5. Bourgeois P, Chales G, Dehais J, et al. Efficacy and tolerability of chondroitin sulfate 1200 mg/day vs chondroitin sulfate 3 × 400 mg/day vs placebo. *Osteoarthritis Cartilage.* 1998;6 suppl A:25-30.
6. Uebelhart D, Thonar EJ, Delmas PD, et al. Effects of oral chondroitin sulfate on the progression of knee osteoarthritis: a pilot study. *Osteoarthritis Cartilage.* 1998;6 suppl A:39-46.
7. Conrozier T. Anti-arthrosis treatments: efficacy and tolerance of chondroitin sulfates (CS 4&6) [translated from French]. *Presse Med.* 1998;27:1862-1865.
8. Mazieres B, Loyau G, Menkes CJ, et al. Chondroitin sulfate in the treatment of gonarthrosis and coxarthrosis. 5-months result of a multicenter double-blind controlled prospective study using placebo [in French; English abstract]. *Rev Rhum Mal Osteoartic.* 1992;59:466-472.
9. Mazieres B, Combe B, Phan Van A, et al. Chondroitin sulfate in osteoarthritis of the knee: a prospective, double blind, placebo controlled multicenter clinical study. *J Rheumatol.* 2001;28:173-181.
10. Morreale P, Manopulo R, Galati M, et al. Comparison of the antiinflammatory efficacy of chondroitin sulfate and diclofenac sodium in patients with knee osteoarthritis. *J Rheumatol.* 1996;23:1385-1391.
11. Verbruggen G, Goemaere S, Veys EM. Chondroitin sulfate: S/DMOAD (structure/disease modifying anti-osteoarthritis drug) in the treatment of finger joint OA. *Osteoarthritis Cartilage.* 1998;6 suppl A:37-38.

12. Uebelhart D, Thonar EJ, Zhang J, et al. Protective effect of exogenous chondroitin 4,6-sulfate in the acute degradation of articular cartilage in the rabbit. *Osteoarthritis Cartilage.* 1998;6 suppl A:6-13.

13. Leffler CT, Philippi AF, Leffler SG, et al. Glucosamine, chondroitin, and manganese ascorbate for degenerative joint disease of the knee or low back: a randomized, double-blind, placebo-controlled pilot study. *Mil Med.* 1999;164:85-91.

14. Moore MG. Promising responses to a new oral treatment for degenerative joint disorders. *Canine Practice.* 1996;21:7-11.

15. McNamara PS, Johnston SA, Todhunter RJ. Slow-acting, disease modifying osteoarthritis agents. *Vet Clin North Am Small Anim Pract.* 1997;27:863-881.

16. Hanson RR, Brawner WR, Hammad TA. The clinical profile of a glucosamine-chondroitin sulfate compound in a double-blinded, placebo-controlled, randomized trial as a selective symptom modifying nutraceutical for navicular syndrome: current data and perspectives [abstract]. *Vet Comp Orthop Traumatol.* 1998;11:A63.

17. Canapp SO Jr, McLaughlin RM Jr, Hoskinson JJ, et al. Scintigraphic evaluation of dogs with acute synovitis after treatment with glucosamine hydrochloride and chondroitin sulfate. *Am J Vet Res.* 1999;60:1552-1557.

18. Das A Jr, Hammad TA. Efficacy of a combination of FCHG49 glucosamine hydrochloride, TRH122 low molecular weight sodium chondroitin sulfate and manganese ascorbate in the management of knee osteoarthritis. *Osteoarthritis Cartilage.* 2000;8:343-350.

19. Nakazawa K. Effect of chondroitin sulfates on *Atherosclerosis.* I. Long term oral administration of chondroitin sulfates to atherosclerotic subjects [in Japanese]. *Nippon Naika Gakkai Zasshi.* 1970;59:1084-1092.

20. Nakazawa K, Murata K. Comparative study of the effects of chondroitin sulfate isomers on atherosclerotic subjects. *ZFA.* 1979;34:153-159.

21. Baggio B, Gambaro G, Marchini F, et al. Correction of erythrocyte abnormalities in idiopathic calcium-oxalate nephrolithiasis and reduction of urinary oxalate by oral glycosaminoglycans. *Lancet.* 1991;338:403-405.

22. Hungerford DS. Treating osteoarthritis with chondroprotective agents. *Orthop Spec Ed.* 1998;4:39-42.

23. Paroli E, Antonilli L, Biffoni M. A pharmacological approach to glycosaminoglycans. *Drugs Exp Clin Res.* 1991;17;9-20.

24. Ronca F, Palmieri L, Panicucci P, et al. Anti-inflammatory activity of chondroitin sulfate. *Osteoarthritis Cartilage.* 1998;6 suppl A:14-21.

Chromium

1. Anderson RA. Chromium, glucose tolerance, and diabetes. *Biol Trace Elem Res.* 1992;32:19-24.

2. Anderson RA. Recent advances in the clinical and biochemical effects of chromium deficiency. *Prog Clin Biol Res.* 1993;380:221-234.

3. Anderson RA. Chromium and parenteral nutrition. *Nutrition.* 1995;11:83-86.

4. Anderson RA, Kozlovsky AS. Chromium intake, absorption, and excretion of subjects consuming self-selected diets. *Am J Clin Nutr.* 1985;41:1177-1183.

5. Davies S, McLaren Howard J, Hunnisett A, et al. Age-related decreases in chromium levels in 51,665 hair, sweat, and serum samples from 40,872 patients: implications for the prevention of cardiovascular disease and type II diabetes mellitus. *Metabolism.* 1997;46:469-473.

6. Schroeder HA. The role of chromium in mammalian nutrition. *Am J Clin Nutr.* 1968;21:230-244.

7. Mertz W. Chromium in human nutrition: a review. *J Nutr.* 1993;123:626-633.

8. Anderson RA, Cheng N, Bryden NA, et al. Elevated intakes of supplemental chromium improve glucose and insulin variables in individuals with type 2 diabetes. *Diabetes.* 1997;46:1786-1791.

9. Bahijiri SM, Mira SA, Mufti AM, et al. The effects of inorganic chromium and brewer's yeast supplementation on glucose tolerance, serum lipids and drug dosage in individuals with type 2 diabetes. *Saudi Med J.* 2000;21:831-837.

10. Ravina A, Slezack L. Chromium in the treatment of clinical diabetes mellitus [translated from Hebrew]. *Harefuah*. 1993;125:142-145.

11. Rabinowitz MB, Gonick HC, Levin SR, et al. Effects of chromium and yeast supplements on carbohydrate and lipid metabolism in diabetic men. *Diabetes Care*. 1983;6:319-327.

12. Trow LG, Lewis J, Greenwood RH, et al. Lack of effect of dietary chromium supplementation on glucose tolerance, plasma insulin and lipoprotein levels in patients with type 2 diabetes. *Int J Vitam Nutr Res*. 2000;70:14-18.

13. Jovanovic L, Gutierrez M, Peterson CM. Chromium supplementation for women with gestational diabetes mellitus. *J Trace Elem Exp Med*. 1999;12:91-97.

14. Kaats GR, Blum K, Fisher JA, et al. Effects of chromium picolinate supplementation on body composition: a randomized, double-masked, placebo-controlled study. *Curr Ther Res*. 1996;57:747-765.

15. Kaats GR, Blum K, Pullin D, et al. A randomized, double-masked, placebo-controlled study of the effects of chromium picolinate supplementation on body composition: a replication and extension of a previous study. *Curr Ther Res*. 1998;59:379-388.

16. Trent LK, Thieding-Cancel D. Effects of chromium picolinate on body composition. *J Sports Med Phys Fitness*. 1995;35:273-280.

17. Clancy SP, Clarkson PM, DeCheke ME, et al. Effects of chromium picolinate supplementation on body composition, strength, and urinary chromium loss in football players. *Int J Sport Nutr*. 1994;4:142-153.

18. Lukaski HC, Bolonchuk WW, Siders WA, et al. Chromium supplementation and resistance training: effects on body composition, strength, and trace element status of men. *Am J Clin Nutr*. 1996;63:954-964.

19. Hallmark MA, Reynolds TH, DeSouza CA, et al. Effects of chromium and resistive training on muscle strength and body composition. *Med Sci Sports Exerc*. 1996;28:139-144.

20. Volpe SL, Huang HW, Larpadisorn K, et al. Effect of chromium supplementation and exercise on body composition, resting metabolic rate, and selected biochemical parameters in moderately obese women following an exercise program. *J Am Coll Nutr*. 2001;20:293-306.

21. Anderson RA, Polansky MM, Bryden NA, et al. Chromium supplementation of human subjects: effects on glucose, insulin, and lipid variables. *Metabolism*. 1983;32:894-899.

22. Wilson BE, Gondy A. Effects of chromium supplementation on fasting insulin levels and lipid parameters in healthy, non-obese young subjects. *Diabetes Res Clin Pract*. 1995;28:179-184.

23. Anderson RA, Polansky MM, Bryden NA, et al. Supplemental-chromium effects on glucose, insulin, glucagon, and urinary chromium losses in subjects consuming controlled low-chromium diets. *Am J Clin Nutr*. 1991;54:909-916.

24. Uusitupa MI, Mykkanen L, Siitonen O, et al. Chromium supplementation in impaired glucose tolerance of elderly: effects on blood glucose, plasma insulin, C-peptide and lipid levels. *Br J Nutr*. 1992;68:209-216.

25. Cefalu WT, Bell-Farrow AD, Stegner J, et al. Effect of chromium picolinate on insulin sensitivity in vivo. *J Trace Elem Exp Med*. 1999;12:71-83.

26. Abraham AS, Brooks BA, Eylath U. The effects of chromium supplementation on serum glucose and lipids in patients with and without non-insulin-dependent diabetes. *Metabolism*. 1992;41:768-771.

27. Press RI, Geller J, Evans GW. The effect of chromium picolinate on serum cholesterol and apolipoprotein fractions in human subjects. *West J Med*. 1990;152:41-45.

28. Lee NA, Reasner CA. Beneficial effect of chromium supplementation on serum triglyceride levels in NIDDM. *Diabetes Care*. 1994;17:1449-1452.

29. Roeback JR Jr, Hla KM, Chambless LE, et al. Effects of chromium supplementation on serum high-density lipoprotein cholesterol levels in men taking beta-blockers: a randomized, controlled trial. *Ann Intern Med*. 1991;115:917-924.

30. Offenbacher EG, Rinko CJ, Pi-Sunyer FX. The effects of inorganic chromium and brewer's yeast on glucose tolerance, plasma lipids, and plasma chromium in elderly subjects. *Am J Clin Nutr*. 1985;42:454-461.

31. Preuss HG, Wallerstedt D, Talpur N, et al. Effects of niacin-bound chromium and grape seed proanthocyanidin extract on the lipid profile of hypercholesterolemic subjects: a pilot study. *J Med.* 2000;31:227-246.
32. Laws A, King AC, Haskell WL, et al. Relation of fasting plasma insulin concentration to high density lipoprotein cholesterol and triglyceride concentrations in men. *Arterioscler Thromb.* 1991;11:1636-1642.
33. Job FP, Wolfertz J, Meyer R, et al. Hyperinsulinism in patients with coronary artery disease. *Coron Artery Dis.* 1994;5:487-490.
34. Fontbonne A, Tchobroutsky G, Eschwege E, et al. Coronary heart disease mortality risk: plasma insulin level is a more sensitive marker than hypertension or abnormal glucose tolerance in overweight males. The Paris Prospective Study. *Int J Obes.* 1988;12:557-565.
35. Despres JP, Lamarche B, Mauriege P, et al. Hyperinsulinemia as an independent risk factor for ischemic heart disease. *N Engl J Med.* 1996;334:952-957.
36. Pyorala K, Savolainen E, Kaukola S, et al. Plasma insulin as coronary heart disease risk factor: relationship to other risk factors and predictive value during 9½-year follow-up of the Helsinki Policemen Study population. *Acta Med Scand Suppl.* 1985;701:38-52.
37. Lamarche B, Tchernof A, Mauriege P, et al. Fasting insulin and apolipoprotein B levels and low-density lipoprotein particle size as risk factors for ischemic heart disease. *JAMA.* 1998;279:1955-1961.
38. Saydah SH, Eberhardt MS, Loria CM, et al. Subclinical states of glucose intolerance and the risk of death in the United States [abstract]. *Diabetes.* 1999;48(suppl 1):A#068.
39. Haffner SM. The importance of hyperglycemia in the nonfasting state to the development of cardiovascular disease. *Endocr Rev.* 1998;19:583-592.
40. Guallar E, Jimenez J, van t' Veer P, et al. The association of chromium with the risk of a first myocardial infaction in men. The EURAMIC Study [abstract]. *Circulation.* 2001;103:1366.
41. Davis JM, Welsh RS, Alerson NA. Effects of carbohydrate and chromium ingestion during intermittent high-intensity exercise to fatigue. *Int J Sport Nutr Exerc Metab.* 2000;10:476-485.
42. Attenburrow MJ, Odontiadis J, Murray BJ, et al. Chromium treatment decreases the sensitivity of 5-HT(2A) receptors. *Psychopharmacology.* 2002;159:432-436.
43. Stearns DM, Silveira SM, Wolf KK, Luke AM. Chromium (III) tris (picolinate) is mutagenic at the hypoxanthine (guanine) phosphoribosyltransferase locus in Chinese hamster ovary cells. *Mutat Res.* 2002;513:135-142.
44. Anderson RA, Bryden NA, Polansky MM. Lack of toxicity of chromium chloride and chromium picolinate in rats. *J Am Coll Nutr.* 1997;16:273-279.
45. Hepburn DD, Vincent JB. In vivo distribution of chromium from chromium picolinate in rats and implications for the safety of the dietary supplement. *Chem Res Toxicol.* 2002;15:93-100.
46. Seaborn CD, Stoecker BJ. Effects of antacid or ascorbic acid on tissue accumulation and urinary excretion of 51-chromium. *Nutr Res.* 1990;10:1401-1407.
47. Anderson RA, Bryden NA, Polansky MM. Lack of toxicity of chromium chloride and chromium picolinate in rats. *J Am Coll Nutr.* 1997;16:273-279.
48. Cerulli J, Grabe DW, Gauthier I, et al. Chromium picolinate toxicity. *Ann Pharmacother.* 1998;32:428-431.
49. Wasser WG, Feldman NS, D'Agati VD. Chronic renal failure after ingestion of over-the-counter chromium picolinate [letter]. *Ann Intern Med.* 1997;126:410.
50. Young PC, Turiansky GW, Bonner MW, et al. Acute generalized exanthematous pustulosis induced by chromium picolinate. *J Am Acad Dermatol.* 1999;41:820-823.
51. Reading SAJ, Wecker L. Chromium picolinate. *J Fla Med Assoc.* 1996;83:29-31.
52. Speetjens JK, Collins RA, Vincent JB, et al. The nutritional supplement chromium (III) tris(picolinate) cleaves DNA. *Chem Res Toxicol.* 1999;12:483-487.
53. Institute of Medicine. *Dietary Reference Intakes for Vitamin A, Vitamin K, Arsenic, Boron, Chromium, Copper, Iodine, Iron, Manganese, Molybdenum, Nickel, Silicon, Vanadium, and Zinc.* Washington DC. National Academy Press; 2001.

54. Committee on Diet and Health. *Diet and Health: Implications for Reducing Chronic Disease Risk*. Washington DC: National Research Council; 1989

55. Bahijri SM Effect of chromium supplementation on glucose tolerance and lipid profile. *Saudi Med J*. 2000;21:45-50.

56. Livolsi JM, Adams GM, Laguna PL. The effect of chromium picolinate on muscular strength and body composition in women athletes. *J Strength Cond Res*. 2001;15: 161-166.

57. Clarkson PM. Effects of exercise on chromium levels. Is supplementation required? *Sports Med*. 1997;23:341-349.

58. Joseph LJO, Farrell PA, Davey SL, et al. Effect of resistance training with or without chromium picolinate supplementation on glucose metabolism in older men and women. *Metabolism*. 1999;48:546-553.

59. Lefavi RG, Anderson RA, Keith RE, et al. Efficacy of chromium supplementation in athletes: emphasis on anabolism. *Int J Sport Nutr*. 1992;2:111-122.

60. Clancy SP, Clarkson PM, DeCheke ME, et al. Effects of chromium picolinate supplementation on body composition, strength, and urinary chromium loss in football players. *Int J Sport Nutr*. 1994;4:142-153.

61. Hallmark MA, Reynolds TH, DeSouza CA, et al. Effects of chromium and resistive training on muscle strength and body composition. *Med Sci Sports Exerc*. 1996;28: 139-144.

62. Campbell WW, Joseph LJ, Davey SL, et al. Effects of resistance training and chromium picolinate on body composition and skeletal muscle in older men. *J Appl Physiol*. 1999;86:29-39.

63. Walker LS, Bemben MG, Bemben DA, et al. Chromium picolinate effects on body composition and muscular performance in wrestlers. *Med Sci Sports Exerc*. 1998;30: 1730-1737.

64. Lukaski HC, Bolonchuk WW, Siders WA, et al. Chromium supplementation and resistance training: effects on body composition, strength and trace element status of men. *Am J Clin Nutr*. 1996;63:954-965.

65. Vincent JB. Elucidating a biological role for chromium at a molecular level. *Acc Chem Res*. 2000;33:503-510.

66. Vincent JB. Quest for the molecular mechanism of chromium action and its relationship to diabetes. *Nutr Rev*. 2000;58:67-72.

67. Vincent, JB. The bioinorganic chemistry of chromium (III). *Polyhedron*. 2001;20:1-26.

Coenzyme Q_{10}

1. Morisco C, Trimarco B, Condorelli M. Effect of coenzyme Q_{10} therapy in patients with congestive heart failure: a long-term multicenter randomized study. *Clin Investig*. 1993;71(8 suppl):S134-S136.

2. Hashiba K, Kuramoto K, Ishimi Z, et al. Coenzyme-Q_{10} for treatment of aneurysm [in Japanese]. *Heart (Japanese)*. 1972;4:1579-1589.

3. Hofman-Bang C, Rehnquist N, Swedberg K, et al. Coenzyme Q_{10} as an adjunctive in treatment of congestive heart failure [abstract]. *J Am Coll Cardiol*. 1992;19:216A.

4. Munkholm H, Hansen HH, Rasmussen K. Coenzyme Q_{10} treatment in serious heart failure. *Biofactors*. 1999;9:285-289.

5. Khatta M, Alexander BS, Krichten CM, et al. Long-term efficacy of coenzyme Q_{10} therapy for congestive heart failure. Presented at: 72nd Scientific Sessions of the American Heart Association; November 7-10, 1999; Atlanta; 1999.

6. Singh RB, Niaz MA, Rastogi SS, et al. Effect of hydrosoluble coenzyme Q_{10} on blood pressures and insulin resistance in hypertensive patients with coronary artery disease. *J Hum Hypertens*. 1999;13:203-208.

7. Digiesi V, Cantini F, Brodbeck B. Effect of coenzyme Q_{10} on essential arterial hypertension. *Curr Ther Res*. 1990;47:841-845.

8. Birnbaum Y, Hale SL, Kloner RA. The effect of coenzyme Q_{10} on infarct size in a rabbit model of ischemia/reperfusion. *Cardiovasc Res*. 1996;32:861-868.

9. Hano O, Thompson-Gorman S, Zweifer J, et al. Coenzyme Q_{10} enhances cardiac functional and metabolic recovery and reduces Ca2+ overload during postischemic reperfusion. *Am J Physiol*. 1994;266:H2174-H2181.

10. Matsushima T, Sueda T, Matsuura Y, et al. Protection by coenzyme Q_{10} of canine myocardial reperfusion injury after preservation. *J Thorac Cardiovasc Surg.* 1992;103: 945-951.
11. Rosenfeldt FL, Pepe S, Ou R, et al. Coenzyme Q_{10} improves the tolerance of the senescent myocardium to aerobic and ischemic stress: studies in rats and in human atrial tissue. *Biofactors.* 1999;9:291-299.
12. Taggart DP, Jenkins M, Hooper J, et al. Effects of short-term supplementation with coenzyme Q_{10} on myocardial protection during cardiac operations. *Ann Thorac Surg.* 1996;61:829-833.
13. Chello M, Mastroroberto P, Romano R, et al. Protection by coenzyme Q_{10} from myocardial reperfusion injury during coronary artery bypass grafting. *Ann Thorac Surg.* 1994;58:1427-1432.
14. Judy WV, Stogsdill WW, Folkers K. Myocardial preservation by therapy with coenzyme Q_{10} during heart surgery. *Clin Investig.* 1993;71(8 Suppl):S155-S161.
15. Chen YF, Lin YT, We SC, et al. Effectiveness of coenzyme Q_{10} on myocardial preservation during hypothermic cardioplegic arrest. *J Thorac Cardiovasc Surg.* 1994;107:242-247.
16. Mortensen SA, Leth A, Agner E, et al. Dose-related decrease of serum coenzyme Q_{10} during treatment with HMG-CoA reductase inhibitors. *Mol Aspects Med.* 1997;18 (suppl):S137-S144.
17. Ghirlanda G, Oradei A, Manto A, et al. Evidence of plasma CoQ_{10}-lowering effect by HMG-CoA reductase inhibitors: a double-blind, placebo-controlled study. *J Clin Pharmacol.* 1993;33:226-229.
18. Folkers K, Langsjoen P, Willis R, et al. Lovastatin decreases coenzyme Q levels in humans. *Proc Natl Acad Sci USA.* 1990;87:8931-8934.
19. Bargossi AM, Battino M, Gaddi A, et al. Exogenous CoQ_{10} preserves plasma ubiquinone levels in patients treated with 3-hydroxy-3-methylglutaryl coenzyme A reductase inhibitors. *Int J Clin Lab Res.* 1994;24:171-176.
20. Kishi T, Kishi H, Watanabe T, Folkers K. Bioenergetics in clinical medicine. XI. Studies on coenzyme Q and diabetes mellitus. *J Med.* 1976;7:307-321.
21. Kishi T, Watanabe T, Folkers K. Bioenergetics in clinical medicine XV. Inhibition of coenzyme Q_{10}-enzymes by clinically used adrenergic blockers of beta-receptors. *Res Commun Chem Pathol Pharmacol.* 1977;17:157-164.
22. Kishi T, Makino K, Okamoto T, et al. Inhibition of myocardial respiration by psychotherapeutic drugs and prevention by coenzyme Q. *Biomed Clin Aspects Coenzyme Q.* 1980;2:139-157.
23. Kishi H, Kishi T, Folkers K. Bioenergetics in clinical medicine. III. Inhibition of coenzyme Q_{10}-enzymes by clinically used anti-hypertensive drugs. *Res Commun Chem Pathol Pharmacol.* 1975;12:533-540.
24. Folkers K. Basic chemical research on coenzyme Q_{10} and integrated clinical research on therapy of diseases. *Biomed Clin Aspects Coenzyme Q.* 1985;5:457-478.
25. Langsjoen PH, Langsjoen PH, Folkers K. A six-year clinical study of therapy of cardiomyopathy with coenzyme Q_{10}. *Int J Tissue React.* 1990;12:169-171.
26. Judy WV. Myocardial effects of coenzyme Q_{10} in primary heart failure. *Biomed Clin Aspects Coenzyme Q.* 1984;4:281-290.
27. Manzoli U, Rossi E, Littarru GP, et al. Coenzyme Q_{10} in dilated cardiomyopathy. *Int J Tissue React.* 1990;12:173-178.
28. Langsjoen PH, Vadhhanavikit S, Folkers K. Response of patients in classes III and IV of cardiomyopathy to therapy in a blind and crossover trial with coenzyme Q_{10}. *Proc Natl Acad Sci.* 1985;82:4240-4244.
29. Permanetter B, Rossy W, Klein G, et al. Ubiquinone (coenzyme Q_{10}) in the long-term treatment of idiopathic dilated cardiomyopathy. *Eur Heart J.* 1992;13:1528-1533.
30. Combs AB, Choe JY, Truong DH, et al. Reduction by coenzyme Q_{10} of the acute toxicity of adriamycin in mice. *Res Commun Chem Pathol Pharmacol.* 1977;18:565-568.
31. Judy WV, Hall JH, Dugan W, et al. Coenzyme Q_{10} reduction of Adriamycin cardiotoxicity. *Biomed Clin Aspects Coenzyme Q.* 1984;4:231-241.

32. Sugiyama S, Yamada K, Hayakawa M, et al. Approaches that mitigate doxorubicin-induced delayed adverse effects on mitochondrial functions in rat hearts: liposome-encapsulated doxorubican or combination therapy with antioxidant. *Biochem Mol Biol Int.* 1995;36:1001-1007.

33. Braun B, Clarkson M, Freedson PS, et al. Effects of coenzyme Q_{10} supplementation on exercise performance, VO2 max and lipid peroxidation in trained cyclists. *Int J Sport Nutr.* 1991;1:353-365.

34. Snider IP, Bazarre TL, Murdoch SD, et al. Effects of coenzyme athletic performance system as an ergogenic aid on endurance performances to exhaustion. *Int J Sport Nutr.* 1992;2:272-286.

35. Porter DA, Costill DL, Zachwieja JJ, et al. The effect of oral coenzyme Q_{10} on the exercise tolerance of middle-aged, untrained men. *Int J Sports Med.* 1995;16:421-427.

36. Malm C, Svensson M, Ekblom B, et al. Effects of ubiquinone-10 supplementation and high intensity training on physical performance in humans. *Acta Physiol Scand.* 1997;161:379-984.

37. Weston SB, Zhou S, Weatherby RP, et al. Does exogenous coenzyme Q_{10} affect aerobic capacity in endurance athletes? *Int J Sport Nutr.* 1997;7:197-206.

38. Zuliani U, Bonetti A, Campana M, et al. The influence of ubiquinone (Co Q_{10}) on the metabolic response to work. *J Sports Med Phys Fitness.* 1989;29:57-62.

39. Ylikoski T, Piirainen J, Hanninen O, et al.. The effect of coenzyme Q_{10} on the exericise performance of cross-country skiers. *Mol Aspects Med.* 1997;18 (suppl):S283-S290.

40. Barbieri B, Lund B, Lundstrom B, et al. Coenzyme Q_{10} administration increases antibody titer in hepatitis B vaccinated volunteers: a single blind placebo-controlled and randomized clinical study. *Biofactors.* 1999;9:351-357.

41. Folkers K, Watanabe T. Bioenergetics in clinical medicine-X: survey of the adjunctive use of coenzyme Q with oral therapy in treating periodontal disease. *J Med.* 1977;8:333-348.

42. Iwamoto Y, Watanabe T, Okamoto H, et al. Clinical effect of coenzyme Q_{10} on periodontal disease. *Biomed Clin Aspects Coenzyme Q.* 1981;3:109-119.

43. Watts TL. Coenzyme Q_{10} and periodontal treatment: is there any beneficial effect? *Br Dent J.* 1995;178:209-213.

44. Folkers K, Simonsen R. Two successful double-blind trials with coenzyme Q_{10} (vitamin Q_{10}) on muscular dystrophies and neurogenic atrophies. *Biochim Biophys Acta.* 1995;1271:281-286.

45. Huntington Study Group. A randomized, placebo-controlled trial of coenzyme Q_{10} and remacemide in Huntington's disease. *Neurology.* 2001;57:397-404.

46. Kitamura N, Yamaguchi A, Otaki M, et al. Myocarial tissue level of coenzyme Q_{10} in patients with cardiac failure. *Biomed Clin Aspects Coenzyme Q.* 1984;4:243-252.

47. Mortensen SA, Vadhanavikit S, Muratsu K, et al. Coenzyme Q_{10}: clinical benefits with biochemical correlates suggesting a scientific breakthrough in the management of chronic heart failure. *Int J Tissue React.* 1990;12:155-162.

48. Weis M, Mortensen SA, Rassing MR, et al. Bioavailability of four oral coenzyme Q_{10} formulations in healthy volunteers. *Mol Aspects Med.* 1994;15(suppl):S273-S280.

49. Baggio E, Gandini R, Plancher AC, et al. Italian multicenter study on the safety and efficacy of coenzyme Q_{10} as adjunctive therapy in heart failure. CoQ$_{10}$ Drug Surveillance Investigators. *Mol Aspects Med.* 1994;15(suppl):S287-S294.

50. Hamada M, Kazatain Y, Ochi T, et al. Correlation between serum CoQ$_{10}$ level and myocardial contractility in hypertensive patients. *Biomed Clin Aspects Coenzyme Q.* 1984;4:263-270.

51. Danysz A, Oledzka K, Bukowska-Kiliszek M. Influence of coenzyme Q-10 on the hypotensive effects of enalapril and nitrendipine in spontaneously hypertensive rats. *Pol J Pharmacol.* 1994;46:457-461.

52. Burke BE, Neuenschwander R, Olson RD. Randomized, double-blind, placebo-controlled trial of coenzyme Q_{10} in isolated systolic hypertension. *South Med J.* 2001;94:1112-1117.

53. Singh RB, Khanna HK, Niaz MA. Randomized, double-blind placebo-controlled trial of coenzyme Q_{10} in chronic renal failure: discovery of a new role. *J Nutr Environ Med.* 2000;10:281-288.

Colostrum

1. Ebina T, Ohta M, Kanamaru Y, et al. Passive immunizations of suckling mice and infants with bovine colostrum containing antibodies to human rotavirus. *J Med Virol.* 1992;38:117-123.
2. Sarker SA, Casswall TH, Mahalanabis D, et al. Successful treatment of rotavirus diarrhea in children with immunoglobulin from immunized bovine colostrum. *Pediatr Infect Dis J.* 1998;17:1149-1154.
3. Mitra AK, Mahalanabis D, Ashraf H, et al. Hyperimmune cow colostrum reduces diarrhoea due to rotavirus: a double-blind, controlled clinical trial. *Acta Paediatr.* 1995;84:996-1001.
4. Ylitalo S, Uhari M, Rasi S, et al. Rotaviral antibodies in the treatment of acute rotaviral gastroenteritis. *Acta Paediatr.* 1998;87:264-267.
5. Okhuysen PC, Chappell CL, Crabb J, et al. Prophylactic effect of bovine anti-*Cryptosporidium* hyperimmune colostrum immunoglobulin in healthy volunteers challenged with *Cryptosporidium parvum*. *Clin Infect Dis.* 1998;26:1324-1329.
6. Greenberg PD, Cello JP. Treatment of severe diarrhea caused by *Cryptosporidium parvum* with oral bovine immunoglobulin concentrate in patients with AIDS. *J Acquir Immune Defic Syndr Hum Retrovirol.* 1996;13:348-354.
7. Plettenberg A, Stoehr A, Stellbrink HJ, et al. A preparation from bovine colostrum in the treatment of HIV-positive patients with chronic diarrhea. *Clin Investig.* 1993;71:42-45.
8. Tacket CO, Binion SB, Bostwick E, et al. Efficacy of bovine milk immunoglobulin concentrate in preventing illness after *Shigella flexneri* challenge. *Am J Trop Med Hyg.* 1992;47:276-283.
9. Tacket CO, Losonsky G, Link H, et al. Protection by milk immunoglobulin concentrate against oral challenge with enterotoxigenic *Escherichia coli*. *N Engl J Med.* 1988;318:1240-1243.
10. Freedman DJ, Tacket CO, Delehanty A, et al. Milk immunoglobulin with specific activity against purified colonization factor antigens can protect against oral challenge with enterotoxigenic *Escherichia coli*. *J Infect Dis.* 1998;177:662-667.
11. Casswall TH, Sarker SA, Albert MJ, et al. Treatment of *Helicobacter pylori* infection in infants in rural Bangladesh with oral immunoglobulins from hyperimmune bovine colostrum. *Aliment Pharmacol Ther.* 1998;12:563-568.
12. Casswall TH, Sarker SA, Faruque SM, et al. Treatment of enterotoxigenic and enteropathogenic *Escherichia coli*–induced diarrhea in children with bovine immunoglobulin milk concentrate from hyperimmunized cows: a double-blind, placebo-controlled, clinical trial. *Scand J Gastroenterol.* 2000;35:711-718.
13. Playford RJ, Floyd DN, Macdonald CE, et al. Bovine colostrum is a health food supplement which prevents NSAID-induced gut damage. *Gut.* 1999;44:653-658.
14. Macdonald CE, Calnan DP, Podas T, et al. Clinical trial of colostrum for protection against NSAID induced enteropathy [abstract]. *Gastroenterology.* 1998;114:G0856.
15. Playford RJ, Macdonald CE, Johnson WS. Colostrum and milk-derived peptide growth factors for the treatment of gastrointestinal disorders. *Am J Clin Nutr.* 2000; 72:5-14.
16. Ashraf H, Mahalanabis D, Mitra AK, et al. Hyperimmune bovine colostrum in the treatment of shigellosis in children: a double-blind, randomized, controlled trial. *Acta Paediatr.* 2001;90:1373-1378.
17. Antonio J, Sanders MS, Van Gammeren D. The effects of bovine colostrum supplementation on body composition and exercise performance in active men and women. *Nutrition.* 2001;17:243-247.

Conjugated Linoleic Acid (CLA)

1. Ferreira M, Kreider R, Wilson M, et al. Effects of conjugated linoleic acid (CLA) supplementation during resistance training on body composition and strength [abstract]. *J Strength Cond Res.* 1997;11:280.
2. Thom E. A pilot study with the aim of studying the efficacy and tolerability of CLA (Tonalin™) on the body composition in humans [unpublished]. July 1997.

3. West DB, Camet PM, Maddus CD, et al. Reduced body fat with conjugated linoleic acid feeding in the mouse [abstract]. *FASEB J*. 1997;11:A599.

4. Blankson H, Stakkestad JA, Fagertun H, et al. Conjugated linoleic acid reduces body fat mass in overweight and obese humans. *J Nutr*. 2000;130:2943-2948.

5. Belury MA, Mahon A, Shi L. Role of conjugated linoleic acid (CLA) in the management of type 2 diabetes: evidence from Zucker diabetic (fa/fa) rats and human subjects. Presented at: 220th ACS National Meeting; August 20-24,2000; Washington, DC; 2000.

6. Ip C, Banni S, Angioni E, et al. Conjugated linoleic acid-enriched butter fat alters mammary gland morphogenesis and reduces cancer risk in the rat. *J Nutr*. 1999;129: 2135-2142.

7. Chajes V, Lavillonniere F, Ferrari P, et al. Conjugated linoleic acid and the risk of breast cancer. Presented at: European Conference on Nutrition & Cancer; June 21-24, 2001; Lyon, France; 2001.

8. Smedman A, Vessby B. Conjugated linoleic acid supplementation in humans; metabolic effects. *Lipids*. 2001;36:773-781.

9. Thom E, Wadstein J, Gudmundsen O. Conjugated linoleic acid reduces body fat in healthy exercising humans. *J Int Med Res* 2001;29:392-396.

10. Riserus U, Berglund L, Vessby B. Conjugated linoleic acid (CLA) reduced abdominal adipose tissue in obese middle-aged men with signs of the metabolic syndrome: a randomized controlled trial. *Int J Obes Relat Metab Disord*. 2001;25:1129-1135.

11. MacDonald HB. Conjugated linoleic acid and disease prevention: a review of current knowledge. *J Am Coll Nutr*. 2000;19:111S-118S.

12. Sebedio JL, Gnaedig S, Chardigny JM. Recent advances in conjugated linoleic acid research. *Curr Opin Clin Nutr Metab Care*. 1999;2:499-506.

Copper

1. Saltman PD, Strause LG. The role of trace minerals in osteoporosis. *J Am Coll Nutr*. 1993;12:384-389.

2. Strause L, Saltman P, Smith KT, et al. Spinal bone loss in postmenopausal women supplemented with calcium and trace minerals. *J Nutr*. 1994;124:1060-1064.

3. Cashman KD, Baker A, Ginty F, et al. No effect of copper supplementation on biochemical markers of bone metabolism in healthy young adult females despite apparently improved copper status. *Eur J Clin Nutr*. 2001;55:525-531.

4. Jones AA, DiSilvestro RA, Coleman M, et al. Copper supplementation of adult men: effects on blood copper enzyme activities and indicators of cardiovascular disease risk. *Metabolism*. 1997;46:1380-1383.

5. Dietary Reference Intakes for Vitamin A, Vitamin K, Arsenic, Boron, Chromium, Copper, Iodine, Iron, Manganese, Molybdenum, Nickel, Silicon, Vanadium, and Zinc (2001). http://www.nap.edu. Accessed October 4, 2001.

6. Fosmire GJ. Zinc toxicity. *Am J Clin Nutr*. 1990;51:225-227.

7. Berg G, Kohlmeier L, Brenner H. Effect of oral contraceptive progestins on serum copper concentration. *Eur J Clin Nutr*. 1998;52:711-715.

8. Milne DB, Johnson PE. Assessment of copper status: effect of age and gender on reference ranges in healthy adults. *Clin Chem*. 1993;39:883-887.

9. Newhouse IJ, Clement DB, Lai C. Effects of iron supplementation and discontinuation on serum copper, zinc, calcium, and magnesium levels in women. *Med Sci Sports Exerc*. 1993;25:562-571.

10. Baum MK, Javier JJ, Mantero-Atienza E, et al. Zidovudine-associated adverse reactions in a longitudinal study of asymptomatic HIV-1-infected homosexual males. *J Acquir Immune Defic Syndr*. 1991;4:1218-1226.

Cranberry

1. Stothers L. A randomized placebo controlled trial to evaluate naturopathic cranberry products as prophylaxis against urinary tract infection in women. Presented at: American Urological Association 2001 Annual Meeting; June 2-7, 2001; Anaheim, CA; 2001.

2. Kontiokari T, Sundqvist K, Nuutinen M, et al. Randomized trial of cranberry-lingonberry juice and *Lactobacillus GG* drink for the prevention of urinary tract infections in women. *BMJ*. 2001;322:1-5.
3. Avorn J, Monane M, Gurwitz JH, et al. Reduction of bacteriuria and pyuria after ingestion of cranberry juice. *JAMA*. 1994;271:751-754.
4. Hopkins WJ, Heisey DM, Jonler M, et al. Reduction of bacteriuria and pyuria using cranberry juice [letter]. *JAMA*. 1994;272:588-589.
5. Katz LM. Reduction of bacteriuria and pyuria using cranberry juice [letter]. *JAMA*. 1994;272:589.
6. Schlager TA, Anderson S, Trudell J, et al. Effect of cranberry juice on bacteriuria in children with neurogenic bladder receiving intermittent catheterization. *J Pediatr.* 1999;135:698-702.
7. Weiss EI, Lev-Dor R, Kashamn Y, et al. Inhibiting interspecies coaggregation of plaque bacteria with a cranberry juice constituent. *JADA.* 1998;129:1719-1723.
8. Howell AB, Vorsa N, Der Marderosian A, et al. Inhibition of the adherence of P-fimbriated *Escherichia coli* to uroepithelial-cell surfaces by proanthocyanidin extracts from cranberries [letter]. *N Engl J Med.* 1998;339:1085-1086.
9. Ofek I, Goldhar J, Zafriri D, et al. Anti–*Escherichia coli* adhesin activity of cranberry and blueberry juices [letter]. *N Engl J Med.* 1991;324:1599.
10. Schmidt DR, Sobota AE. An examination of the anti-adherence activity of cranberry juice on urinary and nonurinary bacterial isolates. *Microbios.* 1988;55:173-181.
11. Sobota AE. Inhibition of bacterial adherence by cranberry juice: potential use for the treatment of urinary tract infections. *J Urol.* 1984;131:1013-1016.
12. Zafriri D, Ofek I, Adar R, et al. Inhibitory activity of cranberry juice on adherence of type 1 and type P fimbriated *Escherichia coli* to eucaryotic cells. *Antimicrob Agents Chemother.* 1989;33:92-98.
13. Habash MB, Van der Mei HC, Busscher HJ, Reid G. The effect of water, ascorbic acid, and cranberry derived supplementation on human urine and uropathogen adhesion to silicone rubber. *Can J Microbiol.* 1999;45:691-694.
14. Schaeffer AJ. Recurrent urinary tract infections in the female patient. *Urology.* 1988;32(suppl):12-15.
15. Terris MK, Issa MM, Tacker JR. Dietary supplementation with cranberry concentrate tablets may increase the risk of nephrolithiasis. *Urology.* 2001;57:26-29.
16. Simpson GM, Khajawall AM. Urinary acidifiers in phencyclidine detoxification. *Hillside J Clin Psychiatry.* 1983;5:161-168.

Creatine

1. Williams MH, Branch JD. Creatine supplementation and exercise performance: an update. *J Am Coll Nutr.* 1998;17:216-234.
2. Balsom PD, Ekblom B, Soderlund K, et al. Creatine supplementation and dynamic high-intensity intermittent exercise. *Scand J Med Sci Sports.* 1993;3:143-149.
3. Mujika I, Padilla S, Ibanez J, et al. Creatine supplementation and sprint performance in soccer players. *Med Sci Sports Exerc.* 2000;32:518-525.
4. Gilliam JD, Hohzorn C, Martin D, et al. Effect of oral creatine supplementation on isokinetic torque production. *Med Sci Sports Exerc.* 2000;32:993-996.
5. Mujika I, Padilla S. Creatine supplementation as an ergogenic acid for sports performance in highly trained athletes: a critical review. *Int J Sports Med.* 1997;18:491-496.
6. Finn JP, Ebert TR, Withers RT, et al. Effect of creatine supplementation on metabolism and performance in humans during intermittent sprint cycling. *Eur J Appl Physiol.* 2001;84:238-243.
7. Kraemer WJ, Volek JS. Creatine supplementation: its role in human performance. *Clin Sports Med.* 1999;18:651-666.
8. Kreider RB, Ferreira M, Wilson P, et al. Effects of creatine supplementation on body composition, strength and sprint performance. *Med Sci Sports Exerc.* 1998;30:73-82.
9. Volek JS, Kraemer WJ, Bush JA, et al. Creatine supplementation enhances muscular performance during high-intensity resistance exercise. *J Am Diet Assoc.* 1997;97:765-770.

10. Vandenberghe K, Goris M, Van Hecke P, et al. Long-term creatine intake is beneficial to muscle performance during resistance training. *J Appl Physiol.* 1997;83:2055-2063.

11. Earnest CP, Snell PG, Rodriguez R, et al. The effect of creatine monohydrate ingestion on anaerobic power indices, muscular strength, and body composition. *Acta Physiol Scand.* 1995;153:207-209.

12. Cooke WH, Grandjean PW, Barnes WS. Effect of oral creatine supplementation on power output and fatigue during bicycle ergometry. *J Appl Physiol.* 1995;78:670-673.

13. Burke LM, Pyne DB, Telford RD. Effect of oral creatine supplementation on single-effort sprint performance in elite swimmers. *Int J Sport Nutr.* 1996;6:222-233.

14. Mujika I, Chatard JC, Lacoste L, et al. Creatine supplementation does not improve sprint performance in competitive swimmers. *Med Sci Sports Exerc.* 1996;28:1435-1441.

15. Gordon A, Hultman E, Kaijser L, et al. Creatine supplementation in chronic heart failure increases skeletal muscle creatine phosphate and muscle performance. *Cardiovasc Res.* 1995;30:413-418.

16. Andrews R, Greenhaff P, Curtis S, et al. The effect of dietary creatine supplementation on skeletal muscle metabolism in congestive heart failure. *Eur Heart J.* 1998;19: 617-622.

17. Earnest CP, Almada AL, Mitchell TL. High-performance capillary electrophoresis-pure creatine monohydrate reduces blood lipids in men and women. *Clin Sci (Colch).* 1996;91:113-118.

18. Wyss M, Felber S, Skladal D, et al. The therapeutic potential of oral creatine supplementation in muscle disease. *Med Hypotheses.* 1998;51:333-336.

19. Pulido SM, Passaquin AC, Leijendekker WJ, et al. Creatine supplementation improves intracellular Ca2+ handling and survival in mdx skeletal muscle cells. *FEBS Lett.* 1998;439:357-362.

20. Walter MC, Lochmuller H, Reilich P, et al. Creatine monohydrate in muscular dystrophies: a double-blind, placebo-controlled clinical study. *Neurology.* 2000;54: 1848-1850.

21. Tarnopolsky M, Martin J. Creatine monohydrate increases strength in patients with neuromuscular disease. *Neurology.* 1999;52:854-857.

22. Vorgerd M, Grehl T, Jager M, et al. Creatine therapy in myophosphorylase deficiency (McArdle disease): a placebo-controlled crossover trial. *Arch Neurol.* 2000;57: 956-963.

23. Tarnopolsky MA, Roy BD, MacDonald JR. A randomized, controlled trial of creatine monohydrate in patients with mitochondrial cytopathies. *Muscle Nerve.* 1997;20: 1502-1509.

24. Borchert A, Wilichowski E, Hanefeld F. Supplementation with creatine monohydrate in children with mitochondrial encephalomyopathies [letter]. *Muscle Nerve.* 1999;22:1299-1300.

25. Klivenyi P, Ferrante RJ, Matthews RT, et al. Neuroprotective effects of creatine in a transgenic animal model of amyotrophic lateral sclerosis. *Nat Med.* 1999;5:347-350.

26. Matthews RT, Yang L, Jenkins BG, et al. Neuroprotective effects of creatine and cyclocreatine in animal models of Huntington's disease. *J Neurosci.* 1998;18:156-163.

27. Stockler S, Hanefeld F, Frahm J. Creatine replacement therapy in guanidinoacetate methyltransferase deficiency: a novel inborn error of metabolism. *Lancet.* 1996;348: 789-790.

28. Schulze A, Hess T, Wevers R, et al. Creatine deficiency syndrome caused by guanidinoacetate methyltransferase deficiency: diagnostic tools for a new inborn error of metabolism. *J Pediatr.* 1997;131:626-631.

29. Casey A, Constantin-Teodosiu D, Howell S, et al. Creatine ingestion favorably affects performance and muscle metabolism during maximal exercise in humans. *Am J Physiol.* 1996;271(1 pt 1):E31-E37.

30. Francaux M, Demeure R, Goudemant JF. Effect of exogenous creatine supplementation on muscle PCr metabolism. *Int J Sport Med.* 2000;21:139-145.

31. Greenhaff PL, Bodin K, Soderlund K, Hultman E. Effect of oral creatine supplementation on skeletal muscle phosphocreatine resynthesis. *Am J Physiol.* 1994;266 (5 pt 1):E725-E730.

32. Harris RC, Soderlund K, Hultman E. Elevation of creatine in resting and exercised muscle of normal subjects by creatine supplementation. *Clin Sci (Lond).* 1992;83: 367-374.

33. Hultman E, Soderlund K, Timmons JA, et al. Muscle creatine loading in men. *J Appl Physiol.* 1996;81:232-237.

34. Volek JS, Kraemer WJ. Creatine supplementation: its effect on human muscular performance and body composition. *J Strength Cond Res.* 1996;10:200-210.

35. Green AL, Hultman E, Macdonald IA, et al. Carbohydrate ingestion augments skeletal muscle creatine accumulation during creatine supplementation in humans. *Am J Physiol.* 1996;271(5 pt 1):E821-E826.

36. Steenge GR, Lambourne J, Casey A, et al. Stimulatory effect of insulin on creatine accumulation in human skeletal muscle. *Am J Physiol.* 1998;275:E974-E979.

37. Nelson AG, Arnall DA, Kokkonen J, et al. Muscle glycogen supercompensation is enhanced by prior creatine supplementation. *Med Sci Sports Exerc.* 2001;33:1096-1100.

38. Juhn MS, Tarnopolsky M. Potential side effects of oral creatine supplementation: a critical review. *Clin J Sport Med.* 1998;8:298-304.

39. Sipila I, Rapola J, Simell O, et al. Supplementary creatine as a treatment for gyrate atrophy of the choroid and retina. *N Engl J Med.* 1981;304:867-870.

40. Graham AS, Hatton RC. Creatine: a review of efficacy and safety. *J Am Pharm Assoc.* 1999;39:803-810.

41. Kreider R, Rasmeussen C, Melton C, et al. Long-term creatine supplementation does not adversely affect clinical markers of health. Presented at: American College of Sports Medicine 2000 Annual Scientific Meeting, May 31-June 3, 2000; Indianapolis, 200.

42. Volek JS, Mazzetti SA, Farquhar WB, et al. Physiological responses to short-term exercise in the heat after creatine loading. *Med Sci Sports Exerc.* 2001;33:1101-1108.

43. Pritchard NR, Kalra PA. Renal dysfunction accompanying oral creatine supplements. *Lancet.* 1998;351:1252-1253.

44. Mihic S, MacDonald JR, McKenzie S, et al. Acute creatine loading increases fat-free mass, but does not affect blood pressure, plasma creatinine, or CK activity in men and women. *Med Sci Sports Exerc.* 2000;32:291-296.

45. Poortmans JR, Francaux M. Long-term oral creatine supplementation does not impair renal function in healthy athletes. *Med Sci Sports Exerc.* 1999;31:1108-1110.

46. Koshy KM, Griswold E, Schneeberger EE. Interstitial nephritis in a patient taking creatine. *N Engl J Med.* 1999;340:814-815.

47. Yu PH, Deng Y. Potential cytotoxic effect of chronic administration of creatine, a nutrition supplement to augment athletic performance. *Med Hypotheses.* 2000;54:726-728.

48. Williams MH, Branch JD (1998). Creatine supplementation and exercise performance: an update. *J Am Coll Nutr.* 17(3):216-234.

49. Bemben MG, Tuttle TD, Bemben DA, et al. Effects of creatine supplementation on isometric force-time curve characteristics. *Med Sci Sports Exerc.* 2001;33:1876-1881

50. Op't Eijnde B, Urso B, Richter EA, et al. Effect of oral creatine supplementation on human muscle GLUT4 protein content after immobilization. *Diabetes.* 2001;50:18-23.

51. Hespel P, Eijnde BO, Van Leemputte M, et al. Oral creatine supplementation facilitates the rehabilitation of disuse atrophy and alters the expression of muscle myogenic factors in humans. *J Physiol.* 2001;536:625-633.

52. Vorgerd M, Zange J, Kley R, et al. Effect of high-dose creatine therapy on symptoms of exercise intolerance in McArdle disease: double-blind, placebo-controlled crossover study. *Arch Neurol.* 2002;59:97-101.

Curcumin

1. Satoskar RR, Shah SJ, Shenoy SG. Evaluation of anti-inflammatory property of curcumin (diferuloyl methane) in patients with postoperative inflammation. *Int J Clin Pharmacol Ther Toxicol.* 1986;24:651-654.

2. Deodhar SD, Sethi R, Srimal RC. Preliminary study on antirheumatic activity of curcumin (diferuloyl methane). *Indian J Med Res.* 1980;71:632-634.

3. Babu PS, Srinivasan K. Hypolipidemic action of curcumin, the active principle of turmeric *(Curcuma longa)* in streptozotocin induced diabetic rats. *Mol Cell Biochem.* 1997;166:169-175.

4. Rao DS, Sekhara NC, Satyanarayana MN, et al. Effect of curcumin on serum and liver cholesterol levels in the rat. *J Nutr.* 1970;100:1307-1316.

5. Srinivasan K, Sambaiah K. The effect of spices on cholesterol 7 alpha-hydroxylase activity and on serum and hepatic cholesterol levels in the rat. *Int J Vitam Nutr Res.* 1991;61:364-369.

6. Soni KB, Kuttan R. Effect of oral curcumin administration on serum peroxides and cholesterol levels in human volunteers. *Indian J Physiol Pharmacol.* 1992;36:273-275.

7. Lal B, Kapoor AK, Asthana OP, et al. Efficacy of curcumin in the management of chronic anterior uveitis. *Phytother Res.* 1999;13:318-322.

8. Lim GP, Chu T, Yang F, et al. The curry spice curcumin reduces oxidative damage and amyloid pathology in an Alzheimer transgenic mouse. *J Neurosci.* 2001;21:8370-8377.

9. Awasthi S, Srivatava SK, Piper JT et al. Curcumin protects against 4-hydroxy-2-trans-nonenal-induced cataract formation in rat lenses. *Am J Clin Nutr.* 1996;64:761-766.

10. Mundell EJ. Curry spice may fight multiple sclerosis: study http:www.vitacost.com/golive/news/newsdetails.cfm?articleid=9A2D4CF1-1E7D-4485-823FA315AC263941, accessed 5/10/02.

11. Ruby AJ, Kuttan G, Babu KD, et al. Anti-tumor and antioxidant activity of natural curcuminoids. *Cancer Lett.* 1995;79-83.

12. Oetari S, Sudibyo M, Commandeur JN, et al. Effects of curcumin on cytochrome P450 and glutathione S-transferase activities in rat liver. *Biochem Pharmacol.* 1996;51:39-45.

13. Shankar TN, Shantha NV, Ramesh HP, et al. Toxicity studies on turmeric *(Curcuma longa):* acute toxicity studies in rats, guinea pigs & monkeys. *Indian J Exp Biol.* 1980;18:73-75

14. Thamlikitkul V, Bunyapraphatsara N, Dechatiwongse T, et al. Randomized double blind study of Curcuma domestica Val. for dyspepsia. *J Med Assoc Thai.* 1989;72:613-620.

15. Van Dau N, Ngoc Ham N, Huy Khac D, et al. The effects of a traditional drug, turmeric *(Curcuma longa)*, and placebo on the healing of duodenal ulcer. *Phytomedicine.* 1998;5:29-34.

16. Kositchaiwat C, Kositchaiwat S, Havanondha J. Curcuma longa Linn. in the treatment of gastric ulcer comparison to liquid antacid: a controlled clinical trial. *J Med Assoc Thai.* 1993;76:601-605.

17. Ammon HP, Wahl MA. Pharmacology of *Curcuma longa. Planta Med.* 1991;57:1-7.

18. Afaq F, Adhami VM, Ahmad N, et al. Botanical antioxidants for chemoprevention of photocarcinogenesis. *Front Biosci.* 2002;7:784-792.

19. Arbiser JL, Klauber N, Rohan R, et al. Curcumin is an in vivo inhibitor of angiogenesis. *Mol Med.* 1998;4:376-383.

20. Cheng AL, Hsu CH, Lin JK, et al. Phase I clinical trial of curcumin, a chemopreventive agent, in patients with high-risk or pre-malignant lesions. *Anticancer Res.* 2001;21:2895-2900.

21. Deshpande SS, Ingle AD, Maru GB. Chemopreventive efficacy of curcumin-free aqueous turmeric extract in 7,12-dimethylbenz(a)anthracene-induced rat mammary tumorigenesis. *Cancer Lett.* 1998;123:35-40.

22. Dorai T, Gehani N, Katz A. Therapeutic potential of curcumin in human prostate cancer. II. Curcumin inhibits tyrosine kinase activity of epidermal growth factor receptor and depletes the protein. *Mol Urol.* 2000;4:1-6.

23. Ireson CR, Jones DJ, Orr S, et al. Metabolism of the cancer chemopreventive agent curcumin in human and rat intestine. *Cancer Epidemiol Biomarkers Prev.* 2002;11:105-111.

24. Krishnaswamy K, Goud VK, Sesikeran B, et al. Retardation of experimental tumorigenesis and reduction in DNA adducts by turmeric and curcumin. *Nutr Cancer.* 1998;30:163-166.

25. Li JK, Lin-Shia SY. Mechanisms of cancer chemoprevention by curcumin. *Proc Natl Sci Counc Repub China B.* 2001;25:59-66.
26. Ruby AJ, Kuttan G, Babu KD et al. Anti-tumor and antioxidant activity of natural curcuminoids. *Cancer Lett.* 1995;79-83.
27. Smith WA, Freeman JW, Gupta RC. Effect of chemopreventive agents on DNA adduction induced by the potent mammary carcinogen dibenzo[a,l]pyrene in the human breast cells MCF-7. *Mutat Res.* 2001;480-481:97-108.
28. Chuang S, Cheng A, Lin J, Kuo M. Inhibition by curcumin of diethylnitrosamine-induced hepatic hyperplasia, inflammation, cellular gene products, and cell-cycle related proteins in rats. *Food Chem Toxicol.* 2000;38(11):991-995.
29. Deshpande UR, Gadre SG, Raste AS, et al. Protective effect of turmeric (*Curcuma longa* L) extract on carbon tetrachloride-induced liver damage in rats. *Indian J Exp Biol.* 1998;36:573-577.
30. Song EK, Cho H, Kim JS, et al. Diarylheptanoids with free radical scavenging and hepatoprotective activity in vitro from Curcuma longa. *Planta Med.* 2001;67:876-877.
31. Venkatesan N. Pulmonary protective effects of curcumin against paraquat toxicity. *Life Sci.* 2000;66:PL21-28.
32. Pilot Projects Symposium 2002. Arizona Center for Phytomedicine Research. http:acprx.pharmacy.arizona.edu/research/pilot/pilotsymp2002.html, accessed 5/25/02.
33. Deshpande S, Lalitha VS, Ingle AD. Subchronic oral toxicity of turmeric and ethanolic turmeric extract in female mice and rats. *Toxicology Letters.* 1998;95:183-193.
34. Kandarkar SV, Sawant SS, Ingle AD, Deshpande SS, Maru GB. Subchronic oral hepatotoxicity of turmeric in mice: histopathological and ultrastructural studies. *Indian J Exp Biol.* 1998;36:675-679.

Damiana

1. Willard T. *The Wild Rose Scientific Herbal.* Calgary, Canada: Wild Rose College of Natural Healing, Ltd.; 1991:104-105.
2. Duke JA. *CRC Handbook of Medicinal Herbs.* Boca Raton, Fla: CRC Press; 1985:492.
3. Newall CA, Anderson LA, Phillipson JD. *Herbal Medicines: A Guide for Health-Care Professionals.* London: Pharmaceutical Press; 1996:94.
4. Tyler VE. Related articles damiana: history of a herbal hoax. *Pharm Hist.* 1983; 25(2):55-60.

Dandelion Root

1. Tita B, Bello U, Faccendini P, et al. *Taraxacum officinale* w.: pharmacological effect of ethanol extract. *Pharmacol Res.* 1993;27(suppl 1):23-24.
2. Mascolo N, Autore G, Capasso F. Biological screening of Italian medicinal plants for anti-inflammatory activity. *Phytother Res.* 1987;1:28-31.
3. European Scientific Cooperative on Phytotherapy. *Taraxaci radix* (dandelion). Exeter, UK: ESCOP; 1996-1997. Monographs on the Medicinal Uses of Plant Drugs, Fascicule 2:1-2.
4. Racz-Kotilla E, Racz G, Solomon A. The action of *Taraxacum officinale* extracts on the body weight and diuresis of laboratory animals. *Planta Med.* 1974;26:212-217.
5. Hook I, McGee A, Henman M. Evaluation of dandelion for diuretic activity and variation in potassium content. *Int J Pharmacol.* 1993;31:29-34.
6. Kuusi T, Pyysalo H, Autio K. The bitterness properties of dandelion. II. Chemical investigations. *Lebensm Wiss Technol.* 1985;18:347-349.
7. Hansel R, Kartarahardja M, Huang JT, et al. Sesquiterpenlacton-beta-D-glucopyranoside as well as an eudesmanolid from *Taraxacum officinale* [in German; English abstract]. *Phytochemistry.* 1980;19:857-861.
8. Guin JD, Skidmore G. Compositae dermatitis in childhood. *Arch Dermatol.* 1987;123:500-502.
9. Blumenthal M, ed. *The Complete German Commission E Monographs, Therapeutic Guide to Herbal Medicines.* Boston, Mass: Integrative Medicine Communications; 1998:119-120.

10. McGuffin M, ed. *American Herbal Products Association's Botanical Safety Handbook*. Boca Raton, Fla: CRC Press; 1997:114.
11. Hirono I, Mori H, Kato K, et al. Safety examination of some edible plants, part 2. *J Environ Pathol Toxicol*. 1977;1:71-74.
12. Hirono I, Shimizu M, Fushmi K, et al. Carcinogenic activity of *Petasites japonicus* MAXIM, a kind of coltsfoot. *Gann*. 1973;64:527-528.
13. Hirono I, Mori H, Culvenor CJ. Carcinogenic activity of coltsfoot, *Tussilago farfara* L. *Gann*. 1976;67:125-129.
14. Matsui AS, Rogers J, Woo YK, et al. Effects of some natural products on fertility in mice. *Med Pharmacol Exp Int J Exp Med*. 1967;16:414-424.
15. Williams CA, Goldstone F, Greenham J. Flavonoids, cinnamic acids and coumarins from the different tissues and medicinal preparations of *Taraxacum officinale*. *Phytochemistry*. 1996;42:121-127.
16. Pyevich D, Bogenschutz MP. Herbal diuretics and lithium toxicity [letter]. *Am J Psychiatry*. 2001;158:1329.

Devil's Claw

1. Gobel H, Heinze A, Ingwersen M, et al. Effects of Harpagophytum procumbens LI 174 (devil's claw) on sensory, motor and vascular muscle reagibility in the treatment of unspecific back pain. *Schmerz*. 2001;15:10-18.
2. European Scientific Cooperative on Phytotherpy. *Harpagophyti radix* (devil's claw). Exeter, UK: ESCOP; 1996-1997. Monographs on the Medicinal Uses of Plant Drugs, Fascicule 2.
3. Leblan D, Chantre P, Fournie B. *Harpagophytum procumbens* in the treatment of knee and hip osteoarthritis. Four-month results of a prospective, multicenter, double-blind trial versus diacerhein. *Joint Bone Spine*. 2000;67:462-467.
4. Chrubasik S, Junck H, Breitschwerdt H, et al. Effectiveness of *Harpagophytum* extract WS 1531 in the treatment of exacerbation of low back pain: a randomized, placebo-controlled, double-blind study. *Eur J Anaesthesiol*. 1999;16:118-129.
5. Chrubasik S, Zimpfer CH, Schutt U, et al. Effectiveness of *Harpagophytum procumbens* in treatment of acute low back pain. *Phytomedicine*. 1996;3:1-10.
6. Schulz V, Hansel R, Tyler VE. *Rational Phytotherapy: A Physicians' Guide to Herbal Medicine*. 3rd ed. Berlin, Germany: Springer-Verlag; 1998:263.
7. Moussard C, Alber D, Toubin MM, et al. A drug used in traditional medicine, *Harpagophytum procumbens*: no evidence for NSAID-like effect on whole blood eicosanoid production in human. *Prostaglandins Leukot Essent Fatty Acids*. 1992;46:283-286.
8. Shaw D, Leon C, Kolev S, et al. Traditional remedies and food supplements: a 5-year toxicological study (1991-1995). *Drug Saf*. 1997;17:342-356.

Dehydroepiandrosterone (DHEA)

1. Mease PJ, Merrill JT, Lahita R, et al. GL701 (prasterone, dehydroepiandrosterone) improves or stabilizes disease activity in systemic lupus erythematosus. Presented at: The Endocrine Society's 82nd Annual Meeting; Toronto; June 21-24, 2000.
2. van Vollenhoven RF, Morabito LM, Engelman EG, et al. Treatment of systemic lupus erythematosus with dehydroepiandrosterone: 50 patients treated up to 12 months. *J Rheumatol*. 1998;25:285-289.
3. van Vollenhoven RF, Park JL, Genovese MC, et al. A double-blind, placebo-controlled, clinical trial of dehydroepiandrosterone in severe systemic lupus erythematosus. *Lupus*. 1999;8:181-187.
4. Robinzon B, Cutolo M. Should dehydroepiandrosterone replacement therapy be provided with glucocorticoids? *Rheumatology (Oxford)*. 1999;38:488-495.
5. Baulieu EE, Thomas G, Legrain S, et al. Dehydroepiandrosterone (DHEA), DHEA sulfate, and aging: contribution of the DHEAge study to a sociobiomedical issue. *Proc Natl Acad Sci*. 2000;97:4279-4284.
6. Piketty C, Jayle D, Leplege A, et al. Double-blind placebo-controlled trial of oral dehydroepiandrosterone in patients with advanced HIV disease *Clin Endocrinol* (Oxf). 2001;55:325-330.

7. Arlt W, Callies F, van Vlijmen JC, et al. Dehydroepiandrosterone replacement in women with adrenal insufficiency. *N Engl J Med.* 1999;341:1013-1020.

8. Hunt PJ, Gurnell EM, Huppert FA, et al. Improvement in mood and fatigue after dehydroepiandrosterone replacement in Addison's disease in a randomized, double blind trial. *J Clin Endocrinol Metab.* 2000;85:4650-4656.

9. Rabkin JG, Ferrando SJ, Wagner GJ, et al. DHEA treatment for HIV+ patients: effects on mood, androgenic and anabolic parameters. *Psychoneuroendocrinology.* 2000;25:53-68.

10. Morales AJ, Nolan JJ, Nelson JC, et al. Effects of replacement dose of dehydroepiandrosterone in men and women of advancing age. *J Clin Endocrinol Metab.* 1994;78:1360-1367.

11. Flynn MA, Weaver-Osterholtz D, Sharpe-Timms KL, et al. Dehydroepiandrosterone replacement in aging humans. *J Clin Endocrinol Metab.* 1999;84:1527-1533.

12. Brown GA, Vukovich MD, Sharp RL, et al. Effect of oral DHEA on serum testosterone and adaptations to resistance training in young men. *J Appl Physiol.* 1999;87:2274-2283.

13. Wallace MB, Lim J, Cutler A, et al. Effects of dehydroepiandrosterone vs androstenedione supplementation in men. *Med Sci Sports Exerc.* 1999;31:1788-1792.

14. Morales AJ, Haubrich RH, Hwang JY, et al. The effect of six months treatment with a 100 mg daily dose of dehydroepiandrosterone (DHEA) on circulating sex steroids, body composition and muscle strength in age-advanced men and women. *Clin Endocrinol (Oxf).* 1998;49:421-432.

15. Wolkowitz OM, Reus VI, Keebler A, et al. Double-blind treatment of major depression with dehydroepiandrosterone. *Am J Psychiatry.* 1999;156:646-649.

16. Barrett-Connor E, von Muhlen D, Laughlin GA, et al. Endogenous levels of dehydroepiandrosterone sulfate, but not other sex hormones, are associated with depressed mood in older women: the Rancho Bernardo Study. *J Am Geriatr Soc.* 1999; 47:685-691.

17. Himmel PB, Seligman TM. A pilot study employing dehydroepiandrosterone (DHEA) in the treatment of chronic fatigue syndrome. *J Clin Rheumatol.* 1999;5:56-59.

18. van Niekerk JK, Huppert FA, Herbert J. Salivary cortisol and DHEA: association with measures of cognition and well-being in normal older men and effects of three months of DHEA supplementation. *Psychoneuroendocrinology.* 2001;26;591-612.

19. Araneo B, Dowell T, Woods ML. DHEAS as an effective vaccine adjuvant in elderly humans: proof-of-principle studies. *Ann NY Acad Sci.* 1995;774:232-248.

20. Evans TG, Judd ME, Dowell T, et al. The use of oral dehydroepiandrosterone sulfate as an adjuvant in tetanus and influenza vaccination of the elderly. *Vaccine.* 1996; 14:1531-1537.

21. Araneo B, Daynes R. Dehydroepiandrosterone functions as more than an antiglucocorticoid in preserving immunocompetence after thermal injury. *Endocrinology.* 1995;136:393-401.

22. Araneo BA, Shelby J, Li G-Z, et al. Administration of dehydroepiandrosterone to burned mice preserves normal immunologic competence. *Arch Surg.* 1993;128:318-325.

23. Kudielka BM, Hellhammer J, Hellhammer DH, et al. Sex differences in endocrine and psychological responses to psychosocial stress in healthy elderly subjects and the impact of a 2-week dehydroepiandrosterone treatment. *J Clin Endocrinol Metab.* 1998;83:1756-1761.

24. Arlt W, Callies F, Koehler I, et al. Dehydroepiandrosterone supplementation in healthy men with an age-related decline of dehydroepiandrosterone secretion *J Clin Endocrinol Metab.* 2001;86:4686-4692.

25. Barrett-Connor E, Goodman-Gruen D. Dehydroepiandrosterone sulfate does not predict cardiovascular death in postmenopausal women. The Rancho Bernardo Study. *Circulation.* 1995;91:1757-1760.

26. Herrington DM, Nanjee N, Achuff SC, et al. Dehydroepiandrosterone and cardiac allograft vasculopathy. *J Heart Lung Transplant.* 1996;15:88-93.

27. Jesse RL, Loesser K, Eich DM, et al. Dehydroepiandrosterone inhibits human platelet aggregation in vitro and in vivo. *Ann NY Acad Sci.* 1995;774:281-290.

28. Barrett-Connor E, Khaw K-T, Yen SSC. A prospective study of dehydroepiandrosterone sulfate, mortality, and cardiovascular disease. *N Engl J Med.* 1986;315:1519-1524.

29. Nafziger AN, Herrington DM, Bush TL. Dehydroepiandrosterone and dehydroepiandrosterone sulfate: their relation to cardiovascular disease. *Epidemiol Rev.* 1991;13:267-293.

30. Barrett-Connor E, Khaw K-T. Absence of an inverse relation of dehydroepiandrosterone sulfate with cardiovascular mortality in postmenopausal women [letter]. *N Engl J Med.* 1987;317:711.

31. Barrett-Connor E, Edelstein SL. A prospective study of dehydroepiandrosterone sulfate and cognitive function in an older population: the Rancho Bernardo Study. *J Am Geriatr Soc.* 1994;42:420-423.

32. Vogiatzi MG, Boeck MA, Vlachopapadopoulou E, et al. Dehydroepiandrosterone in morbidly obese adolescents: effects on weight, body composition, lipids, and insulin resistance. *Metabolism.* 1996;45:1011-1015.

33. Wolf OT, Naumann E, Hellhammer DH, et al. Effects of dehydroepiandrosterone replacement in elderly men on event-related potentials, memory, and well-being. *J Gerontol.* 1998;53:M385-M390.

34. Ebeling P, Koivisto VA. Physiological importance of dehydroepiandrosterone. *Lancet.* 1994;343:1479-1481.

35. Daynes RA, Araneo BA. Natural regulators of T-cell lymphokine production in vivo. *J Immunother.* 1992;12:174-179.

36. Daynes RA, Dudley DJ, Araneo BA. Regulation of murine lymphokine production in vivo. II. Dehydroepiandrosterone is a natural enhancer of interleukin 2 synthesis by helper T cells. *Eur J Immunol.* 1990;20:793-802.

37. Daynes RA, Araneo BA, Dowell TA, et al. Regulation of murine lymphokine production in vivo. III. The lymphoid tissue microenvironment exerts regulatory influences over T helper cell function. *J Exp Med.* 1990;171:979-996.

38. Suzuki T, Suzuki N, Daynes RA, Engleman EG. Dehydroepiandrosterone enhances IL2 production and cytotoxic effector function of human T cells. *Clin Immunol Immunopathol.* 1991;61(2 pt 1):202-211.

39. Van Vollenhoven RF, McGuire JL. Estrogen, progesterone, and testosterone: can they be used to treat autoimmune diseases? *Cleve Clin J Med.* 1994;61:276-284.

40. Jungers P, Nahoul K, Pelissier C, et al. Low plasma androgens in women with active or quiescent systemic lupus erythematosus. *Arthritis Rheum.* 1982;25:454-457.

41. Lahita RG, Bradlow HL, Ginzler E, et al. Low plasma androgens in women with systemic lupus erythematosus. *Arthritis Rheum.* 1987;30:241-248.

42. Regelson W, Kalimi M. Dehydroepiandrosterone (DHEA) the multifunctional steroid. II. Effects on the CNS, cell proliferation, metabolic and vascular, clinical and other effects. Mechanism of action? *Ann NY Acad Sci.* 1994;719:564-575.

43. Regelson W, Loria R, Kalimi M. Dehydroepiandrosterone (DHEA)—the "mother steroid." I. Immunological action. *Ann NY Acad Sci.* 1994;719:553-563.

44. Casson PR, Santoro N, Elkind-Hirsch K, et al. Postmenopausal deydroepiandrosterone administration increases free insulin-like growth factor-I and decreases high-density lipoprotein: a six-month trial. *Fertil Steril.* 1998;70:107-110.

45. van Vollenhoven RF, Engleman EG, McGuire JL. Dehydroepiandrosterone in systemic lupus erythematosus: results of a double-blind, placebo-controlled, randomized clinical trial. *Arthritis Rheum.* 1995;38:1826-1831.

46. Gatto V, Aragno M, Gallo M, et al. Dehydroepiandrosterone inhibits the growth of DMBA-induced rat mammary carcinoma via the androgen receptor. *Oncol Rep.* 1998;5:241-243.

47. Orner GA, Mathews C, Hendricks JD, et al. Dehydroepiandrosterone is a complete hepatocarcinogen and potent tumor promoter in the absence of peroxisome proliferation in rainbow trout. *Carcinogenesis.* 1995;16:2893-2898.

48. Shibata M, Hasegawa R, Imaida K, et al. Chemoprevention by dehydroepiandrosterone and indomethacin in a rat multiorgan carcinogenesis model. *Cancer Res.* 1995;55:4870-4874.

49. Simile M, Pascale RM, De Miglio MR, et al. Inhibition by dehydroepiandrosterone of growth and progression of persistent liver nodules in experimental rat liver carcinogenesis. *Int J Cancer.* 1995;62:210-215.
50. Barrett-Connor E, Friedlander NJ, Khaw K-T. Dehydroepiandrosterone sulfate and breast cancer risk. *Cancer Res.* 1990;50:6571-6574.
51. Helzlsouer KJ, Alberg AJ, Gordon GB, et al. Serum gonadotropins and steroid hormones and the development of ovarian cancer. *JAMA.* 1995;274:1926-1930.
52. Kahn AJ, Haloran B. Dehydroepiandrosterone supplementation and bone turnover in middle-aged to elderly men. *J Clin Endocrinol Metab.* 2002;87:1544-1549.
53. Reiter WJ, Pycha A, Schatzl G, et al. Dehydroepiandrosterone in the treatment of erectile dysfunction: a prospective, double-blind, randomized, placebo-controlled study. *Urology.* 1999;53:590-595.
54. Labrie F, Diamond P, Cusan L, et al. Effect of 12-month dehydroepiandrosterone replacement therapy on bone, vagina and endometrium in postmenopausal women. *J Clin Endocrinol Metab.* 1997;82:3498-3505.
55. van Vollenhoven RF. Dehydroepiandrosterone for the treatment of systemic lupus erythematosus. *Expert Opin Pharmacother.* 2002;3(1):23-31.
56. Meston CM, Heiman JR. Acute dehydroepiandrosterone effects on sexual arousal in premenopausal women. *J Sex Marital Ther.* 2002;28:53-60.
57. Hackbert L, Heiman JR. Acute dehydroepiandrosterone (DHEA) effects on sexual arousal in postmenopausal women. *J Womens Health Gend Based Med.* 2002;11:155-162.

Diosmin/Hesperidin

1. Godeberge P. Daflon 500 mg in the treatment of hemorrhoidal disease: a demonstrated efficacy in comparison with placebo. *Angiology.* 1994;45:574-578.
2. Cospite M. Double-blind, placebo-controlled evaluation of clinical activity and safety of Daflon 500 mg in the treatment of acute hemorrhoids. *Angiology.* 1994;45:566-573.
3. Misra MC, Parshad R. Randomized clinical trial of micronized flavonoids in the early control of bleeding from acute internal haemorrhoids. *Br J Surg.* 2000;87:868-872.
4. Ho YH, Tan M, Seow-Choen F. Micronized purified flavonidic fraction compared favorably with rubber band ligation and fiber alone in the management of bleeding hemorrhoids: randomized controlled trial. *Dis Colon Rectum.* 2000;43:66-69.
5. Thanapongsathorn W, Vajrabukka T. Clinical trial of oral diosmin (Daflon®) in the treatment of hemorrhoids. *Dis Colon Rectum.* 1992;35:1085-1088.
6. Guilhou JJ, Dereure O, Marzin L, et al. Efficacy of Daflon 500 mg in venous leg ulcer healing: a double-blind, randomized, controlled versus placebo trial in 107 patients. *Angiology.* 1997;48:77-85.
7. Galley P, Thiollet M. A double-blind, placebo-controlled trial of a new veno-active flavonoid fraction (S 5682) in the treatment of symptomatic capillary fragility. *Int Angiol.* 1993;12:69-72.
8. Pecking AP, Fevrier B, Wargon C, et al. Efficacy of Daflon 500 mg in the treatment of lymphedema (secondary to conventional therapy of breast cancer). *Angiology.* 1997;48:93-98.
9. Meyer OC. Safety and security of Daflon 500 mg in venous insufficiency and in hemorrhoidal disease. *Angiology.* 1994;45:579-584.
10. Buckshee K, Takkar D, Aggarwal N. Micronized flavonoid therapy in internal hemorrhoids of pregnancy. *Int J Gynaecol Obstet.* 1997;57:145-151.
11. Laurent R, Gilly R, Frileux C. Clinical evaluation of a venotropic drug in man. Example of Daflon 500 mg. *Int Angiol.* 1988;7:39-43.
12. Danielsson G, Jungbeck C, Peterson K, et al. A randomized controlled trial of micronised purified flavonoid fraction vs placebo in patients with chronic venous disease. *Eur J Vasc Endovasc Surg.* 2002;23:73-76.

Dong Quai

1. Nortier JL, Martinez MC, Schmeiser HH, et al. Urothelial carcinoma associated with the use of a Chinese herb (*Aristolochia fangchi*). *N Engl J Med.* 2000;342:1686-1692.
2. Nagourney R. 93rd Annual Meeting of the American Association for Cancer Research. San Francisco, 2002.

3. Chang HM, But PP, eds. *Pharmacology and Application of Chinese Materia Medica.* Singapore: World Scientific; 1986:248.
4. Igarashi M. Efficacy of Kampo medicines in obstetrical and gynecological diseases. In Satellite Meeting on Kampo (Japanese Herbal) Medicines (1987: Aukland, N.Z.). *Recent Advances in the Pharmacology of Kampo (Japanese Herbal) Medicines: Proceedings of the Satellite Meeting on Kampo (Japanese Herbal) Medicines of the 10th International Congress of Pharmacology, Auckland, New Zealand, Aug. 19-21, 1987.* New York, NY: Excerpta Medica; 1987:141-143.
5. Hirata JD, Swiersz LM, Zell B, et al. Does dong quai have estrogenic effects in post-menopausal women? A double-blind, placebo controlled trial. *Fertil Steril.* 1997;68:981-986.
6. Zava DT, Dollbaum CM, Blen M. Estrogen and progestin bioactivity of foods, herbs, and spices. *Proc Soc Exp Biol Med.* 1998;217:369-378.
7. Zhu D. Dong quai. *Am J Chin Med.* 1987;15:117-125.
8. Goh SY, Loh KC. Gynaecomastia and the herbal tonic "Dong Quai." *Singapore Med J.* 2001;42:115-116.
9. Nambiar S, Schwartz RH, Constantino A. Hypertension in mother and baby linked to ingestion of Chinese herbal medicine [letter]. *West J Med.* 1999;171:152.
10. Page RL II, Lawrence JD. Potentiation of warfarin by dong quai. *Pharmacotherapy.* 1999;19:870-876.
11. Zava DT, Dollbaum CM, Blen M. Estrogen and progestin bioactivity of foods, herbs, and spices. *Proc Soc Exp Biol Med.* 1998;217:369-378.
12. Hirata JD, Swiersz LM, Zell B, et al. Does dong quai have estrogenic effects in post-menopausal women? A double-blind placebo controlled trial. *Fertil Steril.* 1997;68:981-986.
13. Amato P, Christophe S, Mellon P. Estrogenic activity of herbs commonly used as remedies for menopausal symptoms. *Menopause.* 2002;9:145-150.
14. Liu J, Burdette JE, Xu H, et al. Evaluation of estrogenic activity of plant extracts for the potential treatment of menopausal symptoms. *J Agric Food Chem.* 2001;49:2472-2479.
15. Lo AC, Chan K, Yeung JH, et al. Danggui *(Angelica sinensis)* affects the pharmaco-dynamics but not the pharmacokinetics of warfarin in rabbits. *Eur J Drug Metab Pharmacokinet.* 1995;20:55-60.

Echinacea

1. Bergner P. Goldenseal and the common cold: the antibiotic myth. *Med Herbalism.* 1996/1997;8(4):1,4-6.
2. Brinkeborn RM, Shah DV, Degenring FH. Echinaforce and other *Echinacea* fresh plant preparations in the treatment of the common cold: a randomized, placebo controlled, double-blind clinical trial. *Phytomedicine.* 1999;6:1-5.
3. Soon SL, Crawford RI. Recurrent erythema nodosum associated with Echinacea herbal therapy. *J Am Acad Dermatol.* 2001;44:298-299.
4. Dorn M, Knick E, Lewith G. Placebo-controlled double-blind study of *Echinacea pallidae* radix in upper respiratory tract infections. *Complement Ther Med.* 1997;5:40-42.
5. Lindenmuth GF, Lindenmuth EB. The efficacy of *Echinacea* compound herbal tea preparation on the severity and duration of upper respiratory and flu symptoms: a randomized, double-blind placebo-controlled study. *J Altern Complement Med.* 2000;6:327-334.
6. Hoheisel O, Sandberg M, Bertram S, et al. Echinagard® treatment shortens the course of the common cold: a double-blind placebo-controlled clinical trial. *Eur J Clin Res.* 1997;9:261-268.
7. Schulten B, Bulitta M, Ballering-Bruhl B, et al. Efficacy of *Echinacea purpurea* in patients with a common cold: a placebo-controlled, randomized, double-blind clinical trial. *Arzneimittelforschung.* 2001;51:563-568.
8. Melchart MD, Linde K, Worku F, et al. Immunomodulation with *Echinacea:* a systemic review of controlled clinical trials. *Phytomedicine.* 1994;1:245-254.

9. Melchart D, Walther E, Linde K, et al. *Echinacea* root extracts for the prevention of upper respiratory tract infections: a double-blind, placebo-controlled randomized trial. *Arch Fam Med.* 1998;7:541-545.

10. Grimm W, Muller HH. A randomized controlled trial of the effect of fluid extract of *Echinacea purpurea* on the incidence and severity of colds and respiratory infections. *Am J Med.* 1999;106:138-143.

11. Schoneberger D. The influence of immune-stimulating effects of pressed juice from *Echinacea purpurea* on the course and severity of colds [translated from German]. *Forum Immunol.* 1992;8:2-12.

12. Chamberlain C. Take echinacea? Bless you (April 27, 1999). ABC News web site. Available at: http://www.abcnews.go.com/sections/living/DailyNews/echinacea 990427.html. Accessed July 15, 2000.

13. Turner RB, Riker DK, Gangemi JD. Ineffectiveness of *Echinacea* for prevention of experimental rhinovirus colds. *Antimicrob Agents Chemother.* 2000;44:1708-1709.

14. Schmidt U, Albrecht M, Schenk N. Immunostimulator decreases the frequency of influenza-like syndromes. Double-blind placebo-controlled trial on 646 students of the University of Cologne [in German; English abstract]. *Natur und Ganzheitsmedizin.* 1990;3:277-281.

15. Vonau B, Chard S, Mandalia S, et al. Does the extract of the plant *Echinacea purpurea* influence the clinical course of recurrent genital herpes? *Int J STD AIDS.* 2001;12:154-158.

16. Coeugniet E, Kuhnast R. Recurrent candidiasis: adjuvant immunotherapy with different formulations of Echinacin® [translated from German]. *Therapiewoche.* 1986;36:3352-3358.

17. Bauer R, Wagner H. *Echinacea* species as potential immunostimulatory drugs. *Econ Med Plant Res.* 1991;5:253-321.

18. Luettig B, Steinmuller C, Gifford GE, et al. Macrophage activation by the polysaccharide arabinogalactan isolated from plant cell cultures of *Echinacea purpurea*. *J Natl Cancer Inst.* 1989;81:669-675.

19. Mose JR. The effect of *Echinacin* on phagocytosis and natural killer cells [in German; English abstract]. *Med Welt.* 1983;34:1463-1467.

20. Stimple M, Proksch A, Wagner H, et al. Macrophage activation and induction of macrophage cytotoxicity by purified polysaccharide fractions from the plant *Echinacea purpurea*. *Infect Immun.* 1984;46:845-849.

21. Vomel T. The effect of a nonspecific immunostimulant on the phagocytosis of erythrocytes and ink by the reticulohistiocyte system in the isolated, perfused liver of rats of various ages [in German; English abstract]. *Arzneimittelforschung.* 1984;34:691-695.

22. Wagner VH, Proksch A, Riess-Maurer I, et al. Immunostimulating polysaccharides (heteroglycans) of higher plants [translated from German]. *Arzneimittelforschung.* 1985;35:1069-1075.

23. Melchart D, Linde K, Worku F, et al. Results of five randomized studies on the immunomodulatory activity of preparations of *Echinacea*. *J Altern Complement Med.* 1995;1:145-160.

24. Rehman J, Dillow JM, Carter SM, et al. Increased production of antigen-specific immunoglobulins G and M following in vivo treatment with the medicinal plants *Echinacea angustifolia* and *Hydrastis canadensis*. *Immunol Lett.* 1999;68:391-395.

25. See DM, Broumand N, Sahl L, et al. In vitro effects of *Echinacea* and ginseng on natural killer cells and antibody-dependent cell cytotoxicity in healthy subjects and chronic fatigue syndrome or acquired immunodeficiency patients. *Immunopharmacology.* 1997;35:229-235.

26. Parnham MJ. Benefit-risk assessment of the squeezed sap of the purple coneflower (*Echinacea purpurea*) for long-term oral immunostimulation. *Phytomedicine.* 1996; 3:95-102.

27. Schulz V, Hansel R, Tyler VE. *Rational Phytotherapy: A Physicians' Guide to Herbal Medicine*, 3rd ed. Berlin, Germany: Springer-Verlag; 1998:276, 278.

28. Mengs U, Clare CB, Poiley JA. Toxicity of *Echinacea purpurea*: acute, subacute and genotoxicity studies. *Arzneimittelforschung.* 1991;41:1076-1081.

29. Blumenthal M, ed. *The Complete Commission E Monographs, Therapeutic Guide to Herbal Medicines.* Boston, Mass: Integrative Medicine Communications; 1998:122.
30. Gallo M, Sarkar M, Au W, et al. Pregnancy outcome following gestational exposure to echinacea: a prospective controlled study. *Arch Intern Med.* 2000;160:3141-3143.
31. Budzinski JW, Foster BC, Vandenhoek S, et al. An in vitro evaluation of human cytochrome P450 3A4 inhibition by selected commercial herbal extracts and tinctures. *Phytomedicine.* 2000;7:273-282.
32. Mullins RJ, Heddle R. Adverse reactions associated with echinacea: the Australian experience. *Ann Allergy Asthma Immunol.* 2002;88:42-51.

Elderberry

1. Zakay-Rones Z, Varsano N, Zlotnik M, et al. Inhibition of several strains of influenza virus and reduction of symptoms by an elderberry extract (*Sambucus nigra* L.) during an outbreak of influenza B Panama. *J Altern Complement Med.* 1995;1:361-369.
2. Shapira-Nahor B, Zakay-Rones Z, Mumcuoglu M. The effect of Sambucol® on HIV infection in vitro. Presented at: Annual Israel Congress of Microbiology; February 6-7, 1995; Jerusalem, Israel.
3. Morag A, Mumcuoglu M, Baybikov T, et al. Inhibition of sensitive and acyclovir-resistant HSV-1 strains by an elderberry extract in vitro [abstract]. *Phylotherapie.* 1997;25:97-98.
4. Barak V, Halperin T, Kalickman I. The effect of Sambucol, a black elderberry-based, natural product, on the production of human cytokines: I. Inflammatory cytokines. *Eur Cytokine Netw.* 2001;12:290-296.

Eleutherococcus

1. Williams M. Immuno-protection against herpes simplex type II infection by *Eleutherococcus* root extract. *Int J Alt Complement Med.* 1995;13:9-12.
2. Farnsworth NR, Kinghorn AD, Soejarto DD, et al. Siberian ginseng (*Eleutherococcus senticosus*): current status as an adaptogen. *Econ Med Plant Res.* 1985;1:156-215.
3. Bohn B, Nebe CT, Birr C. Flow-cytometric studies with *Eleutherococcus senticosus* extract as an immunomodulatory agent. *Arzneimittelforschung.* 1987;37:1193-1196.
4. Dowling EA, Redondo DR, Branch JD, et al. Effect of *Eleutherococcus senticosus* on submaximal and maximal exercise performance. *Med Sci Sports Exerc.* 1996;28:482-489.
5. Eschbach LF, Webster MJ, Boyd JC, et al. The effect of Siberian ginseng (*Eleutherococcus senticosus*) on substrate utilization and performance. *Int J Sport Nutr Exerc Metab.* 2000;10:444-451.
6. Newall CA, Anderson LA, Phillipson JD. *Herbal Medicines: A Guide for Health-Care Professionals.* London, England: The Pharmaceutical Press; 1996:143.
7. McRae S. Elevated serum digoxin levels in a patient taking digoxin and Siberian ginseng. *CMAJ.* 1996;155:293-295.
8. Gaffney BT, Hugel HM, Rich PA. The effects of *Eleutherococcus senticosus* and *Panax ginseng* on steroidal hormone indices of stress and lymphocyte subset numbers in endurance athletes. *Life Sci.* 2001;70:431-442.
9. Szolomicki J, Samochowiec L, Wojcicki J, et al. The influence of active components of *Eleutherococcus senticosus* on cellular defence and physical fitness in man. *Phytother Res.* 2000;14:30-35.
10. Bohn B, Nebe CT, Birr C. Flow-cytometric studies with *Eleutherococcus senticosus* extract as an immunomodulatory agent. *Arzneimittelforschung.* 1987;37(10):1193-1196.

Ephedra

1. Astrup A, Breum L, Toubro S, et al. The effect and safety of an ephedrine/caffeine compound compared to ephedrine, caffeine and placebo in obese subjects on an energy restricted diet: a double-blind trial. *Int J Obes Relat Metab Disord.* 1992;16:269-277.
2. Molnar D, Torok K, Erhardt E, et al. Safety and efficacy of treatment with an ephedrine/caffeine mixture: the first double-blind placebo-controlled pilot study in adolescents. *Int J Obes Relat Metab Disord.* 2000;24:1573-1578.

3. Breum L, Pedersen JK, Ahlstrom F, et al. Comparison of an ephedrine/caffeine combination and dexfenfluramine in the treatment of obesity: a double-blind multi-centre trial in general practice. *Int J Obes Relat Metab Disord.* 1994;18:99-103.
4. Boozer CN, Nasser JA, Heymsfield SB, et al. An herbal supplement containing Ma Huang-Guarana for weight loss: a randomized, double-blind trial. *Int J Obes Relat Metab Disord.* 2001;25:316-324.
5. Norregaard J, Jorgensen S, Mikkelsen KL, et al. The effect of ephedrine plus caffeine on smoking cessation and postcessation weight gain. *Clin Pharmacol Ther.* 1996; 60:679-686.
6. Astrup A, Breum L, Toubro S. Pharmacological and clinical studies of ephedrine and other thermogenic agonists. *Obes Res.* 1995;3:537S-540S.
7. Gurley BJ, Gardner SF, Hubbard MA. Content versus label claims in ephedra-containing dietary supplements. *Am J Health Syst Pharm.* 2000;57:963-969.
8. MedscapeWire. No association between reported adverse events and ephedra when consumed as directed. Available at: http://www.medscape.com/MedscapeWire/2000/0800/medwire.0816.No.html. Accessed August 16, 2000.
9. Haller CA, Benowitz NL. Adverse cardiovascular and central nervous system events associated with dietary supplements containing ephedra alkaloids. *N Engl J Med.* 2000;343:1833-1838.
10. *PDR for Herbal Medicines.* Montvale, NJ: Medical Economics Company; 1998:827.
11. Blumenthal M, King P. Ma huang: ancient herb, modern medicine, regulatory dilemma. A review of the botany, chemistry, medicinal uses, safety concerns, and legal status of ephedra and its alkaloids. *HerbalGram.* 1995;34:22-57.
12. Nadir A, Agrawal S, King PD, Marshall JB. Acute hepatitis associated with the use of a Chinese herbal product, ma-huang. *Am J Gastroenterol.* 1996;91:1436-1438.
13. Samenuk D, Link MS, Homoud MK, et al. Adverse cardiovascular events temporally associated with ma huang, an herbal source of ephedrine. *Mayo Clin Proc.* 2002;77:12-16.

Estriol

1. Lemon HM, Kumar PF, Peterson C, et al. Inhibition of radiogenic mammary carcinoma in rats by estriol or tamoxifen. *Cancer.* 1989;63:1685-1692.
2. Lemon HM, Wotiz HH, Parsons L, et al. Reduced estriol excretion in patients with breast cancer prior to endocrine therapy. *JAMA.* 1966;196:1128-1136.
3. Lemon HM. Pathophysiologic considerations in the treatment of menopausal patients with oestrogens; the role of oestriol in the prevention of mammary carcinoma. *Acta Endocrinol Suppl (Copenh).* 1980;233:17-27.
4. Hayashi T, Ito I, Kano H, et al. Estriol (E3) replacement improves endothelial function and bone mineral density in very elderly women. *J Gerontol A Biol Sci Med Sci.* 2000;55:B183-B190.
5. Takahashi K, Manabe A, Okada M, et al. Efficacy and safety of oral estriol for managing postmenopausal symptoms. *Maturitas.* 2000;34:169-177.
6. Minaguchi H, Uemura T, Shirasu K, et al. Effect of estriol on bone loss in postmenopausal Japanese women: a multicenter prospective open study. *J Obstet Gynaecol Res.* 1996;22:259-265.
7. Itoi H, Minakami H, Sato I. Comparison of the long-term effects of oral estriol with the effects of conjugated estrogen, 1-alpha-hydroxyvitamin D3 and calcium lactate on vertebral bone loss in early menopausal women. *Maturitas.* 1997;28:11-17.
8. Dugal R, Hesla K, Sordal T, et al. Comparison of usefulness of estradiol vaginal tablets and estriol vagitories for treatment of vaginal atrophy. *Acta Obstet Gynecol Scand.* 2000;79:293-297.
9. Raz R, Stamm WE. A controlled trial of intravaginal estriol in postmenopausal women with recurrent urinary tract infections. *N Engl J Med.* 1993;329:753-756.
10. van der Linden MC, Gerretsen G, Brandhorst MS, et al. The effect of estriol on the cytology of urethra and vagina in postmenopausal women with genito-urinary symptoms. *Eur J Obstet Gynecol Reprod Biol.* 1993;51:29-33.

11. Holland EF, Leather AT, Studd JW. Increase in bone mass of older postmenopausal women with low mineral bone density after one year of percutaneous oestradiol implants. *Br J Obstet Gynaecol.* 1995;102:238-242.

12. Nozaki M, Hashimoto K, Inoue Y, et al. Usefulness of estriol for the treatment of bone loss in postmenopausal women [in Japanese; English abstract]. *Nippon Sanka Fujinka Gakkai Zasshi.* 1996;48:83-88.

13. Lippman M, Monaco ME, Bolan G. Effects of estrone, estradiol and estriol on hormone-responsive human breast cancer in long-term tissue culture. *Cancer Res.* 1977;37:1901-1907.

14. Granberg S, Ylostalo P, Wikland M, et al. Endometrial sonographic and histologic findings in women with and without hormonal replacement therapy suffering from postmenopausal bleeding. *Maturitas.* 1997;27:35-40.

15. Weiderpass E, Baron JA, Adami HO, et al. Low-potency oestrogen and risk of endometrial cancer: a case-control study. *Lancet.* 1999;353:1824-1828.

16. Montoneri C, Zarbo G, Garofalo A, et al. Effects of estriol administration on human postmenopausal endometrium. *Clin Exp Obstet Gynecol.* 1987;14:178-181.

17. Punnonen R, Soderstrom KO. The effect of oral estriol succinate therapy on the endometrial morphology in postmenopausal women: the significance of fractionation of the dose. *Eur J Obstet Gynecol Reprod Biol.* 1983;14:217-224.

18. Vooijs GP, Geurts TB. Review of the endometrial safety during intravaginal treatment with estriol. *Eur J Obstet Gynecol Reprod Biol.* 1995;62:101-106.

Eyebright

1. Duke JA. *CRC Handbook of Medicinal Herbs.* Boca Raton, Fla: CRC Press; 1985:141.

Fenugreek

1. Sharma RD, Raghuram TC, Rao NS. Effect of fenugreek seeds on blood glucose and serum lipids in type I diabetes. *Eur J Clin Nutr.* 1990;44:301-306.

2. Sharma RD, Sarkar A, Hazra DK, et al. Use of fenugreek seed powder in the management of non-insulin dependent diabetes mellitus. *Nutr Res.* 1996;16:1331-1339.

3. Madar Z, Abel R, Samish S, et al. Glucose-lowering effect of fenugreek in non-insulin dependent diabetics. *Eur J Clin Nutr.* 1988;42:51-54.

4. Madar Z. New sources of dietary fibre. *Int J Obes.* 1987;11(suppl 1):57-65.

5. Leung AY, Foster S. *Encyclopedia of Common Natural Ingredients Used in Food, Drugs, and Cosmetics.* New York, NY: John Wiley & Sons; 1996:243-244.

6. Gupta A, Gupta R, Lal B. Effect of Trigonella foenum-graecum (fenugreek) seeds on glycaemic control and insulin resistance in type 2 diabetes mellitus: a double blind placebo controlled study. *J Assoc Physicians India.* 2001;49:1057-1061.

7. Bhardwaj PK, Dasgupta DJ, Prashar BS, et al. Control of hyperglycaemia and hyperlipidaemia by plant product. *J Assoc Physicians India.* 1994;42:33-35.

8. Evans AJ, Hood RL, Oakenfull DG, et al. Relationship between structure and function of dietary fibre: a comparative study of the effects of three galactomannans on cholesterol metabolism in the rat. *Br J Nutr.* 1992;68(1):217-229.

9. Sauvaire Y, Ribes G, Baccou JC, et al. Implication of steroid saponins and sapogenins in the hypocholesterolemic effect of fenugreek. *Lipids.* 1991;26(3):191-197.

10. Sowmya P, Rajyalakshmi P. Hypocholesterolemic effect of germinated fenugreek seeds in human subjects. *Plant Foods Hum Nutr.* 1999;53(4):359-365.

11. Stark A, Madar Z. The effect of an ethanol extract derived from fenugreek (Trigonella foenum-graecum) on bile acid absorption and cholesterol levels in rats. *Br J Nutr.* 1993;69(1):277-287.

12. Valette G, Sauvaire Y, Baccou JC, et al. Hypocholesterolaemic effect of fenugreek seeds in dogs. *Atherosclerosis.* 1984;50:105-111.

13. Muralidhara, Narasimhamurthy K, Viswanatha S, et al. Acute and subchronic toxicity assessment of debitterized fenugreek powder in the mouse and rat. *Food Chem Toxicol.* 1999;37:831-838.

14. Lambert JP, Cormier A. Potential interaction between warfarin and boldo-fenugreek. *Pharmacotherapy.* 2001;21:509-512.

Feverfew

1. Murphy JJ, Heptinstall S, Mitchell JRA. Randomized double-blind placebo-controlled trial of feverfew in migraine prevention. *Lancet.* 1988;23:189-192.
2. Palevitch DG, Earon G, Carasso R. Feverfew *(Tanacetum parthenium)* as a prophylactic treatment for migraine: a double-blind placebo-controlled study. *Phytother Res.* 1997;11:508-511.
3. Johnson ES, Kadam NP, Hylands DM, et al. Efficacy of feverfew as a prophylactic treatment of migraine. *Br Med J (Clin Res Ed).* 1985;291:569-573.
4. De Weerdt CJ, Bootsma HPR, Hendriks H. Herbal medicines in migraine prevention: randomized double-blind placebo-controlled crossover trial of a feverfew preparation. *Phytomedicine.* 1996;3:225-230.
5. Pfaffenrath V, Fischer M, Friede M, et al. Clinical dose-response study for the investigation of efficacy and tolerability of *Tanacetum parthenium* in migraine prophylaxis. Presented at: Deutscher Schmerzkongress; October 20-24, 1999; Munich, Germany.
6. Pattrick M, Heptinstall S, Doherty M. Feverfew in rheumatoid arthritis: a double blind, placebo controlled study. *Ann Rheum Dis.* 1989;48:547-549.
7. Collier HO, Butt NM, McDonald-Gibson WJ, et al. Extract of feverfew inhibits prostaglandin biosynthesis [letter]. *Lancet.* 1980;2:922-923.
8. Sumner H, Salan U, Knight DW, Hoult JR. Inhibition of 5-lipoxygenase and cyclo-oxygenase in leukocytes by feverfew: involvement of sesquiterpene lactones and other components. *Biochem Pharmacol.* 1992;43:2313-2320.
9. Williams CA, Hoult JRS, Harborne JB, et al. A biologically active lipophilic flavonol from *Tanacetum parthenium. Phytochemistry.* 1995;38:267-270.
10. Baldwin CA, Anderson LA, Philipson JD. What pharmacists should know about feverfew. *Pharm J.* 1987;239:237-238.
11. Heptinstall S, White A, Williamson L, et al. Extracts of feverfew inhibit granule secretion in blood platelets and polymorphonuclear leucocytes. *Lancet.* 1985;8437:1071-1074.
12. Makheja AN, Bailey JM. The active principle in feverfew [letter]. *Lancet.* 1981;2:1054.
13. Groenewegen WA, Knight DW, Heptinstall S. Progress in the medicinal chemistry of the herb feverfew. *Prog Med Chem.* 1992;29:217-238.
14. Biggs MJ, Johnson ES, Persaud NP, et al. Platelet aggregation in patients using feverfew for migraine [letter]. *Lancet.* 1982;2:776.

Fish Oil

1. James MJ, Cleland LG. Dietary N-3 fatty acids and therapy for rheumatoid arthritis. *Semin Arthritis Rheum.* 1997;27:85-97.
2. Volker D, Fitzgerald P, Major G, et al. Efficacy of fish oil concentrate in the treatment of rheumatoid arthritis. *J Rheumatol.* 2000;27:2343-2346.
3. Harris WS. N-3 fatty acids and serum lipoproteins: human studies. *Am J Clin Nutr.* 1997;65(suppl):1645S-1654S.
4. Cobiac L, Clifton PM, Abbey M, et al. Lipid, lipoprotein, and hemostatic effects of fish vs fish-oil n-3 fatty acids in mildly hyperlipidemic males. *Am J Clin Nutr.* 1991;53:1210-1216.
5. Harris WS. N-3 fatty acids and lipoproteins: comparison of results from human and animal studies. *Lipids.* 1996;31:243-252.
6. Nenseter MS, Osterud B, Larsen T, et al. Effect of Norwegian fish powder on risk factors for coronary heart disease among hypercholesterolemic individuals. *Nutr Metab Cardiovasc Dis.* 2000;10:323-330.
7. Durrington PN, Bhatnagar D, Mackness MI, et al. An omega-3 polyunsaturated fatty acid concentrate administered for one year decreased triglycerides in simvastatin treated patients with coronary heart disease and persisting hypertriglyceridaemia. *Heart.* 2001;85:544-548.
8. van Dam M, Stalenhoef AF, Wittekoek J, et al. Efficacy of concentrated n-3 fatty acids in hypertriglyceridaemia: a comparison with gemfibrozil. *Clin Drug Invest.* 2001;21:175-181.

9. Dyerberg J. N-3 fatty acids and coronary artery disease: potentials and problems. *Omega-3, Lipoproteins, and Atherosclerosis.* 1996;27:251-258. Cited by: Werbach MR. *Nutritional Influences on Illness* [book on CD-ROM]. Tarzana, Calif: Third Line Press; 1998.

10. Lungershausen YK, Abbey M, Nestel PJ, et al. Reduction of blood pressure and plasma triglycerides by omega-3 fatty acids in treated hypertensives. *J Hypertens.* 1994;12:1041-1045.

11. Radack K, Deck C, Huster G. The effects of low doses of n-3 fatty acid supplements on blood pressure in hypertensive subjects. *Arch Intern Med.* 1991;151:1173-1180.

12. Singer P, Jaeger W, Wirth M, et al. Lipid and blood pressure-lowering effect of mackerel diet in man. *Atherosclerosis.* 1983;49:99-108.

13. Singer P, Melzer S, Goschel M, et al. Fish oil amplifies the effect of propranolol in mild essential hypertension. *Hypertension.* 1990;16:682-691.

14. Appel LJ, Miller ER III, Seidler AJ, et al. Does supplementation of diet with 'fish oil' reduce blood pressure? A meta-analysis of controlled clinical trials. *Arch Intern Med.* 1993;153:1429-1438.

15. Whelton PK, Kumanyika SK, Cook NR, et al. Efficacy of nonpharmacologic interventions in adults with high-normal blood pressure: results from phase 1 of the Trials of Hypertension Prevention. *Am J Clin Nutr.* 1997;65 (suppl):S652-S660.

16. Holm T, Andreassen AK, Aukrust P, et al. Omega-3 fatty acids improve blood pressure control and preserve renal function in hypertensive heart transplant recipients. *Eur Heart J.* 2001;22:428-436.

17. Mori TA, Bao DQ, Burke V, et al. Docosahexaenoic acid but not eicosapentaenoic acid lowers ambulatory blood pressure and heart rate in humans. *Hypertension.* 1999;34:253-260.

18. Guallar E, Hennekens CH, Sacks FM, et al. A prospective study of plasma fish oil levels and incidence of myocardial infarction in U.S. male physicians. *J Am Coll Cardiol.* 1995;25:387-394.

19. Iso H, Rexrode KM, Stampfer MJ, et al. Intake of fish and omega-3 fatty acids and risk of stroke in women. *JAMA.* 2001;285:304-312.

20. Kromhout D, Bosschieter EB, de Lezenne Coulander C. The inverse relation between fish consumption and 20-year mortality from coronary heart disease. *N Engl J Med.* 1985;312:1205-1209.

21. Shekelle RB, Missell LV, Paul O, et al. Fish consumption and mortality from coronary heart disease [letter]. *N Engl J Med.* 1985;313:820-821.

22. Dolecek TA, Grandits G. Dietary polyunsaturated fatty acids and mortality in the Multiple Risk Factor Intervention Trial (MRFIT). *World Rev Nutr Diet.* 1991;66:205-216.

23. Kromhout D, Feskens EJM, Bowles CH. The protective effect of a small amount of fish on coronary heart disesae mortality in an elderly population. *Int J Epidemiol.* 1995;24:340-345.

24. Vollset SE, Heuch I, Bjelke E. Fish consumption and mortality from coronary heart disease [letter]. *N Engl J Med.* 1985;313:820-821.

25. Curb JD, Reed DM. Fish consumption and mortality from coronary heart disease [letter]. *N Engl J Med.* 1985;313:821-822.

26. Burr ML, Fehily AM, Gilbert JF, et al. Effects of changes in fat, fish, and fibre intakes on death and myocardial reinfarction: diet and reinfarction trial (DART). *Lancet.* 1989;2:757-761.

27. Ascherio A, Rimm EB, Stampfer MJ, et al. Dietary intake of marine n-3 fatty acids, fish intake, and the risk of coronary disease among men. *N Engl J Med.* 1995;332:977-982.

28. Leaf A, Jorgensen MB, Jacobs AK, et al. Do fish oils prevent restenosis after coronary angioplasty? *Circulation.* 1994;90:2248-2257.

29. Sacks FM, Stone PH, Gibson CM, et al. Controlled trial of fish oil for regression of human coronary atherosclerosis: HARP Research Group. *J Am Coll Cardiol.* 1995;25:1492-1498.

30. Meier R, Wettstein A, Drewe J, et al. Fish oil (Eicosapen) is less effective than metronidazole in combination with pantoprazole and clarithromycin for *Helicobacter pylori* eradication *Aliment Pharmacol Ther.* 2001;15:851-855.

31. de Lorgeril M, Renaud S, Mamelle N, et al. Mediterranean alpha-linolenic acid-rich diet in secondary prevention of coronary heart disease. *Lancet.* 1994;343:1454-1459.

32. Siscovick DS, Raghunathan TE, King I, et al. Dietary intake and cell membrane levels of long-chain N-3 polyunsaturated fatty acids and the risk of primary cardiac arrest. *JAMA.* 1995;274:1363-1367.

33. Billman GE, Hallaq H, Leaf A. Prevention of ischemia-induced ventricular fibrillation by omega 3 fatty acids. *Proc Natl Acad Sci USA.* 1994;91:4427-4430.

34. Sellmayer A, Witzgall H, Lorenz RL, et al. Effects of dietary fish oil on ventricular premature complexes. *Am J Cardiol.* 1995;76:974-977.

35. Nilsen DW, Albrektsen G, Landmark K, et al. Effects of a high-dose concentrate of n-3 fatty acids or corn oil introduced early after an acute myocardial infarction on serum triacylglycerol and HDL cholesterol. *Am J Clin Nutr.* 2001;74:50-56.

36. Harel Z, Biro FM, Kottenhahn RK, et al. Supplementation with omega-3 polyunsaturated fatty acids in the management of dysmenorrhea in adolescents. *Am J Obstet Gynecol.* 1996;174:1335-1338.

37. Deutch B, Jorgensen EB, Hansen JC. Menstrual discomfort in Danish women reduced by dietary supplements of omega-3 PUFA and B_{12} (fish oil or seal oil capsules). *Nutr Res.* 2000;20:621-631.

38. Stoll AL, Severus WE, Freeman MP, et al. Omega 3 fatty acids in bipolar disorder: a preliminary double-blind, placebo-controlled trial. *Arch Gen Psychiatry.* 1999;56:407-412.

39. DiGiacomo RA, Kremer JM, Shah DM. Fish-oil dietary supplementation in patients with Raynaud's phenomenon: a double-blind, controlled, prospective study. *Am J Med.* 1989;86:158-164.

40. Ringer TV, Hughes GS, Spillers. Fish oil blunts the pain response to cold pressor testing in normal males [abstract]. *J Am Coll Nutr.* 1989;8:435.

41. Walton AJ, Snaith ML,Locniskar M. Dietary fish oil and the severity of symptoms in patients with systemic lupus erythematosus. *Ann Rheum Dis.* 1991;50:463-466.

42. Tomer A, Kasey S, Connor WE, et al. Reduction of pain episodes and prothrombotic activity in sickle cell disease by dietary n-3 fatty acids. *Thromb Haemost.* 2001;85:966-974.

43. Donadio JV Jr, Grande JP, Bergstralh EJ, et al. The long-term outcome of patients with IgA nephropathy treated with fish oil in a controlled trial. Mayo Nephrology Collaborative Group. *J Am Soc Nephrol.* 1999;10:1772-1777.

44. Peet M, Brind J, Ramchand CN, et al. Two double-blind placebo-controlled pilot studies of eicosapentaenoic acid in the treatment of schizophrenia. *Schizophr Res.* 2001;49:243-251.

45. Bittiner SB, Tucker WF, Cartwright I, et al. A double-blind, randomized, placebo-controlled trial of fish oil in psoriasis. *Lancet.* 1988;1:378-380.

46. Soyland E, Funk J, Rajka G, et al. Effect of dietary supplementation with very-long-chain n-3 fatty acids in patients with psoriasis. *N Engl J Med.* 1993;328:1812-1816.

47. Halsted CH, Ghandi G, Tamura T. Sulfasalazine inhibits the absorption of folates in ulcerative colitis. *N Engl J Med.* 1981;305:1513-1517.

48. Aslan A, Triadafilopoulos G. Fish oil fatty acid supplementation in active ulcerative colitis: a double-blind, placebo-controlled, crossover study. *Am J Gastroenterol.* 1992;87:432-437.

49. Almallah YZ, El-Tahir A, Heys SD, et al. Distal procto-colitis and n-3 polyunsaturated fatty acids: the mechanism(s) of natural cytotoxicity inhibition. *Eur J Clin Invest.* 2000;30:58-65.

50. Stenson WF, Cort D, Rodgers J, et al. Dietary supplementation with fish oil in ulcerative colitis. *Ann Intern Med.* 1992;116:609-614.

51. Hawthorne AB, Daneshmend TK, Hawkey CJ, et al. Treatment of ulcerative colitis with fish oil supplementation: a prospective 12-month randomized controlled trial. *Gut.* 1992;33:922-928.

52. Belluzzi A, Brignola C, Campieri M, et al. Effect of an enteric-coated fish-oil preparation on relapses in Crohn's disease. *N Engl J Med.* 1996;334:1557-1560.

53. Lorenz-Meyer H, Bauer P, Nicolay C, et al. Omega-3 fatty acids and low carbohydrate diet for maintenance of remission in Crohn's disease: a randomized controlled multicenter trial. Study Group Members (German Crohn's Disease Study Group). *Scand J Gastroenterol.* 1996;31:778-785.

54. Lorenz R, Weber PC, Szimnau P, et al. Supplementation with n-3 fatty acids from fish oil in chronic inflammatory bowel disease—a randomized, placebo-controlled, double-blind cross-over trial. *J Intern Med Suppl.* 1989;225:225-232.

55. Greenfield SM, Green AT, Teare JP, et al. A randomized controlled study of evening primrose oil and fish oil in ulcerative colitis. *Aliment Pharmacol Ther.* 1993;7:159-166.

56. Loeschke K, Ueberschaer B, Pietsch A, et al. N-3 fatty acids only delay early relapse of ulcerative colitis in remission. *Dig Dis Sci.* 1996;41:2087-2094.

57. Carlson SE, Werkman SH, Rhodes PG, et al. Visual-acuity development in healthy preterm infants: effect of marine-oil supplementation. *Am J Clin Nutr.* 1993;58:35-42.

58. Hibbeln JR, Salem N Jr. Dietary polyunsaturated fatty acids and depression: when cholesterol does not satisfy. *Am J Clin Nutr.* 1995;62:1-9.

59. Olsen SF, Sorensen JD, Secher NJ, et al. Randomized controlled trial of effect of fish-oil supplementation on pregnancy duration. *Lancet.* 1992;339:1003-1007.

60. Buck AC, Jenkins A, Lingam K, et al. The treatment of idiopathic recurrent urolithiasis with fish oil (EPA) and evening primrose oil (GLA)—a double blind study. *J Urol.* 1993;149:253A.

61. Norrish AE, Skeaff CM, Arribas GLB, et al. Prostate cancer risk and consumption of fish oils: a dietary biomarker-based case-control study. *Br J Cancer.* 1999;81:1238-1242.

62. Behan PO, Behan WM, Horrobin D. Effect of high doses of essential fatty acids on the postviral fatigue syndrome. *Acta Neurol Scand.* 1990;82:209-216.

63. Warren G, McKendrick M, Peet M. The role of essential fatty acids in chronic fatigue syndrome. A case-controlled study of red-cell membrane essential fatty acids (EFA) and a placebo-controlled treatment study with high dose of EFA. *Acta Neurol Scand.* 1999;99:112-116.

64. Gerbi A, Maixent JM, Ansaldi JL, et al. Fish oil supplementation prevents diabetes-induced nerve conduction velocity and neuroanatomical changes in rats. *J Nutr.* 1999;129:207-213.

65. Nightingale S, Woo E, Smith AD, et al. Red blood cell and adipose tissue fatty acids in mild inactive multiple sclerosis. *Acta Neurol Scand.* 1990;82:43-50.

66. Cunnane SC, Ho SY, Dore-Duffy P, et al. Essential fatty acid and lipid profiles in plasma and erythrocytes in patients with multiple sclerosis. *Am J Clin Nutr.* 1989;50:801-806.

67. Gallai V, Sarchielli P, Trequattrini A, et al. Cytokine secretion and eicosanoid production in the peripheral blood mononuclear cells of MS patients undergoing dietary supplementation with N-3 polyunsaturated fatty acids. *J Neuroimmunol.* 1995;56:143-153.

68. Goldberg P, Fleming MC, Picard EH. Multiple sclerosis: decreased relapse rate through dietary supplementation with calcium, magnesium and vitamin D. *Med Hypotheses.* 1986;21:193-200.

69. Bates D. Dietary lipids and multiple sclerosis. *Ups J Med Sci Suppl.* 1990;48:173-187.

70. Conquer JA, Martin JB, Tummon I, et al. Effect of DHA supplementation on DHA status and sperm motility in asthenozoospermic males. *Lipids.* 2000;35:149-154.

71. Voigt RG, Llorente AM, Jensen CL, et al. A randomized, double-blind, placebo-controlled trial of docosahexaenoic acid supplementation in children with attention-deficit/hyperactivity disorder. *J Pediatr.* 2001;139:189-196.

72. Woods RK, Thien FC, Abramson MJ. Dietary marine fatty acids (fish oil) for asthma. *Cochrane Database Syst Rev.* 2000;(4):1-12.

73. Montori VM, Farmer A, Wollan PC, et al. Fish oil supplementation in type 2 diabetes: a quantitative systematic review. *Diabetes Care.* 2000;23:1407-1415.

74. Thies F, Nebe-Von-Caron G, Powell JR, et al. Dietary supplementation with eico-sapentaenoic acid, but not with other long-chain N-3 or N-6 polyunsaturated fatty acids, decreases natural killer cell activity in healthy subjects aged >55 y. *Am J Clin Nutr*. 2001;73:539-548.

75. Kinrys G. Hypomania associated with omega-3 fatty acids and their role in depressive disorders [abstract]. *Int J Neuropsychopharmcol*. 2000;3(suppl 1):S298.

76. Bucher HC, Hengstler P, Schindler C, et al. N-3 polyunsaturated fatty acids in coronary heart disease: a meta-analysis of randomized controlled trials. *Am J Med*. 2002; 112:298-304.

77. Yam D, Bott-Kanner G, Genin I, et al. The effect of omega-3 fatty acids on risk factors for cardiovascular diseases. *Harefuah*. 2001;140:1156-1158.

78. Angerer P, Stork S, Kothny W, et al. Effect of marine omega-3 fatty acids on peripheral atherosclerosis in patients with coronary artery disease—a randomized 2 year intervention trial [abstract]. *Eur Heart J*. 2001;22(suppl):162.

79. Gruppo Italiano per lo Studio della Sopravvivenza nell'Infarto miocardico. Dietary supplementation with n-3 polyunsaturated fatty acids and vitamin E after myocardial infarction: results of the GISSI-Prevenzione trial. *Lancet*. 1999;354:447-455

80. Singh RB, Niaz MA, Sharma JP, et al. Randomized, double-blind, placebo-controlled trial of fish oil and mustard oil in patients with suspected acute myocardial infarction: the Indian experiment of infarct survival. 4. *Cardiovasc Drugs Ther*. 1997;11:485-491.

81. Nemets B, Stahl Z, Belmaker RH. Addition of omega-3 fatty acid to maintenance medication treatment for recurrent unipolar depressive disorder. *Am J Psychiatry*. 2002;159:477-479.

82. Fenton WS, Dickerson F, Boronow J, et al. A placebo-controlled trial of omega-3 fatty acid (ethyl eicosapentaenoic acid) supplementation for residual symptoms and cognitive impairment in schizophrenia. *Am J Psychiatry*. 2001;158:2071-2074.

83. Pradalier A, Bakouche P, Baudesson G, et al. Failure of omega-3 polyunsaturated fatty acids in prevention of migraine: a double-blind study versus placebo. *Cephalalgia*. 2001;21:818-822.

Flaxseed

1. Blumenthal M, ed. (1998). *The Complete German Commission E Monographs, Therapeutic Guide to Herbal Medicine*. Boston, Mass: Integrative Medicine Communications; 1998:132 [footnote].

2. Tarpila S, Kivinen A. Ground flaxseed is an effective hypolipidemic bulk laxative [abstract]. *Gastroenterology*. 1997;112:A836.

3. Arjmandi BH, Khan DA, Juma S, et al. Whole flaxseed consumption lowers serum LDL-cholesterol and lipoprotein (a) concentrations in postmenopausal women. *Nutr Res*. 1998;18:1203-1214.

4. Jenkins DJ, Kendall CW, Vidgen E, et al. Health aspects of partially defatted flaxseed, including effects on serum lipids, oxidative measures, and ex vivo androgen and progestin activity: a controlled crossover trial. *Am J Clin Nutr*. 1999;69:395-402.

5. Tarpila S, Kivinen A. Ground flaxseed is an effective hypolipidemic bulk laxative [abstract]. *Gastroenterology*. 1997;112:A836.

6. Adlercreutz H, Mazur W. Phyto-oestrogens and Western diseases. *Ann Med*. 1997; 29:95-120.

7. Thompson LU. Experimental studies on lignans and cancer. *Baillieres Clin Endocrinol Metab*. 1998;12:691-705.

8. Thompson LU, Rickard SE, Orcheson LJ, et al. Flaxseed and its lignan and oil components reduce mammary tumor growth at a late stage of carcinogenesis. *Carcinogenesis*. 1996;17:1373-1376.

9. Serraino M, Thompson LU. The effect of flaxseed supplementation on the initiation and promotional stages of mammary tumorigenesis. *Nutr Cancer*. 1992;17:153-159.

10. Yan L, Yee JA, Li D, et al. Dietary flaxseed supplementation and experimental metastasis of melanoma cells in mice. *Cancer Lett*. 1998;124:181-186.

11. Adlercreutz H, Mazur W. Phyto-oestrogens and Western diseases. *Ann Med*. 1997; 29:95-120.

12. Sung MK, Lautens M, Thompson LU. Mammalian lignans inhibit the growth of estrogen-independent human colon tumor cells. *Anticancer Res.* 1998;18:1405-1408.

13. Demark-Wahnefried W, Price DT, Polascik TJ, et al. Pilot study of dietary fat restriction and flaxseed supplementation in men with prostate cancer before surgery: exploring the effects on hormonal levels, prostate-specific antigen, and histopathologic features. *Urology.* 2001;58:47-52.

14. Clark WF, Parbtani A, Huff MW, et al. Flaxseed: a potential treatment for lupus nephritis. *Kidney Int.* 1995;48:475-480.

15. Ogborn MR, Nitschmann E, Bankovic-Calic N, et al. The effect of dietary flaxseed supplementation on organic anion and osmolyte content and excretion in rat polycystic kidney disease. *Biochem Cell Biol.* 1998;76:553-559.

16. Prasad K. Hydroxyl radical-scavenging property of secoisolariciresinol diglucoside (SDG) isolated from flax-seed. *Mol Cell Biochem.* 1997;168:117-123.

17. Yuan YV, et al. Short-term feeding of flaxseed or its lignan has minor influence on in vivo hepatic antioxidant status in young rats. *Nutr Res.* 1999;19:1233-1243.

18. European Scientific Cooperative on Phytotherapy. *Lini semen,* linseed. Exeter, UK: ESCOP; 1996-1997. Monographs on the Medicinal Uses of Plant Drugs, Fascicule 1:1-5.

19. Wanasundara PK, Shahidi F. Process-induced compositional changes of flaxseed. *Adv Exp Med Biol.* 1998;434:307-325.

20. Tou JCL, Chen J, Thompson LU. Flaxseed and its lignan precursor, secoisolariciresinol diglycoside, affect pregnancy outcome and reproductive development in rats. *J Nutr.* 1998;128:1861-1868.

21. Lucas EA, Wild RD, Hammond LJ, et al. Flaxseed improves lipid profile without altering biomarkers of bone metabolism in postmenopausal women. *J Clin Endocrinol Metab.* 2002;87:1527-1532.

22. Hutchins AM, Martini MC, Olson BA, et al. Flaxseed consumption influences endogenous hormone concentrations in postmenopausal women. *Nutr Cancer.* 2001; 39:58-65.

Flaxseed Oil

1. Nordstrom DC, Honkanen VE, Nasu Y, et al. Alpha-linolenic acid in the treatment of rheumatoid arthritis: a double-blind, placebo-controlled and randomized study: flaxseed vs. safflower seed. *Rheumatol Int.* 1995;14:231-234.

2. Thompson LU. Experimental studies on lignans and cancer. *Baillieres Clin Endocrinol Metab.* 1998;12:691-705.

3. Singer P, Jaeger W, Berger I, et al. Effects of dietary oleic, linoleic, and alpha-linolenic acids on blood pressure, serum lipids, lipoproteins and the formation of eicosanoid precursors in patients with mild essential hypertension. *J Hum Hypertens.* 1990;4:227-233.

4. Thompson LU, Rickard SE, Orcheson LJ, et al. Flaxseed and its lignan and oil components reduce mammary tumor growth at a late stage of carcinogenesis. *Carcinogenesis.* 1996;17:1373-1376.

5. Bougnoux P, Koscielny S, Chajes V, et al. Alpha-linolenic acid content of adipose breast tissue: a host determinant of the risk of early metastasis in breast cancer. *Br J Cancer.* 1994;70:330-334.

6. Rose DP. Dietary fatty acids and cancer. *Am J Clin Nutr.* 1997;66(suppl):998S-1003S.

7. Stoll AL, Locke CA, Marangell LB, et al. Omega-3 fatty acids and bipolar disorder: a review. *Prostaglandins Leukot Essent Fatty Acids.* 1999;60:329-337.

Folate

1. Cembrowski GS, Zhang MM, Prosser CI, Higgins T. Folate is not what it is cracked up to be. *Arch Intern Med.* 1999;159:2747-2748.

2. Green TJ, Houghton LA, Donovan U, et al. Oral contraceptives did not affect biochemical folate indexes and homocysteine concentrations in adolescent females. *J Am Diet Assoc.* 1998;98:49-55.

3. Russell RM, Dutta SK, Oaks EV, et al. Impairment of folic acid absorption by oral pancreatic extracts. *Dig Dis Sci.* 1980;25:369-373.

4. Werler MM, Shapiro S, Mitchell AA. Periconceptional folic acid exposure and risk of occurrent neural tube defects. *JAMA*. 1993;269:1257-1261.
5. Milunsky A, Jick H, Jick SS, Bruell CL, et al. Multivitamin/folic acid supplementation in early pregnancy reduces the prevalence of neural tube defects. *JAMA*. 1989;262:2847-2852.
6. Coppen A, Bailey J. Enhancement of the antidepressant action of fluoxetine by folic acid: a randomized, placebo controlled trial. *J Affect Disord*. 2000;60:121-130.
7. Rimm EB, Willett WC, Hu FB, et al. Folate and vitamin B_6 from diet and supplements in relation to risk of coronary heart disease among women. *JAMA*. 1998; 279:359-364.
8. Graham IM, Daly LE, Refsum HM, et al. Plasma homocysteine as a risk factor for vascular disease. The European Concerted Action Project. *JAMA*. 1997;277:1775-1781.
9. Moghadasian MH, McManus B, Frohlich JJ. Homocyst(e)ine and coronary artery disease: clinical evidence and genetic and metabolic background. *Arch Intern Med*. 1997;157:2299-2308.
10. Ubbink JB, van der Merwe A, Vermaak WJH, et al. Hyperhomocysteinemia and the response to vitamin supplementation. *Clin Investig*. 1993;71:993-998.
11. den Heijer M, Brouwer IA, Bos GM, et al. Vitamin supplementation reduces blood homocysteine levels: a controlled trial in patients with venous thrombosis and healthy volunteers. *Arterioscler Thromb Vasc Biol*. 1998;18:356-361.
12. Ward M, McNulty H, McPartlin J. Plasma homocysteine, a risk factor for cardiovascular disease, is lowered by physiological doses of folic acid. *Q J Med*. 1997;90: 519-524.
13. Wald NJ, Watt HC, Law MR, et al. Homocysteine and ischemic heart disease: results of a prospective study with implications regarding prevention. *Arch Intern Med*. 1998;158:862-867.
14. Homocysteine Lowering Trialists' Collaboration. Lowering blood homocysteine with folic acid based supplements: meta-analysis of randomized trials. *BMJ*. 1998; 316:894-898.
15. Wald DS, Bishop L, Wald NJ, et al. Randomized trial of folic acid supplementation and serum homocysteine levels. *Arch Intern Med*. 2001;161:695-700.
16. Butterworth CE II. Effect of folate on cervical cancer: synergism among risk factors. *Ann NY Acad Sci*. 1992;669:293-299.
17. Kim YI, Mason JB. Folate, epithelial dysplasia, and colon cancer. *Proc Assoc Am Physicians*. 1995;107:218-227.
18. Heimburger DC. Localized deficiencies of folic acid in aerodigestive tissues. *Ann NY Acad Sci*. 1992;669:87-95.
19. Zhang S, Hunter D, Hankinson S, et al. A prospective study of folate intake and the risk of breast cancer. *JAMA*. 1999;281:1632-1637.
20. Stolzenberg-Solomon RZ, Pietinen P, Barrett MJ, et al. Dietary and other methyl-group availability factors and pancreatic cancer risk in a cohort of male smokers. *Am J Epidemiol*. 2001;153:680-687.
21. Giovannucci E, Stampfer MJ, Colditz GA, et al. Folate, methionine, and alcohol intake and risk of colorectal adenoma. *J Natl Cancer Inst*. 1993;85:875-884.
22. Giovannucci E, Stampfer MJ, Colditz GA, et al. Multivitamin use, folate, and colon cancer in women in the Nurses' Health Study. *Ann Intern Med*. 1998;129:517-524.
23. Baron JA, Sandler RS, Haile RW, et al. Folate intake, alcohol consumption, cigarette smoking, and risk of colorectal adenomas. *J Natl Cancer Inst*. 1998;90:57-62.
24. Butterworth CE II, Hatch KD, Gore H, et al. Improvement in cervical dysplasia associated with folic acid therapy in users of oral contraceptives. *Am J Clin Nutr*. 1982;35:73-82.
25. Butterworth CE II, Hatch KD, Soong SJ, et al. Oral folic acid supplementation for cervical dysplasia: a clinical intervention trial. *Am J Obstet Gynecol*. 1992;166:803-809.
26. Gori T, Burstein JM, Ahmed S, et al. Folic acid prevents nitroglycerin-induced nitric oxide synthase dysfunction and nitrate tolerance: a human in vivo study. *Circulation*. 2001;104:1119-1123.

27. Snowdon DA, Tully CL, Smith CD, et al. Serum folate and the severity of atrophy of the neocortex in Alzheimer disease: findings from the Nun Study. *Am J Clin Nutr.* 2000;71:993-998.

28. Oster KA. Evaluation of serum cholesterol reduction and xanthine oxidase inhibition in the treatment of atherosclerosis. *Recent Adv Stud Cardiac Struct Metab.* 1973;3:73-80.

29. Boss GR, Ragsdale RA, Zettner A, et al. Failure of folic acid (pteroylglutamic acid) to affect hyperuricemia. *J Lab Clin Med.* 1980;96:783-789.

30. Flouvier B, Devulder B. Folic acid, xanthine oxidase, and uric acid [letter]. *Ann Intern Med.* 1978;88:269.

31. Alpert JE, Fava M. Nutrition and depression: the role of folate. *Nutr Rev.* 1997; 55:145-149.

32. Passeri M, Cucinotta D, Abate G, et al. Oral 5′-methyltetrahydrofolic acid in senile organic mental disorders with depression: results of a double-blind multicenter study. *Aging (Milano).* 1993;5:63-71.

33. Godfrey PS, Toone BK, Carney MW, et al. Enhancement of recovery from psychiatric illness by methylfolate. *Lancet.* 1990;336:392-395.

34. Heseker H, Kubler W, Pudel V, et al. Psychological disorders as early symptoms of a mild-to-moderate vitamin deficiency. *Ann NY Acad Sci.* 1992;669:352-357.

35. Crellin R, Bottiglieri T, Reynolds EH. Folates and psychiatric disorders: clinical potential. *Drugs.* 1993;45:623-636.

36. Brattstrom LE, Hultberg BL, Hardebo JE. Folic acid responsive postmenopausal homocysteinemia. *Metabolism.* 1985;34:1073-1077.

37. Botez MI. Folate deficiency and neurological disorders in adults. *Med Hypotheses.* 1976;2:135-140.

38. Coppen A, Swade C, Jones SA, et al. Depression and tetrahydrobiopterin: the folate connection. *J Affect Disord.* 1989;16:103-107.

39. Flynn MA, Irvin W, Krause G. The effect of folate and cobalamin on osteoarthritic hands. *J Am Coll Nutr.* 1994;13:351-356.

40. Kremer JM, Bigaouette J. Nutrient intake of patients with rheumatoid arthritis is deficient in pyridoxine, zinc, copper, and magnesium. *J Rheumatol.* 1996;23:990-994.

41. Montes LF, Diaz ML, Lajous J, et al. Folic acid and vitamin B_{12} in vitiligo: a nutritional approach. *Cutis.* 1992;50:39-42.

42. O'Keeffe ST. Restless legs syndrome: a review. *Arch Intern Med.* 1996;156:243-248.

43. Coppen A, Abou-Saleh MT. Plasma folate and affective morbidity during long-term lithium therapy. *Br J Psychiatry.* 1982;141:87-89.

44. Coppen A, Chaudhry S, Swade C. Folic acid enhances lithium prophylaxis. *J Affect Disord.* 1986;10:9-13.

45. Callaghan TJ. The effect of folic acid on seborrheic dermatitis. *Cutis.* 1967;3:583-588.

46. Juhlin L, Olsson MJ. Improvement of vitiligo after oral treatment with vitamin B_{12} and folic acid and the importance of sun exposure. *Acta Derm Venereol (Stockh).* 1997;77:460-462.

47. Kim SM, Kim YK, Hann S-K. Serum levels of folic acid and vitamin B_{12} in Korean patients with vitiligo. *Yonsei Med J.* 1999;40:195-198.

48. Dietary Reference Intakes for Thiamin, Riboflavin, Niacin, Vitamin B_6, Folate, Vitamin B_{12}, Panothenic Acid, Biotin, and Choline (1998). Available at: http://www.nap.edu. Accessed October 4, 2001.

49. Butterworth CE II, Tamura T. Folic acid safety and toxicity: a brief review. *Am J Clin Nutr.* 1989;50:353-358.

50. Lewis DP, Van Dyke DC, Willhite LA, et al. Phenytoin-folic acid interaction. *Ann Pharmacother.* 1995;29:726-735.

51. Morgan SL, Baggott JE, Vaughn WH, et al. Supplementation with folic acid during methotrexate therapy for rheumatoid arthritis: a double-blind, placebo-controlled trial. *Ann Intern Med.* 1994;121:833-841.

52. Duhra P. Treatment of gastrointestinal symptoms associated with methotrexate therapy for psoriasis. *J Am Acad Dermatol.* 1993;28:466-469.

53. Hunt PG, Rose CD, McIlvain-Simpson G, et al. The effects of daily intake of folic acid on the efficacy of methotrexate therapy in children with juvenile rheumatoid arthritis: a controlled study. *J Rheumatol.* 1997;24:2230-2232.

54. Griffith SM, Fisher J, Clarke S, et al. Do patients with rheumatoid arthritis established on methotrexate and folic acid 5 mg daily need to continue folic acid supplements long term? *Rheumatology (Oxford).* 2000;39:1102-1109.

55. Jackson RC. Biological effects of folic acid antagonists with antineoplastic activity. *Pharmacol Ther.* 1984;25:61-82.

56. Omer A, Mowat AG. Nature of anaemia in rheumatoid arthritis. IX. Folate metabolism in patients with rheumatoid arthritis. *Ann Rheum Dis.* 1968;27:414-424.

57. van Ede AE, Laan RF, Rood MJ, et al. Effect of folic or folinic acid supplementation on the toxicity and efficacy of methotrexate in rheumatoid arthritis: a forty-eight week, multicenter, randomized, double-blind, placebo-controlled study. *Arthritis Rheum.* 2001;44:1515-1524.

58. Hoppner K, Lampi B. Bioavailability of folate following ingestion of cholestyramine in the rat. *Int J Vitam Nutr Res.* 1991;61:130-134.

59. West RJ, Lloyd JK. The effect of cholestyramine on intestinal absorption. *Gut.* 1975;16:93-98.

60. Hendel J, Dam M, Gram L, et al. The effects of carbamazepine and valproate on folate metabolism in man. *Acta Neurol Scand.* 1984;69:226-231.

61. Reynolds EH, Milner G, Matthews DM, et al. Anticonvulsant therapy, megaloblastic haemopoiesis and folic acid metabolism. *QJM.* 1966;35:521-537.

62. Lewis DP, Van Dyke DC, Stumbo PJ, et al. Drug and environmental factors associated with adverse pregnancy outcomes. I. Antiepileptic drugs, contraceptives, smoking, and folate. *Ann Pharmacother.* 1998;32:802-817.

63. Berg MJ, Stumbo PJ, Chenard CA, et al. Folic acid improves phenytoin pharmacokinetics. *J Am Diet Assoc.* 1995;95:352-356.

64. Ono H, Sakamoto A, Eguchi T, et al. Plasma total homocysteine concentrations in epileptic patients taking anticonvulsants. *Metabolism.* 1997;46:959-962.

65. Kishi T, Fujita N, Eguchi T, et al. Mechanism for reduction of serum folate by antiepileptic drugs during prolonged therapy. *J Neurol Sci.* 1997;145:109-112.

66. Biale Y, Lewenthal H. Effect of folic acid supplementation on congenital malformations due to anticonvulsive drugs. *Eur J Obstet Gynecol Reprod Biol.* 1984;18:211-216.

67. Baum CL, Selhub J, Rosenberg IH. Antifolate actions of sulfasalazine on intact lymphocytes. *J Lab Clin Med.* 1981;97:779-784.

68. Selhub J, Dhar GJ, Rosenberg IH. Inhibition of folate enzymes by sulfasalazine. *J Clin Invest.* 1978;61:221-224.

69. Krogh Jensen M, Ekelund S, Svendsen L. Folate and homocysteine status and haemolysis in patients treated with sulphasalazine for arthritis. *Scand J Clin Lab Invest.* 1996;56:421-429.

70. Baggott JE, Morgan SL, Ha T, et al. Inhibition of folate-dependent enzymes by nonsteroidal anti-inflammatory drugs. *Biochem J.* 1992;282(pt 1):197-202.

71. Lawrence VA, Loewenstein JE, Eichner ER. Aspirin and folate binding: in vivo and in vitro studies of serum binding and urinary excretion of endogenous folate. *J Lab Clin Med.* 1984;103:944-948.

72. Lieberman FL, Bateman JR. Megaloblastic anemia possibly induced by triamterene in patients with alcoholic cirrhosis. *Ann Intern Med.* 1968;68:168-173.

73. Mason JB, Zimmerman J, Otradovec CL, et al. Chronic diuretic therapy with moderate doses of triamterene is not associated with folate deficiency. *J Lab Clin Med.* 1991;117:365-369.

74. Amos RJ, Amess JA, Hinds CJ, et al. Investigations into the effect of nitrous oxide anaesthesia on folate metabolism in patients receiving intensive care. *Chemioterapia.* 1985;4:393-399.

75. Ermens AA, Refsum H, Rupreht J, et al. Monitoring cobalamin inactivation during nitrous oxide anesthesia by determination of homocysteine and folate in plasma and urine. *Clin Pharmacol Ther.* 1991;49:385-393.

76. Amos RJ, Amess JA, Hinds CJ, et al. Incidence and pathogenesis of acute megaloblastic bone-marrow change in patients receiving intensive care. *Lancet.* 1982;2:835-838.

77. Koblin DD, Tomerson BW, Waldman FM, et al. Effect of nitrous oxide on folate and vitamin B_{12} metabolism in patients. *Anesth Analg.* 1990;71:610-617.

78. Nunn JF, Chanarin I, Tanner AG, et al. Megaloblastic bone marrow changes after repeated nitrous oxide anaesthesia: reversal with folinic acid. *Br J Anaesth.* 1986;58: 1469-1470.

79. Kahn SB, Fein SA, Brodsky I. Effects of trimethoprim on folate metabolism in man. *Clin Pharmacol Ther.* 1968;9:550-560.

80. Vinnicombe HG, Derrick JP. Dihydropteroate synthase from *Streptococcus pneumoniae:* characterization of substrate binding order and sulfonamide inhibition. *Biochem Biophys Res Commun.* 1999;258:752-757.

81. Russell RM, Golner BB, Krasinski SD, et al. Effect of antacid and H_2 receptor antagonists on the intestinal absorption of folic acid. *J Lab Clin Med.* 1988;112:458-463.

82. Stumm W, Morgan JJ. *Aquatic Chemistry: An Introduction Emphasizing Chemical Equilibria in Natural Waters.* 2nd ed. New York, NY: John Wiley & Sons; 1981:240.

83. Hernandez-Diaz S, Werler MM, Walker AM, et al. Folic acid antagonists during pregnancy and the risk of birth defects. *N Engl J Med.* 2000;343:1608-1614.

84. Steegers-Theunissen RPM, Van Rossum JM, Steegers EAP, et al. Sub-50 oral contraceptives affect folate kinetics. *Gynecol Obstet Invest.* 1993;36:230-233.

85. Mooij PN, Thomas CM, Doesburg WH, et al. Multivitamin supplementation in oral contraceptive users. *Contraception.* 1991;44:277-288.

Gamma-Linolenic Acid (GLA)

1. Keen H, Payan J, Allawi J, et al. Treatment of diabetic neuropathy with gamma-linolenic acid: the gamma-linolenic acid multicenter trial group. *Diabetes Care.* 1993;16:8-15.

2. Jamal GA, Carmichael H. The effect of gamma-linolenic acid on human diabetic peripheral neuropathy: a double-blind placebo-controlled trial. *Diabet Med.* 1990;7: 319-323.

3. Zurier RB, Rossetti RG, Jacobson EW, et al. Gamma-linolenic acid treatment of rheumatoid arthritis: a randomized, placebo-controlled trial. *Arthritis Rheum.* 1996; 39:1808-1817.

4. Leventhal LJ, Boyce EG, Zurier RB. Treatment of rheumatoid arthritis with gamma-linolenic acid. *Ann Intern Med.* 1993;119:867-873.

5. Leventhal LJ, Boyce EG, Zurier RB. Treatment of rheumatoid arthritis with black-currant seed oil. *Br J Rheumatol.* 1994;33:847-852.

6. Rothman D, DeLuca P, Zurier RB. Botanical lipids: effects on inflammation, immune responses, and rheumatoid arthritis. *Semin Arthritis Rheum.* 1995;25:87-96.

7. Belch JJ, Ansell D, Madhok R, et al. Effects of altering dietary essential fatty acids on requirements for non-steroidal anti-inflammatory drugs in patients with rheumatoid arthritis: a double blind placebo controlled study. *Ann Rheum Dis.* 1988;47:96-104.

8. Horrobin DF. Nutritional and medical importance of gamma-linolenic acid. *Prog Lipid Res.* 1992;31:163-194.

9. Pashby NL, Mansel RE, Hughes LE, et al. A clinical trial of evening primrose oil in mastalgia [abstract]. *Br J Surg.* 1981;68:801.

10. Mansel RE, Gateley CA, Harrison BJ, et al. Effects and tolerability of n-6 essential fatty acid supplementation in patients with recurrent breast cysts: a randomized double-blind placebo-controlled trial. *J Nutr Med.* 1990;1:195-200.

11. Mansel RE, Harrison BJ, Melhuish J, et al. A randomized trial of dietary intervention with essential fatty acids in patients with categorized cysts. *Ann NY Acad Sci.* 1990; 586:288-294.

12. Kollias J, Macmillan RD, Sibbering DM, et al. Effect of evening primrose oil on clinically diagnosed fibroadenomas. *Breast.* 2000;9:35-36.

13. Budeiri D, Li Wan Po A, Dornan JC. Is evening primrose oil of value in the treatment of premenstrual syndrome? *Control Clin Trials.* 1996;17:60-68.

14. Henz BM, Jablonska S, van de Kerkhof PC, et al. Double-blind, multicentre analysis of the efficacy of borage oil in patients with atopic eczema. *Br J Dermatol.* 1999;140:685-688.

15. Hederos CA, Berg A. Epogam evening primrose oil treatment in atopic dermatitis and asthma. *Arch Dis Child.* 1996;75:494-497.

16. Berth-Jones J, Graham-Brown RAC. Placebo-controlled trial of essential fatty acid supplementation in atopic dermatitis. *Lancet.* 1993;341:1557-1560.

17. Morse PF, Horrobin DF, Manku MS, et al. Meta-analysis of placebo-controlled studies of the efficacy of Epogam in the treatment of atopic eczema: relationship between plasma essential fatty acid changes and clinical response. *Br J Dermatol.* 1989;121:75-90.

18. Biagi PL, Bordoni A, Hrelia S, et al. The effect of gamma-linolenic acid on clinical status, red cell fatty acid composition and membrane microviscosity in infants with atopic dermatitis. *Drugs Exp Clin Res.* 1994;20:77-84.

19. Haslett C, Douglas JG, Chalmers SR, et al. A double-blind evaluation of evening primrose oil as an antiobesity agent. *Int J Obes.* 1983;7:549-553.

20. Garcia CM, Carter J, Chou A. Gamma linolenic acid causes weight loss and lower blood pressure in overweight patients with family history of obesity. *Swed J Biol Med.* 1986;4:8-11.

21. Behan PO, Behan WMH, Horrobin D. Effect of high doses of essential fatty acids on the postviral fatigue syndrome. *Acta Neurol Scand.* 1990;82:209-216.

22. Warren G, McKendrick M, Peet M. The role of essential fatty acids in chronic fatigue syndrome: a case-controlled study of red-cell membrane essential fatty acids (EFA) and a placebo-controlled treatment study with high dose of EFA. *Acta Neurol Scand.* 1999;99:112-116.

23. Belch JJ, Shaw B, O'Dowd A, et al. Evening primrose oil (Efamol) in the treatment of Raynaud's phenomenon: a double blind study. *Thromb Haemost.* 1985;54:490-494.

24. Barre DE, Holub BJ, Chapkin RS. The effect of borage oil supplementation on human platelet aggregation, thromboxane B_2, prostaglandin E_1, and E_2 formation. *Nutr Res.* 1993;13:739-751.

25. Horrobin DF. The use of gamma-linolenic acid in diabetic neuropathy. *Agents Actions Suppl.* 1992;37:120-144.

26. Horrobin DF. Gamma linolenic acid: an intermediate in essential fatty acid metabolism with potential as an ethical pharmaceutical and as a food. *Rev Contemp Pharmacother.* 1990;1:1-41.

27. Horrobin DF, Manku M, Brush M, et al. Abnormalities in plasma essential fatty acid levels in women with premenstrual syndrome and with nonmalignant breast disease. *J Nutr Med.* 1991;2:259-264.

28. Manku MS, Horrobin DF, Morse NL, et al. Essential fatty acids in the plasma phospholipids of patients with atopic eczema. *Br J Dermatol.* 1984;110:643-648.

29. Cameron NE, Cotter MA, Horrobin DH, et al. Effects of alpha-lipoic acid on neurovascular function in diabetic rats: interaction with essential fatty acids. *Diabetologia.* 1998;41:390-399.

30. Hounsom L, Horrobin DF, Tritschler H, et al. A lipoic acid-gamma linolenic acid conjugate is effective against multiple indices of experimental diabetic neuropathy. *Diabetologia.* 1998;41:839-843.

31. Reddy P, Lokesh BR. Dietary unsaturated fatty acids, vitamin E, curcumin and eugenol alter serum and liver lipid peroxidation in rats. *Nutr Res.* 1994;14:1423-1437.

32. Vaddadi KS. The use of gamma-linolenic acid and linoleic acid to differentiate between temporal lobe epilepsy and schizophrenia. *Prostaglandins Med.* 1981;6:375-379.

33. Aman MG, Mitchell EA, Turbott SH. The effects of essential fatty acid supplementation by Efamol in hyperactive children. *J Abnorm Child Psychol.* 1987;15:75-90.

34. Arnold LE, Kleykamp D, Votolato NA, et al. Gamma-linolenic acid for attention-deficit hyperactivity disorder: placebo-controlled comparison to D-amphetamine. *Biol Psychiatry.* 1989; 25:222-228.

35. Kast RE. Borage oil reduction of rheumatoid arthritis activity may be mediated by increased cAMP that suppresses tumor necrosis factor-alpha. *Int Immunopharmacol.* 2001;1:2197-2199.

Garlic

1. Koscielny J, Klussendorf D, Latza R, et al. The antiatherosclerotic effect of *Allium sativum*. *Atherosclerosis.* 1999;144:237-249.

2. Breithaupt-Grogler K, Ling M, Boudoulas H, et al. Protective effect of chronic garlic intake on elastic properties of aorta in the elderly. *Circulation.* 1997;96:2649-2655.

3. Bordia A. Garlic and coronary heart disease. The effects of garlic extract therapy over three years on the reinfarction and mortality rate [translated from German]. *Dtsch Apoth Ztg.* 1989;129(suppl 15):16-17.
4. Warshafsky S, Kamer RS, Sivak SL. Effect of garlic on total serum cholesterol: a meta-analysis. *Ann Intern Med.* 1993;119:599-605.
5. Mader FH. Treatment of hyperlipidaemia with garlic-powder tablets: evidence from the German Association of General Practitioners' multicentric placebo-controlled double-blind study. *Arzneimittelforschung.* 1990;40:1111-1116.
6. Steiner M, Khan AH, Holbert D, et al. A double-blind crossover study in moderately hypercholesterolemic men that compared the effect of aged garlic extract and placebo administration on blood lipids. *Am J Clin Nutr.* 1996;64:866-870.
7. Holzgartner H, Schmidt U, Kuhn U. Comparison of the efficacy and tolerance of a garlic preparation vs. bezafibrate. *Arzneimittelforschung.* 1992;42:1473-1477.
8. Neil HA, Silagy CA, Lancaster T, et al. Garlic powder in the treatment of moderate hyperlipidaemia: a controlled trial and meta-analysis. *J R Coll Physicians Lond.* 1996;30:329-334.
9. Simons LA, Balasubramaniam S, von Konigsmark M, et al. On the effect of garlic on plasma lipids and lipoproteins in mild hypercholesterolaemia. *Atherosclerosis.* 1995; 113:219-225.
10. Superko HR, Krauss RM. Garlic powder, effect on plasma lipids, postprandial lipemia, low-density lipoprotein particle size, high-density lipoprotein subclass distribution and lipoprotein (a). *J Am Coll Cardiol.* 2000;35:321-326.
11. Isaacsohn JL, Moser M, Stein EA, et al. Garlic powder and plasma lipids and lipoproteins: a multicenter, randomized, placebo-controlled trial. *Arch Intern Med.* 1998; 158:1189-1194.
12. Gardner CD, Chatterjee LM, Carlson JJ. The effect of a garlic preparation on plasma lipid levels in moderately hypercholesterolemic adults. *Atherosclerosis.* 2001;154:213-220.
13. Kannar D, Wattanapenpaiboon N, Savige GS, et al. Hypocholesterolemic effect of an enteric-coated garlic supplement. *J Am Coll Nutr.* 2001;20:225-231.
14. Stevinson C, Pittler MH, Ernst E. Garlic for treating hypercholesterolemia: a meta-analysis of randomized clinical trials. *Ann Intern Med.* 2000;133:420-429.
15. Silagy CA, Neil HA. A meta-analysis of the effect of garlic on blood pressure. *J Hypertens.* 1994;12:463-468.
16. Auer W, Eiber A, Hertkorn E, et al. Hypertension and hyperlipidaemia: garlic helps in mild cases. *Br J Clin Pract Suppl.* 1990;69:3-6.
17. Kiesewetter H, Jung F, Pindur G, et al. Effect of garlic on thrombocyte aggregation, microcirculation, and other risk factors. *Int J Clin Pharmacol Ther Toxicol.* 1991;29: 151-155.
18. Steiner M, Lin RS. Changes in platelet function and susceptibility of lipoproteins to oxidation associated with administration of aged garlic extract. *J Cardiovasc Pharmacol.* 1998;31:904-908.
19. Reuter HD. *Allium sativum* and *Allium ursinum.* 2. Pharmacology and medicinal application. *Phytomedicine.* 1995;2:73-91.
20. Agarwal KC. Therapeutic actions of garlic constituents. *Med Res Rev.* 1996;16:111-124.
21. Dausch JG, Nixon DW. Garlic: a review of its relationship to malignant disease. *Prev Med.* 1990;19:346-361.
22. Dorant E, van den Brandt PA, Goldbohm RA, et al. Garlic and its significance for the prevention of cancer in humans: a critical view. *Br J Cancer.* 1993;67:424-429.
23. Lau BH, Tadi PP, Tosk JM. *Allium sativum* (garlic) and cancer prevention. *Nutr Res.* 1990;10:937-948.
24. Steinmetz KA, Kushi LH, Bostick RM, et al. Vegetables, fruit, and colon cancer in the Iowa Women's Health Study. *Am J Epidemiol.* 1994;139:1-15.
25. You WC, Blot WJ, Chang YS, et al. *Allium* vegetables and reduced risk of stomach cancer. *J Natl Cancer Inst.* 1989;81;162-164.
26. Ernst E. Can *Allium* vegetables prevent cancer? *Phytomedicine.* 1997;4:79-83.
27. Stjernberg L, Berglund J. Garlic as an insect repellent [letter]. *JAMA.* 2000;284:831.

28. Ghannoum MA. Studies on the anticandidal mode of action of *Allium sativum* (garlic). *J Gen Microbiol.* 1988;134:2917-2924.

29. Hughes BG, Lawson LD. Antimicrobial effects of *Allium sativum* L. (garlic), *Allium ampeloprasum* L. (elephant garlic), and *Allium cepa* L. (onion), garlic compounds and commercial garlic supplement products. *Phytother Res.* 1991;5:154-158.

30. Sandhu DK, Warraich MK, Singh S. Sensitivity of yeasts isolated from cases of vaginitis to aqueous extracts of garlic. *Mykosen.* 1980;23:691-698.

31. Chowdhury AKA, Ahsan M, Islam SN, et al. Efficacy of aqueous extract of garlic & allicin in experimental shigellosis in rabbits. *Indian J Med Res.* 1991;93:33-36.

32. Sharma VD, Sethi MS, Kumar A, et al. Antibacterial property of *Allium sativum* Linn: in vivo & in vitro studies. *Indian J Exp Biol.* 1977;15:466-468.

33. Sivam GP. Protection against *Helicobacter pylori* and other bacterial infections by garlic. *J Nutr.* 2001;131(3 suppl):1106S-1108S.

34. Graham DY, Anderson SY, Lang T. Garlic or jalapeno peppers for treatment of *Helicobacter pylori* infection. *Am J Gastroenterol.* 1999;94:1200-1202.

35. Aydin A, Ersoz G, Tekesin O, et al. Garlic oil and *Helicobacter pylori* infection [letter]. *Am J Gastroenterol.* 2000;95:563-564.

36. Das I, Khan NS, Sooranna SR. Potent activation of nitric oxide synthase by garlic: a basis for its therapeutic applications. *Curr Med Res Opin.* 1995;13:257-263.

37. Gebhardt R. Multiple inhibitory effects of garlic extracts on cholesterol biosynthesis in hepatocytes. *Lipids.* 1993;28:613-619.

38. Gebhardt R, Beck H, Wagner KG. Inhibition of cholesterol biosynthesis by allicin and ajoene in rat hepatocytes and HepG2 cells. *Biochim Biophys Acta.* 1994;1213:57-62.

39. Gebhardt R, Beck H. Differential inhibitory effects of garlic-derived organosulfur compounds on cholesterol biosynthesis in primary rat hepatocyte cultures. *Lipids.* 1996;31:1269-1276.

40. Qureshi AA, Abuirmeileh N, Din ZZ, et al. Inhibition of cholesterol and fatty acid biosynthesis in liver enzymes and chicken hepatocytes by polar fractions of garlic. *Lipids.* 1983;18:343-348.

41. Yeh YY, Yeh SM. Garlic reduces plasma lipids by inhibiting hepatic cholesterol and triacylglycerol synthesis. *Lipids.* 1994;29:189-193.

42. Yeh YY, Liu L. Cholesterol-lowering effect of garlic extracts and organosulfur compounds: human and animal studies. *J Nutr.* 2001;131:989S-993S.

43. Ip C, Lisk DJ. Efficacy of cancer prevention by high-selenium garlic is primarily dependent on the action of selenium. *Carcinogenesis.* 1995;16:2649-2652.

44. Das T, Roychoudhury A, Sharma A, et al. Modification of clastogenicity of three known clastogens by garlic extract in mice in vivo. *Environ Mol Mutagen.* 1993;21:383-388.

45. Lawson LD, Wang ZJ, Hughes BG. Identification and HPLC quantitation of the sulfides and dialk(en)yl thiosulfinates in commercial garlic products. *Planta Med.* 1991;57:363-370.

46. Garty BZ. Garlic burns. *Pediatrics.* 1993;91:658-659.

47. Sumiyoshi H, Kanezawa A, Masamoto K, et al. Chronic toxicity test of garlic extract in rats [in Japanese; English abstract]. *J Toxicol Sci.* 1984;9:61-75.

48. Abraham SK, Kesavan PC. Genotoxicity of garlic, turmeric and asafoetida in mice. *Mutat Res.* 1984;136:85-88.

49. Yoshida S, Hirao Y, Nakagawa S. Mutagenicity and cytotoxicity tests of garlic [in Japanese; English abstract]. *J Toxicol Sci.* 1984;9:77-86.

50. Beck E, Grunwald J. *Allium sativum* in der Stufentherapie der Hyperlipidamie. Studie mit 1997 Patienten belegt Wirksamkeit und Vertraglichkeit [English abstract]. *Med Welt.* 1993;44:516-520.

51. Schulz V, Hansel R, Tyler VE. *Rational Phytotherapy: A Physicians' Guide to Herbal Medicine.* 3rd ed. Berlin, Germany: Springer-Verlag; 1998:112, 115, 121.

52. Rose KD, Croissant PD, Parliament CF, et al. Spontaneous spinal epidural hematoma with associated platelet dysfunction from excessive garlic ingestion: a case report. *Neurosurgery.* 1990;26:880-882.

53. Burnham BE. Garlic as a possible risk for postoperative bleeding [letter]. *Plast Reconstr Surg.* 1995;95:213.

54. European Scientific Cooperative on Phytotherapy. *Allii sativi bulbus* (garlic). Exeter, UK: ESCOP; 1996-1997. Monographs on the Medicinal Uses of Plant Drugs, Fascicule 3:4-5.
55. German K, Kumar U, Blackford HN. Garlic and the risk of TURP bleeding. *Br J Urol.* 1995;76:518.
56. Sunter WH. Warfarin and garlic [letter]. *Pharmacol J.* 1991;246:722.
57. Piscitelli SC, Burstein AH, Welden N, et al. The effect of garlic supplements on the pharmacokinetics of saquinavir. *Clin Infect Dis.* 2002;34:234-238.
58. Piscitelli SC. Use of complementary medicines by patients with HIV: full sail into uncharted waters. *Medscape HIV/AIDS.* 2000;6(3).
59. Ackermann RT, Mulrow CD, Ramirez G, et al. Garlic shows promise for improving some cardiovascular risk factors. *Arch Intern Med.* 2001;161:813-824.
60. Josling P. Preventing the common cold with a garlic supplement: a double-blind, placebo-controlled survey. *Adv Ther.* 2001;18(4):189-193.
61. Morcos NC, Camilo K. Acute and chronic toxicity study of fish oil and garlic combination. *Int J Vitam Nutr Res.* 2001;71:306-312.

Genistein

1. Fanti O, Faugere MC, Gang Z, et al. Systematic administration of genistein partially prevents bone loss in ovariectomized rats in a nonestrogen-like mechanism [abstract]. *Am J Clin Nutr.* 1998;68(suppl):1517S-1518S.
2. Anderson JJ, Ambrose WW, Garner SC. Biphasic effects of genistein on bone tissue in the ovariectomized, lactating rat model. *Proc Soc Exp Biol Med.* 1998;217:345-350.
3. Fanti P, Monier-Faugere MC, Geng Z, et al. The phytoestrogen genistein reduces bone loss in short-term ovariectomized rats. *Osteoporos Int.* 1998;8:274-281.
4. Messina MJ, Persky V, Setchell KDR, et al. Soy intake and cancer risk: a review of the in vitro and in vivo data. *Nutr Cancer.* 1994;21:113-131.
5. Alhasan SA, Ensley JF, Sarkar FH. Genistein induced molecular changes in a squamous cell carcinoma of the head and neck cell line. *Int J Oncol.* 2000;16:333-338.
6. Wei H, Bowen R, Cai Q, et al. Antioxidant and antipromotional effects of the soybean isoflavone genistein. *Proc Soc Exp Biol Med.* 1995;208:124-130.
7. Tham DM, Gardner CD, Haskell WL. Clinical review 97: potential health benefits of dietary phytoestrogens: a review of the clinical, epidemiological, and mechanistic evidence. *J Clin Endocrinol Metab.* 1998;83:2223-2235.
8. Crouse JR III, Morgan T, Terry JG, et al. A randomized trial comparing the effect of casein with that of soy protein containing varying amounts of isoflavones on plasma concentrations of lipids and lipoproteins. *Arch Intern Med.* 1999;159:2070-2076.
9. Trieu VN, Uckun FM. Genistein is neuroprotective in murine models of familial amyotrophic lateral sclerosis and stroke. *Biochem Biophys Res Commun.* 1999;258:685-688.
10. Wei H, Bowen R, Cai Q, et al. Antioxidant and antipromotional effects of the soybean isoflavone genistein. *Proc Soc Exp Biol Med.* 1995;208:124-130.
11. Crowell JA, Levine BS, Page JG, et al. Preclinical safety studies of isoflavones [abstract]. *J Nutr.* 2000;130(suppl):677S.
12. Petrakis NL, Barnes S, King EB, et al. Stimulatory influence of soy protein isolate on breast secretion in pre- and post-menopausal women. *Cancer Epidemiol Biomarkers Prev.* 1996;5:785-794.
13. McMichael-Phillips DL, Harding C, Morton M, et al. Effects of soy-protein supplementation on epithelial proliferation in the histologically normal human breast. *Am J Clin Nutr.* 1998;68 (suppl):1431S-1436S.
14. Divi RL, Chang HC, Doerge DR. Anti-thyroid isoflavones from soybean: isolation, characterization, and mechanisms of action. *Biochem Pharmacol.* 1997;54:1087-1096.
15. Hilakivi-Clarke L, Cho E, Onojafe I, et al. Maternal exposure to genistein during pregnancy increases carcinogen-induced mammary tumorigenesis in female rat offspring. *Oncol Rep.* 1999;6:1089-1095.
16. Martini MC, Dancisak BB, Haggans CJ, et al. Effects of soy intake on sex hormone metabolism in premenopausal women. *Nutr Cancer.* 1999;34:133-139.
17. Scambia G, Mango D, Signorile PG, et al. Clinical effects of a standardized soy extract in postmenopausal women: a pilot study. *Menopause.* 2000;7:105-111.

Ginger

1. Grontved A, Brask T, Kambskard J, et al. Ginger root against seasickness: a controlled trial on the open sea. *Acta Otolaryngol (Stockh)*. 1988;105:45-49.
2. Riebenfeld D, Borzone L. Randomized double-blind study comparing ginger (Zintona®) and dimenhydrinate in motion sickness. *Healthnotes Rev*. 1999;6:98-101.
3. Careddu P. Motion sickness in children: results of a double-blind study with ginger (Zintona®) and dimenhydrinate. *Healthnotes Rev*. 1999;6:102-107.
4. Mowrey DB, Clayson DE. Motion sickness, ginger, and psychophysics. *Lancet*. 1982;1:655-657.
5. Schmid R, Schick T, Steffen R, et al. Comparison of seven commonly used agents for prophylaxis of seasickness. *J Travel Med*. 1994;1:203-206.
6. Stewart JJ, Wood MJ, Wood CD, et al. Effects of ginger on motion sickness susceptibility and gastric function. *Pharmacology*. 1991;42:111-120.
7. Stott JR, Hubble MP, Spencer MB. A double-blind comparative trial of powdered ginger root, hyoscine hydrobromide, and cinnarizine in the prophylaxis of motion sickness induced by cross coupled stimulation. *AGARD Conf Proc*. 1985;372:1-6.
8. Wood CD, Manno JE, Wood MJ, et al. Comparison of efficacy of ginger with various antimotion sickness drugs. *Clin Res Pract Drug Regul Aff*. 1988;6:129-136.
9. Vutyavanich T, Kraisarin T, Ruangsri R. Ginger for nausea and vomiting in pregnancy: randomized, double-masked, placebo-controlled trial. *Obstet Gynecol*. 2001;97:577-582.
10. Fischer-Rasmussen W, Kjaer SK, Dahl C, et al. Ginger treatment of hyperemesis gravidarum. *Eur J Obstet Gynecol Reprod Biol*. 1991;38:19-24.
11. Bone ME, Wilkinson DJ, Young JR, et al. Ginger root: a new antiemetic. The effect of ginger root on postoperative nausea and vomiting after major gynaecological sugery. *Anaesthesia*. 1990;45:669-671.
12. Phillips S, Ruggier R, Hutchinson SE, et al. *Zingiber officinale* (ginger): an antiemetic for day case surgery. *Anaesthesia*. 1993;48:715-717.
13. Arfeen Z, Owen H, Plummer JL, et al. A double-blind randomized controlled trial of ginger for the prevention of postoperative nausea and vomiting. *Anaesth Intensive Care*. 1995;23:449-452.
14. Visalyaputra S, Petchpaisit N, Somcharoen K, et al. The efficacy of ginger root in the prevention of postoperative nausea and vomiting after outpatient gynaecological laparoscopy. *Anaesthesia*. 1998;53:506-510.
15. Meyer K, Schwartz J, Crater D, et al. *Zingiber officinale* (ginger) used to prevent 8-Mop associated nausea. *Dermatol Nurs*. 1995;7:242-244.
16. Bliddal H, Rosetzsky A, Schlichting P, et al. A randomized, placebo-controlled, crossover study of ginger extracts and ibuprofen in osteoarthritis. *Osteoarthritis Cartilage*. 2000;8:9-12.
17. Holtmann S, Clarke AH, Scherer H, et al. The anti-motion sickness mechanism of ginger: a comparative study with placebo and dimenhydrinate. *Acta Otolaryngol*. 1989;108:168-174.
18. Phillips S, Hutchinson S, Ruggier R. *Zingiber officinale* does not affect gastric emptying rate: a randomized, placebo-controlled, crossover trial. *Anaesthesia*. 1993;48:393-395.
19. Qian D-S, Liu Z-S. Pharmacologic studies of antimotion sickness actions of ginger [in Chinese; English abstract]. *Chung Kuo Chung Hsi I Chieh Ho Tsa Chih*. 1992;12:95-98.
20. Mascolo N, Jain R, Jain SC, et al. Ethnopharmacologic investigation of ginger (*Zingiber officinale*). *J Ethnopharmacol*. 1989;27:129-140.
21. Kada T, Morita K, Inoue T. Anti-mutagenic action of vegetable factor(s) on the mutagenic principle of tryptophan pyrolysate. *Mutat Res*. 1978;53:351-353.
22. Nakamura H, Yamamoto T. Mutagen and anti-mutagen in ginger, *Zingiber officinale*. *Mutat Res*. 1982;103:119-126.
23. Nagabhushan M, Amonkar AJ, Bhide SV. Mutagenicity of gingerol and shogaol and antimutagenicity of zingerone in *Salmonella*/microsome assay. *Cancer Lett*. 1987;36:221-233.

24. European Scientific Cooperative on Phytotherapy. *Zingiberis rhizoma* (ginger). Exeter, UK: ESCOP; 1996-1997. Monographs on the Medicinal Uses of Plant Drugs, Fascicule 1:1, 5.

25. Kiuchi F, Shibuya M, Sankawa U. Inhibitors of prostaglandin biosynthesis from ginger. *Chem Pharm Bull (Tokyo)*. 1982;30:754-757.

26. Kiuchi F, Iwakami S, Shibuya M, et al. Inhibition of prostaglandin and leukotriene biosynthesis by gingerols and diarylheptanoids. *Chem Pharm Bull (Tokyo)*. 1992; 40:387-391.

27. Srivastava KC. Effects of aqueous extracts of onion, garlic and ginger on platelet aggregation and metabolism of arachidonic acid in the blood vascular system: in vitro study. *Prostaglandins Leukot Med*. 1984;13:227-235.

28. Srivastava KC. Isolation and effects of some ginger components on platelet aggregation and eicosanoid biosynthesis. *Prostaglandins Leukot Med*. 1986;25:187-198.

29. Srivastava KC. Effect of onion and ginger consumption on platelet thromboxane production in humans. *Prostaglandins Leukot Essent Fatty Acids*. 1989;35:183-185.

30. Bordia A, Verma SK, Srivastava KC. Effect of ginger (*Zingiber officinale* rosc.) and fenugreek (*Trigonella foenumgraecum* L.) on blood lipids, blood sugar and platelet aggregation in patients with coronary artery disease. *Prostaglandins Leukot Essent Fatty Acids*. 1997;56:379-384.

31. Janssen PL, Meyboom S, van Staveren WA, et al. Consumption of ginger (*Zingiber officinale* roscoe) does not affect ex vivo platelet thromboxane production in humans. *Eur J Clin Nutr*. 1996;50:772-774.

32. Lumb AB. Effect of dried ginger on human platelet function. *Thromb Haemost*. 1994;71:110-111.

33. Altman RD, Marcussen KC. Effects of a ginger extract on knee pain in patients with osteoarthritis. *Arthritis Rheum*. 2001;44:2531-2538.

Ginkgo

1. Le Bars PL, Katz MM, Berman N, et al. A placebo-controlled, double-blind, randomized trial of an extract of *Ginkgo biloba* for dementia. North American EGb Study Group. *JAMA*. 1997;278:1327-1332.

2. Hofferberth B. The efficacy of EGb 761 in patients with senile dementia of the Alzheimer type, a double-blind, placebo-controlled study on different levels of investigation. *Hum Psychopharmacol*. 1994;9:215-222.

3. Kanowski S, Herrmann WM, Stephan K, et al. Proof of efficacy of the *Ginkgo biloba* special extract Egb 761 in outpatients suffering from mild to moderate primary degenerative dementia of the Alzheimer type or multi-infarct dementia. *Pharmacopsychiatry*. 1996;29:47-56.

4. Kleijnen J, Knipschild P. *Ginkgo biloba* for cerebral insufficiency. *Br J Clin Pharmacol*. 1992;34:352-358.

5. van Dongen MC, van Rossum E, Kessels AG, et al. The efficacy of *Ginkgo* for elderly people with dementia and age-associated memory impairment: new results of a randomized clinical trial. *J Am Geriatr Soc*. 2000;48:1183-1194.

6. Brautigam MR, Blommaert FA, Verleye G, et al. Treatment of age-related memory complaints with *Ginkgo biloba* extract: a randomized double-blind placebo-controlled study. *Phytomedicine*. 1998;5:425-434.

7. Mix JA, Crews WD Jr. An examination of the efficacy of *Ginkgo biloba* extract EGb 761 on the neuropsychologic functioning of cognitively intact older adults. *J Altern Complement Med*. 2000;6:219-229.

8. Winther K, Randlov C, Rein E, et al. Effects of *Ginkgo biloba* extract on cognitive function and blood pressure in elderly subjects. *Curr Ther Res*. 1998;59:881-888.

9. Rai GS, Shovlin C, Wesnes KA. A double-blind, placebo controlled study of *Ginkgo biloba* extract ('Tanakan™') in elderly outpatients with mild to moderate memory impairment. *Curr Med Res Opin*. 1991;12:350-355.

10. Rigney U, Kimber S, Hindmarch I. The effects of acute doses of standardized *Ginkgo biloba* extract on memory and psychomotor performance in volunteers. *Phytotherapy Res*. 1999;13:408-415.

11. Allain H, Raoul P, Lieury A, et al. Effect of two doses of *Ginkgo biloba* extract (EGb 761) on the dual-coding test in elderly subjects. *Clin Ther.* 1993;15:549-558.

12. Kennedy DO, Scholey AB, Wesnes KA. The dose-dependent cognitive effects of acute administration of *Ginkgo biloba* to healthy young volunteers. *Psychopharmacology (Berl).* 2000;151:416-423.

13. Hindmarch I. Activity of *Ginkgo biloba* extract on short term memory [in French; English abstract]. *Presse Med.* 1986;15:1592-1594.

14. Warot D, Lacomblez L, Danjou P, et al. Comparative effects of *Ginkgo biloba* extracts on psychomotor performances and memory in healthy subjects [in French; English abstract]. *Therapie.* 1991;46:33-36.

15. Moulton PL, Boyko LN, Fitzpatrick JL, et al. The effect of Ginkgo biloba on memory in healthy male volunteers. *Physiol Behav.* 2001;73:659-665.

16. Pittler MH, Ernst E. *Ginkgo biloba* extract for the treatment of intermittent claudication: a meta-analysis of randomized trials. *Am J Med.* 2000;108:276-281.

17. Peters H, Kieser M, Holscher U. Demonstration of the efficacy of *Ginkgo biloba* special extract EGb 761 on intermittent claudication—a placebo-controlled, double-blind multicenter trial. *Vasa.* 1998;27:106-110.

18. Blume J, Kieser M, Holscher U. Placebo-controlled double-blind study of the effectiveness of *Ginkgo biloba* special extract EGb 761 in trained patients with intermittent claudication [translated from German]. *Vasa.* 1996;25:265-274.

19. Schweizer J, Hautmann C. Comparison of two dosages of *Ginkgo biloba* extract EGb 761 in patients with peripheral arterial occlusive disease Fontaine's stage IIb: a randomized, double-blind, multicentric clinical trial. *Arzneimittelforschung.* 1999;49: 900-904.

20. Tamborini A, Taurell R. Value of standardized *Ginkgo biloba* extract (Egb 761) in the management of congestive symptoms of premenstrual syndrome [translated from French]. *Rev Fr Gynecol Obstet.* 1993;88:447-457.

21. Ernst E, Stevinson C. *Ginkgo biloba* for tinnitus: a review. *Clin Otolaryngol.* 1999;24: 164-167.

22. Holgers KM, Axelsson A, Pringle I. *Ginkgo biloba* extract for the treatment of tinnitus. *Audiology.* 1994;33:85-92.

23. Meyer B. Multicenter randomized double-blind drug vs. placebo study of the treatment of tinnitus with *Ginkgo biloba* extract [translated from French]. *Presse Med.* 1986;15:1562-1564.

24. Morgenstern C, Biermann E. Long-term tinnitus therapy with ginkgo special extract EGb 761 [translated from German]. *Fortschr Med.* 1997;115(29):57-58.

25. Drew S, Davies E. Effectiveness of *Ginkgo biloba* in treating tinnitus: double blind, placebo controlled trial. *BMJ.* 2001;322:73-75.

26. Schubert H, Halama P. Depressive episode primarily unresponsive to therapy in elderly patients: efficacy of *Ginkgo biloba* extract EGb 761 in combination with antidepressants [translated from German]. *Geriatr Forsch.* 1993;3:45-53.

27. Eckmann F. Cerebral insufficiency—treatment with *Ginkgo-biloba* extract. Time of onset of effect in a double-blind study with 60 inpatients [translated from German]. *Fortschr Med.* 1990;108:557-560.

28. Haguenauer JP, Cantenot F, Koskas H, et al. Treatment of equilibrium disorders with *Ginkgo biloba* extract: a multicenter double-blind drug vs. placebo study [translated from French]. *Presse Med.* 1986;15:1569-1572.

29. Burschka MA, Hassan HA, Reineke T, et al. Effect of treatment with *Ginkgo biloba* extract EGb 761 (oral) on unilateral idiopathic sudden hearing loss in a prospective randomized double-blind study of 106 outpatients. *Eur Arch Otorhinolaryngol.* 2001;258:213-219.

30. Roncin JP, Schwartz F, D'Arbigny P. EGb 761 in control of acute mountain sickness and vascular reactivity to cold exposure. *Aviat Space Environ Med.* 1996;67:445-452.

31. Lebuisson DA, Leroy L, Rigal G. Treatment of senile macular degeneration with *Ginkgo biloba* extract: a preliminary double-blind, drug versus placebo study [translated from French]. *Presse Med.* 1986;15:1556-1558.

32. Cohen A. Treatment of antidepressant-induced sexual dysfunction with *Ginkgo biloba* extract. Presented at: 149th Annual Meeting of the American Psychiatric Association, May 5-8, 1996; New York, NY. Abstract no. 716.

33. Cohen A. Long term safety and efficacy of *Ginkgo biloba* extract in the treatment of anti-depressant-induced sexual dysfunction (1997). Priory Lodge Education web site. Available at: http://www.priory.com/pharmol/gingko.htm. Accessed July 1, 1997. (Please note variant spelling of "ginkgo.")

34. Cohen AJ, Bartlik B. *Ginkgo biloba* for antidepressant-induced sexual dysfunction. *J Sex Marital Ther.* 1998;24:139-143.

35. Cohen A, Bartlik B. Treatment of sexual dysfunction with *Ginkgo biloba* extract [scientific reports]. Presented at: 150th Annual Meeting of the American Psychiatric Association; May 18-21, 1997; San Diego, Calif.

36. McCann B. Botanical could improve sex life of patients on SSRIs. *Drug Topics.* 1997; 141:33.

37. De Feudis FV. Ginkgo biloba *Extract (EGb 761): Pharmacological and Clinical Applications.* Paris, France: Elsevier; 1991:143-146.

38. Sikora R, Sohn M, Deutz FJ, et al. *Ginkgo biloba* extract in the therapy of erectile dysfunction [abstract]. *J Urol.* 1989;141:188A.

39. Hauns B, Haring B, Kohler S, et al. Phase II study with 5-fluorouracil and *Ginkgo biloba* extract (GBE 761 ONC) in patients with pancreatic cancer. *Arzneimittel-forschung.* 1999;49:1030-1034.

40. Liu P, Luo H-C, Shen Y-C, et al. Combined use of *Ginkgo biloba* extracts on the efficacy and adverse reactions of various antipsychotics [translated from Chinese]. *Chin J Clin Pharmacol.* 1997;13:193-198.

41. Funfgeld EW. *Rokan* (Ginkgo biloba): *Recent Results in Pharmacology and Clinic.* New York, NY: Springer-Verlag; 1988.

42. Kleijnen J, Knipschild P. *Ginkgo biloba. Lancet.* 1992;340:1136-1139.

43. Klein J, Chatterjee SS, Loffelholz K. Phospholipid breakdown and choline release under hypoxic conditions: inhibition by bilobalide, a constituent of *Ginkgo biloba. Brain Res.* 1997;755:347-350.

44. Rapin JR, Zaibi M, Drieu K. In vitro and in vivo effects of an extract of *Ginkgo biloba* (EGb 761), ginkgolide B, and bilobalide on apoptosis in primary cultures of rat hippocampal neurons. *Drug Res.* 1998;45:23-29.

45. Schulz V, Hansel R, Tyler VE. *Rational Phytotherapy: A Physicians' Guide to Herbal Medicine,* 3rd ed. Berlin, Germany: Springer-Verlag; 1998: 40, 43, 46-47, 126.

46. White HL, Scates PW, Cooper BR. Extracts of *Ginkgo biloba* leaves inhibit monoamine oxidase. *Life Sci.* 1996;58:1315-1321.

47. Ramassamy C, Clostre F, Christen Y, et al. Prevention by a *Ginkgo biloba* extract (GBE 761) of the dopaminergic neurotoxicity of MPTP. *J Pharm Pharmacol.* 1990;42:785-789.

48. Paick JS, Lee JH. An experimental study of the effect of *Ginkgo biloba* extract on the human and rabbit corpus cavernosum tissue. *J Urol.* 1996;156:1876-1880.

49. Blumenthal M, ed. *The Complete German Commission E Monographs, Therapeutic Guide to Herbal Medicines.* Boston, Mass: Integrative Medicine Communications; 1998:136.

50. Rowin J, Lewis SL. Spontaneous bilateral subdural hematomas associated with chronic *Ginkgo biloba* ingestion. *Neurology.* 1996;46:1775-1776.

51. Siegers CP. Cytotoxicity of alkylphenols from *Ginkgo biloba. Phytomedicine.* 1999; 6:281-283.

52. Arenz A, Klein M, Fiehe K, et al. Occurrence of neurotoxic 4'-O-methylpyridoxine in *Ginkgo biloba* leaves, ginkgo medications and Japanese ginkgo food. *Planta Med.* 1996;62:548-551.

53. Kudolo GB. The effect of 3-month ingestion of *Ginkgo biloba* extract on pancreatic beta-cell function in response to glucose loading in normal glucose tolerant individuals. *J Clin Pharmacol.* 2000;40:647-654.

54. Duche JC, Barre J, Guinot P, et al. Effect of *Ginkgo biloba* extract on microsomal enzyme induction. *Int J Clin Pharmacol Res.* 1989;9:165-168.

55. Le Bars P. Conflicting results on ginkgo research. *Forsch Komplementarmed Klass Naturheilkd.* 2002;9:19-20.

56. Stough C, Clark J, Lloyd J, et al. Neuropsychological changes after 30-day *Ginkgo biloba* administration in healthy participants. *Int J Neuropsychopharm.* 2001;4:131-134.

57. Reisser CH, Weidauer H. Ginkgo biloba extract EGb 761® or pentoxifylline for the treatment of sudden deafness: a randomized reference-controlled double-blind study. *Acta Otolaryngol.* 2001; 121:579-584.

58. Ashton AK, Ahrens K, Gupta S, et al. Antidepressant-induced sexual dysfunction and Ginkgo biloba [letter]. *Am J Psychiatry.* 2000;157:836-837.

59. Zhang XY, Zhou DF, Zhang PY, et al. A double-blind, placebo-controlled trial of extract of Ginkgo biloba added to haloperidol in treatment-resistant patients with schizophrenia. *J Clin Psychiatry.* 2001;62:878-883.

60. DeFeudis FV. Ginkgo biloba *Extract (EGb 761): Pharmacological Activities and Clinical Applications.* Paris, France: Elsevier Science; 1991:143-146.

61. Granger AS. Ginkgo biloba precipitating epileptic seizures. *Age Ageing.* 2001;30: 523-525.

62. Gregory PJ. Seizure associated with Ginkgo biloba? [letter]. *Ann Intern Med.* 2001; 134:344.

63. Davydov L, Sterling AL. Stevens-Johnson syndrome with Ginkgo biloba. *J Herbal Pharmacother.* 2001; 1:65-69.

Ginseng

1. Scaglione F, Cattaneo G, Alessandria M, et al. Efficacy and safety of the standardised Ginseng extract G115 for potentiating vaccination against the influenza syndrome and protection against the common cold. *Drugs Exp Clin Res.* 1996;22:65-72.

2. Sorenson H, Sonne J. A double-masked study of the effects of ginseng on cognitive functions. *Curr Ther Res.* 1996;57:959-968.

3. Forgo I, Kayasseh L, Staub JJ. Effect of a standardized ginseng extract on general well-being, reaction time, lung function and gonadal hormones [translated from German]. *Med Welt.* 1981;32:751-756.

4. Siegl C, Siegl HJ. The possible revision of impaired mental abilities in old age: a double-blind study with *Panax ginseng* [translated from German]. *Therapiewoche.* 1979;29:4206, 4209-4216.

5. Sandberg F, Dencker L. Experimental and clinical tests on ginseng. *Z Phytother.* 1994;15:38-42.

6. D'Angelo L, Grimaldi R, Caravaggi M, et al. A double-blind, placebo-controlled clinical study on the effect of a standardized ginseng extract on psychomotor performance in healthy volunteers. *J Ethnopharmacol.* 1986;16:15-22.

7. Wesnes KA, Faleni RA, Hefting NR, et al. The cognitive, subjective, and physical effects of a *Ginkgo biloba/Panax ginseng* combination in healthy volunteers with neurasthenic complaints. *Psychopharmacol Bull.* 1997;33:677-683.

8. Sotaniemi EA, Haapakoski E, Rautio A. Ginseng therapy in non-insulin-dependent diabetic patients. *Diabetes Care.* 1995;18:1373-1375.

9. Vuksan V, Sievenpiper JL, Koo VY, et al. American ginseng (*Panax quinquefolius* L) reduces postprandial glycemia in nondiabetic subjects and subjects with type 2 diabetes mellitus. *Arch Intern Med.* 2000;160:1009-1013.

10. Vuksan V, Xu Z, Jenkins AL, et al. American ginseng (*Panax quinquefolium* L.) improves long term glycemic control in type 2 diabetes. Presented at: 60th Scientific Sessions of the American Diabetes Association; June 9-13, 2000; San Antonio, Tex.

11. Vuksan V, Sievenpiper JL, Wong J, et al. American ginseng (*Panax quinquefolius* L.) attenuates postprandial glycemia in a time-dependent but not dose-dependent manner in healthy individuals. *Am J Clin Nutr.* 2001;73:753-758.

12. Cherdrungsi P, Rungroeng K. Effects of standardized ginseng extract and exercise training on aerobic and anaerobic capacities in humans. *Korean J Ginseng Sci.* 1995;19:93-100.

13. Forgo I. Effect of drugs on physical exertion and the hormonal system of athletes. 2 [translated from German]. *MMW Munch Med Wochenschr.* 1983;125:822-824.

14. McNaughton LG, Egan G, Caelli G. A comparison of Chinese and Russian ginseng as ergogenic aids to improve various facets of physical fitness. *Int J Clin Nutr Rev.* 1989;9:32-35.

15. Engels HJ, Wirth JC. No ergogenic effects of ginseng (*Panax ginseng* C.A. Meyer) during graded maximal aerobic exercise. *J Am Diet Assoc.* 1997;97:1110-1115.

16. Allen JD, McLung J, Nelson AG, et al. Ginseng supplementation does not enhance healthy young adults' peak aerobic exercise performance. *J Am Coll Nutr.* 1998;17: 462-466.

17. Engels HJ, Said JM, Wirth JC. Failure of chronic ginseng supplementation to affect work performance and energy metabolism in healthy adult females. *Nutr Res.* 1996;16:1295-1306.

18. Kolokouri I, Engels H-J, Cieslak T, et al. Effect of chronic ginseng supplementation on short duration, supramaximal exercise test performance [abstract]. *Med Sci Sports Exerc.* 1999;31(5 suppl):S117.

19. Lifton B, Otto RM, Wygand J. The effect of ginseng on acute maximal aerobic exercise [abstract]. *Med Sci Sports Exerc.* 1997;29(5 suppl):S249.

20. Morris AC, Jacobs I, McLellan TM, et al. No ergogenic effect of ginseng ingestion. *Int J Sport Nutr.* 1996;6:263-271.

21. Teves MA, Wright JE, Welch MJ, et al. Effects of ginseng on repeated bouts of exhaustive exercise [abstract]. *Med Sci Sports Exerc.* 1983;15:162.

22. Bittles AH, Fulder SJ, Grant EC, et al. The effect of ginseng on the lifespan and stress responses in mice. *Gerontology.* 1979;25:125-131.

23. Brekhman II, Dardymov IV. Pharmacological investigation of glycosides from Ginseng and *Eleutherococcus. Lloydia.* 1969;32:46-51.

24. Dua PR, Shanker G, Srimal RC, et al. Adaptogenic activity of Indian *Panax pseudo-ginseng. Indian J Exp Biol.* 1989;27:631-634.

25. Grandhi A, Mujumdar AM, Patwardhan B. A comparative pharmacological investigation of ashwagandha and ginseng. *J Ethnopharmacol.* 1994;44:131-135.

26. Hiai S, Yokoyaa H, Oura H. Features of ginseng saponin induced corticosterone secretion. *Endocrinol Jpn.* 1979;26:737-740.

27. Newall CA, et al. *Herbal Medicines: A Guide for Health-Care Professionals.* London, England: Pharmaceutical Press; 1996: 146-148.

28. Oura HS, Hiai S, Nabetani S, et al. Effect of ginseng extract on endoplasmic reticulum and ribosome. *Planta Med.* 1975;28:76-88.

29. Ramachandran U, Divekar HM, Grover SK, et al. New experimental model for the evaluation of adaptogenic products. *J Ethnopharmacol.* 1990;29:275-281.

30. Schulz V, Hansel R, Tyler VE. *Rational Phytotherapy: A Physicians' Guide to Herbal Medicine.* 3rd ed. Berlin, Germany: Springer-Verlag; 1998:271-278.

31. Singh VK, George CX, Singh N. Combined treatment of mice with *Panax ginseng* extract and interferon inducer: amplification of host resistance to Semliki forest virus. *Planta Med.* 1983;47:234-236.

32. Singh VK, Agarwal SS, Gupta BM. Immunomodulatory activity of *Panax ginseng* extract. *Planta Med.* 1984;50:462-465.

33. Song ZJ, Moser C, Wu H, et al. Ginseng treatment induces a Th1 cytokine response in a mouse model of *Pseudomonas aeruginosa* lung infection. Poster presented at: 100th General Meeting American Society for Microbiology, Los Angeles, California; May 21-25, 2000.

34. Avakian EV, Evonuk E. Effect of *Panax ginseng* extract on tissue glycogen and adrenal cholesterol depletion during prolonged exercise. *Planta Med.* 1979;36:43-48.

35. Scaglione F, Ferrara F, Dugnani S, et al. Immunomodulatory effects of two extracts of *Panax ginseng* C.A. Meyer. *Drugs Exp Clin Res.* 1990;16:537-542.

36. Caso Marasco A, Vargas Ruiz R, Salas Villagomez A, et al. Double-blind study of a multivitamin complex supplemented with ginseng extract. *Drugs Exp Clin Res.* 1996;22:323-329.

37. Cardinal BJ, Engels HJ. Ginseng does not enhance psychological well-being in healthy, young adults: results of a double-blind placebo-controlled, randomized clinical trial. *J Am Diet Assoc.* 2001;101:655-660.

38. Wiklund IK, Mattsson LA, Lindgren R, et al. Effects of a standardized ginseng extract on quality of life and physiological parameters in symptomatic postmenopausal women: a double-blind, placebo-controlled trial. *Int J Clin Pharmacol Res.* 1999; 19:89-99.

39. Quiroga HA. A comparative double-blind study of the action of Ginsana G115 and Hydergine on cerebrovascular deficit [translated from Spanish]. *Orientacion Medica.* 1982;(1281):201-202.

40. Sievenpiper JL, Stavro MP, Leiter LA, et al. Variable effects of ginseng: American Ginseng (*Panax quinquefolius* L.) with a low ginsenoside content does not affect postprandial glycemia in normal subjects [abstract]. *Diabetes.* 2001;50(suppl 2):Abst no. 1771-PO.

41. Baldwin CA, Anderson LA, Phillipson JD. What pharmacists should know about ginseng. *Pharm J.* 1986;237:583-586.

42. Hess FG, Parent RA, Cox GE, et al. Reproduction study in rats of ginseng extract G115. *Food Chem Toxicol.* 1982;20:189-192.

43. Sonnenborn U, Proppert Y. Ginseng (*Panax ginseng* C.A. Meyer). *Br J Phytother.* 1991;2:3-14.

44. Greenspan EM. Ginseng and vaginal bleeding [letter]. *JAMA.* 1983;249:2018.

45. Hammond TG, Whitworth JA. Adverse reactions to ginseng [letter]. *Med J Aust.* 1981;1:492.

46. Palmer BV, Montgomery AC, Monteiro JC. Ginseng and mastalgia [letter]. *Br Med J.* 1978;1:1284.

47. Punnonen R, Lukola A. Oestrogen-like effect of ginseng. *Br Med J.* 1980;281:1110.

48. Ryu SJ, Chien YY. Ginseng-associated cerebral arteritis. *Neurology.* 1995;45:829-830.

49. Cui J, Garle M, Eneroth P, et al. What do commercial ginseng preparations contain? [letter]. *Lancet.* 1994;344:134.

50. Tyler VE. *Herbs of Choice: The Therapeutic Use of Phytochemicals.* New York, NY: Pharmaceutical Products Press; 1994:172.

51. Jones BD, Runikis AM. Interaction of ginseng with phenelzine [letter]. *J Clin Psychopharmacol.* 1987;7:201-202.

52. Kroll D. University of Colorado School of Pharmacy, unpublished communication. 1998.

53. Janetzky K, Morreale AP. Probable interaction between warfarin and ginseng. *Am J Health Syst Pharm.* 1997;54:692-693.

54. Zhu M, Chan W, Ng S, et al. Possible influences of ginseng on the pharmacokinetics and pharmacodynamics of warfarin in rats. *J Pharm Pharmacol.* 1999;51:175-180.

55. McRae S. Elevated serum digoxin levels in a patient taking digoxin and Siberian ginseng. *CMAJ.* 1996;155:293-295.

56. Gaffney BT, Hugel HM, Rich PA. The effects of *Eleutherococcus senticosus* and *Panax ginseng* on steroidal hormone indices of stress and lymphocyte subset numbers in endurance athletes. *Life Sci.* 2001;70:431-442.

57. Ellis JM, Reddy P. Effects of Panax ginseng on quality of life. *Ann Pharmacother.* 2002;36:375-379.

58. Choi HK, et al. Clinical efficacy of Korean red ginseng for erectile dysfunction. *Int J Impotence Res.* 1995;7:181-186.

59. Salvati G, Genovesi G, Marcellini L, et al. Effects of Panax Ginseng C.A. Meyer saponins on male fertility. *Panminerva Med.* 1996;38;249-254.

60. Scaglione F, Weiser K, Allessandria M. Effects of the standardised ginseng extract G115 in patients with chronic bronchitis. *Clin Drug Invest.* 2001;21:41-45.

61. Fugh-Berman A. Herb-drug interactions. *Lancet.* 2000;355:134-138.

62. Amato P, Christophe S, Mellon P. Estrogenic activity of herbs commonly used as remedies for menopausal symptoms. *Menopause.* 2002;9:145-150.

63. Engels H-J, et al. Effects of ginseng supplementation on supramaximal exercise performance and short-term recovery. *J Strength Conditioning Res.* 2001;15:290-295.

Glucosamine

1. Noack W, Fischer M, Forster KK, et al. Glucosamine sulfate in osteoarthritis of the knee. *Osteoarthritis Cartilage.* 1994;2:51-59.

2. Crolle G, D'Este E. Glucosamine sulphate for the management of arthrosis: a controlled clinical investigation. *Curr Med Res Opin.* 1980;7:104-109.

3. D'Ambrosio E, Casa B, Bompani R, et al. Glucosamine sulphate: a controlled clinical investigation in arthrosis. *Pharmatherapeutica.* 1981;2:504-508.

4. Drovanti A, Bignamini AA, Rovati AL. Therapeutic activity of oral glucosamine sulfate in osteoarthrosis: a placebo-controlled double-blind investigation. *Clin Ther.* 1980;3:260-272.

5. Rindone JP, Hiller D, Collacott E, et al. Randomized, controlled trial of glucosamine for treating osteoarthritis of the knee. *West J Med.* 2000;172:91-94.

6. Houpt JB, McMillian R, Wein C, et al. Effect of glucosamine hydrochloride in the treatment of pain and osteoarthritis of the knee. *J Rheumatol.* 1999;26:2423-2430.

7. Muller-Fassbender H, Bach GL, Haase W, et al. Glucosamine sulfate compared to ibuprofen in osteoarthritis of the knee. *Osteoarthritis Cartilage.* 1994;2:61-69.

8. Qiu GX, Gao SN, Giacovelli G, et al. Efficacy and safety of glucosamine sulfate versus ibuprofen in patients with knee osteoarthritis. *Arzneimittelforschung.* 1998;48: 469-474.

9. Thie NM, Prasad NG, Major PW. Evaluation of glucosamine sulfate compared to ibuprofen for the treatment of temporomandibular joint osteoarthritis: a randomized double blind controlled 3 month clinical trial. *J Rheumatol.* 2001;28:1347-1355.

10. Rovati LC, Giacovelli G, Annefeld M, et al. A large, randomized, placebo controlled, double-blind study of glucosamine sulfate vs piroxicam and vs their association, on the kinetics of the symptomatic effect in knee osteoarthritis [abstract]. *Osteoarthritis Cartilage.* 1994;2(suppl 1):56.

11. Reginster JY, Deroisy R, Rovati L, et al. Long-term effects of glucosamine sulphate on osteoarthritis progression: a randomized, placebo-controlled clinical trial. *Lancet.* 2001;357:251-256.

12. Hellio MP. The effects of glucosamine on human osteoarthritic chondrocytes. Presented at: The Ninth EULAR Symposium; October 7-10, 1996; Madrid, Spain.

13. Jimenez SA. The effects of glucosamine on human chondrocyte gene expression. Presented at: The Ninth EULAR Symposium; October 7-10, 1996; Madrid, Spain.

14. Piperno M, Reboul P, Hellio Le Graverand MP, et al. Glucosamine sulfate modulates dysregulated activities of human osteoarthritic chondrocytes in vitro. *Osteoarthritis Cartilage.* 2000;8:207-212.

15. Setnikar I, Pacini MA, Revel L. Antiarthritic effects of glucosamine sulfate studied in animal models. *Arzneimittelforschung.* 1991;41:542-545.

16. Setnikar I. Antireactive properties of "chondroprotective" drugs. *Int J Tissue React.* 1992;14:253-261.

17. Reichelt A, Forster KK, Fischer M, et al. Efficacy and safety of intramuscular glucosamine sulfate in osteoarthritis of the knee: a randomized, placebo-controlled, double-blind study. *Arzneimittelforschung.* 1994;44:75-80.

18. Lopes Vaz A. Double-blind clinical evaluation of the relative efficacy of ibuprofen and glucosamine sulphate in the management of osteoarthrosis of the knee in out-patients. *Curr Med Res Opin.* 1982;8:145-149.

19. Lippiello L, Woodward J, Karpman R, et al. In vivo chondroprotection and metabolic synergy of glucosamine and chondroitin sulfate. *Clin Orthop.* 2000;381: 229-240.

20. Lippiello L, Karpman RR, Hammad T. Synergistic effect of glucosamine HCL and chondroitin sulfate on in vitro proteoglycan synthesis by bovine chondrocytes. Presented at: American Academy of Orthopaedic Surgeons 67th Annual Meeting; March 15-19, 2000; Orlando, Fla.

21. Setnikar I, Giacchetti C, Zanolo G. Pharmacokinetics of glucosamine in the dog and in man. *Arzneimittelforschung.* 1986;36:729-735.

22. Setnikar I, Palumbo R, Canali S, et al. Pharmacokinetics of glucosamine in man. *Arzneimittelforschung.* 1993;43:1109-1113.

23. Tapadinhas MJ, Rivera IC, Bignamini AA. Oral glucosamine sulphate in the management of arthrosis: report on a multi-centre open investigation in Portugal. *Pharmatherapeutica.* 1982;3:157-168.

24. Almada AL, Harvey PW, Platt KJ. Effect of chronic oral glucosamine sulfate upon fasting insulin resistance index (FIRI) in nondiabetic individuals [abstract]. *FASEB J.* 2000;14:A750.

25. Head K. Personal communication of case reports. 1999.

26. Patti ME, Virkamaki A, Landaker EJ, et al. Activation of the hexosamine pathway by glucosamine in vivo induces insulin resistance of early postreceptor insulin signaling events in skelatal muscle. *Diabetes.* 1999;48:1562-1571.
27. Shankar RR, Zhu JS, Baron AD. Glucosamine infusion in rats mimics the beta-cell dysfunction of non-insulin-dependant diabetes mellitus. *Metabolism.* 1998;47:573-577.
28. Virkamaki A, Yki-Jarvinen H. Allosteric regulation of glycogen synthase and hexokinase by glucosamine-6-phosphate during glucosamine-induced insulin resistance in skeletal muscle and heart. *Diabetes.* 1999;48:1101-1107.
29. Pouwels MJ, Jacobs JR, Span PN, et al. Short-term glucosamine infusion does not affect insulin sensitivity in humans. *J Clin Endocrinol Metab.* 2001;86:2099-2103.
30. Monauni T, Zenti MG, Cretti A, et al. Effects of glucosamine infusion on insulin secretion and insulin action in humans. *Diabetes.* 2000;49:926-935.
31. Ajiboye R, Harding JJ. The non-enzymic glycosylation of bovine lens proteins by glucosamine and its inhibition by aspirin, ibuprofen and glutathione. *Exp Eye Res.* 1989;49:31-41.
32. Lippiello L, Woodward J, Karpman R, et al. In vivo chondroprotection and metabolic synergy of glucosamine and chondroitin sulfate. *Clin Orthop.* 2000;(381):229-240.
33. Lippiello L, Karpman RR, Hammad T. Synergistic effect of glucosamine HCL and chondroitin sulfate on in vitro proteoglycan synthesis by bovine chondrocytes. Presented at: American Academy of Orthopaedic Surgeons 67th Annual Meeting; March 15-19, 2000: Orlando, Fla.
34. McAlindon TE, LaValley MP, Gulin JP, et al. Glucosamine and chondroitin for treatment of osteoarthritis: a systematic quality assessment and meta-analysis. *JAMA.* 2000;283:1469-1475.
35. Hughes R, Carr A. A randomized, double-blind, placebo-controlled trial of glucosamine sulphate as an analgesic in osteoarthritis of the knee. *Rheumatology (Oxford).* 2002;41:279-284.

Glutamine

1. Castell LM, Newsholme EA. Glutamine and the effects of exhaustive exercise upon the immune response. *Can J Physiol Pharmacol.* 1998;76:524-532.
2. Rohde T, MacLean DA, Hartkopp A, et al. The immune system and serum glutamine during a triathalon. *Eur J Appl Physiol.* 1996;74:428-434.
3. Rowbottom DG, Keast D, Morton AR, et al. The emerging role of glutamine as an indicator of exercise stress and overtraining. *Sports Med.* 1996;21:80-97.
4. Castell LM, Newsholme EA. The effects of oral glutamine supplementation on athletes after prolonged, exhaustive exercise. *Nutrition.* 1997;13:738-742.
5. Mackinnon LT, Hooper SL. Plasma glutamine and upper respiratory tract infection during intensified training in swimmers. *Med Sci Sports Exerc.* 1996;28:285-290.
6. Castell LM, Poortmans JR, Newsholme EA. Does glutamine have a role in reducing infections in athletes? *Eur J Appl Physiol Occup Physiol.* 1996;73:488-490.
7. Griffiths RD, Jones C, Palmer TEA. Six-month outcome of critically ill patients given glutamine-supplemented parenteral nutrition. *Nutrition.* 1997;13:295-302.
8. van der Hulst RR, van Kreel BK, von Meyenfeldt MF, et al. Glutamine and the preservation of gut integrity. *Lancet.* 1993;341:1363-1365.
9. Zoli G, Care M, Falco F, et al. Effect of oral glutamine on intestinal permeability and nutritional status in Crohn's disease [abstract]. *Gastroenterology.* 1995;108:A766.
10. Bozzetti F, Biganzoli L, Gavazzi C, et al. Glutamine supplementation in cancer patients receiving chemotherapy: a double-blind randomized study. *Nutrition.* 1997;13:748-751.
11. Den Hond E, Hiele M, Peeters M, et al. Effect of long-term oral glutamine supplements on small intestinal permeability in patients with Crohn's disease. *JPEN J Parenter Enteral Nutr.* 1999;23:7-11.
12. Daniele B, Perrone F, Gallo C, et al. Oral glutamine in the prevention of fluorouracil induced intestinal toxicity: a double blind, placebo controlled, randomized trial. *Gut.* 2001;48:28-33.

13. Mebane AH. L-glutamine and mania [letter]. *Am J Psychiatry*. 1984;141:1302-1303.
14. Krzywkowski K, et al. Effect of glutamine supplementation on exercise-induced changes in lymphocyte function. *Am J Physiol Cell Physiol*. 2001;281:C1259-C1265.
15. Khogali SE, Pringle SD, Weryk BV, et al. Is glutamine beneficial in ischemic heart disease? *Nutrition*. 2002;18:123-126.
16. Candow DG, Chilibeck PD, Burke DG, et al. Effect of glutamine supplementation combined with resistance training in young adults. *Eur J Appl Physiol*. 2001;86:142-149.
17. Antonio J, Sanders MS, Kalman D, et al. The effects of high-dose glutamine ingestion on weightlifting performance. *J Strength Cond Res*. 2002;16:157-160.

Glycine

1. Gusev EI, Skvortsova VI, Komissarova IA, et al. Neuroprotective effects of glycine in the acute period of ischemic stroke [translated from Russian]. *Zh Nevrol Psikhiatr Im S S Korsakova*. 1999;99:12-20.
2. Heresco-Levy U, Javitt DC, Ermilov M, et al. Efficacy of high-dose glycine in the treatment of enduring negative symptoms of schizophrenia. *Arch Gen Psychiatry*. 1999;56:29-36.
3. Heresco-Levy U, Javitt DC, Ermilov M, et al. Double-blind, placebo-controlled, crossover trial of glycine adjuvant therapy for treatment-resistant schizophrenia. *Br J Psychiatry*. 1996;169:610-617.
4. Javitt DC, Zylberman I, Zukin SR, et al. Amelioration of negative symptoms in schizophrenia by glycine. *Am J Psychiatry*. 1994;151:1234-1236.
5. Semba J. Glycine therapy of schizophrenia; its rationale and a review of clinical trials [translated from Japanese]. *Nihon Shinkei Seishin Yakurigaku Zasshi*. 1998;18:71-80.
6. Evins AE, Fitzgerald SM, Wine L, et al. Placebo-controlled trial of glycine added to clozapine in schizophrenia. *Am J Psychiatry*. 2000;157:826-828.
7. Fries MH, Rinaldo P, Schmidt-Sommerfeld E, et al. Isovaleric acidemia: response to a leucine load after three weeks of supplementation with glycine, L-carnitine, and combined glycine-carnitine therapy. *J Pediatr*. 1996;129:449-452.
8. Itoh T, Ito T, Ohba S, et al. Effect of carnitine administration on glycine metabolism in patients with isovaleric acidemia: significance of acetylcarnitine determination to estimate the proper carnitine dose. *Tohoku J Exp Med*. 1996;179:101-109.
9. de Koning TJ, Duran M, Dorland L, et al. Beneficial effects of L-serine and glycine in the management of seizures in 3-phosphoglycerate dehydrogenase deficiency. *Ann Neurol*. 1998;44:261265.
10. Yin M, Ikejima K, Arteel GE, et al. Glycine accelerates recovery from alcohol-induced liver injury. *J Pharmacol Exp Ther*. 1998;286:1014-1019.
11. Thurman RG, Zhong Z, von Frankenberg M, et al. Prevention of cyclosporine-induced nephrotoxicity with dietary glycine. *Transplantation*. 1997;63:1661-1667.
12. Zhong Z, Arteel GE, Connor HD, et al. Cyclosporin A increases hypoxia and free radical production in rat kidneys: prevention by dietary glycine. *Am J Physiol*. 1998;275:F595-F604.
13. Rose ML, Cattley RC, Dunn C, et al. Dietary glycine prevents the development of liver tumors caused by the peroxisome proliferator WY-14,643. *Carcinogenesis*. 1999;20:2075-2081.
14. Rose ML, Madren J, Bunzendahl H, et al. Dietary glycine inhibits the growth of B16 melanoma tumors in mice. *Carcinogenesis*. 1999;20:793-798.
15. Javitt DC. Management of negative symptoms of schizophrenia. *Curr Psychiatry Rep*. 2001;3:413-417.
16. File SE, Fluck E, Fernandes C. Beneficial effects of glycine (Bioglycin) on memory and attention in young and middle-aged adults. *J Clin Psychopharmacol*. 1999;19:506-512.
17. Sopala M, Schweizer S, Schafer N, et al. Neuroprotective activity of a nanoparticulate formulation of the glycine B site antagonist MRZ 2/576 in transient focal ischaemia in rats. *Arzneimittelforschung*. 2002;52:168-174.
18. Tatlisumak T, Takano K, Meiler MR, et al. A glycine site antagonist ZD9379 reduces number of spreading depressions and infarct size in rats with permanent middle cerebral artery occlusion. *Acta Neurochir Suppl*. 2000;76:331-333.

Goldenrod

1. Blumenthal M, ed. *The Complete German Commission E Monographs, Therapeutic Guide to Herbal Medicines.* Boston, Mass: Integrative Medicine Communications; 1998: 139-140.
2. European Scientific Cooperative on Phytotherapy. *Solidaginis virgaureae herba* (goldenrod). Exeter, UK: ESCOP; 1996-1997. Monographs on the Medicinal Uses of Plant Drugs, Fascicule 2:1-3.
3. Pyevich D, Bogenschutz MP. Herbal diuretics and lithium toxicity [letter]. *Am J Psychiatry.* 2001;158:1329.

Goldenseal

1. Budzinski JW, Foster BC, Vandenhoek S, et al. An in vitro evaluation of human cytochrome P450 3A4 inhibition by selected commercial herbal extracts and tinctures. *Phytomedicine.* 2000;7:273-282.
2. Amin AH, Subbaiah TV, Abbasi KM. Berberine sulfate: antimicrobial activity, bioassay, and mode of action. *Can J Microbiol.* 1969;15:1067-1076.
3. Hahn FE, Ciak J. Berberine. *Antibiotics.* 1976;3:577-584.
4. Kaneda Y, Torii M, Tanaka T, et al. In vitro effects of berberine sulphate on the growth and structure of *Entamoeba histolytica, Giardia lamblia* and *Trichomonas vaginalis. Ann Trop Med Parasitol.* 1991;85:417-425.
5. Rabbani GH, Butler T, Knight J, et al. Randomized controlled trial of berberine sulfate therapy for diarrhea due to enterotoxigenic *Escherichia coli* and *Vibrio cholerae. J Infect Dis.* 1987;155:979-984.
6. Khin-Maung-U, Myo-Khin, Nyunt-Nyunt-Wai, et al. Clinical trial of berberine in acute watery diarrhoea. *Br Med J (Clin Res Ed).* 1985;291:1601-1605.
7. Choudhry VP, Sabir M, Bhide VN. Berberine in giardiasis. *Indian Pediatr.* 1972; 9:143-146.
8. Gupte S. Use of berberine in treatment of giardiasis. *Am J Dis Child.* 1975;129:866.
9. Babbar OP, Chhatwal VK, Ray IB, et al. Effect of berberine chloride eye drops on clinically positive trachoma patients. *Indian J Med Res.* 1982;76(suppl):83-88.
10. Mohan M, Pant CR, Angra SK, et al. Berberine in trachoma (a clinical trial). *Indian J Ophthalmol.* 1982;30:69-75.
11. Sun D, Abraham SN, Beachey EH. Influence of berberine sulfate on synthesis and expression of Pap fimbrial adhesin in uropathogenic *Escherichia coli. Antimicrob Agents Chemother.* 1988;32:1274-1277.
12. Foster S. *Botanical Series No. 309—Goldenseal.* Austin, Tex: American Botanical Council; 1991:5-6.
13. Smet PA de, et al, eds. *Adverse Effects of Herbal Drugs.* Vol. I. Berlin, Germany: Springer-Verlag; 1992:97-104.
14. Chan E. Displacement of bilirubin from albumin by berberine. *Biol Neonat.* 1993;63:201-208.

Gotu Kola

1. Pointel JP, Boccalon H, Cloarec M, et al. Titrated extract of *Centella asiatica* (TECA) in the treatment of venous insufficiency of the lower limbs. *Angiology.* 1987;38:46-50.
2. Cesarone MR, Laurora G, De Sanctis MT, et al. The microcirculatory activity of *Centella asiatica* in venous insufficiency: a double-blind study [translated from Italian]. *Minerva Cardioangiol.* 1994;42:299-304.
3. Belcaro GV, Rulo A, Grimaldi R. Capillary filtration and ankle edema in patients with venous hypertension treated with TTFCA. *Angiology.* 1990;41:12-18.
4. Allegra C, Pollari G, Criscuolo A, et al. *Centella asiatica* extract in venous disorders of the lower limbs. Comparative clinico-instrumental studies with a placebo [in Italian; English abstract]. *Clin Ter.* 1981;99:507-513.
5. Barletta S, Borgioli A, Corsi C, et al. Results with *Centella asiatica* in chronic venous insufficiency [in Italian; English abstract]. *Gazz Med Ital.* 1981;140:33-35.

6. Cospite M, Ferrara F, Milio G, et al. Study about pharmacologic and clinical activity of *Centella asiatica* titrated extract in the chronic venous deficiency of the lower limbs: valuation with strain gauge plethismography [in Italian; English abstract]. *G Ital Angiol.* 1984;4:200-205.

7. Frausini G, Rotatori P, Oliva S, et al. Controlled trial on clinical-dynamic effects of three treatments in chronic venous insufficiency [in Italian; English abstract]. *G Ital Angiol.* 1985;5:147-151.

8. Cesarone MR, Laurora G, De Sanctis MT, et al. Activity of *Centella asiatica* in venous insufficiency [in Italian; English abstract]. *Minerva Cardioangiol.* 1992;40:137-143.

9. Kartnig T. Clinical applications of *Centella asiatica* (L.). *Herbs Spices Med Plants.* 1988;3:146-173.

10. Bosse JP, Papillon J, Frenette G, et al. Clinical study of a new antikeloid agent. *Ann Plast Surg.* 1979;3:13-21.

11. Nalini K, Aroor AR, Karanth KS, et al. Effects of *Centella asiatica* fresh leaf aqueous extract on learning and memory and biogenic amine turnover in albino rats. *Fitoterapia.* 1992;63:232-237.

12. Bradwejn J, Zhou Y, Koszycki D, et al. A double-blind, placebo-controlled study on the effects of gotu kola *(Centella asiatica)* on acoustic startle response in healthy subjects. *J Clin Psychopharmacol.* 2000;20:680-684.

13. Tenni R, Zanaboni G, de Agostini MP, et al. Effect of the triterpenoid fraction of *Centella asiatica* on macromolecules of the connective matrix in human skin fibroblast cultures. *Ital J Biochem.* 1988;37:69-77.

14. Boiteau P, Ratsimamanga AR. Asiaticoside extracted from *Centella asiatica*, its therepautic uses in the healing of experimental or refractory wounds, leprosy, skin tuberculosis, and lupus [in French]. *Therapie.* 1956;11:125-149.

15. Laerum OD, Iversen OH. Reticuloses and epidermal tumors in hairless mice after topical skin applications of cantharidin and asiaticoside. *Cancer Res.* 1972;32:1463-1469.

16. Basellini A, Agus GB, Antonucci E, et al. Varices in pregnancy (an up-date) [translated from Italian]. *Ann Ostet Ginecol Med Perinat.* 1985;106:337-341.

Grass Pollen Extract

1. Becker H, Ebeling L. Conservative therapy of benign prostatic hyperplasia (BPH) with Cernilton® N [translated from German]. *Urologe B.* 1988;28:301-306.

2. Buck AC, Cox R, Rees RWM, et al. Treatment of outflow tract obstruction due to benign prostatic hyperplasia with the pollen extract, Cernilton: a double-blind, placebo-controlled study. *Br J Urol.* 1990;66:398-404.

3. Rugendorff EW, Weidner W, Ebeling L, et al. Results of treatment with pollen extract (Cernilton N) in chronic prostatitis and prostatodynia. *Br J Urol.* 1993; 71:433-438.

4. Buck AC, Rees RWM, Ebeling L. Treatment of chronic prostatitis and prostatodynia with pollen extract. *Br J Urol.* 1989;64:496-499.

5. Suzuki T, Kurokawa K, Mashimo T, et al. Clinical effect of Cernilton in chronic prostatitis [in Japanese; English abstract]. *Hinyokika Kiyo.* 1992;38:489-494.

6. Habib FK, Ross M, Buck AC, et al. In vitro evaluation of the pollen extract, cernitin T-60, in the regulation of prostate cell growth. *Br J Urol.* 1990;66:393-397.

7. Roberts KP, Iyer RA, Prasad G, et al. Cyclic hydroxamic acid inhibitors of prostate cancer cell growth: selectivity and structure activity relationships. *Prostate.* 1998;34:92-99.

8. Zhang X, Habib FK, Ross M, et al. Isolation and characterization of a cyclic hydroxamic acid from a pollen extract, which inhibits cancerous cell growth in vitro. *J Med Chem.* 1995;38:735-738.

9. Wojcicki J, Samochowiec L, Bartlomowicz B, et al. Effect of pollen extract on the development of experimental atherosclerosis in rabbits. *Atherosclerosis.* 1986;62:39-45.

10. Loschen G, Ebeling L. Inhibition of the arachidonate metabolism by an extract of rye pollen [in German; English abstract]. *Arzneimittelforschung.* 1991;41:162-167.

11. Schulz V, Hansel R, Tyler VE. *Rational Phytotherapy: A Physicians' Guide to Herbal Medicine.* 3rd ed. Berlin, Germany: Springer-Verlag; 1998:231.

Green Tea

1. Krahwinkel T, Willershausen B. The effect of sugar-free green tea chew candies on the degree of inflammation of the gingiva. *Eur J Med Res.* 2000;5;463-467.
2. Stoner GD, Mukhtar H. Polyphenols as cancer chemopreventive agents. *J Cell Biochem.* 1995;22(suppl):169-180.
3. Imai K, Suga K, Nakachi K. Cancer-preventive effects of drinking green tea among a Japanese population. *Prev Med.* 1997;26:769-775.
4. Kohlmeier L, Weterings KG, Steck S, et al. Tea and cancer prevention: an evaluation of the epidemiologic literature. *Nutr Cancer.* 1997;27:1-13.
5. Tsubono Y, Nishino Y, Komatsu S, et al. Green tea and the risk of gastric cancer in Japan. *N Engl J Med.* 2001;344:632-666.
6. Galanis DJ, Kolonel LN, Lee J, et al. Intakes of selected foods and beverages and the incidence of gastric cancer among the Japanese residents of Hawaii: a prospective study. *Int J Epidemiol.* 1998;27:173-180.
7. Imai K, Nakachi K. Cross sectional study of effects of drinking green tea on cardio-vascular and liver diseases. *BMJ.* 1995;310:693-696.
8. Kono S, Shinchi K, Ikeda N, et al. Green tea consumption and serum lipid profiles: a cross-sectional study in Northern Kyushu, Japan. *Prev Med.* 1992;21:526-531.
9. Tsubono Y, Tsugane S. Green tea intake in relation to serum lipid levels in middle-aged Japanese men and women. *Ann Epidemiol.* 1997;7:280-284.
10. van het Hof KH, de Boer HSM, Wiseman SA, et al. Consumption of green or black tea does not increase resistance of low-density lipoprotein to oxidation in humans. *Am J Clin Nutr.* 1997;66:1125-1132.
11. Katiyar SK, Matsui MS, Elmets CA, et al. Polyphenolic antioxidant (−)-epigallo-catechin-3-gallate from green tea reduces UVB-induced inflammatory responses and infiltration of leukocytes in human skin. *Photochem Photobiol.* 1999;69:148-153.
12. Katiyar SK, Elmets CA, Agarwal R, et al. Protection against ultraviolet-B radiation-induced local and systemic suppression of contact hypersensitivity and edema re-sponses in C3H/HeN mice by green tea polyphenols. *Photochem Photobiol.* 1995;62:855-861.
13. Elmets CA, Singh D, Tubesing K, et al. Cutaneous photoprotection from ultravio-let injury by green tea polyphenols. *J Am Acad Dermatol.* 2001;44:425-432.
14. Hegarty VM, May HM, Khaw KT. Tea drinking and bone mineral density in older women. *Am J Clin Nutr.* 2000;71:1003-1007.
15. Geleijnse JM, Launer LJ, Hofman A, et al. Tea flavonoids may protect against ath-erosclerosis: the Rotterdam Study. *Arch Intern Med.* 1999;159:2170-2174.
16. Snow JM. *Camellia sinensis* (L.) Kuntze (Theaceae). *Protocol J Bot Med.* 1995; Autumn:28-32.
17. Cao Y, Cao R. Angiogenesis inhibited by drinking tea [letter]. *Nature.* 1999;398:381.
18. Taylor JR, Wilt VM. Probable antagonism of warfarin by green tea. *Ann Pharmacother.* 1999;33:426-428.

Guggul

1. Singh RB, Niaz MA, Ghosh S. Hypolipidemic and antioxidant effects of *Commiphora mukul* as an adjunct to dietary therapy in patients with hypercholesterolemia. *Cardiovasc Drugs Ther.* 1994;8:659-664.
2. Verma SK, Bordia A. Effect of *Commiphora mukul* (gum guggulu) in patients of hy-perlipidemia with special reference to HDL-cholesterol. *Indian J Med Res.* 1988; 87:356-360.
3. Nityanand S, Srivastava JS, Asthana OP. Clinical trials with gugulipid: a new hypo-lipidaemic agent. *J Assoc Physicians India.* 1989;37:323-328.
4. Thappa DM, Dogra J. Nodulocystic acne: oral gugulipid versus tetracycline. *J Dermatol.* 1994;21:729-731.
5. Subramaniam A, Stocker C, Sennitt MV, et al. Guggul lipid reduces insulin resis-tance and body weight gain in C57B1/6 lep/lep mice [abstract]. *Int J Obes Relat Metab Disord.* 2001;25(suppl 2):S24.

6. Antonio J, Colker CM, Torina GC, et al. Effects of a standardized guggulsterone phosphate supplement on body composition in overweight adults: a pilot study. *Curr Ther Res.* 1999;60:220-227.
7. Nityanand S, Srivastava JS, Asthana OP. Clinical trials with gugulipid: a new hypolipidaemic agent. *J Assoc Physicians India.* 1989;37:323-328.
8. Agarwal RC, Singh SP, Saran RK, et al. Clinical trial of gugulipid—a new hyperlipidemic agent of plant origin in primary hyperlipidemia. *Indian J Med Res.* 1986; 84:626-634.

Gymnema

1. Shanmugasundaram ERB, Rajeswari G, Baskaran K, et al. Use of gymnema sylvestre leaf extract in the control of blood glucose in insulin-dependent diabetes mellitus. *J Ethnopharmacol.* 1990;30:281-294.
2. Baskaran K, Kizar Ahamath B, Radha Shanmugasundaram K, et al. Antidiabetic effect of a leaf extract from *Gymnema sylvestre* in non-insulin-dependent diabetes mellitus patients. *J Ethnopharmacol.* 1990;30:295-305.
3. Shanmugasundaram ERB, et al. Effect on an isolate of *Gymnema sylvestre* R.Br. in the control of diabetes mellitus and the associated pathological changes. *Anc Sci Life.* 1988;8:163-194.
4. Shanmugasundaram ER, Gopinath KL, Radha Shanmugasundaram K, et al. Possible regeneration of the islets of Langerhans in streptozotocin-diabetic rats given *Gymnema sylvestre* leaf extracts. *J Ethnopharmacol.* 1990;30:265-279.

Hawthorn

1. Schulz V, Hansel R, Tyler VE. *Rational Phytotherapy: A Physicians' Guide to Herbal Medicine.* 3rd ed. Berlin, Germany: Springer-Verlag; 1998:93, 94, 95.
2. Leuchtgens VH. Crataegus special extract WS 1442 in NYHA II heart failure: a placebo controlled randomized double-blind study [in German; English abstract]. *Fortschr Med.* 1993;111:352-354.
3. Schmidt U, Kuhn U, Ploch M, et al. Efficacy of the hawthorn *(Crataegus)* preparation LI 132 in 78 patients with chronic congestive heart failure defined as NYHA functional class II. *Phytomedicine.* 1994;1:17-24.
4. Tauchert M, Siegel G, Schulz V. Hawthorn extract as plant medication for the heart; a new evaluation of its therapeutic effectiveness [translated from German]. *MMW Munch Med Wochenschr.* 1994;136(suppl 1):S3-S5.
5. Zapfe jun G. Clinical efficacy of crataegus extract WS 1442 in congestive heart failure NYHA class II. *Phytomedicine.* 2001;8:262-266.
6. Hanak T, Bruckel MH. The treatment of mild stable forms of angina pectoris using Crategutt® novo [in German; English abstract]. *Therapiewoche.* 1983;33:4331-4333.
7. Joseph G, Zhao Y, Klaus W. Pharmacologic profile of crataegus extract compared to epinephrine, amrinone, milrinone and digoxin in isolated guinea pig hearts [in German; English abstract]. *Arzneimittelforschung.* 1995;45:1261-1265.
8. Popping S, Rose H, Ionescu I, et al. Effect of a hawthorn extract on contraction and energy turnover of isolated rat cardiomyocytes. *Arzneimittelforschung.* 1995;45: 1157-1161.
9. Al Makdessi S, Sweidan H, Dietz K, et al. Protective effect of *Crataegus oxyacantha* against reperfusion arrhythmias after global no-flow ischemia in the rat heart. *Basic Res Cardiol.* 1999;94:71-77.
10. Krzeminski T, Chatterjee SS. Ischemia and early reperfusion induced arrhythmias: beneficial effects of an extract of *Crataegus oxyacantha* L. *Pharm Pharmacol Lett.* 1993;3:45-48.
11. Kurcok A. Ischemia and reperfusion-induced cardiac injury: effects of two flavonoid containing plant extracts possessing radical scavenging properties [abstract]. *Naunyn Schmiedebergs Arch Pharmacol.* 1992;345(suppl 1):R81.
12. Muller A, Linke W, Klaus W. *Crataegus* extract blocks potassium currents in guinea pig ventricular cardiac myocytes. *Planta Med.* 1999;65:335-339.
13. Bahorun T, Trotin F, Pommery J, et al. Antioxidant activities of *Crataegus monogyna* extracts. *Planta Med.* 1994;60:323-328.

14. Petkov E, Nikolov N, Uzunov P. Inhibitory effect of some flavonoids and falvonoid mixtures on cyclic AMP phosphodiesterase activity of rat heart. *Planta Med.* 1981; 43:183-186.
15. Siegel G, Casper U, Schnalke F. Molecular physiological effector mechanisms of hawthorn extract in cardiac papillary muscle and coronary vascular smooth muscle. *Phytother Res.* 1996;10:S195-S198.
16. Uchida S, Ikari N, Ohta H, et al. Inhibitory effects of condensed tannins on angiotensin converting enzyme. *Jpn J Pharmacol.* 1987;43:242-246.
17. Schwinger RH, Pietsch M, Frank K, et al. Crataegus special extract WS 1442 increases force of contraction in human myocardium cAMP-independently. *J Cardiovasc Pharmacol.* 2000;35:700-707.
18. Siegel G, Casper U, Walter A, et al. Concentration-response study with the Crataegus extract LI 132 on membrane potential and tone of human coronary arteries and canine papillary muscle [in German; English abstract]. *MMW Munch Med Wochenschr.* 1994;136(suppl 1):S47-S56.
19. Siegel G, et al. *Crataegi folium* cum flore. In: Lowe D, Rietbrock N, eds. *Phytopharmaka in Forschung und klinischer Anwendung.* Darmstadt, Germany: Steinkopff Verlag; 1995:1-14. Cited by: Schulz V, Hansel R, Tyler VE. *Rational Phytotherapy: A Physicians' Guide to Herbal Medicine,* 3rd ed. Berlin, Germany: Springer-Verlag; 1998:91-93.
20. Mavers VWH, Hensel H. Changes in local myocardial blood flow following oral administration of a crataegus extract to non-anesthetized dogs [in German; English abstract]. *Arzneimittelforschung.* 1974;24:783-785.
21. Nasa Y, Hashizume H, Hoque AN, et al. Protective effect of crataegus extract on the cardiac mechanical dysfunction in isolated perfused working rat heart. *Arzneimittelforschung.* 1993;43:945-949.
22. Bahorun T, Gressier B, Trotin F, et al. Oxygen species scavenging activity of phenolic extracts from hawthorn fresh plant organs and pharmaceutical preparations. *Arzneimittelforschung.* 1996;46:1086-1089.
23. Ammon HPT, Handel M. *Crataegus,* toxicology and pharmacology. I. Toxicity [translated from German]. *Planta Med.*1981;43:105-120.
24. Ammon HP, Handel M. *Crataegus,* toxicology and pharmacology. II. Pharmacodynamics [translated from German]. *Planta Med.* 1981;43:209-239.
25. Rietbrock N, Hamel M, Hempel B, et al. Efficacy of a standardized extract of fresh Crataegus berries on exercise tolerance and quality of life in patients with congestive heart failure (NYHA II) [in German; English abstract]. *Arzneimittelforschung.* 2001;51:793-798.
26. Ammon HPT, Handel M. Crataegus, toxicology and pharmacology. I, II, and III [translated from German]. *Planta Med.* 1981;43:105-120, 209-239, 313-322.
27. Walker AF, Marakis G, Morris AP, et al. Promising hypotensive effect of hawthorn extract: a randomized double-blind pilot study of mild, essential hypertension. *Phytother Res.* 2002;16:48-54.

Hops

1. Lee KM, Jung JS, Song DK, et al. Effects of *Humulus lupulus* extract on the central nervous system in mice [abstract]. *Planta Med.* 1993;59(7 suppl):A691.
2. Schulz V, Hansel R, Tyler VE. *Rational Phytotherapy: A Physicians' Guide to Herbal Medicine,* 3rd ed. Berlin, Germany: Springer-Verlag; 1998:82-83.
3. Duncan KL, Hare WR, Buck WB. Malignant hyperthermia-like reaction secondary to ingestion of hops in five dogs. *J Am Vet Med Assoc.* 1997;210:51-54.
4. Coldham NG, Sauer MJ. Identification, quantitation and biological activity of phytoestrogens in a dietary supplement for breast enhancement. *Food and Chemical Toxicology.* 2001;39:1211-1224.
5. Milligan SR, Kalita JC, Heyerick A, et al. Identification of a potent phytoestrogen in hops *(Humulus lupulus L.)* and beer. *J Clin Endocrinol Metab.* 1999;83(6):2249-2252.
6. Zava DT, Dollbaum CM, Blen M. Estrogen and progestin bioactivity of foods, herbs, and spices. *Proc Soc Exp Biol Med.* 1998; 217: 369-378.

7. Milligan S, Kalita J, Pocock V, et al. Oestrogenic activity of the hop phyto-oestrogen, 8-prenylnaringenin. *Reproduction.* 2002;123:235-242.

Horse Chestnut

1. Bisler H, Pfeifer R, Kluken N, et al. Effects of horse-chestnut seed extract on transcapillary filtration in chronic venous insufficiency. *Dtsch Med Wochenschr.* 1986; 111:1321-1329.
2. Lohr E, Garanin G, Jesau P, et al. Anti-edemic therapy in chronic venous insufficiency with tendency to formation of edema [translated from German]. *MMW Munch Med Wochenschr.* 1986;128:579-581.
3. Rudofsky G, Neiss A, Otto K, et al. Antiedematous effects and clinical effectiveness of horse chestnut seed extract in double blind studies [translated from German]. *Phlebol Proktol.* 1986;15:47-54.
4. Steiner M, Hillemanns HG. Investigation of the anti-edemic efficacy of Venostasin® retard [translated from German]. *MMW Munch Med Wochenschr.* 1986;128:551-552.
5. Diehm C, Vollbrecht D, Amendt K, Comberg HU. Medical edema protection—clinical benefit in patients with chronic deep vein incompetence: a placebo controlled double blind study. *Vasa.* 1992;21:188-192.
6. Friederich HC, Vogelsberg H, Neiss A. Evaluation of internally effective venous drugs [translated from German]. *Z Hautkr.* 1978;53:369-374.
7. Neiss A, Bohm C. Proof of the efficacy of horse chestnut seed extract in the treatment of varicose syndrome [translated from German]. *MMW Munch Med Wochenschr.* 1976;118:213-216.
8. Diehm C. The role of edema protective drugs in the treatment of chronic venous insufficiency: a review of evidence based on placebo-controlled clinical trials with regard to efficacy and tolerance. *Phlebology.* 1996;11:23-29.
9. Wilhelm K, Feldmeier C. Thermometric investigations about the efficacy of Beta-escin to reduce postoperative edema [in German; English abstract]. *Med Klin.* 1977;72:128-134.
10. Hitzenberger G. The therapeutic effectiveness of chestnut extract [translated from German]. *Wien Med Wochenschr.* 1989;139:385-389.
11. Kreysel HW, Nissen HP, Enghofer E. A possible role of lysosomal enzymes in the pathogenesis of varicosis and the reduction in their serum activity by Venostasin®. *Vasa.* 1983;12:377-382.
12. Newall CA, Anderson LA, Phillipson JE. *Herbal Medicines: A Guide for Health-Care Professionals.* London, England: The Pharmaceutical Press; 1996:166-167.
13. Bougelet C, Roland IH, Ninane N, et al. Effect of aescine on hypoxia-induced neutrophil adherence to umbilical vein endothelium. *Eur J Pharmacol.* 1998;345:89-95.
14. Chandler RF. Horse chestnut. *Can Pharm J.* 1993;126:297-300, 306.
15. Hansel R, Keller K, Rimpler H, et al. *Hagers Handbuch der Pharmazeutischen. Band 5: Drogen E-O.* Berlin, Germany: Springer Verlag; 1993:108-122.
16. Grasso A, Corvaglia E. Two cases of suspected toxic tubulonephrosis due to escine [in Italian; English abstract]. *Gazz Med Ital.* 1976;135:581-584.
17. Reynolds JE, ed. *Martindale: The Extra Pharmacopeia,* 29th ed. London, England: The Pharmaceutical Press; 1989:1539-1540.
18. Rothkopf M, Vogel G, Lang W, et al. Animal experiments on the question of the renal toleration of the horse chestnut saponin aescin. *Arzneimittelforschung.* 1977;27:598-605.
19. Takegoshi K, Tohyama T, Okuda K, et al. A case of Venoplant-induced hepatic injury. *Gastroenterol Jpn.* 1986;21:62-65.
20. Alter H. Drug therapy of varicosis [translated from German]. *Z Allgemeinmed.* 1973;49:1301-1304.

Huperzine A

1. Cheng DH, Tang XC. Comparative studies of huperzine A, E2020, and tacrine on behavior and cholinesterase activities. *Pharmacol Biochem Behav.* 1998;60:377-386.
2. Cheng DH, Ren H, Tang XC. Huperzine A, a novel promising acetylcholinesterase inhibitor. *Neuroreport.* 1996;8:97-101.

3. Xiong ZQ, Tang XC. Effect of huperzine A, a novel acetylcholinesterase inhibitor, on radial maze performance in rats. *Pharmacol Biochem Behav.* 1995;51:415-419.

4. Zhi QX, Yi FH, Xi CT. Huperzine A ameliorates the spatial working memory impairments induced by AF64A. *Neuroreport.* 1995;6:2221-2224.

5. Zhu XD, Giacobini E. Second generation cholinesterase inhibitors: effect of (L)-huperzine-A on cortical biogenic amines. *J Neurosci Res.* 1995;41:828-835.

6. Zhang GB, Wang MY, Zheng JQ, et al. Facilitation of cholinergic transmission by huperzine A in toad paravertebral ganglia in vitro. *Zhongguo Yao Li Xue Bao.* 1994; 15:158-161.

7. Laganiere S, Corey J, Tang XC, et al. Acute and chronic studies with the anti-cholinesterase huperzine A: effect on central nervous system cholinergic parameters. *Neuropharmacology.* 1991;30:763-768.

8. Tang XC, DeSarno P, Sugaya K, et al. Effect of huperzine A, a new cholinesterase inhibitor, on the central cholinergic system of the rat. *J Neurosci Res.* 1989;24:276-285.

9. Tang XC, Han YF, Chen XP, et al. Effects A huperzine A on learning and the retrieval process of discrimination performance in rats. *Zhongguo Yao Li Xue Bao.* 1986;7:507-511.

10. Guan LC, Chen SS, Lu WH, et al. Effect of huperzine A on electroencephalography power spectrum in rabbits [in Chinese; English abstract]. *Acta Pharm Sin.* 1989;10: 496-500.

11. Lu WH, Shou J, Tang XC. Improving effect of huperzine A on discrimination performance in aged rats and adult rats with experimental cognitive impairment. *Zhongguo Yao Li Xue Bao.* 1988;9:11-15.

12. Wang YE, Feng J, Lu WH, et al. Pharmacokinetics of huperzine A in rats and mice. *Zhongguo Yao Li Xue Bao.* 1988;9:193-196.

13. Wang YE, Yue DX, Tang XC. Anti-cholinesterase activity of huperzine A. *Zhongguo Yao Li Xue Bao.* 1986;7:110-113.

14. Zhu XD, Tang XC. Improvement of impaired memory in mice by huperzine A and huperzine B. *Zhongguo Yao Li Xue Bao.* 1988;9:492-497.

15. Zhu XD, Tang XC. Facilitatory effects of huperzine A and B on learning amd memory of spatial discrimination in mice. *Yao Xue Xue Bao.* 1987;22:812-817.

16. Yan XF, Lu WH, Lou WJ, Tang XC. Effects of huperzine A and B on skeletal muscle and the electroencephalogram. *Zhongguo Yao Li Xue Bao.* 1987;8:117-123.

17. Xu SS, Gao ZX, Weng Z, et al. Efficacy of tablet huperzine-A on memory, cognition, and behavior in Alzheimer's disease. *Zhongguo Yao Li Xue Bao.* 1995;16:391-395.

18. Wang LM, Han YF, Tang XC. Huperzine A improves cognitive deficits caused by chronic cerebral hypoperfusion in rats. *Eur J Pharmacol.* 2000;398:65-72.

19. Zhang RW, Tang XC, Han YY, et al. Drug evaluation of huperzine A in the treatment of senile memory disorders. *Zhongguo Yao Li Xue Bao.* 1991;12:250-252.

20. Xu SS, Cai ZY, Qu ZW, et al. Huperzine-A in capsules and tablets for treating patients with Alzheimer disease. *Zhongguo Yao Li Xue Bao.* 1999;20:486-490.

21. Sun QQ, Xu SS, Pan JL, et al. Huperzine-A capsules enhance memory and learning performance in 34 pairs of matched adolescent students. *Zhongguo Yao Li Xue Bao.* 1999;20:601-603.

22. Raves ML, Harel M, Pang YP, et al. Structure of acetylcholinesterase complexed with the nootropic alkaloid, (−)-huperzine A. *Nat Struct Biol.* 1997;4:57-63.

23. Ashani Y, Peggins JO III, Doctor BP. Mechanism of inhibition of cholinesterases by huperzine A. *Biochem Biophys Res Commun.* 1992;184:719-726.

24. Pang YP, Kozikowski AP. Prediction of the binding sites of huperzine A in acetylcholinesterase by docking studies. *J Comput Aided Mol Des.* 1994;8:669-681.

Hydroxycitric Acid

1. Heymsfield SB, Allison DB, Vasselli JR, et al. *Garcinia cambogia* (hydroxycitric acid) as a potential antiobesity agent: a randomized controlled trial. *JAMA.* 1998;280: 1596-1600.

2. Kriketos AD, Thompson HR, Greene H, et al. (−)-Hydroxycitric acid does not affect energy expenditure and substrate oxidation in adult males in a post-absorptive state. *Int J Obes Relat Metab Disord.* 1999;23:867-873.

3. Mattes RD, Bormann L. Effects of (−)-hydroxycitric acid on appetitive variables. *Physiol Behav.* 2000;71:87-94.
4. Greenwood MR, Cleary MP, Gruen R, et al. Effect of (−)-hydroxycitrate on development of obesity in the Zucker obese rat. *Am J Physiol.* 1981;240:E72-E78.
5. Sullivan C, Triscari J. Metabolic regulation as a control for lipid disorders. I. Influence of (−)-hydroxycitrate on experimentally induced obesity in the rodent. *Am J Clin Nutr.* 1977;30:767-776.
6. Sullivan AC, Triscari J, Hamilton JG, et al. Effect of (−)-hydroxycitrate upon the accumulation of lipid in the rat. I. Lipogenesis. *Lipids.* 1974;9:121-128.
7. Sullivan AC, Triscari J, Hamilton JG, et al. Effect of (−)-hydroxycitrate upon the accumulation of lipid in the rat. II. Appetite. *Lipids.* 1974;9:129-134.
8. Sergio W. A natural food, the malabar tamarind, may be effective in the treatment of obesity. *Medical Hypothesis.* 1988;27:39-40.
9. Lowenstein JM. Effect of (−)-hydroxycitrate on fatty acid synthesis by rat liver in vivo. *J Biol Chem.* 1971;246:629-632.
10. Triscari J, Sullivan AC. Comparative effects of (−)-hydroxycitrate and (+)-allo-hydroxycitrate on acetyl CoA carboxylase and fatty acid and cholesterol synthesis in vivo. *Lipids.* 1977;12:357-363.
11. Cheema-Dhadli S, Halperin ML, Leznoff CC. Inhibition of enzymes which interact with citrate by (−)hydroxycitrate and 1,2,3,-tricarboxybenzene. *Eur J Biochem.* 1973;38:98-102.
12. Sullivan AC, Hamilton JG, Miller ON, et al. Inhibition of lipogenesis in rat liver by (−)-hydroxycitrate. *Arch Biochem Biophys.* 1972;150:183-190.
13. Thom E. Hydroxycitrate (HCA) in the treatment of obesity [abstract]. *Int J Obes Relat Metab Disord.* 1996;20(suppl 4):75.
14. Badmaev V, Majeed M, Conte AA, et al. *Garcinia cambogia* for weight loss [letter]. *JAMA.* 1999;282:233-234.
15. Kovacs EM, Westerterp-Plantenga MS, Saris WH. The effects of 2-week ingestion of (−)-hydroxycitrate and (−)-hydroxycitrate combined with medium-chain triglycerides on satiety, fat oxidation, energy expenditure and body weight. *Int J Obes Relat Metab Disord.* 2001;25:1087-1094.

Hydroxymethyl Butyrate (HMB)

1. Ostaszewski P, Kostiuk S, Balasinska B, et al. The effect of leucine metabolite 3-hydroxy-3-methylbutyrate (HMB) on muscle protein synthesis and protein breakdown in chick and rat muscle [abstract]. *J Anim Sci.* 1996;74(suppl 1):138.
2. Nissen S, Sharp R, Ray M, et al. Effect of leucine metabolite beta-hydroxy-beta-methylbutyrate on muscle metabolism during resistance-exercise training. *J Appl Physiol.* 1996;81:2095-2104.
3. Nissen S, Panton L, Fuller J, et al. Effect of feeding beta-hydroxy-beta-methylbutyrate (HMB) on body composition and strength of women [abstract]. *FASEB J.* 1997;11:A150.
4. Kreider RB. Dietary supplements and the promotion of muscle growth with resistance exercise. *Sports Med.* 1999; 27:97-110.
5. Panton LB, Rathmacher JA, Baier S, et al. Nutritional supplementation of the leucine metabolite beta-hydroxy beta-methylbutyrate (HMB) during resistance training. *Nutrition.* 2000;16:734-739.
6. Gallagher PM, Carrithers JA, Godard MP, et al. Beta-hydroxy-beta-methylbutyrate ingestion. I. Effects on strength and fat free mass. *Med Sci Sports Exerc.* 2000;32:2109-2115.
7. Slater GJ, Jenkins D. Beta-hydroxy-beta-methylbutyrate (HMB) supplementation and the promotion of muscle growth and strength. *Sports Med.* 2000;30:105-116.
8. Vukovich MD, Stubbs NB, Bohlken RM. Body composition in 70-year-old adults responds to dietary beta-hydroxy-beta-methylbutyrate similarly to that of young adults. *J Nutr.* 2001;131:2049-2052.
9. Jowko E, Ostaszewski P, Jank M, et al. Creatine and beta-hydroxy-beta-methylbutyrate (HMB) additively increase lean body mass and muscle strength during a weight-training program. *Nutrition.* 2001;17:558-566.

10. Knitter AE, Panton L, Rathmacher JA, et al. Effects of beta-hydroxy-beta-methyl-butyrate on muscle damage after a prolonged run. *J Appl Physiol.* 2000;89:1340-1344.
11. Abumrad N, Flakoll P. The efficacy and safety of CaHMB (beta-hydroxy-beta-methylbutyrate) in humans. Vanderbilt University Medical Center Annual Report, 1991.
12. Nissen S, Sharp RL, Panton L, et al. Beta-hydroxy-beta-methylbutyrate (HMB) supplementation in humans is safe and may decrease cardiovascular risk factors. *J Nutr.* 2000;130:1937-1945.
13. Slater G, Jenkins D, Logan P, et al. Beta-hydroxy-beta-methylbutyrate (HMB) supplementation does not affect changes in strength or body composition during resistance training in trained men. *Int J Sport Nutr Exerc Metab.* 2001;11:384-396.

Inosine

1. Starling RD, Trappe TA, Short KR, et al. Effect of inosine supplementation on aerobic and anaerobic cycling performance. *Med Sci Sports Exerc.* 1996;28:1193-1198.
2. Dragan I, Baroga M, Eremia N, et al. Studies regarding some effects of inosine in elite weightlifters. *Rom J Physiol.* 1993;30:47-50.
3. Williams MH, Kreider RB, Hunter DW, et al. Effect of inosine supplementation on 3-mile treadmill run performance and VO$_2$ peak. *Med Sci Sports Exerc.* 1990;22:517-522.
4. Rosenbloom C, Millard-Stafford M, Lathrop J. Contemporary ergogenic aids used by strength/power athletes. *J Am Diet Assoc.* 1992;92:1264-1266.
5. McNaughton L, Dalton B, Tarr J. Inosine supplementation has no effect on aerobic or anaerobic cycling performance. *Int J Sport Nutr.* 1999;9:333-344.
6. Juhasz-Nagy A, Aviado DM. Inosine as a cardiotonic agent that reverses adrenergic beta blockade. *J Pharmacol Exp Ther.* 1977;202:683-695.
7. Kipshidze NN, Korotkov AA, Chapidze GE, et al. Indications for the use of inosine in myocardial infarct [in Russian; English abstract]. *Kardiologiia.* 1978;18:18-28.
8. Cheng Y, Jiang DH. The therapeutic effect of inosine in Tourette syndrome and its possible mechanism of action [in Chinese;English abstract]. *Chung Hua Shen Ching Ching Shen Ko Tsa Chih.* 1990;23:126-127.
9. Akerblom O, de Verdier CH, Garby L, et al. Restoration of defective oxygen-transport function of stored red blood cells by addition of inosine. *Scand J Clin Lab Invest.* 1968;21:245-248.
10. de Verdier CH, Westman M. Intravenous infusion of inosine in man: effect on erythrocyte 2,3-diphosphoglycerate concentration and on blood oxygen affinity. *Scand J Clin Lab Invest.* 1973;32:205-210.
11. Smiseth OA, Gunnes P, Sand T, Mjos OD. Inosine causing insulin release and increased myocardial uptake of carbohydrates relative to free fatty acids in dogs. *Clin Physiol.* 1989;9:27-38.
12. Powers FM, Sobotka PA, Thomas JX Jr. Effect of inosine in the normal and reperfused rat heart. *J Cardiovasc Pharmacol.* 1990;15:862-867.

Inositol (Vitamin B$_8$)

1. Levine J, Barak Y, Kofman O, et al. Follow-up and relapse analysis of an inositol study of depression. *Isr J Psychiatry Relat Sci.* 1995;32:14-21.
2. Levine J. Controlled trials of inositol in psychiatry. *Eur Neuropsychopharmacol.* 1997;7:147-155.
3. Benjamin J, Agam G, Levine J, et al. Inositol treatment in psychiatry. *Psychopharmacol Bull.* 1995;31:167-175.
4. Nemets B, Mishory A, Levine J, et al. Inositol addition does not improve depression in SSRI treatment failures. *J Neural Transm.* 1999;106:795-798.
5. Chengappa KN, Levine J, Gershon S, et al. Inositol as an add-on treatment for bipolar depression. *Bipolar Disord.* 2000;2:47-55.
6. Benjamin J, Levine J, Fux M, et al. Double-blind, placebo-controlled, crossover trial of inositol treatment for panic disorder. *Am J Psychiatry.* 1995;152:1084-1086.

7. Palatnik A, Frolov K, Fux M, et al. Double-blind, controlled, crossover trial of ino-sitol versus fluvoxamine for the treatment of panic disorder. *J Clin Psychopharmacol.* 2001;21:335-339.
8. Gelber D, Levine J, Belmaker RH. Effect of inositol on bulimia nervosa and binge eating. *Int J Eat Disord.* 2001;29:345-348.
9. Fux M, Levine J, Aviv A, et al. Inositol treatment of obsessive-compulsive disorder. *Am J Psychiatry.* 1996;153:1219-1221.
10. Fux M, Benjamin J, Belmaker RH. Inositol versus placebo augmentation of serotonin reuptake inhibitors in the treatment of obsessive-compulsive disorder: a double-blind cross-over study. *Int J Neuropsychopharmcol.* 1999;2:193-195.
11. Salway JG, Finnegan JA, Barnett D, et al. Effect of myo-inositol on peripheral-nerve function in diabetes. *Lancet.* 1978;2:1282-1284.
12. Gregersen G, Bertelsen B, Harbo H, et al. Oral supplementation of myoinositol: ef-fects on peripheral nerve function in human diabetics and on the concentration in plasma, erythrocytes, urine and muscle tissue in human diabetics and normals. *Acta Neurol Scand.* 1983;67:164-172.
13. Wattenberg LW. Chemoprevention of pulmonary carcinogenesis by myo-inositol. *Anticancer Res.* 1999;19:3659-3661.
14. Dong Z, Huang C, Ma WY. PI-3 kinase in signal transduction, cell transformation, and as a target for chemoprevention of cancer. *Anticancer Res.* 1999;19:3743-3747.
15. Yang GY, Shamsuddin AM. IP6-induced growth inhibition and differentiation of HT-29 human colon cancer cells: involvement of intracellular inositol phosphates. *Anticancer Res.* 1995;15:2479-2487.
16. Ishikawa T, Nakatsuru Y, Zarkovic M, et al. Inhibition of skin cancer by IP6 in vivo: initiation-promotion model. *Anticancer Res.* 1999;19(5A):3749-3752.
17. Shamsuddin AM. Metabolism and cellular functions of IP6: a review. *Anticancer Res.* 1999;19(5A):3733-3736.
18. Shamsuddin AM, Vucenik I. Mammary tumor inhibition by IP6: a review. *Anticancer Res.* 1999;19(5A):3671-3674.
19. Vucenik I, Kalebic T, Tantivejkul K, et al. Novel anticancer function of inositol hexa-phosphate: inhibition of human rhabdomyosarcoma in vitro and in vivo. *Anticancer Res.* 1998;18(3A):1377-1384.
20. Shamsuddin AM, Vucenik I, Cole KE. IP6: a novel anti-cancer agent. *Life Sci.* 1997;61:343-354.
21. Levine J, Witztum E, Greenberg BD, et al. Inositol-induced mania? [letter]. *Am J Psychiatry.* 1996;153:839.

Ipriflavone

1. Agnusdei D, Zacchei F, Bigazzi S, et al. Metabolic and clinical effects of ipriflavone in established post-menopausal osteoporosis. *Drugs Exp Clin Res.* 1989;15:97-104.
2. Agnusdei D, Adami S, Cervetti R, et al. Effects of ipriflavone on bone mass and calcium metabolism in postmenopausal osteoporosis. *Bone Miner.* 1992;19(suppl 1): S43-S48.
3. Agnusdei D, Crepaldi G, Isaia G, et al. A double blind, placebo-controlled trial of ipriflavone for prevention of postmenopausal spinal bone loss. *Calcif Tissue Int.* 1997;61:142-147.
4. Gambacciani M, Spinetti A, Piaggesi L, et al. Ipriflavone prevents the bone mass re-duction in premenopausal women treated with gonadotropin hormone-releasing hormone agonists. *Bone Miner.* 1994;26:19-26.
5. Gambacciani M, Cappagli B, Piaggesi L, et al. Ipriflavone prevents the loss of bone mass in pharmacological menopause induced by GnRH-agonists. *Calcif Tissue Int.* 1997;61:S15-S18.
6. Gennari C, Adami S, Agnusdei D, et al. Effect of chronic treatment with ipriflavone in postmenopausal women with low bone mass. *Calcif Tissue Int.* 1997;61:S19-S22.
7. Kovacs AB. Efficacy of ipriflavone in the prevention and treatment of post-menopausal osteoporosis. *Agents Actions.* 1994;41:86-87.

8. Maugeri D, Panebianco P, Russo MS, et al. Ipriflavone-treatment of senile osteo-porosis: results of a multicenter, double-blind clinical trial of 2 years. *Arch Gerontol Geriatr.* 1994;19:253-263.

9. Passeri M, Biondi M, Costi D, et al. Effects of 2-year therapy with ipriflavone in elderly women with established osteoporosis. *Ital J Miner Electrolyte Metab.* 1995;9:137-144.

10. Valente M, Bufalino L, Castiglione GN, et al. Effects of 1-year treatment with ipri-flavone on bone in postmenopausal women with low bone mass. *Calcif Tissue Int.* 1994;54:377-380.

11. Alexandersen P, Toussaint A, Christiansen C, et al. Ipriflavone in the treatment of postmenopausal osteoporosis: a randomized controlled trial. *JAMA.* 2001;285:1482-1488.

12. Melis GB, Paoletti AM, Cagnacci A. Ipriflavone prevents bone loss in post-menopausal women. *Menopause.* 1996;3:27-32.

13. Moscarini M, Patacchiola F, Spacca G, et al. New perspectives in the treatment of postmenopausal osteoporosis: ipriflavone. *Gynecol Endocrinol.* 1994;8:203-207.

14. Scali G, Mansanti P, Zurlo A, et al. Analgesic effect of ipriflavone versus sCalcitonin in the treatment of osteoporotic vertebral pain. *Curr Ther Res.* 1991;49:1004-1010.

15. Mazzuoli G, Romagnoli E, Carnevale V, et al. Effects of ipriflavone on bone re-modeling in primary hyperparathyroidism. *Bone Miner.* 1992;19(suppl 1):S27-S33.

16. Yamazaki I, Shino A, Shimizu Y, et al. Effect of ipriflavone on glucocorticoid-in-duced osteoporosis in rats. *Life Sci.* 1986;38:951-958.

17. Agnusdei D, Gennari C, Bufalino L. Prevention of early postmenopausal bone loss using low doses of conjugated estrogens and the non-hormonal, bone-active drug ipriflavone. *Osteoporos Int.* 1995;5:462-466.

18. Choi YK, Han IK, Yoon HK. Ipriflavone for the treatment of osteoporosis. *Osteoporos Int.* 1997;7(suppl 3):S174-S178.

19. de Aloysio D, Gambacciani M, Altieri P, et al. Bone density changes in post-menopausal women with the administration of ipriflavone alone or in association with low-dose ERT. *Gynecol Endocrinol.* 1997;11:289-293.

20. Gambacciani M, Ciaponi M, Cappagli B, et al. Effects of combined low dose of the isoflavone derivative ipriflavone and estrogen replacement on bone mineral density and metabolism in postmenopausal women. *Maturitas.* 1997;28:75-81.

21. Melis GB, Paoletti AM, Bartolini R, et al. Ipriflavone and low doses of estrogens in the prevention of bone mineral loss in climacterium. *Bone Miner.* 1992;19(suppl 1):S49-S56.

22. Nozaki M, Hashimoto K, Inoue Y, et al. Treatment of bone loss in oophorectomized women with a combination of ipriflavone and conjugated equine estrogen. *Int J Gynaecol Obstet.* 1998;62:69-75.

23. Hanabayashi T, Imai A, Tamaya T. Effects of ipriflavone and estriol on post-menopausal osteoporotic changes. *Int J Gynaecol Obstet.* 1995;51:63-64.

24. Ushiroyama T, Okamura S, Ikeda A, et al. Efficacy of ipriflavone and 1 alpha vitamin D therapy for the cessation of vertebral bone loss. *Int J Gynaecol Obstet.* 1995;48:283-288.

25. Agnusdei D, Camporeale A, Gonnelli S, et al. Short-term treatment of Paget's dis-ease of bone with ipriflavone. *Bone Miner.* 1992;19(suppl 1):S35-S42.

26. Benvenuti S, Petilli M, Frediani U, et al. Binding and bioeffects of ipriflavone on a human preosteoclastic cell line. *Biochem Biophys Res Commun.* 1994;201:1084-1089.

27. Bonucci E, Silvestrini G, Ballanti P, et al. Cytological and ultrastructural investiga-tion on osteoblastic and preosteoclastic cells grown in vitro in the presence of ipri-flavone: preliminary results. *Bone Miner.* 1992;19(suppl):S15-S25.

28. Cecchini MG, Fleisch H, Muhibauer RC. Ipriflavone inhibits bone resorption in in-tact and ovariectomized rats. *Calcif Tissue Int.* 1997;61(suppl 1):S9-S11.

29. Brandi ML. Ipriflavone influences the osteoblastic phenotype in vitro. *Osteoporos Int.* 1993;3(suppl 1):226-229.

30. Cheng SL, Zhang SF, Nelson TL, et al. Stimulation of human osteoblast differenti-ation and function by ipriflavone and its metabolites. *Calcif Tissue Int.* 1994;55:356-362.

31. Shibano K, Watanabe J, Iwamoto M, et al. Culture of stromal cells derived from medullary cavity of human long bone in the presence of 1,25-dihydroxyvitamin D_3, recombinant human bone morphogenetic protein-2, or ipriflavone. *Bone*. 1998;22: 251-258.

32. Kakai Y, Kawase T, Nakano T, et al. Effect of ipriflavone and estrogen on the differentiation and proliferation of osteogenic cells. *Calcif Tissue Int*. 1992;51(suppl 1):S11-S15.

33. Sziklai I, Ribari O. The effect of flavone treatment on human otosclerotic ossicle organ cultures. *Arch Otorhinolaryngol*. 1985;242:67-70.

34. Civitelli R. In vitro and in vivo effects of ipriflavone on bone formation and bone biomechanics. *Calcif Tissue Int*. 1997;61(suppl 1):S12-S14.

35. Rondelli I, Acerbi D, Ventura P. Steady-state pharmacokinetics of ipriflavone and its metabolites in patients with renal failure. *Int J Clin Pharmacol Res*. 1991;11:183-192.

36. Matsuoka M, Yoshida Y, Hayakawa K, et al. Gastrojejunal fistula caused by gastric ulcer. *J Gastroenterol*. 1998;33:267-271.

37. Agnusdei D, Bufalino L. Efficacy of ipriflavone in established osteoporosis and long-term safety. *Calcif Tissue Int*. 1997;61:2327.

38. Kuiper GG, Lemmen JG, Carlsson B, et al. Interaction of estrogenic chemicals and phytoestrogens with estrogen receptor beta. *Endocrinology*. 1998;139:4252-4263.

39. Petilli M, Fiorelli G, Benvenuti S, et al. Interactions between ipriflavone and the estrogen receptor. *Calcif Tissue Int*. 1995;56:160-165.

40. Caltagirone S, Ranelletti FO, Rinelli A, et al. Interaction with type II estrogen binding sites and antiproliferative activity of tamoxifen and quercetin in human non-small-cell lung cancer. *Am J Respir Cell Mol Biol*. 1997;17:51-59.

41. Ferrandina G, Almadori G, Maggiano N, et al. Growth-inhibitory effect of tamoxifen and quercetin and presence of type II estrogen binding sites in human laryngeal cancer cell lines and primary laryngeal tumors. *Int J Cancer*. 1998;77:747-754.

42. Monostory K, Vereczkey L. Interaction of theophylline and ipriflavone at the cytochrome P450 level. *Eur J Drug Metab Pharmacokinet*. 1995;20:43-47.

43. Takahashi J, Kawakatsu K, Wakayama T, et al. Elevation of serum theophylline levels by ipriflavone in a patient with chronic obstructive pulmonary disease. *Eur J Clin Pharmacol*. 1992;43:207-208.

44. Monostory K, Vereczkey L, Levai F, et al. Ipriflavone as an inhibitor of human cytochrome P450 enzymes. *Br J Pharmacol*. 1998;123:605-610.

45. Yamazaki I, Shino A, Shimizu Y, et al. Effect of ipriflavone on glucocorticoid-induced osteoporosis in rats. *Life Sci*. 1986;38:951-958.

46. Petilli M, Fiorelli G, Benvenuti S, et al. Interactions between ipriflavone and the estrogen receptor. *Calcif Tissue Int*. 1995;56:160-165.

47. Cecchini MG, Fleisch H, Muhibauer RC. Ipriflavone inhibits bone resorption in intact and ovariectomized rats. *Calcif Tissue Int*. 1997;61(suppl 1):S9-S11.

Iron

1. Shils ME, Olson JA, Shike M, eds. *Modern Nutrition in Health and Disease*. 9th ed. Baltimore, Md: Williams & Wilkins; 1999:210, 860, 1422, 1424, 1772.

2. Nelson M, Ash R, Mulvhill C, et al. Iron status, diet and cognitive function in British adolescent girls. Presented at: The Nutrition Society's Nutrition 2000—Research Themes for the New Millenium; June 26-30, 2000; Cork, Ireland.

3. Hinton PS, Giordano C, Brownlie T, et al. Iron supplementation improves endurance after training in iron-depleted, nonanemic women. *J Appl Physiol*. 2000;88: 1103-1111.

4. Friedmann B, Weller E, Mairbaurl H, et al. Effects of iron repletion on blood volume and performance capacity in young athletes. *Med Sci Sports Exerc*. 2001;33:741-746.

5. Taymor ML, Sturgis SH, Yahia C. The etiological role of chronic iron deficiency in production of menorrhagia. *JAMA*. 1964;187:323-327.

6. O'Keefe ST. Restless legs syndrome: A review. *Arch Intern Med*. 1996;156:243-248.

7. Sun ER, Chen CA, Ho G, et al. Iron and the restless legs syndrome. *Sleep*. 1998; 21:371-377.

8. O'Keefe ST, Gavin K, Lavan JN. Iron status and restless legs syndrome in the elderly. *Age Ageing.* 1994;23:200-203.
9. Davis BJ, Rajput A, Rajput ML, et al. A randomized, double-blind placebo-controlled trial of iron in restless legs syndrome. *Eur Neurol.* 2000;43:70-75.
10. Castaldo A, Tarallo L, Palomba E, et al. Iron deficiency and intestinal malabsorption in HIV disease. *J Pediatr Gastroenterol Nutr.* 1996;22:359-363.
11. Abrams B, Duncan D, Hertz-Picciotto I. A prospective study of dietary intake and acquired immune deficiency syndrome in HIV-seropositive homosexual men. *J Acquir Immune Defic Syndr.* 1993;6:949-958.
12. Lee SC, Park SW, Kim DK, et al. Iron supplementation inhibits cough associated with ACE inhibitors. *Hypertension.* 2001;38:166-170.
13. Dietary Reference Intakes for Vitamin A, Vitamin K, Arsenic, Boron, Chromium, Copper, Iodine, Manganese, Molybdenum, Nickel, Silicon, Vanadium, and Zinc (2001). Available at: http://www.nap.edu. Accessed October 4, 2001.
14. Hallberg L. Does calcium interfere with iron absorption? *Am J Clin Nutr.* 1998;68:3-4.
15. Cook JD, Dassenko SA, Whittaker P. Calcium supplementation: effect on iron absorption. *Am J Clin Nutr.* 199153:106-111.
16. Dawson-Hughes B, Seligson FH, Hughes VA. Effects of calcium carbonate and hydroxyapatite on zinc and iron retention in postmenopausal women. *Am J Clin Nutr.* 1986;44:83-88.
17. Sokoll LJ, Dawson-Hughes B. Calcium supplementation and plasma ferritin concentrations in premenopausal women. *Am J Clin Nutr.* 1992;56:1045-1048.
18. Hallberg L, Rossander L, Skanberg AB. Phytates and the inhibitory effects of bran on iron absorption in man. *Am J Clin Nutr.* 1987;45:988-996.
19. Sandstrom B, Davidsson L, Cederblad A, et al. Oral iron, dietary ligands and zinc absorption. *J Nutr.* 1985;115:411-414.
20. Haschke F, Ziegler EE, Edwards BB, et al. Effect of iron fortification of infant formula on trace mineral absorption. *J Pediatr Gastroenterol Nutr.* 1986;5:768-773.
21. Freeland-Graves JH. Manganese: an essential nutrient for humans. *Nutr Today.* 1988;23:13-19.
22. Aronow WS, Ahn C. Three-year follow-up shows no association of serum ferritin levels with incidence of new coronary events in 577 persons aged $\geq$ 62 years. *Am J Cardiol.* 1996;78:678-679.
23. Danesh J, Appleby P. Coronary heart disease and iron status: meta-analyses of prospective studies. *Circulation.* 1999;99:852-854.
24. Kiechl S, Willeit J, Egger G, et al. Body iron stores and the risk of carotid atherosclerosis: prospective results from the Bruneck study. *Circulation.* 1997;96:3300-3307.
25. Magnusson MK, Sigfusson N, Sigvaldason H, et al. Low iron-binding capacity as a risk factor for myocardial infarction. *Circulation.* 1994;89:102-108.
26. Manttari M, Manninen V, Huttunen JK, et al. Serum ferritin and ceruloplasmin as coronary risk factors. *Eur Heart J.* 1994;15:1599-1603.
27. Meyers DG. The iron hypothesis—does iron cause atherosclerosis? *Clin Cardiol.* 1996;19:925-929.
28. Salonen JT, Nyyssonen K, Korpela H, et al. High stored iron levels are associated with excess risk of myocardial infarction in Eastern Finnish men. *Circulation.* 1992;86:803-811.
29. Salonen JT, Tuomainen TP, Salonen R, et al. Donation of blood is associated with reduced risk of myocardial infarction. The Kuopio Ischaemic Heart Disease Risk Factor Study. *Am J Epidemiol.* 1998;148:445-451.
30. Sempos CT, Looker AC, Gillum RF. Iron and heart disease: the epidemiologic data. *Nutr Rev.* 1996;54:73-84.
31. Sullivan JL. Iron versus cholesterol—perspectives on the iron and heart disease debate. *J Clin Epidemiol.* 1996;49:1345-1352.
32. Tuomainen TP, Punnonen K, Nyyssonen K, et al. Association between body iron stores and the risk of acute myocardial infarction in men. *Circulation.* 1998;97:1461-1466.
33. Yuan XM, Brunk UT. Iron and LDL-oxidation in atherogenesis. *APMIS.* 1998; 106:825-842.

34. Sempos CT, Looker AC, Gillum RE, et al. Serum ferritin and death from all causes and cardiovascular disease: the NHANES II Mortality Study. *Ann Epidemiol.* 2000;10:441-448.

35. Davolos A, Castillo J, Marrugat J, et al. Body iron stores and early neurologic deterioration in acute cerebral infarction. *Neurology.* 2000;54:1568-1574.

36. Lao TT, Tam K, Chan LY. Third trimester iron status and pregnancy outcome in non-anaemic women; pregnancy unfavourably affected by maternal iron excess. *Hum Reprod.* 2000;15:1843-1848.

37. Maskos Z, Koppenol WH. Oxyradicals and multivitamin tablets. *Free Radic Biol Med.* 1991;11:609-610.

38. Conrad ME, Schade SG. Ascorbic acid chelates in iron absorption: a role for hydrochloric acid and bile. *Gastroenterology.* 1968;55:35-45.

39. Brise H, Hallberg L. Effect of ascorbic acid on iron absorption. *Acta Med Scand.* 1962;171(suppl 376):51.

40. Lynch SR, Cook JD. Interaction of vitamin C and iron. *Ann NY Acad Sci.* 1980;355: 32-44.

41. Hunt JR, Gallagher SK, Johnson LK. Effect of ascorbic acid on apparent iron absorption by women with low iron stores. *Am J Clin Nutr.* 1994;59:1381-1385.

42. Diplock AT. Safety of antioxidant vitamins and beta-carotene. *Am J Clin Nutr.* 1995;62(suppl 6):1510S-1516S.

43. Hoffman KE, Yanelli K, Bridges KR. Ascorbic acid and iron metabolism: alterations in lysosomal function. *Am J Clin Nutr.* 1991;54(suppl 6):1188S-1192S.

44. Siegenberg D, Baynes RD, Bothwell TH, et al. Ascorbic acid prevents the dose-dependent inhibitory effects of polyphenols and phytates on nonheme-iron absorption. *Am J Clin Nutr.* 1991;53:537-541.

45. Kara M, Hasinoff BB, McKay DW, et al. Clinical and chemical interactions between iron preparations and ciprofloxacin. *Br J Clin Pharmacol.* 1991;31:257-261.

46. Polk RE, Healy DP, Sahai J, et al. Effect of ferrous sulfate and multivitamins with zinc on absorption of ciprofloxacin in normal volunteers. *Antimicrob Agents Chemother.* 1989;33:1841-1844.

47. Campbell NR, Kara M, Hasinoff BB, et al. Norfloxacin interaction with antacids and minerals. *Br J Clin Pharmacol.* 1992;33:115-116.

48. Lehto P, Kivisto KT. Different effects of products containing metal ions on the absorption of lomefloxacin. *Clin Pharmacol Ther.* 1994;56:477-482.

49. Lehto P, Kivisto KT, Neuvonen PJ. The effect of ferrous sulphate on the absorption of norfloxacin, ciprofloxacin and ofloxacin. *Br J Clin Pharmacol.* 1994;37:82-85.

50. Neuvonen PJ. Interactions with the absorption of tetracyclines. *Drugs.* 1976;11:45-54.

51. Campbell NR, Hasinoff BB. Iron supplements: a common cause of drug interactions. *Br J Clin Pharmacol.* 1991;31:251-255.

52. Heinrich HC, Oppitz KH, Gabbe EE. Inhibition of iron absorption in man by tetracycline [in German]. *Klin Wochenschr.* 1974;52:493-498.

53. Campbell N, Paddock V, Sundaram R. Alteration of methyldopa absorption, metabolism, and blood pressure control caused by ferrous sulfate and ferrous gluconate. *Clin Pharmacol Ther.* 1988;43:381-386.

54. Osman MA, Patel RB, Schuna A, et al. Reduction in oral penicillamine absorption by food, antacid, and ferrous sulfate. *Clin Pharmacol Ther.* 1983;33:465-470.

55. Campbell NR, Hasinoff BB, Stalts H, et al. Ferrous sulfate reduces thyroxine efficacy in patients with hypothyroidism. *Ann Intern Med.* 1992;117:1010-1013.

56. Champagne ET. Low gastric hydrochloric acid secretion and mineral bioavailability. *Adv Exp Med Biol.* 1989;249:173-184.

Isoflavones

1. Anderson JW, Johnstone BM, Cook-Newell ME. Meta-analysis of the effects of soy protein intake on serum lipids. *N Engl J Med.* 1995;333:276-282.

2. Baum J, Teng H, Eerdman JW Jr, et al. Long-term intake of soy protein improves blood lipid profiles and increases mononuclear cell low-density-lipoprotein receptor messenger RNA in hypercholesterolemic, postmenopausal women. *Am J Clin Nutr.* 1998;68:545-551.

3. Wangen KE, Duncan AM, Xu X, et al. Soy isoflavones improve plasma lipids in nor-mocholesterolemic and mildly hypercholesterolemic postmenopausal women. *Am J Clin Nutr.* 2001;73:225-231.

4. Crouse JR III, Morgan T, Terry JG, et al. A randomized trial comparing the effect of casein with that of soy protein containing varying amounts of isoflavones on plasma concentrations of lipids and lipoproteins. *Arch Intern Med.* 1999;159:2070-2076.

5. Anthony MS, Clarkson TB, Hughes CL Jr, et al. Soybean isoflavones improve car-diovascular risk factors without affecting the reproductive system of peripubertal rhesus monkeys. *J Nutr.* 1996;126:43-50.

6. Sirtori CR, Gianazza E, Manzoni C, et al. Role of isoflavones in the cholesterol re-duction by soy proteins in the clinic [letter]. *Am J Clin Nutr.* 1997;65:166-167.

7. Greaves KA, Parks JS, Williams JK, et al. Intact dietary soy protein, but not adding an isoflavone-rich soy extract to casein, improves plasma lipids in ovariectomized cynomolgus monkeys. *J Nutr.* 1999;129:1585-1592.

8. Simons LA, von Konigsmark M, Simons J, et al. Phytoestrogens do not influence lipoprotein levels or endothelial function in healthy, postmenopausal women. *Am J Cardiol.* 2000;85:1297-1301.

9. Mackey R, Ekangaki A, Eden JA. The effects of soy protein in women and men with elevated plasma lipids. *Biofactors.* 2000;12:251-257.

10. Setchell KD, Brown NM, Desai P, et al. Bioavailability of pure isoflavones in healthy humans and analysis of commercial soy isoflavone supplements. *J Nutr.* 2001;131(4 suppl):1362S-1375S.

11. Howes JB, Sullivan D, Lai N, et al. The effects of dietary supplementation with isoflavones from red clover on the lipoprotein profiles of post menopausal women with mild to moderate hypercholesterolaemia. *Atherosclerosis.* 2000;152:143-147.

12. Albertazzi P, Pansini F, Bonaccorsi G, et al. The effect of dietary soy supplementa-tion on hot flashes. *Obstet Gynecol.* 1998;91:6-11.

13. Duncan AM, Underhill KEW, Xu X, et al. Modest hormonal effects of soy isoflavones in postmenopausal women. *J Clin Endocrinol Metab.* 1999;84:3479-3484.

14. Xu X, Duncan AM, Merz BE, Kurzer MS. Effects of soy isoflavones on estrogen and phytoestrogen metabolism in premenopausal women. *Cancer Epidemiol Biomarkers Prev.* 1998;7:1101-1108.

15. Kumar NB, Cantor A, Allen K, et al. The specific role of isoflavones on estrogen metabolism in premenopausal women. *Cancer.* 2002;94:1166-1174.

16. St. Germain A, Peterson CT, Robinson JG, et al. Isoflavone-rich or isoflavone-poor soy protein does not reduce menopausal symptoms during 24 weeks of treatment. *Menopause.* 2001;8:17-26.

17. Baber RJ, Templeman C, Morton T, et al. Randomized placebo-controlled trial of an isoflavone supplement and menopausal symptoms in women. *Climacteric.* 1999;2:85-92.

18. Knight DC, Howes JB, Eden JA. The effect of Promensil(tm), an isoflavone extract, on menopausal symptoms. *Climacteric.* 1999;2:79-84.

19. Potter SM, Baum JA, Teng H, et al. Soy protein and isoflavones: their effects on blood lipids and bone density in postmenopausal women. *Am J Clin Nutr.* 1998;68(6 suppl):1375S-1379S.

20. Alekel DL, Germain AS, Peterson CT, et al. Isoflavone-rich soy protein isolate at-tenuates bone loss in the lumbar spine of perimenopausal women. *Am J Clin Nutr.* 2000;72:844-852.

21. Harrison E, Adjei A, Ameho C, et al. The effect of soybean protein on bone loss in a rat model of postmenopausal osteoporosis. *J Nutr Sci Vitaminol.* 1998;44:257-268.

22. Fanti O, Faugere MC, Gang Z, et al. Systematic administration of genistein par-tially prevents bone loss in ovariectomized rats in a nonestrogen-like mechanism [abstract]. *Am J Clin Nutr.* 1998;68(suppl):1517S-1518S.

23. Arjmandi BH, Alekel L, Hollis BW, et al. Dietary soybean protein prevents bone loss in an ovariectomized rat model of osteoporosis. *J Nutr.* 1996;126:161-167.

24. Fanti P, Monier-Faugere MC, Geng Z, et al. The phytoestrogen genistein reduces bone loss in short-term ovariectomized rats. *Osteoporos Int.* 1998;8:274-281.

25. Anderson JJ, Ambrose WW, Garner SC. Biphasic effects of genistein on bone tissue in the ovariectomized, lactating rat model. *Proc Soc Exp Biol Med.* 1998;217:345-350.

26. Arjmandi BH, Birnbaum R, Goyal NV, et al. Bone-sparing effect of soy protein in ovarian hormone-deficient rats is related to its isoflavone content. *Am J Clin Nutr.* 1998;68(6 suppl):1364S-1368S.

27. Lees CJ, Ginn TA. Soy protein isolate diet does not prevent increased cortical bone turnover in ovariectomized macaques. *Calcif Tissue Int.* 1998;62:557-558.

28. Jayo MJ. Dietary soy isoflavones and bone loss: a study in ovariectomized monkeys [abstract]. *J Bone Miner Res.* 1996;11:S228.

29. Gallagher JC, Rafferty K, Haynatzka V, et al. The effect of soy protein on bone metabolism [abstract]. *J Nutr.* 2000;130:667S.

30. Dalais F, Teede HJ, Kotsopoulos D, et al. The effects of dietary soy protein containing phytoestrogens on lipids and indices of bone turnover in postmenopausal women. Presented at: 83rd Annual Meeting of the Endocrine Society; June 20-23, 2001; Denver, Colo.

31. Messina MJ, Persky V, Setchell KD, et al. Soy intake and cancer risk: a review of the in vitro and in vivo data. *Nutr Cancer.* 1994;21:113-131.

32. Adlercreutz H, Mazur W. Phyto-oestrogens and Western diseases. *Ann Med.* 1997; 29:95-120.

33. Stoll BA. Eating to beat breast cancer: potential role for soy supplements. *Ann Oncol.* 1997;8:223-225.

34. Day NE. Phyto-oestrogens and hormonally dependent cancers [abstract]. *Pathol Biol (Paris).* 1994;42:1090.

35. Barnes S, Peterson TG, Coward L. Rationale for the use of genistein-containing soy matrices in chemoprevention trials for breast and prostate cancer. *J Cell Biochem Suppl.* 1995;22:181-187.

36. Ingram D, Sanders K, Kolybaba M, et al. Case-control study of phyto-oestrogens and breast cancer. *Lancet.* 1997;350:990-994.

37. Goodman MT, Wilkens LR, Hankin JH, et al. Association of soy and fiber consumption with the risk of endometrial cancer. *Am J Epidemiol.* 1997;146:294-306.

38. Hodgson JM, Puddey IB, Beilin LJ, et al. Effects of isoflavonoids on blood pressure in subjects with high-normal ambulatory blood pressure levels: a randomized controlled trial. *Am J Hypertens.* 1999;12:47-53.

39. Wei H, Bowen R, Cai Q, et al. Antioxidant and antipromotional effects of the soybean isoflavone genistein. *Proc Soc Exp Biol Med.* 1995;208:124-130.

40. Tham DM, Gardner CD, Haskell WL. Clinical review 97: Potential health benefits of dietary phytoestrogens: a review of the clinical, epidemiological, and mechanistic evidence. *J Clin Endocrinol Metab.* 1998;83:2223-2235.

41. Crowell JA, Levine BS, Page JG, et al. Preclinical safety studies of isoflavones [abstract]. *J Nutr.* 2000;130(suppl):677S.

42. Petrakis NL, Barnes S, King EB, et al. Stimulatory influence of soy protein isolate on breast secretion in pre- and postmenopausal women. *Cancer Epidemiol Biomarkers Prev.* 1996;5:785-794.

43. McMichael-Phillips DL, Harding C, Morton M, et al. Effects of soy-protein supplementation on epithelial proliferation in the histologically normal human breast. *Am J Clin Nutr.* 1998;68(suppl):1431S-1436S.

44. Divi RL, Chang HC, Doerge DR. Anti-thyroid isoflavones from soybean: isolation, characterization, and mechanisms of action. *Biochem Pharmacol.* 1997;54:1087-1096.

45. Chorazy PA, Himelhoch S, Hopwood NJ, et al. Persistent hypothyroidism in an infant receiving a soy formula: a case report and review of the literature. *Pediatrics.* 1995;96:148-150.

46. Jabbar MA, Larrea J, Shaw RA. Abnormal thyroid function tests in infants with congenital hypothyroidism: the influence of soy-based formula. *J Am Coll Nutr.* 1997;16: 280-282.

47. Maskarinec G, Williams AE, Inouye JS, et al. A randomized isoflavone intervention among premenopausal women. *Cancer Epidemiol Biomarkers Prev.* 2002;11:195-201.

48. Teede HJ, Dalais FS, Kotsopoulos D, et al. Dietary soy has both beneficial and potentially adverse cardiovascular effects: a placebo-controlled study in men and postmenopausal women. *J Clin Endocrinol Metab.* 2001;86:3053-3060.

49. [No authors listed]. Third International Symposium on the Role of Soy in Preventing and Treating Chronic Disease; October 31-November 3, 1999; Washington DC. Proceedings and abstracts. *J Nutr.* 2000;130(suppl):653S-711S.
50. Hilakivi-Clarke L, Cho E, Onojafe I, et al. Maternal exposure to genistein during pregnancy increases carcinogen-induced mammary tumorigenesis in female rat offspring. *Oncol Rep.* 1999;6:1089-1095.
51. Martini MC, Dancisak BB, Haggans CJ, et al. Effects of soy intake on sex hormone metabolism in premenopausal women. *Nutr Cancer.* 1999;34:133-139.
52. Dewell A, Hollenbeck CB, Bruce B. The effects of soy-derived phytoestrogens on serum lipids and lipoproteins in moderately hypercholesterolemic postmenopausal women. *J Clin Endocrinol Metab.* 2002;87:118-121.
53. Kotsopoulos D, Dalais FS, Liang YL, et al. The effects of soy protein containing phytoestrogens on menopausal symptoms in postmenopausal women. *Climacteric.* 2000;3:161-167.
54. Allred CD, Allred KF, Ju YH, et al. Soy diets containing varying amounts of genistein stimulate growth of estrogen-dependent (MCF-7) tumors in a dose-dependent manner. *Cancer Res.* 2001;61:5045-5050.
55. Brzezinski A, Adlercreutz H, Shaoul R, et al. Short-term effects of phytoestrogen-rich diet on postmenopausal women. *Menopause.* 1997;4:89-94.
56. Washburn S, Burke GL, Morgan T, et al. Effect of soy protein supplementation on serum lipoproteins, blood pressure, and menopausal symptoms in perimenopausal women. *Menopause.* 1999;6:7-13.
57. Ju YH, Allred CD, Allred KF, et al. Physiological concentrations of dietary genistein dose-dependently stimulate growth of estrogen-dependent human breast cancer (MCF-7) tumors implanted in athymic nude mice. *J Nutr.* 2001;131:2957-2962.
58. Van Patten CL, Olivotto IA, Chambers GK, et al. Effect of soy phytoestrogens on hot flashes in postmenopausal women with nreast cancer: a randomized, controlled clinical trial. *J Clin Oncol.* 2002;20:1449-1455.
59. Ingram DM, Hickling C, West L, et al. A double-blind randomized controlled trial of isoflavones in the treatment of cyclical mastalgia. *Breast.* 2002;11:170-174.
60. Persky VW, et al. Effect of soy protein on endogenous hormones in postmenopausal women. *Am J Clin Nutr.* 2002;75:145-153.
61. Lu LJW, Anderson KE, Grady JJ, Nagamani M. Effects of soya consumption for one month on steroid hormones in premenopausal women: implications for breast cancer risk reduction. *Cancer Epidemiol Biomarkers Prev.* 1996;5:63-70.
62. Allred CD, Ju YH, Allred KF, et al. Dietary genistin stimulates growth of estrogen-dependent breast cancer tumors similar to that observed with genistein. *Carcinogenesis.* 2001;22:1667-1673.
63. Han KK, Soares JM Jr, Haidar MA, et al. Benefits of soy isoflavone therapeutic regimen on menopausal symptoms. *Obstet Gynecol.* 2002;99(3):389-394.

Kava

1. Volz HP, Kieser M. Kava-kava extract WS 1490 versus placebo in anxiety disorders—a randomized placebo-controlled 25-week outpatient trial. *Pharmacopsychiatry.* 1997;30:1-5.
2. Warnecke G. Psychosomatic disorders in the female climacterium, clinical efficacy and tolerance of kava extract WS 1490 [translated from German]. *Fortschr Med.* 1991;109:119-122.
3. Warnecke G, Pfaender H, Gerster G, et al. Efficacy of an extract of kava root in patients with climacteric syndrome: a double blind study with a new mono-preparation [translated from German]. *Z Phytother.* 1990;11:81-86.
4. Kinzler E, Kromer J, Lehmann E. Effect of a special kava extract in patients with anxiety-, tension-, and excitation states of non-psychotic genesis: double blind study with placebos over 4 weeks [translated from German]. *Arzneimittelforschung.* 1991;41:584-588.
5. Malsch U, Kieser M. Efficacy of kava-kava in the treatment of non-psychotic anxiety following pretreatment with benzodiazepines. *Psychopharmacology (Berl).* 2001; 157:277-283.

6. Woelk H, Kapoula O, Lehrl S, et al. The treatment of patients with anxiety. A double-blind study: kava extract WS 1490 versus benzodiazepine [translated from German]. *Z Allgemeinmed.* 1993;69:271-277.

7. Lindenberg D, Pitule-Schodel HD. L-Kavain in comparison with oxazepam in anxiety disorders: a double-blind study of clinical effectiveness [translated from German]. *Fortschr Med.* 1990;108:48-54.

8. Scholing WE, Clausen HD. On the effect of D,L-kavain: experience with Neuronika® [in German; English abstract]. *Med Klin.* 1977;72:1301-1306.

9. Schulz V, Hansel R, Tyler VE. *Rational Phytotherapy: A Physicians' Guide to Herbal Medicine.* 3rd ed. Berlin, Germany: Springer-Verlag; 1998:67-68, 70-72.

10. Munte TF, Heinze HJ, Matzke M, et al. Effects of oxazepam and an extract of kava roots *(Piper methysticum)* on event-related potentials in a word recognition task. *Neuropsychobiology.* 1993;27:46-53.

11. Heinze HJ, Munthe TF, Steitz J, et al. Pharmacopsychological effects of oxazepam and kava-extract in a visual search paradigm assessed with event-related potentials. *Pharmacopsychiatry.* 1994;27:224-230.

12. Gessner B, Cnota P. Extract of the kava-kava rhizome in comparison with diazepam and placebo [in German; English abstract]. *Z Phytother.* 1994;15:30-37.

13. Saletu B, Grunberger J, Linzmayer L, et al. EEG-brain mapping, psychometric and psychophysiological studies on central effects of Kavain—a kava plant derivative. *Hum Psychopharmacol.* 1989;4:169-190.

14. Emser W, Bartylla K. Improvement in sleep quality: effect of kava extract WS 1490 on the sleep pattern in healthy subjects [in German, English abstract]. *Neurol Psychiatr.* 1991;5:636-642.

15. Bruggemann VF, Meyer HJ. Studies on the analgesic efficacy of the kava constituents dihydrokavain (DHK) and dihydromethysticin (DHM) [in German; English abstract]. *Arzneimittelforschung.* 1963;13:407-409.

16. Jamieson DD, Duffield PH. Positive interaction of ethanol and kava resin in mice. *Clin Exp Pharmacol Physiol.* 1990;17:509-514.

17. Klohs MW, Keller F, Williams RE, et al. A chemical and pharmacological investigation of *Piper methysticum* Forst. *J Med Pharm Chem.* 1959;1:95-103.

18. Meyer HJ, Kretzschmar R. Kava pyrones—a new substance class of central muscle relaxants of the mephenesin type [translated from German]. *Klin Wochenschr.* 1966;44:902-903.

19. Meyer HJ. Pharmacology of the active compounds of the kava rhizomel *(Piper methysticum* Forst) [translated from German]. *Arch Int Pharmacodyn Ther.* 1962; 138:505-536.

20. Singh YN. Effects of kava on neuromuscular transmission and muscle contractility. *J Ethnopharmacol.* 1983;7:267-276.

21. Meyer HJ, May HU. Local anaesthetic properties of natural Kava pyrones [translated from German]. *Klin Wochenschr.* 1964;42:407.

22. Davies LP, Drew CA, Duffield P, et al. Kava pyrones and resin: studies on GABAA, GABAB and benzodiazepine binding sites in rodent brain. *Pharmacol Toxicol.* 1992;71:120-126.

23. Gleitz J, Friese J, Beile A, et al. Anticonvulsive action of (±)-kavain estimated from its properties on stimulated synaptosomes and Na+ channel receptor sites. *Eur J Pharmacol.* 1996;315:89-97.

24. Magura EI, Kopanitsa MV, Gleitz J, et al. Kava extract ingredients, (+)-methysticin and (±)-kavain inhibit voltage-operated Na(+)-channels in rat CA1 hippocampal neurons. *Neuroscience.* 1997;81:345-351.

25. Jussofie A, Schmiz A, Hiemke C. Kavapyrone enriched extract from *Piper methysticum* as modulator of the GABA binding site in different regions of rat brain. *Psychopharmacology (Berl).* 1994;116:469-474.

26. Boonen G, Haberlein H. Influence of genuine kavapyrone enantiomers on the GABA-A binding site. *Planta Med.* 1998;64:504-506.

27. Boonen G, Pramanik A, Rigler R, et al. Evidence for specific interactions between kavain and human cortical neurons monitored by fluorescence correlation spectroscopy. *Planta Med.* 2000;66:7-10.

28. Norton SA, Ruze P. Kava dermopathy. *J Am Acad Dermatol.* 1994;31:89-97.
29. Mathews JD, Riley MD, Fejo L, et al. Effects of the heavy usage of kava on physical health: summary of a pilot survey in an Aboriginal community. *Med J Aust.* 1988; 148:548-555.
30. Kraft M, Spahn TW, Menzel J, et al. Fulminant liver failure after administration of the herbal antidepressant Kava-Kava [in German; English abstract]. *Dtsch Med Wochenschr.* 2001;126(36):970-972.
31. Strahl S, Ehret V, Dahm HH, Maier KP. Necrotizing hepatitis after taking herbal remedies. *Dtsch Med Wochenschr.* 1998;123:1410-1414.
32. Prescott J, Jamieson D, Emdur N, et al. Acute effects of kava on measures of cognitive performance, physiological function and mood. *Drug Alcohol Rev.* 1993;12:49-57.
33. Russell PN, Bakker D, Singh NN. The effects of kava on alerting and speed of access of information from long-term memory. *Bull Psychonomic Soc.* 1987;25:236-237.
34. Duffield PH, Jamieson D. Development of tolerance to kava in mice. *Clin Exp Pharmacol Physiol.* 1991;18:571-578.
35. Schelosky L, Raffauf C, Jendroska K, et al. Kava and dopamine antagonism [letter]. *J Neurol Neurosurg Psychiatry.* 1995;58:639-640.
36. Almeida JC, Grimsley EW. Coma from the health food store: interaction between kava and alprazolam [letter]. *Ann Intern Med.* 1996;125:940-941.
37. De Leo V, la Marca A, Morgante G, et al. Evaluation of combining kava extract with hormone replacement therapy in the treatment of postmenopausal anxiety. *Maturitas.* 2001;39:185-188.
38. Veh I, Chatterjee SS, Kiianmaa K, et al. Reduction of voluntary ethanol intake in alcohol-preferring AA-rats by kava extract. Presented at International Congress and 49th Meeting of the Society for Medicinal Plant Research; September 2-6 2001; Erlangen, Germany.
39. Strahl S, Ehret V, Dahm HH, Maier KP. Necrotizing hepatitis after taking herbal remedies. *Dtsch Med Wochenschr.* 1998;123:1410-1414.
40. Escher M, Desmeules J, Giostra E, et al. Hepatitis associated with Kava a herbal remedy for anxiety. *BMJ.* 2001;322:139.
41. Russmann S, Lauterburg BH, Helbling A. Kava hepatotoxicity [letter]. *Ann Intern Med.* 2001;135:68-69.

Kelp

1. Kathan RH. Kelp extracts as antiviral substances. *Ann NY Acad Sci.* 1965;130:390-397.
2. Carlucci MJ, Ciancia M, Matulewicz MC, et al. Antiherpetic activity and mode of action of natural carrageenans of diverse structural types. *Antiviral Res.* 1999;43:93-102.
3. Lee JB, Hayashi K, Hayashi T, et al. Antiviral activities against HSV-1, HCMV, and HIV-1 of rhamnan sulfate from *Monostroma latissimum. Planta Med.* 1999;65:439-441.
4. Chida K, Yamamoto I. Antitumor activity of a crude fucoidan fraction prepared from the roots of kelp (*Laminaria* species). *Kitasato Arch Exp Med.* 1987;60:33-39.
5. Maruyama H, Watanabe K, Yamamoto I. Effect of dietary kelp on lipid peroxidation and glutathione peroxidase activity in livers of rats given breast carcinogen DMBA. *Nutr Cancer.* 1991;15:221-228.
6. Teas J. The dietary intake of *Laminaria*, a brown seaweed, and breast cancer prevention. *Nutr Cancer.* 1983;4:217-222.
7. Funahashi H, Imai T, Tanaka Y, et al. Wakame seaweed suppresses the proliferation of 7,12-dimethylbenz(a)-anthracene-induced mammary tumors in rats. *Jpn J Cancer Res.* 1999;90:922-927.
8. Shan BE, Yoshida Y, Kuroda E, Yamashita U. Immunomodulating activity of seaweed extract on human lymphocytes in vitro. *Int J Immunopharmacol.* 1999;21:59-70.
9. Ohno Y, Yoshida O, Oishi K, et al. Dietary beta-carotene and cancer of the prostate: a case-control study in Kyoto, Japan. *Cancer Res.* 1988;48:1331-1336.
10. Chiu KW, Fung AY. The cardiovascular effects of green beans (*Phaseolus aureus*), common rue (*Ruta graveolens*), and kelp (*Laminaria japonica*) in rats. *Gen Pharmacol.* 1997;29:859-862.

11. Norman JA, Pickford J, Sanders TW, et al. Human intake of arsenic and iodine from seaweed-based food supplements and health foods available in the UK. *Food Addit Contam.* 1988;5:103-109.

12. Konno N, Makita H, Yuri K, et al. Association between dietary iodine intake and prevalence of subclinical hypothyroidism in the coastal regions of Japan. *J Clin Endocrinol Metab.* 1994;78:393-397.

13. Eliason BC. Transient hyperthyroidism in a patient taking dietary supplements containing kelp. *J Am Board Fam Pract.* 1998;11:478-480.

14. Shilo S, Hirsch HJ. Iodine-induced hyperthyroidism in a patient with a normal thyroid gland. *Postgrad Med J.* 1986;62:661-662.

15. Okamura K, Inoue K, Omae T. A case of Hashimoto's thyroiditis with thyroid immunological abnormality manifested after habitual ingestion of seaweed. *Acta Endocrinol (Copenh).* 1978;88:703-712.

16. Tajiri J, Higashi K, Morita M, et al. Studies of hypothyroidism in patients with high iodine intake. *J Clin Endocrinol Metab.* 1986;63:412-417.

17. Yamaguchi K, Fukushima H, Uzawa H, et al. A case of iodide myxedema observed for 3 years under a low iodide diet—especially on the restoration of the mechanism of escape from the Wolf-Chaikoff effect. *Nippon Naibunpi Gakkai Zasshi.* 1984;60:79-88.

18. Ishizuki Y, Yamauchi K, Miura Y. Transient thyrotoxicosis induced by Japanese kombu. *Nippon Naibunpi Gakkai Zasshi.* 1989;65:91-98.

19. Harrell BL, Rudolph AH. Letter: Kelp diet: a cause of acneiform eruption. *Arch Dermatol.* 1976;112:560.

20. Pye KG, Kelsey SM, House IM, et al. Severe dyserythropoiesis and autoimmune thrombocytopenia associated with indigestion of kelp supplements [letter]. *Lancet.* 1992;339:1540.

21. Walkiw O, Douglas DE. Health food supplements prepared from kelp—a source of elevated urinary arsenic. *Clin Toxicol.* 1975;8:325-331.

22. Norman JA, Pickford J, Sanders TW, et al. Human intake of arsenic and iodine from seaweed-based food supplements and health foods available in the UK. *Food Addit Contam.* 1988;5:103-109.

Kudzu

1. Keung WM, Vallee BL. Daidzin and daidzein suppress free-choice ethanol intake by Syrian golden hamsters. *Proc Natl Acad Sci USA.* 1993;90:10008-10012.

2. Shebek J, Rindone JP. A pilot study exploring the effect of kudzu root on the drinking habits of patients with chronic alcoholism. *J Altern Complement Med.* 2000;6:45-48.

3. Keung WM, Vallee BL. Kudzu root: an ancient Chinese source of modern antidipsotropic agents. *Phytochemistry.* 1998;47:499-506.

Lapacho

1. Li CJ, Averboukh L, Pardee AB. Beta-lapachone, a novel DNA topoisomerase I inhibitor with a mode of action different from camptothecin. *J Biol Chem.* 1993;268: 22463-22468.

2. Guiraud P, Steiman R, Campos-Takaki GM, et al. Comparison of antibacterial and antifungal activities of lapachol and beta-lapachone. *Planta Med.* 1994;60:373-374.

3. Chau YP, Shiah SG, Don MJ, et al. Involvement of hydrogen peroxide in topoisomerase inhibitor beta-lapachone-induced apoptosis and differentiation in human leukemia cells. *Free Radic Biol Med.* 1998;24:660-670.

4. Pink JJ, Planchon SM, Tagliarino C, et al. NAD(P)H:Quinone oxidoreductase activity is the principal determinant of beta-lapachone cytotoxicity. *J Biol Chem.* 2000;275:5416-5424.

5. Oswald EH. Lapacho. *Br J Phytother.* 1993/1994;3:112-117.

Lemon Balm

1. Wolbling RH, Leonhardt K. Local therapy of herpes simplex with dried extract from *Melissa officinalis. Phytomedicine.* 1994;1:25-31.

2. Koytchev R, Alken RG, Dundarov S. Balm mint extract (Lo-701) for topical treatment of recurring herpes labialis. *Phytomedicine.* 1999;6:225-230.

3. Dressing H, Riemann D, Low H, et al. Insomnia: are valerian/balm combinations of equal value to benzodiazepines? [translated from German]. *Therapiewoche.* 1992;42: 726-736.

4. Chlabicz J, Galasinski W. The components of *Melissa officinalis* L. that influence protein biosynthesis in-vitro. *J Pharm Pharmacol.* 1986;38:791-794.

5. Schimmer O, Kruger A, Paulini H, et al. An evaluation of 55 commercial plant extracts in the Ames mutagenicity test. *Pharmazie.* 1994;49:448-451.

6. Soulimani R, Fleurentin J, Mortier F, et al. Neurotropic action of the hydroalcoholic extract of *Melissa officinalis* in the mouse. *Planta Med.* 1991;57:105-109.

Licorice

1. Newall CA, et al. *Herbal Medicines: A Guide for Health-Care Professionals.* London, England: Pharmaceutical Press; 1996:183-184.

2. Fujita H, Sakurai T, Yoshida M, et al. Antiinflammatory effect of glycyrrhizinic acid: effects of glycyrrhizinic acid against carrageenin-induced edema, UV-erythema and skin reaction sensitised with DNCB [in Japanese; English abstract]. *Pharmacometrics.* 1980;19:481-484.

3. Pompei R, Pani A, Flore O, et al. Antiviral activity of glycyrrhizic acid. *Experientia.* 1980;36:304.

4. Mitscher LA, Park YH, Clark D, et al. Antimicrobial agents from higher plants: antimicrobial isoflavonoids and related substances from *Glycyrrhiza glabra* L. var. *typica. J Nat Prod.* 1980;43:259-269.

5. Chandler RF. Licorice, more than just a flavour. *Can Pharm J.* 1985;118:421-424.

6. Amagaya S, Sugishita E, Ogihara Y, et al. Separation and quantitative analysis of 18-alpha-glycrrhetinic acid and 18-beta-glyrrhetinic acid in *Glycyrrhizae radix* by gas-lipid chromarography. *J Chromatogr.* 1985;320:430-434.

7. Aida K, Tawata M, Shindo H, et al. Isoliquiritigenin: a new aldose reductase inhibitor from *Glycyrrhizae radix. Planta Med.* 1990;56:254-258.

8. Zava DT, Dollbaum CM, Blen M. Estrogen and progestin bioactivity of foods, herbs, and spices. *Proc Soc Exp Biol Med.* 1998;217:369-378.

9. Kumagai A, Nanaboshi M, Asanuma Y, et al. Effects of glycyrrhizin on thymolytic and immunosupressive action of cortisone. *Endocrinol Jpn.* 1967;14:39-42.

10. Tamura Y, Nishikawa T, Yamada K, et al. Effects of glycyrrhetinic acid and its derivatives on delta-4-5-alpha- and 5-beta-reductase in rat liver. *Arzneimittelforschung.* 1979;29:647-649.

11. Teelucksingh S, Mackie ADR, Burt D, et al. Potentiation of hydrocortisone activity in skin by glycyrrhetinic acid. *Lancet.* 1990;335:1060-1063.

12. Strandberg TE, Jarvenpaa AL, Vanhanen H, et al. Birth outcome in relation to licorice consumption during pregnancy. *Am J Epidemiol.* 2001;153:1085-1088.

13. Kassir ZA. Endoscopic controlled trial of four drug regimens in the treatment of chronic duodenal ulceration. *Ir Med J.* 1985;78:153-156.

14. Morgan AG, Pacsoo C, McAdam WAF. Maintenance therapy: a two-year comparison between caved-S and cimetidine treatment in the prevention of symptomatic gastric ulcer recurrence. *Gut.* 1985;26:599-602.

15. Rees WD, Rhodes J, Wright JE, et al. Effect of deglycyrrhizinated liquorice on gastric mucosal damage by aspirin. *Scand J Gastroenterol.* 1979;14:605-607.

16. Peterson PK, Pheley A, Schroeppel J, et al. A preliminary placebo-controlled crossover trial of fludrocortisone for chronic fatigue syndrome. *Arch Intern Med.* 1998;158:908-914.

17. Conn JW, Rovner DR, Cohen EL. Licorice-induced pseudoaldosteronism: hypertension, hypokalemia, aldosteronopenia, and suppressed plasma renin activity. *JAMA.* 1968;205:492-496.

18. Epstein MT, Espiner EA, Donald RA, et al. Liquorice toxicity and the renin-angiotensin-aldosterone axis in man. *Br Med J.* 1977;1:209-210.

19. Mantero F. Exogenous mineralocorticoid-like disorders. *Clin Endocrinol Metab.* 1981;10:465-478.

20. Sigurjonsdottir HA, Franzson L, Manhem K, et al. Liquorice-induced rise in blood pressure: a linear dose-response relationship. *J Hum Hypertens.* 2001;15:549-552.

21. Stewart PM, Wallace AM, Valentino R, et al. Mineralocorticoid activity of liquorice: 11-beta-hydroxysteroid dehydrogenase deficiency comes of age. *Lancet.* 1987;2: 821-824.

22. Forslund T, Fyhrquist F, Froseth B. Effects of licorice on plasma atrial natriuretic peptide in healthy volunteers. *J Intern Med.* 1989;225:95-99.

23. Pompei R, Pani A, Flore O, et al. Antiviral activity of glycyrrhizic acid. *Experientia.* 1980;36:304.

24. Kiso Y, Tohkin M, Hikino H, et al. Mechanism of antihepatotoxic activity of glycyrrhizin. I. Effect on free radical generation and lipid peroxidation. *Planta Med.* 1984;50:298-302.

25. Guslandi M. Ulcer-healing drugs and endogenous prostaglandins. *Int J Clin Pharmacol Ther Toxicol.* 1985;23:398-402.

26. Schulz V, Hansel R, Tyler VE. *Rational Phytotherapy: A Physicians' Guide to Herbal Medicine.* 3rd ed. Berlin, Germany: Springer-Verlag; 1998:160.

27. Armanini D, Bonanni G, Palermo M. Reduction of serum testosterone in men by licorice [letter]. *N Engl J Med.* 1999;341:1158.

28. Budzinski JW, Foster BC, Vandenhoek S, et al. An in vitro evaluation of human cytochrome P450 3A4 inhibition by selected commercial herbal extracts and tinctures. *Phytomedicine.* 2000;7:273-282.

29. Strandberg TE, Jarvenpaa AL, Vanhanen H, et al. Birth outcome in relation to licorice consumption during pregnancy. *Am J Epidemiol.* 2001;153:1085-1088.

30. van Rossum TG, de Jong FH, Hop WC, et al. 'Pseudo-aldosteronism' induced by intravenous glycyrrhizin treatment of chronic hepatitis C patients. *J Gastroenterol Hepatol.* 2001; 16:789-795.

31. Teelucksingh S, Mackie AD, Burt D, et al. Potentiation of hydrocortisone activity in skin by glycyrrhetinic acid. *Lancet.* 1990;335:1060-1063.

32. Ploeger B, Mensinga T, Sips A, et al. The pharmacokinetics of glycyrrhizic acid evaluated by physiologically based pharmacokinetic modeling. *Drug Metab Rev.* 2001;33:125-147.

33. Sato H, Goto W, Yamamura J, et al. Therapeutic basis of glycyrrhizin on chronic hepatitis B. *Antiviral Res.* 1996;30:171-177.

34. Abe Y, Ueda T, Kato T, et al. Effectiveness of interferon, glycyrrhizin combination therapy in patients with chronic hepatitis C *Nippon Rinsho.* 1994;52:1817-1822.

35. Sigurjonsdottir HA, Franzson L, Manhem K, et al. Liquorice-induced rise in blood pressure: a linear dose-response relationship. *J Hum Hypertens.* 2001;15:549-552.

36. van Gelderen CE, Bijlsma JA, van Dokkum W, et al. Glycyrrhizic acid: the assessment of a no effect level. *Hum Exp Toxicol.* 2000;19:434-439.

Lignans

1. Sung MK, Lautens M, Thompson LU. Mammalian lignans inhibit the growth of estrogen-independent human colon tumor cells. *Anticancer Res.* 1998;18(3A):1405-1408.

2. Jenkins DJ, Kendall CW, Vidgen E, et al. Health aspects of partially defatted flaxseed, including effects on serum lipids, oxidative measures, and ex vivo androgen and progestin activity: a controlled crossover trial. *Am J Clin Nutr.* 1999;69:395-402.

3. Arjmandi BH, Khan DA, Juma S, et al. Whole flaxseed consumption lowers serum LDL-cholesterol and lipoprotein (a) concentrations in postmenopausal women. *Nutr Res.* 1998;18:1203-1214.

4. Prasad K. Dietary flax seed in prevention of hypercholesterolemic *Atherosclerosis. Atherosclerosis.* 1997;132:69-76.

5. Prasad K. Reduction of serum cholesterol and hypercholesterolemic atherosclerosis in rabbits by secoisolariciresinol diglucoside isolated from flaxseed. *Circulation.* 1999;99:1355-1362.

6. Adlercreutz H, Mazur W. Phyto-oestrogens and Western diseases. *Ann Med.* 1997; 29:95-120.

7. Clark WF, Parbtani A, Huff MW, et al. Flaxseed: a potential treatment for lupus nephritis. *Kidney Int.* 1995;48:475-480.

8. Ogborn MR, Nitschmann E, Bankovic-Calic N, et al. The effect of dietary flaxseed supplementation on organic anion and osmolyte content and excretion in rat poly-cystic kidney disease. *Biochem Cell Biol.* 1998;76:553-559.

9. Thompson LU, Rickard SE, Orcheson LJ, et al. Flaxseed and its lignan and oil com-ponents reduce mammary tumor growth at a late stage of carcinogenesis. *Carcino-genesis.* 1996;17:1373-1376.

10. Serraino M, Thompson LU. The effect of flaxseed supplementation on the initiation and promotional stages of mammary tumorigenesis. *Nutr Cancer.* 1992;17:153-159.

11. Yan L, Yee JA, Li D, et al. Dietary flaxseed supplementation and experimental metas-tasis of melanoma cells in mice. *Cancer Lett.* 1998;124:181-186.

12. Tarpila S, Kivinen A. Ground flaxseed is an effective hypolipidemic bulk laxative [ab-stract]. *Gastroenterology.* 1997;112:A836.

13. Griffiths K, Morton MS, Denis L. Certain aspects of molecular endocrinology that relate to the influence of dietary factors on the pathogenesis of prostate cancer. *Eur Urol.* 1999;35:443-455.

14. Tou JCL, Chen J, Thompson LU. Flaxseed and its lignan precursor, secoisolari-ciresinol diglycoside, affect pregnancy outcome and reproductive development in rats. *J Nutr.* 1998;128:1861-1868.

15. Hutchins AM, Martini MC, Olson BA, et al. Flaxseed consumption influences en-dogenous hormone concentrations in postmenopausal women. *Nutr Cancer.* 2001; 39:58-65.

Lipoic Acid

1. Ziegler D, Hanefeld M, Ruhnau KJ, et al. Treatment of symptomatic diabetic polyneuropathy with the antioxidant alpha-lipoic acid: a 7-month multicenter ran-domized controlled trial (ALADIN III Study). ALADIN III Study Group. Alpha-Lipoic Acid in Diabetic Neuropathy. *Diabetes Care.* 1999;22:1296-1301.

2. Ziegler D, Hanefeld M, Ruhnau KJ, et al. Treatment of symptomatic diabetic pe-ripheral neuropathy with the anti-oxidant alpha-lipoic acid: a 3-week multicentre randomized controlled trial (ALADIN Study). *Diabetologia.* 1995;38:1425-1433.

3. Kahler W, Kuklinski B, Ruhlmann C, et al. Diabetes mellitus—a free radical-associated disease: results of an adjuvant antioxidant supplementation [in German; English abstract]. *Z Gesamte Inn Med.* 1993;48:223-232.

4. Packer L. Antioxidant properties of lipoic acid and its therapeutic effects in preven-tion of diabetes complications and cataracts. *Ann NY Acad Sci.* 1994;738:257-264.

5. Ziegler D, Gries FA. Alpha-lipoic acid in the treatment of diabetic peripheral and cardiac autonomic neuropathy. *Diabetes.* 1997;46(suppl 2):S62-S66.

6. Jacob S, Henriksen EJ, Schiemann AL, et al. Enhancement of glucose disposal in patients with type 2 diabetes by alpha-lipoic acid. *Arzneimittelforschung.* 1995;45: 872-874.

7. Jacob S, Ruus P, Hermann R, et al. Oral administration of RAC-alpha-lipoic acid modulates insulin sensitivity in patients with type-2 diabetes mellitus: a placebo-controlled pilot trial. *Free Radic Biol Med.* 1999;27:309-314.

8. Kawabata T, Packer L. Alpha-lipoate can protect against glycation of serum albu-min, but not low density lipoprotein. *Biochem Biophys Res Commun.* 1994;203:99-104.

9. Nagamatsu M, Nickander KK, Schmelzer JD, et al. Lipoic acid improves nerve blood flow, reduces oxidative stress, and improves distal nerve conduction in exper-imental diabetic neuropathy. *Diabetes Care.* 1995;18:1160-1167.

10. Suzuki YJ, Tsuchiya M, Packer L. Lipoate prevents glucose-induced protein modi-fications. *Free Radical Res Commun.* 1992;17:211-217.

11. Kilic F, Handelman GJ, Serbinova E, et al. Modelling cortical cataractogenesis 17: in vitro effect of a-lipoic acid on glucose-induced lens membrane damage, a model of diabetic cataractogenesis. *Biochem Mol Biol Int.* 1995;37:361-370.

12. Fuchs J, Schofer H, Milbradt R, et al. Studies on lipoate effects on blood redox state in human immunodeficiency virus infected patients. *Arzneimittelforschung.* 1993;43: 1359-1362.

13. Kagan VE, Shvedova A, Serbinova E, et al. Dihydrolipoic acid: a universal antioxidant both in the membrane and in the aqueous phase. *Biochem Pharmacol.* 1992; 44:1637-1649.
14. Biewenga GP, Haenen GR, Bast A. The pharmacology of the antioxidant lipoic acid. *Gen Pharmacol.* 1997;29:315-331.
15. Salonen JT, Nyyssonen K, Tuomainen TP, et al. Increased risk of non-insulin dependent diabetes mellitus at low plasma vitamin E concentrations: a four year follow-up study in men. *Br Med J.* 1995;311:1124-1127.
16. Packer L, Tritschler HJ, Wessel K. Neuroprotection by the metabolic antioxidant alpha-lipoic acid. *Free Radic Biol Med.* 1997;22:359-378.
17. Podda M, Tritschler HJ, Ulrich H, et al. Alpha-lipoic acid supplementation prevents symptoms of vitamin E deficiency. *Biochem Biophys Res Commun.* 1994;204:98-104.
18. Cameron NE, Cotter MA, Horrobin DH, et al. Effects of alpha-lipoic acid on neurovascular function in diabetic rats: interaction with essential fatty acids. *Diabetologia.* 1998;41:390-399.
19. Hounsom L, Horrobin DF, Tritschler H, et al. A lipoic acid-gamma linolenic acid conjugate is effective against multiple indices of experimental diabetic neuropathy. *Diabetologia.* 1998;41:839-843.

Lutein

1. Mares-Perlman JA, Brady WE, Klein BE, et al. Diet and nuclear lens opacities. *Am J Epidemiol.* 1995;141:322-334.
2. Hankinson S, Stampfer M, Seddon J, et al. Nutrient intake and cataract extraction in women: a prospective study. *BMJ.* 1992;305:335-339.
3. Brown L, Rimm EB, Seddon JM, et al. A prospective study of carotenoid intake and risk of cataract extraction in US men. *Am J Clin Nutr.* 1999;70:517-524.
4. Chasan-Taber L, Willett WC, Seddon JM, et al. A prospective study of carotenoid and vitamin A intakes and risk of cataract extraction in US women. *Am J Clin Nutr.* 1999;70:509-516.
5. Landrum JT, Bone RA, Kilburn MD. The macular pigment: a possible role in protection from age-related macular degeneration. *Adv Pharmacol.* 1997;38:537-556.
6. Hammond BR Jr, Wooten BR, Snodderly DM. Density of the human crystalline lens is related to the macular pigment carotenoids, lutein and zeaxanthin. *Optom Vis Sci.* 1997;74:499-504.
7. Mares-Perlman JA, Fisher AI, Klein R, et al. Lutein and zeaxanthin in the diet and serum and their relation to age-related maculopathy in the third national health and nutrition examination survey. *Am J Epidemiol.* 2001;153:424-432.
8. Hassan K, Hough G, Wang X, et al. Dietary lutein markedly reduces atherosclerotic lesion formation in apolipoprotein null mouse [abstract]. *FASEB J.* 1999;13:A176.

Lycopene

1. Giovannucci E, Ascherio A, Rimm EB, et al. Intake of carotenoids and retinol in relation to risk of prostate cancer [articles]. *J Natl Cancer Inst.* 1995;87:1767-1776.
2. Giovannucci E, Clinton SK. Tomatoes, lycopene, and prostate cancer. *Proc Soc Exp Biol Med.* 1998;218:129-139.
3. Franceschi S, Bidoli E, LaVecchia C, et al. Tomatoes and risk of digestive-tract cancers. *Int J Cancer.* 1994;59:181-184.
4. Kim DJ, Takasuka N, Kim JM, et al. Chemoprevention by lycopene of mouse lung neoplasia after combined initiation treatment with DEN, MNU and DMH. *Cancer Lett.* 1997;120:15-22.
5. Okajima E, Tsutsumi M, Ozono S, et al. Inhibitory effect of tomato juice on rat urinary bladder carcinogenesis after N-butyl-N-(4-hydroxybutyl) nitrosamine initiation. *Jpn J Cancer Res.* 1998;89:22-26.
6. Gann PH, Ma J, Giovannucci E, et al. Lower prostate cancer risk in men with elevated plasma lycopene levels: results of a prospective analysis. *Cancer Res.* 1999; 59:1225-1230.
7. Giovannucci E. Tomatoes, tomato-based products, lycopene, and cancer: review of the epidemioilogic literature [review]. *J Natl Cancer Inst.* 1999;91:317-331.

8. Key TJA, Silcocks PB, Davey GK, et al. A case-control study of diet and prostate cancer. *Br J Cancer.* 1997;76:678-687.
9. Nomura AM, Stemmermann GN, Lee J, et al. Serum micronutrients and prostate cancer in Japanese Americans in Hawaii. *Cancer Epidemiol Biomarkers Prev.* 1997; 6:487-491.
10. Mares-Perlman JA, Brady WE, Klein R, et al. Serum antioxidants and age-related macular degeneration in a population-based case-control study. *Arch Ophthalmol.* 1995;113:1518-1523.
11. Kucuk O, Sarkar FH, Sakr W, et al. Phase II randomized clinical trial of lycopene supplementation before radical prostatectomy. *Cancer Epidemiol Biomarkers Prev.* 2001;10:861-868.
12. Kumar R, Gupta NP. Lycopene therapy in idiopathic male infertility: results of a clinical trial. Presented at: 34th Annual Conference of the Urological Society of India. January 18-21, 2001; Nagpur, India. Abstract no. 102.
13. New Management Alternative for Those at Risk for Heart Disease. Press Release from LycoRed Natural Products Industries Ltd., P.O.B. 320, Beer-Sheva 84102, Israel.
14. New Research Shows Combination of Tomato Phytonutrients Effectively Combats Breast Cancer. Press Release from LycoRed Natural Products Industries Ltd., P.O.B. 320, Beer-Sheva 84102, Israel.

Lysine

1. Griffith RS, Walsh DE, Myrmel KH, et al. Success of L-lysine therapy in frequently recurrent herpes simplex infection: treatment and prophylaxis. *Dermatologica.* 1987;175:183-190.
2. McCune MA, Perry HO, Muller SA, et al. Treatment of recurrent herpes simplex infections with L-lysine monohydrochloride. *Cutis.* 1984;34:366-373.
3. Milman N, Scheibel J, Jessen O. Lysine prophylaxis in recurrent herpes simplex labialis: a double-blind, controlled crossover study. *Acta Derm Venereol.* 1980;60:85-87.
4. DiGiovanna JJ, Blank H. Failure of lysine in frequently recurrent herpes simplex infection: treatment and prophylaxis. *Arch Dermatol.* 1984;120:48-51.
5. Milman N, Scheibel J, Jessen O. Failure of lysine treatment in recurrent herpes simplex labialis [letter]. *Lancet.* 1978;2:942.
6. Griffith RS, DeLong DC, Nelson JD. Relation of arginine-lysine antagonism to herpes simplex growth in tissue culture. *Chemotherapy.* 1981;27:209-213.
7. Kritchevsky D, Weber MM, Klurfeld DM. Gallstone formation in hamsters: influence of specific amino acids. *Nutr Rep Int.* 1984;29:117-121.
8. Leszczynski DE, Kummerow FA. Excess dietary lysine induces hypercholesterolemia in chickens. *Experientia.* 1982;38:266-267.

Magnesium

1. Kelepouris E, Agus ZS. Hypomagnesemia: renal magnesium handling. *Semin Nephrol.* 1998;18:58-73.
2. al-Ghamdi SM, Cameron EC, Sutton RA. Magnesium deficiency: pathophysiologic and clinical overview. *Am J Kidney Dis.* 1994;24:737-752.
3. Lewis NM, Marcus MS, Behling AR, et al. Calcium supplements and milk: effects on acid-base balance and on retention of calcium, magnesium, and phosphorus. *Am J Clin Nutr.* 1989;49:527-533
4. Andon MB, Ilich JZ, Tzagournis MA, et al. Magnesium balance in adolescent females consuming a low- or high-calcium diet. *Am J Clin Nutr.* 1996;63:950-953.
5. *Drug Evaluations Annual.* Vol. 2. Milwaukee, Wis: American Medical Association; 1994.
6. Zuccaro P, Pacifici R, Pichini S, et al. Influence of antacids on the bioavailability of glibenclamide. *Drugs Exp Clin Res.* 1989;15:165-169.
7. Attias J, Weisz G, Almog S, et al. Oral magnesium intake reduces permanent hearing loss induced by noise exposure. *Am J Otolaryngol.* 1994;15:26-32.

8. Shechter M, Sharir M, Labrador MJ, et al. Oral magnesium therapy improves endothelial function in patients with coronary artery disease. *Circulation.* 2000; 102:2353-2358.

9. Shechter M, Merz CN, Paul-Labrador M, et al. Beneficial antithrombotic effects of the association of pharmacological oral magnesium therapy with aspirin in coronary heart disease patients. *Magnes Res.* 2000;13:275-284.

10. Seifert B, Wagler P, Dartsch S, et al. Magnesium—an alternative in treatment of primary dysmenorrhoea [translated from German]. *Zentralbl Gynakol.* 1989;111: 755-760.

11. Fontana-Klaiber H, Hogg B. Therapeutic effects of magnesium in dysmenorrhea [in German; English abstract]. *Schweiz Rundsch Med Prax.* 1990;79:491-494.

12. Facchinetti F, Borella P, Sances G, et al. Oral magnesium successfully relieves premenstrual mood changes. *Obstet Gynecol.* 1991;78:177-181.

13. Facchinetti F, Sances G, Borella P, et al. Magnesium prophylaxis of menstrual migraine: effects on intracellular magnesium. *Headache.* 1991;31:298-301.

14. De Souza MC, Walker AF, Robinson PA, et al. A synergistic effect of a daily supplement for 1 month of 200 mg magnesium plus 50 mg vitamin B_6 for the relief of anxiety-related premenstrual symptoms: a randomized, double-blind, crossover study. *J Womens Health Gend Based Med.* 2000;9:131-139.

15. Peikert A, Wilimzig C, Kohne-Volland R. Prophylaxis of migraine with oral magnesium: results from a prospective, multicenter, placebo-controlled and double-blind randomized study. *Cephalalgia.* 1996;16:257-263.

16. Taubert K. Magnesium in the treatment of migraine: result of a multicenter pilot study [in German; English abstract]. *Fortschr Med.* 1994;112:328-330.

17. Pfaffenrath V, Wessely P, Meyer C, et al. Magnesium in the prophylaxis of migraine: a double-blind, placebo-controlled study. *Cephalalgia.* 1996;16:436-440.

18. Gaby AR. Aluminum: the ubiquitous poison contributing to Alzheimer's and osteoporosis, with advice on avoiding exposure. *Nutr Healing.* 1997;4:3-4, 11.

19. Li MK, Blacklock NJ, Garside J. Effects of magnesium on calcium oxalate crystallization. *J Urol.* 1985;133:123-125.

20. Parivar F, Low RK, Stoller ML. The influence of diet on urinary stone disease. *J Urol.* 1996;155:432-440.

21. Johansson G, Backman U, Danielson BG, et al. Biochemical and clinical effects of the prophylactic treatment of renal calcium stones with magnesium hydroxide. *J Urol.* 1980;124:770-774.

22. Ettinger B, Citron JT, Livermore B, et al. Chlorthalidone reduces calcium oxalate calculous recurrence but magnesium hydroxide does not. *J Urol.* 1988;139:679-684.

23. Frick M, Darpo B, Ostergren J, et al. The effect of oral magnesium, alone or as an adjuvant to sotalol, after cardioversion in patients with persistent atrial fibrillation. *Eur Heart J.* 2000;21:1177-1185.

24. Sanjuliani AF, de Abreu Fagundes VG, Francischetti EA. Effects of magnesium on blood pressure and intracellular ion levels of Brazilian hypertensive patients. *Int J Cardiol.* 1996;56:177-183.

25. Witteman JCM, Grobbee DE, Derkx FH, et al. Reduction of blood pressure with oral magnesium supplementation in women with mild to moderate hypertension. *Am J Clin Nutr.* 1994;60:129-135.

26. Dyckner T, Wester PO. Effect of magnesium on blood pressure. *Br Med J (Clin Res Ed).* 1983;286:1847-1849.

27. Henderson DG, Schierup J, Schodt T. Effect of magnesium supplementation on blood pressure and electrolyte concentrations in hypertensive patients receiving long term diuretic treatment. *Br Med J (Clin Res Ed).* 1986;293:664-665.

28. Sibai BM, Villar MA, Bray E. Magnesium supplementation during pregnancy: a double-blind randomized controlled clinical trial. *Am J Obstet Gynecol.* 1989;161:115-119.

29. Kovacs L, Molnar BG, Huhn E, et al. Magnesium substitution in pregnancy: a prospective, randomized double-blind study [translated from German]. *Geburtsh Frauenheilk.* 1988;48:595-600.

30. Elamin A, Tuvemo T. Magnesium and insulin-dependent diabetes mellitus. *Diabetes Res Clin Pract.* 1990;10:203-209.

31. Tosiello L. Hypomagnesemia and diabetes mellitus: a review of clinical implications. *Arch Intern Med.* 1996;156:1143-1148.

32. Eibl NL, Kopp HP, Nowak HR, et al. Hypomagnesemia in type II diabetes: effect of a 3-month replacement therapy. *Diabetes Care.* 1995;18:188-192.

33. Martineau J, Barthelemy C, Garreau B, et al. Vitamin B_6, magnesium, and combined B_6-Mg: therapeutic effects in childhood autism. *Biol Psychiatry.* 1985;20:467-478.

34. Pfeiffer SI, Norton J, Nelson L, et al. Efficacy of vitamin B_6 and magnesium in the treatment of autism: a methodology review and summary of outcomes. *J Autism Dev Disord.* 1995;25:481-493.

35. Barthelemy C, Garreau B, Leddet I, et al. Behavioral and biological effects of oral magnesium, vitamin B_6, and combined magnesium-B_6 administration in autistic children. *Magnes Bull.* 1981;2:150-153.

36. Lelord G, Callaway E, Muh JP. Clinical and biological effects of high doses of vitamin B_6 and magnesium on autistic children. *Acta Vitaminol Enzymol.* 1982;4:27-44.

37. Lelord G, Muh JP, Barthelemy C, et al. Effects of pyridoxine and magnesium on autistic symptoms—initial observations. *J Autism Dev Disord.* 1981;11:219-230.

38. Martineau J, Garreau B, Barthelemy C, et al. Effects of vitamin B_6 on averaged evoked potentials in infantile autism. *Biol Psychiatry.* 1981;16:627-641.

39. Rimland B, Callaway E, Dreyfus P. The effect of high doses of vitamin B_6 on autistic children: a double-blind crossover study. *Am J Psychiatry.* 1978;135:472-475.

40. Cook R, Botting D. Use of orthomolecular therapy for those with behavioural problems and mental handicap: a review. *Complement Ther Med.* 1997;5:228-232.

41. Rimland B. Controversies in the treatment of autistic children: vitamin and drug therapy. *J Child Neurol.* 1988;3(suppl):S68-S72.

42. Rimland B. Vitamin B_6 versus fenfluramine: a case-study in medical bias. *J Nutr Med.* 1991;2:321-322.

43. Kummerow FA, Zhou Q, Mahfouz MM. Effect of trans fatty acids on calcium influx into human arterial endothelial cells. *Am J Clin Nutr.* 1999;70:832-838.

44. Bernstein WK, Khastgir T, Khastgir A, et al. Lack of effectiveness of magnesium in chronic stable asthma. A prospective, randomized, double-blind, placebo-controlled, crossover trial in normal subjects and in patients with chronic stable asthma. *Arch Intern Med.* 1995;155:271-276.

45. Finstad EW, Newhouse IJ, Lukaski HC, et al. The effects of magnesium supplementation on exercise performance. *Med Sci Sports Exerc.* 2001;33:493-498.

46. Brilla LR, Haley TF. Effect of magnesium supplementation on strength training in humans. *J Am Coll Nutr.* 1992;11:326-329.

47. Weller E, Bachert P, Meinck HM, et al. Lack of effect of oral Mg-supplementation on Mg in serum, blood cells, and calf muscle. *Med Sci Sports Exerc.* 1998;30:1584-1591.

48. Ripari P, Pieralisi G, Giamberardino MA, et al. Effects of magnesium pidolate on some cardiorespiratory submaximal effort parameters [abstract]. *Magnes Res.* 1989;2:70.

49. Brilla LR, Gunter KB. Effect of magnesium supplementation on exercise time to exhaustion. *Med Exerc Nutr Health.* 1995;4:230-233.

50. Terblanche S, Noakes TD, Dennis SC, et al. Failure of magnesium supplementation to influence marathon running performance or recovery in magnesium-replete subjects. *Int J Sport Nutr.* 1992;2:154-164.

51. Dragani L, Giamberardino MA, Vecchiet L. Effects of magnesium administration on muscle damage from physical exercise. In: Vecchiet L, ed. *Magnesium and Physical Activity.* New York, NY: Parthenon Publishing Group; 1994:253-260.

52. Ruddel H, Werner C, Ising H. Impact of magnesium supplementation on performance data in young swimmers. *Magnes Res.* 1990;3:103-107.

53. Kivisto KT, Neuvonen PJ. Effect of magnesium hydroxide on the absorption and efficacy of tolbutamide and chlorpropamide. *Eur J Clin Pharmacol.* 1992;42:675-679.

54. Devane J, Ryan MP. The effects of amiloride and triamterene on urinary magnesium excretion in conscious saline-loaded rats. *Br J Pharmacol.* 1981;72:285-289.

55. Institute of Medicine. *Dietary Reference Intakes for Calcium, Phosphorus, Magnesium, Vitamin D and Fluoride.* Washington, DC: National Academy Press; 2001.

56. Spencer H, Norris C, Williams D. Inhibitory effects of zinc on magnesium balance and magnesium absorption in man. *J Am Coll Nutr.* 1994;13:479-484.

57. Dietary Reference Intakes for Calcium, Phosphorus, Magnesium, Vitamin D, and Fluoride (1997). Available at: http://www.nap.edu. Accessed October 4, 2001.

58. McGuire JK, Kulkarni MS, Baden HP. Fatal hypermagnesemia in a child treated with megavitamin/megamineral therapy. *Pediatrics.* 2000;105:E18.

59. Tatro D, ed. *A to Z Drug Facts.* St Louis, Mo: Facts and Comparisons; 1999.

60. Lomaestro BM, Bailie GR. Quinolone-cation interactions: a review. *DICP.* 1991; 25:1249-1258.

61. Nix DE, Wilton JH, Ronald B, et al. Inhibition of norfloxacin absorption by antacids. *Antimicrob Agents Chemother.* 1990;34:432-435.

62. Grasela TH Jr, Schentag JJ, Sedman AJ, et al. Inhibition of enoxacin absorption by antacids or ranitidine. *Antimicrob Agents Chemother.* 1989;33:615-617.

63. Shimada J, Shiba K, Oguma T, et al. Effect of antacid on absorption of the quinolone lomefloxacin. *Antimicrob Agents Chemother.* 1992;36:1219-1224.

64. Teng R, Dogolo LC, Willavize SA, et al. Effect of Maalox and omeprazole on the bioavailability of trovafloxacin. *J Antimicrob Chemother.* 1997;39(suppl B):93-97.

65. Shiba K, Sakamoto M, Nakazawa Y, Sakai O. Effects of antacid on absorption and excretion of new quinolones. *Drugs.* 1995;49(suppl 2):360-361.

66. Naggar VF, Khalil SA. Effect of magnesium trisilicate on nitrofurantoin absorption. *Clin Pharmacol Ther.* 1979;25:857-863.

67. Mannisto P. The effect of crystal size, gastric content and emptying rate on the absorption of nitrofurantoin in healthy human volunteers. *Int J Clin Pharmacol Biopharm.* 1978;16:223-228.

68. Osman MA, Patel RB, Schuna A, et al. Reduction in oral penicillamine absorption by food, antacid, and ferrous sulfate. *Clin Pharmacol Ther.* 1983;33:465-470.

69. Martin BJ, Milligan K. Diuretic-associated hypomagnesemia in the elderly. *Arch Intern Med.* 1987;147:1768-1771.

70. Elisaf M, Bairaktari E, Kalaitzidis R, Siamopoulos K. Hypomagnesemia in alcoholic patients. *Alcohol Clin Exp Res.* 1998;22:244-246.

Maitake

1. Kidd PM. The use of mushroom glucans and proteoglycans in cancer treatment. *Altern Med Rev.* 2000;5:4-27.

2. Nanba H, Yamasaki P, Shirota M, et al. Immunostimulant activity (in vivo) and anti-HIV activity (in vitro) of 3 branched B 1.6 glucan extracted from maitake mushroom *(Grifola frondosa)* [abstract]. VIII International Conference on AIDS/III STD World Congress, Amsterdam, The Netherlands, July 19-24, 1992. London, England: Wellcome Foundation; 1992:30.

3. Kubo K, Nanba H. Anti-hyperliposis effect of maitake fruit body *(Grifola frondosa).* I. *Biol Pharm Bull.* 1997;20:781-785.

4. Kubo K, Aoki H, Nanba H. Anti-diabetic activity present in the fruit body of *Grifola frondosa* (Maitake). I. *Biol Pharm Bull.* 1994;17:1106-1110.

5. Fullerton SA, Samadi AA, Tortorelis DG, et al. Induction of apoptosis in human prostatic cancer cells with beta-glucan (Maitake mushroom polysaccharide). *Mol Urol.* 2000;4:7-13.

Malic Acid

1. Russell IJ, Michalek JE, Flechas JD, et al. Treatment of fibromyalgia syndrome with Super Malic: a randomized, double blind, placebo controlled, crossover pilot study. *J Rheumatol.* 1995;22:953-958.

2. Abraham GE, Flechas JD. Management of fibromyalgia: rationale for the use of magnesium and malic acid. *J Nutr Med.* 1992;3:49-59.

Manganese

1. National Institute of Medicine. *Dietary Reference Intakes for Vitamin A, Vitamin K, Arsenic, Boron, Chromium, Copper, Iodine, Iron, Manganese, Molybdenum, Nickel, Silicon, Vanadium, and Zinc.* Washington, DC: National Academic Press; 2001.

2. Davidsson L, Cederblad A, Lonnerdal B, et al. The effect of individual dietary components on manganese absorption in humans. *Am J Clin Nutr.* 1991;54:1065-1070.

3. Freeland-Graves JH, Lin PH. Plasma uptake of manganese as affected by oral loads of manganese, calcium, milk, phosphorous, copper, and zinc. *J Am Coll Nutr.* 1991; 10:38-43.
4. Akram M, Sullivan C, Mack G, et al. What is the clinical significance of reduced manganese and zinc levels in treated epileptic patients [letter]. *Med J Aust.* 1989;151:113.
5. Kosenko LG. The content of some trace elements in the blood of patients suffering from diabetes mellitus [in Russian; English abstract]. *Klin Med (Mosk).* 1964;42: 113-116.
6. Dietary Reference Intakes for Vitamin A, Vitamin K, Arsenic, Boron, Chromium, Copper, Iodine, Iron, Manganese, Molybdenum, Nickel, Silicon, Vanadium, and Zinc (2001). Available at: http://www.nap.edu. Accessed October 4, 2001.

Medium-Chain Triglycerides

1. Craig GB, Darnell BE, Weinsier RL, et al. Decreased fat and nitrogen losses in patients with AIDS receiving medium-chain-triglyceride-enriched formula vs those receiving long-chain-triglyceride-containing formula. *J Am Diet Assoc.* 1997;97:605-611.
2. Wanke CA, Pleskow D, Degirolami PC, et al. A medium chain triglyceride-based diet in patients with HIV and chronic diarrhea reduces diarrhea and malabsorption: a prospective, controlled trial. *Nutrition.* 1996;12:766-771.
3. Caliari S, Benini L, Sembenini C, et al. Medium-chain triglyceride absorption in patients with pancreatic insufficiency. *Scand J Gastroenterol.* 1996;31:90-94.
4. Yost TJ, Eckel RH. Hypocaloric feeding in obese women: metabolic effects of medium-chain triglyceride substitution. *Am J Clin Nutr.* 1989;49:326-330.
5. Tsuji H, Kasai M, Takeuchi H, et al. Dietary medium-chain triacylglycerols suppress accumulation of body fat in a double-blind controlled trial in healthy men and women. *J Nutr.* 2001;131:2853-2859.
6. Baba N, Bracco EF, Hashim SA. Enhanced thermogenesis and diminished deposition of fat in response to overfeeding with diet containing medium chain triglyceride. *Am J Clin Nutr.* 1982; 35:678-682.
7. Scalfi L, Coltorti A, Contaldo F. Postprandial thermogenesis in lean and obese subjects after meals supplemented with medium-chain and long-chain triglycerides. *Am J Clin Nutr.* 1991;53:1130-1133.
8. Mak SC, Chi CS, Wan CJ. Clinical experience of ketogenic diet on children with refractory epilepsy. *Acta Paediatr Taiwan.* 1999;40:97-100.
9. Lefevre F, Aronson N. Ketogenic diet for the treatment of refractory epilepsy in children: a systematic review of efficacy. *Pediatrics.* 2000;105:E46.
10. Rosenthal E, Weissman B, Kyllonen K. Use of parenteral medium-chain triglyceride emulsion for maintaining seizure control in a 5-year-old girl with intractable diarrhea. *JPEN J Parenter Enteral Nutr.* 1990;14:543-545.
11. Bach AC, Babayan VK. Medium-chain triglycerides: an update. *Am J Clin Nutr.* 1982;36:950-962.
12. Traul KA, Driedger A, Ingle DL, et al. Review of the toxicologic properties of medium-chain triglycerides. *Food Chem Toxicol.* 2000;38:79-98.
13. Anderson O. Putting medium-chain triglycerides in your sports drink can increase your endurance. *Nutr Sci News.* 1994;6:6-7.
14. Jeukendrup AE, Saris WHM, Schrauwen P, et al. Oxidation of orally ingested medium chain triglyceride (MCT) during prolonged exercise [abstract]. *Med Sci Sports Exerc.* 1995;27(suppl 5):S101.
15. Jeukendrup AE, Thielen JJ, Wagenmakers AJ, et al. Effect of medium-chain triacylglycerol and carbohydrate ingestion during exercise on substrate utilization and subsequent cycling performance. *Am J Clin Nutr.* 1998;67:397-404.
16. Misell LM, Lagomarcino ND, Schuster V, et al. Chronic medium-chain triacylglycerol consumption and endurance performance in trained runners. *J Sports Med Phys Fitness.* 2001;41:210-215.
17. Satabin P, Portero P, Defer G, et al. Metabolic and hormonal responses to lipid and carbohydrate diets during exercise in man. *Med Sci Sports Exerc.* 1987;19:218-223.

18. Van Zyl CG, Lambert EV, Hawley JA, et al. Effects of medium-chain triglyceride ingestion on fuel metabolism and cycling performance. *J Appl Physiol.* 1996;80: 2217-2225.

19. Krotkiewski M. Value of VLCD supplementation with medium chain triglycerides. *Int J Obes Relat Metab Disord.* 2001;25:1393-1400.

20. Seaton TB, Welle SL, Warenko MK, et al. Thermic effect of medium-chain and long-chain triglycerides in man. *Am J Clin Nutr.* 1986;44:630-634.

Melatonin

1. Suhner A, Schlagenhauf P, Johnson R, et al. Comparative study to determine the optimal melatonin dosage form for the alleviation of jet lag. *Chronobiol Int.* 1998; 15:655-666.

2. Petrie K, Dawson AG, Thompson L, et al. A double-blind trial of melatonin as a treatment for jet lag in international cabin crew. *Biol Psychiatry.* 1993;33:526-530.

3. Petrie K, Conaglen JV, Thompson L, et al. Effect of melatonin on jet lag after long haul flights. *BMJ.* 1989;298:705-707.

4. Claustrat B, Brun J, David M, et al. Melatonin and jet lag: confirmatory result using a simplified protocol. *Biol Psychiatry.* 1992;32:705-711.

5. Suhner A, Schlagenhauf P, Hofer I, et al. Effectiveness and tolerability of melatonin and zolpidem for the alleviation of jet lag. *Aviat Space Environ Med.* 2001;72:638-646.

6. Spitzer RL, Terman M, Williams JB, et al. Jet lag: clinical features, validation of a new syndrome-specific scale, and lack of response to melatonin in a randomized, double-blind trial. *Am J Psychiatry.* 1999;156:1392-1396.

7. Edwards BJ, Atkinson G, Waterhouse J, et al. Use of melatonin in recovery from jet-lag following an eastward flight across 10 time-zones. *Ergonomics.* 2000;43:1501-1513.

8. Smits MG, Nagtegaal EE, van der Heijden J, et al. Melatonin for chronic sleep on-set insomnia in children: a randomized placebo-controlled trial. *J Child Neurol.* 2001;16:86-92.

9. Dodge NN, Wilson GA. Melatonin for treatment of sleep disorders in children with developmental disabilities. *J Child Neurol.* 2001;16:581-584.

10. Yang CM, Spielman AJ, D'Ambrosio P, et al. A single dose of melatonin prevents the phase delay associated with a delayed weekend sleep pattern. *Sleep.* 2001;24:272-281.

11. Garfinkel D, Zisapel N, Wainstein J, et al. Facilitation of benzodiazepine discontin-uation by melatonin: a new clinical approach. *Arch Intern Med.* 1999;159:2456-2460.

12. Garfinkel D, Wainstein J, Halabe A, et al. Beneficial effect of controlled release mela-tonin on sleep quality and hemoglobin A1C in type 2 diabetic patients. Presented at: World Congress of Gerontology; July 1-6, 2001; Vancouver, Canada.

13. Fraschini F, Cesarani A, Alpini D, et al. Melatonin influences human balance. *Biol Signals Recept.* 1999;8:111-119.

14. Shamir E, Laudon M, Barak Y, et al. Melatonin improves sleep quality of patients with chronic schizophrenia. *J Clin Psychiatry.* 2000;61:373-377.

15. Kayumov L, Brown G, Jindal R, et al. A randomized, double-blind, placebo-con-trolled crossover study of the effect of exogenous melatonin on delayed sleep phase syndrome. *Psychosom Med.* 2001;63:40-48.

16. Shamir E, Barak Y, Shalman I, et al. Melatonin treatment for tardive dyskinesia: a double-blind, placebo-controlled, crossover study. *Arch Gen Psychiatry.* 2001;58: 1049-1052.

17. Zhdanova IV, Wurtman RJ, Regan MM, et al. Melatonin treatment for age-related insomnia. *J Clin Endocrinol Metab.* 2001;86:4727-4730.

18. Garfinkel D, Laudon M, Zisapel N. Improvement of sleep quality by controlled-release melatonin in benzodiazepine-treated elderly insomniacs. *Arch Gerontol Geriatr.* 1997;24:223-231.

19. Haimov I, Lavie P, Laudon M, et al. Melatonin replacement therapy of elderly in-somniacs. *Sleep.* 1995;18:598-603.

20. Folkard S, Arendt J, Clark M. Can melatonin improve shift workers' tolerance of the night shift? Some preliminary findings. *Chronobiol Int.* 1993;10:315-320.

21. Dawson D, Encel N, Lushington K. Improving adaptation to simulated night shift: timed exposure to bright light versus daytime melatonin administration. *Sleep.* 1995;18:11-21.

22. Wright SW, Lawrence LM, Wrenn KD, et al. Randomized clinical trial of melatonin after night-shift work: efficacy and neuropsychologic effects. *Ann Emerg Med.* 1998;32:334-340.

23. Naguib M, Samarkandi AH. Premedication with melatonin: a double-blind, placebo-controlled comparison with midazolam. *Br J Anaesth.* 1999;82:875-880.

24. Naguib M, Samarkandi AH. The comparative dose-response effects of melatonin and midazolam for premedication of adult patients: a double-blinded, placebo-controlled study. *Anesth Analg.* 2000;91:473-479.

25. Lissoni P, Meregalli S, Nosetto L, et al. Increased survival time in brain glioblastomas by a radioneuroendocrine strategy with radiotherapy plus melatonin compared to radiotherapy alone. *Oncology.* 1996;53:43-46.

26. Lissoni P, Paolorossi F, Ardizzoia A, et al. A randomized study of chemotherapy with cisplatin plus etoposide versus chemoendocrine therapy with cisplatin, etoposide and the pineal hormone melatonin as a first-line treatment of advanced non-small cell lung cancer patients in a poor clinical state. *J Pineal Res.* 1997;23:15-19.

27. Neri B, De Leonardis V, Gemelli MT, et al. Melatonin as biological response modifier in cancer patients. *Anticancer Res.* 1998;18:1329-1332.

28. Lissoni P, Tancini G, Barni S, et al. Treatment of cancer chemotherapy-induced toxicity with the pineal hormone melatonin. *Support Care Center.* 1997;5:126-129.

29. Lissoni P, Barni S, Mandala M, et al. Decreased toxicity and increased efficacy of cancer chemotherapy using the pineal hormone melatonin in metastatic solid tumour patients with poor clinical status. *Eur J Cancer.* 1999;35:1688-1692.

30. Waldhauser F, Weiszenbacher G, Tatzer E, et al. Alterations in nocturnal serum melatonin levels in humans with growth and aging. *J Clin Endocrinol Metab.* 1988; 66:648-652.

31. Sack RL, Lewy AJ, Erb DL, et al. Human melatonin production decreases with age. *J Pineal Res.* 1986;3:379-388.

32. Carnazzo G, Paternó-Raddusa F, Travali S, et al. Variations of melatonin incretion in elderly patients affected by cerebral deterioration. *Arch Gerontol Geriatr.* 1991; (suppl 2):123-126.

33. Oaknin-Bendahan S, Anis Y, Nir I, et al. Effects of long-term administration of melatonin and a putative antagonist on the aging rat. *Neuroreport.* 1995;6:785-788.

34. Zeitzer JM, Daniels JE, Duffy JF, et al. Do plasma melatonin concentrations decline with age? *Am J Med.* 1999;107:432-436.

35. Leibenluft E, Feldman-Naim S, Turner EH, et al. Effects of exogenous melatonin administration and withdrawal in five patients with rapid-cycling bipolar disorder. *J Clin Psychiatry.* 1997;58:383-388.

36. Fauteck J-D, Schmidt H, Lerchl A, et al. Melatonin in epilepsy: first results of replacement therapy and first clinical results. *Biol Signals Recept.* 1999;8:105-110.

37. Molina-Carballo A, Munoz-Hoyos A, Reiter RJ, et al. Utility of high doses of melatonin as adjunctive anticonvulsant therapy in a child with severe myoclonic epilepsy: two years' experience. *J Pineal Res.* 1997;23:97-105.

38. Pappolla MA, Chyan YJ, Poeggeler B, et al. An assessment of the antioxidant and the antiamyloidogenic properties of melatonin: implications for Alzheimer's disease. *J Neural Transm.* 2000;107:203-231.

39. Nelson RJ, Demas GE. Role of melatonin in mediating seasonal energetic and immunologic adaptations. *Brain Res Bull.* 1997;44:423-430.

40. Shamir E, Barak Y, Plopsky I, et al. Is melatonin treatment effective for tardive dyskinesia? *J Clin Psychiatry.* 2000;61:556-558.

41. Sack RL, Hughes RJ, Edgar DM, et al. Sleep-promoting effects of melatonin: at what dose, in whom, under what conditions, and by what mechanisms? *Sleep.* 1997;20:908-915.

42. Molis TM, Spriggs LL, Jupiter Y, et al. Melatonin modulation of estrogen-regulated proteins, growth factors, and proto-oncogenes in human breast cancer. *J Pineal Res.* 1995;18:93-103.

43. Neri B, De Leonardis V, Gemelli MT, et al. Melatonin as biological response modifier in cancer patients. *Anticancer Res.* 1998;18:1329-1332.

44. Jan JE, Hamilton D, Seward N, et al. Clinical trials of controlled-release melatonin in children with sleep-wake cycle disorders. *J Pineal Res.* 2000;29:34-39.

45. Graw P, Werth E, Krauchi K, et al. Early morning melatonin administration impairs psychomotor vigilance. *Behav Brain Res.* 2001;121:167-172.

46. Seabra ML V, Bignotto M, Pinto LR Jr, et al. Randomized, double-blind clinical trial, controlled with placebo, of the toxicology of chronic melatonin treatment. *J Pineal Res.* 2000;29:193-200.

47. Cagnacci A, Arangino S, Renzi A, et al. Influence of melatonin administration on glucose tolerance and insulin sensitivity of postmenopausal women. *Clin Endocrinol (Oxf).* 2001;54:339-346.

48. Ninomiya T, Iwatani N, Tomoda A, et al. Effects of exogenous melatonin on pituitary hormones in humans. *Clin Physiol.* 2001;21:292-299.

49. McIntyre IM, Norman TR, Burrows GD, et al. Alterations to plasma melatonin and cortisol after evening alprazolam administration in humans. *Chronobiol Int.* 1993;10:205-213.

50. McIntyre IM, Burrows GD, Norman TR. Suppression of plasma melatonin by a single dose of the benzodiazepine alprazolam in humans. *Biol Psychiatry.* 1988;24: 108-112.

51. Paul MA, Brown G, Buguet A, et al. Melatonin and zopiclone as pharmacologic aids to facilitate crew rest. *Aviat Space Environ Med.* 2001;72:974-984.

52. Hughes RJ, Sack RL, Lewy AJ. The role of melatonin and circadian phase in agerelated sleep-maintenance insomnia: assessment in a clinical trial of melatonin replacement. *Sleep.* 1998;21:52-68.

53. Chase JE, Gidal BE. Melatonin: therapeutic use in sleep disorders. *Ann Pharmacother.* 1997;31: 1218-1226.

54. Sharkey KM, Fogg LF, Eastman CI. Effects of melatonin administration on daytime sleep after simulated night shift work. *J Sleep Res.* 2001;10:181-192.

55. James M, Tremea MO, Jones JS, et al. Can melatonin improve adaptation to night shift? *Am J Emerg Med.* 1998;16:367-370.

56. Garfinkel D, Laudon M, Nof D, et al. Improvement of sleep quality in elderly people by controlled-release melatonin. *Lancet.* 1995;346:541-544.

Methyl Sulfonyl Methane (MSM)

1. Lawrence R, Sanchez D, Grosman M. Lignisul MSM (methylsulfonylmethane) in the treatment of acute athletic injuries [unpublished]. http:www.msm.com/msmresearch.cfm#. Accessed May 14, 2002.

2. Lawrence R. Lignisul MSM (methylsulfonylmethane: a double-blind study of its use in degenerative arthritis. http:www.msm.com/msmresearch.cfm. Accessed October 30, 2001.

3. Murav'ev IuV, Venikova MS, Pleskovskaia GN, et al. Effect of dimethyl sulfoxide and dimethyl sulfone on a destructive process in the joints of mice with spontaneous arthritis [in Russian; English abstract]. *Patol Fiziol Eksp Ter.* 1991;2:37-39.

4. Childs SJ. Dimethyl sulfone (DMSO[2]) in the treatment of interstitial cystitis. *Urol Clin North Am.* 1994;21:85-88.

5. Lawrence R. The effectiveness of the use of oral lignisul MSM (methylsulfonylmethane) supplementation on hair & nail health [unpublished]. http:www.msm.com/msmresearch.cfm#. Accessed May 15, 2002.

6. McCabe D. Polar solvents in the chemoprevention of dimethylbenzanthracene-induced rat mammary cancer. *Arch Surg.* 1986;121:1455-1459.

7. O'Dwyer PJ, McCabe DP, Sickle-Santanello BJ, et al. Use of polar solvents in chemoprevention of 1,2-dimethylhydrazine-induced colon cancer. *Cancer.* 1988;62: 944-948.

8. Jacob SW, Herschler R. Dimethyl sulfoxide after twenty years. *Ann NY Acad Sci.* 1983;411:13-17.

9. Morton JI, Siegel BV. Effects of oral dimethyl sulfoxide and dimethyl sulfone on murine autoimmune lymphoproliferative disease. *Proc Soc Exp Biol Med.* 1986;183: 227-230.
10. Jacob SW. The current status on the use of a new pharmacologic approach (dimethyl sulfone) for the relief of snoring. Oregon Health Sciences University [unpublished].

Milk Thistle

1. Salmi HA, Sarna S. Effect of silymarin on chemical, functional, and morphological alterations of the liver: a double-blind controlled study. *Scand J Gastroenterol.* 1982;17:517-521.
2. Feher J, Deak G, Muzes G, et al. Liver-protective action of silymarin therapy in chronic alcoholic liver diseases [in Hungarian]. *Orv Hetil.* 1989;130:2723-2727.
3. Fintelmann V, Albert A. Proof of the therapeutic efficacy of Legalon® for toxic liver illnesses in a double-blind trial [translated from German]. *Therapiewoche.* 1980; 30:5589-5594.
4. Trinchet J, Coste T, Levy VG, et al. Treatment of alcoholic hepatitis with silymarin: a double-blind comparative study in 116 patients [translated from French]. *Gastroenterol Clin Biol.* 1989;13:120-124.
5. Bunout D, Hirsch S, Petermann M, et al. The controlled study of the effect of sily-marin on alcholic liver disease [translated from Spanish]. *Rev Med Chil.* 1992;120: 1370-1376.
6. Ferenci P, Dragosics B, Dittrich H, et al. Randomized controlled trial of silymarin treatment in patients with cirrhosis of the liver. *J Hepatol.* 1989;9:105-113.
7. Benda L, Dittrich H, Ferenzi P, et al. The influence of therapy with silymarin on the survival rate of patients with liver cirrhosis [translated from German]. *Wien Klin Wochenschr.* 1980;92:678-683.
8. Pares A, Planas R, Torres M, et al. Effects of silymarin in alcoholic patients with cir-rhosis of the liver: results of a controlled, double-blind, randomized and multicenter trial. *J Hepatol.* 1998;28:615-621.
9. Lang I, Nekam K, Gonzalez-Cabello R, et al. Hepatoprotective and immunological effects of antioxidant drugs. *Tokai J Exp Clin Med.* 1990;15:123-127.
10. Lang I, Nekan K, Deak G, et al. Immunomodulatory and hepatoprotective effects of in vivo treatment with free radical scavengers. *Ital J Gastroenterol Hepatol.* 1990;22: 283-287.
11. Berenguer J, Carrasco D. Double-blind trial of silymarin vs. placebo in the treat-ment of chronic hepatitis. *MMW Munch Med Wochenschr.* 1977;119:240-260.
12. Buzzelli G, Moscarella S, Giusti A, et al. A pilot study on the liver protective effect of silybinphosphatidylcholine complex (IdB1016) in chronic active hepatitis. *Int J Clin Pharmacol Ther Toxicol.* 1993;31:456-460.
13. Lirussi F, Okolicsanyi L. Cytoprotection in the nineties: experience with ur-sodeoxycholic acid and silymarin in chronic liver disease. *Acta Physiol Hung.* 1992; 80:363-367.
14. Magliulo E, Gagliardi B, Fiori GP. Results of a double blind study on the effect of silymarin in the treatment of acute viral hepatitis, carried out at two medical centres [translated from German]. *Med Klin.* 1978;73:1060-1065.
15. Bode JC, Schmidt U, Durr HK. Silymarin for the treatment of acute viral hepatitis? Report of a controlled trial [translated from German]. *Med Klin.* 1977;72:513-518.
16. Allain H, Schuck S, Lebreton S, et al. Aminotransferase levels and silymarin in de novo tacrine-treated patients with Alzheimer's disease. *Dement Geriatr Cogn Disord.* 1999;10:181-185.
17. Muriel P, Garciapina T, Perez-Alvarez V, et al. Silymarin protects against paraceta-mol-induced lipid peroxidation and liver damage. *J Appl Toxicol.* 1992;12:439-442.
18. Paulova J, Dvorak M, Kolouch F, et al. Evaluation of the hepatoprotective and ther-apeutic effects of silymarin in an experimental carbon tetrachloride intoxication of liver in dogs [in Czech; English abstract]. *Vet Med (Praha).* 1990;35:629-635.
19. Rui YC. Advances in pharmacological studies of silymarin. *Mem Inst Oswaldo Cruz.* 1991;86(suppl 2):79-85.

20. Skakun NP, Moseichuk IP. Clinical pharmacology of legalon [in Russian]. *Vrach Delo.* 1988;5:5-10.
21. Tuchweber B, Sieck R, Trost W. Prevention of silybin of phalloidin-induced acute hepatoxicity. *Toxicol Appl Pharmacol.* 1979;51:265-275.
22. Boari C, Montanari FM, Galletti GP, et al. Toxic occupational liver diseases: therapeutic effects of silymarin [in Italian; English abstract]. *Minerva Med.* 1981;72:2679-2688.
23. Szilard S, Szentgyorgyi D, Demeter I. Protective effect of Legalon in workers exposed to organic solvents. *Acta Med Hung.* 1988;45:249-256.
24. Hruby K, Fuhrmann M, Csomos G, et al. Pharmacotherapy of *Amanita phalloides* poisoning using silybin [in German; English abstract]. *Wien Klin Wochenschr.* 1983;95:225-231.
25. Schulz V, Hansel R, Tyler VE. *Rational Phytotherapy: A Physicians' Guide to Herbal Medicine.* 3rd ed. Berlin, Germany: Springer-Verlag; 1998:215-216, 218.
26. Nassuato G, Iemmolo RM, Strazzabosco M, et al. Effect of silibinin on biliary lipid composition: experimental and clinical study. *J Hepatol.* 1991;12:290-295.
27. Sonnenbichler J, Scalera F, Sonnenbichler I, et al. Stimulatory effects of silibinin and silicristin from the milk thistle *Silybum marianum* on kidney cells. *J Pharmacol Exp Ther.* 1999;290:1375-1383.
28. Bokemeyer C, Fels LM, Dunn T, et al. Silibinin protects against cisplatin-induced nephrotoxicity without compromising cisplatin or ifosfamide anti-tumour activity. *Br J Cancer.* 1996;74:2036-2041.
29. Sonnenbichler J, Zetl I. Biochemical effects of the flavonolignane silibinin on RNA, protein and DNA synthesis in rat livers. *Prog Clin Biol Res.* 1986;213:319-331.
30. Muzes G, Deak G, Lang I, et al. Effects of silymarin (Legalon) therapy on the antioxidant defense mechanism and lipid peroxidation in alcoholic liver disease [in Hungarian; English abstract]. *Orv Hetil.* 1990;131:863-866.
31. Hikino H, Kiso Y. Natural products for liver disease. *Econ Med Plant Res.* 1988;2:39-72.
32. Comoglio A, Tomasi A, Malandrino S, et al. Scavenging effect of silipide, a new silybin-phospholipid complex, on ethanol-derived free radicals. *Biochem Pharmacol.* 1995;50:1313-1316.
33. Dehmlow C, Erhard J, de Groot H. Inhibition of Kupffer cell functions as an explanation for the hepatoprotective properties of silibinin. *Hepatology.* 1996;23:749-754.
34. Lorenz D, Lucker PW, Mennicke WH, et al. Pharmacokinetic studies with silymarin in human serum and bile. *Methods Find Exp Clin Pharmacol.* 1984;6:655-661.
35. Kim DH, Jin YH, Park JB, et al. Silymarin and its components are inhibitors of beta-glucuronidase. *Biol Pharm Bull.* 1994;17:443-445.
36. Barzaghi N, Crema F, Gatti G, et al. Pharmacokinetic studies on IdB 1016, a silybin-phosphatidylcholine complex, in healthy human subjects. *Eur J Drug Metab Pharmacokinet.* 1990;15:333-338.
37. Schandalik R, Gatti G, Perucca E. Pharmacokinetics of silybin in bile following administration of silipide and silymarin in cholecystectomy patients. *Arzneimittelforschung.* 1992;42:964-968.
38. Awang D. Milk thistle. *Can Pharm J.* 1993;126:403-404.
39. Albrecht M, Frerick H, Kuhn U, et al. Therapy of toxic liver pathologies with Legalon® [in German; English abstract]. *Z Klin Med.* 1992;47:87-92.
40. Adverse Drug Reactions Advisory Committee. An adverse reaction to the herbal medication milk thistle *(Silybum marianum). MJA.* 1999;170:218-219.
41. Giannola C, Buogo F, Forestiere G, et al. A two-center study on the effects of silymarin in pregnant women and adult patients with so-called minor hepatic insufficiency [in Italian; English abstract]. *Clin Ter.* 1985;114:129-135.
42. Lucena MI, Andrade RJ, de la Cruz JP, et al. Effects of silymarin MZ-80 on oxidative stress in patients with alcoholic cirrhosis: results of a randomized, double-blind, placebo-controlled clinical study. *Int J Clin Pharmacol Ther.* 2002;40:2-8.

N-Acetyl Cysteine (NAC)

1. Grandjean EM, Berthet P, Ruffmann R, et al. Efficacy of oral long-term N-acetyl-cysteine in chronic bronchopulmonary disease: a meta-analysis of published double-blind, placebo-controlled clinical trials. *Clin Ther.* 2000;22:209-221.
2. Hansen NC, Skriver A, Brorsen-Riis L, et al. Orally administered N-acetylcysteine may improve general well-being in patients with mild chronic bronchitis. *Respir Med.* 1994;88:531-535.
3. Grassi C, Casali L, Rossi A, et al. A comparison between different methods for detecting bronchial hyperreactivity. Bronchial hyperreactivity: methods of study. *Eur J Respir Dis Suppl.* 1980;106:19-27.
4. Grassi C, Morandini GC. A controlled trial of intermittent oral acetylcysteine in the long-term treatment of chronic bronchitis. *Eur J Clin Pharmacol.* 1976;9:393-396.
5. Riise GC, Larsson S, Larsson P et al. The intrabronchial microbial flora in chronic bronchitis patients: a target for N-acetylcsteine therapy? *Eur Respir J.* 1994;7:94-101.
6. Rasmussen JB, Glennow C. Reduction in days of illness after long-term treatment with N-acetylcysteine controlled-release tablets in patients with chronic bronchitis. *Eur Respir J.* 1988;1:351-355.
7. Parr GD, Huitson A. Oral Fabrol (oral N-acetyl-cysteine) in chronic bronchitis. *Br J Dis Chest.* 1987;81:341-348.
8. Boman G, Backer U, Larsson S, et al. Oral acetylcysteine reduces exacerbation rate in chronic bronchitis: report of a trial organized by the Swedish Society for Pulmonary Diseases. *Eur J Respir Dis.* 1983;64:405-415.
9. Verstraeten JM. Mucolytic treatment in chronic obstructive pulmonary disease: double-blind comparative clinical trial with N-acetylcysteine, bromhexine and placebo. *Acta Tuberc Pneumol Belg.* 1979;70:71-80.
10. Ardissino D, Merlini PA, Savonitto S, et al. Effect of transdermal nitroglycerin or N-acetylcysteine, or both, in the long-term treatment of unstable angina pectoris. *J Am Coll Cardiol.* 1997;29:941-947.
11. Iversen HK. N-acetylcysteine enhances nitroglycerin-induced headache and cranial arterial responses. *Clin Pharmacol Ther.* 1992;52:125-133.
12. Pizzulli L, Hagendorff A, Zirbes M, et al. N-acetylcysteine attenuates nitroglycerin tolerance in patients with angina pectoris and normal left ventricular function. *Am J Cardiol.* 1997;79:28-33.
13. Hogan JC, Lewis MJ, Henderson AH. Chronic administration of N-acetylcysteine fails to prevent nitrate tolerance in patients with stable angina pectoris. *Br J Clin Pharmacol.* 1990;30:573-577.
14. Bernard GR, Wheeler AP, Arons MM, et al. A trial of antioxidants N-acetylcysteine and procysteine in ARDS. *Chest.* 1997;112:164-172.
15. Rank N, Michel C, Haertel C, et al. N-acetylcysteine increases liver blood flow and improves liver function in septic shock patients: results of a prospective, randomized, double-blind study. *Crit Care Med.* 2000;28:3799-3807.
16. Badawy AH, Abd El Aal SF, Samour SA. Liver injury associated with N-acetylcysteine administration. *J Egypt Soc Parasitol.* 1989;19:563-571.
17. Adair JC, Knoefel JE, Morgan N. Controlled trial of N-acetylcysteine for patients with probable Alzheimer's disease. *Neurology.* 2001;57:1515-1517.

Neem

1. Stix G. Village pharmacy: the neem tree yields products from pesticides to soap. *Sci Am.* 1992;266:132.
2. Neem Foundation web site. Available at: http://www.neemfoundation.org. Accessed November 20, 2000.
3. Awasthy, KS, Charuasia OP, Sinha SP. Prolonged murine genotoxic effecs of crude extracted from neem. *Phytother Res.* 1999;13:81-83.

Nettle

1. Dathe G, Schmid H. Phytotherapy of benign prostate hyperplasia (BPH); double-blind study with stinging nettle root extract (*Extractum Radicis Urticae*—ERU) [translated from German]. *Urologe B.* 1987;27:223-226.

2. European Scientific Cooperative on Phytotherapy. *Urticae radix.* Exeter, UK: ESCOP; 1996-1997. Monographs on the Medicinal Uses of Plant Drugs, Fascicule 2:2-4.

3. Vontobel HP, Herzog R, Rutishauser G, et al. Results of a double-blind study on the effectiveness of ERU *(Extractum radicis Urticae)* capsules in conservative treatment of benign prostatic hyperplasia [translated from German]. *Urologe A.* 1985;24:49-51.

4. Mittman P. Randomized, double-blind study of freeze-dried *Urtica dioica* in the treatment of allergic rhinitis. *Planta Med.* 1990;56:44-47.

5. Hryb DJ, Khan MS, Romas NA, et al. The effect of extracts of the roots of the stinging nettle *(Urtica dioica)* on the interaction of SHBG with its receptor on human prostatic membranes. *Planta Med.* 1995;61:31-32.

6. Wagner H, Willer F, Samtleben R, et al. Search for the antiprostatic principle of stinging nettle *(Urtica dioica)* roots. *Phytomedicine.* 1994;1:213-224.

7. Schulz V, Hansel R, Tyler VE. *Rational Phytotherapy: A Physicians' Guide to Herbal Medicine.* 3rd ed. Berlin, Germany: Springer-Verlag; 1998:229.

8. Konrad L, Muller HH, Lenz C, et al. Antiproliferative effect on human prostate cancer cells by a stinging nettle root *(Urtica dioica)* extract. *Planta Med.* 2000;66:44-47.

9. Hartmann RW, Mark M, Soldati F. Inhibition of 5-alpha-reductase and aromatase by PHL-00801 (Prostatonin®), a combination of PY 102 *(Pygeum africanum)* and UR 102 *(Urtica dioica)* extracts. *Phytomedicine.* 1996;3:121-128.

10. Krzeski T, Kazon M, Borkowski A, et al. Combined extracts of *Urtica dioica* and *Pygeum africanum* in the treatment of benign prostatic hyperplasia: double-blind comparison of two doses. *Clin Ther.* 1993;15:1011-1020.

11. Newall CA, Anderson LA, Phillipson JD. *Herbal Medicines: A Guide for Health-Care Professionals.* London, England: Pharmaceutical Press; 1996:201-202.

Nicotinamide Adenine Dinucleotide (NADH)

1. Kay GG, Viirre E, Clark J. Stabilized NADH as a countermeasure for jet lag. Presented at: 48th International Congress of Aviation and Space Medicine; September 17-21, 2000; Rio de Janeiro, Brazil.

2. Forsyth LM, Preuss HG, MacDowell AL, et al. Therapeutic effects of oral NADH on the symptoms of patients with chronic fatigue syndrome. *Ann Allergy Asthma Immunol.* 1999;82:185-191.

3. Birkmayer JG, Vrecko C, Volc D, et al. Nicotinamide adenine dinucleotide (NADH)—a new therapeutic approach to Parkinson's disease. Comparison of oral and parenteral application. *Acta Neurol Scand Suppl.* 1993;146:32-35.

4. Birkmayer JG, Birkmayer W. The coenzyme nicotinamide adenine dinucleotide (NADH) as biological antidepressive agent. *New Trends Clin Neuropharmacol.* 1991; 5:19-25.

5. Birkmayer JG. Coenzyme nicotinamide adenine dinucleotide—new therapeutic approach for improving dementia of the Alzheimer type. *Ann Clin Lab Sci.* 1996;26:1-9.

6. Dizdar N, Kagedal B, Lindvall B. Treatment of Parkinson's disease with NADH. *Acta Neurol Scand.* 1994;90:345-347.

Noni

1. Elkins R. *Hawaiian Noni:* (Morinda citrifolia). Pleasant Grove, Utah: Woodland Publishing; 1998.

2. Hirazumi A, Furusawa E, Chou SC, et al. Anticancer activity of *Morinda citrifolia* (noni) on intraperitoneally implanted Lewis lung carcinoma in syngeneic mice. *Proc West Pharmacol Soc.* 1994;37:145-146.

3. Hirazumi A, Furusawa E, Chou SC, et al. Immunomodulation contributes to the anticancer activity of *Morinda citrifolia* (noni) fruit juice. *Proc West Pharmacol Soc.* 1996;39:7-9.

4. Hirazumi A, Furusawa E. An immunomodulatory polysaccharide-rich substance from the fruit juice of *Morinda citrifolia* (noni) with antitumour activity. *Phytother Res.* 1999;13:380-387.

5. Hiwasa T, Arase Y, Chen Z, et al. Stimulation of ultraviolet-induced apoptosis of human fibroblast UVr-1 cells by tyrosine kinase inhibitors. *FEBS Lett.* 1999;444: 173-176.

6. Hiramatsu T, Imoto M, Koyano T, et al. Induction of normal phenotypes in ras-transformed cells by damnacanthal from *Morinda citrifolia. Cancer Lett.* 1993;73:161-166.
7. Younos C, Rolland A, Fleurentin J, et al. Analgesic and behavioural effects of *Morinda citrifolia. Planta Med.* 1990;56:430-434.
8. Heinicke RM. The pharmacologically active ingredient of noni. HyperMedia Technologies web site. Available at: http://www.hmt.com/noni/active.html. Accessed January 10, 2001.
9. Mueller BA, Scott MK, Sowinski KM, et al. Noni juice *(Morinda citrifolia):* hidden potential for hyperkalemia? *Am J Kidney Dis.* 2000;35:310-312.

Oligomeric Proanthocyanidin Complexes (OPCs)

1. Thebaut JF, Thebaut P, Vin F. Study of Endotelon® in functional manifestations of peripheral venous insufficiency: results of a double-blind study of 92 patients [translated from French]. *Gaz Med.* 1985;92:96-100.
2. Arcangeli P. Pycnogenol® in chronic venous insufficiency. *Fitoterapia.* 2000;71:236-244.
3. Henriet JP. Exemplary study for a phlebotropic substance, the EIVE Study [translated from French]. Fairfield, Conn: Primary Source; not dated.
4. Petrassi C, Mastromarino A, Spartera C. Pycnogenol® in chronic venous insufficiency. *Phytomedicine.* 2000;7:383-388.
5. Delacroix P. Double-blind study of Endotelon® in chronic venous insufficiency [translated from French]. *La Revue de Medecine.* 1981;22:1793-1802.
6. Pecking A, Desprez-Curely JP, Megret G. Oligomeric grape flavonols (Endotelon®) in the treatment of secondary upper limb lymphedemas [translated from French]. Paris, France: Association de Lymphologie de Lange Francaise Hopital Saint-Louis; 1989:69-73.
7. Baruch J. Effect of Endotelon® in postoperative edema: results of a double-blind study versus placebo in 32 female patients [translated from French]. *Ann Chir Plast Esthet.* 1984;29:393-395.
8. Parienti JJ, Parienti-Amsellem J. Post traumatic edemas in sports: a controlled test of Endotelon® [translated from French]. *Gaz Med Fr.* 1983;90:231-235.
9. Gendre PM, Laparra J, Barraud E. Procyanidolic oligomer preventive action on experimental lathyrism in the rat [in French; English abstract]. *Ann Pharm Fr.* 1985;43:61-71.
10. Schwitters B, Masquelier J. *OPC in Practice.* Rome, Italy: Alfa Omega; 1993.
11. Uchida S, Edamatsu R, Hiramatsu M, et al. Condensed tannins scavenge active oxygen free radicals. *Med Sci Res.* 1987;15:831-832.
12. Wegrowski J, Robert AM, Moczar M. The effect of procyanidolic oligomers on the composition of normal and hypercholesterolemic rabbit aortas. *Biochem Pharmacol.* 1984;33:3491-3497.
13. Putter M, Grotemeyer KH, Wurthwein G, et al. Inhibition of smoking-induced platelet aggregation by aspirin and pycnogenol. *Thromb Res.* 1999;95:155-161.
14. Hertog MG, Feskens EJ, Hollman PC, et al. Dietary antioxidant flavonoids and risk of coronary heart disease: the Zutphen Elderly Study. *Lancet.* 1993;342:1007-1011.
15. Lesbre FX, Tigaud JD. Effect of Endotelon® on the capillary fragility index of a specific controlled group: cirrhosis patients [translated from French]. *Gaz Med Fr.* 1983;90:2333-2337.
16. Boissin JP, Corbe C. Siou A. Chorioretinal circulation and dazzling: use of procyanidol oligomers [in French; English abstract]. *Bull Soc Ophtalmol Fr.* 1988;88:173-174, 177-179.
17. Corbe C, Boissin JP, Siou A. Light vision and chorioretinal circulation: study of the effect of procyanidolic oligomers [translated from French]. *J Fr Ophtalmol.* 1988;11:453-460.
18. Bernstein CK, Deng C, Shuklah R, et al. Double blind placebo controlled (DBPC) study of grapeseed extract in the treatment of seasonal allergic rhinitis (SAR) [abstract]. *J Allergy Clin Immunol.* 2001;107:abstr 1018.

19. Preuss HG, Wallerstedt D, Talpur N, et al. Effects of niacin-bound chromium and grape seed proanthocyanidin extract on the lipid profile of hypercholesterolemic subjects: a pilot study. *J Med.* 2000;31:227-246.
20. Maffei Facino R, Carini M, Aldini G, et al. Free radicals scavenging action and anti-enzyme activities of procyanidines from *Vitis vinifera:* a mechanism for their capillary protective action. *Arzneimittelforschung.* 1994;44:592-601.
21. Kuttan R, Donnelly RV, Di Ferrante N. Collagen treated with (+)-catechin becomes resistant to the action of mammalian collagenase. *Experientia.* 1981;37:221-223.
22. Masquelier J. Procyanidolic oligomers (Leucocyanidins) [translated from French]. *Parfums Cosmetiques Aromes.* 1990;95:89-97.
23. Masquelier J, Dumon MC, Dumas J. Stabilization of collagen by procyanidolic oligomers [in French; English abstract]. *Acta Ther.* 1981;7:101-105.
24. Tixier JM, Godeau G, Robert AM, et al. Evidence in vivo in vitro studies that binding of pycnogenols to elastin affects its rate of degradation by elastases. *Biochem Pharmacol.* 1984;33:3933-3939.
25. Chang WC, Hsu FL. Inhibition of platelet aggregation and arachidonate metabolism in platelets by procyanidins. *Prostaglandins Leukot Essent Fatty Acids.* 1989;38:181-188.
26. Schulz V, Hansel R, Tyler VE. *Rational Phytotherapy: A Physicians' Guide to Herbal Medicine.* 3rd ed. Berlin, Germany: Springer-Verlag; 1998:282-284.
27. Hosseini S, et al. Pycnogenol in the management of asthma. *J Medicinal Food.* 2001; 4:201-210.
28. Stefanescu M, et al. Pycnogenol efficacy in the treatment of systemic lupus erythe-matosus patients. *Phytother Res.* 2001;15:698-704.
29. Spadea L, Balestrazzi E. Treatment of vascular retinopathies with Pycnogenol. *Phytother Res.* 2001;15:219-223.
30. Hosseini S, Lee J, Sepulveda RT, et al. A randomized double-blind placebo-controlled prospective 16-week crossover study to determine the role of Pycnogenol in modifying blood pressure in mildly hypertensive patients. *Nutr Res.* 2001; 21: 1251-1260.

Oregon Grape

1. Wiesenauer M, Ludtke R. *Mahonia aquifolium* in patients with psoriasis vulgaris—an intraindividual study. *Phytomedicine.* 1996;3:231-235.
2. Augustin M, Andrees U, Grimme H, et al. Effects of *Mahonia aquifolium* ointment on the expression of adhesion, proliferation, and activation markers in the skin of pa-tients with psoriasis. *Forsch Komplementarmed.* 1999;6 (suppl 2):19-21.
3. McCutcheon AR, Ellis SM, Hancock REW, et al. Antifungal screening of medicinal plants of British Columbian native peoples. *J Ethnopharmacol.* 1994;44:157-169.
4. Galle K, Muller-Jakic B, Proebstle A, et al. Analytical and pharmacological studies on *Mahonia aquifolium.* *Phytomedicine.* 1994;1:59-62.
5. Muller K, Ziereis K. The antipsoriatic *Mahonia aquifolium* and it active constituents. I. Pro- and antioxidant properties and inhibition of 5-lipoxygenase. *Planta Med.* 1994;60:421-424.
6. Gieler U, von der Weth A, Heger M. *Mahonia aquifolium*—a new type of topical treatment for psoriasis. *J Dermatol Treat.* 1995;6:31-34.
7. Smet PA de, ed. *Adverse Effects of Herbal Drugs.* Berlin, Germany: Springer-Verlag; 1992:97-104.
8. Chan E. Displacement of bilirubin from albumin by berberine. *Biol Neonat.* 1993;63:201-208.

Ornithine Alpha-Ketoglutarate (OKG)

1. Donati L, Ziegler F, Pongelli G, et al. Nutritional and clinical efficacy of ornithine alpha-ketoglutarate in severe burn patients. *Clin Nutr.* 1999;18:307-311.
2. Bucci LR, Hickson JF Jr, Wolinsky I, et al. Ornithine supplementation and insulin release in bodybuilders. *Int J Sport Nutr.* 1992;2:287-291.
3. Lambert MI, Hefer JA, Millar RP, et al. Failure of commercial oral amino acid sup-plements to increase serum growth hormone concentrations in male body-builders. *Int J Sport Nutr.* 1993;3:298-305.

4. De Bandt JP, Cynober LA. Amino acids with anabolic properties. *Curr Opin Clin Nutr Metab Care.* 1998;1:263-172.

5. Brocker P, Vellas B, Albarede J, et al. A two-centre, randomized, double-blind trial of ornithine oxoglutarate in 194 elderly, ambulatory, convalescent subjects. *Age Aging.* 1994;23:303-306.

6. Coudray-Lucas C, Le Bever H, Cynober L, De Bandt JP, Carsin H. Ornithine alpha-ketoglutarate improves wound healing in severe burn patients: a prospective randomized double-blind trial versus isonitrogenous controls. *Crit Care Med.* 2000;28: 1772-1776.

7. Cynober LA. The use of alpha-ketoglutarate salts in clinical nutrition and metabolic care. *Curr Opin Clin Nutr Metab Care.* 1999;2(1):33-37.

8. Neu J, DeMarco V, Li N. Glutamine: clinical applications and mechanisms of action. *Curr Opin Clin Nutr Metab Care.* 2002;5:69-75.

9. Reynolds TM. The future of nutrition and wound healing. *J Tissue Viability.* 2001; 11(1):5-13.

10. Elam RP, Hardin DH, Sutton RA, et al. Effects of arginine and ornithine on strength, lean body mass and urinary hydroxyproline in adult males. *J Sports Med Phys Fitness.* 1989;29:52-56.

11. Bucci L, Hickson JF, Pivarnik JM, et al. Ornithine ingestion and growth hormone release in bodybuilders. *Nutr Res.* 1990;10:239-245.

12. Fogelholm GM, Naveri HK, Kiilavuori KT, et al. Low-dose amino acid supplementation: no effects on serum human growth hormone and insulin in male weightlifters. *Int J Sport Nutr.* 1993;3:290-297.

Oxerutins

1. Wadworth AN, Faulds D. Hydroxyethylrutosides: a review of its pharmacology, and therapeutic efficacy in venous insufficiency and related disorders. *Drugs.* 1992; 44:1013-1032.

2. Pulvertaft TB. General practice treatment of symptoms of venous insufficiency with oxerutins: results of a 660 patient multicentre study in the UK. *Vasa.* 1983;12:373-376.

3. Unkauf M, Rehn D, Klinger J, et al. Investigation of the efficacy of oxerutins compared to placebo in patients with chronic venous insufficiency treated with compression stockings. *Arzneimittelforschung.* 1996;46:478-482.

4. MacLennan WJ, Wilson J, Rattenhuber V, et al. Hydroxyethylrutosides in elderly patients with chronic venous insufficiency: its efficacy and tolerability. *Gerontology.* 1994;40:45-52.

5. Rehn D, Brunnauer H, Diebschlag W, et al. Investigation of the therapeutic equivalence of different galenical preparations of O-(beta-hydroxyethyl)-rutosides following multiple dose peroral administration. *Arzneimittelforschung.* 1996;46:488-492.

6. Rehn D, Unkauf M, Klein P, et al. Comparative clinical efficacy and tolerability of oxerutins and horse chestnut extract in patients with chronic venous insufficiency. *Arzneimittelforschung.* 1996;46:483-487.

7. Balmer A, Limoni C. Clinical, placebo-controlled double-blind study of venoruton in the treatment of chronic venous insufficiency: importance of the selection of patients [in German; English abstract]. *Vasa.* 1980;9:76-82.

8. Bergqvist D, Hallbook T, Lindblad B, et al. A double-blind trial of O-(beta-Hydroxyethyl)-Rutoside in patients with chronic venous insufficiency. *Vasa.* 1981; 10:253-260.

9. Anderson JH, Geraghty JG, Wilson YT, et al. Paroven© and graduated compression hosiery for superficial venous insufficiency. *Phlebology.* 1990;5:271-276.

10. van Cauwenberge H. Double blind study of the efficacy of O(beta-hydroxyethyl)-rutosides in the treatment of venous conditions [in French]. *Med Hyg (Geneve).* 1978;36:4175-4177.

11. de Jongste AB, Jonker JJ, Huisman MV, et al. A double blind three center clinical trial on the short-term efficacy of 0-(beta-hydroxyethyl)-rutosides in patients with post-thrombotic syndrome. *Thromb Haemost.* 1989;62:826-829.

12. Prerovsky I, Roztocil K, Hlavova A, et al. The effect of hydroxyethylrutosides after acute and chronic oral administration in patients with venous diseases: a double-blind study. *Angiologica.* 1972;9:408-414.

13. Cappelli R, Pecchi S, Oberhausser V, et al. Efficacy of O-(beta-hydroxyethy)-rutosides at high dosages in counteracting the unwanted activity of oral contraceptives on venous function. *Int J Clin Pharmacol Res.* 1987;7:291-299.

14. Bergstein NA. Clinical study on the efficacy of O-(beta-hydroxyethyl)rutoside (HR) in varicosis of pregnancy. *J Int Med Res.* 1975;3:189-193.

15. Stegmann W, Hubner K, Deichmann B, et al. The efficacy of O-(beta-hydroxy-ethyl)-rutosides in the treatment of venous leg ulcers [in French; English abstract]. *Phlebologie.* 1987;40:149-156.

16. Wright DD, Franks PJ, Blair SD, et al. Oxerutins in the prevention of recurrence in chronic venous ulceration: randomized controlled trial. *Br J Surg.* 1991;78:1269-1270.

17. Wijayanegara H, Mose JC, Achmad L, et al. A clinical trial of hydroxyethylrutosides in the treatment of haemorrhoids of pregnancy. *J Int Med Res.* 1992;20:54-60.

18. Mortimer PS, Badger C, Clarke I, et al. A double-blind, randomized, parallel-group, placebo-controlled trial of O-(beta-hydroxyethyl)-rutosides in chronic arm edema resulting from breast cancer treatment. *Phlebology.* 1995;10:51-55.

19. Piller NB, Morgan RG, Casley-Smith JR. A double-blind, cross-over trial of O-(beta-hydroxyethyl)-rutosides (benzo-pyrones) in the treatment of lymphedema of the arms and legs. *Br J Plast Surg.* 1988;41:20-27.

20. Taylor HM, Rose KE, Twycross RG. A double-blind clinical trial of hydroxyethyl-rutosides in obstructive arm lymphedema. *Phlebology.* 1993;(suppl 1):22-28.

21. Fassina A, Rubinacci A. Post-traumatic edema: a controlled study into the activity of hydroxyethyl rutoside [translated from Italian]. *Gazz Med Ital Arch Sci.* 1987;146: 103-109.

22. Moser M, Ranacher G, Wilmot TJ, et al. A double-blind clinical trial of hydroxy-ethylrutosides in Meniere's disease. *J Laryngol Otol.* 1984;98:265-272.

23. Sohn C, Jahnichen C, Bastert G. Effectiveness of beta-hydroxyethylrutoside in patients with varicose veins in pregnancy [in German; English abstract]. *Zentralbl Gynakol.* 1995;117:190-197.

Pantethine

1. Gaddi A, Descovich GC, Noseda G, et al. Controlled evaluation of pantethine, a natural hypolipidemic compound, in patients with different forms of hyperlipoproteinemia. *Atherosclerosis.* 1984;50:73-83.

2. Angelico M, Pinto G, Ciaccheri C, et al. Improvement in serum lipid profile in hy-perlipoproteinaemic patients after treatment with pantethine: a crossover, double-blind trial versus placebo. *Curr Ther Res.* 1983;33:1091-1097.

3. Bertolini S, Donati C, Elicio N, et al. Lipoprotein changes induced by pantethine in hyperlipoproteinemic patients: adults and children. *Int J Clin Pharmacol Ther Toxicol.* 1986;24:630-637.

4. Rubba R, Postiglione A, DeSimone B, et al. Comparative evaluation of the lipid-lowering effects of fenofibrate and pantethine in type II hyperlipoproteinemia. *Curr Ther Res.* 1985;38:719-727.

5. Da Col PG, Cattin L, Fonda M, et al. Pantethine in the treatment of hypercholes-terolemia: a randomized double-blind trial versus tiadenol. *Curr Ther Res.* 1984; 36:314-322.

Passion Flower

1. Speroni E, Billi R, Mercati V, et al. Sedative effects of crude extract of *Passiflora in-carnata* after oral administration. *Phytother Res.* 1996;10(suppl):S92-S94.

2. Speroni E, Minghetti A. Neuropharmacological activity of extracts from *Passiflora incarnata. Planta Med.* 1988;54:488-491.

3. Aoyagi N, Kimura R, Murata T. Studies on *Passiflora incarnata* dry extract. I. Isolation of maltol and pharmacological action of maltol and ethyl maltol. *Chem Pharm Bull (Tokyo).* 1974;22:1008-1013.

4. Newall CA, Anderson LA, Phillipson JD. *Herbal Medicines: A Guide for Health-Care Professionals.* London, England: Pharmaceutical Press; 1996:206.
5. Solbakken AM, Rorbakken G, Gundersen T. Nature medicine as intoxicant [in Norwegian; English abstract]. *Tidsskr Nor Laegeforen.* 1997;117:1140-1141.
6. Dhawan K, Kumar S, Sharma A. Anxiolytic activity of aerial and underground parts of *Passiflora incarnata. Fitoterapai.* 2001;72:922-926
7. Akhondzadeh S, Naghavi HR, Vazirian M, et al. Passionflower in the treatment of generalized anxiety: a pilot double-blind randomized controlled trial with oxazepam. *J Clin Pharm Ther.* 2001; 26:363-367.
8. Akhondzadeh S, Kashani L, Mobaseri M, et al. Passionflower in the treatment of opiates withdrawal: a double-blind randomized controlled trial. *J Clin Pharm Ther.* 2001;26:369-373.

PC-SPES

1. Hsieh T, Chen SS, Wang X, et al. Regulation of androgen receptor (AR) and prostate specific antigen (PSA) expression in the androgen-responsive human prostate LNCaP cells by ethanolic extracts of the Chinese herbal preparation, PC-SPES. *Biochem Mol Biol Int.* 1997;42:535-544.
2. Halicka HD, Ardelt B, Juan G, et al. Apoptosis and cell cycle effects induced by extracts of the Chinese herbal preparation PC-SPES. *Int J Oncol.* 1997;11:437-448.
3. Hsieh TC, Ng C, Chang CC, et al. Induction of apoptosis and down-regulation of bcl-6 in Mutu I cells treated with ethanolic extracts of the Chinese herbal supplement PC-SPES. *Int J Oncol.* 1998;13:1199-1202.
4. de la Taille A, Hayek OR, Buttyan R, et al. Effects of a phytotherapeutic agent, PC-SPES, on prostate cancer: a preliminary investigation on human cell lines and patients. *BJU Int.* 1999;84:845-850.
5. Tiwari RK, Geliebter J, Garikapaty VPS, et al. Anti-tumor effects of PC-SPES, an herbal formulation in prostate cancer. *Int J Oncol.* 1999;14:713-719.
6. Weinrobe MC, Montgomery B. Acquired bleeding diathesis in a patient taking PC-SPES [letter]. *N Engl J Med.* 2001;345:1213-1214.
7. Oh WK, George DJ, Hackmann K, et al. Activity of the herbal combination, PC-SPES, in the treatment of patients with androgen-independent prostate cancer. *Urology.* 2001;57:122-126.
8. Pfeifer BL, Pirani JF, Hamann SR, et al. PC-SPES, a dietary supplement for the treatment of hormone-refractory prostate cancer. *BJU Int.* 2000;85:481-485.
9. Kameda H, Small EJ, Reese DM, et al. A phase II study of PC-SPES, an herbal compound, for the treatment of advanced prostate cancer (Pca). Presented at: 35th Annual Meeting of the American Society of Clinical Oncology; May 15-18, 1999; Atlanta, Ga.
10. Moyad MA, Pienta KJ, Montie JE. Use of PC-SPES, a commercially available supplement for prostate cancer, in a patient with hormone-naïve disease. *Urology.* 1999;54:319-324.
11. Nagourney R. 93rd Annual Meeting of the American Association for Cancer Research. San Francisco, Calif: 2002.

Peppermint

1. Rees WD, Evans BK, Rhodes J. Treating irritable bowel syndrome with peppermint oil. *Br Med J.* 1979;2:835-836.
2. Dew MJ, Evans BK, Rhodes J. Peppermint oil for the irritable bowel syndrome: a multicentre trial. *Br J Clin Pract.* 1984;38:394, 398.
3. Liu JH, Chen GH, Yeh HZ. Enteric-coated peppermint-oil capsules in the treatment of irritable bowel syndrome: a prospective, randomized trial. *J Gastroenterol.* 1997;32:765-768.
4. Kline RM, Kline JJ, Di Palma J, et al. Enteric-coated, pH-dependent peppermint oil capsules for the treatment of irritable bowel syndrome in children. *J Pediatr.* 2001;138:125-128.

5. Carling L, Svedberg LE, Hulten S, et al. Short-term treatment of the irritable bowel syndrome: a placebo-controlled trial of peppermint oil against hyoscyamine. *Opusc Med.* 1989;34:55-57.
6. Nash P, Gould SR, Barnardo DE. Peppermint oil does not relieve the pain of irritable bowel syndrome. *Br J Clin Pract.* 1986;40:292-293.
7. Lawson MJ, Knight RE, Tran K, et al. Failure of enteric-coated peppermint oil in the irritable bowel syndrome: a randomized, double-blind crossover study. *J Gastroenterol Hepatol.* 1988;3:235-238.
8. Sparks MJ, O'Sullivan P, Herrington AA, et al. Does peppermint oil relieve spasm during barium enema? *Br J Radiol.* 1995;68:841-843.
9. Somerville KW, Ellis WR, Whitten BH, et al. Stones in the common bile duct: experience with medical dissolution therapy. *Postgrad Med J.* 1985;61:313-316.
10. Tate S. Peppermint oil: a treatment for postoperative nausea. *J Adv Nurs.* 1997; 26:543-549.
11. Gunn JW. The carminative action of volatile oils. *J Pharmacol Exp Ther.* 1920;16:39-47.
12. Taylor BA, Luscombe DK, Duthie HL. Inhibitory effect of peppermint oil on gastrointestinal smooth muscle [abstract]. *Gut.* 1983;24:A992.
13. Hawthorn M, Ferrante J, Luchowski E, et al. The actions of peppermint oil and menthol on calcium channel dependent processes in intestinal, neuronal, and cardiac preparations. *Aliment Pharmacol Ther.* 1988;2:101-118.
14. Spindler P, Madsen C. Subchronic toxicity study of peppermint oil in rats. *Toxicol Lett.* 1992;62:215-220.
15. European Scientific Cooperative on Phytotherapy. *Menthae piperitae aetheroleum* (peppermint oil). Exeter, UK: ESCOP; 1996-1997. Monographs on the Medicinal Uses of Plant Drugs, Fascicule 3:1-6.
16. Pittler MH, Ernst E. Peppermint oil for irritable bowel syndrome: a critical review and meta-analysis. *Am J Gastroenterol.* 1998;93:1131-1135.

Phenylalanine

1. Heller B. Pharmacological and clinical effects of D-phenylalanine in depression and Parkinson's disease. In: Mosnaim AD, Wolf ME, eds. *Noncatecholic Phenylethylamines. Part 1. Phenylethylamine: Biological Mechanisms and Clinical Aspects.* New York, NY: Marcel Dekker; 1978:397-417.
2. Beckmann H, Athen D, Olteanu M, et al. DL-phenylalanine versus imipramine: a double-blind controlled study. *Arch Psychiatr Nervenkr.* 1979;227:49-58.
3. Balagot RC, Ehrenpreis S, Kubota K, et al. Analgesia in mice and humans by D-phenylalanine: relation to inhibition of enkephalin degradation and enkephalin levels. *Adv Pain Res Ther.* 1983;5:289-293.
4. Budd K. Use of D-phenylalanine, an enkephalinase inhibitor, in the treatment of intractable pain. *Adv Pain Res Ther.* 1983;5:305-308.
5. Walsh NE, Ramamurthy S, Schoenfeld LS, et al. D-Phenylalanine was not found to exhibit opiate receptor mediated analgesia in monkeys [letter]. *Pain.* 1986;26:409-410.
6. Walsh NE, Ramamurthy S, Schoenfeld L, et al. Analgesic effectiveness of D-phenylalanine in chronic pain patients. *Arch Phys Med Rehabil.* 1986;67:436-439.
7. Heller B, Fischer E, Martin R. Therapeutic action of D-phenylalanine in Parkinson's disease. *Arzneimittelforschung.* 1976;26:577-579.
8. Janssen PA, Leysen JE, Megens AA, Awouters FH. Does phenylethylamine act as an endogenous amphetamine in some patients? *Int J Neuropsychopharmacol.* 1999; 2:229-240.
9. Sabelli HC, Javaid JI. Phenylethylamine modulation of affect: therapeutic and diagnostic implications. *J Neuropsychiatry Clin Neurosci.* 1995;7:6-14.
10. Gardos G, Cole JO, Matthews JD, et al. The acute effects of a loading dose of phenylalanine in unipolar depressed patients with and without tardive dyskinesia. *Neuropsychopharmacology.* 1992;6:241-247.
11. Winter A. New treatment for multiple sclerosis. *Neurol Orthoped J Med Surg.* 1984;5:39-43.
12. Zametkin AJ, Koroum F, Rapoport JL. Treatment of hyperactive children with D-phenylalanine. *Am J Psychiatry.* 1987;144:792-794.

13. Wood DR, Reimherr FW, Wender PH. Treatment of attention deficit disorder with DL-phenylalanine. *Psychiatry Res.* 1985;16:21-26.
14. Mosnik DM, Spring B, Rogers K, et al. Tardive dyskinesia exacerbated after ingestion of phenylalanine by schizophrenic patients. *Neuropsychopharmacology.* 1997;16: 136-146.
15. Richardson MA. *Amino Acids in Psychiatric Disease.* Washington, DC: American Psychiatric Press; 1990.

Phosphatidylcholine

1. Misra S, Ahn C, Ament ME, et al. Plasma choline concentrations in children requiring long-term home parenteral nutrition: a case control study. *JPEN J Parenter Enteral Nutr.* 1999;23:305-308.
2. Buchman AL, Dubin M, Jenden D, et al. Lecithin increases plasma free choline and decreases hepatic steatosis in long-term total parenteral nutrition patients. *Gastroenterology.* 1992;102:1363-1370.
3. Zeisel SH, Da Costa KA, Franklin PD, et al. Choline, an essential nutrient for humans. *FASEB J.* 1991;5:2093-2098.
4. Tayek JA, Bistrian B, Sheard NF, et al. Abnormal liver function in malnourished patients receiving total parenteral nutrition: a prospective randomized study. *J Am Coll Nutr.* 1990;9:76-83.
5. Zeisel SH. Choline: an important nutrient in brain development, liver function and carcinogenesis. *J Am Coll Nutr.* 1992;11:473-481.
6. Burt ME, Hanin I, Brennan MF. Choline deficiency associated with total parenteral nutrition [letter]. *Lancet.* 1980;2:638-639.
7. Niederau C, Strohmeyer G, Heintges T, et al. Polyunsaturated phosphatidyl-choline and interferon alpha for treatment of chronic hepatitis B and C: a multi-center, randomized, double-blind, placebo-controlled trial. Leich Study Group. *Hepatogastroenterology.* 1998;45:797-804.
8. Jenkins PJ, Portmann BP, Eddleston F, et al. Use of polyunsaturated phosphatidyl-choline in HBsAg negative chronic active hepatitis: results of prospective double-blind controlled trial. *Liver.* 1982;2:77-81.
9. Guan R, Ho KY, Kang JY, et al. The effect of polyunsaturated phosphatidyl choline in the treatment of acute viral hepatitis. *Aliment Pharmacol Ther.* 1995;9:699-703.
10. Lieber CS, Robins SJ, Li J, et al. Phosphatidylcholine protects against fibrosis and cirrhosis in the baboon. *Gastroenterology.* 1994;106:152-159.
11. Lieber CS, DeCarli LM, Mak KM. Attenuation of alcohol-induced hepatic fibrosis by polyunsaturated lecithin. *Hepatology.* 1990;12:1390-1398.
12. Lieber CS, Leo MA, Mak KM, et al. Choline fails to prevent liver fibrosis in ethanol-fed baboons but causes toxicity. *Hepatology.* 1985;5:561-572.
13. Lieber CS, Rubin E. Alcoholic fatty liver. *N Engl J Med.* 1969;280:705-708.
14. Schuller-Perez A, Gonzalez San Martin F. A controlled study with polyunsaturated phosphatidylcholine compared to placebo in alcoholic steatosis of the liver [translated from German]. *Med Welt.* 1985;36:517-521.
15. Knuchel F. A double-blind study of patients with a fatty liver caused by the toxic effects of alcohol: effect of essential phospholipids on enzyme behavior and lipid composition of the serum [translated from German]. *Med Welt.* 1979;30:411-416.
16. Heyman A, Schmechel D, Wilkinson W, et al. Failure of long term high-dose lecithin to retard progression of early-onset Alzheimer's disease. *J Neurol Transm Suppl.* 1987;24:279-286.
17. Weintraub S, Mesulan MM, Auty R, et al. Lecithin in the treatment of Alzheimer's disease [letter]. *Arch Neurol.* 1983;40:527-528.
18. Etienne P, Dastoor D, Gauthier S, et al. Alzheimer disease: lack of effect of lecithin treatment for 3 months. *Neurology.* 1981;31:1552-1554.
19. Gauthier S, Bouchard R, Bacher Y, et al. Progress report on the Canadian Multicentre Trial of tetrahydroaminoacridine with lecithin in Alzheimer's disease. *Can J Neurol Sci.* 1989;16:543-546.
20. Leathwood PD, Schlosser B. Phosphatidylcholine, choline and cholinergic function. *Int J Vitam Nutr Res Suppl.* 1986;29:49-67.

21. Sanchez CJ, Hooper E, Garry PJ, et al. The relationship between dietary intake of choline, choline serum levels, and cognitive function in healthy elderly persons. *J Am Geriatr Soc.* 1984;32:208-212.

22. Harris CM, Dysken MW, Fovall P, et al. Effect of lecithin on memory in normal adults. *Am J Psychiatry.* 1983;140:1010-1012.

23. Stoll AL, Sachs GS, Cohen BM, et al. Choline in the treatment of rapid-cycling bipolar disorder: clinical and neurochemical findings in lithium-treated patients. *Biol Psychiatry.* 1996;40:382-388.

24. Cohen BM, Lipinski JF, Altesman RI. Lecithin in the treatment of mania: double-blind, placebo-controlled trials. *Am J Psychiatry.* 1982;139:1162-1164.

25. Gelenberg AJ, Dorer DJ, Wojcik JD, et al. A crossover study of lecithin treatment of tardive dyskinesia. *J Clin Psychiatry.* 1990;51:149-153.

26. Domino EF, May WW, Demetriou S, et al. Lack of clinically significant improvement of patients with tardive dyskinesia following phosphatidylcholine therapy. *Biol Psychiatry.* 1985;20:1189-1196.

27. Davis KL, Berger PA. Pharmacological investigations of the cholinergic imbalance hypotheses of movement disorders and psychosis. *Biol Psychiatry.* 1978;13:23-49.

28. Brook JG, Linn S, Aviram M. Dietary soya lecithin decreases plasma triglyceride levels and inhibits collagen- and ADP-induced platelet aggregation. *Biochem Med Metab Biol.* 1986;35:31-39.

29. Wojcicki J, Pawlik A, Samochowiec L, et al. Clinical evaluation of lecithin as a lipid-lowering agent. *Phytother Res.* 1995;9:597-599.

30. Oosthuizen W, Vorster HH, Vermaak WJ, et al. Lecithin has no effect on serum lipoprotein, plasma fibrinogen and macro molecular protein complex levels in hyper-lipidaemic men in a double-blind controlled study. *Eur J Clin Nutr.* 1998;52:419-424.

31. Singh NK, Prasad RC. A pilot study of polyunsaturated phosphatidyl choline in fulminant and subacute hepatic failure. *J Assoc Physicians India.* 1998;46:530-532.

32. Newberne PM. Lipotropic factors and oncogenesis. *Adv Exp Med Biol.* 1986;206:223-251.

33. Wainfan E, Poirier LA. Methyl groups in carcinogenesis: effects on DNA methylation and gene expression. *Cancer Res.* 1992;52:2071S-2077S.

34. Rogers AE. Methyl donors in the diet and responses to chemical carcinogens. *Am J Clin Nutr.* 1995;61:659S-665S.

35. Olszewski AJ, Szostak WB, Bialkowska M, et al. Reduction of plasma lipid and homocysteine levels by pyridoxine, folate, cobalamin, choline, riboflavin, and troxerutin in atherosclerosis. *Atherosclerosis.* 1989;75:1-6.

36. Dudman NP, Wilcken DE, Wang J, et al. Disordered methionine/homocysteine metabolism in premature vascular disease: its occurrence, cofactor therapy, and enzymology. *Arterioscler Thromb.* 1993;13:1253-1260.

37. Hirsch MJ, Growdon JH, Wurtman RJ. Relations between dietary choline or lecithin intake, serum choline levels, and various metabolic indices. *Metabolism.* 1978;27:953-960.

38. Wood JL, Allison RG. Effects of consumption of choline and lecithin on neurological and cardiovascular systems. *Fed Proc.* 1982;41:3015-3021.

39. Russell RW. Continuing the search for cholinergic factors in cognitive dysfunction. *Life Sci.* 1996;58:1965-1970.

40. Wurtman RJ, Growdon JH. Dietary enhancement of CNS neurotransmitters. *Hosp Pract.* 1978;13:71-77.

41. Zeisel SH. Dietary influences on neurotransmission. *Adv Pediatr.* 1986;33:23-47.

42. Schmidt DE, Wecker L. CNS effects of choline administration: evidence for temporal dependence. *Neuropharmacology.* 1981;20:535-539.

43. Wecker L. Neurochemical effects of choline supplementation. *Can J Physiol Pharmacol.* 1986;64:329-333.

44. Wecker L. Dietary choline: a limiting factor for the synthesis of acetylcholine by the brain. *Adv Neurol.* 1990;51:139-145.

45. [No authors listed]. Choline: a conditionally essential nutrient for humans. *Nutr Rev.* 1992;50:112-114.

Phosphatidylserine

1. Cenacchi T, Bertoldin T, Farina C, et al. Cognitive decline in the elderly: a double-blind, placebo-controlled multicenter study on efficacy of phosphatidylserine administration. *Aging (Milano)*. 1993;5:123-133.
2. Amaducci L, the SMID Group. Phosphatidylserine in the treatment of Alzheimer's disease: results of a multicenter study. *Psychopharmacol Bull.* 1988;24:130-134.
3. Crook T, Petrie W, Wells C, et al. Effects of phosphatidylserine in Alzheimer's disease. *Psychopharmacol Bull.* 1992;28:61-66.
4. Delwaide PJ, Gyselynck-Mambourg AM, Hurlet A, et al. Double-blind randomized controlled study of phosphatidylserine in senile demented patients. *Acta Neurol Scand.* 1986;73:136-140.
5. Engel RR, Satzger W, Gunther W, et al. Double-blind cross-over study of phosphatidylserine vs. placebo in patients with early dementia of the Alzheimer type. *Eur Neuropsychopharmacol.* 1992;2:149-155.
6. Funfgeld EW, Baggen M, Nedwidek P, et al. Double-blind study with phosphatidylserine (PS) in Parkinsonian patients with senile dementia of Alzheimer's type (SDAT). *Prog Clin Biol Res.* 1989;317:1235-1246.
7. Palmieri G, Palmieri R, Inzoli MR, et al. Double-blind controlled trial of phosphatidylserine in patients with senile mental deterioration. *Clin Trials J.* 1987;24:73-83.
8. Villardita C, Grioli S, Salmeri G, et al. Multicentre clinical trial of brain phosphatidylserine in elderly patients with intellectual deterioration. *Clin Trials J.* 1987;24:84-93.
9. Crook TH, Tinklenberg J, Yesavage J, et al. Effects of phosphatidylserine in age-associated memory impairment. *Neurology.* 1991;41:644-649.
10. Maggioni M, Picotti GB, Bondiolotti GP, et al. Effects of phosphatidylserine therapy in geriatric patients with depressive disorders. *Acta Psychiatr Scand.* 1990;81:265-270.
11. Fahey TD, Pearl MS. The hormonal and perceptive effects of phosphatidylserine administration during two weeks of resistive exercise-induced overtraining. *Biol Sport.* 1998;15:135-144.
12. Monteleone P, Beinat L, Tanzillo C, et al. Effects of phosphatidylserine on the neuroendocrine response to physical stress in humans. *Neuroendocrinology.* 1990;52:243-248.
13. Monteleone P, Maj M, Beinat L, et al. Blunting by chronic phosphatidylserine administration of the stress-induced activation of the hypothalamo-pituitary-adrenal axis in healthy men. *Eur J Clin Pharmacol.* 1992;41:385-388.
14. Casamenti F, Mantovani P, Amaducci L, et al. Effect of phosphatidylserine on acetylcholine output from the cerebral cortex of the rat. *J Neurochem.* 1979;32:529-533.
15. Calderini G, Bellini F, Consolazione A, et al. Reparative processes in aged brain. *Gerontology.* 1987;33:227-233.
16. Martin SJ, Reutelingsperger CP, McGahon AJ, et al. Early redistribution of plasma membrane phosphatidylserine is a general feature of apoptosis regardless of the initiating stimulus: inhibition by overexpression of Bcl-2 and Abl. *J Exp Med.* 1995;182:1545-1556.
17. Palatini P, Viola G, Bigon E, et al. Pharmacokinetic characterization of phosphatidylserine liposomes in the rat. *Br J Pharmacol.* 1991;102:345-350.
18. Mantovani P, Pepeu G, Amaducci L. Investigations into the relationship between phospholipids and brain acetylcholine. *Adv Exp Med Biol.* 1976;72:285-292.
19. Toffano G, Leon A, Benvegnu D, et al. Effect of brain cortex phospholipids on catecholamine content of mouse brain. *Pharmacol Res Commun.* 1976;8:581-590.
20. Blokland A, Honig W, Brouns F, et al. Cognition-enhancing properties of subchronic phosphatidylserine (PS) treatment in middle-aged rats: comparison of bovine cortex PS with egg PS and soybean PS. *Nutrition.* 1999;15:778-783.
21. Cenacchi B, Baggio C, Palm E. Human tolerability of oral phosphatidylserine assessed through laboratory examinations. *Clin Trials J.* 1987;24:125-130.
22. Heywood R, Cozens DD, Richold M. Toxicology of a phosphatidylserine preparation from bovine brain (BC-PS). *Clin Trials J.* 1987;24:25-32.
23. van den Besselaar AM. Phosphatidylethanolamine and phosphatidylserine synergistically promote heparin's anticoagulant effect. *Blood Coagul Fibrinolysis.* 1995;6:239-244.

Phyllanthus

1. Calixto JB, Santos AR, Cechinel Filho V, et al. A review of the plants of the genus *Phyllanthus:* their chemistry, pharmacology, and therapeutic potential. *Med Res Rev.* 1998;18:225-258.
2. Thyagarajan SP, Subramanian S, Thirunalasundar T, et al. Effect of *Phyllanthus amarus* on chronic carriers of hepatitis B virus. *Lancet.* 1988;2:764-766.
3. Berk L, de Man RA, Schalm SW, et al. Beneficial effects of *Phyllanthus amarus* for chronic hepatitis B, not confirmed. *J Hepatol.* 1991;12:405-406.
4. Leelarasamee A, Trakulsomboon S, Maunwongyathi P, et al. Failure of *Phyllanthus amarus* to eradicate hepatitis B surface antigen from symptomless carriers [letter]. *Lancet.* 1990;335:1600-1601.
5. Thyagarajan SP, Jayaram S, Valliammai T, et al. *Phyllanthus amarus* and hepatitis B [letter]. *Lancet.* 1990;336:949-950.
6. Thamlikitkul V, Wasuwat S, Kanchanapee P. Efficacy of *Phyllanthus amarus* for eradication of hepatitis B virus in chronic carriers. *J Med Assoc Thai.* 1991;74:381-385.
7. Doshi JC, Vaidya AB, Antarkar DS, et al. A two-stage clinical trial of *Phyllanthus amarus* in hepatitis B carriers: failure to eradicate the surface antigen. *Indian J Gastroenterol.* 1994;13:7-8.
8. Milne A, Hopkirk N, Lucas CR, et al. Failure of New Zealand hepatitis B carriers to respond to Phyllanthus amarus. *NZ Med J.* 1994;107:243.
9. Narendranathan M, Remla A, Mini PC, et al. A trial of *Phyllanthus amarus* in acute viral hepatitis. *Trop Gastroenterol.* 1999;20:164-166.

Policosanol

1. Mas R. D-002; beeswax alcohols, BWA, Abexol®. *Drugs Future.* 2001;26(8):731-744.
2. Aneiros E, Calderon B, Mas R, et al. Effect of successive dose increases of policosanol on the lipid profile and tolerability of treatment. *Curr Ther Res.*1993:54:304-312.
3. Aneiros E, Mas R, Calderon B, et al. Effect of policosanol in lowering cholesterol levels in patients with Type II hypercholesterolemia. *Curr Ther Res.* 1995;56:176-182.
4. Castano G, Canetti M, Moreira M, et al. Efficacy and tolerability of policosanol in elderly patients with type II hypercholesterolemia: a 12-month study. *Curr Ther Res.* 1995;56:819-828.
5. Castano G, Mas R, Nodase M, et al. One-year study of the efficacy and safety of policosanol (5 mg twice daily) in the treatment of type II hypercholesterolemia. *Curr Ther Res.* 1995;56:296-304.
6. Castano G, Tula L, Canetti M, et al. Effects of policosanol in hypertensive patients with type II hypercholesterolemia. *Curr Ther Res.* 1996;57:691-699.
7. Castano G, Mas R, Fernandez L, et al. Effects of policosanol on postmenopausal women with type II hypercholesterolemia. *Gynecol Endocrinol.* 2000;14:187-195.
8. Crespo N, Alvarez M, Mas R, et al. Effect of policosanol on patients with non-insulin-dependent diabetes mellitus and hypercholesterolemia: a pilot study. *Curr Ther Res.* 1997;58:44-51.
9. Mas R., Castano G, Illnait J, et al. Effects of policosanol in patients with type II hypercholesterolemia and additional coronary risk factors. *Clin Pharmacol Ther.* 1999;65:439-447.
10. Mirkin A, Mas R, Matinto M, et al. Efficacy and tolerability of policosanol in hypercholesterolemic postmenopausal women. *Int J Clin Pharm Res.* 2001;21:31-34 .
11. Pons P, Mas R, Illnait J, et al. Efficacy and safety of policosanol in patients with primary hypercholesterolemia. *Curr Ther Res.* 1992;52:507-513.
12. Pons P, Rodriguez M, Robaina C, et al. Effects of successive dose increases of policosanol on the lipid profile of patients with type II hypercholesterolaemia and tolerability to treatment. *Int J Clin Pharmacol Res.* 1994;14:27-33.
13. Pons P, Rodriquez M, Mas R, et al. One-year efficacy and safety of policosanol in patients with type II hypercholesterolemia. *Curr Ther Res.* 1994;55:1084-1092.
14. Pons P, Jimenez A, Rodriquez M, et al. Effects of policosanol in elderly hypercholesterolemic patients. *Curr Ther Res.* 1993;53:265-269.
15. Torres O, Agramonte AJ, Illnait J, et al. Treatment of hypercholesterolemia in NIDDM with policosanol. *Diabetes Care.* 1995;18:393-397.

16. Zardoya R, Tula L, Castano G, et al. Effects of policosanol on hypercholesterolemic patients with abnormal serum biochemical indicators of hepatic function. *Curr Ther Res*.1996;57:568-577.

17. Alcocer L, Fernandez L, Campos E, et al. A comparative study of policosanol versus acipimox in patients with type II hypercholesterolemia. *Int J Tissue React*.1999;21:85-92.

18. Benitez M, Romero C, Mas R. et al. A comparative study of policosanol versus pravastatin in patients with type II hypercholesterolemia. *Curr Ther Res*. 1997;58: 859-867.

19. Castano G, Mas R, Arruzazabala M, et al. Effects of policosanol and pravastatin on lipid profile, platelet aggregation and endothelemia in older hypercholesterolemic patients. *Int J Clin Pharmacol Res*. 1999;19:105-116.

20. Castano G, Mas R, Fernando JC, et al. Efficacy and tolerability of policosanol compared with lovastatin in patients with type II hypercholesterolemia and concomitant coronary risk factors. *Curr Ther Res*. 2000;61:137-146.

21. Crespo N, Illnait J, Mas R, et al. Comparative study of the efficacy and tolerability of policosanol and lovastatin in patients with hypercholesterolemia and noninsulin dependent diabetes mellitus. *Int J Clin Pharmacol Res*. 1999;19:117-127.

22. Fernandez JC, Mas R, Castano G, et al. Comparison of the efficacy, safety and tolerability of policosanol versus fluvastatin in elderly hypercholesterolaemic women. *Clin Drug Invest*. 2001; 21:103-113.

23. Ortensi G, Gladstein A, Valle H, et al. A comparative study of policosanol versus simvastatin in elderly patients with hypercholesterolemia. *Curr Ther Res*. 1997; 58:390-401.

24. Castano G, Mas Ferreiro R, Fernandez L, et al. A long-term study of policosanol in the treatment of intermittent claudication. *Angiology*. 2001;52:115-125.

25. Saint-John M, McNaughton L. Octacosanol ingestion and its effects on metabolic responses to submaximal cycle ergometry, reaction time and chest and grip strength. *Int Clin Nutr Rev*. 1986;6:81-87.

26. Snider SR. Octacosanol in parkinsonism [letter]. *Ann Neurol*. 1984;16:723.

27. Norris FH, Denys EH, Fallat RJ. Trial of octacosanol in amyotrophic lateral sclerosis. *Neurology*. 1986;36:1263-1264.

28. Menendez R, Arruzazabala L, Mas R, et al. Cholesterol-lowering effect of policosanol on rabbits with hypercholesterolaemia induced by a wheat starch-casein diet. *Br J Nutr*. 1997;77:923-932.

29. Arruzazabala ML, Mas R, Molina V, et al. Effect of policosanol on platelet aggregation in type II hypercholesterolemic patients. *Int J Tissue React*. 1998;20:119-124.

30. Arruzazabala ML, Valdes S, Mas R, et al. Effect of policosanol successive dose increases on platelet aggregation in healthy volunteers. *Pharmacol Res*. 1996;34:181-185.

31. Menendez R, Fraga V, Amor AM, et al. Oral administration of policosanol inhibits in vitro copper ion-induced rat lipoprotein peroxidation. *Physiol Behav*. 1999;67:1-7.

32. Fraga V, Menendez R, Amor AM, et al. Effect of policosanol on in vitro and in vivo rat liver microsomal lipid peroxidation. *Arch Med Res*. 1997;28:355-360.

33. Fernandez L, Mas R, Illnait J, et al. Policosanol: results of a postmarketing surveillance control on 27,879 patients. *Curr Ther Res*. 1998;59:717-722.

34. Rodriguez-Echenique C, Mesa R, Mas R, et al. Effects of policosanol chronically administered in male monkeys *(Macaca arctoides)*. *Food Chem Toxicol*. 1994;32:565-575.

35. Mesa AR, Mas R, Noa M, et al. Toxicity of policosanol in beagle dogs: one-year study. *Toxicol Lett*. 1994;73:81-90.

36. Aleman CL, Mas R, Hernandez C, et al. A 12-month study of policosanol oral toxicity in Sprague Dawley rats. *Toxicol Lett*. 1994;70:77-87.

37. Rodriguez MD, Garcia H. Teratogenic and reproductive studies of policosanol in the rat and rabbit. *Teratog Carcinog Mutagen*. 1994;14:107-113.

38. Castano G, Mas R, Roca J, et al. A double-blind, placebo-controlled study of the effects of policosanol in patients with intermittent claudication. *Angiology*. 1999; 50:123-130.

39. Arruzazabala ML, Valdes S, Mas R, et al. Comparative study of policosanol, aspirin and the combination therapy policosanol-aspirin on platelet aggregation in healthy volunteers. *Pharmacol Res*. 1997;36:293-297.

40. Gamez R, et al. A 6-month study on the toxicity of high doses of policosanol orally administered to Sprague-Dawley rats. *J Med Food.* 2001;4:57-65.
41. Arruzazabala ML, Carbajal D, Mas R, et al. Pharmacological interaction between policosanol and nitroprusside in rats. *J Med Food.* 2001;4:67-70.

Pregnenolone

1. Meldrum D, Davidson BJ, Tataryn IV, et al. Changes in circulating steroids with aging in postmenopausal women. *Obstet Gynecol.* 1981;57:624-628.
2. Flood JF, Morley JE, Roberts E. Pregnenolone sulfate enhances post-training memory processes when injected in very low doses into limbic system structures: the amygdala is by far the most sensitive. *Proc Natl Acad Sci USA.* 1995;92:10806-10810.
3. Flood JF, Morley JE, Roberts E. Memory-enhancing effects in male mice of pregnenolone and steroids metabolically derived from it. *Proc Natl Acad Sci USA.* 1992; 89:1567-1571.

Probiotics

1. Oksanen PJ, Salminen S, Saxelin M, et al. Prevention of travellers' diarrhoea by *Lactobacillus GG. Ann Med.* 1990;22:53-56.
2. Kirchhelle VA, Fruhwein N, Toburen D. Treatment of persistent diarrhea with *S. boulardii* in returning travelers: results of a prospective study [in German; English abstract]. *Fortschr Med.* 1996;114:136-140.
3. Kollaritsch H, Holst H, Grobara P, et al. Prevention of traveler's diarrhea with *Saccharomyces boulardii:* results of a placebo-controlled double-blind study [translated from German]. *Fortschr Med.* 1993;111:152-156.
4. Elmer GW, Surawicz CM, McFarland LV. Biotherapeutic agents: a neglected modality for the treatment and prevention of selected intestinal and vaginal infections. *JAMA.* 1996;275:870-876.
5. Scarpignato C, Rampal P. Prevention and treatment of traveler's diarrhea: a clinical pharmacological approach. *Chemotherapy.* 1995;41:48-81.
6. Hilton E, Kolakowski P, Singer C, et al. Efficacy of *Lactobacillus GG* as a diarrheal preventive in travelers. *J Travel Med.* 1997;4:41-43.
7. Guandalini S, Pensabene L, Zikri MA, et al. *Lactobacillus GG* administered in oral rehydration solution to children with acute diarrhea: a multicenter European trial. *J Pediatr Gastroenterol Nutr.* 2000;30:54-60.
8. Isolauri E, Juntunen M, Rautanen T, et al. A human *Lactobacillus* strain (*Lactobacillus casei* sp strain GG) promotes recovery from acute diarrhea in children. *Pediatrics.* 1991;88:90-97.
9. Shornikova AV, Casas IA, Mykkanen H, et al. Bacteriotherapy with *Lactobacillus reuteri* in rotavirus gastroenteritis. *Pediatr Infect Dis J.* 1997;16:1103-1107.
10. Simakachorn N, Pichaipat V, Rithipornpaisarn P, et al. Clinical evaluation of the addition of lyophilized, heat-killed *Lactobacillus acidophilus* LB to oral rehydration therapy in the treatment of acute diarrhea in children. *J Pediatr Gastroenterol Nutr.* 2000;30:68-72.
11. De Francesco V, Stoppino V, Sgarro C, et al. Lactobacillus acidophilus administration added to omeprazole/amoxycillin-based double therapy in *Helicobacter pylori* eradication. *Dig Liver Dis.* 2000;32:746-747.
12. Szajewska H, Kotowska M, Mrukowicz JZ, et al. Efficacy of *Lactobacillus GG* in prevention of nosocomial diarrhea in infants. *J Pediatr.* 2001;138:361-365.
13. Oberhelman RA, Gilman RH, Sheen P, et al. A placebo-controlled trial of *Lactobacillus GG* to prevent diarrhea in undernourished Peruvian children. *J Pediatr.* 1999;134:15-20.
14. Saavedra JM, Bauman NA, Oung I, et al. Feeding of *Bifidobacterium bifidum* and *Streptococcus thermophilus* to infants in hospital for prevention of diarrhoea and shedding of rotavirus. *Lancet.* 1994;344:1046-1049.
15. Pedone C, Bernabeu A, Postaire E, et al. The effect of supplementation with milk fermented by *Lactobacullus casei* (strain DN-114 001) on acute diarrhoea in children attending daycare centres. *Int J Clin Pract.* 1999;53:179-184.

16. Rembacken BJ, Snelling AM, Hawkey PM, et al. Non-pathogenic *Escherichia coli* versus mesalazine for the treatment of ulcerative colitis: a randomized trial. *Lancet.* 1999;354:635-639.

17. Faubion WA, Sandborn WJ. Probiotic therapy with *E. coli* for ulcerative colitis: take the good with the bad. *Gastroenterology.* 2000;118:630-631.

18. Gionchetti P, Rizzello F, Venturi A, et al. Oral bacteriotherapy as maintenance treatment in patients with chronic pouchitis: a double-blind, placebo-controlled trial. *Gastroenterology.* 2000;119:305-309.

19. Colombel JF, Cortot A, Neut C, et al. Yoghurt with *Bifidobacterium longum* reduces erythromycin-induced gastrointestinal effects [letter]. *Lancet.* 1987;2:43.

20. Surawicz CM, Elmer GW, Speelman P, et al. Prevention of antibiotic-associated diarrhea by *Saccharomyces boulardii*: a prospective study. *Gastroenterology.* 1989;96:981-988.

21. Surawicz CM, McFarland LV, Elmer G, et al. Treatment of recurrent *Clostridium difficile* colitis with vancomycin and *Saccharomyces boulardii*. *Am J Gastroenterol.* 1989; 84:1285-1287.

22. Arvola T, Laiho K, Torkkeli S, et al. Prophylactic *Lactobacillus GG* reduces antibiotic-associated diarrhea in children with respiratory infections: a randomized study. *Pediatrics.* 1999;104:e64.

23. Thomas MR, Litin SC, Osmon DR, et al. Lack of effect of *Lactobacillus GG* on antibiotic-associated diarrhea: a randomized, placebo-controlled trial. *Mayo Clin Proc.* 2001;76:883-889.

24. Siitonen S, Vapaatalo H, Salminen S, et al. Effect of *Lactobacillus GG* yoghurt in prevention of antibiotic associated diarrhoea. *Ann Med.* 1990;22:57-59.

25. Vanderhoof JA, Whitney DB, Antonson DL, et al. *Lactobacillus GG* in the prevention of antibiotic-associated diarrhea in children. *J Pediatr.* 1999;135:564-568.

26. McFarland LV, Surawicz CM, Greenberg RN, et al. Prevention of beta-lactam-associated diarrhea by *Saccharomyces boulardii* compared with placebo. *Am J Gastroenterol.* 1995;90:439-448.

27. Canducci F, Armuzzi A, Cremonini F, et al. A lyophilized and inactivated culture of *Lactobacillus acidophilus* increases *Helicobacter pylori* eradication rates. *Aliment Pharmacol Ther.* 2000;14:1625-1629.

28. Nobaek S, Johansson M-L, Molin G, et al. Alteration of intestinal microflora is associated with reduction in abdominal bloating and pain in patients with irritable bowel syndrome. *Am J Gastroenterol.* 2000;95:1231-1238.

29. Armuzzi A, Cremonini F, Ojetti V, et al. Effect of *Lactobacillus GG* supplementation on antibiotic-associated gastrointestinal side effects during *Helicobacter pylori* eradication therapy: a pilot study. *Digestion.* 2001;63:1-7.

30. Kalliomaki M, Salminen S, Arvilommi H, et al. Probiotics in primary prevention of atopic disease: a randomized placebo-controlled trial. *Lancet.* 2001;357:1076-1079.

31. Isolauri E, Arvola T, Sutas Y, et al. Probiotics in the management of atopic eczema. *Clin Exp Allergy.* 2000;30:1604-1610.

32. Majamaa H, Isolauri E. Probiotics: a novel approach in the management of food allergy. *J Allergy Clin Immunol.* 1997;99:179-185.

33. Hatakka K, Savilahti E, Ponka A, et al. Effect of long term consumption of probiotic milk on infections in children attending day care centres: double blind, randomized trial. *BMJ.* 2001;322:1-5.

34. Meydani SN, Ha WK. Immunological effects of yogurt. *Am J Clin Nutr.* 2000; 71:861-872.

35. Arunachalam K, Gill HS, Chandra RK. Enhancement of natural immune function by dietary consumption of *Bifidobacterium lactis*. *Eur J Clin Nutr.* 2000;54:263-267.

36. Chiang BL, Sheih YH, Wang LH, et al. Enhancing immunity by dietary consumption of a probiotic lactic acid bacterium (*Bifidobacterium lactis* HN019): optimization and definition of cellular immune responses. *Eur J Clin Nutr.* 2000;54:849-855.

37. Reid G, Bruce AW, McGroarty JA, et al. Is there a role for *Lactobacilli* in prevention of urogenital and intestinal infections. *Clin Microbiol Rev.* 1990;3:335-344.

38. McGroarty JA. Probiotic use of *Lactobacilli* in the human female urogenital tract. *FEMS Immunol Med Microbiol.* 1993;6:251-264.

39. Hilton E, Rindos P, Isenberg HD. *Lactobacillus GG* vaginal suppositories and vaginitis [letter]. *J Clin Microbiol.* 1995;33:1433.

40. Friedlander A, Druker MM, Schachter A. *Lactobacillus acidophilus* and vitamin B complex in the treatment of vaginal infection. *Panminerva Med.* 1986;28:51-53.

41. Hilton E, Isenberg HD, Alperstein P, et al. Ingestion of yogurt containing *Lactobacillus acidophilus* as prophylaxis for candidal vaginitis. *Ann Intern Med.* 1992;116: 353-357.

42. Kontiokari T, Sundqvist K, Nuutinen M, et al. Randomized trial of cranberry-lingonberry juice and *Lactobacillus GG* drink for the prevention of urinary tract infections in women. *BMJ.* 2001;322:1-5.

43. Urbancsek H, Kazar T, Mezes I, et al. Results of a double-blind, randomized study to evaluate the efficacy and safety of *Antibiophilus* in patients with radiation-induced diarrhoea. *Eur J Gastroenterol Hepatol.* 2001;13:391-396.

44. Unger C, Haring B, Kruse A, et al. Double-blind randomized placebo-controlled phase III study of an *E. coli* extract plus 5-fluorouracil versus 5-fluorouracil in patients with advanced colorectal cancer. *Arzneimittelforschung.* 2001;51:332-338.

45. Armuzzi A, Cremonini F, Bartolozzi F, et al. The effect of oral administration of *Lactobacillus GG* on antibiotic-associated gastrointestinal side-effects during *Helicobacter pylori* eradication therapy. *Aliment Pharmacol Ther.* 2001;15:163-169.

46. Agerholm-Larsen L, Raben A, Haulrik N, et al. Effect of 8 week intake of probiotic milk products on risk factors for cardiovascular diseases. *Eur J Clin Nutr.* 2000; 54:288-297.

47. Anderson JW, Gilliland SE. Effect of fermented milk (yogurt) containing *Lactobacillus acidophilus* L1 on serum cholesterol in hypercholesterolemic humans. *J Am Coll Nutr.* 1999;18:43-50.

48. Agerbaek M, Gerdes LU, Richelsen B. Hypocholesterolaemic effect of a new fermented milk product in healthy middle-aged men. *Eur J Clin Nutr.* 1995;49:346-352.

49. Bertolami MC, Faludi AA, Batlouni M. Evaluation of the effects of a new fermented milk product (Gaio) on primary hypercholesterolemia. *Eur J Clin Nutr.* 1999;53: 97-101.

50. Agerholm-Larsen L, Bell ML, Grunwald GK, et al. The effect of a probiotic milk product on plasma cholesterol: a meta-analysis of short-term intervention studies. *Eur J Clin Nutr.* 2000;54:856-860.

51. Richelsen B, Kristensen K, Pedersen SB. Long-term (6 months) effect of a new fermented milk product on the level of plasma lipoproteins—a placebo-controlled and double blind study. *Eur J Clin Nutr.* 1996;50(12):811-815.

52. Pelto L, Isolauri E, Lilius EM, et al. Probiotic bacteria down-regulate the milk-induced inflammatory response in milk-hypersensitive subjects but have an immunostimulatory effect in healthy subjects. *Clin Exp Allergy.* 1998;28:1474-1479.

53. Isolauri E. Probiotics in human disease. *Am J Clin Nutr.* 2001;73(suppl):1142S-1146S.

54. Kaila M, Isolauri E, Soppi E, et al. Enhancement of the circulating antibody secreting cell response in human diarrhea by a human *Lactobacillus* strain. *Pediatr Res.* 1992; 32:141-144.

55. Hughes VL, Hillier SL. Microbiologic characteristics of *Lactobacilllus* products used for colonizaton of the vagina. *Obstet Gynecol.* 1990;75:244-248.

56. Le Blay G, Michel C, Blottiere HM, et al. Prolonged intake of fructo-oligosaccharides induces a short-term elevation of lactic acid-producing bacteria and a persistent increase in cecal butyrate in rats. *J Nutr.* 1999;129:2231-2235.

57. Szajewska H, Mrukowicz JZ. Probiotics in the treatment and prevention of acute infectious diarrhea in infants and children: a systematic review of published randomized double-blind placebo-controlled trials. *J Pediatr Gastroenterol Nutr.* 2001;33 (4 suppl):S17-S25.

58. Tankanow RM, Ross MB, Ertel IJ, et al. A double-blind placebo-controlled study of the efficacy of Lactinex in the prophylaxis of amoxicillin-induced diarrhea. *DICP.* 1990;24:382-384

59. Niedzielin K, Kordecki H, Birkenfeld B. A controlled, double-blind, randomized study on the efficacy of Lactobacillus plantarum 299V in patients with irritable bowel syndrome. *Eur J Gastroenterol Hepatol.* 2001;13:1143-1147.

60. Michetti P, Dorta G, Wiesel PH, et al. Effect of whey-based culture supernatant of *Lactobacillus acidophilus* (johnsonii) La1 on *Helicobacter pylori* infection in humans. *Digestion.* 1999;60:203-209.

61. O'Sullivan MA, et al. Bacterial supplementation in the irritable bowel syndrome: a randomized double-blind placebo-controlled crossover study. *Digest Liver Dis.* 2000;32:294-301.

62. Roos K, Hakansson EG,Holm S. Effect of recolonisation with interfering alpha streptococci on recurrences of acute and secretory otitis media in children: randomized placebo controlled trial. *BMJ.* 2001;322:210-212.

63. Tano K, Grahn Hakansson E, Holm SE, et al. A nasal spray with alpha-haemolytic streptococci as long term prophylaxis against recurrent otitis media. *Int J Pediatr Otorhinolaryngol.* 2002;62:17-23.

64. Aiba Y, Suzuki N, Kabir AM, et al. Lactic acid-mediated suppression of *Helicobacter pylori* by the oral administration of *Lactobacillus salivarius* as a probiotic in a gnotobiotic murine model. *Am J Gastroenterol.* 1998;93(11):2097-2101.

65. Sakamoto I, Igarashi M, Kimura K, et al. Suppressive effect of *Lactobacillus gasseri* OLL 2716 (LG21) on *Helicobacter pylori* infection in humans. *J Antimicrob Chemother.* 2001;47:709-710.

66. Wendakoon CN, Thomson AB, Ozimek L. Lack of therapeutic effect of a specially designed yogurt for the eradication of *Helicobacter pylori* infection. *Digestion.* 2002; 65:16-20.

67. Felley CP, Corthesy-Theulaz I, Rivero JL, et al. Favourable effect of an acidified milk (LC-1) on *Helicobacter pylori* gastritis in man. *Eur J Gastroenterol Hepatol.* 2001; 13:25-29.

Progesterone Cream

1. Leonetti HB, Longo S, Anasti JN. Transdermal progesterone cream for vasomotor symptoms and postmenopausal bone loss. *Obstet Gynecol.* 1999;94:225-228.

2. Prior JC. Progesterone as a bone-trophic hormone. *Endocr Rev.* 1990;11:386-398.

3. Verhaar HJ, Damen CA, Duursma SA, et al. A comparison of the action of progestins and estrogen on the growth and differentiation of normal adult human osteoblast-like cells in vitro. *Bone.* 1994;15:307-311.

4. Lee JR. Is natural progesterone the missing link in osteoporosis prevention and treatment? *Med Hypotheses.* 1991;35:316-318.

5. Lee JR. Osteoporosis reversal with transdermal progesterone [letter]. *Lancet.* 1990; 336:1327.

6. Lee JR. Osteoporosis reversal, the role of progesterone. *Int Clin Nutr Rev.* 1990; 10:384-391.

7. Writing Group for the PEPI Trial. Effects of hormone replacement therapy on endometrial histology in postmenopausal women: the postmenopausal estrogen/progestin interventions (PEPI) trial. *JAMA.* 1996;275:370-375.

8. Wren BG, McFarland K, Edwards L. Micronised transdermal progesterone and endometrial response. *Lancet.* 1999;354:1447-1448.

9. *Physicians' Desk Reference: PDR.* 53rd ed. Montvale, NJ: Medical Economics Co; 1999:125.

Proteolytic Enzymes

1. Zatuchni GI, Colombi DJ. Bromelains therapy for the prevention of episiotomy pain. *Obstet Gynecol.* 1967;29:275-278.

2. Howat RC, Lewis GD. The effect of bromelain therapy on episiotomy wounds—a double-blind controlled clinical trial. *J Obstet Gynaecol Br Commonw.* 1972;79:951-953.

3. Soule SD, Wasserman HC, Burstein R. Oral proteolytic enzyme therapy (Chymoral) in episiotomy patients. *Am J Obstet Gynecol.* 1966;95:820-823.

4. Cameron IW. An investigation into some of the factors concerned in the surgical removal of the impacted lower wisdom tooth, including a double blind trial of chymoral. *Br J Oral Surg.* 1980;18:112-124.

5. Seltzer AP. Minimizing post-operative edema and ecchymoses by the use of an oral enzyme preparation (bromelain): a controlled study of 53 rhinoplasty cases. *Eye Ear Nose Throat Mon.* 1962;41:813-817.

6. Tassman GC, Zafran JN, Zayon GM. Evaluation of a plant proteolytic enzyme for the control of inflammation and pain. *J Dent Med.* 1964;19:73-77.

7. Gylling U, Rintala A, Taipale S, et al. The effect of a proteolytic enzyme combinate (bromelain) on the postoperative edema by oral application: a clinical and experimental study. *Acta Chir Scand.* 1966;131:193-196.

8. Spaeth GL. The effect of bromelains on the inflammatory response caused by cataract extraction: a double-blind study. *Eye Ear Nose Throat Mon.* 1968;47:634-639.

9. Rahn H-D. Efficacy of hydrolytic enzymes in surgery. Presented at: Symposium on Enzyme Therapy in Sports Injuries: XXIV FIMS World Congress of Sport Medicine; May 29 1990; Amsterdam, the Netherlands.

10. Vinzenz K. Treatment of edema with hydrolytic enzymes in oral surgical procedures [translated from German]. *Quintessenz.* 1991;42:1053-1064.

11. Baumuller M. The application of hydrolytic enzymes in blunt wounds to the soft tissue and distortion of the ankle joint - a double-blind clinical trial [translated from German]. *Allgemeinmedizin.* 1990;19:178-182.

12. Zuschlag JM. Double-blind clinical study using certain proteolytic enzyme mixtures in karate fighters. Gerestsried, Germany: Mucos Pharma GmbH; 1988.

13. Rathgeber WF. The use of proteolytic enzymes (chymoral) in sporting injuries. *S Afr Med J.* 1971;45:181-183.

14. Deitrick RE. Oral proteolytic enzymes in the treatment of athletic injuries: a double-blind study. *Pa Med.* 1965;68:35-37.

15. Kleine MW, Pabst H. The effect of an oral enzyme therapy on experimentally produced hematomas [translated from German]. *Forum des Prakt und Allgemeinarztes.* 1988;27:42, 45-46, 48.

16. Shaw PC. The use of a trypsin-chymotrypsin formulation in fractures of the hand. *Br J Clin Pract.* 1969;23:25-26.

17. Blonstein JL. Control of swelling in boxing injuries. *Practitioner.* 1969;203:206.

18. Billigmann P. Enzyme therapy—an alternative in treatment of herpes zoster: a controlled study of 192 patients [translated from German]. *Fortschr Med.* 1995;113:43-48.

19. Gibson T, Dilke TF, Grahame R. Chymoral in the treatment of lumbar disc prolapse. *Rheumatol Rehabil.* 1975;14:186-190.

20. Felton GE. Fibrinolytic and antithrombotic action of bromelain may eliminate thrombosis in heart patients. *Med Hypotheses.* 1980;6:1123-1133.

21. Bodi T. Modifications of tissue permeability by orally administered proteolytic enzymes in man. *Exp Med Surg.* 1965;23(suppl):51-62.

22. Taussig SJ. The mechanism of the physiological action of bromelain. *Med Hypotheses.* 1980;6:99-104.

23. Taussig SJ, Batkin S. Bromelain, the enzyme complex of pineapple (*Ananas comosus*) and its clinical application: an update. *J Ethnopharmacol.* 1988;22:191-203.

24. Lotz-Winter H. On the pharmacology of bromelain: an update with special regard to animal studies on dose-dependent effects. *Planta Med.* 1990;56:249-253.

25. Vellini M, Desideri D, Milanese A, et al. Possible involvement of eicosanoids in the pharmacological action of bromelain. *Arzneimittelforschung.* 1986;36:110-112.

26. Kumakura S, Yamashita M, Tsurufuji S. Effect of bromelain on kaolin-induced inflammation in rats. *Eur J Pharmacol.* 1988;150:295-301.

27. Ako H, Cheung AHS, Matsuura PK. Isolation of a fibrinolysis enzyme activator from commercial bromelain (1). *Arch Int Pharmacodyn Ther.* 1981;254:157-167.

28. Petry JJ. Surgically significant nutritional supplements. *Plast Reconstr Surg.* 1996; 97:233-240.

29. Desser L, Rehberger A, Paukovits W. Proteolytic enzymes and amylase induce cytokine production in human peripheral blood mononuclear cells in vitro. *Cancer Biother.* 1994;9:253-263.

30. Shaw D, Leon C, Kolev S, et al. Traditional remedies and food supplements: a 5-year toxicological study (1991-1995). *Drug Saf.* 1997;Nov 17:342-356.
31. Russell RM, Dutta SK, Oaks EV, et al. Impairment of folic acid absorption by oral pancreatic extracts. *Dig Dis Sci.* 1980;25:369-373.
32. Frank SC. Use of chymoral as an anti-inflammatory agent following surgical trauma. *J Am Podiatr Assoc.* 1965;55:706-709.
33. Tilscher H, Keusch R, Neumann K. Results of a double-blind randomized comparative study of Wobenzym®-placebo in patients with cervical syndrome [translated from German]. *Wien Med Wochenschr.*1996;146:91-95.
34. Singer F, Oberleitner H. Drug therapy of activated arthrosis: on the effectiveness of an enzyme mixture versus Diclofenac® [translated from German]. *Wien Med Wochenschr.* 1996;146:55-58.
35. Klein G, Kullich W. Reducing pain by oral enzyme therapy in rheumatic diseases [translated from German]. *Wien Med Wochenschr.* 1999;149:577-580.
36. Kolac C, Streichhan P, Lehr CM. Oral bioavailability of proteolytic enzymes. *Eur J Pharm Biopharm.* 1996;42:222-232.
37. Sakalova A, Kunze R, Holomanova D, et al. Density of adhesive proteins after oral administration of proteolytic enzymes in multiple myeloma [in Slovak; English abstract]. *Vnitr Lek.* 1995;41:822-826.
38. Brakebusch M, Wintergerst U, Petropoulou T, et al. Bromelain is an accelerator of phagocytosis respiratory burst and killing of *Candida albicans* by human granulocytes and monocytes. *Eur J Med Res.* 2001;6:193-200.
39. Tilscher H, Keusch R, Neumann K. Results of a double-blind randomized comparative study of Wobenzym®-placebo in patients with cervical syndrome [translated from German]. *Wien Med Wochenschr.* 1996;146:91-95.
40. Moss JN, et al. Bromelains: the pharmacology of the enzymes. *Arch Int Pharmacodyn Ther.* 1963;145:166-188.
41. Taussig SJ, et al. Bromelain: a proteolytic enzyme and its clinical application. A review. *Hiroshima J Med Sci.* 1975;24:185-193.
42. Baur X. Studies on the specificity of human IgE-antibodies to the plant proteases papain and bromelain. *Clin Allergy.* 1979;9:451-457.
43. Baur X, Fruhmann G. Allergic reactions, including asthma, to the pineapple protease bromelain following occupational exposure. *Clin Allergy.* 1979;9:443-450.
44. Gailhofer G, et al. Asthma caused by bromelain: an occupational allergy. *Clin Allergy.* 1988;18:445-450.
45. Gall H, et al. Kiwi fruit allergy: a new birch pollen-associated food allergy. *J Allergy Clin Immunol.* 1994;94:70-76.
46. Pike RN, et al. Immunological cross-reactivity of the major allergen from perennial ryegrass *(Lolium perenne):* lop pI, and the cysteine proteinase, bromelain. *Int Arch Allergy Immunol.* 1997;112:412-414.
47. Tanabe S, Tasake S, Watanabe M, et al. Cross-reactivity between bromelain and soluble fraction from wheat flour [in Japanese; English abstract]. *Arerugi.* 1997;46:1170-1173.
48. Gutfreund AE, Taussig SJ, Morris AK, et al. Effect of oral bromelain on blood pressure and heart rate of hypertensive patients. *Hawaii Med J.* 1978;37:143-146.
49. Cirelli MG, Smyth RD. Effects of bromelain anti-edema therapy on coagulation, bleeding, and prothrombin times. *J New Drugs.* 1963;3:37-39.

Pygeum

1. Del Vaglio B. Use of a new drug in the treatment of chronic prostatitis [in Italian]. *Minerva Urol.* 1974;26:81-94.
2. Carani C, Salvioli V, Scuteri A, et al. Urological and sexual evaluation of treatment of benign prostatic disease using *Pygeum africanum* at high doses [in Italian; English abstract]. *Arch Ital Urol Nefrol Androl.* 1991;63:341-345.
3. Menchini-Fabris GF, Giorgi P, Andreini F, et al. New perspectives on the use of *Pygeum africanum* in prostato-bladder pathology [in Italian; English abstract]. *Arch Ital Urol Nefrol Androl.* 1988;60:313-322.

4. Andro MC, Riffaud JP. *Pygeum africanum* extract for the treatment of patients with benign prostatic hyperplasia: a review of 25 years of published experience. *Curr Ther Res.* 1995;56:796-817.
5. Breza J, Dzurny O, Borowka A, et al. Efficacy and acceptability of Tadenan® (*Pygeum africanum* extract) in the treatment of benign prostatic hyperplasia (BPH): a multicentre trial in central Europe. *Curr Med Res Opin.* 1998;14:127-139.
6. Barlet A, Albrecht J, Aubert A, et al. Efficacy of *Pygeum africanum* extract in the treatment of micturitional disorders due to benign prostatic hyperplasia: evaluation of objective and subjective parameters. A multicenter, placebo-controlled double-blind trial [translated from German]. *Wien Klin Wochenschr.* 1990;102:667-673.
7. Schulz V, Hansel R, Tyler VE. *Rational Phytotherapy: A Physicians' Guide to Herbal Medicine.* 3rd ed. Berlin, Germany: Springer-Verlag; 1998:232-234.
8. Kozai K, Miyake Y, Kohda H, et al. Inhibition of glucosyltranferase from *Streptococcus mutans* by oleanolic acid and ursolic acid. *Caries Res.* 1987;21:104-108.
9. Yablonsky F, Nicolas V, Riffaud JP, et al. Antiproliferative effect of *Pygeum africanum* extract on rat prostatic fibroblasts. *J Urol.* 1997;157:2381-2387.
10. Rhodes L, Primka RL, Berman C, et al. Comparison of finasteride (Proscar®), a 5-alpha reductase inhibitor, and various commercial plant extracts in In vitro and In vivo 5-alpha reductase inhibition. *Prostate.* 1993;22:43-51.
11. Chatelain C, Autet W, Brackman F. Comparison of once and twice daily dosage forms of *Pygeum africanum* extract in patients with benign prostatic hyperplasia: a randomized, double-blind study, with long-term open label extension. *Urology.* 1999;54:473-478.
12. Hartmann RW, Mark M, Soldati F. Inhibition of 5-alpha-reductase and aromatase by PHL-00801 (Prostatonin®), a combination of PY 102 *(Pygeum africanum)* and UR 102 *(Urtica dioica)* extracts. *Phytomedicine.* 1996;3:121-128.
13. Krzeski T, Kazon M, Borkowski A, et al. Combined extracts of *Urtica dioica* and *Pygeum africanum* in the treatment of benign prostatic hyperplasia: double-blind comparison of two doses. *Clin Ther.* 1993;15:1011-1020.
14. Bombardelli E, Morazonni P. *Prunus africana* (Hook. F.) Kalkm. *Fitoterapia.* 1997; 68:205-218.

Pyruvate

1. Kalman D, Colker CM, Stark S, et al. Effect of pyruvate supplementation on body composition and mood. *Curr Ther Res.* 1998;59:793-802.
2. Stanko RT, Reynolds HR, Hoyson R, et al. Pyruvate supplementation of a low-cholesterol, low-fat diet: effects on plasma lipid concentration and body composition in hyperlipidemic patients. *Am J Clin Nutr.* 1994;59:423-427.
3. Stanko RT, Tietze DL, Arch JE. Body composition, energy utilization, and nitrogen metabolism with a 4.25-MJ/d low-energy diet supplemented with pyruvate. *Am J Clin Nutr.* 1992;56:630-635.
4. Stanko RT, Arch JE. Inhibition of regain in body weight and fat with addition of 3-carbon compound to the diet with hyperenergetic refeeding after weight reduction. *Int J Obes Relat Metab Disord.* 1996;20:925-930.
5. Stanko RT, Tietze DL, Arch JE. Body composition, energy utilization, and nitrogen metabolism with a severely restricted diet supplemented with dihydroxyacetone and pyruvate. *Am J Clin Nutr.* 1992;55:771-772.
6. Kalman D, Colker CM, Wilets I, et al. The effects of pyruvate supplementation on body composition in overweight individuals. *Nutrition.* 1999;15:337-340.
7. Ivy JL. Effect of pyruvate and dihydroxyacetone on metabolism and aerobic endurance capacity. *Med Sci Sports Exerc.* 1998;30:837-843.
8. Stanko RT, Robertson RJ, Galbreath RW, et al. Enhanced leg exercise endurance with a high-carbohydrate diet and dihydroxyacetone and pyruvate. *J Appl Physiol.* 1990;69:1651-1656.
9. Stanko RT, Robertson RJ, Spina RJ, et al. Enhancement of arm exercise endurance capacity with dihydroxyacetone and pyruvate. *J Appl Physiol.* 1990;68:119-124.
10. Morrison MA, Spriet LL, Dyck DJ. Pyruvate ingestion for 7 days does not improve aerobic performance in well-trained individuals. *J Appl Physiol.* 2000;89:549-556.

11. Stanko RT, Adibi SA. Inhibition of lipid accumulation and enhancement of energy expenditure by the addition of pyruvate and dihydroxyacetone to a rat diet. *Metabolism.* 1986;35:182-186.
12. Stanko RT, Ferguson TL, Newman CW, et al. Reduction of carcass fat in swine with dietary addition of dihydroxyacetone and pyruvate. *J Anim Sci.* 1989;67:1272-1278.
13. Stanko RT, Mendelow H, Shinozuka H, et al. Prevention of alcohol-induced fatty liver by natural metabolites and riboflavin. *J Lab Clin Med.* 1978;91:228-235.
14. Cortez MY, Torgan CE, Brozinick JT Jr, et al. Effects of pyruvate and dihydroxy-acetone consumption on the growth and metabolic state of obese Zucker rats. *Am J Clin Nutr.* 1991;53:847-853.

Quercetin

1. Shoskes DA, Zeitlin SI, Shahed A, et al. Quercetin in men with category III chronic prostatitis: a preliminary prospective, double-blind, placebo-controlled trial. *Urology.* 1999;54:960-963.
2. Ogasawara H, Middleton E Jr. Effect of selected flavonoids on histamine release (HR) and hydrogen peroxide (H_2O_2) generation by human leukocytes [abstract]. *J Allergy Clin Immunol.* 1985;75(suppl 1 pt 2):184.
3. Middleton E Jr. Effect of flavonoids on basophil histamine release and other secretory systems. *Prog Clin Biol Res.* 1986;213:493-506.
4. Yoshimoto T, Furukawa M, Yamamoto S, et al. Flavonoids: potent inhibitors of arachidonate 5-lipoxygenase. *Biochem Biophys Res Commun.* 1983;116:612-618.
5. Rodriguez LV, Janzen N, Raz S, et al. Treatment of interstitial cystitis with a quercetin containing compound: a preliminary, double-blind placebo control trial. Presented at: American Urological Association 2001 Annual Meeting; June 2-7, 2001; Anaheim, Calif.
6. Frankel EN, Waterhouse AL, Kinsella JE. Inhibition of human LDL oxidation by resveratrol [letter]. *Lancet.* 1993;341:1103-1104.
7. Alliangana DM. Effects of beta-carotene, flavonoid quercetin and quinacrine on cell proliferation and lipid peroxidation breakdown products in BHK-21 cells. *East Afr Med J.* 1996;73:752-757.
8. Cross HJ, Tilby M, Chipman JK, et al. Effect of quercetin on the genotoxic potential of cisplatin. *Int J Cancer.* 1996;66:404-408.
9. Hoffman R, Graham L, Newlands ES. Enhanced anti-proliferative action of busulphan by quercetin on the human leukaemia cell line K562. *Br J Cancer.* 1989;59: 347-348.
10. El Attar TM, Virji AS. Modulating effect of resveratrol and quercetin on oral cancer cell growth and proliferation. *Anticancer Drugs.* 1999;10:187-193.
11. Yoshida M, Yamamoto M, Nikaido T. Quercetin arrests human leukemic T-cells in late G1 phase of cell cycle. *Cancer Res.* 1992;52:6676-6681.
12. Balasubramanian S, Govindasamy S. Inhibitory effect of dietary flavonol quercetin on 7,12-dimethylbenz[a]anthracene-induced hamster buccal pouch carcinogenesis. *Carcinogenesis.* 1996;17:877-879.
13. Kaul TN, Middleton E Jr, Ogra PL. Antiviral effect of flavonoids on human viruses. *J Med Virol.* 1985;15:71-79.
14. Mucsi I, Pragai BM. Inhibition of virus multiplication and alteration of cyclic AMP level in cell cultures by flavonoids. *Experientia.* 1985;41:930-931.
15. Hayek T, Fhurman B, Vaya J, et al. Reduced progression of atherosclerosis in apolipoprotein E-deficient mice following consumption of red wine, or its polyphenols quercetin or catechin, is associated with reduced susceptibility of LDL to oxidation and aggregation. *Arterioscler Thromb Vasc Biol.* 1997;17:2744-2752.
16. Varma SD, Mizuno A, Kinoshita JH. Diabetic cataracts and flavonoids. *Science.* 1977;195:205-206.
17. Sesink AL, O'Leary KA, Hollman PC. Quercetin glucuronides but not glucosides are present in human plasma after consumption of quercetin-3-glucoside or quercetin-4'-glucoside. *J Nutr.* 2001;131:1938-1941.
18. Stavric B. Quercetin in our diet: from potent mutagen to probable anticarcinogen. *Clin Biochem.* 1994;27:245-248.

19. Friedman M, Smith GA. Factors which facilitate inactivation of quercetin mutagenicity. *Adv Exp Med Biol.* 1984;177:527-544.
20. Pignatelli P, Pulcinelli FM, Celestini A, et al. The flavonoids quercetin and catechin synergistically inhibit platelet function by antagonizing the intracellular production of hydrogen peroxide. *Am J Clin Nutr.* 2000;72:1150-1155.
21. Strick R, Strissel PL, Borgers S, et al. Dietary bioflavonoids induce cleavage in the MLL gene and may contribute to infant leukemia. *Proc Natl Acad Sci USA.* 2000; 97:4790-4795.
22. Gabor M. Anti-inflammatory and anti-allergic properties of flavonoids. *Prog Clin Biol Res.* 1986;213:471-480.
23. Pearce FL, et al. Mucosal mast cells. III. Effect of quercetin and other flavonoids on antigen-induced histamine secretion from rat intestinal mast cells. *J Allergy Clin Immunol.* 1984;73:819-823.
24. Orhan H, Marol S, Hepsen IF, Sahin G. Effects of some probable antioxidants on selenite-induced cataract formation and oxidative stress-related parameters in rats. *Toxicology.* 1999;139:219-232.
25. Sanderson J, McLauchlan WR, Williamson G. Quercetin inhibits hydrogen peroxide-induced oxidation of the rat lens. *Free Radic Biol Med.* 1999;26:639-645.
26. McLauchlan WR, Sanderson J, Williamson G. Quercetin protects against hydrogen peroxide–induced cataract. *Biochem Soc Trans.* 1997;25:S581.
27. Crespy V, Morand C, Besson C, et al. Quercetin, but not its glycosides, is absorbed from the rat stomach. *J Agric Food Chem.* 2002;50:618-621.

Red Clover

1. Cassady JM, Zennie TM, Chae YH, et al. Use of a mammalian cell culture benzo(a)pyrene metabolism assay for the detection of potential anticarcinogens from natural products: inhibition of metabolism by biochanin A, an isoflavone from *Trifolium pratense* L. *Cancer Res.* 1988;48:6257-6261.
2. Yanagihara K, Ito A, Toge T, et al. Antiproliferative effects of isoflavones on human cancer cell lines established from the gastrointestinal tract. *Cancer Res.* 1993;53:5815-5821.
3. Alhasan SA, Ensley JF, Sarkar FH. Genistein induced molecular changes in a squamous cell carcinoma of the head and neck cell line. *Int J Oncol.* 2000;16:333-338.
4. Wei H, Bowen R, Cai Q, et al. Antioxidant and antipromotional effects of the soybean isoflavone genistein. *Proc Soc Exp Biol Med.* 1995;208:124-130.
5. Tham DM, Gardner CD, Haskell WL. Clinical review 97: potential health benefits of dietary phytoestrogens: a review of the clinical, epidemiological, and mechanistic evidence. *J Clin Endocrinol Metab.* 1998;83:2223-2235.
6. Baber RJ, Templeman C, Morton T, et al. Randomized placebo-controlled trial of an isoflavone supplement and menopausal symptoms in women. *Climacteric.* 1999;2:85-92.
7. Knight DC, Howes JB, Eden JA. The effect of Promensil™, an isoflavone extract, on menopausal symptoms. *Climacteric.* 1999;2:79-84.
8. Howes JB, Sullivan D, Lai N, et al. The effects of dietary supplementation with isoflavones from red clover on the lipoprotein profiles of post menopausal women with mild to moderate hypercholesterolaemia. *Atherosclerosis.* 2000;152:143-147.
9. Olesek WA, Jurzysta M. Isolation, chemical and biological activity of red clover (*Trifolium pratense* L.) root saponins. *Acta Soc Bot Pol.* 1986;55: 247-252.
10. Newall CA, Anderson LA, Phillipson JD. *Herbal Medicines: A Guide for Health-Care Professionals.* London, England: Pharmaceutical Press; 1996:227.
11. Hale G. A double-blind randomized study on the effects of red clover isoflavones on the endometrium. *Menopause.* 2001;8:338-346.

Red Yeast Rice

1. Heber D, Yip I, Ashley JM, et al. Cholesterol-lowering effects of a proprietary Chinese red-yeast-rice dietary supplement. *Am J Clin Nutr.* 1999;69:231-236.
2. Rippe J, Bonovich K, Colfer H, et al. A multi-center, self-controlled study of Cholestin™ in subjects with elevated cholesterol [abstract]. *Circulation.* 1999; 99:1123.

3. Wang J, Lu Z, Chi J, et al. Multicenter clinical trial of the serum lipid-lowering effects of a *Monascus purpureus* (red yeast) rice preparation from traditional Chinese medicine. *Curr Ther Res.* 1997;58:964-978.
4. Chang M. *Cholestin: Health-Care Professional Product Guide.* Provo, Utah: Pharmanex; 1998:1-6.
5. Heber D, Lembertas A, Lu QY, et al. An analysis of nine proprietary Chinese red yeast rice dietary supplements: implications of variability in chemical profile and contents. *J Altern Complement Med.* 2001;7:133-139.
6. Ghirlanda G, Oradei A, Manto A, et al. Evidence of plasma CoQ$_{10}$-lowering effect by HMG-CoA reductase inhibitors: a double-blind, placebo-controlled study. *J Clin Pharmacol.* 1993;33:226-229.
7. Mortensen SA, Leth A, Agner E, et al. Dose-related decrease of serum coenzyme Q$_{10}$ during treatment with HMG-CoA reductase inhibitors. *Mol Aspects Med.* 1997;18(suppl):S137-S144.
8. Folkers K, Langsjoen P, Willis R, et al. Lovastatin decreases coenzyme Q levels in humans. *Proc Natl Acad Sci USA.* 1990;87:8931-8934.
9. Bargossi AM, Battino M, Gaddi A, et al. Exogenous CoQ$_{10}$ preserves plasma ubiquinone levels in patients treated with 3-hydroxy-3-methylglutaryl coenzyme A reductase inhibitors. *Int J Clin Lab Res.* 1994;24:171-176.

Reishi

1. Eo SK, Kim YS, Lee CK, et al. Antiherpetic activities of various protein bound polysaccharides isolated from *Ganoderma lucidum*. *J Ethnopharmacol.* 1999;68:175-181.
2. Eo SK, Kim YS, Lee CK, et al. Antiviral activities of various water and methanol soluble substances isolated from *Ganoderma lucidum*. *J Ethnopharmacol.* 1999;68:129-136.
3. Chiu SW, Wang ZM, Leung TM, et al. Nutritional value of ganoderma extract and assessment of its genotoxicity and antigenotoxicity using comet assays of mouse lymphocytes. *Food Chem Toxicol.* 2000;38:173-178.

Ribose

1. Pliml W, von Arnim T, Stablein A, et al. Effects of ribose on exercise-induced ischaemia in stable coronary artery disease. *Lancet.* 1992;340:507-510.
2. Tullson PC, Terjung RL. Adenine nucleotide synthesis in exercising and endurance-trained skeletal muscle. *Am J Physiol.* 1991;261:C342-C347.
3. Zollner N et al. Myoadenylate deaminase deficiency: successful symptomatic therapy by high dose oral administration of ribose. *Klin Wochenschr.* 1986;64:1281-1290.
4. Wagner DR, Gresser U, Zollner N. Effects of oral ribose on muscle metabolism during bicycle ergometer in AMPD-deficient patients. *Ann Nutr Metab.* 1991;35:297-302.
5. Steele IC, Patterson VH, Nicholls DP. A double blind, placebo controlled, crossover trial of D-ribose in McArdle's disease. *J Neurol Sci.* 1996;136:174-177.
6. Griffiths RD, Cady EB, Edwards RH, et al. Muscle energy metabolism in Duchenne dystrophy studied by 31P-NMR: controlled trials show no effect of allopurinol or ribose. *Muscle Nerve.* 1985;8:760-767.
7. Op 't Eijnde B, Van Leemputte M, Brouns F, et al. No effects of oral ribose supplementation on repeated maximal exercise and de novo ATP resynthesis. *J Appl Physiol.* 2001;91:2275-2281.

S-Adenosylmethionine (SAMe)

1. Stramentinoli G. Pharmacologic aspects of S-adenosylmethionine: pharmacokinetics and pharmacodynamics. *Am J Med.* 1987;83(5A):35-42.
2. di Padova C. S-adenosylmethionine in the treatment of osteoarthritis: review of the clinical studies. *Am J Med.* 1987;83(5A):60-65.
3. Caruso I, Pietrogrande V. Italian double-blind multicenter study comparing S-adenosylmethionine, naproxen, and placebo in the treatment of degenerative joint disease. *Am J Med.* 1987;83(5A):66-71.

4. Glorioso S, Todesco S, Mazzi A, et al. Double-blind multicentre study of the activity of S-adenosylmethionine in hip and knee osteoarthritis. *Int J Clin Pharmacol Res.* 1985;5:39-49.

5. Muller-Fassbender H. Double-blind clinical trial of S-adenosylmethionine versus ibuprofen in the treatment of osteoarthritis. *Am J Med.* 1987;83(5A):81-83.

6. Maccagno A, Di Giorgio EE, Caston OL, et al. Double-blind controlled clinical trial of oral S-adenosylmethionine versus piroxicam in knee osteoarthritis. *Am J Med.* 1987;83(5A):72-77.

7. Jacobsen S, Danneskiold-Samsoe B, Andersen RB. Oral S-adenosylmethionine in primary fibromyalgia: double-blind clinical evaluation. *Scand J Rheumatol.* 1991;20: 294-302.

8. Tavoni A, Vitali C, Bombardieri S, et al. Evaluation of S-adenosylmethionine in primary fibromyalgia: a double-blind crossover study. *Am J Med.* 1987;83(5A):107-110.

9. Bressa GM. S-adenosyl-l-methionine (SAMe) as antidepressant: meta-analysis of clinical studies. *Acta Neurol Scand Suppl.* 1994;154:7-14.

10. Salmaggi P, Bressa GM, Nicchia G, et al. Double-blind, placebo-controlled study of S-adenosyl-L-methionine in depressed postmenopausal women. *Psychother Psychosom.* 1993;59:34-40.

11. Cerutti R, Sichel MP, Perin M, et al. Psychological distress during puerperium: a novel therapeutic approach using S-adenosylmethionine. *Curr Ther Res.* 1993;53: 707-716.

12. Kagan BL, Sultzer DL, Rosenlicht N, et al. Oral S-adenosylmethionine in depression: a randomized, double-blind, placebo-controlled trial. *Am J Psychiatry.* 1990;147: 591-595.

13. Fava M, Rosenbaum JF, Birnbaum R, et al. The thyrotropin response to thyrotropin-releasing hormone as a predictor of response to treatment in depressed outpatients. *Acta Psychiatr Scand.* 1992;86:42-45.

14. Delle Chiaie R, Pancheri P. Combined analysis of two controlled, multicentric, double-blind studies to assess efficacy and safety of Sulfo-Adenosyl-Methionine (SAMe) vs. placebo (MC1) and SAMe vs. clomipramine (MC2) in the treatment of major depression [in Italian; English abstract]. *G Ital Psicopatol.* 1999;5:1-16.

15. Delle Chiaie R, Pancheri P, Scapicchio P. MC3: Multicentre, controlled efficacy and safety trial of oral S-adenosyl-methionine (SAMe) vs. oral imipramine in the treatment of depression [abstract]. *Int J Neuropsychopharmcol.* 2000;3(suppl 1):S230.

16. De Vanna M, Rigamonti R. Oral S-adenosyl-L-methionine in depression. *Curr Ther Res.* 1992;52:478-485.

17. Bell KM, Potkin SG, Carreon D, et al. S-adenosylmethionine blood levels in major depression: changes with drug treatment. *Acta Neurol Scand Suppl.* 1994;154:15-18.

18. Echols JC, Naidoo U, Salzman C. SAMe (S-adenosylmethionine). *Harv Rev Psychiatry.* 2000;8:84-90.

19. Delle Chiaie R, Pancheri P, Scapicchio P. MC4: Multicentre, controlled efficacy and safety trial of intramuscular S-adenosyl-methionine (SAMe) vs. oral imipramine in the treatment of depression [abstract]. *Int J Neuropsychopharmcol.* 2000;3(suppl 1):S230.

20. Liu X, Lamango N, Charlton C. L-dopa depletes S-adenosylmethionine and increases S-adenosyl homocysteine: relationship to the wearing-off effects [abstract]. *Abstr Soc Neurosci.* 1998;24:1469.

21. Bottiglieri T, Hyland K, Reynolds EH. The clinical potential of ademetionine (S-adenosylmethionine) in neurological disorders. *Drugs.* 1994;48:137-152.

22. Carrieri PB, Indaco A, Gentile S, et al. S-adenosylmethionine treatment of depression in patients with Parkinson's disease: a double-blind, crossover study versus placebo. *Curr Ther Res.* 1990;48:154-160.

23. Mato JM, Camara J, Fernandez de Paz J, et al. S-adenosylmethionine in alcoholic liver cirrhosis: a randomized, placebo-controlled, double-blind, multicenter clinical trial. *J Hepatol.* 1999;30:1081-1089.

24. Bombardieri G, Milani A, Bernardi L, et al. Effects of S-adenosyl-methionine (SAMe) in the treatment of Gilbert's syndrome. *Curr Ther Res.* 1985;37:580-585.

25. Frezza M, Pozzato G, Chiesa L, et al. Reversal of intrahepatic cholestasis of pregnancy in women after high dose S-adenosyl-L-methionine administration. *Hepatology.* 1984;4:274-278.

26. Frezza M, Pozzato G, Pison G, et al. S-adenosylmethionine counteracts oral contraceptive hepatotoxicity in women. *Am J Med Sci.* 1987;293:234-238.

27. Nicastri PL, Diaferia A, Tartagni M, et al. A randomized placebo-controlled trial of ursodeoxycholic acid and S-adenosylmethionine in the treatment of intrahepatic cholestasis of pregnancy. *Br J Obstet Gynaecol.* 1998;105:1205-1207.

28. Gatto G, Caleri d, Michelacci S, et al. Analgesizing effect of a methyl donor (S-adenosylmethionine) in migraine: an open clinical trial. *Int J Clin Pharmacol Res.* 1986;6:15-17.

29. Harmand MF, Vilamitjana J, Maloche E, et al. Effects of S-adenosylmethionine on human articular chondrocyte differentiation: an in vitro study. *Am J Med.* 1987; 83(5A):48-54.

30. Konig B. A long-term (two years) clinical trial with S-adenosylmethionine for the treatment of osteoarthritis. *Am J Med.* 1987;83(5A):89-94.

31. Barcelo HA, Wiemeyer JC, Sagasta CL, et al. Experimental osteoarthritis and its course when treated with S-adenosyl-L-methionine [in Spanish; English abstract]. *Rev Clin Esp.* 1990;187:74-78.

32. Kalbhen DA, Jansen G. Pharmacologic studies on the antidegenerative effect of ademetionine in experimental arthritis in animals [in German; English abstract]. *Arzneimittelforschung.* 1990;40:1017-1021.

33. Fava M, Rosenbaum JF, MacLaughlin R, et al. Neuroendocrine effects of S-adenosyl-L-methionine, a novel putative antidepressant. *J Psychiatr Res.* 1990;24:177-184.

34. Baldessarini RJ. Neuropharmacology of S-adenosyl-L-methionine. *Am J Med.* 1987;83(5A):95-103.

35. Reynolds EH, Carney MW, Toone BK. Methylation and mood. *Lancet.* 1984;2:196-198.

36. Bottiglieri T, Laundy M, Martin R, et al. S-adenosylmethionine influences monoamine metabolism [letter]. *Lancet.* 1984;2:224.

37. Bottiglieri T. Ademetionine (S-adenosylmethionine) neuro-pharmacology: implications for drug therapies in psychiatric and neurological disorders. *Expert Opin Investig Drugs.* 1997;6:417-426.

38. Parnetti L, Bottiglieri T, Lowenthal D. Role of homocysteine in age-related vascular and non-vascular diseases. *Aging (Milano).* 1997;9:241-257.

39. Spillmann M, Fava M. S-Adenosylmethionine (ademetionine) in psychiatric disorders: historical perspective and current status. *CNS Drugs.* 1996;6:416-425.

40. Morana A, Di Lernia I, Carteni M, et al. Synthesis and characterisation of a new class of stable S-adenosyl-L-methionine salts. *Int J Pharmacol.* 2000;194:61-68.

41. Cozens DD, Barton SJ, Clark R, et al. Reproductive toxicity studies of ademetionine. *Arzneimittelforschung.* 1988;38:1625-1629.

42. Pezzoli C, Galli-Kienle M, Stramentinoli G. Lack of mutagenic activity of ademetionine in vitro and in vivo. *Arzneimittelforschung.* 1987;37:826-829.

43. Berger R, Nowak H. A new medical approach to the treatment of osteoarthritis. Report of an open phase IV study with ademetionine (Gumbaral). *Am J Med.* 1987; 83(5A):84-88.

44. Carney MW, Chary TK, Bottiglieri T, et al. Switch and S-adenosylmethionine. *Ala J Med Sci.* 1988;25:316-319.

45. Carney MW, Chary TK, Bottiglieri T, et al. The switch mechanism and the bipolar/unipolar dichotomy. *Br J Psychiatry.* 1989;154:48-51.

46. Frezza M, Centini G, Cammareri G, et al. S-adenosylmethionine for the treatment of intrahepatic cholestasis of pregnancy: results of a controlled clinical trial. *Hepatogastroenterology.* 1990;37(suppl 2):122-125.

47. Reicks M, Hathcock JN. Effects of methionine and other sulfur compounds on drug conjugations. *Pharmacol Ther.* 1988;37:67-79.

48. Iruela LM, Minguez L, Merino J, et al. Toxic interaction of S-adenosylmethionine and clomipramine [letter]. *Am J Psychiatry.* 1993;150:522.

Saw Palmetto

1. Boccafoschi S, Annoscia S. Comparison of *Serenoa repens* extract with placebo by controlled clinical trial in patients with prostatic adenomatosis [in Italian]. *Urolgia*. 1983;50:1257-1268.

2. Champault G, Patel JC, Bonnard AM. A double-blind trial of an extract of the plant *Serenoa repens* in benign prostatic hyperplasia [letter]. *Br J Clin Pharmacol*. 1984; 18:461-462.

3. Descotes JL, Rambeaud JJ, Deschaseaux P, et al. Placebo-controlled evaluation of the efficacy and tolerability of Permixon® in benign prostatic hyperplasia after exclusion of placebo responders. *Clin Drug Invest*. 1995;9:291-297.

4. Emili E, Lo Cigno M, Petrone U. Clinical trial of a new drug for treating hypertrophy of the prostate (Permixon®) [in Italian]. *Urolgia*. 1983;50:1042-1048.

5. Mattei FM, Capone M, Acconcia A. *Serenoa repens* extract in the medical treatment of benign prostatic hypertrophy [in Italian]. *Urolgia*. 1988;55:547-552.

6. Reece Smith H, Memon A, Smart CJ, et al. The value of Permixon® in benign prostatic hypertrophy. *Br J Urol*. 1986;58:36-40.

7. Tasca A, Barulli M, Cavazzana A, et al. Treatment of obstruction in prostatic adenoma using an extract of *Serenoa repens:* double-blind clinical test v. placebo [in Italian; English abstract]. *Minerva Urol Nefrol*. 1985;37:87-91.

8. Bach D, Schmitt M, Ebeling L. Phytopharmaceutical and synthetic agents in the treatment of benign prostatic hyperplasia (BPH). *Phytomedicine*. 1996-1997;3:309-313.

9. Bracher F. Phytotherapy in the treatment of benign proststic hyperplasia [in German; English abstract]. *Urologe A*. 1997;36:10-17.

10. Plosker GL, Brogden RN. *Serenoa repens* (Permixon®): a review of its pharmacology and therapeutic efficacy in benign prostatic hyperplasia. *Drugs Aging*. 1996;9:379-395.

11. Carraro JC, Raynaud JP, Koch G, et al. Comparison of phytotherapy (Permixon) with finasteride in the treatment of benign prostate hyperplasia: a randomized international study of 1,098 patients. *Prostate*. 1996;29:231-240.

12. Boyle P, Gould AL, Roehrborn CG. Prostate volume predicts outcome of treatment of benign prostatic hyperplasia with finasteride: meta-analysis of randomized clinical trials. *Urology*. 1996;48:398-405.

13. Gormley GJ, Stoner E, Bruskewitz RC, et al. The effect of finasteride in men with benign prostatic hyperplasia. *N Engl J Med*. 1992;327:1185-1191.

14. Sokeland J. Combined sabal and urtica extract compared with finasteride in men with benign prostatic hyperplasia: analysis of prostate volume and therapeutic outcome. *BJU Int*. 2000;86:439-442.

15. Debruyne F. Phytotherapy (LSESR) vs an alpha-blocker for treatment of lower urinary tract symptoms secondary to benign prostate enlargement: a randomized comparative study. Presented at: American Urological Association 2001 Annual Meeting; June 2-7, 2001; Anaheim, Calif.

16. Marks LS, Partin AW, Epstein JI, et al. Effects of a saw palmetto herbal blend in men with symptomatic benign prostatic hyperplasia. *J Urol*. 2000;163:1451-1456.

17. Kuznetsov DD, Gerber GS, Burstein JD. Randomized, double blind, placebo-controlled study of saw palmetto in men with lower urinary tract symptoms (LUTS). Presented at: American Urological Association 2001 Annual Meeting; June 2-7, 2001; Anaheim, Calif.

18. Volpe MA, Cabelin M, Te AE, et al. A prospective trial using saw palmetto versus finasteride in the treatment of chronic nonbacterial prostatitis (CP). Presented at: American Urological Association 2001 Annual Meeting; June 2-7, 2001; Anaheim, Calif.

19. Braeckman J. The extract of *Serenoa repens* in the treatment of benign prostatic hyperplasia: a multicenter open study. *Curr Ther Res*. 1994;55:776-785.

20. Nickel JC. Placebo therapy of benign prostatic hyperplasia: a 25-month study. Canadian PROSPECT Study Group. *Br J Urol*. 1998;81:383-387.

21. Romics I, Schmitz H, Frang D. Experience in treating benign prostatic hypertrophy with *Sabal serrulata* for one year. *Int Urol Nephrol*. 1993;25:565-569.

22. Niederprum HJ, Schweikert HU, Zanker KS. Testosterone 5-alpha-reductase inhibition by free fatty acids from *Sabal serrulata* fruits. *Phytomedicine*. 1994;1:127-133.

23. Strauch G, Perles P, Vergult G, et al. Comparison of finasteride (Proscar®) and *Serenoa repens* (Permixon®) in the inhibition of 5-alpha reductase in healthy male voulunteers. *Eur Urol.* 1994;26:247-252.

24. Di Silverio F, Sciarra A, D'Eramo G, et al. Response of tissue androgen and epidermal growth factor concentrations to the long-term administration of finasteride, flutamide and *Serenoa repens* in patients with benign prostatic hyperplasia (BHP) [abstract]. *Eur Urol.* 1996;30(suppl 2):96.

25. Carilla E, Briley M, Fauran F, et al. Binding of Permixon, a new treatment for prostatic benign hyperplasia, to the cytosolic androgen receptor in the rat prostate. *J Steroid Biochem.* 1984;20:521-523.

26. Sultan C, Terraza A, Devillier C, et al. Inhibition of androgen metabolism and binding by a liposterolic extract of "*Serenoa repens* B" in human foreskin fibroblasts. *J Steroid Biochem.* 1984;20:515-519.

27. Paubert-Braquet M, Mencia Huerta JM, Cousse H, et al. Effect of the lipidic lipidosterolic extract of *Serenoa repens* (Permixon®) on the ionophore A23187-stimulated production of leukotriene B4 (LTB4) from human polymorphonuclear neutrophils. *Prostaglandins Leukot Essent Fatty Acids.* 1997;57:299-304.

28. Gutierrez M, Garcia de Boto MJ, Cantabrana B, et al. Mechanisms involved in the spasmolytic effect of extracts from *Sabal serrulata* fruit on smooth muscle. *Gen Pharmacol.* 1996;27:171-176.

29. Gutierrez M, Hidalgo A, Cantabrana B. Spasmolytic activity of a lipidic extract from *Sabal serrulata* fruits: further study of the mechanisms underlying this activity. *Planta Med.* 1996;62:507-511.

30. Bombardelli I. *Serenoa repens* (Bartram) J. K. Small. *Fitoterapia.* 1997;68:99-113.

31. Goepel M, Dinh L, Mitchell A, et al. Do saw palmetto extracts block human alpha(1)-adrenoceptor subtypes in vivo? *Prostate.* 2001;46:226-232.

32. Braeckman J, Bruhwyler J, Vandekerckhove K, et al. Efficacy and safety of the extract of *Serenoa repens* in the treatment of benign prostatic hyperplasia: the therapeutic equivalence between twice and once daily dosage forms. *Phytother Res.* 1997;11:558-563.

33. Stepanov VN, Siniakova LA, Sarrazin B, et al. Efficacy and tolerability of the lipidosterolic extract of *Serenoa repens* (Permixon®) in benign prostatic hyperplasia: a double-blind comparison of two dosage regimens. *Adv Ther.* 1999;16:231-241.

34. Cheema P, El-Mefty O, Jazieh AR. Intraoperative haemorrhage associated with the use of extract of Saw Palmetto herb: a case report and review of literature. *J Intern Med.* 2001:250;167-169.

Schisandra

1. Hancke JL, Burgos RA, Ahumada F. *Schisandra chinensis* (Turcz.) Baill. *Fitoterapia.* 1999;70:451-471.

2. Volicer L, Sramka M, Janku I, et al. Some pharmacological effects of *Schizandra chinensis.* *Arch Int Pharmacodyn Ther.* 1966;163:249-262.

3. Bao TT, Xu GF, Liu GT, et al. A comparison of the pharmacological actions of seven constituents isolated from *Fructus Schizandrae* [in Chinese; English abstract]. *Acta Pharm Sin.* 1979;14:1-7.

4. Pao TT, Hsu KF, Liu KT, et al. Protective action of schizandrin B on hepatic injury in mice. *Chin Med J (Engl).* 1977;3:173-179.

5. Li XY. Bioactivity of neolignans from Fructus Schizandrae. *Mem Inst Oswaldo Cruz.* 1991;86:31-37.

6. Liu GT Pharmacological actions and clinical use of *Fructus Schizandrae.* *Chin Med J (Engl).* 1989;102:740-749.

7. Ahumada F, Hermosilla J, Hola R, et al. Studies on the effect of *Schizandra chinensis* extract on horses submitted to exercise and maximum effort. *Pytother Res.* 1989; 3:175-179.

8. Ahumada F, Hola R, Wikman G, et al. Effect of *Schizandra chinensis* extract on thoroughbreds in sprint races. *Equine Athlete.* 1991;4:1, 4-5.

9. Hancke J, Burgos R, Caceres D, et al. Reduction of serum hepatic transaminases and CPK in sport horses with poor performance treated with a standardized *Schizandra chinensis* fruit extract. *Phytomedicine.* 1996;3:237-240.

10. Liu J, Xiao PG. Recent advances in the study of antioxidative effects of Chinese medicinal plants. *Pytother Res.* 1994;8:445-451.
11. McGuffin M, ed. *American Herbal Products Association's Botanical Safety Handbook.* Boca Raton, Fla: CRC Press; 1997:104.

Selenium

1. Clark LC. The epidemiology of selenium and cancer. *Fed Proc.* 1985;44:2584-2589.
2. Guo W, Li J-Y, Blot WJ, et al. Correlations of dietary intake and blood nutrient levels with esophageal cancer mortality in China. *Nutr Cancer.* 1990;13:121-127.
3. Clark LC, Combs GF Jr, Turnbull BW, et al. Effects of selenium supplementation for cancer prevention in patients with carcinoma of the skin: a randomized controlled trial. Nutritional Prevention of Cancer Study Group. *JAMA.* 1996;276:1957-1963.
4. Yu SY, Zhu YJ, Li WG. Protective role of selenium against hepatitis B virus and primary liver cancer in Qidong. *Biol Trace Elem Res.* 1997;56:117-124.
5. van den Brandt PA, Goldbohm RA, van 't Veer P, et al. A prospective cohort study on selenium status and the risk of lung cancer. *Cancer Res.* 1993;53:4860-4865.
6. Garland M, Morris S, Stampfer MJ, et al. Prospective study of toenail selenium levels and cancer among women. *J Natl Cancer Inst.* 1995;87:497-505.
7. van den Brandt PA, Goldbohm RA, van 't Veer P, et al. Toenail selenium levels and the risk of breast cancer. *Am J Epidemiol.* 1994;140:20-26.
8. Tarp U. Selenium in rheumatoid arthritis: a review. *Analyst.* 1995;120:877-881.
9. Tarp U, Overvad K, Hansen JC, et al. Low selenium level in severe rheumatoid arthritis. *Scand J Rheumatol.* 1985;14:97-101.
10. Knekt P, Heliovaara M, Aho K, et al. Serum selenium, serum alpha-tocopherol, and the risk of rheumatoid arthritis. *Epidemiology.* 2000;11:402-405.
11. Peretz A, Neve J, Duchateau J, et al. Adjuvant treatment of recent onset rheumatoid arthritis by selenium supplementation: preliminary observations [letter]. *Br J Rheumatol.* 1992;31:281-286.
12. Neve J. Selenium as a risk factor for cardiovascular diseases. *J Cardiovasc Risk.* 1996;3:42-47.
13. Kardinaal AFM, Kok FJ, Kohlmeier L, et al. Association between toenail selenium and risk of acute myocardial infarction in European men: the EURAMIC study. *Am J Epidemiol.* 1997;145:373-379.
14. Beaglehole R, Jackson R, Watkinson J, et al. Decreased blood selenium and risk of myocardial infarction. *Int J Epidemiol.* 1990;19:918-922.
15. Kok FJ, Hofman A, Witteman JCM, et al. Decreased selenium levels in acute myocardial infarction. *JAMA.* 1989;261:1161-1164.
16. Salonen JT, Alfthan G, Huttunen JK. Association between cardiovascular death and myocardial infarction and serum selenium in a matched-pair longitudinal study. *Lancet.* 1982;2:175-179.
17. Korpela H, Kumpulainen J, Jussila E, et al. Effect of selenium supplementation after acute myocardial infarction. *Res Commun Chem Pathol Pharmacol.* 1989;65:249-252.
18. Ip C, Lisk DJ. Modulation of phase I and phase II xenobiotic-metabolizing enzymes by selenium-enriched garlic in rats. *Nutr Cancer.* 1997;28:184-188.
19. Kiremidjian-Schumacher L, Roy M, Wishe HI, et al. Supplementation with selenium and human immune cell functions. II. Effect on cytotoxic lymphocytes and natural killer cells. *Biol Trace Elem Res.* 1994;41:115-127.
20. Patterson BH, Levander OA. Naturally occurring selenium compounds in cancer chemoprevention trials: a workshop summary. *Cancer Epidemiol Biomarkers Prev.* 1997;6:63-69.
21. Roy M, Kiremidjian-Schumacher L, Wishe HI, et al. Supplementation with selenium restores age-related decline in immune cell function. *Proc Soc Exp Biol Med.* 1995;209:369-375.
22. Harrison PR, Lanfear J, Wu L, et al. Chemopreventive and growth inhibitory effects of selenium. *Biomed Environ Sci.* 1997;10:235-245.
23. Spallholz JE. Free radical generation by selenium compounds and their prooxidant toxicity. *Biomed Environ Sci.* 1997;10:260-270.

24. Sinha R, Medina D. Inhibition of cdk2 kinase activity by methylselenocysteine in synchronized mouse mammary epithelial tumor cells. *Carcinogenesis.* 1997;18:1541-1547.
25. Andersen O, Nielsen JB. Effects of simultaneous low-level dietary supplementation with inorganic and organic selenium on whole-body, blood, and organ levels of toxic metals in mice. *Environ Health Perspect.* 1994;102 (suppl 3):321-324.
26. Contempre B, Duale NL, Dumont JE, et al. Effect of selenium supplementation on thyroid hormone metabolism in an iodine and selenium deficient population. *Clin Endocrinol.* 1992;36:579-583.
27. Dietary Reference Intakes for Vitamin C, Vitamin E, Selenium, and Carotenoids (2000). Available at: http://www.nap.edu. Accessed October 4, 2001.
28. Fan AM, Kizer KW. Selenium: nutritional, toxicologic, and clinical aspects. *West J Med.* 1990;153:160-167.
29. Karunanithy R, Roy AC, Ratnam SS. Selenium status in pregnancy: studies in amniotic fluid from normal pregnant women. *Gynecol Obstet Invest.* 1989;27:148-150.
30. Hu YJ, Chen Y, Zhang YQ, et al. The protective role of selenium on the toxicity of cisplatin-contained chemotherapy regimen in cancer patients. *Biol Trace Elem Res.* 1997;56:331-341.
31. Peretz AM, Neve JD, Famaey JPP. Selenium in rheumatic diseases. *Semin Arthritis Rheum.* 1991;20:305-316.
32. Peretz A, Siderova V, Neve J. Selenium supplementation in rheumatoid arthritis investigated in a double blind placebo-controlled trial. *Scand J Rheumatol.* 2001; 30:208-212.
33. Petersson I, Majberger E, Palm S, et al. Treatment of rheumatoid arthritis with selenium and vitamin E [abstract]. *Scand J Rheumatol.* 1991;20:218.
34. Jantti J, Vapaatalo H, Seppala E, et al. Treatment of rheumatoid arthritis with fish oil selenium vitamins A and E and placebo [abstract]. *Scand J Rheumatol.* 1991;20:225.

Soy Protein

1. Anderson JW, Johnstone BM, Cook-Newell ME. Meta-analysis of the effects of soy protein intake on serum lipids. *N Engl J Med.* 1995;333:276-282.
2. Baum J, Teng H, Eerdman JW Jr, et al. Long-term intake of soy protein improves blood lipid profiles and increases mononuclear cell low-density-lipoprotein receptor messenger RNA in hypercholesterolemic, postmenopausal women. *Am J Clin Nutr.* 1998;68:545-551.
3. Teede HJ, Dalais FS, Kotsopoulos D, et al. Dietary soy has both beneficial and potentially adverse cardiovascular effects: a placebo-controlled study in men and postmenopausal women. *J Clin Endocrinol Metab.* 2001;86:3053-3060.
4. Han KK, Soares JM Jr, Haidar MA, et al. Benefits of soy isoflavone therapeutic regimen on menopausal symptoms. *Obstet Gynecol.* 2002;99(3):389-394.
5. Maskarinec G, Williams AE, Inouye JS, et al. A randomized isoflavone intervention among premenopausal women. *Cancer Epidemiol Biomarkers Prev.* 2002;11:195-201.
6. Kumar NB, Cantor A, Allen K, et al. The specific role of isoflavones on estrogen metabolism in premenopausal women. *Cancer.* 2002;94:1166-1174.
7. Xu X, Duncan AM, Merz BE, Kurzer MS. Effects of soy isoflavones on estrogen and phytoestrogen metabolism in premenopausal women. *Cancer Epidemiol Biomarkers Prev.* 1998;7:1101-1108.
8. Duncan AM, Underhill KEW, Xu X, Lavalleur J, Phipps WR, Kurzer MS. Modest hormonal effects of soy isoflavones in postmenopausal women. *J Clin Endocrinol Metab.* 1999;84:3479-3484.
9. Potter SM, Baum JA, Teng H, et al. Soy protein and isoflavones: their effects on blood lipids and bone density in postmenopausal women. *Am J Clin Nutr.* 1998;68 (6 suppl):1375S-1379S.
10. Alekel DL, Germain AS, Peterson CT, et al. Isoflavone-rich soy protein isolate attenuates bone loss in the lumbar spine of perimenopausal women. *Am J Clin Nutr.* 2000;72:844-852.
11. Harrison E, Adjei A, Ameho C, et al. The effect of soybean protein on bone loss in a rat model of postmenopausal osteoporosis. *J Nutr Sci Vitaminol.* 1998;44:257-268.

12. Fanti O, Faugere MC, Gang Z, et al. Systematic administration of genistein partially prevents bone loss in ovariectomized rats in a nonestrogen-like mechanism [abstract]. *Am J Clin Nutr.* 1998;68(suppl):1517S-1518S.

13. Arjmandi BH, Alekel L, Hollis BW, et al. Dietary soybean protein prevents bone loss in an ovariectomized rat model of osteoporosis. *J Nutr.* 1996;126:161-167.

14. Fanti P, Monier-Faugere MC, Geng Z, et al. The phytoestrogen genistein reduces bone loss in short-term ovariectomized rats. *Osteoporos Int.* 1998;8:274-281.

15. Anderson JJ, Ambrose WW, Garner SC. Biphasic effects of genistein on bone tissue in the ovariectomized, lactating rat model. *Proc Soc Exp Biol Med.* 1998;217:345-350.

16. Malochet S, Picherit C, Horcajada-Molteni MN, et al. Do endurance training and soy isoflavones exhibit additive effects on ovariectomy-induced osteopenia in the rat? [abstract]. *J Bone Miner Res.* 1999;14(suppl 1):S536.

17. Arjmandi BH, Birnbaum R, Goyal NV, et al. Bone-sparing effect of soy protein in ovarian hormone-deficient rats is related to its isoflavone content. *Am J Clin Nutr.* 1998;68(suppl):1364S-1368S.

18. Lees CJ, Ginn TA. Soy protein isolate diet does not prevent increased cortical bone turnover in ovariectomized macaques. *Calcif Tissue Int.* 1998;62:557-558.

19. Jayo MJ. Dietary soy isoflavones and bone loss: a study in ovariectomized monkeys [abstract]. *J Bone Miner Res.* 1996;11:S228.

20. Gallagher JC, Rafferty K, Haynatzka V, et al. The effect of soy protein on bone metabolism [abstract]. *J Nutr.* 2000;130:666S-669S.

21. Dalais F, Teede HJ, Kotsopoulos D, et al. The effects of dietary soy protein containing phytoestrogens on lipids and indices of bone turnover in postmenopausal women. Presented at: 83rd Annual Meeting of the Endocrine Society; June 20-23, 2001; Denver, Colo.

22. Goodman MT, Wilkens LR, Hankin JH, et al. Association of soy and fiber consumption with the risk of endometrial cancer. *Am J Epidemiol.* 1997;146:294-306.

23. Messina MJ, Persky V, Setchell KD, et al. Soy intake and cancer risk: a review of the in vitro and in vivo data. *Nutr Cancer.* 1994;21:113-131.

24. Barnes S, Peterson TG, Coward L. Rationale for the use of genistein-containing soy matrices in chemoprevention trials for breast and prostate cancer. *J Cell Biochem Suppl.* 1995;22:181-187.

25. Ingram D, Sanders K, Kolybaba M, et al. Case-control study of phyto-oestrogens and breast cancer. *Lancet.* 1997;350:990-994.

26. Adlercreutz H, Mazur W. Phyto-oestrogens and Western diseases. *Ann Med.* 1997; 29:95-120.

27. Day NE. Phyto-oestrogens and hormonally dependent cancers [abstract]. *Pathol Biol (Paris).* 1994;42:1090.

28. Nagata C, Kabuto M, Kurisu Y, et al. Decreased serum estradiol concentration associated with high dietary intake of soy products in premenopausal Japanese women. *Nutr Cancer.* 1997;29:228-233.

29. Nagata C, Takatsuka N, Inaba S, et al. Effect of soymilk consumption on serum estrogen concentrations in premenopausal Japanese women. *J Natl Cancer Inst.* 1998; 90:1830-1835.

30. Baber RJ, Templeman C, Morton T, et al. Randomized placebo-controlled trial of an isoflavone supplement and menopausal symptoms in women. *Climacteric.* 1999;2:85-92.

31. Knight DC, Howes JB, Eden JA. The effect of Promensil™, an isoflavone extract, on menopausal symptoms. *Climacteric.* 1999;2:79-84.

32. Crouse JR III, Morgan T, Terry JG, et al. A randomized trial comparing the effect of casein with that of soy protein containing varying amounts of isoflavones on plasma concentrations of lipids and lipoproteins. *Arch Intern Med.* 1999;159:2070-2076.

33. Greaves KA, Parks JS, Williams JK, et al. Intact dietary soy protein, but not adding an isoflavone-rich soy extract to casein, improves plasma lipids in ovariectomized cynomolgus monkeys. *J Nutr.* 1999;129:1585-1592.

34. Simons LA, von Konigsmark M, Simons J, et al. Phytoestrogens do not influence lipoprotein levels or endothelial function in healthy, postmenopausal women. *Am J Cardiol.* 2000;85:1297-1301.

35. Wangen KE, Duncan AM, Xu X, et al. Soy isoflavones improve plasma lipids in nor-mocholesterolemic and mildly hypercholesterolemic postmenopausal women. *Am J Clin Nutr.* 2001;73:225-231.

36. Anthony MS, Clarkson TB, Hughes CL Jr, et al. Soybean isoflavones improve car-diovascular risk factors without affecting the reproductive system of peripubertal rhesus monkeys. *J Nutr.* 1996;126:43-50.

37. Mackey R, Ekangaki A, Eden JA. The effects of soy protein in women and men with elevated plasma lipids. *Biofactors.* 2000;12:251-257.

38. Sirtori CR, Gianazza E, Manzoni C, et al. Role of isoflavones in the cholesterol re-duction by soy proteins in the clinic [letter]. *Am J Clin Nutr.* 1997;65:166-167.

39. Wei H, Bowen R, Cai Q, et al. Antioxidant and antipromotional effects of the soy-bean isoflavone genistein. *Proc Soc Exp Biol Med.* 1995;208:124-130.

40. Tham DM, Gardner CD, Haskell WL. Clinical review 97: potential health benefits of dietary phytoestrogens: a review of the clinical, epidemiological, and mechanistic evidence. *J Clin Endocrinol Metab.* 1998;83:2223-2235.

41. Werbach MR. *Foundations of Nutritional Medicine: A Sourcebook of Clinical Research.* Tarzana, Calif: Third Line Press; 1997:202.

42. Hallberg L, Rossander L, Skanberg AB. Phytates and the inhibitory effects of bran on iron absorption in man. *Am J Clin Nutr.* 1987;45:988-996.

43. Heaney RP, Weaver CM, Fitzsimmons ML. Soybean phytate content effects on cal-cium absorption. *Am J Clin Nutr.* 1991;53:745-747.

44. Divi RL, Chang HC, Doerge DR. Anti-thyroid isoflavones from soybean: isolation, characterization, and mechanisms of action. *Biochem Pharmacol.* 1997;54:1087-1096.

45. Chorazy PA, Himelhoch S, Hopwood NJ, et al. Persistent hypothyroidism in an in-fant receiving a soy formula: a case report and review of the literature. *Pediatrics.* 1995;96:148-150.

46. Jabbar MA, Larrea J, Shaw RA. Abnormal thyroid function tests in infants with con-genital hypothyroidism: the influence of soy-based formula. *J Am Coll Nutr.* 1997;16:280-282.

47. Lu LJW, Anderson KE, Grady JJ, Nagamani M. Effects of soya consumption for one month on steroid hormones in premenopausal women: implications for breast cancer risk reduction. *Cancer Epidemiol Biomarkers Prev.* 1996;5:63-70.

48. Massey LK, Palmer RG, Horner HT. Oxalate content of soybean seeds (Glycine max: Leguminosae), soyfoods, and other edible legumes. *J Agric Food Chem.* 2001; 49:4262-4266.

49. Martini MC, Dancisak BB, Haggans CJ, et al. Effects of soy intake on sex hormone metabolism in premenopausal women. *Nutr Cancer.* 1999;34:133-139.

50. Persky VW, et al. Effect of soy protein on endogenous hormones in postmenopausal women. *Am J Clin Nutr.* 2002;75:145-153.

51. Van Patten CL, Olivotto IA, Chambers GK, et al. Effect of soy phytoestrogens on hot flashes in postmenopausal women with breast cancer: a randomized, controlled clinical trial. *J Clin Oncol.* 2002;20:1449-1455.

52. St. Germain A, Peterson CT, Robinson JG, et al. Isoflavone-rich or isoflavone-poor soy protein does not reduce menopausal symptoms during 24 weeks of treatment. *Menopause.* 2001;8:17-26.

53. Washburn S, Burke GL, Morgan T, et al. Effect of soy protein supplementation on serum lipoproteins, blood pressure, and menopausal symptoms in perimenopausal women. *Menopause.* 1999;6:7-13.

54. Brzezinski A, Adlercreutz H, Shaoul R, et al. Short-term effects of phytoestrogen-rich diet on postmenopausal women. *Menopause.* 1997;4:89-94.

55. Albertazzi P, Pansini F, Bonaccorsi G, et al. The effect of dietary soy supplementa-tion on hot flushes. *Obstet Gynecol.* 1998;91:6-11.

56. Kotsopoulos D, Dalais FS, Liang YL, et al. The effects of soy protein containing phytoestrogens on menopausal symptoms in postmenopausal women. *Climacteric.* 2000;3:161-167.

57. Dewell A, Hollenbeck CB, Bruce B. The effects of soy-derived phytoestrogens on serum lipids and lipoproteins in moderately hypercholesterolemic postmenopausal women. *J Clin Endocrinol Metab.* 2002;87:118-121.

58. Setchell KD, Brown NM, Desai P, et al. Bioavailability of pure isoflavones in healthy humans and analysis of commercial soy isoflavone supplements. *J Nutr.* 2001;131 (4 suppl):1362S-1375S.

Spirulina

1. Dillon JC, Phuc AP, Dubacq JP. Nutritional value of the alga *Spirulina. World Rev Nutr Diet.* 1995;77:32-46.
2. Merchant RE, Andre CA. A review of recent clinical trials of the nutritional supplement *Chlorella pyrenoidosa* in the treatment of fibromyalgia, hypertension, and ulcerative colitis. *Altern Ther Health Med.* 2001;7:79-80, 82-91.
3. Iwata K, Inayama T, Kato T. Effects of *Spirulina platensis* on plasma lipoprotein lipase activity in fructose-induced hyperlipidemic rats. *J Nutr Sci Vitaminol.* 1990;36: 165-171.
4. Gonzalez de Rivera C, Miranda-Zamora R, Diaz-Zagoya JC, et al. Preventive effect of *Spirulina maxima* on the fatty liver induced by a fructose-rich diet in the rat, a preliminary report. *Life Sci.* 1993;53:57-61.
5. Nakaya N, Homma Y, Goto Y. Cholesterol lowering effect of *Spirulina. Nutr Rep Int.* 1988;37:1329-1337.
6. Schwartz J, Shklar G, Reid S, et al. Prevention of experimental oral cancer by extracts of *Spirulina-Dunaliella* algae. *Nutr Cancer.* 1988;11:127-134.
7. Mathew B, Sankaranarayanan R, Nair PP, et al. Evaluation of chemoprevention of oral cancer with *Spirulina fusiformis. Nutr Cancer.* 1995;24:197-202.
8. Mishima T, Murata J, Toyoshima M, et al. Inhibition of tumor invasion and metastasis by calcium spirulan (Ca-SP), a novel sulfated polysaccharide derived from a blue-green alga, *Spirulina platensis. Clin Exp Metastasis.* 1998;16:541-550.
9. Ayehunie S, Belay A, Baba TW, et al. Inhibition of HIV-1 replication by an aqueous extract of *Spirulina platensis (Arthrospira platensis). J Acquir Immune Defic Syndr Hum Retrovirol.* 1998;18:7-12.
10. Hayashi K, Hayashi T, Kojima I. A natural sulfated polysaccharide, calcium spirulan, isolated from *Spirulina platensis:* in vitro and ex vivo evaluation of anti-herpes simplex virus and anti-human immunodeficiency virus activities. *AIDS Res Hum Retro-viruses.* 1996;12:1463-1471.
11. Baeten JM, Mostad SB, Hughes MP, et al. Selenium deficiency is associated with shedding of HIV-1-infected cells in the female genital tract. *J Acquir Immune Defic Syndr.* 2001;26:360-364.
12. Qureshi MA, Ali RA. *Spirulina platensis* exposure enhances macrophage phagocytic function in cats. *Immunopharmacol Immunotoxicol.* 1996;18:457-463.
13. Qureshi MA, Garlich JD, Kidd MT. Dietary *Spirulina platensis* enhances humoral and cell-mediated immune functions in chickens. *Immunopharmacol Immunotoxicol.* 1996;18:465-476.
14. Hayashi O, Katoh T, Okuwaki Y. Enhancement of antibody production in mice by dietary *Spirulina platensis. J Nutr Sci Vitaminol.* 1994;40:431-441.
15. Kim HM, Lee EH, Cho HH, et al. Inhibitory effect of mast cell-mediated immediate-type allergic reactions in rats by spirulina. *Biochem Pharmacol.* 1998;55:1071-1076.
16. Yang HN, Lee EH, Kim HM. *Spirulina platensis* inhibits anaphylactic reaction. *Life Sci.* 1997;61:1237-1244.
17. Torres-Duran PV, Miranda-Zamora R, Paredes-Carbajal MC, et al. *Spirulina maxima* prevents induction of fatty liver by carbon tetrachloride in the rat. *Biochem Mol Biol Int.* 1998;44:787-793.
18. Vadiraja BB, Gaikwad NW, Madyastha KM. Hepatoprotective effect of C-phycocyanin: protection for carbon tetrachloride and R-(+)-pulegone-mediated hepatotoxicity in rats. *Biochem Biophys Res Commun.* 1998;249:428-431.
19. Becker EW, Jakober B, Luft D, et al. Clinical and biochemical evaluations of the alga *Spirulina* with regard to its application in the treatment of obesity: a double-blind cross-over study. *Nutr Rep Int.* 1986;33:565-574.
20. Salazar M, Chamorro GA, Salazar S, et al. Effect of *Spirulina maxima* consumption on reproduction and peri- and postnatal development in rats. *Food Chem Toxicol.* 1996;34:353-359.

21. Chamorro GA, Herrera G, Salazar M, et al. Short-term toxicity study of *Spirulina* in F3b generation rats. *J Toxicol Clin Exp.* 1988;8:163-167.
22. *Review of Natural Products.* St. Louis Mo: Facts and Comparisons; 1998: *Spirulina* monograph.
23. Johnson PE, Shubert LE. Accumulation of mercury and other elements by spirulina *(Cyanophyceae). Nutr Rep Int.* 1986;34:1063-1070.
24. Slotton DG, Goldman CR, Franke A. Commercially grown spirulina found to contain low levels of mercury and lead. *Nutr Rep Int.* 1989;40:1165-1171.
25. Pouria S, de Andrade A, Barbosa J, et al. Fatal microcystin intoxication in haemodialysis unit in Caruaru, Brazil. *Lancet.* 1998;352:21-26.
26. Gilroy DJ, Kauffman KW, Hall RA, et al. Assessing potential health risks from microcystin toxins in blue-green algae dietary supplements. *Environ Health Perspect.* 2000;108:435-439.
27. Islam MS, Rahim Z, Alam MJ, et al. Association of *Vibrio cholerae* O1 with the cyanobacterium, *Anabaena sp.,* elucidated by polymerase chain reaction and transmission electron microscopy. *Trans R Soc Trop Med Hyg.* 1999;93:36-40.

St. John's Wort

1. Laakmann G, Schule C, Baghai T, et al. St. John's wort in mild to moderate depression: the relevance of hyperforin for the clinical efficacy. *Pharmacopsychiatry.* 1998;31(suppl 1):54-59.
2. Schrader E, Meier B, Brattstrom A. *Hypericum* treatment of mild-moderate depression in a placebo-controlled study: a prospective, double-blind, randomized, placebo-controlled, multicentre study. *Hum Psychopharmacol.* 1998;13:163-169.
3. Schrader E. Equivalence of St John's wort extract (Ze 117) and fluoxetine: a randomized, controlled study in mild-moderate depression. *Int Clin Psychopharmacol.* 2000;15:61-68.
4. Harrer G, Schmidt U, Kuhn U, et al. Comparison of equivalence between the St. John's wort extract LoHyp-57 and fluoxetine. *Arzneimittelforschung.* 1999;49:289-296.
5. Brenner R, Azbel V, Madhusoodanan S, et al. Comparison of an extract of *Hypericum* (LI 160) and sertraline in the treatment of depression: a double-blind, randomized pilot study. *Clin Ther.* 2000;22:411-419.
6. Philipp M, Kohnen R, Hiller KO. *Hypericum* extract versus imipramine or placebo in patients with moderate depression: randomized multicentre study of treatment for eight weeks. *BMJ.* 1999;319:1534-1539.
7. Woelk H. Comparison of St John's wort and imipramine for treating depression: randomized controlled trial. *BMJ.* 2000;321:536-539.
8. Hansgen KD, Vesper J. Antidepressant efficacy of a high-dose *Hypericum* extract [translated from German]. *MMW Munch Med Wochenschr.* 1996;138:29-33.
9. Linde K, Ramirez G, Mulrow CD, et al. St John's wort for depression—an overview and meta-analysis of randomized clinical trials. *BMJ.* 1996;313:253-258.
10. Kalb R, Trautmann-Sponsel RD, Kieser M. Efficacy and tolerability of *Hypericum* extract WS 5572 versus placebo in mildly to moderately depressed patients: a randomized double-blind multicenter clinical trial. *Pharmacopsychiatry.* 2001;34:96-103.
11. Shelton RC, Keller MB, Gelenberg A, et al. Effectiveness of St. John's wort in major depression: a randomized controlled trial. *JAMA.* 2001;285:1978-1986.
12. Vorbach EU, Arnoldt KH, Hubner WD. Efficacy and tolerability of St. John's wort extract LI 160 vs. imipramine in patients with severe depressive episodes according to ICD-10. *Pharmacopsychiatry.* 1997;30(suppl 2):81-85.
13. Sindrup SH, Madsen C, Bach FW, et al. St. John's wort has no effect on pain in polyneuropathy. *Pain.* 2001;91:361-365.
14. Martinez B, Kasper S, Ruhrmann S, et al. *Hypericum* in the treatment of seasonal affective disorders. *J Geriatr Psychiatry Neurol.* 1994;7(suppl 1):S29-S33.
15. Werth W. Psychotonin® M versus imipramine in surgery [in German]. *Der Kassenarzt.* 1989;15:64-68.
16. Hubner W-D, Lande S, Podzuweit H. *Hypericum* treatment of mild depressions with somatic symptons. *J Geriatr Psychiatry Neurol.* 1994;7(suppl 1):S12-S14.

17. Stevinson C, Ernst E. A pilot study of *Hypericum perforatum* for the treatment of premenstrual syndrome. *Br J Obstet Gynaecol.* 2000;107:870-876.

18. Grube B, Walper A, Wheatley D. St. John's Wort extract: efficacy for menopausal symptoms of psychological origin. *Adv Ther.* 1999;16:177-186.

19. Schulz H, Jobert M. The influence of *Hypericum* extract on the sleep EEG in older volunteers [in German; English abstract]. *Nervenheilkunde.* 1993;12:323-327.

20. Gulick RM, McAuliffe V, Holden-Wiltse J, et al. Phase I studies of hypericin, the active compound in St. John's wort, as an antiretroviral agent in HIV-infected adults. AIDS Clinical Trials Group Protocols 150 and 258. *Ann Intern Med.* 1999;130:510-514.

21. Suzuki O, Satsumata Y, Oya M, et al. Inhibition of monoamine oxidase by hypericin. *Planta Med.* 1984;50:272-274.

22. Bladt S, Wagner H. Inhibition of MAO by fractions and constituents of *Hypericum* extract. *J Geriatr Psychiatry Neurol.* 1994;7(suppl 1):S57-S59.

23. Thiede HM, Walper A. Inhibition of MAO and COMT by *Hypericum* extracts and hypericin. *J Geriatr Psychiatry Neurol.* 1994;7(suppl 1):S54-S56.

24. Muller WE, Kasper S. *Hypericum* extract (Li 160) as a herbal antidepressant. *Pharmacopsychiatry.* 1997;30(suppl 2):71-134.

25. Muller WE, Singer A, Wonnemann M, et al. Hyperforin represents the neurotransmitter reuptake inhibiting constituent of *Hypericum* extract. *Pharmacopsychiatry.* 1998;31(suppl 1):16-21.

26. Muller WEG, Rossol R. Effects of *Hypericum* extract on the expression of serotonin receptors. *J Geriatr Psychiatry Neurol.* 1994;7(suppl 1):S63-S64.

27. Teufel-Mayer R, Gleitz J. Effects of long-term administration of hypericum extracts on the affinity and density of the central serotonergic 5-HT1 A and 5-HT2 A receptors. *Pharmacopsychiatry.* 1997;30(suppl):113-116.

28. Butterweck V, Winterhoff H, Herkenham M. St John's wort, hypericin, and imipramine: a comparative analysis of mRNA levels in brain areas involved in HPA axis control following short-term and long-term administration in normal and stressed rats. *Mol Psychiatry.* 2001;6:547-564.

29. Bhattacharya SK, Chakrabarti A, Chatterjee SS. Activity profiles of two hyperforin-containing *Hypericum* extracts in behavioral models. *Pharmacopsychiatry.* 1998;31 (suppl 1):22-29.

30. Baureithel KH, Buter KB, Engesser A, et al. Inhibition of benzodiazepine binding in vitro by amentoflavone, a constituent of various species of *Hypericum*. *Pharm Acta Helv.* 1997;72:153-157.

31. Cott JM. In vitro receptor binding and enzyme inhibition by *Hypericum perforatum* extract. *Pharmacopsychiatry.* 1997;30(suppl 2):108-112.

32. Butterweck V, Jurgenliemk G, Nahrstedt A, et al. Flavonoids from *Hypericum perforatum* show antidepressant activity in the forced swimming test. *Planta Med.* 2000;66:3-6.

33. Dimpfel W, Schober F, Mannel M. Effects of a methanolic extract and a hyperforin-enriched CO_2 extract of St. John's wort *(Hypericum perforatum)* on intracerebral field potentials in the freely moving rat (Tele-Stereo-EEG). *Pharmacopsychiatry.* 1998;31(suppl):30-35.

34. Woelk H, Burkard G, Grunwald J. Benefits and risks of the *Hypericum* extract LI 160: drug monitoring study with 3250 patients. *J Geriatr Psychiatry Neurol.* 1994;7(suppl 1):S34-S38.

35. Hubner WD, Arnoldt KH. St John's wort: a one year treatment study [in German; English abstract]. *Z Phytother.* 2000;21:306-310.

36. Schulz V, Hansel R, Tyler VE. *Rational Phytotherapy: A Physicians' Guide to Herbal Medicine.* 3rd ed. Berlin, Germany: Springer-Verlag; 1998:52, 54-56.

37. Vukovic-Gacic B, Simic D. Identification of natural antimutagens with modulating effects on DNA repair. *Basic Life Sci.* 1993;61:269-277.

38. Miskovsky P, Chinsky L, Wheeler GV, et al. Hypericin site specific interactions within polynucleotides used as DNA model compounds. *J Biomol Struct Dyn.* 1995;13:547-552.

39. Nierenberg AA, Burt T, Matthews J, et al. Mania associated with St. John's wort. *Biol Psychiatry.* 1999;46:1707-1708.

40. Barbenel DM, Yusufi B, O'Shea D, et al. Mania in a patient receiving testosterone replacement postorchidectomy taking St John's wort and sertraline. *J Psychopharmacol.* 2000;14:84-86.

41. Brockmoller J, Reum T, Bauer S, et al. Hypericin and pseudohypericin: pharmacokinetics and effects on photosensitivity in humans. *Pharmacopsychiatry.* 1997;30 (suppl):94-101.

42. Lane-Brown MM. Photosensitivity associated with herbal preparations of St John's wort *(Hypericum perforatum)* [letter]. *Med J Aust.* 2000;172:302.

43. Roberts JE, Wang RH, Tan IP, et al. Hypericin (active ingredients in St. John's wort) photooxidation of lens proteins [abstract]. *Photochem Photobiol.* 1999;69(suppl):42S.

44. Ellis KA, Stough C, Vitetta L, et al. An investigation into the acute nootropic effects of *Hypericum perforatum* L. (St. John's wort) in healthy human volunteers. *Behav Pharmacol.* 2001;12:173-182.

45. Rayburn WF, Gonzalez CL, Christensen HD, et al. Effect of prenatally administered *Hypericum* (St John's wort) on growth and physical maturation of mouse offspring. *Am J Obstet Gynecol.* 2001;184:191-195.

46. Breidenbach T, Kliem V, Burg M, et al. Profound drop of cyclosporin A whole blood trough levels caused by St. John's wort *(Hypericum perforatum)* [letter]. *Transplantation.* 2000;69:2229-2230.

47. Jobst K, McIntyre M, St George D, et al. Safety of St. John's wort *(Hypericum perforatum)* [letters]. *Lancet.* 2000;355:575-577.

48. Johne A, Brockmuller J, Bauer S, et al. Pharmacokinetic interaction of digoxin with an herbal extract from St. John's wort *(Hypericum perforatum).* *Clin Pharmacol Ther.* 1999;66:338-345.

49. Maurer A, Johne A, Bauer S, et al. Interaction of St. John's wort extract with phenprocoumon [abstract]. *Eur J Clin Pharmacol.* 1999;55:A22.

50. Nebel A, Schneider BJ, Baker R, et al. Potential metabolic interaction between St. John's wort and theophylline [letter]. *Ann Pharmacother.* 1999;33:502.

51. Piscitelli SC, Burstein AH, Chaitt D, et al. Indinavir concentrations and St. John's wort [letter]. *Lancet.* 2000;355:547-548.

52. Ruschitzka F, Meier PJ, Turina M, et al. Acute heart transplant rejection due to St. John's wort [letter]. *Lancet.* 2000;355:548-549.

53. Dresser GK, Schwarz UI, Wilkinson GR, et al. St. John's wort induces intestinal and hepatic CYP3A4 and P-glycoprotein in healthy volunteers [abstract]. *Clin Pharmacol Ther.* 2001;69:P23.

54. Barone GW, Gurley BJ, Ketel BL, et al. Drug interaction between St. John's wort and cyclosporine. *Ann Pharmacother.* 2000;34:1013-1016.

55. Obach RS. Inhibition of human cytochrome P450 enzymes by constituents of St. John's wort, an herbal preparation used in the treatment of depression. *J Pharmacol Exp Ther.* 2000;294:88-95.

56. Moore LB, Goodwin B, Jones SA, et al. St. John's wort induces hepatic drug metabolism through activation of the pregnane X receptor. *Proc Natl Acad Sci USA.* 2000;97:7500-7502.

57. Baker RK, Brandt TL, Siegel D, et al. Inhibition of human DNA topoisomerase II-alpha by the naphtha-di-anthrone, hypericin [abstract]. *Proc Annu Meet Am Assoc Cancer Res.* 1998;39:422.

58. DeMott K. St. John's wort tied to serotonin syndrome. *Clin Psychiatry News.* 1998; 26(3):28.

59. Gordon JB. SSRIs and St. John's wort: possible toxicity? [letter]. *Am Fam Physician.* 1998;57:950, 953.

60. Lantz MS, Buchalter E, Giambanco V. St. John's wort and antidepressant drug interactions in the elderly. *J Geriatr Psychiatry Neurol.* 1999;12:7-10.

61. Mirossay A, Mirossay L, Tothova J, et al. Potentiation of hypericin and hypocrellin-induced phototoxicity by omeprazole. *Phytomedicine.* 1999;6:311-317.

62. Hypericum Depression Trial Study Group. Effect of *Hypericum perforatum* (St. John's wort) in major depressive disorder: a randomized controlled trial. *JAMA.* 2002; 287:1807-1814.

63. Randlov C, Thomsen C, Winther K, et al. Effects of hypericum in mild to moderately depressed outpatients—a placebo-controlled clinical trial [abstract]. *Altern Ther Health Med.* 2001;7:108.

64. Behnke K, Jensen GS, Graubaum HJ, et al. *Hypericum perforatum* versus fluoxetine in the treatment of mild to moderate depression. *Adv Ther.* 2002;19:43-52.

65. Siegers CP, Biel S, Wilhelm KP. Phototoxicity caused by hypericum [translated from German]. *Nervenheilkunde.* 1993;12:320-322.

66. Schempp CM, et al. Single-dose and steady-state administration of *Hypericum perforatum* extract (St. John's wort) does not influence skin sensitivity to UV radiation, visible light, and solar-simulated radiation. *Arch Dermatol.* 2001;137:512-513.

67. Parker V, Wong AH, Boon HS, et al. Adverse reactions to St John's wort. *Can J Psychiatry.* 2001; 46:77-79.

68. Laird RD, Webb M. Psychotic episode during use of St. John's wort. *J Herbal Pharmacother.* 2001;1:81-87.

69. Hubner WD, Kirste T. Experience with St John's wort *(Hypericum perforatum)* in children under 12 years with symptoms of depression and psychovegetative disturbances. *Phytother Res.* 2001;15:367-370.

70. Dresser GK, Schwarz UI, Wilkinson GR, et al. St. John's wort induces intestinal and hepatic CYP3A4 and P-glycoprotein in healthy volunteers [abstract]. *Clin Pharmacol Ther.* 2001;69:P23.

71. Gorski JC, Hamman MA, Wang Z, et al. The effect of St. John's wort on the efficacy of oral contraception. American Society for Clinical Pharmacology and Therapeutics Annual Meeting, March 24-27, 2002, Atlanta, Ga; abstract MPI-80.

72. Sugimoto Ki K, Ohmori M, Tsuruoka S, et al. Different effects of St John's wort on the pharmacokinetics of simvastatin and pravastatin. *Clin Pharmacol Ther.* 2001; 70:518-524.

73. Durr D, Stieger B, Kullak-Ublick GA, et al. St John's wort induces intestinal P-glycoprotein/MDR1 and intestinal and hepatic CYP3A4. *Clin Pharmacol Ther.* 2000;68:598-604.

74. de Maat MM, Hoetelmans RM, Mathot RA, et al. Drug interaction between St. John's wort and nevirapine [letter]. *AIDS.* 2001;15:420-421.

75. Mai I, Kruger H, Budde K, et al. Hazardous pharmacokinetic interaction of Saint John's wort *(Hypericum perforatum)* with the immunosuppressant cyclosporin. *Int J Clin Pharmacol Ther.* 2000;38:500-502.

76. Roots I, Johne A, Schmider J, et al. Interaction of a herbal extract from St. John's wort with amitriptyline and its metabolites [abstract]. *Clin Pharmacol Ther.* 2000; 67:159.

77. Diminished effect of birth control pill with concurrent use of SJW has led to unwanted pregnancy. http://www.mpa.se/. Accessed June 10, 2002.

Taurine

1. Azuma J, Sawamura A, Awata N, et al. Double-blind randomized crossover trial of taurine in congestive heart failure. *Curr Ther Res.* 1983;34:543-557.

2. Azuma J, Sawamura A, Awata N, et al. Therapeutic effect of taurine in congestive heart failure: a double-blind crossover trial. *Clin Cardiol.* 1985;8:276-282.

3. Azuma J, Takihara K, Awata N, et al. Taurine and failing heart: experimental and clinical aspects. *Prog Clin Biol Res.* 1985;179:195-213.

4. Azuma J, Hasegawa H, Sawamura A, Awata N, et al. Therapy of congestive heart failure with orally administered taurine. *Clin Ther.* 1983;5:398-408.

5. Takihara K, Azuma J, Awata N, et al. Beneficial effect of taurine in rabbits with chronic congestive heart failure. *Am Heart J.* 1986;112:1278-1284.

6. Azuma J, Takihara K, Awata N, et al. Beneficial effect of taurine on congestive heart failure induced by chronic aortic regurgitation in rabbits. *Res Commun Chem Pathol Pharmacol.* 1984;45:261-270.

7. Azuma J, Sawamura A, Awata N. Usefulness of taurine in chronic congestive heart failure and its prospective application. *Jpn Circ J.* 1992;56:95-99.

8. Matsuyama Y, Morita T, Higuchi M, et al. The effect of taurine administration on patients with acute hepatitis. *Prog Clin Biol Res.* 1983;125:461-468.

9. Podda M, Ghezzi C, Battezzati PM, et al. Effects of ursodeoxycholic acid and taurine on serum liver enzymes and bile acids in chronic hepatitis. *Gastroenterology.* 1990; 98:1044-1050.
10. Yamori Y, et al. Studies on stroke prevention in animal models, and their supportable epidemiological evidence. In: Barnett HJ, ed. *Cerebrovascular Diseases: New Trends in Surgical and Medical Aspects.* Amsterdam, the Netherlands: Elsevier/North Holland Biomedical Press; 1981;47-62.
11. Franconi F, Bennardini F, Mattana A, et al. Plasma and platelet taurine are reduced in subjects with insulin-dependent diabetes mellitus: effects of taurine supplementation. *Am J Clin Nutr.* 1995;61:1115-1119.
12. Marchesi GF, Quattrini A, Scarpino O, et al. Therapeutic effects of taurine in epilepsy: a clinical and polyphysiographic study [in Italian; English abstracts]. *Riv Patol Nerv Ment.* 1975;96:166-184.
13. Fukuyama Y, Ochiai Y. Therapeutic trial by taurine for intractable childhood epilepsies. *Brain Dev.* 1982;4:63-69.

Tea Tree Oil

1. May J, Chan CH, King A, et al. Time-kill studies of tea tree oils on clinical isolates. *J Antimicrob Chemother.* 2000;45:639-643.
2. Tong MM, Altman PM, Barnetson RS. Tea tree oil in the treatment of tinea pedis. *Australas J Dermatol.* 1992;33:145-149.
3. Bassett IB, Pannowitz DL, Barnetson RS. A comparative study of tea-tree oil versus benzoylperoxide in the treatment of acne. *Med J Aust.* 1990;153:455-458.
4. Pena EF. Melaleuca alternifolia oil: its use for trichomonal vaginitis and other vaginal infections. *Obstet Gynecol.* 1962;19:793-795.
5. Vazquez JA, Vaishampayan J, Arganoza MT, et al. Use of an over-the-counter product, Breathaway (Melaleuca Oral Solution), as an alternative agent for refractory oropharyngeal candidiasis in AIDS patients [abstract]. *Int Conf AIDS.* 1996;11:109.
6. Lippert U, Walter A, Hausen B, et al. Increasing incidence of contact dermatitis to tea tree oil [abstract]. *J Allergy Clin Immunol.* 2000;105(1 pt 2):A127.
7. Carson CF, Ashton L, Dry L, et al. *Melaleuca alternifolia* (tea tree) oil gel (6%) for the treatment of recurrent *herpes labialis. J Antimicrob Chemother.* 2001;48:450-451.

Thymus Extract

1. Fiocchi A, Borella E, Riva E, et al. A double-blind clinical trial for the evaluation of the therapeutical effectiveness of a calf thymus derivative (thymomodulin) in children with recurrent respiratory infections. *Thymus.* 1986;8:331-339.
2. Garagiola U, Buzzetti M, Cardella E. Immunological patterns during regular intensive training in athletes: quantification and evaluation of a preventive pharmacological approach. *J Int Med Res.* 1995;23:85-95.
3. Civeira MP, Castilla A, Morte S, et al. A pilot study of thymus extract in chronic non-A, non-B hepatitis. *Aliment Pharmacol Ther.* 1989;3:395-401.
4. Bortolotti F, Cadrobbi P, Crivellaro C, et al. Effect of an orally administered thymic derivative, thymomodulin, in chronic type B hepatitis in children. *Curr Ther Res.* 1988;43:67-72.
5. Galli M, Crocchiolo P, Negri C, et al. Attempt to treat acute type B hepatitis with an orally administered thymic extract (thymomodulin): preliminary results. *Drugs Exp Clin Res.* 1985;11:665-669.
6. Raymond RS, Fallon MB, Abrams GA. Oral thymic extract for chronic hepatitis C in patients previously treated with interferon: a randomized, double-blind, placebo-controlled trial. *Ann Intern Med.* 1998;129:797-800.
7. Cavagni G, Piscopo E, Rigoli E, et al. Food allergy in children: an attempt to improve the effects of the elimination diet with an immunomodulating agent (thymomodulin). A double-blind clinical trial. *Immunopharmacol Immunotoxicol.* 1989;11:131-142.
8. Bagnato A, Brovedani P, Comina P, et al. Long-term treatment with thymomodulin reduces airway hyperresponsiveness to methacholine. *Ann Allergy.* 1989;62:425-428.
9. Skotnicki AB. Therapeutic application of calf thymus extract (TFX). *Med Oncol Tumor Pharmacother.* 1989;6:31-43.

10. Leung DY, Hirsch RL, Schneider L, et al. Thymopentin therapy reduces the clinical severity of atopic dermatitis. *J Allergy Clin Immunol.* 1990;85:927-933.
11. Beall G, Kruger S, Morales F, et al. A double-blind, placebo-controlled trial of thymostimulin in symptomatic HIV-infected patients. *AIDS.* 1990;4:679-681.
12. Harper JI, Mason UA, White TR, et al. A double-blind placebo-controlled study of thymostimulin (TP-1) for the treatment of atopic eczema. *Br J Dermatol.* 1991;125: 368-372.
13. Roullet E, Cesaro P, Simon-Lavoine N, et al. Nonathymulin treatment of multiple sclerosis: double-blind pilot study. *Acta Neurol Scand.* 1989;80:575-578.
14. Fransen L, Anthoons J, Hoogewijs G, et al. Thymopentin treatment in genital warts of long duration. *Cancer Detect Prev.* 1988;12:503-509.
15. Malaise M, Franchimont P, Hauwaert C, et al. Confirmative study of the effectiveness of thymopentin in active rheumatoid arthritis. *Surv Immunol Res.* 1985;4(suppl 1):87-93.
16. Bolla K, Djawari D, Kokoschka EM, et al. Prevention of recurrences in frequently relapsing herpes labialis with thymopentin: a randomized double-blind placebo-controlled multicenter study. *Surv Immunol Res.* 1985;4(suppl 1):37-47.
17. Kouttab NM, Prada M, Cazzola P. Thymomodulin: biological properties and clinical applications. *Med Oncol Tumor Pharmacother.* 1989;6:5-9.
18. Norton SA. Raw animal tissues and dietary supplements [letter]. *N Engl J Med.* 2000;343:304-305.

Tribulus

1. Wang B, Ma L, Liu T. 406 cases of angina pectoris in coronary heart disease treated with saponin of *Tribulus terrestris* [in Chinese; English abstract]. *Zhong Xi Yi Jie He Za Zhi.* 1990;10:68,85-87.
2. Anand R, Patnaik GK, Kulshreshtha DK, et al. Activity of certain fractions of *Tribulus terrestris* fruits against experimentally induced urolithiasis in rats. *Indian J Exp Biol.* 1994;32:548-552.
3. Antonio J, Uelmen J, Rodriguez R, et al. The effects of *Tribulus terrestris* on body composition and exercise performance in resistance-trained males. *Int J Sport Nutr Exerc Metab.* 2000;10:208-215.
4. Bourke CA, Stevens GR, Carrigan MJ. Locomotor effects in sheep of alkaloids identified in Australian *Tribulus terrestris*. *Aust Vet J.* 1992;69:163-165.
5. Bourke CA. Staggers in sheep associated with the ingestion of *Tribulus terrestris*. *Aust Vet J.* 1984;61:360-363.
6. Bourke CA. A novel nigrostriatal dopaminergic disorder in sheep affected by *Tribulus terrestris* staggers. *Res Vet Sci.* 1987;43:347-350.
7. Kumanov F, Bozadzhieva E, Andreeva M, et al. Clinical trial of the drug "Tribestan." *Savr Med.* 1982;4:211-215.
8. Protich M, Tsvetkov D, Nalbanski B, et al. Clinical trial of the preparation Tribestan in infertile men. *Akush Ginekol.* 1983;22(4):326-329.
9. Tanev G, Zarkova S. Toxicological studies on Tribestan. Cited in Zarkova S. *Tribestan: Experimental and Clinical Investigations.* Sofia, Bulgaria: Chemical Pharmaceutical Research Institute; 1985.
10. Viktorov IV, Kaloyanov AL, Lilov L, et al. Clinical investigation on Tribestan in males with disorders in the sexual function. *Med-Biol Inf.* 1982. Cited in Zarkova S. *Tribestan: Experimental and Clinical Investigations.* Sofia, Bulgaria. Chemical Pharmaceutical Research Institute, 1982.
11. Zarkova S. *Tribestan: Experimental and Clinical Investigations.* Sofia, Bulgaria: Chemical Pharmaceutical Research Institute; 1983.
12. Wang B, Ma L, Liu T. 406 cases of angina pectoris in coronary heart disease treated with saponin of *Tribulus terrestris*. *Chung His I Chieh Ho Tsa Chih.* 1990;10(2):85-87.
13. Adaikan PG, Gauthaman K, Prasad RN, Ng SC. Proerectile pharmacological effects of *Tribulus terrestris* extract on the rabbit corpus cavernosum. *Ann Acad Med Singapore.* 2000;29:22-26.
14. Li M, Qu W, Chu S, et al. Effect of the decoction of *Tribulus terrestris* on mice gluconeogenesis. *Zhong Yao Cai.* 2001;24:586-588.

15. Arcasoy HB, Erenmemisoglu A, Tekol Y, et al. Effect of *Tribulus terrestris* L. saponin mixture on some smooth muscle preparations: a preliminary study. *Boll Chim Farm.* 1998;137:473-475.

16. Sangeeta D, Sidhu H, Thind SK, et al. Effect of *Tribulus terrestris* on oxalate metabolism in rats. *J Ethnopharmacol.* 1994;44:61-66.

Tylophora

1. Shivpuri DN, Singhal SC, Parkash D. Treatment of asthma with an alcoholic extract of *Tylophora indica*: a cross-over, double-blind study. *Ann Allergy.* 1972;30:407-412.

2. Shivpuri DN, Menon MP, Prakash D. A crossover double-blind study on *Tylophora indica* in the treatment of asthma and allergic rhinitis. *J Allergy.* 1969;43:145-150.

3. Mathew KK, Shivpuri DN. Treatment of asthma with alkaloids of *Tylophora indica*: a double-blind study. *Aspects Allergy Appl Immunol.* 1974;7:166-179.

4. Gupta S, George P, Gupta V, et al. *Tylophora indica* in bronchial asthma—a double blind study. *Indian J Med Res.* 1979;69:981-989.

5. Gopalakrishnan C, Shankaranarayanan D, Nazimudeen SK, et al. Effect of tylophorine, a major alkaloid of *Tylophora indica*, on immunopathological and inflammatory reactions. *Indian J Med Res.* 1980;71:940-948.

6. Udupa AL, Udupa SL, Guruswamy MN. The possible site of anti-asthmatic action of *Tylophora asthmatica* on pituitary-adrenal axis in albino rats. *Planta Med.* 1991; 57:409-413.

7. Nandi M. Physical, chemical and biological assay of *Tylophora indica* mother tincture—a comparative study. *Br Homeopath J.* 1999;88:161-165.

8. Wagner H. Search for new plant constituents with potential antiphlogistic and antiallergic activity. *Planta Med.* 1989;55:235-241.

9. Dikshith TS, Raizada RB, Mulchandani NB. Toxicity of pure alkaloid of *Tylophora asthamatica* in male rat. *Indian J Exp Biol.* 1990;28:208-212.

Tyrosine

1. Neri DF, Wiegmann D, Stanny RR, et al. The effects of tyrosine on cognitive performance during extended wakefulness. *Aviat Space Environ Med.* 1995;120:313-319.

2. Gibson CJ, Gelenberg A. Tyrosine for the treatment of depression. *Adv Biol Psychiatry.* 1983;10:148-159.

3. Gelenberg AJ, Wojcik JD, Falk WE, et al. Tyrosine for depression: a double-blind trial. *J Affect Disord.* 1990;19:125-132.

4. Eisenberg J, Asnis GM, van Praag HM, et al. Effect of tyrosine on attention deficit disorder with hyperactivity. *J Clin Psychiatry.* 1988;49:193-195.

5. Reimherr FW, Wender PH, Wood DR, et al. An open trial of L-tyrosine in the treatment of attention deficit disorder, residual type. *Am J Psychiatry.* 1987;144:1071-1073.

6. Wood DR, Reimherr FW, Wender PH. Amino acid precursors for the treatment of attention deficit disorder, residual type. *Psychopharmacol Bull.* 1985;21:146-149.

7. Deijen JB, Wientjes CJ, Vullinghs HF, et al. Tyrosine improves cognitive performance and reduces blood pressure in cadets after one week of a combat training course. *Brain Res Bull.* 1999;48:203-209.

Uva Ursi

1. Larsson B, Jonasson A, Fianu S. Prophylactic effect of UVA-E in women with recurrent cystitis: a preliminary report. *Curr Ther Res.* 1993;53:441-443.

2. Frohne D. The urinary disinfectant effect of extract from leaves *Uva-Ursi* [in German; English abstract]. *Planta Med.* 1970;18:1-25.

3. Schulz V, Hansel R, Tyler VE. *Rational Phytotherapy: A Physicians' Guide to Herbal Medicine.* 3rd ed. Berlin, Germany: Springer-Verlag; 1998:223, 224.

4. European Scientific Cooperative on Phytotherapy. *Uvae ursi folium* (bearberry leaf). Exeter, UK: ESCOP; 1996-1997. Monographs on the Medicinal Uses of Plant Drugs, Fascicule 5:1, 5.

5. Tyler VE. *Herbs of Choice: The Therapeutic Use of Phytochemicals.* New York, NY: Pharmaceutical Products Press; 1994.

Valerian

1. Vorbach EU, Goetelmeyer R, Bruening J. Therapy for insomniacs: effectiveness and tolerance of valerian preparations [translated from German]. *Psychopharmakotherapie*. 1996;3:109-115.

2. Leathwood PD, Chauffard F, Heck E, et al. Aqueous extract of valerian root (*Valeriana officinalis* L.) improves sleep quality in man. *Pharmacol Biochem Behav*. 1982;17:65-71.

3. Kamm-Kohl AV, Jansen W, Brockmann P. Modern valerian therapy for nervous disorders in old age [translated from German]. *Med Welt*. 1984;35:1450-1454.

4. Lindahl O, Lindwall L. Double blind study of a valerian preparation. *Pharmacol Biochem Behav*. 1989;32:1065-1066.

5. Schulz H, Stolz C, Muller J. The effect of valerian extract on sleep polygraphy in poor sleepers: a pilot study. *Pharmacopsychiatry*. 1994;27:147-151.

6. Donath F, Quispe S, Diefenbach K. Critical evaluation of the effect of valerian extract on sleep structure and sleep quality. *Pharmacopsychiatry*. 2000;33:47-53.

7. Dorn M. Efficacy and tolerability of *Baldrian* versus oxazepam in non-organic and non-psychiatric insomniacs: a randomized, double-blind, clinical, comparative study [translated from German]. *Forsch Komplementarmed Klass Naturheilkd*. 2000;7:79-84.

8. Cerny A, Schmid K. Tolerability and efficacy of valerian/lemon balm in healthy volunteers (a double-blind, placebo-controlled, multicentre study). *Fitoterapia*. 1999; 70:221-228.

9. Hendriks H, Bos R, Woerdenbag HJ, et al. Central nervous depressant activity of valerenic acid in the mouse. *Planta Med*. 1985;1:28-31.

10. Dressing H, Riemann D, Low H, et al. Insomnia: are valerian/balm combinations of equal value to benzodiazepines? [translated from German]. *Therapiewoche*. 1992; 42:726-736.

11. Kohnen R, Oswald WD. The effects of valerian, propranolol, and their combination on activation, performance and mood of healthy volunteers under social stress conditions. *Pharmacopsychiatry*. 1988;21:447-448.

12. Andreatini R, Leite JR. Effect of valepotriates on the behavior of rats in the elevated plus-maze during diazepam withdrawal. *Eur J Pharmacol*. 1994;260:233-235.

13. European Scientific Cooperative on Phytotherapy. *Valeriana radix* (valerian root). Exeter, UK: ESCOP; 1996-1997. Monographs on the Medicinal Uses of Plant Drugs, Fascicule 4:2, 6.

14. Tyler VE. *Herbs of Choice: The Therapeutic Use of Phytochemicals*. New York, NY: Pharmaceutical Products Press; 1994:118.

15. Holzl J, Godau P. Receptor bindings studies with *Valeriana officinalis* on the benzodiazepine receptor [abstract]. *Planta Med*. 1989;55(7 spec no):642.

16. Mennini T, Bernasconi P, Bombardelli E, et al. In vitro study on the interaction of extracts and pure compounds from *Valeriana officinalis* roots with GABA, benzodiazepine and barbiturate receptors in rat brain. *Fitoterapia*. 1993;64:291-300.

17. Santos MS, Ferreira F, Cunha AP, et al. Synaptosomal GABA release as influenced by valerian root extract—involvement of the GABA carrier. *Arch Int Pharmacodyn Ther*. 1994;327:220-231.

18. Santos MS, Ferreira F, Cunha AP, et al. An aqueous extract of valerian influences the transport of GABA in synaptosomes [letter]. *Planta Med*. 1994;60:278-279.

19. Cavadas C, Araujo I, Cotrim MD, et al. In vitro study on the interaction of *Valeriana officinalis* L. extracts and their amino acids on GABAA receptor in rat brain. *Arzneimittelforschung*. 1995;45:753-755.

20. Santos MS, Ferreira F, Faro C, et al. The amount of GABA present in aqueous extracts of valerian is sufficient to account for [3H]GABA release in synaptosomes. *Planta Med*. 1994;60:475-476.

21. Schulz V, Hansel R, Tyler VE. *Rational Phytotherapy: A Physicians' Guide to Herbal Medicine*. 3rd ed. Berlin, Germany: Springer-Verlag; 1998:76-77, 81.

22. Bounthanh C, Bergmann C, Beck JP, et al. Valepotriates, a new class of cytotoxic and antitumor agents. *Planta Med*. 1981;41:21-28.

23. Houghton PJ. The biological activity of *Valerian* and related plants. *J Ethnopharmacol*. 1988;22:121-142.

24. von der Hude W, Scheutwinkel-Reich M, Braun R. Bacterial mutagenicity of the tranquilizing constituents in *Valerianaceae* roots. *Mutat Res.* 1986;169:23-27.

25. Willey LB, Mady SP, Cobaugh DJ, et al. Valerian overdose: a case report. *Vet Hum Toxicol.* 1995;37:364-365.

26. Rosecrans JA, Defeo JJ, Youngken HW Jr. Pharmacological investigation of certain *Valeriana officinalis* L. extracts. *J Pharm Sci.* 1961;50:240-244.

27. MacGregor FB, Abernethy VE, Dahabra S, et al. Hepatotoxicity of herbal remedies. *BMJ.* 1989;299:1156-1157.

28. Chan TY, Tang CH, Critchley JA. Poisoning due to an over-the-counter hypnotic, Sleep-Qik™ (hyoscine, cyproheptadine, valerian). *Postgrad Med J.* 1995;71:227-228.

29. Chan TY. An assessment of the delayed effects associated with valerian overdose [letter]. *Int J Clin Pharmacol Ther.* 1998;36:569.

30. Albrecht M, Berger W, Laux P, et al. Psychopharmaceuticals and traffic safety: the effect of Euvegal® Dragees Forte on driving ability and combination effects with alcohol [translated from German]. *Z Allgemeinmed.* 1995;71:1215-1218, 1221-1222, 1225.

31. Gerhard U, Linnenbrink N, Georghiadou C, et al. Vigilance-decreasing effects of 2 plant-derived sedatives [in German; English abstract]. *Schweiz Rundsch Med Prax.* 1996;85:473-481.

32. Kuhlmann J, Berger W, Podzuweit H, et al. The influence of valerian treatment on "reaction time, alertness and concentration" in volunteers. *Pharmacopsychiatry.* 1999;32:235-241.

33. Garges HP, Varia I, Doraiswamy PM. Cardiac complications and delirium associated with valerian root withdrawal [letter]. *JAMA.* 1998;280:1566-1567.

34. Sakamoto T, Mitani Y, Nakajima K. Psychotropic effects of Japanese valerian root extract. *Chem Pharm Bull (Tokyo).* 1992;40:758-761.

35. Leuschner J, Muller J, Rudmann M. Characterisation of the central nervous depressant activity of a commercially available valerian root extract. *Arzneimittelforschung.* 1993;43:638-641.

36. Hiller KO, Zetler G. Neuropharmacological studies on ethanol extracts of *Valeriana officinalis* L: behavioural and anticonvulsant properties. *Phytother Res.* 1996;10:145-151.

Vanadium

1. Matsumoto J. Vanadate, moluybate and tungstate for orthomolecular medicine. *Med Hypotheses.* 1994;43:177-182.

2. Shamberger RJ. The insulin-like effects of vanadium. *J Adv Med.* 1996;9:121-131.

3. Ramanadham S, Mongold JJ, Brownsey RW, et al. Oral vanadyl sulfate in treatment of diabetes mellitus in rats. *Am J Physiol.* 1989;257:H904-H911.

4. Brichard SM, Okitolonda W, Henquin JC. Long term improvement of glucose homeostasis by vanadate treatment in diabetic rats. *Endocrinology.* 1988;123:2048-2053.

5. Kanthasamy A, Sekar N, Govindasamy S. Vanadate substitutes insulin role in chronic experimental diabetes. *Indian J Exp Biol.* 1988;26:778-780.

6. Shechter Y. Perspectives in diabetes. Insulin-mimetic effects of vanadate: possible implications for future treatment of diabetes. *Diabetes;*1990;39:1-5.

7. Challiss RAJ, Leighton B, Lozeman FJ, et al. Effects of chronic administration of vanadate to the rat on the sensitivity of glycolysis and glycogen synthesis in skeletal muscle to insulin. *Biochem Pharmacol.* 1987;36:357-361.

8. Sakurai H, Tsuchiya K, Nakatsuka M, et al. Insulin-like effect of vanadyl ion on streptozocin-induced diabetic rats. *J Endocrinol.* 1990;126:451-459.

9. Pederson RA, Ramanadham S, Buchan AMJ, et al. Long-term effects of vanadyl treatment on streptozotocin-induced diabetes in rats. *Diabetes.* 1989;38:1390-1395.

10. Meyerovitch J, Farfel A, Sack J, et al. Oral administration of vanadate normalizes blood glucose levels in streptozotocin-treated rats: characterization and mode of action. *J Biol Chem.* 1987;262:6658-6662.

11. Heyliger CE, Tahiliani AG, McNeill JH. Effect of vanadate on elevated blood glucose and depressed cardiac performance of diabetic rats. *Science.* 1985;227:1474-1476.

12. Crans DC. Chemistry and insulin-like properties of vanadium(IV) and vanadium(V) compounds. *J Inorg Biochem.* 2000;80:123-131.

13. Boden G, Chen X, Ruiz J, et al. Effects of vanadyl sulfate on carbohydrate and lipid metabolism in patients with non-insulin-dependent diabetes mellitus. *Metabolism.* 1996;45:1130-1135.

14. Cohen N, Halberstam M, Shlimovich P, et al. Oral vanadyl sulfate improves hepatic and peripheral insulin sensitivity in patients with non-insulin-dependent diabetes mellitus. *J Clin Invest.* 1995;95:2501-2509.

15. Goldfine AB, Folli F, Patti PE, et al. Effects of sodium vanadate on in vivo and in vitro insulin action in diabetes [abstract]. *Clin Res.* 1994;42:116A.

16. Halberstam M, Cohen N, Shlimovich P, et al. Oral vanadyl sulfate improves insulin sensitivity in NIDDM but not in obese nondiabetic subjects. *Diabetes.* 1996;45:659-666.

17. Goldfine AB, Patti ME, Zuberi L, et al. Metabolic effects of vanadyl sulfate in humans with non-insulin-dependent diabetes mellitus: in vivo and in vitro studies. *Metabolism.* 2000;49:400-410.

18. Srivastava AK. Anti-diabetic and toxic effects of vanadium compounds. *Mol Cell Biochem.* 2000;206:177-182.

19. Fawcett JP, Farquhar SJ, Walker RJ, et al. The effect of oral vanadyl sulfate on body composition and performance in weight-training athletes. *Int J Sport Nutr.* 1996; 6:382-390.

20. Amano R, Enomoto S, Nobuta M. Bone uptake of vanadium in mice: simultaneous tracting of V, Se, Sr, Y, Zr, Ru and Rh using a radioactive multitracer. *J Trace Elem Med Biol.* 1996;10:145-148.

21. Harland BF, Harden-Williams BA. Is vanadium of human nutritional importance yet? *J Am Diet Assoc.* 1994;94:891-894.

22. Dietary Reference Intakes for Vitamin A, Vitamin K, Arsenic, Boron, Chromium, Copper, Iodine, Iron, Manganese, Molybdenum, Nickel, Silicon, Vanadium, and Zinc (2001). Available at: http://www.nap.edu. Accessed October 4, 2001.

23. Domingo JL, Gomez M, Llobet JM, et al. Oral vanadium administration to streptozotocin-diabetic rats has marked negative side effects which are independent of the form of vanadium used. *Toxicology.* 1991;66:279-287.

24. Sanchez DJ, Colomina MT, Domingo JL. Effects of vanadium on activity and learning in rats. *Physiol Behav.* 1998;63:345-350.

25. Domingo JL. Vanadium: a review of the reproductive and developmental toxicity. *Reprod Toxicol.* 1996;10:175-182.

Vinpocetine

1. Hindmarch I, Fuchs HH, Erzigkeit H. Efficacy and tolerance of vinpocetine in ambulant patients suffering from mild to moderate organic psychosyndromes. *Int Clin Psychopharmacol.* 1991;6:31-43.

2. Balestreri R, Fontana L, Astengo F. A double-blind placebo controlled evaluation of the safety and efficacy of vinpocetine in the treatment of patients with chronic vascular senile cerebral dysfunction. *J Am Geriatr Soc.* 1987;35:425-430.

3. Dragunow M, Faull RL. Neuroprotective effects of adenosine. *Trends Pharmacol Sci.* 1988;9:193-194.

4. Fenzl E, et al. Efficacy and tolerance of vinpocetine administered intravenously, in addition of standard therapy, to patients suffering from an apoplectic insult. In: Krieglstein J, ed. *Pharmacology of Cerebral Ischaemia: Proceedings of the International Symposium on Pharmacology of Cerebral Ischemia, held in Marburg (FRG) on 16-17 July 1986.* New York, NY: Elsevier Science Publishers; 1986:430-434.

5. Manconi E, Binaghi F, Pitzus F. A double-blind clinical trial of vinpocetine in the treatment of cerebral insufficiency of vascular and degenerative origin. *Curr Ther Res.* 1986;40:702-709.

6. Peruzza M, DeJacobis M. A double-blind placebo controlled evaluation of the efficacy and safety of vinpocetine in the treatment of patients with chronic vascular or degenerative senile cerebral dysfunction. *Adv Ther.* 1986;3:201-209.

7. Blaha L, et al. Clinical evidence of the effectiveness of vinpocetine in the treatment of organic psychosyndrome. *Hum Psychopharmacol.* 1989;4:103-111. Cited by: Hindmarch I, Fuchs HH, Erzigkeit H. Efficacy and tolerance of vinpocetine in ambulant patients suffering from mild to moderate organic psychosyndromes. *Int Clin Psychopharmacol.* 1991;6:31-43.

8. Feigin VL, Doronin BM, Popova TF, et al. Vinpocetine treatment in acute ischaemic stroke: a pilot single-blind randomized clinical trial. *Eur J Neurol.* 2001;8:81-85.

9. Bereczki D, Fekete I. A systematic review of vinpocetine therapy in acute ischaemic stroke. *Eur J Clin Pharmacol.* 1999;55:349-352.

10. Kiss B, Karpati E. Mechanism of action of vinpocetine [in Hungarian; English abstract]. *Acta Pharm Hung.* 1996;66:213-224.

11. Miyazaki M. The effect of a cerebral vasodilator, vinpocetine, on cerebral vascular resistance evaluated by the Doppler ultrasonic technique in patients with cerebrovascular diseases. *Angiology.* 1995;46:53-58.

12. Lohmann A, Dingler E, Sommer W, et al. Bioavailability of vinpocetine and interference of the time of application with food intake. *Arzneimittelforschung.* 1992;42:914-917.

13. Shimizu Y, Saitoh K, Nakayama M, et al. Agranulocytosis induced by vinpocetine. *Int J Med.* [serial online]. Available at: http://www.priory.com/med.htm. Accessed December 7, 2000.

14. Hitzenberger G, Sommer W, Grandt R. Influence of vincpocetine on warfarin-induced inhibition of coagulation. *Int J Clin Pharmacol Ther Toxicol.* 1990;28:323-328.

15. Wollschlaeger B. Efficacy of vinpocetine in the management of cognitive impairment and memory loss. *J Am Nutraceutical Assoc.* 2001;4:25-30.

Vitamin A

1. Combs GF. *The Vitamins: Fundamental Aspects in Nutrition and Health.* 2nd ed. San Diego, Calif: Academic Press; 1998:5-6.

2. Martinoli L, Di Felice M, Seghieri G, et al. Plasma retinol and alpha-tocopherol concentrations in insulin-dependent diabetes mellitus: their relationship to microvascular complications. *Int J Vitam Nutr Res.* 1993;63:87-92.

3. Singh RB, Ghosh S, Niaz MA, et al. Dietary intake and plasma levels of antioxidant vitamins in health and disease: a hospital-based case-control study. *J Nutr Environ Med.* 1995;5:235-242.

4. Basualdo CG, Wein EE, Basu TK. Vitamin A (retinol) status of First Nation adults with non-insulin-dependent diabetes mellitus. *J Am Coll Nutr.* 1997;16:39-45.

5. Straub RH, Rokitzki L, Schumacher T, et al. No evidence of deficiency of vitamins A, E, beta-carotene, B_1, B_2, B_6, B_{12} and folate in neuropathic Type II diabetic women. *Int J Vitam Nutr Res.* 1993;63:239-240.

6. Glasziou PP, Mackerras DE. Vitamin A supplementation in infectious diseases: a meta-analysis. *BMJ.* 1993;306:366-370.

7. Wright JP, Mee AS, Parfitt A, et al. Vitamin A therapy in patients with Crohn's disease. *Gastroenterology.* 1985;88:512-514.

8. Bresee JS, Fischer M, Dowell SF, et al. Vitamin A therapy for children with respiratory syncytial virus infection: a multicenter trial in the United States. *Pediatr Infect Dis J.* 1996;15:777-782.

9. Stoesser AV, Lloyd S, Nelson LS. Synthetic vitamin A in treatment of eczema in children. *Ann Allergy.* 1952;10:703-704.

10. Kligman AM, Mills OH Jr, Leyden JJ, et al. Oral vitamin A in acne vulgaris: preliminary report. *Int J Dermatol.* 1981;20:278-285.

11. Marrakchi S, Kim I, Delaporte E, et al. Vitamin A and E blood levels in erythrodermic and pustular psoriasis associated with chronic alcoholism. *Acta Derm Venereol.* 1994;74:298-301.

12. Brenner S, Horwitz C. Possible nutrient mediators in psoriasis and seborrheic dermatitis. II. Nutrient mediators: essential fatty acids; vitamins A, E and D; vitamins B_1, B_2, B_6, niacin and biotin; vitamin C selenium; zinc; iron. *World Rev Nutr Diet.* 1988;55:165-182.

13. Lithgow DM, Politzer WM. Vitamin A in the treatment of menorrhagia. *S Afr Med J.* 1977;51:191-193.
14. Leo MA, Lieber CS. Alcohol, vitamin A, and beta-carotene: adverse interactions, including hepatotoxicity and carcinogenicity. *Am J Clin Nutr.* 1999;69:1071-1085.
15. Melhus H, Michaelsson K, Kindmark A, et al. Excessive dietary intake of vitamin A is associated with reduced bone mineral density and increased risk for hip fracture. *Ann Intern Med.* 1998;129:770-778.
16. Dietary Reference Intakes for Vitamin A, Vitamin K, Arsenic, Boron, Chromium, Copper, Iodine, Iron, Manganese, Molybdenum, Nickel, Silicon, Vanadium, and Zinc (2001). Available at: http://www.nap.edu. Accessed October 4, 2001.
17. Nau H, Tzimas G, Mondry M, et al. Antiepileptic drugs alter endogenous retinoid concentrations: a possible mechanism of teratogenesis of anticonvulsant therapy. *Life Sci.* 1995;57:53-60.
18. Harris JE. Interaction of dietary factors with oral anticoagulants: review and applications. *J Am Diet Assoc.* 1995;95:580-584.
19. West RJ, Lloyd JK. The effect of cholestyramine on intestinal absorption. *Gut.* 1975;16:93-98.
20. Johansson S, Melhus H. Vitamin A antagonizes calcium response to vitamin D in man. *J Bone Miner Res.* 2001;16:1899-1905.

Vitamin B$_1$

1. Brady JA, Rock CL, Horneffer MR. Thiamin status, diuretic medications, and the management of congestive heart failure. *J Am Diet Assoc.* 1995;95:541-544.
2. Shimon I, Almog S, Vered Z, et al. Improved left ventricular function after thiamine supplementation in patients with congestive heart failure receiving long-term furosemide therapy. *Am J Med.* 1995;98:485-490.
3. Gold M, Hauser RA, Chen MF. Plasma thiamine deficiency associated with Alzheimer's disease but not Parkinson's disease. *Metab Brain Dis.* 1998;13:43-53.
4. Bettendorff L, Mastrogiacomo F, Wins P, et al. Low thiamine diphosphate levels in brains of patients with frontal lobe degeneration of the non-Alzheimer's type. *J Neurochem.* 1997;69:2005-2010.
5. Mimori Y, Katsuoka H, Nakamura S. Thiamine therapy in Alzheimer's disease. *Metab Brain Dis.* 1996;11:89-94.
6. Meador K, Loring D, Nichols M, et al. Preliminary findings of high-dose thiamine in dementia of Alzheimer's type. *J Geriatr Psychiatry Neurol.* 1993;6:222-229.
7. Nolan KA, Black RS, Sheu KF, et al. A trial of thiamine in Alzheimer's disease. *Arch Neurol.* 1991;48:81-83.

Vitamin B$_2$

1. Powers HJ, Thurnham DI. Riboflavin deficiency in man: effects on haemoglobin and reduced glutathione in erythrocytes of different ages. *Br J Nutr.* 1981;46:257-266.
2. Elsborg L, Nielsen JA, Bertram U, et al. The intake of vitamins and minerals by the elderly at home. *Int J Vitam Nutr Res.* 1983;53:321-329.
3. Lopez R, Schwartz JV, Cooperman JM. Riboflavin deficiency in an adolescent population in New York City. *Am J Clin Nutr.* 1980;33:1283-1286.
4. Southon S, Bailey AL, Wright AJA, et al. Micronutrient undernutrition in British schoolchildren. *Pro Nutr Soc.* 1993;52:155-163.
5. Schoenen J, Jacquy J, Lenaerts M. Effectiveness of high-dose riboflavin in migraine prophylaxis: a randomized controlled trial. *Neurology.* 1998;50:466-470.
6. Ajayi OA, George BO, Ipadeola T. Clinical trial of riboflavin in sickle cell disease. *East Afr Med J.* 1993;70:418-421.
7. Webb JL. Nutritional effects of oral contraceptive use. *J Reprod Med.* 1980;25:150-156.
8. Larsson-Cohn U. Oral contraceptives and vitamins: a review. *Am J Obstet Gynecol.* 1975;121:84-90.
9. Wynn V. Vitamins and oral contraceptive use. *Lancet.* 1975;1:561-564.

Vitamin B₃

1. Illingworth DR, Stein EA, Mitchel YB, et al. Comparative effects of lovastatin and niacin in primary hypercholesterolemia: a prospective trial. *Arch Intern Med.* 1994;154:1586-1595.
2. Guyton JR, Goldberg AC, Kreisberg RA, et al. Effectiveness of once-nightly dosing of extended-release niacin alone and in combination for hypercholesterolemia. *Am J Cardiol.* 1998;82:737-743.
3. Vega GL, Grundy SM. Lipoprotein responses to treatment with lovastatin, gemfibrozil, and nicotinic acid in normolipidemic patients with hypoalphalipoproteinemia. *Arch Intern Med.* 1994;154:73-82.
4. Lal SM, Hewett JE, Petroski GF, et al. Effects of nicotinic acid and lovastatin in renal transplant patients: a prospective, randomized, open-labeled crossover trial. *Am J Kidney Dis.* 1995;25:616-622.
5. Jacobsen TA, Amorosa LF. Combination therapy with fluvastatin and niacin in hypercholesterolemia: a preliminary report on safety. *Am J Cardiol.* 1994;73:25D-29D.
6. Kashyap ML, Evans R, Simmons PD, et al. New combination niacin/statin formulation shows pronounced effects on major lipoproteins and is well tolerated [abstract]. *J Am Coll Cardiol.* 2000;35(suppl A):326.
7. Canner PL, Berge KG, Wenger NK, et al. Fifteen year mortality in Coronary Drug Project patients: long-term benefit with niacin. *J Am Coll Cardiol.* 1986;8:1245-1255.
8. Elam MB, Hunninghake DB, Davis KB, et al. Effect of niacin on lipid and lipoprotein levels and glycemic control in patients with diabetes and peripheral arterial disease. The ADMIT Study: a randomized trial. *JAMA.* 2000;284:1263-1270.
9. O'Hara J, Jolly PN, Nicol CG. The therapeutic efficacy of inositol nicotinate (Hexopal) in intermittent claudication: a controlled trial. *Br J Clin Pract.* 1988;42:377-383.
10. Kiff RS, Quick CRG. Does inositol nicotinate (Hexopal) influence intermittent claudication? A controlled trial. *Br J Clin Pract.* 1988;42:141-145.
11. Head A. Treatment of intermittent claudication with inositol nicotinate. *Practitioner.* 1986;230:49-54.
12. Tyson VC. Treatment of intermittent claudication. *Practitioner.* 1979;223:121-126.
13. Jonas WB, Rapoza CP, Blair WF. The effect of niacinamide on osteoarthritis: a pilot study. *Inflamm Res.* 1996;45:330-334.
14. Sunderland GT, Belch JJ, Sturrock RD, et al. A double blind randomized placebo controlled trial of hexopal in primary Raynaud's disease. *Clin Rheumatol.* 1988;7:46-49.
15. Elliott RB, Pilcher CC, Fergusson DM, et al. A population based strategy to prevent insulin-dependent diabetes using nicotinamide. *J Pediatr Endocrinol Metab.* 1996; 9:501-509.
16. Pozzilli P, Visalli N, Signore A, et al. Double blind trial of nicotinamide in recent-onset IDDM (the IMDIAB III study). *Diabetologia.* 1995;38:848-852.
17. Lampeter EF, Klinghammer A, Scherbaum WA, et al. The Deutsche Nicotinamide Intervention Study: an attempt to prevent type 1 diabetes. *Diabetes.* 1998;47:980-984.
18. Shalita AR, Smith JG, Parish LC, et al. Topical nicotinamide compared with clindamycin gel in the treatment of inflammatory acne vulgaris. *Int J Dermatol.* 1995; 34:434-437.
19. Neumann R, Rappold E, Pohl-Markl H. Treatment of polymorphous light eruption with nicotinamide: a pilot study. *Br J Dermatol.* 1986;115:77-80.
20. Gibbons LW, Gonzalez V, Gordon N, et al. The prevalence of side effects with regular and sustained-release nicotinic acid. *Am J Med.* 1995;99:378-385.
21. *Physicians' Desk Reference: PDR.* 53rd ed. Montvale, NJ: Medical Economics Co; 1999:1507.
22. Dietary Reference Intakes for Thiamin, Riboflavin, Niacin, Vitamin B₆, Folate, Vitamin B₁₂, Pantothenic Acid, Biotin, and Choline (1998). Available at: http://www.nap.edu. Accessed October 4, 2001.
23. Bourgeois BFD, Dodson WE, Ferrendelli JA. Interactions between primidone, carbamazepine, and nicotinamide. *Neurology.* 1982;32:1122-1126.

24. Wolfe ML, Vartanian SF, Ross JL, et al. Safety and effectiveness of Niaspan when added sequentially to a statin for treatment of dyslipidemia. *Am J Cardiol.* 2001; 87:476-479.

25. DiLorenzo PA. Pellagra-like syndrome associated with isoniazid therapy. *Acta Derm Venereol.* 1967;47:318-322.

26. Ishii N, Nishihara Y. Pellagra encephalopathy among tuberculous patients: its relation to isoniazid therapy. *J Neurol.* 1985;48:628-634.

27. Wink J, Giacoppe G, King J. Effect of very-low-dose niacin on high-density lipoprotein in patients undergoing long-term statin therapy. *Am Heart J.* 2002;143:514-518.

Vitamin B$_6$

1. Kant AK, Block G. Dietary vitamin B-6 intake and food sources in the US population: NHANES II, 1976-1980. *Am J Clin Nutr.* 1990;52:707-716.

2. van der Wielen RPJ, de Groot LCPGM, van Staveren WA. Dietary intake of water soluble vitamins in elderly people living in a Western society (1980-1993). *Nutr Res.* 1994;14:605-638.

3. Albertson AM, Tobelmann RC, Engstrom A, et al. Nutrient intakes of 2- to 10-year-old American children: 10-year trends. *J Am Diet Assoc.* 1992;92:1492-1496.

4. Vutyavanich T, Wongtra-ngan S, Ruangsri R. Pyridoxine for nausea and vomiting of pregnancy: a randomized, double-blind, placebo-controlled trial. *Am J Obstet Gynecol.* 1995;173:881-884.

5. Rimm EB, Willett WC, Hu FB, et al. Folate and vitamin B$_6$ from diet and supplements in relation to risk of coronary heart disease among women. *JAMA.* 1998; 279:359-364.

6. Folsom AR, Nieto FJ, McGovern PG, et al. Prospective study of coronary heart disease incidence in relation to fasting total homocysteine, related genetic polymorphisms, and B vitamins: the Atherosclerosis Risk in Communities (ARIC) study. *Circulation.* 1998;98:204-210.

7. Vermeulen EG, Stehouwer CD, Twisk JW, et al. Effect of homocysteine-lowering treatment with folic acid plus vitamin B$_6$ on progression of subclinical atherosclerosis: a randomized, placebo-controlled trial. *Lancet.* 2000;355:517-522.

8. Booth GL, Wang EE. Preventive health care, 2000 update: screening and management of hyperhomocysteinemia for the prevention of coronary artery disease events: the Canadian Task Force on Preventive Health Care. *CMAJ.* 2000;163:21-29.

9. McKinley MC, McNulty H, McPartlin J, et al. Low-dose vitamin B-6 effectively lowers fasting plasma homocysteine in healthy elderly persons who are folate and riboflavin replete. *Am J Clin Nutr.* 2001;73:759-764.

10. Collipp PJ, Goldzier S III, Weiss N, et al. Pyridoxine treatment of childhood bronchial asthma. *Ann Allergy.* 1975;35:93-97.

11. Sur S, Camara M, Buchmeier A, et al. Double-blind trial of pyridoxine (vitamin B$_6$) in the treatment of steroid-dependent asthma. *Ann Allergy.* 1993;70:147-152.

12. Ellis JM. Vitamin B$_6$ deficiency in patients with a clinical syndrome including the carpal tunnel defect: biochemical and clinical response to therapy with pyridoxine. *Res Commun Chem Pathol Pharmacol.* 1976;13:743-757.

13. Franzblau A, Rock CL, Werner RA, et al. The relationship of vitamin B$_6$ status to median nerve function and carpal tunnel syndrome among active industrial workers. *J Occup Environ Med.* 1996;38:485-491.

14. Stransky M, Rubin A, Lava NS, et al. Treatment of carpal tunnel syndrome with vitamin B$_6$: a double-blind study. *South Med J.* 1989;82:841-842.

15. Spooner GR, Desai HB, Angel JF, et al. Using pyridoxine to treat carpal tunnel syndrome: randomized control trial. *Can Fam Physician.* 1993;39:2122-2127.

16. Wyatt KM, Dimmock PW, Jones PW, et al. Efficacy of vitamin B$_6$ in the treatment of premenstrual syndrome: systematic review. *BMJ.* 1999;318:1375-1381.

17. Kleijnen J, Ter Riet G, Knipschild P. Vitamin B$_6$ in the treatment of premenstrual syndrome—a review. *Br J Obstet Gynaecol.* 1990;97:847-852.

18. Diegoli MS, da Fonseca AM, Diegoli CA, et al. A double-blind trial of four medications to treat severe premenstrual syndrome. *Int J Gynaecol Obstet.* 1998;62:63-67.

19. De Souza MC, Walker AF, Robinson PA, et al. A synergistic effect of a daily supplement for 1 month of 200 mg magnesium plus 50 mg vitamin B_6 for the relief of anxiety-related premenstrual symptoms: a randomized, double-blind, crossover study. *J Womens Health Gend Based Med.* 2000;9:131-139.
20. Cohen KL, Gorecki GA, Silverstein SB, et al. Effect of pyridoxine (vitamin B_6) on diabetic patients with peripheral neuropathy. *J Am Podiatr Assoc.* 1984;74:394-397.
21. McCann VJ, Davis RE. Pyridoxine and diabetic neuropathy: a double-blind controlled study [letter]. *Diabetes Care.* 1983;6:102-103.
22. Levin ER, Hanscom TA, Fisher M, et al. The influence of pyridoxine in diabetic peripheral neuropathy. *Diabetes Care.* 1981;4:606-609.
23. Effersoe H. The effect of topical application of pyridoxine ointment on the rate of sebaceous secretion in patients with seborrheic dermatitis. *Acta Derm Venereol.* 1954;3:272-278.
24. Bell IR, Edman JS, Morrow FD, et al. Brief communication: Vitamin B_1, B_2, and B_6 augmentation of tricyclic antidepressant treatment in geriatric depression with cognitive dysfunction. *J Am Coll Nutr.* 1992;11:159-163.
25. Bennink HJ, Schreurs WH. Improvement of oral glucose tolerance in gestational diabetes by pyridoxine. *Br Med J.* 1975;3:13-15.
26. Lerner V, Miodownik C, Kaptsan A, et al. Vitamin B(6) in the treatment of tardive dyskinesia: a double-blind, placebo-controlled, crossover study. *Am J Psychiatry.* 2001;158:1511-1514.
27. DeVeaugh-Geiss J, Manion L. High-dose pyridoxine in tardive dyskinesia. *J Clin Psychiatry.* 1978;39:573-575.
28. Sandyk R, Pardeshi R. Pyridoxine improves drug-induced parkinsonism and psychosis in a schizophrenic patient. *Int J Neurosci.* 1990;52:225-232.
29. Lerner V, Kaptsan A, Miodownik C, Kotler M. Vitamin B_6 in treatment of tardive dyskinesia: a preliminary case series study. *Clin Neuropharmacol.* 1999;22:241-243.
30. Ross JB, Moss MA. Relief of the photosensitivity of erythropoietic protoporphyria by pyridoxine. *J Am Acad Dermatol.* 1990;22(2 pt 2):340-342.
31. Parivar F, Low RK, Stoller ML. The influence of diet on urinary stone disease. *J Urol.* 1996;155:432-440.
32. Murthy MS, Farooqui S, Talwar HS, et al. Effect of pyridoxine supplementation on recurrent stone formers. *Int J Clin Pharmacol Ther Toxicol.* 1982;20:434-437.
33. Curhan GC, Willett WC, Speizer FE, et al. Intake of vitamins B_6 and C and the risk of kidney stones in women. *J Am Soc Nephrol.* 1999;10:840-845.
34. Curhan GC, Willett WC, Rimm EB, et al. A prospective study of the intake of vitamins C and B_6, and the risk of kidney stones in men. *J Urol.* 1996;155:1847-1851.
35. Pfeiffer SI, Norton J, Nelson L, et al. Efficacy of vitamin B_6 and magnesium in the treatment of autism: a methodology review and summary of outcomes. *J Autism Dev Disord.* 1995;25:481-493.
36. Barthelemy C, Garreau B, Leddet I, et al. Behavioral and biological effects of oral magnesium, vitamin B_6, and combined magnesium-B_6 administration in autistic children. *Magnes Bull.* 1981;2:150-153.
37. Lelord G, Callaway E, Muh JP. Clinical and biological effects of high doses of vitamin B_6 and magnesium on autistic children. *Acta Vitaminol Enzymol.* 1982;4:27-44.
38. Lelord G, Muh JP, Barthelemy C, et al. Effects of pyridoxine and magnesium on autistic symptoms—initial observations. *J Autism Dev Disord.* 1981;11:219-230.
39. Martineau J, Barthelemy C, Garreau B, et al. Vitamin B_6, magnesium, and combined B_6-Mg: therapeutic effects in childhood autism. *Biol Psychiatry.* 1985;20:467-478.
40. Martineau J, Garreau B, Barthelemy C, et al. Effects of vitamin B_6 on averaged evoked potentials in infantile autism. *Biol Psychiatry.* 1981;16:627-641.
41. Hansen CM, Shultz TD, Kwak HK, et al. Assessment of vitamin B-6 status in young women consuming a controlled diet containing four levels of vitamin B-6 provides an estimated average requirement and recommended dietary allowance. *J Nutr.* 2001; 131:1777-1786.
42. Parry GJ, Bredesen DE. Sensory neuropathy with low-dose pyridoxine. *Neurology.* 1985;35:1466-1468.

43. Sherertz EF. Acneiform eruption due to "megadose" vitamins B_6 and B_{12}. *Cutis.* 1991;48:119-120.
44. Braun-Falco O, Lincke H. The problem of vitamin B_6/B_{12} acne: a contribution on acne medicamentosa [in German; English abstract]. *MMW Munch Med Wochenschr.* 1976;118:155-160.
45. Dietary Reference Intakes for Thiamin, Riboflavin, Niacin, Vitamin B_6, Folate, Vitamin B_{12}, Pantothenic Acid, Biotin, and Choline (1998). Available at: http://www. nap.edu. Accessed October 4, 2001.
46. Lim D, McKay M. Food-drug interactions. *Drug Inf Bull.* 1995;15(2).
47. Yahr MD, Duvoisin RC. Pyridoxine and levodopa in the treatment of Parkinsonism. *JAMA.* 1972;220:861.
48. Leon AS, Spiegel HE, Thomas G, et al. Pyridoxine antagonism of levodopa in parkinsonism. *JAMA.* 1971;218:1924-1927.
49. Vidrio H. Interaction with pyridoxal as a possible mechanism of hydralazine hypotension. *J Cardiovasc Pharmacol.* 1990;15:150-156.
50. Rumsby PC, Shepherd DM. The effect of penicillamine on vitamin B_6 function in man. *Biochem Pharmacol.* 1981;30:3051-3053.
51. Delport R, Ubbink JB, Serfontein WJ, et al. Vitamin B_6 nutritional status in asthma: the effect of theophylline therapy on plasma pyridoxal-5'-phosphate and pyridoxal levels. *Int J Vitam Nutr Res.* 1988;58:67-72.
52. Ubbink JB, Vermaak WJ, Delport R, et al. The relationship between vitamin B_6 metabolism, asthma, and theophylline therapy. *Ann NY Acad Sci.* 1990;585:285-294.
53. Delport R, Ubbink JB, Vermaak WJH, et al. Theophylline increases pyridoxal kinase activity independently from vitamin B_6 nutritional status. *Res Commun Chem Pathol Pharmacol.* 1993;79:325-333.
54. Ubbink JB, Delport R, Bissbort S, et al. Relationship between vitamin B_6 status and elevated pyridoxal kinase levels induced by theophylline therapy in humans. *J Nutr.* 1990;120:1352-1359.
55. Shimizu T, Maeda S, Mochizuki H, et al. Theophylline attenuates circulating vitamin B_6 levels in children with asthma. *Pharmacology.* 1994;49:392-397.
56. Heller CA, Friedman PA. Pyridoxine deficiency and peripheral neuropathy associated with long-term phenelzine therapy. *Am J Med.* 1983;75:887-888.
57. Goldman AL, Braman SS. Isoniazid: a review with emphasis on adverse effects. *Chest.* 1972;62:71-77.
58. Biehl JP, Vilter RW. Effect of isoniazid on vitamin B_6 metabolism; its possible significance in producing isoniazid neuritis. *Proc Soc Exp Biol Med.* 1954;85:389-392.
59. Snider DE Jr. Pyridoxine supplementation during isoniazid therapy. *Tubercle.* 1980;61:191-196.
60. Bartel PR, Ubbink JB, Delport R, et al. Vitamin B-6 supplementation and theophylline-related effects in humans. *Am J Clin Nutr.* 1994;60:93-99.
61. Villegas-Salas E, Ponce de Leon R, Juarez-Perez MA, et al. Effect of vitamin B_6 on the side effects of a low-dose combined oral contraceptive. *Contraception.* 1997;55: 245-248.
62. Mabin DC, Hollis S, Lockwood J, et al. Pyridoxine in atopic dermatitis. *Br J Dermatol.* 1995;133:764-767.

Vitamin B_{12}

1. Carmel R, Gott P, Degiorgio C, et al. Abnormal P300 event-related potentials in mild, preclinical cobalamin deficiency [abstract]. *Int J Hematol.* 2000;72(suppl 1):207.
2. Kumamoto Y, Maruta H, Ishigami J, et al. Clinical efficacy of mecobalamin in treatment of oligozoospermia: results of double-blind comparative clinical study [in Japanese; English abstract]. *Hinyokika Kiyo.* 1988;34:1109-1132.
3. Rule SA, Hooker M, Costello C, et al. Serum vitamin B_{12} and transcobalamin levels in early HIV disease. *Am J Hematol.* 1994;47:167-171.
4. Richman DD, Fischl MA, Grieco MH, et al. The toxicity of azidothymidine (AZT) in the treatment of patients with AIDS and AIDS-related complex: a double-blind, placebo-controlled trial. *N Engl J Med.* 1987;317:192-197.

5. Wright J. Vitamin B_{12}: powerful protection against asthma. *Int Clin Nutr Rev.* 1989;9:185-188.

6. Ide H, Fujiya S, Asanuma Y, et al. Clinical usefulness of intrathecal injection of methylcobalamin in patients with diabetic neuropathy. *Clin Ther.* 1987;9:183-192.

7. Yaqub BA, Siddique A, Sulimani R. Effects of methylcobalamin on diabetic neuropathy. *Clin Neurol Neurosurg.* 1992;94:105-111.

8. Kira J, Tobimatsu S, Goto I. Vitamin B_{12} metabolism and massive-dose methyl vitamin B_{12} therapy in Japanese patients with multiple sclerosis. *Int Med.* 1994;33:82-86.

9. Goodkin DE, Jacobsen DW, Galvez N, et al. Serum cobalamin deficiency is uncommon in multiple sclerosis. *Arch Neurol.* 1994;51:1110-1114.

10. Baig SM, Qureshi GA, Minami M. The interrelation between the deficiency of vitamin B_{12} and neurotoxicity of homocysteine with nitrite in some neurologic disorders. *Biogenic Amines.* 1998;14:1-14.

11. Reynolds EH. Multiple sclerosis and vitamin B_{12} metabolism. *J Neuroimmunol.* 1992;40:225-230.

12. Simpson CA, Newell DJ, Miller H. The treatment of multiple sclerosis with massive doses of hydroxycobalamin. *Neurology.* 1965;15:599-603.

13. O'Keeffe ST. Restless legs syndrome: a review. *Arch Intern Med.* 1996;156:243-248.

14. Silber MH. Restless legs syndrome. *Mayo Clin Proc.* 1997;72:261-264.

15. Shemesh Z, Attias J, Ornan M, et al. Vitamin B_{12} deficiency in patients with chronic-tinnitus and noise-induced hearing loss. *Am J Otolaryngol.* 1993;14:94-99.

16. Montes LF, Diaz ML, Lajous J, et al. Folic acid and vitamin B_{12} in vitiligo: a nutritional approach. *Cutis.* 1992;50:39-42.

17. Juhlin L, Olsson MJ. Improvement of vitiligo after oral treatment with vitamin B_{12} and folic acid and the importance of sun exposure. *Acta Derm Venereol.* 1997;77: 460-462.

18. Kim SM, Kim YK, Hann SK. Serum levels of folic acid and vitamin B_{12} in Korean patients with vitiligo. *Yonsei Med J.* 1999;40:195-198.

19. Kwok T, Tang C, Woo J, et al. Randomized trial of the effect of supplementation on the cognitive function of older people with subnormal cobalamin levels. *Int J Geriatr Psychiatry.* 1998;13:611-616.

20. Teunisse S, Bollen AE, van Gool WA, et al. Dementia and subnormal levels of vitamin B_{12}: effects of replacement therapy on dementia. *J Neurol.* 1996;243:522-529.

21. Elia M. Oral or parenteral therapy for B_{12} deficiency. *Lancet.* 1998;352:1721-1722.

22. McIntyre PA, Hahn R, Masters JM, et al. Treatment of pernicious amenia with orally administered cyanocobalamin (vitamin B_{12}). *Arch Intern Med.* 1960;106:280-292.

23. Waife SO, Jansen J II, Crabtree RE, et al. Oral vitamin B_{12} without intrinsic factor in the treatment of pernicious anemia. *Ann Intern Med.* 1963;58:810-817.

24. Berlin H, Berlin R, Brante G. Oral treatment of pernicious anemia with high doses of vitamin B_{12} without intrinsic factor. *Acta Med Scand.* 1968;184:247-258.

25. Saltzman JR, Kemp JA, Golner BB, et al. Effect of hypochlorhydria due to omeprazole treatment or atrophic gastritis on protein-bound vitamin B_{12} absorption. *J Am Coll Nutr.* 1994;13:584-591.

26. van Goor L, Woiski MD, Lagaay AM, et al. Review: cobalamin deficiency and mental impairment in elderly people. *Age Ageing.* 1995;24:536-542.

27. Pennypacker LC, Allen RH, Kelly JP, et al. High prevalence of cobalamin deficiency in elderly outpatients. *J Am Geriatr Soc.* 1992;40:1197-1204.

28. Yao Y, Yao SL, Yao SS, et al. Prevalence of vitamin B_{12} deficiency among geriatric outpatients. *J Fam Pract.* 1992;35:524-528.

29. Marcuard SP, Albernaz L, Khazanie PG. Omeprazole therapy causes malabsorption of cyanocobalamin (vitamin B_{12}). *Ann Intern Med.* 1994;120:211-215.

30. Streeter AM, Goulston KJ, Bathur FA, et al. Cimetidine and malabsorption of cobalamin. *Dig Dis Sci.* 1982;27:13-16.

31. Aymard JP, Aymard B, Netter P, et al. Haematological adverse effects of histamine H_2-receptor antagonists. *Med Toxicol Adverse Drug Exp.* 1988;3:430-448.

32. Salom IL, Silvis SE, Doscherholmen A. Effect of cimetidine on the absorption of vitamin B_{12}. *Scand J Gastroenterol.* 1982;17:129-131.

33. Belaiche J, Zittoun J, Marquet J, et al. Effect of ranitidine on secretion of gastric intrinsic factor and absorption of vitamin B_{12} [translated from French]. *Gastroenterol Clin Biol.* 1983;7:381-384.

34. Sherertz EF. Acneiform eruption due to "megadose" vitamins B_6 and B_{12}. *Cutis.* 1991; 48:119-120.

35. Braun-Falco O, Lincke H. The problem of vitamin B_6/B_{12} acne: a contribution on acne medicamentosa [in German; English abstract]. *MMW Munch Med Wochenschr.* 1976;118:155-160.

36. Webb DI, Chodos RB, Mahar CQ, et al. Mechanism of vitamin B_{12} malabsorption in patients receiving colchicine. *N Engl J Med.* 1968;279:845-850.

37. Adams JF, Clark JS, Ireland JT, et al. Malabsorption of vitamin B_{12} and intrinsic factor secretion during biguanide therapy. *Diabetologia.* 1983;24:16-18.

38. Flippo TS, Holder WD Jr. Neurologic degeneration associated with nitrous oxide anesthesia in patients with vitamin B_{12} deficiency. *Arch Surg.* 1993;128:1391-1395.

39. Baum MK, Javier JJ, Mantero-Atienza E, et al. Zidovudine-associated adverse reactions in a longitudinal study of asymptomatic HIV-1-infected homosexual males. *J Acquir Immune Defic Syndr.* 1991;4:1218-1226.

40. *Drug Evaluations Annual.* (Subscription edition, section 19, chapter 5). Vol. 3. Chicago, Ill: American Medical Association. Division of Drugs and Toxicology; Spring 1993.

41. Mauro GL, Martorana U, Cataldo P, et al. Vitamin B_{12} in low back pain: a randomized double-blind placebo-controlled study. *Eur Rev Med Pharmacol Sci.* 2000;4:53-58.

42. Oren DA, Teicher MH, Schwartz PJ, et al. A controlled trial of cyanocobalamin (vitamin B_{12}) in the treatment of winter seasonal affective disorder. *J Affect Disord.* 1994;32:197-200.

Vitamin C

1. Hemila H. Does vitamin C alleviate the symptoms of the common cold? A review of current evidence. *Scand J Infect Dis.* 1994;26:1-6.

2. Hemila H. Vitamin C and the common cold. *Br J Nutr.* 1992;67:3-16.

3. Hemila H. Vitamin C supplementation and common cold symptoms: factors affecting the magnitude of the benefit. *Med Hypotheses.* 1999;52:171-178.

4. Peters EM, Goetzsche JM, Grobbelaar B, et al. Vitamin C supplementation reduces the incidence of postrace symptoms of upper-respiratory-tract infection in ultramarathon runners. *Am J Clin Nutr.* 1993;57:170-174.

5. Hemila H. Vitamin C and common cold incidence: a review of studies with subjects under heavy physical stress. *Int J Sports Med.* 1996;17:379-383.

6. Hemila H. Vitamin C intake and susceptibility to the common cold. *Br J Nutr.* 1997;77:59-72.

7. Zollinger PE, Tuinebreijer WE, Kreis RW, et al. Effect of vitamin C on frequency of reflex sympathetic dystrophy in wrist fractures: a randomized trial. *Lancet.* 1999;354:2025-2028.

8. Schorah CJ, Tormey WP, Brooks GH, et al. The effect of vitamin C supplements on body weight, serum proteins, and general health of an elderly population. *Am J Clin Nutr.* 1981;34:871-876.

9. Duffy SJ, Gokce N, Holbrook M, et al. Treatment of hypertension with ascorbic acid. *Lancet.* 1999;354:2048-2049.

10. Osilesi O, Trout DL, Ogunwole JO, et al. Blood pressure and plasma lipids during ascorbic acid supplementation in borderline hypertensive and normotensive adults. *Nutr Res.* 1991;11:405-412.

11. Fotherby MD, Williams JC, Forster LA, et al. Effect of vitamin C on ambulatory blood pressure and plasma lipids in older persons. *J Hypertens.* 2000;18:411-415.

12. Ghosh SK, Ekpo EB, Shah IU, et al. A double-blind, placebo-controlled parallel trial of vitamin C treatment in elderly patients with hypertension. *Gerontology.* 1994;40:268-272.

13. Lovat LB, Lu Y, Palmer AJ, et al. Double-blind trial of vitamin C in elderly hypertensives. *J Hum Hypertens.* 1993;7:403-405.

14. Mackerras D, Irwig L, Simpson JM, et al. Randomized double-blind trial of beta-carotene and vitamin C in women with minor cervical abnormalities. *Br J Cancer.* 1999;79:1448-1453.
15. Taylor TV, Rimmer S, Day B, et al. Ascorbic acid supplementation in the treatment of pressure-sores. *Lancet.* 1974;2:544-546.
16. Dolske MC, Spollen J, McKay S, et al. A preliminary trial of ascorbic acid as supplemental therapy for autism. *Prog Neuropsychopharmacol Biol Psychiatry.* 1993;17:765-774.
17. McAlindon TE, Jacques P, Zhang Y, et al. Do antioxidant micronutrients protect against the development and progression of knee osteoarthritis? *Arthritis Rheum.* 1996;39:648-656.
18. Schwartz ER. The modulation of osteoarthritic development by vitamins C and E. *Int J Vitam Nutr Res Suppl.* 1984;26:141-146.
19. Khaw KT, Bingham S, Welch A, et al. Relation between plasma ascorbic acid and mortality in men and women in EPIC-Norfolk prospective study: a prospective population study. *Lancet.* 2001;357:657-663.
20. Shibata A, Paganini-Hill A, Ross RK, et al. Intake of vegetables, fruits, beta-carotene, vitamin C and vitamin supplements and cancer incidence among the elderly: a prospective study. *Br J Cancer.* 1992;66:673-679.
21. Cohen M, Bhagavan HN. Ascorbic acid and gastrointestinal cancer. *J Am Coll Nutr.* 1995;14:565-578.
22. Esteve J, Riboli E, Pequignot G, et al. Diet and cancers of the larynx and hypopharynx: the IARC multi-center study in southwestern Europe. *Cancer Causes Control.* 1996;7:240-252.
23. Flagg EW, Coates RJ, Greenberg RS. Epidemiologic studies of antioxidants and cancer in humans. *J Am Coll Nutr.* 1995;14:419-427.
24. Block G. Epidemiologic evidence regarding vitamin C and cancer. *Am J Clin Nutr.* 1991;54(suppl 6):1310S-1314S.
25. Hankinson S, Stampfer M, Seddon J, et al. Nutrient intake and cataract extraction in women: a prospective study. *BMJ.* 1992;305:335-339.
26. Jacques PF, Taylor A, Hankinson SE, et al. Long-term vitamin C supplement use and prevalence of early age-related lens opacities. *Am J Clin Nutr.* 1997;66:911-916.
27. Will JC, Byers T. Does diabetes mellitus increase the requirement for vitamin C? *Nutr Rev.* 1996;54:193-202.
28. Mares-Perlman JA, Klein R, Klein BEK, et al. Relationships between age-related maculopathy and intake of vitamin and mineral supplements [abstract]. *Invest Ophthalmol Vis Sci.* 1993;34:1133.
29. Mares-Perlman JA, Klein R, Klein BEK, et al. Association of zinc and antioxidant nutrients with age-related maculopathy. *Arch Ophthalmol.* 1996;114:991-997.
30. Age Related Macular Degeneration Study Group. Multicenter ophthalmic and nutritional age-related macular degeneration study. 2. Antioxidant intervention and conclusions. *J Am Optom Assoc.* 1996;67:30-49.
31. Simon JA, Hudes ES. Serum ascorbic acid and gallbladder disease prevalence among US adults: the Third National Health and Nutrition Examination Survey (NHANES III). *Arch Intern Med.* 2000;160:931-936.
32. Masaki KH, Losonczy KG, Izmirlian G, et al. Association of vitamin E and C supplement use with cognitive function and dementia in elderly men. *Neurology.* 2000;54:1265-1272.
33. Chappell LC, Seed PT, Briley AL, et al. Effect of antioxidants on the occurrence of pre-eclampsia in women at increased risk: a randomized trial. *Lancet.* 1999;354:810-816.
34. van Rooij J, Schwartzenberg SG, Mulder PG, et al. Oral vitamins C and E as additional treatment in patients with acute anterior uveitis: a randomized double masked study in 145 patients. *Br J Ophthalmol.* 1999;83:1277-1282.
35. Eberlein-Konig B, Placzek M, Przybilla B. Protective effect against sunburn of combined systemic ascorbic acid (vitamin C) and d-alpha-tocopherol (vitamin E). *J Am Acad Dermatol.* 1998;38:45-48.

36. Fuchs J, Kern H. Modulation of UV-light-induced skin inflammation by D-alpha-tocopherol and L-ascorbic acid: a clinical study using solar simulated radiation. *Free Radic Biol Med.* 1998;25:1006-1012.

37. Darr D, Dunston S, Faust H, et al. Effectiveness of antioxidants (vitamin C and E) with and without sunscreens as topical photoprotectants. *Acta Derm Venereol.* 1996; 76:264-268.

38. Trevithick JR, Shum DT, Redae S, et al. Reduction of sunburn damage to skin by topical application of vitamin E acetate following exposure to ultraviolet B radiation: effect of delaying application or of reducing concentration of vitamin E acetate applied. *Scanning Microsc.* 1993;7:1269-1281.

39. Trevithick JR, Xiong H, Lee S, et al. Topical tocopherol acetate reduces post-UVB, sunburn-associated erythema, edema, and skin sensitivity in hairless mice. *Arch Biochem Biophys.* 1992;296:575-582.

40. Werninghaus K, Meydani M, Bhawan J, et al. Evaluation of the photoprotective effect of oral vitamin E supplementation. *Arch Dermatol.* 1994;130:1257-1261.

41. Traikovich SS. Use of topical ascorbic acid and its effects on photodamaged skin topography. *Arch Otolaryngol Head Neck Surg.* 1999;125:1091-1098.

42. Darr D, Combs S, Dunston S, et al. Topical vitamin C protects porcine skin from ultraviolet radiation-induced damage. *Br J Dermatol.* 1992;127:247-253.

43. Rougier A, Humbert P, Zahouani H, et al. Clinical and biological effects of topical vitamin C in the treatment of skin aging. Presented at: 2nd World Congress of the International Academy of Cosmetic Dermatology; November 9-11, 2000; Rio de Janeiro, Brazil.

44. Bielory L, Gandhi R. Asthma and vitamin C. *Ann Allergy.* 1994;73:89-96.

45. Bucca C, Rolla G, Oliva A, et al. Effect of vitamin C on histamine bronchial responsiveness of patients with allergic rhinitis. *Ann Allergy.* 1990;65:311-314.

46. Bellioni P, Artuso A, Di Luzio Paparatti U, et al. Histaminic provocation in allergy: the role of ascorbic acid [in Italian]. *Riv Eur Sci Med Farmacol.* 1987;9:419-422.

47. Fortner BR II, Danziger RE, Rabinowitz PS, et al. The effect of ascorbic acid on cutaneous and nasal response to histamine and allergen. *J Allergy Clin Immunol.* 1982; 69:484-488.

48. Dawson EB, Harris WA, Rankin WE, et al. Effect of ascorbic acid on male fertility. *Ann NY Acad Sci.* 1987;498:312-323.

49. Rolf C, Cooper T, Yeung C, et al. Antioxidant treatment of patients with asthenozoospermia of moderate oligoasthenozoospermia with high-dose vitamin C and vitamin E: a randomized, placebo-controlled, double-blind study. *Hum Reprod.* 1999;14:1028-1033.

50. Lykkesfeldt J, Christen S, Wallock LM, et al. Ascorbate is depleted by smoking and repleted by moderate supplementation: a study in male smokers and nonsmokers with matched dietary antioxidant intakes. *Am J Clin Nutr.* 2000;71:530-536.

51. Blanchard J, Tozer TN, Rowland M. Pharmacokinetic perspectives on megadoses of ascorbic acid. *Am J Clin Nutr.* 1997;66:1165-1171.

52. Levine M, Wang Y, Padayatty SJ, et al. A new recommended dietary allowance of vitamin C for healthy young women. *Proc Natl Acad Sci USA.* 2001;98:9842-9846.

53. Gerster H. No contribution of ascorbic acid to renal calcium oxalate stones. *Ann Nutr Metab.* 1997;41:269-282.

54. Traxer O, Adams-Huet B, Pak CY, et al. Risk of calcium oxalate stone formation with ascorbic acid ingestion. Presented at: American Urological Association 2001 Annual Meeting; June 2-7, 2001; Anaheim, Calif.

55. Curhan GC, Willett WC, Speizer FE, et al. Intake of vitamins B_6 and C and the risk of kidney stones in women. *Am Soc Nephrol.* 1999;10:840-845.

56. Curhan GC. A prospective study of the intake of vitamin C and vitamin B_6 and the risk of kidney stones in men. *J Urol.* 1996;155:1847-1851.

57. Simon JA, Hudes ES. Relation of serum ascorbic acid to serum vitamin B_{12}, serum ferritin, and kidney stones in US adults. *Arch Intern Med.* 1999;159:619-624.

58. Auer BL, Auer D, Rodgers AL. Relative hyperoxaluria, crystalluria and haematuria after megadose ingestion of vitamin C. *Eur J Clin Invest.* 1998;28:695-700.

59. Owen CA, Tyce GM, Flock EV, et al. Heparin-ascorbic acid antagonism. *Mayo Clin Proc.* 1970;45:140-145.

60. Rosenthal G. Interaction of ascorbic acid and warfarin [letter]. *JAMA.* 1971; 215:1671.

61. Harris JE. Interaction of dietary factors with oral anticoagulants: review and applications. *J Am Diet Assoc.* 1995;95:580-584.

62. Smith EC, Skalski RJ, Johnson GC, et al. Interaction of ascorbic acid and warfarin. *JAMA.* 1972;221:1166.

63. Houston JB, Levy G. Drug biotransformation interactions in man. VI. Acetaminophen and ascorbic acid. *J Pharm Sci.* 1976;65:1218-1221.

64. Coffey G, Wilson CM. Ascorbic acid deficiency and aspirin-induced haematemesis [letter]. *Br Med J.* 1975;1:208.

65. Das N, Nebioglu S. Vitamin C aspirin interactions in laboratory animals. *J Clin Pharm Ther.* 1992;17:343-346.

66. Molloy TP, Wilson CW. Protein-binding of ascorbic acid. 2. Interaction with acetylsalicylic acid. *Int J Vitam Nutr Res.* 1980;50:387-392.

67. Rivers JM, Devine MM. Plasma ascorbic acid concentrations and oral contraceptives. *Am J Clin Nutr.* 1972;25:684-689.

68. Webb JL. Nutritional effects of oral contraceptive use. *J Reprod Med.* 1980;25:150-156.

69. Larsson-Cohn U. Oral contraceptives and vitamins: a review. *Am J Obstet Gynecol.* 1975;121:84-90.

70. Wynn V. Vitamins and oral contraceptive use. *Lancet.* 1975;1:561-564.

71. Briggs M, Briggs M. Vitamin C requirements and oral contraceptives. *Nature.* 1972;238:277.

72. Weijl NI, Cleton FJ, Osanto S. Free radicals and antioxidants in chemotherapy-induced toxicity. *Cancer Treat Rev.* 1997;23:209-240.

73. Kurbacher CM, Wagner U, Kolster B, et al. Ascorbic acid (vitamin C) improves the antineoplastic activity of doxorubicin, cisplatin, and paclitaxel in human breast carcinoma cells in vitro. *Cancer Lett.* 1996;103:183-189.

74. Milne DB, Klevay LM, Hunt JR. Effects of ascorbic acid supplements and a diet marginal in copper on indices of copper nutriture in women. *Nutr Res.* 1988;8:865-873.

75. Finley EB, Cerklewski FL. Influence of ascorbic acid supplementation on copper status in young adult men. *Am J Clin Nutr.* 1983;37:553-556.

76. Jacob RA, Skala JH, Omaye ST, et al. Effect of varying ascorbic acid intakes on copper absorption and ceruloplasmin levels of young men. *J Nutr.* 1987;117:2109-2115.

77. Harris ED, Percival SS. A role for ascorbic acid in copper transport. *Am J Clin Nutr.* 1991;54(6 suppl):1193S-1197S.

78. Maskos Z, Koppenol WH. Oxyradicals and multivitamin tablets. *Free Radic Biol Med.* 1991;11:609-610.

79. Conrad ME, Schade SG. Ascorbic acid chelates in iron absorption: a role for hydrochloric acid and bile. *Gastroenterology.* 1968;55:35-45.

80. Brise H, Hallberg L. Effect of ascorbic acid on iron absorption. *Acta Med Scand Suppl.* 1962;171:51-58.

81. Lynch SR, Cook JD. Interaction of vitamin C and iron. *Ann NY Acad Sci.* 1980; 355:32-44.

82. Hunt JR, Gallagher SK, Johnson LK. Effect of ascorbic acid on apparent iron absorption by women with low iron stores. *Am J Clin Nutr.* 1994;59:1381-1385.

83. Diplock AT. Safety of antioxidant vitamins and beta-carotene. *Am J Clin Nutr.* 1995;62 (6 suppl):1510S-1516S.

84. Hoffman KE, Yanelli K, Bridges KR. Ascorbic acid and iron metabolism: alterations in lysosomal function. *Am J Clin Nutr.* 1991;54(6 suppl):1188S-1192S.

85. Siegenberg D, Baynes RD, Bothwell TH, et al. Ascorbic acid prevents the dose-dependent inhibitory effects of polyphenols and phytates on nonheme-iron absorption. *Am J Clin Nutr.* 1991;53:537-541.

86. Bassenge E, Fink N, Skatchkov M, et al. Dietary supplement with vitamin C prevents nitrate tolerance. *J Clin Invest.* 1998;31:67-71.

87. Watanabe H, Kakihana M, Ohtsuka S, et al. Randomized, double-blind, placebo-controlled study of the preventive effect of supplemental oral vitamin C on attenuation of development of nitrate tolerance. *J Am Coll Cardiol.* 1998;31:1323-1329.
88. Blee TH, Cogbill TH, Lambert PJ. Hemorrhage associated with vitamin C deficiency in surgical patients. *Surgery.* 2002;131:408-412.
89. Audera C, Patulny RV, Sander BH, et al. Mega-dose vitamin C in treatment of the common cold: a randomized controlled trial. *Med J Aust.* 2001;175:359-362.

Vitamin D

1. Utiger R. The need for more vitamin D. *N Engl J Med.* 1998;338:828-829.
2. Semba RD, Garrett E, Johnson BA, et al. Vitamin D deficiency among older women with and without disability. *Am J Clin Nutr.* 2000;72:1529-1534.
3. Mezquita-Raya P, Munoz-Torres M, De Dios Luna J, et al. Relation between vitamin D insufficiency, bone density, and bone metabolism in healthy postmenopausal women. *J Bone Miner Res.* 2001;16:1408-1415.
4. Dawson-Hughes B, Dallal GE, Krall EA. Effect of vitamin D supplementation on wintertime and overall bone loss in healthy postmenopausal women. *Ann Intern Med.* 1991;115:505-512.
5. Dawson-Hughes B, Harris SS, Krall EA, et al. Effect of calcium and vitamin D supplementation on bone density in men and women 65 years of age or older. *N Engl J Med.* 1997;337:670-676.
6. Dawson-Hughes B, Harris SS, Krall EA, et al. Effect of withdrawal of calcium and vitamin D supplements on bone mass in elderly men and women. *Am J Clin Nutr.* 2000;72:745-750.
7. Homik J, Suarez-Almazor ME, Shea B, et al. Calcium and vitamin D for corticosteroid-induced osteoporosis. *Cochrane Database Syst Rev.* 2000;30:1-9.
8. LeBoff MS, Kohlmeier L, Hurwitz S, et al. Occult vitamin D deficiency in postmenopausal US women with acute hip fracture. *JAMA.* 1999;281:1505-1511.
9. Lips P, Graafmans WC, Ooms ME, et al. Vitamin D supplementation and fracture incidence in elderly persons: a randomized, placebo-controlled clinical trial. *Ann Intern Med.* 1996;124:400-406.
10. Hunter D, Major P, Arden N, et al. A randomized controlled trial of vitamin D supplementation on preventing postmenopausal bone loss and modifying bone metabolism using identical twin pairs. *J Bone Miner Res.* 2000;15:2276-2283.
11. Garland FC, Garland CF, Gorham ED, et al. Geographic variation in breast cancer mortality in the United States: a hypothesis involving exposure to solar radiation. *Prev Med.* 1990;19:614-622.
12. Martinez ME, Giovannucci EL, Colditz GA, et al. Calcium, vitamin D, and the occurrence of colorectal cancer among women. *J Natl Cancer Inst.* 1996;88:1375-1382.
13. Kearney J, Giovannucci E, Rimm E, et al. Calcium, vitamin D, and dairy foods and the occurrence of colon cancer in men. *Am J Epidemiol.* 1996;143:907-917.
14. James SY, Mackay AG, Colston KW. Effects of 1,25 dihydroxyvitamin D_3 and its analogues on induction of apoptosis in breast cancer cells. *J Steroid Biochem Mol Biol.* 1996;58:395-401.
15. Taylor JA, Hirvonen A, Watson M, et al. Association of prostate cancer with vitamin D receptor gene polymorphism. *Cancer Res.* 1996;56:4108-4110.
16. Douglas WC. Vitamin D scores again. *Second Opin.* 1997;7(7):4-5.
17. Fuller KE, Casparian JM. Vitamin D: balancing cutaneous and systematic considerations. *South Med J.* 2001;94:58-64.
18. Gilchrest BA, Eller MS, Geller AC, et al. The pathogenesis of melanoma induced by ultraviolet radiation. *N Engl J Med.* 1999;340:1341-1348.
19. Studzinski GP, Moore DC. Sunlight—can it prevent as well as cause cancer? *Cancer Res.* 1995;55:4014-4022.
20. Blutt SE, Weigel NL. Vitamin D and prostate cancer. *Proc Soc Exp Biol Med.* 1999;221:89-98.
21. Vandewalle B, Hornez L, Wattez N, et al. Vitamin-D_3 derivatives and breast-tumor cell growth: effect on intracellular calcium and apoptosis. *Int J Cancer.* 1995;61:806-811.

22. Hofer H, Ho GM, Peterlik M, et al. Biological effects of 1alpha-hydroxy- and 1beta-(hydroxymethyl)-vitamin D compounds relevant for potential colorectal cancer therapy. *J Pharmacol Exp Ther.* 1999;291:450-455.

23. Tong WM, Kallay E, Hofer H, et al. Growth regulation of human colon cancer cells by epidermal growth factor and 1,25-dihydroxyvitamin D_3 is mediated by mutual modulation of receptor expression. *Eur J Cancer.* 1998;34:2119-2125.

24. Ekman P. Genetic and environmental factors in prostate cancer genesis: identifying high-risk cohorts. *Eur Urol.* 1999;35:362-369.

25. Peehl DM. Vitamin D and prostate cancer risk. *Eur Urol.* 1999;35:392-394.

26. Hanchette CL, Schwartz GG. Geographic patterns of prostate cancer mortality: evidence for a protective effect of ultraviolet radiation. *Cancer.* 1992;70:2861-2869.

27. Moffatt KA, Johannes WU, Miller GJ. 1Alpha,25dihydroxyvitamin D_3 and platinum drugs act synergistically to inhibit the growth of prostate cancer cell lines. *Clin Cancer Res.* 1999;5:695-703.

28. Danielsson C, Torma H, Vahlquist A, et al. Positive and negative interaction of 1,25-dihydroxyvitamin D_3 and the retinoid CD437 in the induction of human melanoma cell apoptosis. *Int J Cancer.* 1999;81:467-470.

29. Evans SR, Houghton AM, Schumaker L, et al. Vitamin D receptor and growth inhibition by 1,25-dihydroxyvitamin D_3 in human malignant melanoma cell lines. *J Surg Res.* 1996;61:127-133.

30. Rostand SG. Ultraviolet light may contribute to geographic and racial blood pressure differences. *Hypertension.* 1997;30(2 pt 1):150-156.

31. Scragg R. Sunlight, vitamin D, and cardiovascular disease. In: Crass MF II, Avioli LV, eds. *Calcium Regulating Hormones and Cardiovascular Function.* Boca Raton, Fla: CRC Press; 1995.

32. O'Connell TD, Simpson RU. 1,25-Dihydroxyvitamin D_3 and cardiac muscle structure and function. In: Crass MF II, Avioli LV, eds. *Calcium-Regulating Hormones and Cardiovascular Function.* Boca Raton, Fla: CRC Press; 1995:191-211.

33. Thys-Jacobs S, Donovan D, Papadopoulos A, et al. Vitamin D and calcium dysregulation in the polycystic ovarian syndrome. *Steroids.* 1999;64:430-435.

34. Kragballe K. Vitamin D_3 analogues in psoriasis [letter]. *Dermatologica.* 1990;180:110-111.

35. Vieth R. Vitamin D supplementation, 25-hydroxyvitamin D concentrations, and safety. *Am J Clin Nutr.* 1999;69:842-856.

36. Holick MF. Sunlight "D"ilemma: risk of skin cancer or bone disease and muscle weakness. *Lancet.* 2001;357:4-6.

37. Glerup H, Mikkelsen K, Poulsen L, et al. Hypovitaminosis D myopathy without biochemical signs of osteomalacic bone involvement. *Calcif Tissue Int.* 2000;66:419-424.

38. Glerup H, Mikkelsen K, Poulsen L, et al. Commonly recommended daily intake of vitamin D is not sufficient if sunlight exposure is limited. *J Intern Med.* 2000;247:260-268.

39. Holick MF. McCollum Award Lecture, 1994: vitamin D—new horizons for the 21st century. *Am J Clin Nutr.* 1994;60:619-630.

40. Malabanan A, Veronikis IE, Holick MF. Redefining vitamin D insufficiency [letter]. *Lancet.* 1998;351:805-806.

41. Moon JC. A brief history of vitamin D toxicity. *J Appl Nutr.* 1997;49:18-31.

42. Dietary Reference Intakes for Calcium, Phosphorus, Magnesium, Vitamin D, and Fluoride (1997). Available at: http://www.nap.edu. Accessed October 4, 2001.

43. Bar-Or D, Gasiel Y. Calcium and calciferol antagonise effect of verapamil in atrial fibrillation. *Br Med J (Clin Res Ed).* 1981;282:1585-1586.

44. Riis B, Christiansen C. Actions of thiazide on vitamin D metabolism: a controlled therapeutic trial in normal women early in the postmenopause. *Metabolism.* 1985;34:421-424.

45. Lemann J Jr, Gray RW, Maierhofer WJ, et al. Hydrochlorothiazide inhibits bone resorption in men despite experimentally elevated serum 1,25-dihydroxyvitamin D concentrations. *Kidney Int.* 1985;28:951-958.

46. Crowe M, Wollner L, Griffiths RA. Hypercalcaemia following vitamin D and thiazide therapy in the elderly. *Practitioner.* 1984;228:312-313.

47. Holmes R, Kummerow F. The relationship of adequate and excessive intake of vitamin D to health and disease. *J Am Coll Nutr.* 1983;2:173-199.
48. Roe DA. *Drug-Induced Nutritional Deficiencies.* 2nd ed. Westport, Conn: AVI Pub. Co; 1985:164-166.
49. Roe D, Campbell T, eds. *Drugs and Nutrients: The Interactive Effects.* New York, NY: Marcel Decker; 1984:505-523.
50. Hodges RE. Drug-nutrient interaction. In: Hodges RE. *Nutrition in Medical Practice.* Philadelphia, Pa: WB Saunders; 1980:323-331.
51. Bengoa JM, Bolt MJ, Rosenberg IH. Hepatic vitamin D 25-hydroxylase inhibition by cimetidine and isoniazid. *J Lab Clin Med.* 1984;104:546-552.
52. Odes HS, Fraser GM, Krugliak P, et al. Effect of cimetidine on hepatic vitamin D metabolism in humans. *Digestion.* 1990;46:61-64.
53. [No authors listed]. Cimetidine inhibits the hepatic hydroxylation of vitamin D. *Nutr Rev.* 1985;43:184-185.
54. Brodie MJ, Boobis AR, Hillyard CJ, et al. Effect of isoniazid on vitamin D metabolism and hepatic monooxygenase activity. *Clin Pharmacol Ther.* 1981;30:363-367.
55. Hahn TJ, Hendin BA, Scharp CR, et al. Effect of chronic anticonvulsant therapy on serum 25-hydroxycalciferol levels in adults. *N Engl J Med.* 1972;287:900-904.
56. Jubiz W, Haussler MR, McCain TA, et al. Plasma 1,25-dihydroxyvitamin D levels in patients receiving anticonvulsant drugs. *J Clin Endocrinol Metab.* 1977;44:617-621.
57. Williams C, Netzloff M, Folkerts L, et al. Vitamin D metabolism and anticonvulsant therapy: effect of sunshine on incidence of osteomalacia. *South Med J.* 1984;77: 834-836.
58. Tomita S, Ohnishi J, Nakano M, et al. The effects of anticonvulsant drugs on vitamin D_3-activating cytochrome P-450-linked monooxygenase systems. *J Steroid Biochem Mol Biol.* 1991;39:479-485.
59. Buckley LM, Leib ES, Cartularo KS, et al. Calcium and vitamin D_3 supplementation prevents bone loss in the spine secondary to low-dose corticosteroids in patients with rheumatoid arthritis: a randomized, double-blind, placebo-controlled study. *Ann Intern Med.* 1996;125:961-968.
60. Aarskog D, Aksnes L, Markestad T, et al. Heparin-induced inhibition of 1,25-dihydroxyvitamin D formation. *Am J Obstet Gynecol.* 1984;148:1141-1142.
61. Haram K, Hervig T, Thordarson H, et al. Osteopenia caused by heparin treatment in pregnancy. *Acta Obstet Gynecol Scand.* 1993;72:674-675.
62. Wise PH, Hall AJ. Heparin-induced osteopenia in pregnancy. *Br Med J.* 1980; 281:110-111.
63. Brodie MJ, Boobis AR, Dollery CT, et al. Rifampicin and vitamin D metabolism. *Clin Pharmacol Ther.* 1980;27:810-814.
64. Williams SE, Wardman AG, Taylor GA, et al. Long term study of the effect of rifampicin and isoniazid on vitamin D metabolism. *Tubercle.* 1985;66:49-54.
65. Perry W, Erooga MA, Brown J, et al. Calcium metabolism during rifampicin and isoniazid therapy for tuberculosis. *J R Soc Med.* 1982;75:533-536.
66. Hypponen E, Laara E, Reunanen A, et al. Intake of vitamin D and risk of type I diabetes: a birth-cohort study. *Lancet.* 2001;358:1500-1503.
67. The EURODIAB Substudy 2 Study Group. Vitamin D supplement in early childhood and risk for Type I (insulin-dependent) diabetes mellitus. *Diabetologia.* 1999; 42:51-54.
68. Johansson S, Melhus H. Vitamin A antagonizes calcium response to vitamin D in man. *J Bone Miner Res.* 2001;16:1899-1905.
69. Stene LC, Ulriksen J, Magnus P, et al. Use of cod liver oil during pregnancy associated with lower risk of Type I diabetes in the offspring. *Diabetologia.* 2000;43:1093-1098.

Vitamin E

1. Heinonen OP, Albanes D, Virtamo J, et al. Prostate cancer and supplementation with alpha-tocopherol and beta-carotene: incidence and mortality in a controlled trial. *J Natl Cancer Inst.* 1998;90:440-446.

2. Albanes D, Heinonen OP, Huttunen JK, et al. Effects of alpha-tocopherol and beta-carotene supplements on cancer incidence in the Alpha-Tocopherol Beta-Carotene Cancer Prevention Study. *Am J Clin Nutr.* 1995;62(suppl):1427S-1430S.

3. White E, Shannon JS, Patterson RE. Relationship between vitamin and calcium supplement use and colon cancer. *Cancer Epidemiol Biomarkers Prev.* 1997;6:769-774.

4. Macready N. Vitamins associated with lower colon-cancer risk. *Lancet.* 1997; 350:1452.

5. Losonczy KG, Harris TB, Havlik RJ. Vitamin E and vitamin C supplement use and risk of all-cause and coronary heart disease mortality in older persons: the Established Populations for Epidemiologic Studies of the Elderly. *Am J Clin Nutr.* 1996;64:190-196.

6. Bostick RM, Potter JD, McKenzie DR, et al. Reduced risk of colon cancer with high intake of vitamin E: the Iowa Women's Health Study. *Cancer Res.* 1993;53:4230-4237.

7. Ocke MC, Bueno-de-Mesquita HB, Feskens EJ, et al. Repeated measurements of vegetables, fruits, beta-carotene, and vitamins C and E in relation to lung cancer: the Zutphen Study. *Am J Epidemiol.* 1997;145:358-365.

8. Giovannucci E, Stampfer MJ, Colditz GA, et al. Multivitamin use, folate, and colon cancer in women in the nurses' health study. *Ann Intern Med.* 1998;129:517-524.

9. Malila N, Virtamo J, Virtanen M, et al. The effect of alpha-tocopherol and beta-carotene supplementation on colorectal adenomas in middle-aged male smokers. *Cancer Epidemiol Biomarkers Prev.* 1999;8:489-493.

10. Hennekens CH, Buring JE, Manson JE, et al. Lack of effect of long-term supplementation with beta carotene on the incidence of malignant neoplasms and cardiovascular disease. *N Engl J Med.* 1996;334:1145-1149.

11. Greenberg ER, Baron JA, Tosteson TD, et al. A clinical trial of antioxidant vitamins to prevent colorectal adenoma. *N Engl J Med.* 1994;331:141-147.

12. Helzlsouer KJ, Huang HY, Alberg AJ, et al. Association between alpha-tocopherol, gamma-tocopherol, selenium, and subsequent prostate cancer. *J Natl Cancer Inst.* 2000;92:2018-2023.

13. Zheng W, Sellers TA, Doyle TJ, et al. Retinol, antioxidant vitamins, and cancers of the upper digestive tract in a prospective cohort study of postmenopausal women. *Am J Epidemiol.* 1995;142:955-960.

14. Esteve J, Riboli E, Pequignot G, et al. Diet and cancers of the larynx and hypopharynx: the IARC multi-center study in southwestern Europe. *Cancer Causes Control.* 1996;7:240-252.

15. Chen J, Geissler C, Parpia B, et al. Antioxidant status and cancer mortality in China. *Int J Epidemiol.* 1992;21:625-635.

16. Meydani SN, Meydani M, Blumberg JB, et al. Vitamin E supplementation and in vivo immune response in healthy elderly subjects: a randomized controlled trial. *JAMA.* 1997;277:1380-1386.

17. Sano M, Ernesto C, Thomas RG, et al. A controlled trial of selegiline, alpha-tocopherol, or both as treatment for Alzheimer's disease. *N Engl J Med.* 1997;336: 1216-1222.

18. Masaki KH, Losonczy KG, Izmirlian G, et al. Association of vitamin E and C supplement use with cognitive function and dementia in elderly men. *Neurology.* 2000; 54:1265-1272.

19. Manzella D, Barbieri M, Ragno E, et al. Chronic administration of pharmacologic doses of vitamin E improves the cardiac autonomic nervous system in patients with type 2 diabetes. *Am J Clin Nutr.* 2001;73:1052-1057.

20. Suleiman SA, Ali EM, Zaki ZMS, et al. Lipid peroxidation and human sperm motility: protective role of vitamin E. *J Androl.* 1996;17:530-537.

21. Rolf C, Cooper T, Yeung C, et al. Antioxidant treatment of patients with asthenozoospermia of moderate oligoasthenozoospermia with high-dose vitamin C and vitamin E: a randomized, placebo-controlled, double-blind study. *Hum Reprod.* 1999; 14;1028-1033.

22. Soares KV, McGrath JJ. The treatment of tardive dyskinesia—a systematic review and meta-analysis. *Schizophr Res.* 1999;39:1-18.

23. Adler LA, Rotrosen J, Edson R, et al. Vitamin E treatment for tardive dyskinesia. *Arch Gen Psychiatry.* 1999;56:836-841.
24. Rimm EB, Stampfer MJ, Ascherio A, et al. Vitamin E consumption and the risk of coronary heart disease in men. *N Engl J Med.* 1993;328:1450-1456.
25. Manson JE, Stampfer MJ, Willitt WC, et al. A prospective study of antioxidant vitamins and incidence of coronary heart disease in women [abstract]. *J Am Coll Nutr.* 1992;11:633.
26. Stampfer MJ, Hennekens CH, Manson JE, et al. Vitamin E consumption and the risk of coronary disease in women. *N Engl J Med.* 1993;328:1444-1449.
27. Bazzano LA, He J, Ogden LG, et al. Dietary vitamin E intake and risk of coronary heart disease in a representative sample of US adults: NHANES I Epidemiologic Follow-up Study [abstract]. *Circulation.* 2001;103:1366.
28. Heart Outcomes Prevention Evaluation Study Investigators. Vitamin E supplementation and cardiovascular events in high-risk patients. *N Engl J Med.* 2000;342: 154-160.
29. Rapola JM, Virtamo J, Ripatti S, et al. Randomized trial of alpha-tocopherol and beta-carotene supplements on incidence of major coronary events in men with previous myocardial infarction. *Lancet.* 1997;349:1715-1720.
30. Rapola JM, Virtamo J, Haukka JK, et al. Effect of vitamin E and beta carotene on the incidence of angina pectoris. *JAMA.* 1996;275;693-698.
31. Tornwall ME, Virtamo J, Haukka JK, et al. Alpha-tocopherol (vitamin E) and beta-carotene supplementation does not affect the risk for large abdominal aortic aneurysm in a controlled trial. *Atherosclerosis.* 2001;157:167-173.
32. Lonn EM, Yusuf S, Dzavik V, et al. Effects of Ramipril and vitamin E on atherosclerosis: the study to evaluate carotid ultrasound changes in patients treated with Ramipril and vitamin E (SECURE). *Circulation.* 2001;103:919-925.
33. Collaborative Group of the Primary Prevention Project (PPP). Low-dose aspirin and vitamin E in people at cardiovascular risk: a randomized trial in general practice. *Lancet.* 2001;357:89-95.
34. Stephens NG, Parsons A, Schofield PM, et al. Randomized controlled trial of vitamin E in patients with coronary disease: Cambridge Heart Antioxidant Study (CHAOS). *Lancet.* 1996;347:781-786.
35. GISSI-Prevenzione Investigators. Dietary supplementation with n-3 polyunsaturated fatty acids and vitamin E after myocardial infarction: results of the GISSI-Prevenzione trial. *Lancet.* 1999;354:447-455.
36. Alpha-Tocopherol, Beta Carotene Cancer Prevention Study Group. The effect of vitamin E and beta-carotene on the incidence of lung cancer and other cancers in male smokers. *N Engl J Med.* 1994;330:1029-1035.
37. Legha SS, Wang YM, Mackay B, et al. Clinical and pharmacologic investigation of the effects of alpha-tocopherol on adriamycin cardiotoxicity. *Ann NY Acad Sci.* 1982;393:411-418.
38. Desnuelle C, Dib M, Garrel C, et al. A double-blind, placebo-controlled randomized clinical trial of alpha-tocopherol (vitamin E) in the treatment of amyotrophic lateral sclerosis: ALS riluzole-tocopherol Study Group. *Amyotroph Lateral Scler Other Motor Neuron Disord.* 2001;2:9-18.
39. Abrams B, Duncan D, Hertz-Picciotto I. A prospective study of dietary intake and acquired immune deficiency syndrome in HIV-seropositive homosexual men. *J Acquir Immune Defic Syndr.* 1993;6:949-958.
40. Allard JP, Aghdassi E, Chau J, et al. Effects of vitamin E and C supplementation on oxidative stress and viral load in HIV-infected subjects. *AIDS.* 1998;12:1653-1659.
41. Edmonds SE, Winyard PG, Guo R, et al. Putative analgesic activity of repeated oral doses of vitamin E in the treatment of rheumatoid arthritis: results of a prospective placebo controlled double blind trial. *Ann Rheum Dis.* 1997;56:649-655.
42. Knekt P, Heliovaara M, Aho K, et al. Serum selenium, serum alpha-tocopherol, and the risk of rheumatoid arthritis. *Epidemiology.* 2000;11:402-405.
43. Tutuncu NB, Bayraktar M, Varli K. Reversal of defective nerve conduction with vitamin E supplementation in type 2 diabetes: a preliminary study. *Diabetes Care.* 1998;21:1915-1918.

44. Kahler W, Kuklinski B, Ruhlmann C, et al. Diabetes mellitus—a free radical-associated disease. Results of an adjuvant antioxidant supplementation [in German; English abstract]. *Z Gesamte Inn Med.* 1993;48:223-232.
45. Bursell S-E, Clermont AC, Aiello LP, et al. High-dose vitamin E supplementation normalizes retinal blood flow and creatinine clearance in patients with type 1 diabetes. *Diabetes Care.* 1999;22:1245-1251.
46. Paolisso G, D'Amore A, Galzerano D, et al. Daily vitamin E supplements improve metabolic control but not insulin secretion in elderly type II diabetic patients. *Diabetes Care.* 1993;16:1433-1437.
47. Paolisso G, Di Maro G, Galzerano D, et al. Pharmacological doses of vitamin E and insulin action in elderly subjects. *Am J Clin Nutr.* 1994;59:1291-1296.
48. Paolisso G, D'Amore A, Giugliano D, et al. Pharmacologic doses of vitamin E improve insulin action in healthy subjects and non-insulin-dependent diabetic patients. *Am J Clin Nutr.* 1993;57:650-656.
49. Tavani A, Negri E, La Vecchia C. Food and nutrient intake and risk of cataract. *Ann Epidemiol.* 1996;6:41-46.
50. Leske MC, Chylack LT Jr, He Q, et al. Antioxidant vitamins and nuclear opacities: the longitudinal study of cataract. *Ophthalmology.* 1998;105:831-836.
51. Teikari JM, Rautalahti M, Haukka J, et al. Incidence of cataract operations in Finnish male smokers unaffected by alpha tocopherol or beta carotene supplements. *J Epidemiol Community Health.* 1998;52:468-472.
52. Seddon JM, Christen WG, Manson JE, et al. The use of vitamin supplements and the risk of cataract among U.S. male physicians. *Am J Public Health.* 1994;84:788-792.
53. Ayres S Jr, Mihan R. "Restless legs" syndrome: response to vitamin E. *J Appl Nutr.* 1973;25:8-15.
54. McBride JM, Kraemer WJ, Triplett-McBride T, et al. Effect of resistance exercise on free radical production. *Med Sci Sports Exerc.* 1998;30:67-72.
55. London RS, Murphy L, Kitlowski KE, et al. Efficacy of alpha-tocopherol in the treatment of the premenstrual syndrome. *J Reprod Med.* 1987;32:400-404.
56. London RS, Sundaram GS, Murphy L, et al. The effect of alpha-tocopherol on premenstrual symptomatology: a double-blind study. *J Am Coll Nutr.* 1983;2:115-122.
57. London RS, Sundaram GS, Murphy L, et al. The effect of vitamin E on mammary dysplasia: a double-blind study. *Obstet Gynecol.* 1985;65:104-106.
58. Parkinson Study Group. Effects of tocopherol and deprenyl on the progression of disability in early Parkinson's disease. *N Engl J Med.* 1993;328:176-183.
59. Kieburtz K, McDermott M, Como P, et al. The effect of deprenyl and tocopherol on cognitive performance in early untreated Parkinson's disease. *Neurology.* 1994;44:1756-1759.
60. Parkinson Study Group. Impact of deprenyl and tocopherol treatment on Parkinson's disease in DATATOP patients requiring levodopa. *Ann Neurol.* 1996;39:37-45.
61. Barton DL, Loprinzi CL, Quella SK, et al. Prospective evaluation of vitamin E for hot flashes in breast cancer survivors. *J Clin Oncol.* 1998;16:495-500.
62. Tornwall ME, Virtamo J, Haukka JK, et al. The effect of alpha-tocopherol and beta-carotene supplementation on symptoms and progression of intermittent claudication in a controlled trial. *Atherosclerosis.* 1999;147:193-197.
63. Kostis JB, Wilson AC, Lacy CR. Hypertension and ascorbic acid [letter]. *Lancet.* 2000;355:1272.
64. Buchman AL, Killip D, Ou CN, et al. Short-term vitamin E supplementation before marathon running: a placebo-controlled trial. *Nutrition.* 1999;15:278-283.
65. Chappell LC, Seed PT, Briley AL, et al. Effect of antioxidants on the occurrence of pre-eclampsia in women at increased risk: a randomized trial. *Lancet.* 1999;354:810-816.
66. Fuchs J, Kern H. Modulation of UV-light-induced skin inflammation by D-alpha-tocopherol and L-ascorbic acid: a clinical study using solar simulated radiation. *Free Radic Biol Med.* 1998;25:1006-1012.

67. Eberlein-Konig B, Placzek M, Przybilla B. Protective effect against sunburn of combined systemic ascorbic acid (vitamin C) and d-alpha-tocopherol (vitamin E). *J Am Acad Dermatol.* 1998;38:45-48.

68. Darr D, Dunston S, Faust H, et al. Effectiveness of antioxidants (vitamin C and E) with and without sunscreens as topical photoprotectants. *Acta Derm Venereol.* 1996;76:264-268.

69. Trevithick JR, Shum DT, Redae S, et al. Reduction of sunburn damage to skin by topical application of vitamin E acetate following exposure to ultraviolet B radiation: effect of delaying application or of reducing concentration of vitamin E acetate applied. *Scanning Microsc.* 1993;7:1269-1281.

70. Trevithick JR, Xiong H, Lee S, et al. Topical tocopherol acetate reduces post-UVB, sunburn-associated erythema, edema, and skin sensitivity in hairless mice. *Arch Biochem Biophys.* 1992;296:575-582.

71. Werninghaus K, Meydani M, Bhawan J, et al. Evaluation of the photoprotective effect of oral vitamin E supplementation. *Arch Dermatol.* 1994;130:1257-1261.

72. Vetrugno M, Maino A, Cardia G, et al. A randomized, double masked, clinical trial of high dose vitamin A and vitamin E supplementation after photorefractive keratectomy. *Br J Ophthalmol.* 2001;85:537-539.

73. van Rooij J, Schwartzenberg SG, Mulder PG, et al. Oral vitamins C and E as additional treatment in patients with acute anterior uveitis: a randomized double masked study in 145 patients. *Br J Ophthalmol.* 1999;83:1277-1282.

74. Meagher EA, Barry OP, Lawson JA, et al. Effects of vitamin E on lipid peroxidation in healthy persons. *JAMA.* 2001;285:1178-1182.

75. Weitzman SA, Lorell F, Carey RW, et al. Prospective study of tocopherol prophylaxis for anthracycline cardiac toxicity. *Curr Ther Res.* 1980;28:682-686.

76. Lenzhofer R, Ganzinger U, Rameis H, et al. Acute cardiac toxicity in patients after doxorubicin treatment and the effect of combined tocopherol and nifedipine pretreatment. *J Cancer Res Clin Oncol.* 1983;106:143-147.

77. Van Vleet JF, Ferrans VJ, Weirich WE. Cardiac disease induced by chronic adriamycin administration in dogs and an evaluation of vitamin E and selenium as cardioprotectants. *Am J Pathol.* 1980;99:13-42.

78. Breed JG, Zimmerman AN, Dormans JA, et al. Failure of the antioxidant vitamin E to protect against adriamycin-induced cardiotoxicity in the rabbit. *Cancer Res.* 1980;40:2033-2038.

79. Van Vleet JF, Ferrans VJ. Evaluation of vitamin E and selenium protection against chronic adriamycin toxicity in rabbits. *Cancer Treat Rep.* 1980;64:315-317.

80. Shinozawa S, Gomita Y, Araki Y. Effect of high dose alpha-tocopherol and alpha-tocopherol acetate pretreatment on Adriamycin (doxorubicin) induced toxicity and tissue distribution. *Physiol Chem Phys Med NMR.* 1988;20:329-335.

81. Hercberg S, Preziosi P, Galan P, et al. Vitamin status of a healthy French population: dietary intakes and biochemical markers. *Int J Vitam Nutr Res.* 1994;64:220-232.

82. Murphy SP, Subar AF, Block G. Vitamin E intakes and sources in the United States. *Am J Clin Nutr.* 1990;52:361-367.

83. Ford E, Sowell A. Serum alpha-tocopherol status in the United States population: findings from the Third National Health and Nutrition Examination Survey. *Am J Epidemiol.* 1999;150:290-300.

84. Dietary Reference Intakes for Vitamin C, Vitamin E, Selenium, and Carotenoids (2000). Available at: http://www.nap.edu. Accessed January 16, 2001.

85. Leppala JM, Virtamo J, Fogelholm R, et al. Controlled trial of alpha-tocopherol and beta-carotene supplements on stroke incidence and mortality in male smokers. *Arterioscler Thromb Vasc Biol.* 2000;20:230-235.

86. Labriola D, Livingston R. Possible interactions between dietary antioxidants and chemotherapy. *Oncology (Huntingt).* 1999;13:1003-1012.

87. Weijl NI, Cleton FJ, Osanto S. Free radicals and antioxidants in chemotherapy-induced toxicity. *Cancer Treat Rev.* 1997;23:209-240.

88. Liede KE, Haukka JK, Saxen LM, et al. Increased tendency towards gingival bleeding caused by joint effect of alpha-tocopherol supplementation and acetylsalicylic acid. *Ann Med.* 1998;30:542-546.

89. Kim JM, White RH. Effect of vitamin E on the anticoagulant response to Warfarin. *Am J Cardiol.* 1996;77:545-546.

90. Kachel DL, Moyer TP, Martin WJ II. Amiodarone-induced injury of human pulmonary artery endothelial cells: protection by alpha-tocopherol. *J Pharmacol Exp Ther.* 1990;254:1107-1112.

91. Gogu SR, Beckman BS, Rangan SR, et al. Increased therapeutic efficacy of zidovudine in combination with vitamin E. *Biochem Biophys Res Commun.* 1989;165:401-407.

92. Ford ES, Sowell A. Serum alpha-tocopherol status in the United States population: findings from the Third National Health and Nutrition Examination Survey. *Am J Epidemiol.* 1999;150:290-300.

93. Ziaei S, Faghihzadeh S, Sohrabvand F, et al. A randomized placebo-controlled trial to determine the effect of vitamin E in treatment of primary dysmenorrhoea. *Br J Obstet Gynaecol.* 2001;108:1181-1183.

94. Brand C, Snaddon J, Bailey M, et al. Vitamin E is ineffective for symptomatic relief of knee osteoarthritis: a six month double blind randomized placebo controlled study. *Ann Rheum Dis.* 2001;60:946-949.

95. Ohrvall M, Sundlof G, Vessby B. Gamma, but not alpha, tocopherol levels in serum are reduced in coronary heart disease patients. *J Intern Med.* 1996;239:111-117.

96. Kristenson M, Zieden B, Kucinskiene Z, et al. Antioxidant state and mortality from coronary heart disease in Lithuanian and Swedish men: concomitant cross sectional study of men aged 50. *BMJ.* 1997;314:629-633.

97. Kontush A, Spranger T, Reich A, et al. Lipophilic antioxidants in blood plasma as markers of atherosclerosis: the role of alpha-carotene and gamma-tocopherol. *Atherosclerosis.* 1999;144:117-122.

98. l-Sohemy A, Baylin A, Spiegelman D, et al. Dietary and adipose tissue gamma-tocopherol and risk of myocardial infarction. *Epidemiology.* 2002;13:216-223.

99. erman EH, Ferrans VJ. Influence of vitamin E and ICRF-187 on chronic doxorubicin cardiotoxicity in miniature swine. *Lab Invest.* 1983;49:69-77.

100. Watanabe H, et al. Randomized, double-blind, placebo-controlled study of supplemental vitamin E on attenuation of the development of nitrate tolerance. *Circulation.* 1997;96:2545-2550.

101. Lenzhofer R, Magometschnigg D, Dudczak R, et al. Indication of reduced doxorubicin-induced cardiac toxicity by additional treatment with antioxidative substances. *Experientia.* 1983;39:62-64.

102. Mimnaugh EG, Siddik ZH, Drew R, et al. The effects of alpha-tocopherol on the toxicity, disposition, and metabolism of Adriamycin in mice. *Toxicol Appl Pharmacol.* 1979;49:119-126.

103. Hermansen K, Wassermann K. The effect of vitamin E and selenium on doxorubicin (Adriamycin) induced delayed toxicity in mice. *Acta Pharmacol Toxicol (Copenh).* 1986;58:31-37.

104. Wang YM, Madanat FF, Kimball JC, et al. Effect of vitamin E against Adriamycin-induced toxicity in rabbits. *Cancer Res.* 1980;40:1022-1027.

105. Milei J, Boveris A, Llesuy S, et al. Amelioration of Adriamycin-induced cardiotoxicity in rabbits by prenylamine and vitamins A and E. *Am Heart J.* 1986;111:95-102.

Vitamin K

1. Avery RA, Duncan WE, Alving BM. Severe vitamin K deficiency induced by occult celiac disease BR96-026 [letter]. *Am J Hematol.* 1996;53:55.

2. Benitez Leon MD, Hernandez Hernandez L, Sanchez Arcos E, et al. Changes in the prothrombin complex as clinical manifestation of celiac sprue in adults [letter] [in Spanish]. *Rev Clin Esp.* 1996;196:492-493.

3. Krasinski SD, Russell RM, Furie BC, et al. The prevalence of vitamin K deficiency in chronic gastrointestinal disorders. *Am J Clin Nutr.* 1985;41:639-643.

4. Krejs GJ. Diarrhea. In: JB Wyngaarden, LH Smith, Jr, eds. *Cecil Textbook of Medicine.* 18th ed. Philadelphia, Pa: Saunders; 1988.

5. Iber FL, Shamszad M, Miller PA, et al. Vitamin K deficiency in chronic alcoholic males. *Alcohol Clin Exp Res.* 1986;10:679-681.

6. Ekelund H, Finnstrom O, Gunnarskog J, et al. Administration of vitamin K to new-born infants and childhood cancer. *BMJ.* 1993;307:89-91.

7. Klebanoff MA, Read JS, Mills JL, et al. The risk of childhood cancer after neonatal exposure to vitamin K. *N Engl J Med.* 1993;329:905-908.

8. Feskanich D, Weber P, Willett WC, et al. Vitamin K intake and hip fractures in women: a prospective study. *Am J Clin Nutr.* 1999;69:74-79.

9. Booth SL, Tucker KL, Chen H, et al. Dietary vitamin K intakes are associated with hip fracture but not with bone mineral density in elderly men and women. *Am J Clin Nutr.* 2000;71:1201-1208.

10. Jie KS, Gijsbers BL, Knapen MH, et al. Effects of vitamin K and oral anticoagulants on urinary calcium excretion. *Br J Haematol.* 1993;83:100-104.

11. Knapen MH, Hamulyak K, Vermeer C. The effect of vitamin K supplementation on circulating osteocalcin (bone Gla protein) and urinary calcium excretion. *Ann Intern Med.* 1989;111:1001-1005.

12. Tomita A, Fujita T, Takatsuki K, et al. 47 Ca kinetic study and vitamin K 2 in post-menopausal osteoporosis [in Japanese]. *Horumon To Rinsho.* 1971;19:731-736.

13. Suttie JW. Vitamin K and human nutrition. *J Am Diet Assoc.* 1992;92:585-590.

14. Gubner R, Ungerleider HE. Vitamin K therapy in menorrhagia: a consideration of the hepatic factor in menstrual disorders. *South Med J.* 1944;37:556-558.

15. Dietary Reference Intakes for Vitamin A, Vitamin K, Arsenic, Boron, Chromium, Copper, Iodine, Iron, Manganese, Molybdenum, Nickel, Silicon, Vanadium, and Zinc (2001). Available at: http://www.nap.edu. Accessed October 4, 2001.

16. Cornelissen M, Steegers-Theunissen R, Kollee L, et al. Increased incidence of neonatal vitamin K deficiency resulting from maternal anticonvulsant therapy. *Am J Obstet Gynecol.* 1993;168(pt 1):923-928.

17. Howe AM, Lipson AH, Sheffield LJ, et al. Prenatal exposure to phenytoin, facial development, and a possible role for vitamin K. *Am J Med Genet.* 1995;58:238-244.

18. Cohen H, Scott SD, Mackie IJ, et al. The development of hypoprothrombinaemia following antibiotic therapy in malnourished patients with low serum vitamin K_1 levels. *Br J Haematol.* 1988;68:63-66.

19. Shearer MJ, Bechtold H, Andrassy K, et al. Mechanism of cephalosporin-induced hypoprothrombinemia: relation to cephalosporin side chain, vitamin K metabolism, and vitamin K status. *J Clin Pharmacol.* 1988;28:88-95.

20. Lipsky JJ. Nutritional sources of vitamin K. *Mayo Clin Proc.* 1994;69:462-466.

21. Goss TF, Walawander CA, Grasela TH, et al. Prospective evaluation of risk factors for antibiotic-associated bleeding in critically ill patients. *Pharmacotherapy.* 1992; 12:283-291.

22. Booth SL, Tucker KL, Chen H, et al. Dietary vitamin K intakes are associated with hip fracture but not with bone mineral density in elderly men and women. *Am J Clin Nutr.* 2000;71:1201-1208.

White Willow

1. Chrubasik S, Eisenberg E, Balan E, et al. Treatment of low back pain exacerbations with willow bark extract: a randomized double-blind study. *Am J Med.* 2000;109:9-14.

2. Schmid B, Ludtke R, Selbmann HK, et al. Efficacy and tolerability of a standard-ized willow bark extract in patients with osteoarthritis: randomized, placebo-controlled, double blind clinical trial [translated from German]. *Z Rheumatol.* 2000; 59:314-320.

3. European Scientific Cooperative on Phytotherapy. *Salicis cortex.* Exeter, UK: ES-COP; 1996-1997. Monographs on the Medicinal Uses of Plant Drugs, Fascicule 4:2.

4. Krivoy N, Pavlotzky E, Chrubasik S, et al. Effect of *Salicic cortex* extract on human platelet aggregation. *Planta Med.* 2001;67:209-212.

Xylitol

1. Gales MA, Nguyen TM. Sorbitol compared with xylitol in prevention of dental caries. *Ann Pharmacother.* 2000;34:98-100.

2. Makinen KK, Bennett CA, Hujoel PP, et al. Xylitol chewing gums and caries rates: a 40-month cohort study. *J Dent Res.* 1995;74:1904-1913.

3. Makinen KK, Hujoel PP, Bennett CA, et al. Polyol chewing gums and caries rates in primary dentition: a 24-month cohort study. *Caries Res.* 1996;30:408-417.
4. Makinen KK, Pemberton D, Makinen PL, et al. Polyol-combinant saliva stimulants and oral health in Veterans Affairs patients—an exploratory study. *Spec Care Dentist.* 1996;16:104-115.
5. Isokangas P, Alanen P, Tiekso J, et al. Xylitol chewing gum in caries prevention: a field study in children. *J Am Dent Assoc.* 1988;117:315-320.
6. Sintes JL, Escalante C, Stewart B, et al. Enhanced anticaries efficacy of a 0.243% sodium fluoride/10% xylitol/silica dentifrice: 3-year clinical results. *Am J Dent.* 1995;8:231-235.
7. Alanen P, Isokangas P, Gutmann K. Xylitol candies in caries prevention: results of a field study in Estonian children. *Community Dent Oral Epidemiol.* 2000;28:218-224.
8. Uhari M, Kontiokari T, Niemela M. A novel use of xylitol sugar in preventing acute otitis media. *Pediatrics.* 1998;102:879-884.
9. Uhari M, Kontiokari T, Koskela M. Xylitol chewing gum in prevention of acute otitis media: double blind randomized trial. *BMJ.* 1996;313:1180-1184.
10. Hildebrandt GH, Sparks BS. Maintaining mutans streptococci suppression with xylitol chewing gum. *J Am Dent Assoc.* 2000;131:909-916.
11. Kontiokari T, Uhari M, Koskela M. Antiadhesive effects of xylitol on otopathogenic bacteria. *J Antimicrob Chemother.* 1998;41:563-565.
12. Soderling E, Isokangas P, Pienihakkinen K, et al. Influence of maternal xylitol consumption on mother-child transmission of mutans streptococci: 6-year follow-up. *Caries Res.* 2001;35:173-177.
13. Isokangas P, Soderling E, Pienihakkinen K, et al. Occurrence of dental decay after maternal consumption of xylitol chewing gum, a follow-up from 0-5 years of age. *J Dent Res.* 2000;79(11):1885-1889.
14. Soderling E, Isokangas P, Peinihakkinen K, et al. Influence of maternal xylitol consumption on acquisition of mutans streptococci by infants. *J Dent Res.* 2000;79(3):882-887.

Yohimbe

1. Riley AJ. Yohimbine in the treatment of erectile disorder. *Br J Clin Pract.* 1994;48:133-136.
2. Charney DA, Heninger GR. Alpha 2-adrenergic and opiate receptor blockade. *Arch Gen Psychiatry.* 1986;43:1037-1041.
3. Charney DS, Heninger GR, Sternberg DE. Assessment of alpha 2 adrenergic autoreceptor function in humans: effects of oral yohimbine. *Life Sci.* 1982;30:2033-2041.
4. Charney DS, Heninger GR, Sternberg DE. Yohimbine induced anxiety and increased noradrenergic function in humans: effects of diazepam and clonidine. *Life Sci.* 1983;33:19-29.
5. Charney DS, Breier A, Jatlow PI, et al. Behavioral, biochemical, and blood pressure responses to alprazolam in healthy subjects: interactions with yohimbine. *Psychopharmacology.* 1986;88:133-140.
6. Charney DS, Price LH, Heninger GR. Desipramine-yohimbine combination treatment of refractory depression: implications for the beta-adrenergic receptor hypothesis of antidepressant action. *Arch Gen Psychiatry.* 1986;43:1155-1161.
7. De Smet PA, Smeets OS. Potential risks of health food products containing yohimbe extracts [letter]. *BMJ.* 1994;309:958.
8. Grossman E, Rosenthal T, Peleg E, et al. Oral yohimbine increases blood pressure and sympathetic nervous outflow in hypertensive patients. *J Cardiovasc Pharmacol.* 1993;22:22-26.
9. Lacomblez L, Bensimon G, Isnard F, et al. Effect of yohimbine on blood pressure in patients with depression and orthostatic hypotension induced by clomipramine. *Clin Pharmacol Ther.* 1989;45:241-251.
10. Murburg MM, Villacres EC, Ko GN, et al. Effects of yohimbine on human sympathetic nervous system function. *J Clin Endocrinol Metab.* 1991;73:861-865.
11. Musso NR, Vergassola C, Pende A, Lotti G. Yohimbine effects on blood pressure and plasma catecholamines in human hypertension. *Am J Hypertens.* 1995;8:565-571.

12. Meston, C. Worcel M. A randomized double-blind, crossover, placebo-controlled clinical trial examining the effects of yohimbine plus L-arginine glutamate on sexual arousal in post-menopausal women with sexual arousal disorder. *Archives of Sexual Behavior* (accepted for publication).
13. Betz JM, White KD. Gas chromatographic determination of yohimbine in commercial yohimbe products. *J AOAC Intl.* 1995;78(5):1189-1194.

Zinc

1. Hirt M, Nobel S, Barron E. Zinc nasal gel for the treatment of common cold symptoms: a double-blind, placebo-controlled trial. *Ear Nose Throat J.* 2000;79:778-781.
2. Eby GA. Linearity in dose-response from zinc lozenges in treatment of common colds. *J Pharm Technol.* 1995;11:110-122.
3. Eby GA. Zinc ion availability—the determinant of efficacy in zinc lozenge treatment of common colds. *J Antimicrob Chemother.* 1997;40:483-493.
4. Belongia EA, Berg R, Liu K. A randomized trial of zinc nasal spray for the treatment of upper respiratory illness in adults. *Am J Med.* 2001;111:103-108.
5. Marshall S. Zinc gluconate and the common cold: review of randomized controlled trials. *Can Fam Physician.* 1998;44:1037-1042.
6. Prasad AS, Fitzgerald JT, Bao B, et al. Duration of symptoms and plasma cytokine levels in patients with the common cold treated with zinc acetate: a randomized, double-blind, placebo-controlled trial. *Ann Intern Med.* 2000;133:245-252.
7. Macknin ML, Piedmonte M, Calendine C, et al. Zinc gluconate lozenges for treating the common cold in children: a randomized controlled trial. *JAMA.* 1998;279: 1962-1967.
8. Godfrey HR, Godfrey NJ, Godfrey JC, et al. A randomized clinical trial on the treatment of oral herpes with topical zinc oxide/glycine. *Altern Ther Health Med.* 2001; 7:49-54,56.
9. Girodon F, Lombard M, Galan P, et al. Effect of micronutrient supplementation on infection in institutionalized elderly subjects: a controlled trial. *Ann Nutr Metab.* 1997;41:98-107.
10. Sugarman B. Zinc and infection. *Rev Infect Dis.* 1983;5:137-147.
11. Bhutta ZA, Black RE, Brown KH, et al. Prevention of diarrhea and pneumonia by zinc supplementation in children in developing countries: pooled analysis of randomized controlled trials. *J Pediatr.* 1999;135:689-697.
12. Sazawal S, Black RE, Jalla S, et al. Zinc supplementation reduces the incidence of acute lower respiratory infections in infants and preschool children: a double-blind, controlled trial. *Pediatrics.* 1998;102:1-5.
13. Gupta VL, Chaubey BS. Efficacy of zinc therapy in prevention of crisis in sickle cell anemia: a double blind, randomized controlled clinical trial. *J Assoc Physicians India.* 1995;43:467-469.
14. Newsome DA, Swartz M, Leone NC, et al. Oral zinc in macular degeneration. *Arch Ophthalmol.* 1988;106:192-198.
15. Stur M, Tittl M, Reitner A, et al. Oral zinc and the second eye in age-related macular degeneration. *Invest Ophthalmol Vis Sci.* 1996;37:1225-1235.
16. Pohit J, Saha KC, Pal B. Zinc status of acne vulgaris patients. *J Appl Nutr.* 1985; 37:18-25.
17. Amer M, Bahgat MR, Tosson Z, et al. Serum zinc in acne vulgaris. *Int J Dermatol.* 1982;21:481-484.
18. Michaelsson G, Vahlquist A, Juhlin L. Serum zinc and retinol-binding protein in acne. *Br J Dermatol.* 1977;96:283-286.
19. Goransson K, Liden S, Odsell L. Oral zinc in acne vulgaris: a clinical and methodological study. *Acta Derm Venereol.* 1978;58:443-448.
20. Verma KC, Saini AS, Dhamija SK. Oral zinc sulphate therapy in acne vulgaris: a double-blind trial. *Acta Derm Venereol.* 1980;60:337-340.
21. Weimar VM, Puhl SC, Smith WH, et al. Zinc sulfate in acne vulgaris. *Arch Dermatol.* 1978;114:1776-1778.
22. Hillstrom L, Pettersson L, Hellbe L, et al. Comparison of oral treatment with zinc sulphate and placebo in acne vulgaris. *Br J Dermatol.* 1977;97:681-684.

23. Michaelsson G, Johlin L, Vahlquist A. Effects of zinc and vitamin A in acne. *Arch Dermatol.* 1977;113:31-36.
24. Weismann K, Wadskov S, Sondergaard J. Oral zinc sulphate therapy for acne vulgaris. *Acta Derm Venereol.* 1977;57:357-360.
25. Orris L, Shalita A, Sibulkin D, et al. Oral zinc therapy of acne: absorption and clinical effect. *Arch Dermatol.* 1978;114:1018-1020.
26. Dreno B, Amblard P, Agache P, et al. Low doses of zinc gluconate for inflammatory acne. *Acta Derm Venereol.* 1989;69:541-543.
27. Michaelsson G, Juhlin L, Ljunghall K. A double-blind study of the effect of zinc and oxytetracycline in acne vulgaris. *Br J Dermatol.* 1977;97:561-566.
28. Cunliffe WJ, Burke B, Dodman B, et al. A double-blind trial of a zinc sulphate/citrate complex and tetracycline in the treatment of acne vulgaris. *Br J Dermatol.* 1979;101:321-325.
29. Meynadier J. Efficacy and safety study of two zinc gluconate regimens in the treatment of inflammatory acne. *Eur J Dermatol.* 2000;10:269-273.
30. Netter A, Hartoma R, Nahoul K. Effect of zinc administration on plasma testosterone, dihydrotestosterone, and sperm count. *Arch Androl.* 1981;7:69-73.
31. Mattingly PC, Mowat AG. Zinc sulphate in rheumatoid arthritis. *Ann Rheum Dis.* 1982;41:456-457.
32. Rasker JJ, Kardaun SH. Lack of beneficial effect of zinc sulphate in rheumatoid arthritis. *Scand J Rheumatol.* 1982;11:168-170.
33. Dixon JS, Martin MF, McKenna F, et al. Biochemical and clinical changes occurring during the treatment of rheumatoid arthritis with novel antirheumatoid drugs. *Int J Clin Pharmacol Res.* 1985;5:25-33.
34. Job C, Menkes CJ, Delbarre F. Zinc sulphate in the treatment of rheumatoid arthritis [letter]. *Arthritis Rheum.* 1980;23:1408-1409.
35. Simkin PA. Treatment of rheumatoid arthritis with oral zinc sulfate. *Agents Actions Suppl.* 1981;8:587-596.
36. Pandey SP, Bhattacharya SK, Sundar S. Zinc in rheumatiod arthritis. *Indian J Med Res.* 1985;81:618-620.
37. Mocchegiani E, Rivabene R, Santini MT. Benefit of oral zinc supplementation as an adjunct to zidovudine (AZT) therapy against opportunistic infections in AIDS. *Int J Immunopharmacol.* 1995;17:719-727.
38. Constantinidis J. Alzheimer's disease and the zinc theory [in French; English abstract]. *Encephale.* 1990;16:231-239.
39. Constantinidis J. The hypothesis of zinc deficiency in the pathogenesis of neurofibrillary tangles. *Med Hypotheses.* 1991;35:319-323.
40. Cuajungco MP, Lees GJ. Zinc metabolism in the brain: relevance to human neurodegenerative disorders. *Neurobiol Dis.* 1997;4:137-169.
41. Lovell MA, Robertson JD, Teesdale WJ, et al. Copper, iron and zinc in Alzheimer's disease senile plaques. *J Neurol Sci.* 1998;158:47-52.
42. Birmingham CL, Goldner EM, Bakan R. Controlled trial of zinc supplementation in anorexia nervosa. *Int J Eat Disord.* 1994;15:251-255.
43. Katz RL, Keen CL, Litt IF, et al. Zinc deficiency in anorexia nervosa. *J Adolesc Health Care.* 1987;8:400-406.
44. Lask B, Fosson A, Rolfe U, et al. Zinc deficiency and childhood-onset anorexia nervosa. *J Clin Psychiatry.* 1993;54:63-66.
45. Roijen SB, Worsaae U, Zlotnik G. Zinc in patients with anorexia nervosa [in Danish; English abstract]. *Ugeskr Laeger.* 1991;153:721-723.
46. Leake A, Chisholm GD, Habib FK. The effect of zinc on the 5-alpha-reduction of testosterone by the hyperplastic human prostate gland. *J Steroid Biochem.* 1984; 20:651-655.
47. Leake A, Chrisholm GD, Busuttil A, et al. Subcellular distribution of zinc in the benign and malignant human prostate: evidence for a direct zinc androgen interaction. *Acta Endocrinol (Copenh).* 1984;105:281-288.
48. Schmidt LE, Arfken CL, Heins JM. Evaluation of nutrient intake in subjects with non-insulin dependent diabetes mellitus. *J Am Diet Assoc.* 1994;94:773-774.

49. Blostein-Fujii A, DiSilvestro RA, Frid D, et al. Short-term zinc supplementation in women with non-insulin-dependent diabetes mellitus: effects on plasma 5'-nucleotidase activities, insulin-like growth factor I concentrations, and lipoprotein oxidation rates in vitro. *Am J Clin Nutr.* 1997;66:639-642.

50. Rauscher AM, Fairweather-Tait SJ, Wilson PD, et al. Zinc metabolism in non-insulin dependent diabetes mellitus. *J Trace Elem Med Biol.* 1997;11:65-70.

51. Sustrova M, Strbak V. Thyroid function and plasma immunoglobulins in subjects with Down's syndrome (DS) during ontogenesis and zinc therapy. *J Endocrinol Invest.* 1994;17:385-390.

52. Licastro F, Mocchegiani E, Masi M, et al. Modulation of the neuroendocrine system and immune functions by zinc supplementation in children with Down's syndrome. *J Trace Elem Electrolytes Health Dis.* 1993;7:237-239.

53. Lockitch G, Puterman M, Godolphin W, et al. Infection and immunity in Down syndrome: a trial of long-term low oral doses of zinc. *J Pediatr.* 1989;114:781-787.

54. Frommer DJ. The healing of gastric ulcers by zinc sulphate. *Med J Aust.* 1975;2: 793-796.

55. Garcia-Plaza A, Arenal JI, Belda O, et al. A multicenter clinical trial: zinc acexamate versus famotidine in the treatment of acute duodenal ulcer [in Spanish; English abstract]. *Rev Esp Enferm Dig.* 1996;88:757-762.

56. Sjogren A, Floren CH, Nilsson A. Evaluation of zinc status in subjects with Crohn's disease. *J Am Coll Nutr.* 1988;7:57-60.

57. Van de Wal Y, Van der Sluys Veer A, Verspaget HW, et al. Effect of zinc therapy on natural killer cell activity in inflammatory bowel disease. *Aliment Pharmacol Ther.* 1993;7:281-286.

58. Mulder TP, van der Sluys Veer A, Verspaget HW, et al. Effect of oral zinc supplementation on metallothionein and superoxide dismutase concentrations in patients with inflammatory bowel disease. *J Gastroenterol Hepatol.* 1994;9:472-477.

59. Dronfield MW, Malone JD, Langman MJ. Zinc in ulcerative colitis: a therapeutic trial and report on plasma levels. *Gut.* 1977;18:33-36.

60. Relea P, Revilla M, Ripoll E, Arribas I, et al. Zinc, biochemical markers of nutrition, and type I osteoporosis. *Age Ageing.* 1995;24:303-307.

61. Neal DE, Kaack MB, Fussell EN, et al. Changes in seminal fluid zinc during experimental prostatitis. *Urol Res.* 1993;21:71-74.

62. Gersdorff M, Robillard T, Stein F, et al. The zinc sulfate overload test in patients suffering from tinnitus associated with low serum zinc. Preliminary report [in French; English abstract]. *Acta Otorhinolaryngol Belg.* 1987;41:498-505.

63. Paaske PB, Pedersen CB, Kjems G, et al. Zinc therapy of tinnitus: a placebo controlled study [in Danish; English abstract]. *Ugeskr Laeger.* 1990;152:2473-2475.

64. Han CM. Changes in body zinc and copper levels in severely burned patients and the effects of oral administration of ZnSO4 by a double-blind method [in Chinese; English abstract]. *Zhonghua Zheng Xing Shao Shang Wai Ke Za Zhi.* 1990;6:83-86, 155.

65. Agren MS, Stromberg HE, Rindby A, et al. Selenium, zinc, iron and copper levels in serum of patients with arterial and venous leg ulcers. *Acta Derm Venereol.* 1986;66:237-240.

66. Floersheim GL, Lais E. Lack of effect of oral zinc sulfate on wound healing in leg ulcer [in German; English abstract]. *Schweiz Med Wochenschr.* 1980;110:1138-1145.

67. Dietary Reference Intakes for Vitamin A, Vitamin K, Arsenic, Boron, Chromium, Copper, Iodine, Iron, Manganese, Molybdenum, Nickel, Silicon, Vanadium, and Zinc (2001). Available at: http://www.nap.edu. Accessed October 4, 2001.

68. Sturniolo GC, Montino MC, Rossetto L, et al. Inhibition of gastric acid secretion reduces zinc absorption in man. *J Am Coll Nutr.* 1991;10:372-375.

69. Campbell NR, Kara M, Hasinoff BB, et al. Norfloxacin interaction with antacids and minerals. *Br J Clin Pharmacol.* 1992;33:115-116.

70. Polk RE, Healy DP, Sahai J, et al. Effect of ferrous sulfate and multivitamins with zinc on absorption of ciprofloxacin in normal volunteers. *Antimicrob Agents Chemother.* 1989;33:1841-1844.

71. Mapp RK, McCarthy TJ. The effect of zinc sulphate and of bicitropeptide on tetracycline absorption. *S Afr Med J.* 1976;50:1829-1830.

72. Neuvonen PJ. Interactions with the absorption of tetracyclines. *Drugs*. 1976;11:45-54.
73. Porea TJ, Belmont JW, Mahoney DH Jr. Zinc-induced anemia and neutropenia in an adolescent. *J Pediatr*. 2000;136:688-690.
74. Hoffman HN II, Phyliky RL, Fleming CR. Zinc-induced copper deficiency. *Gastroenterology*. 1988;94:508-512.
75. Sandstead HH. Requirements and toxicity of essential trace elements, illustrated by zinc and copper. *Am J Clin Nutr*. 1995;61(suppl.):621S-624S.
76. Fosmire GJ. Zinc toxicity. *Am J Clin Nutr*. 1990;51:225-227.
77. Neuvonen PJ. Interactions with the absorption of tetracyclines. *Drugs*. 1976;11:45-54.
78. *Drug Evaluations Annual*. Vol. 2. Milwaukee, Wis: American Medical Association; 1993.
79. Andersson KE, Bratt L, Dencker H, et al. Inhibition of tetracycline absorption by zinc. *Eur J Clin Pharmacol*. 1976;10:59-62.
80. Reyes AJ, Olhaberry JV, Leary WP, et al. Urinary zinc excretion, diuretics, zinc deficiency and some side-effects of diuretics. *S Afr Med J*. 1983;64:936-941.
81. Wester PO. Urinary zinc excretion during treatment with different diuretics. *Acta Med Scand*. 1980;208:209-212.
82. Reyes AJ, Leary WP, Lockett CJ, et al. Diuretics and zinc. *S Afr Med J*. 1982;62:373-375.
85. Polk RE, Healy DP, Sahai J, et al. Effect of ferrous sulfate and multivitamins with zinc on absorption of ciprofloxacin in normal volunteers. *Antimicrob Agents Chemother*. 1989;33:1841-1844.
86. Lim D, McKay M. Food-drug interactions. *Drug Information Bulletin* (UCLA Dept. of Pharmaceutical Services). 1995;15(2).
87. Spencer H, Kramer L, Norris C, et al. Effect of calcium and phosphorus on zinc metabolism in man. *Am J Clin Nutr*. 1984;40:1213-1218.
88. Dawson-Hughes B, Seligson FH, Hughes VA. Effects of calcium carbonate and hydroxyapatite on zinc and iron retention in postmenopausal women. *Am J Clin Nutr*. 1986;44: 83-88.
89. Pecoud A, Donzel P, Schelling JL. Effect of foodstuffs on the absorption of zinc sulfate. *Clin Pharmacol Ther*. 1975;17: 469-474.
90. Hwang SJ, Lai YH, Chen HC, Tasi JH. Comparisons of the effects of calcium carbonate and calcium acetate on zinc tolerance test in hemodialysis patients. *Am J Kidney Dis*. 1992; 19:57-60.
91. Argiratos V, Samman S. The effect of calcium carbonate and calcium citrate on the absorption of zinc in healthy female subjects. *Eur J Clin Nutr*. 1994;126:161-167.
92. Golik A, Zaidenstein R, Dishi V, et al. Effects of captopril and enalapril on zinc metabolism in hypertensive patients. *J Am Coll Nutr*. 1998;17:75-78.
93. Golik A, Modai D, Averbukh Z, et al. Zinc metabolism in patients treated with captopril versus enalapril. *Metabolism*. 1990;39:665-667.
94. Campbell NR, Hasinoff BB. Iron supplements: a common cause of drug interactions. *Br J Clin Pharmacol*. 1991;31:251-255.
95. Hambidge M. Human zinc deficiency. *J Nutr*. 2000;130(5S suppl):1344S-1349S.
96. Prasad AS. Role of zinc in human health. *Bol Asoc Med PR*. 1991;83:558-560.
97. Sandstead HH. Is zinc deficiency a public health problem? *Nutrition*. 1995;11:87-92.
98. Goldenberg RL, Tamura T, Neggers Y, et al. The effect of zinc supplementation on pregnancy outcome. *JAMA*. 1995;274:463-468.
99. Lukaski HC. Magnesium, zinc, and chromium nutriture and physical activity. *Am J Clin Nutr*. 2000;72:585S-593S.
100. Ma J, Betts NM. Zinc and copper intakes and their major food sources for older adults in the 1994-96 continuing survey of food intakes by individuals (CSFII). *J Nutr*. 2000;130:2838-2843.
101. Prasad AS. Zinc deficiency in women, infants, and children. *J Am Coll Nutr*. 1996; 15:113-120.
102. Stang J, Story MT, Harnack L, et al. Relationships between vitamin and mineral supplement use, dietary intake, and dietary adequacy among adolescents. *J Am Diet Assoc*. 2000;100:905-910.

103. Zemel BS, Kawchak DA, Fung EB, et al. Effect of zinc supplementation on growth and body composition in children with sickle cell disease. *Am J Clin Nutr.* 2002; 75:300-307.

104. Age-Related Eye Disease Study Research. Group A randomized placebo-controlled clinical trial of high-dose supplementation with vitamins C and E beta carotene and zinc for age-related macular degeneration and vision loss: AREDS Report no. 8. *Arch Ophthalmol.* 2001;119:1417-1436.

105. Birmingham CL, Goldner EM, Bakan R. Controlled trial of zinc supplementation in anorexia nervosa. *Int J Eat Disord.* 1994;15:251-255.

106. Ewing CI, Gibbs AC, Ashcroft C, et al. Failure of oral zinc supplementation in atopic eczema. *Eur J Clin Nutr.* 1991;45:507-510.

107. Su JC, Birmingham CL. Zinc supplementation in the treatment of anorexia nervosa. *Eat Weight Disord.* 2002;7:20-22.

108. Peretz A, Neve J, Jeghers O, et al. Zinc distribution in blood components, inflammatory status, and clinical indexes of disease activity during zinc supplementation in inflammatory rheumatic diseases. *Am J Clin Nutr.* 1993;57:690-694.

109. Simkin PA. Oral zinc sulphate in rheumatoid arthritis. *Lancet.* 1976;2:539-542.

INDEX

Turmeric. *See also* Curcumin
  for dysmenorrhea, 108, 109
  for dyspepsia, 113, 114
  for gallstones, 57, 58
  for hyperlipidemia, 160
  for osteoarthritis, 226, 231
  for peptic ulcer disease, 251, 253
  for rheumatoid arthritis, 293, 296
Turnera diffusa. See Damiana
Tussilago farfara. See Coltsfoot
Tylophora, 37, 38, 903-905
  for allergies, 904
  for asthma, 903-904
  for dysentery, 904
  for joint pain, 904
  for respiratory infections, 904
Tylophora spp. *See* Tylophora
Tyrosine, 906-908
  for ADHD, 42, 44, 907
  for cognition, 907
  for depression, 92, 97, 906, 907
  for sleep deprivation, alterness
    during, 906
  for weight loss, 353

U

Ulcerative colitis, 327-330
  approach to the patient, 327
  biotin for, 395
  blue-green algae for, 329
  boswellia for, 327, 329, 414
  bromelain for, 327, 329, 422
  calcium for, 327
  colostrum for, 484
  copper for, 327
  drug interactions, 329-330
  EPO for, 328
  essential fatty acids for, 327, 328
  fish oil for, 328-329, 556
  folate for, 327
  GAGs for, 327, 329
  glutamine for, 327, 329, 614, 615
  iron for, 327
  magnesium for, 327
  main discussion, 327-330
  principal proposed natural therapies,
    327
  probiotics for, 327, 328, 819, 820,
    821
  protein for, 327
  selenium for, 327
  vitamin A for, 327
  vitamin B₁₂ for, 327
  vitamin C for, 327
  vitamin D for, 327
  vitamin E for, 327
  vitamin K for, 327, 967
  zinc for, 327, 984

Ulcers. *See also* Apthous ulcers; Peptic
  ulcer disease
  colostrum for chemotherapy-
    induced mouth ulcers, 484
Ulmus rubra. See Slippery elm
Umbrella leaves. *See* Butterbur
Una de gato. *See* Cat's claw
Uncaria tomentosa. See Cat's claw
Upper respiratory infections. *See*
  Respiratory infections (minor)
Urinary tract infection (UTI). *See*
  Cystitis
Urinary tract stones. *See* Urolithiasis
URIs. *See* Respiratory infections
  (minor)
Urolithiasis, 331-335
  approach to the patient, 331-332
  asparagus for, 333
  birch leaf for, 333
  bishop's weed fruit for, 333
  butterbur for, 333
  calcium for, 331, 334, 435
  calcium safety issues, 334, 435
  chondroitin sulfate for, 466
  citrate for, 331, 332-333
  couch grass for, 333
  cranberry for, 331
  drug interactions, 334-335
  fish oil for, 331, 334, 556
  GAGs for, 334
  GLA for, 331, 334
  goldenrod for, 331, 333, 622
  horsetail for, 333
  lovage for, 333
  magnesium for, 331, 333, 728
  main discussion, 331-335
  nettle for, 333
  parsley for, 333
  principal proposed natural therapies,
    331
  tribulus for, 901
  vitamin A for, 331, 334
  vitamin B₆ for, 331, 333, 936, 939
  vitamin C for, 331
  vitamin C safety issues, 334, 952
Urticaria, 336-337
  colon cleansing for, 336
  detoxification for, 336
  ginseng for, 336
  quercetin for, 336
  vitamin B₁₂ for, 336
  vitamin C for, 336
Urtica spp. *See* Nettle
Uterine cancer. *See also* Cancer
  boron safety issues, 412
  estriol safety issues, 543
Uterine inflammation, blue cohosh for,
  404